BIOACTIVE FOODS IN PROMOTING HEALTH: PROBIOTICS AND PREBIOTICS

BIOACTIVE FOODS IN PROMOTING HEALTH: PROBIOTICS AND PREBIOTICS

Edited by

RONALD ROSS WATSON
College of Public Health,
University of Arizona,
Tucson, Arizona, USA

VICTOR R. PREEDY
Department of Nutrition and Dietetics,
King's College London,
London, UK

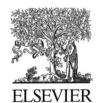

ELSEVIER

AMSTERDAM • BOSTON • HEIDELBERG • LONDON
NEW YORK • OXFORD • PARIS • SAN DIEGO
SAN FRANCISCO • SINGAPORE • SYDNEY • TOKYO

Academic Press is an imprint of Elsevier

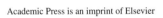

Academic Press is an imprint of Elsevier

32 Jamestown Road, London NW1 7BY, UK
30 Corporate Drive, Suite 400, Burlington, MA 01803, USA
525 B Street, Suite 1900, San Diego, CA 92101-4495, USA

First edition 2010

British Library Cataloguing-in-Publication Data
A catalogue record for this book is available from the British Library

Library of Congress Cataloging-in-Publication Data
A catalog record for this book is available from the Library of Congress

ISBN : 978-0-12-374938-3

For information on all Academic Press publications
visit our website at www.elsevierdirect.com

Typeset by Macmillan Publishing Solutions
www.macmillansolutions.com

Printed and bound in United States of America
10 11 12 13 14   10 9 8 7 6 5 4 3 2 1

Working together to grow
libraries in developing countries

www.elsevier.com | www.bookaid.org | www.sabre.org

ELSEVIER   BOOK AID
International   Sabre Foundation

Contents

Section D
PROBIOTICS AND HEALTH

Section E
ANIMAL MODELS TO STUDY PROBIOTICS

Preface

By use of probiotics people can dramatically expand their exposure to protective chemicals and thus readily reduce their risk of multiple diseases. Specific foods, individual fruits or vegetables and their by-products are biomedicines with expanded understanding and use. However, which bacteria and their metabolism of bio-molecules in the diet are best to prevent with disease or promote health? How can their growth be stimulated? What dietary supplements will help the bacteria proper and provide health benefits? This book focuses on probiotics and their role in bio-modulation of natural products to produce active agents from inactive molecules in dietary fruits and vegetables.

This book brings together experts working on the different aspects of supplementation, foods, and bacterial preparations, in health promotion and disease prevention. Their expertise and experience provide the most current knowledge to promote future research. Dietary habits need to be altered, for most people. Therefore, the conclusions and recommendations from the various chapters will provide a basis for change.

Probiotics and prebiotics are dietary supplements. They are now a multi-billion-dollar business which is built upon limited but growing research data. For example the U.S. Food and Drug Administration is pushing the whole dietary supplement industry, with the support of Congress, to base its claims and products on scientific research. Since common dietary bacterial preparations are over-the-counter and readily available, this book will be useful to laymen who apply it to modify their lifestyles, as well as to the growing nutrition, food science, and natural product community. This book focuses on the growing body of knowledge on the role of various bacteria in reducing disease.

Expert reviews define and support the actions of bacteria; materials that promote gastrointestinal organisms, bacteria modified bio-molecules they make as well as modified from other materials that are part of the diet. As such probiotic bacteria with health-promoting activities may have biological activity. Therefore, their role is a major emphasis, along with discussions of which agents may be the active components.

The overall goal is the most current, concise, scientific appraisal of the efficacy of key foods and constituent bacteria and their growth promoting food sources, in preventing disease and improving the quality of life. This book reviews and often presents new hypotheses and conclusions on the effects of different bioactive components of probiotics to prevent disease and improve the health of various populations.

Acknowledgments

The work of editorial assistant, Bethany L. Stevens, in communicating with authors, working with the manuscripts and the publisher was critical to the successful completion of the book and is much appreciated. Her daily responses to queries and collection of manuscripts and documents were extremely helpful. Support for her work was graciously provided by the National Health Research Institute as part of its mission to communicate to scientists about bioactive foods and dietary supplements was vital (http://www.naturalhealthresearch.org). This was part of their efforts to educate scientists and the lay public on the health and economic benefits of nutrients in the diet as well as supplements. Finally Nguyen T. Nga and Mari Stoddard of the Arizona Health Sciences library was instrumental in finding the authors and their addresses in the early stages of the book's preparation.

Abbreviations

3′, 5′-cyclic adenosine monophosphate	cAMP
Acidic oligosaccharides	AOS
Active hexose correlated compound	AHCC
Alginates containing high percentages of mannuronic acid polymers	High-M alginates
Alternating IBS	(IBS-A)
Antibiotic-associated diarrhea	AAD
Atopic eczema	AE
Bacterial translocation	BT
Bifidobacterium Mixed Species	BSM
Blood–brain barrier	BBB
Body mass index	BMI
Branched-chains fatty acids	BCFA
Clostridium difficile-associated diarrhea	CDAD
Center of Disease Control (in China), The	CDC
Cerebrospinal fluid	CSF
Chromium-labeled ethylenediaminetetraacetic acid	CrEDTA
Clostridium difficile-associated diarrhea	CDAD
Colitis ulcerosa (ulcerative colitis)	UC
Colony-forming units	CFU
Conditional pathogens	CP
Conditional susceptibility	CS
Confederation of the Food and Drink Industries of the EU (in French)	CIAA
Constipation-predominant IBS	(IBS-C)
Cow milk allergy	CMA
Crohn's disease	CD
Denaturing gradient gel electrophoresis	DGGE
Derjaguin, Landau, Verwey and Overbeek Theory	DLVO theory
Dextran sulfate sodium	DSS
Diarrhea-predominant IBS	(IBS-D)
Dietary fibers	DF
Dinitrobenzene sulfonic acid	DNBS
Double-blind, placebo-controlled, randomized intervention trial	DBRCT
Enterohemorrhagic *Escherichia coli*	EHEC
Enteroinvasive *Escherichia coli*	EIEC
Enteropathogenic *Escherichia coli*	EPEC
Enterotoxigenic *Escherichia coli*	ETEC
European Food Safety Authority	EFSA

Fluorescence *in situ* hybridization — FISH
Food for Specified Health Uses (in Japan) — FOSHU
Food with Health Claims (in Japan) — FHC
Food with Nutrient Function Claims (in Japan) — FNFC
Fructo-oligosaccharides — FOS

Gastrointestinal tract — GIT
Gastrointestinal — GI
Generally Recognised As Safe — GRAS
Genetically modified organisms — GMOs
Germinated barley foodstuff — GBF
Global symptom scores — GSS
Glutathione peroxidase — GPO
Group B Streptococcus — GBS
Gut-associated lymphoid tissue — GALT

Human intestinal epithelial cell line from colorectal adenocarcinoma — Caco-2
Human intestinal epithelial cell line from colorectal carcinoma — T84
Human milk oligosaccharides — HMOS

Immunoglobulin M — IgM
Inducible nitric oxide synthase — iNOS
Infant milk formula — IMF
Inflammatory bowel diseases — IBD
Inhibitory protein κB — IκB
Interleukin — IL
International Life Science Institutes — ILSI
Irritable bowel syndrome — IBS

Joint Health Claims Initiative (in UK) — JHCI

Lactic acid bacteria — LAB
Lactobacillus rhamnosus strain GG — LLG
Lipopolysaccharide — LPS

Mesenteric lymph nodes — MLN
Microentrapment — ME
Minimal inhibitory concentration — MIC
Ministry of Health, Labor and Welfare (in Japan) — MHLW
Mitogen-activated protein kinase — MAPK
Mucin — MUC
Myeloperoxidase — MPO

National Health Surveillance Agency (in Brazil) — ANVISA
Necrotizing enterocolitis — NEC
Neonatal sepsis and meningitis — NSM
Non-digestible oligosaccharides — NDOs
Non-pathogenic microbiota — NP
Non-susceptibility — NS

No-observed-adverse-effect level	NOAEL
Nuclear factor κB	NFκB
Nucleotide oligomerization domain	NOD
Nutrition and Health Claim	NHC
Oligofructose	OF
Oligosaccharides	OS
Oral rehydration solution	ORS
Peptidoglycan	PGN
Phosphatidylinositol 3-kinase	PI3K
Phosphoenolpyruvate transport system	PTS
Phosphotransferase system	PTS
Polydextrose	PDX
Polyethylene glycol	PEG
Protein kinase C	PKC
Qualified Perception of Safety	QPS
Qualified Presumption of Safety	QPS
Randomized control trial	RCT
Raw potato starch	RPS
Reactive oxygen species	ROS
Resistant starches	RS
Scientific Committee on Animal Nutrition	SCAN
Scientific Committee on Food	SCF
Scoring index for atopic dermatitis	SCORAD
Senescence-accelerated mouse	SAM
Severe combined immunodeficiency	SCID
Sexually transmitted diseases	STD
Short-chain fructo-oligosaccharides	SC-FOS
Short circuit current	I_{sc}
Short-chain fatty acids	SCFAs
Small intestinal bacterial overgrowth	SIBO
Soluble dietary fiber	SDF
Spontaneous bacterial peritonitis	SBP
Spray coating	SC
State Food and Drug Administration (in China), The	SFDA
Superoxide dismutases	SODs
Systemic inflammatory response syndrome	SIRS
Technical Scientific Commission on Functional Foods and Novel Foods (in Brazil)	CTCAF
Tight junction	TJ
Toll-like receptors	TLRs
(trans-)galacto-oligosaccharides	TOS or GOS
Transgalactosylated oligosaccharides	TOS

Transepithelial electrical resistance TEER
Trinitrobenzene sulfonic acid TNBS
Tumor necrosis factor TNF

Unconditional pathogens UP
Unconditional susceptibility US

Very low birth weight VLBW

Water availability a_w
Widespread antibiotic use WAU

Xylo-oligosaccharides XOS

Zonula occludens proteins 1, 2, 3 ZO-1, -2, -3

Contributors

Alighieri, Giovanni Catholic University of the Sacred Heart, Division of Neonatology, Largo Agostino Gemelli 8, Rome 00168, Italy

Anadón, Arturo Department of Toxicology and Pharmacology, Faculty of Veterinary Medicine, Universidad Complutense de Madrid, Madrid, Spain

Bibas Bonet, María Eugenia Institute of Microbiology, Tucuman University, Ayacucho 471. 4000, San Miguel de Tucuman, Argentina

Brunser, Oscar Gastroenterology Unit and Laboratory of Microbiology and Probiotics, Institute of Nutrition and Food Technology (INTA), University of Chile, Santiago, Chile

Budak, Alicja Department of Pharmaceutical Microbiology Jagiellonian University, Medical College, Krakow, Poland

Buddendick, Kirsten Department of Dermatology, University Hospital Münster, Münster, Germany

Bunselmeyer, Britta Department of Dermatology, University Hospital Münster, Münster, Germany

Caballero, Virginia Department of Toxicology and Pharmacology, Faculty of Veterinary Medicine, Universidad Complutense de Madrid, Madrid, Spain

Cao, Hong Department of Microbiology, School of Public Health and Tropical Medicine, Southern Medical University, Guangzhou, China

Carey, Christine M. Agriculture and Agri-Food Canada Guelph, Food Research Centre, 93 Stone Road West, Guelph, Ontario, Canada

Castellano, Victor Department of Toxicology and Pharmacology, Faculty of Veterinary Medicine, Universidad Complutense de Madrid, Madrid, Spain

Champagne, Claude Food Research and Development Centre, Agriculture and Agri-Food Canada, Saint-Hyacinthe, Quebec, Canada

Chen, Jian Jun Shanghai Rundo Biotech Japan Co. Ltd., Kobe KIMEC Center Bldg 8F, Minotojima-minamimachi 1-5-2, Chio-ku, Kobe, Hyogo, 650-0047, Japan

Collado, Maria Carmen Instituto de Agroquimica y Tecnologia de los Alimentos (IATA-CSIC), Valencia, Spain and Functional Food Forum, University of Turku, Turku, Finland

Comalada, Mònica Department of Physiology, University of Veterinary, Ramon y Cajal Program of the Spanish Ministry of Science and Technology, Barcelona, Spain

de Aguilar-Nascimento, José Eduardo Department of Surgery, Medical Sciences School, Federal University of Mato Grosso, Cuiaba, Brazil

de Marco, Guido Internal Medicine, Catholic University of Rome, Rome, Italy

de Moreno de LeBlanc, Alejandra Centro de Referencia para Lactobacilos (CERELA-CONICET), Chacabuco 145 San Miguel de Tucumán, Argentina

de Vrese, Michael Institute of Physiology and Biochemistry of Nutrition, Federal Dairy Research Center, Kiel, Germany

Dowhower Karpa, Kelly Department of Pharmacology, Mail Code R130, Penn State College of Medicine, Hershey, PA, USA

Farnworth, Edward R. Food Research and Development Centre, Agriculture and Agri-Food Canada, Saint-Hyacinthe, Quebec, Canada

Feleszko, Wojciech Department of Pediatric Pneumology and Allergy, The Medical University of Warsaw, The Medical University Children's Hospital, Warszawa, Poland

Fernández-López, Juana Departamento de Tecnología Agroalimentaria, Universidad Miguel Hernández de Elche, Orihuela (Alicante), Spain

Fitzpatrick, Leo R. Department of Pharmacology, Penn State College of Medicine, 1214 Research Boulevard, Hummelstown, PA, USA

Franceschi, Francesco Internal Medicine, Catholic University of Rome, Rome, Italy

Fukushima, Yoichi Nestlé Research Center, PO Box 44, Vers-chez-les-Blanc, CH-1000 Lausanne 26, Switzerland

Gálvez, Julio Department of Pharmacology, School of Pharmacy, University of Granada, Campus Universitario de Cartuja s/n, 18071-Granada Spain

Gasbarrini, Antonio Internal Medicine, Catholic University of Rome, Rome, Italy

Gatesoupe, Joel UMR 1067 NuAGe, Nutrition, Aquaculture et Genomique, INRA-IFREMER IFREMER, Centre de Brest, BP 70, F-29280 PLOUZANÉ, France

Gérard, Philippe Unité d'Ecologie et Physiologie du Système Digestif, INRA, CR JOUY, Domaine de Vilvert, Bâtiment 440 78352 Jouy-en-Josas, France

Gigante, Giovanni Internal Medicine, Catholic University of Rome, Rome, Italy

Giupponi, Bianca Internal Medicine, Catholic University of Rome, Rome, Italy

Gotteland, Martin Gastroenterology Unit and Laboratory of Microbiology and Probiotics Institute of Nutrition and Food Technology (INTA), University of Chile, Casilla 138-11 — Macul, Santiago, Chile

Gueimonde, Miguel Instituto de Productos Lácteos de Asturias, (IPLA-CSIC), Asturias, Spain

Hanning, Irene B. Center for Food Safety-IFSE and Food Science Department, 2650 Young Ave., University of Arkansas, Fayetteville, AR, USA

Hirayama, Kazuhiro Laboratory of Veterinary Public Health, The University of Tokyo, Bunkyo, Tokyo 113-8657, Japan

Huang, Sheng-He Saban Research Institute of Childrens Hospital Los Angeles, Department of Pediatrics, University of Southern California, Los Angeles, CA, USA

Hurt, Eva CT-Regulatory, Nestec Ltd. Avenue Nestlé 55, CH-1800 Vevey, Switzerland

Jaworska, Joanna Department of Pediatric Pneumology and Allergy, The Medical University of Warsaw, The Medical University Children's Hospital, Warszawa, Poland

Jong, Ambrose Saban Research Institute of Childrens Hospital Los Angeles, Department of Pediatrics, University of Southern California, Los Angeles, CA, USA

Kelly Dowhower Karpa Pennsylvania State University College of Medicine, Department of Pharmacology, Hershey, PA, USA

Kostrzynska, Magdalena Research Scientist, Agriculture and Agri-Food Canada, Guelph Food Research Centre, 93 Stone Road West, Guelph, Ontario, Canada

Lara-Villaslada, Federico Department of Immunology and Animal Sciences. Puleva Biotech, Granada, Spain

LeBlanc, Jean Guy CONICET (Consejo Nacional de Investigaciones Científicas y Técnicas), CERELA-CONICET, Chacabuco 145. 4000, San Miguel de Tucuman, Argentina

Lingbeck, Jody M. Center for Food Safety-IFSE and Food Science Department, 2650 Young Ave., University of Arkansas, Fayetteville, AR, USA

Lodemann, Ulrike Institute of Veterinary Physiology, Department of Veterinary Medicine, Freie Universität Berlin, Berlin, Germany

Looijer-van Langen, Mirjam Division of Gastroenterology, Department of Medicine, University of Alberta, Edmonton, Alberta, Canada

Macfarlane, Sandra University of Dundee, Micro-biology and Gut Biology Group, Ninewells Hospital Medical School, Dundee, UK

Mach, Tomasz Department of Gastroenterology and Hepatology, Jagiellonian University, Medical College, Krakow, Poland

Madsen, Karen Division of Gastroenterology, Department of Medicine, University of Alberta, Edmonton, Alberta, Canada

Martínez-Larrañaga, Maria Rosa Department of Toxicology and Pharmacology, Faculty of

Veterinary Medicine, Universidad Complutense de Madrid, Madrid, Spain

Moreno-Villares, Jose M. Nutrition Unit, Department of Pediatrics, Hospital Universitario 12 de Octubre, Madrid, Spain

Nomoto, Koji Yakult Central Institute for Microbiological Research, Kunitachi-shi, Tokyo, Japan

Offick, B. Institute of Physiology and Biochemistry of Nutrition, Federal Dairy Research Center, Kiel, Germany

Olivares, Mónica Department of Nutrition and Health, Puleva Biotech, Granada, Spain

Parkes, Gareth C. Nutritional Sciences Division, King's College London, 150 Stamford Street, London, SE1 9NH, UK

Perdigón, Gabriela Institute of Microbiology, Tucuman University, Ayacucho 471, Centro de Referencia para Lactobacilos (CERELA-CONICET), Chacabuco 145, San Miguel de Tucuman, Argentina

Pérez-Alvarez, José Angel Departamento de Tecnología Agroalimentaria, Universidad Miguel Hernández de Elche, Orihuela (Alicante), Spain

Pupin, Antonio Marcos CT-Regulatory, Nestec Ltd., Avenue Nestlé 55, CH-1800 Vevey, Switzerland

Rabot, Sylvie Institut National de la Recherche Agronomique, UR 910-Ecologie et Physiologie du Système Digestif, Bâtiment Jacques Poly, 78352 Jouy-en-Josas Cedex, France

Ricke, Steven C. IFSE Food Science Dept., Division of Agriculture, University of Arkansas, 2650 North Young Avenue, Fayetteville, AR, USA

Roccarina, Davide Internal Medicine, Catholic University of Rome, Rome, Italy

Sai, Ika Shanghai Rundo Biotech Japan Co., Ltd. Kobe KIMEC Center Bldg 8F, Minotojima-minami-machi 1-5-2, Chio-ku, Kobe, Hyogo, 650-0047, Japan

Salminen, Seppo Functional Food Forum, University of Turku, Turku, Finland

Salvatore, Silvia Clinica Pediatrica, Università dell'Insubria, Ospedale 'F. Del Ponte', Varese, Italy

Santacruz, Arlette Microbial Ecophysiology and Nutrition Group, Institute of Agrochemistry and Food Technology (CSIC), Burjassot, Valencia, Spain

Sanz, Yolanda Microbial Ecophysiology and Nutrition Group, Institute of Agrochemistry and Food Technology (CSIC), Burjassot, Valencia, Spain

Sayas-Barberá, Estrella Departamento de Tecnología Agroalimentaria, Universidad Miguel Hernández de Elche, Orihuela (Alicante), Spain

Scorrano, Antonio Catholic University of the Sacred Heart, Division of Neonatology, Largo Agostino Gemelli 8, Rome 00168, Italy

Sendra Nadal, Esther Departamento de Tecnología Agroalimentaria, Universidad Miguel Hernández de Elche, Orihuela (Alicante), Spain

Sesma, Fernando CONICET (Consejo Nacional de Investigaciones Científicas y Técnicas), CERELA-CONICET, Chacabuco 145. 4000, San Miguel de Tucuman, Argentina

Sleator, Roy D. Department of Biological Sciences, Cork Institute of Technology, Rossa Avenue, Bishopstown, Cork, Ireland

Smolyansky, Julie Lifeway Foods, Morton Grove, IL, USA

Trois, Livia Ottawa, Ontario, Canada

Vandenplas, Yvan Department of Pediatrics, Universitair Ziekenhuis Kinderen Brussel, Vrije Universiteit Brussel, Brussels, Belgium

Veereman-Wauters, Gigi Pediatric Gastroenterology & Nutrition, Queen Paola Children's Hospital – ZNA and University Hospital Antwerp, Antwerp, Belgium

Xaus, Jordi Drug Development & Clinical Research, Palau Pharma, Palau-solità i Plegamans, Barcelona, Spain

Zuppa, Antonio Alberto Catholic University of the Sacred Heart, Division of Neonatology, Largo Agostino, Gemelli 8, Rome 00168, Italy

Zwolińska-Wcislo, Malgorzata Department of Gastroenterology and Hepatology, Jagiellonian University, Medical College, Poland

INTRODUCTION AND OVERVIEW

1

Production of Probiotic Cultures and Their Incorporation into Foods

Edward R. Farnworth and Claude Champagne
Food Research and Development Centre, Agriculture and Agri-Food Canada
Saint-Hyacinthe, Quebec, Canada

1. INTRODUCTION

Our understanding of the population of bacteria that inhabit the gastrointestinal tract is increasing, and it is becoming more evident that the makeup of this large diverse bacterial community impacts on our digestion, metabolism and health [1, 2]. The chapters in this book illustrate the many and varied ways in which human health might be improved by the consumption of live bacteria.

Many experiments involving the feeding of probiotic bacteria have used the organism of interest either alone, or added to milk or yogurt [3–8]. However, as the number of bacteria identified with beneficial properties has grown, there has been increasing interest in expanding the type of foods into which these beneficial bacteria could be added. However, live bacteria often have strict nutrient requirements for growth, and their viability can be dependent on the environment (food matrix) in which they are located.

A commonly accepted definition of probiotics is that they are 'live microorganisms which, when administered in adequate amounts, confer a health benefit on the host' [9]. This implies that cells must be alive when consumed, and explains why the focus of this chapter is on the delivery of viable cells. However, there are instances where a beneficial effect derived from a probiotic culture does not need live cells [10]. We shall address this aspect and introduce the concept of 'probioactives.'

Furthermore, in the definition of probiotics given above, the efficacy of probiotic-carrying foods can only be assured when: a) beneficial bacteria have been added to foods and beverages in sufficient numbers; b) means have been found to minimize harmful/food matrix interaction; and c) viability has been maintained during manufacture, storage and consumption. This chapter will detail the challenges that face food manufacturers who wish to add bacteria to their probiotic products, and outline some of the solutions that have allowed for the development of an ever-growing diverse line of probiotic foods.

3

2. PRODUCTION OF PROBIOTIC CULTURES FOR FOODS OR FOOD SUPPLEMENTS

The technology related to the production of probiotic cultures by specialized suppliers has already been reviewed [11]. Therefore, this section will not focus on the production parameters that affect the biomass yields. Rather, emphasis is placed on production parameters as they pertain to subsequent viability of the cultures in stressful conditions. The more cells are able to survive stressful conditions in food processing and storage, and/or the stomach, the greater is their viability once they reach to the intestines.

A summary of the production parameters that impact on the ability of probiotic bacteria to survive challenges in the food and the gastrointestinal tract (GIT) are presented in Table 1.1. The first parameter, strain selection, is arguably the most important. Lactic cultures are notorious for variability (even within a given species) of their abilities to grow on food matrices as well as survive heating, freezing, or storage in acid environments [12]. In the past, probiotic cultures destined for addition to foods were chosen, therefore, mainly on their technological properties [13]. However, the requirement for demonstrated health effects has resulted in this parameter increasingly being the principal element of strain selection for food applications.

TABLE 1.1   Parameters during the production of the commercial probiotic cultures that affect their ability to survive stress conditions in foods or in the gastrointestinal tract (GIT)

Stage	Parameter	Basis of effect
Cultures selection	Strain	Variations in the nature and quantity of genetically-determined cell components.
Fermentation	1. Above optimal growth temperature 2. Sub-optimal growth temperature 3. Sub-optimal pH 4. Presence of oxygen	1, 3 and 4. Induce stress responses evidenced by specific proteins. 2. Some stains have enhanced exopolysaccharide production. 1 and 2. Change the lipid composition of cell membranes.
Concentration	Pumping during ultrafiltration. Pressure during centrifugation	Damage to cell walls reduce their ability to subsequently resist the stress. Temporary only, if a 'repair' period is allowed before exposure to the stress.
Stabilization	Freezing or drying	Freezing and drying generate damage to cell wall, membranes and intracellular components. Freeze-dried cells are thus generally more damaged that frozen only. Fresh liquid cultures generally are more resistant to food or GIT stresses than free. Temporary only, if a 'repair' period is allowed before exposure to the stress.
Encapsulation	Technique used: microentrapment (ME) in alginate beads or spray-coating (SC) with fats	Free cells are more rapidly exposed to a stressful environment than SC or ME cultures (SC initially better than ME for this effect). Free cells distribute rather evenly in the matrix but not SC and ME which remain in a capsule microenvironment (ME better than SC for this effect).
Shipping	Temperature	The lower the temperature (even in the frozen state) the more the cells are stable.

In this situation, production and food processing parameters must be adapted to prevent lethal or sub-lethal damages to cells.

Production parameters of probiotic cultures can be adapted at the fermentation, concentration, stabilization, or storage levels (Table 1.1). For example, fermentation temperature modifies the composition of bacterial membranes [14]. A first concept that must be emphasized is that cells can have sub-lethal damage due to processing parameters. This damage can be to the cell wall or the membranes [15]. Presumably, denaturation of internal cell components (for example enzymes) would also generate such sub-lethal damage. It is easy to visualize how high pressures, freezing, and drying can have such effects on cells, and how they result in cultures having lower subsequent resistance to detrimental environmental conditions [16]. But it is less obvious how the fermentation conditions can damage the cells. For example, with lactic cultures, it is well known that extensive over-incubation of a starter with [17] or without [18] pH control, will result in lower specific acidifying activity. A second concept that warrants mention is that applying limited controlled stresses can actually increase the ability of cultures to survive subsequent harsh conditions. As an example, when *Lactobacillus delbrueckii* ssp. *bulgaricus* cells were submitted to a heat pre-treatment at 50°C or to a hyper-osmotic pre-treatment, the viability of cells to a lethal temperature challenge (65°C) increased [19]. A small heat pre-treatment can also improve survival to freeze-drying [20]. Other data show how sub-lethal acid shocks improve viability to heating [21] or freezing [22]. From these two concepts it is clear that biomass production parameters modify the resulting cells; sometimes to their disadvantage, sometimes to their benefit. This requires research and a stringent process control to successfully produce probiotic cultures with an improved ability to be delivered in a viable state in foods following harsh processing conditions.

3. ENSURING DELIVERY OF VIABLE CULTURES IN FOODS AND SUPPLEMENTS

3.1. Delivering as Food Supplements

Supplements are typically delivered in caplets or capsules. The ability of the products to deliver probiotics is mainly set at the production level and, for consumers, storage then becomes the main issue for viability. There are three principal factors which influence the viability of probiotics during storage: temperature, oxygen and relative humidity.

As a rule, cultures, even dried, should be kept refrigerated. In traditional freeze-drying processes, increasing the storage temperature from 4 to 25°C results in a ten-fold reduction of stability [23]. Some commercial products can be kept at room temperature over a few months and do not suffer losses in viability greater than 1 log. However, highly specific and controlled manufacturing conditions are required to obtain such products. As a result, there are reports of products, often inappropriately stored on the shelves, that do not have the claimed populations [24]. Another problem is the fact that strains do not die at the same rate during storage [23]. Thus, the 'total' population in the product might be correct, but the strain ratios could be significantly modified during storage.

Moisture is the second parameter to consider. As a rule, dried cultures should have a water activity (a_w) content of 0.1, and high losses in viability occur above an a_w of 0.3 [25]. During storage it is imperative that the moisture in the air be able to increase the a_w of the culture powder. To prevent exposure of the cultures to water during storage, two actions are taken by companies: 1) packaging in water-impermeable bottles or films; and 2) addition of small moisture-binding sachets in bottles. These strategies work well until the packaging is opened. From this point on, the stability of the culture will depend on the amount of water that is absorbed by the product, especially when the packaging bottle is repeatedly opened.

Finally, oxygen is detrimental to the viability of probiotics during storage. To enhance stability during storage, companies typically add anti-oxidants in the drying medium. Oxygen binders also exist in sachets, but they are not used nearly as much as the water-absorbing ones. As for moisture, this protection is reduced when the product is opened.

All of these elements point to desirable practices for consumers who wish to receive the maximum delivery of probiotics through caplet or capsule supplements:

1. Keep products refrigerated, even if the label states that the cultures are stable at room temperature.
2. Close the bottle as rapidly as possible once the supplement is taken, in order to reduce the entrance of oxygen and moisture into the bottle.
3. If water-absorbing or oxygen-binding sachets are present in the bottle, do not remove them.

3.2. Delivering by Processed Foods

The first foods with probiotic bacteria were yogurts, and fermented milks are still the most important food vehicle for the delivery of probiotic bacteria. However, other foods have now appeared which carry probiotic bacteria. Numerous entries in the functional food market are linked to beverages, such as unfermented milk and fruit juices. Cheese is also gaining acceptance in the market. In addition to these commercial products, many research projects have been carried out which propose the addition of probiotics to chocolate, sausages, cereal products, dried products and vegetables. A multitude of food products contain lactic cultures and are subject to enrichment by probiotic bacteria [26]. Therefore, the potential of delivery of probiotic bacteria by foods is immense.

The first question, with respect to delivering probiotics in foods, is 'how do we add the cultures to the food matrix?' With the exception of very large companies, probiotic cultures are not prepared at the food processing plant but, rather, added directly to the vat. This is some-times called 'direct to the vat inoculation' (DVI). Various reasons explain this [27], but mostly it is for greater flexibility, and to better standard-ize the delivery of the cultures. DVI can be car-ried out by simply opening the sealed packaging and adding the frozen or dried culture to the food matrix. Although it appears easy, if done inappropriately it can lead to substantial losses in viability. Indeed, how a culture is thawed or hydrated can result in a ten-fold variation in colony-forming units (CFU). With respect to fro-zen cultures, the thawing temperature needs to be selected, but few other thawing parameters seem to require specific adjustments. This makes inoculation with frozen cultures rather easy, and few mistakes can be made. This is not the case with the freeze-dried cultures. Although dried cultures are much easier to ship and store than frozen ones, their use in the food processing plant is more difficult. In addition to the plat-ing medium itself, four rehydration parameters influence CFU counts following addition of a powder in a food matrix (Table 1.2). It should be mentioned that these data could also be applied to clinicians wishing to provide probiotics to patients through foods. Rehydration of a powder into a cold fruit juice and drunk immediately, for example, introduces three conditions (low tem-perature, high acidity, no recovery period) which potentially generates viability losses. A question thus arises: 'could probiotic preparation tech-niques be responsible for wide variations of inoc-ulation level and, hence, variable clinical effects?'

The second point to consider is 'can the probiotic cultures survive the processing steps?' Processing of foods requires various techno-logical steps, and many are detrimental to the viability of probiotic bacteria. Examples are presented in Table 1.3. It can be seen that viability losses sometimes reach 6 logs. Reviews of the challenges which occur during food processing have been published [12, 28], and the reader is referred to these publications for examples of applications. To prevent viability losses during processing, two main strategies have proven successful:

1. Modify the food matrix
   a. pH (neutral pH preferable)
   b. addition of antioxidants
   c. addition of growth factors (prebiotics, plant or yeast extracts)
   d. selection of non-toxic ingredients (flavours, preservatives).
2. Modify the process
   a. lower temperatures
   b. include vacuum or nitrogen flushing
   c. modify the fermentation parameters (selection of compatible starter culture, inoculation rate, enzymes)
   d. adapt cells by applying sub-lethal stresses (thermal, pH, osmotic).

Although adapting media and processing conditions may seem easy, it is not. As an example, in the development of a new fermented milk containing probiotic bacteria, 21 parameters can be considered (Table 1.4).

A third point to consider is storage. Unfortunately, processing parameters are not the only elements which affect the delivery of

TABLE 1.2 Factors that affect the viable counts of lactic or probiotic cultures following rehydration

Factor	Effect	Reference
Rehydration medium composition	Viability in milk > peptone > water	[85, 86]
Solids level in rehydration medium	Lower CFU in diluted media	[87]
Rehydration temperature	Highest CFU at optimum growth temperature	[85, 88]
Rehydration time	Less than 10 or longer than 30 minutes detrimental to CFU counts in highly concentrated cultures	[87]
Plating medium	Very variable	[89]

TABLE 1.3 Examples of how food processing conditions affect the viability of probiotic bacteria

Process	Food	Loss of viability		Reference
		Species	Effect	
Addition to the food matrix	Cranberry juice concentrate	L. rhamnosus	↓ 0.7 to 2.3 logs	[90]
Addition of ingredients	Flavours in dairy products	Lactobacilli and Bifidobacteria	Many fruit extracts cause ↓	[91]
Addition of starter cultures	Fermented milks	Bifidobacteria	Viable counts 1 log lower in mixed cultures	[92]
Blending/pumping	Edible spread	B. infantis	↓ of up to 4 logs during processing	[93]
Pasteurization	Peptone broth	Lactobacilli	↓ of 6 logs to 65°C for 30 min	[94]
Freezing	Ice cream	L. bulgaricus	↓ of 1 log	[95]

↓ = Reduction in viability.

TABLE 1.4 Parameters that need to be considered in the development of a probiotic-containing yogurt

Milk blend	Fermentation	Storage
• animal source • pre-processing storage time of raw milk • non-fat solids • fat content • growth supplements • sugar level • flavours and fruits • preservatives • heating parameters • redox level	• compatible starter • form of starter or probiotic (liquid, DVI) • if dried DVI, rehydration parameters (solids, temperature, time) • inoculation level of starter or probiotic (CFU/mL) • moment of inoculation of probiotic • fermentation temperature • fermentation time	• pH (yogurt and after fruit addition) • moment of inoculation of the probiotic • *L. bulgaricus* content and activity (H_2O_2, over acidification) • redox level, addition of antioxidants • packaging, particularly with respect to oxygen permeability • encapsulation

Reproduced with permission from Champagne [96].

TABLE 1.5 Effect of storage in a fruit juice blend for 35 days at 4°C on subsequent viability losses of four probiotic cultures to conditions simulating gastrointestinal stresses

Culture condition	Strain	Viability loss (log CFU/mL) after treatment[1]		
		Acid (pH 2)	Bile (0.25%)	Pancreatic enzymes
Fresh	*L. acidophilus* LB3	2.8	1.2	0
culture	*L. rhamnosus* LB11	2.8	0.3	0
	L. reuteri LB38	2.7	0.1	0
	L. plantarum LB42	2.6	0.2	0
Stored	*L. acidophilus* LB3	5.0	0	0
(35 days)	*L. rhamnosus* LB11	4.5	0	0.1
	L. reuteri LB38	3.2	0	0.2
	L. plantarum LB42	3.7	0	0

Reproduced with permission from Champagne and Gardner [97].

[1]In reference to control treatment (Base medium at pH 6.0).

viable cells to consumers in foods. As was the case for supplements, viability losses occur during storage. Again temperature, moisture and oxygen constitute factors which affect the extent of population losses. However, in foods, additional factors must be mentioned: nature of the starter culture, pH, redox level, type of packaging. Storage also not only affects the viability of cells *per se*, but also the ability of the viable cells to survive the harsh environment of the GIT following consumption. Thus, cultures of lactobacilli were much more sensitive to low pH similar to that in the stomach, when they had been stored for 35 days in a fruit juice blend (Table 1.5). Fortunately, the ability to survive exposure to bile salts was not affected by this 35-day storage period in the juice (Table 1.5). Little is known on how storage can affect the subsequent functionality of probiotic bacteria, and more research is needed in this area.

Finally, the question of how viability can be affected at consumers' homes has received little attention. With beverages in large containers (greater than 1 L), bottles are opened, a portion is taken (typically 250 mL), and the remainder is replaced in the refrigerator. Since some probiotic bacteria are quite sensitive to oxygen [29], a concern can be raised on the detrimental effect of oxygen on the cells found in the remaining beverage. With *L. rhamnosus* R0011 this has not been found to be a problem [30], but studies on other cultures, particularly bifidobacteria, seem warranted.

4. ADDITION OF PROBIOTICS TO FOODS—ENSURING EFFICACY

4.1. Effective Dose

Consumers who are looking to add probiotic bacteria to their diet have several questions to ask themselves. The first question is—'which bacteria to consume?' The science behind the beneficial effects of consuming probiotic bacteria is expanding. Although there have been a large number of diseases/health conditions that have been the target of probiotic treatment studies, a consensus on the effectiveness of probiotics for specific uses in humans is limited to a few applications at the present time. This reality is emphasized by the fact that, to date, very few probiotic products have received health claims approved by health regulatory bodies [31–33].

The second and equally important question is that of dose and duration of the consumption. Because of the lack of clear scientific evidence to show the level of consumption to ensure efficacy, the industrial strategy appears to have been to add as many live bacteria to a food product as is technically and economically realistic [34]. This inevitably results in the conclusion on the part of the consumer that 'more is better.' It is difficult to find published data for

proposed probiotic bacteria to satisfy the major part of the probiotic definition—'...*administered in adequate amounts* confer a health benefit...' [9]—a definition that clearly requires demonstration of the effective dose.

It has to be emphasized that the minimum number will vary depending on the bacteria (at the species and sub-species level) being used, the form in which it is consumed (as part of a food or in a capsule or pill), and the application it is being used for. The scientific literature contains a large range for the number of bacteria that have been suggested to produce a probiotic effect; 10^5 colony-forming units (CFU) as a 'therapeutic minimum' [35] to 10^{11} [36]. Unlike studies of new drugs, dose response studies for probiotic bacteria are not common [36–38].

The Fermented Milks and Lactic Acid Bacteria Beverages Association in Japan have set a minimum of 10^7 bifidobacteria/g or mL for fermented milk products in Japan [39]. CODEX has set a minimum of 10^6 CFU/g for microorganisms added (in addition to those added to produce the product) to fermented milk and yogurt [40]. Recommendations for foods other than fermented milk are not evident at this time.

Although there is still much work to be done in establishing the effective dose for bacteria for specific applications, there is universal agreement that probiotics need to be consumed daily. This arises from the fact that probiotic bacteria presently available, even those from human sources, do not establish themselves in the human gastrointestinal tract. The endogenous population becomes established early on in life. Even though some potential probiotic bacteria have been shown to have the ability to adhere to intestinal cells and mucus soon after the cessation of consumption, they cannot be found in fecal samples, indicating their inability to implant, grow and multiply in the GI tract [41–44].

Some, but not all, definitions of a probiotic bacteria emphasize the need for the bacteria to be alive when they are consumed/administered [45]. However, there appears to be some

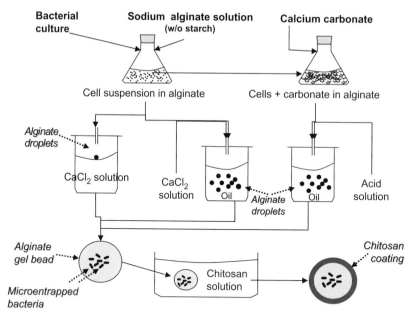

FIGURE 1.1 Three methodologies based on extrusion or emulsion to obtain alginate beads (Reproduced with permission from Claude Champagne).

beneficial effects that do not necessarily require that the bacteria are in fact alive when consumed (see below).

4.2. Effect of Food Matrix

In addition to the effect of storage on the ability of a probiotic culture to survive a simulated gastric environment (Table 1.5), the nature of the food matrix itself has an effect. Data from Saxelin et al. [46] show an increased recovery of *L. rhamnosus* in human stools resulting from the following delivery matrices: powder < juice or fermented milk < unfermented milk < cheese. The buffering ability of the food matrix is arguably a critical factor. But the presence of a fermentable carbohydrate also improves a culture's ability to survive a simulated gastric environment [47]. In this instance, the carbohydrate provides the cell with the ability to produce ATP, which is required for pumping out

acid from the cytoplasm. Not surprisingly, the fibre/carbohydrate content of the food matrix strongly affects the stability of probiotic bacteria during storage in a fruit juice [48].

4.3. Using Encapsulation

The most important recent advance in improving the delivery of probiotics has been encapsulation. There are various techniques available [49], but two have retained the most attention (Table 1.1; Figures 1.1 and 1.2). The microentrapment (ME) technology has been applied mostly to alginate (Figure 1.1), but many other polymers can be used, such as carrageenan, pectin, whey proteins. A further advantage of the alginate ME technology is that it enables a novel biomass production method [50] that can prevent many of the damages to cells which occur during the traditional process (Table 1.1). Although ME with alginate has

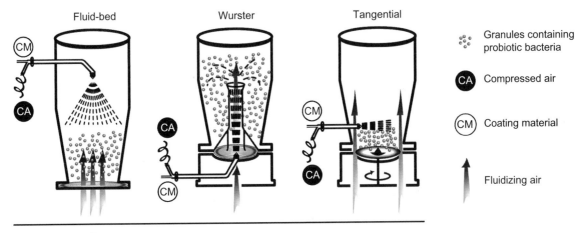

Spray-coating units

FIGURE 1.2 Various methodologies of spray-coating (Reproduced with permission from Claude Champagne).

obtained wide interest in the academic community, its industrial acceptance has been limited. Rather, industry has preferred spray-coating (SC) (Figure 1.2). Cultures encapsulated with the SC technology have much slower rehydration properties than the ME cultures or the standard free-cell cultures. This is very helpful when short exposure to a very stressful environment, such as stomach acid, is required. Accordingly, the cultures prepared for the supplement market are encapsulated by SC rather than ME.

There are reviews on the benefits of encapsulation in the delivery of probiotics in dairy products [51] and other foods [52].

In summary, MEs increase the resistance of probiotic bacteria to rehydration in the presence of spices, heating, freezing, pumping/blending, and storage in yogurt. ME in alginate (Figure 1.1) has often been found to improve survival to the gastric environment [53–57]. However, there are also reports with negative data [58, 59]. The reasons for these discrepancies could be the bead production method or coating method (Figure 1.1), particle size or cell load [51, 60]. Although ME is effective in protecting cells in simulated stomach conditions, SC is probably even more effective at that level.

4.4. Simulated Gastrointestinal Tract Conditions

There are many examples where probiotic bacteria need to arrive alive at the site of action in the gastrointestinal tract. It is commonly believed that the lower GIT, viz. the colon, is the target. Even when product formulation procedures that ensure viability during production and storage have been used as described above, the live bacteria must survive transit of the upper GIT. Ethics, cost, and complexity of tests prevent the testing of foods containing probiotics using human feeding trials. *In vitro* tests, using models of the GIT, can be used to provide data about the ability of bacteria to survive the harsh conditions of the upper GIT.

Many studies that have used test-tube experiments to simulate the acidic conditions in the stomach, and exposure to bile salts and digestive enzymes that occur in the small intestine, have been reported [61–63]. However, such tests cannot replicate the dynamic conditions that occur in the human GIT, and are limited to testing the actual bacteria as opposed to testing the (as eaten) food product. The effects of absorption of nutrients, interaction with undigested and partially digested food, and peristalsis cannot be studied in such simple systems.

Several dynamic *in vitro* models simulating both the events that occur in the stomach and the small intestine of the human GIT have been published [64–66]. Using gravity, pump or mechanical peristalsis, samples move from one chamber to the next and are exposed sequentially to HCl (stomach), bile salts (intestine) and digestive enzymes (intestine). The TNO system [64] also contains porous filters that allow small molecules to pass out of the model, thus simulating absorption. Samples can be taken along the artificial GIT to study how bacteria survive and how the food matrix can protect them (e.g., buffering effects). Such information allows food manufacturers to change conditions in their products that ensure adequate numbers of probiotic bacteria to arrive at their site of action.

In spite of their sophistication, even these dynamic *in vitro* systems are still limited to liquid or puréed samples. However, such *in vitro* GIT simulators have been used to test the protective characteristics of potential encapsulation techniques [67].

5. CONCEPT OF PROBIOACTIVE

The beneficial effects resulting from the consumption of probiotic bacteria are believed to be dependent upon the administered/consumed bacteria still being alive [68, 69]. Interactions between the probiotic bacteria and the intestinal wall cells and resulting changes to the host's immune system are possible [70]. However, in cases where bacteria have been added to a food matrix, and a fermentation has occurred, it is not always evident that the bacteria in the product are the responsible agents [31, 71]. During fermentation, bioactives could have been generated due to the action of the probiotic bacteria on the food matrix. It is also possible that the probiotic bacteria produce metabolites that are bioactive, as they grow in the food matrix. In both cases, once these 'probioactives' have

been formed, there would be no further need to have live bacteria in the product. Figure 1.3 shows how these two types of probioactives could be found in probiotic foods. This concept of probioactives is more inclusive, and more clearly defines the different origins of beneficial ingredients in fermented foods than the term biogenics [72].

5.1. Probioactives from the Food Matrix

During bacterial fermentation of many foods, the action of the bacteria on the food matrix can produce a wide variety of compounds from the initial constituents of the food. In some cases, it is the generation of these bioactive compounds or probioactives that give the fermented food its health benefits.

The most common matrix for probiotic bacteria is cows' milk, although a wide variety of fermented foods believed to be beneficial to health can be found around the world [73]. It has been shown that, through bacterial hydrolytic enzyme activity on cows' milk, a variety of peptides can be produced that have biologic effects including antihypertension (from angiotensin conversion enzyme (ACE) inhibition peptides), opioid agonism, antidiarrheal effects (from casomorhin production), and induction of protective immunity against infections and some tumors (from immunomodulatory peptides) [74, 75]. The release of free amino acids is also possible depending on the bacteria involved and their protease/peptidase activity. Milk glutamic acid is the source of γ-aminobutyric acid (GABA) in cheese due to the action of lactic acid bacteria; GABA has been shown to be useful in improving brain metabolic function and hypertension [76].

Bioconversion of the isoflavone glucosides (daidzin, genistin) into their corresponding bioactive aglycones (daidzein, genistein) has been reported during soymilk fermentation [77, 78].

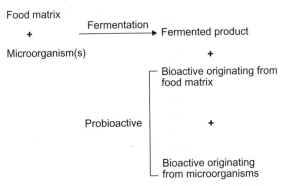

FIGURE 1.3 The production of probioactives in foods.

Included in the list of probioactives would be the short-chain fatty acid butyric acid found in many cheeses [79]. During the production of cheese, bacterial action on the milk fats can result in high levels of butyric acid; butyric acid has been recognized as an anticancer agent and may be implicated in the regulation of cholesterol metabolism [80].

As the development of fermented functional foods expands to include an ever-increasing number of food matrices, and the number of bacteria used to carry out the fermentation of these foods grows, new probioactives will be generated (Figure 1.3).

5.2. Probioactives from Bacterial Metabolism

Microorganisms use the milieu/media that surround them to produce a wide variety of metabolites as they grow and reproduce. These metabolites serve many purposes including contributing to the structure of the cell's wall, carrying out digestion of nutrients required by the bacteria, providing protection for the bacteria against other bacteria, and allowing the bacteria to survive in its environment/niche. Some of these metabolites are found on the outside of the cell wall, some are excreted into the surrounding milieu, while others are only liberated after the

bacterial cell's wall is ruptured. Some bacterial metabolites could be bioactive and have beneficial effects on the host through which the probiotic bacteria are passing.

β-galactosidase is the enzyme responsible for the hydrolysis of lactose into its two constituent sugars, glucose and galactose; insufficient β-galactosidase activity in the brush border membrane on the mucosa in the small intestine leads to lactose maldigestion. Some bacteria also produce this enzyme, and it has been found that lactose maldigestion can be overcome by eating yogurt that contains bacteria which synthesize β-galactosidase. However, it has been reported that lactose hydrolysis is the same if the bacteria (producing β-galactosidase) consumed are alive or not [81]. It is the bacterial enzyme that is the probioactive element.

Bacteria have a wide variety of enzymes, and therefore the careful selection of bacteria to be added to a food could target specific metabolic or digestive problems in the host. Bacteria are capable of producing a wide variety of exopolysaccharides that serve many purposes [82]. Several of these complex carbohydrates have also been shown to have potential beneficial effects including—antitumor properties, immunostimulatory properties, and possible effects on cholesterol metabolism [83, 84]. These beneficial effects are due to the exopolysaccharides and not the bacteria that produced them.

5.3. Protection of Probioactives

It is apparent that the health benefits of fermented foods can be attributed to probioactives derived from the initial food matrix or that can be the result of bacterial metabolism during fermentation. In either case, the bioactive action of the food would not require that the responsible bacteria be alive when consumed. However, to retain their bioactive effect, food producers will have to find ways to protect probioactives during production and storage up to the time of consumption.

6. CONCLUSION

Consumers eager to include probiotics in their diet need to be aware that the ingredients responsible for the health benefits—be they live bacteria or probioactives—are easily killed or destroyed during production, packaging, and storage. Only products produced by companies that have the knowledge and capability to produce such sensitive foods should be eaten. Products need to be formulated so that the live bacteria or probioactives arrive at the site of action in sufficient numbers to be effective. Consumers should read labels carefully to ensure that the product they have purchased has the bacteria (identified to the species or subspecies level) that will produce the effect they want. In the future, more foods will contain live bacteria, as technologies such as encapsulation become widely used in the food industry.

References

1. Guarner, F., & Malagelada, J.-R. (2003). Gut flora in health and disease. *The Lancet*, *360*, 512–519.
2. Saavedra, J. M. (2007). Use of probiotics in pediatrics: rationale, mechanisms of action, and practical aspects. *Nutrition in Clinical Practice*, *22*, 351–365.
3. Biasco, G., Paganelli, G. M., Brandi, G., et al. (1991). Effect of *Lactobacillus acidophilus* and *Bifidobacterium bifidum* on rectal cell kinetics and fecal pH. *Italian Journal of Gastroenterology*, *23*, 142.
4. Orrhage, K., Lidbeck, A., & Nord, C. E. (1991). Effect of *Bifidobacterium longum* supplements on the human fecal microflora. *Microbial Ecology in Health and Disease*, *4*, 265–270.
5. Goldin, B. R., Gorbach, S. L., Saxelin, M., et al. (1992). Survival of Lactobacillus species (strain GG) in human gastrointestinal tract. *Digestive Diseases and Sciences*, *37*, 121–128.
6. de Roos, N. M., Schouten, G., & Katan, M. B. (1999). Yogurt enriched with *Lactobacillus acidophilus* does not lower blood lipids in healthy men and women with normal to borderline high serum cholesterol levels. *European Journal of Clinical Nutrition*, *53*, 277–280.
7. Gardiner, G. E., Heinemann, C., Baroja, M. L., et al. (2002). Oral administration of the probiotic combination *Lactobacillus rhamnosus* GR-1 and *L. Fermentum* RC-14 for human intestinal applications. *International Dairy Journal*, *12*, 191–196.
8. Bonorden, M. J. L., Greany, K. A., Wangen, K. E., et al. (2004). Consumption of *Lactobacillus acidophilus* and *Bifidobacterium longum* do not alter urinary equol excretion and plasma reproductive hormones in premenopausal women. *European Journal of Clinical Nutrition*, *58*, 1635–1642.
9. WHO /FAO. (2002). Report of a Joint FAO/WHO Working Group 'Guidelines for the Evaluation of Probiotics in Food' London, Ont. Canada. <http://www.who.int/ foodsafety/fs_management/en/probiotic_guidelines. pdf/>
10. Ouwehand, A. C., & Salminen, S. J. (1998). The health effects of cultured milk products with viable and nonviable bacteria. *International Dairy Journal*, *8*, 749–758.
11. Champagne, C. P., & Møllgaard, H. (2008). Production of probiotic cultures and their addition in fermented foods. Chapter 19. In E. R. Farnworth (Ed.), *Handbook of Fermented Functional Foods* (2nd edn.) (pp. 513–532). Boca Raton, FL: CRC Press (Taylor and Francis).
12. Champagne, C. P., Gardner, N., & Roy, D. (2005). Challenges in the addition of probiotic cultures to foods. *Critical Reviews in Food Science and Nutrition*, *45*, 61–84.
13. Marr, A. G., & Ingraham, J. L. (1962). Effect of temperature on the composition of fatty acids in *Escherichia coli*. *Journal of Bacteriology*, *84*, 1260–1267.
14. Piuri, M., Sanchez-Rivas, C., & Ruzal, S. M. (2005). Cell wall modifications during osmotic stress in Lactobacillus *casei*. *Journal of Applied Microbiology*, *98*, 84–95.
15. Castro, H. P., Teixeira, P. M., & Kirby, R. (1997). Evidence of membrane damage in *Lactobacillus bulgaricus* following freeze drying. *Journal of Applied Microbiology*, *82*, 87–94.
16. Ananta, E., Volkert, M., & Knorr, D. (2005). Cellular injuries and storage stability of spray-dried *Lactobacillus rhamnosus* GG. *International Dairy Journal*, *15*, 399–409.
17. Champagne, C. P., Piette, M., & St. Gelais, D. (1995). Characteristics of lactococci cultures produced on commercial media. *Journal of Industrial Microbiology*, *15*, 472–479.
18. Ross, G. D. (1980). Observations on the effect of inoculum pH on the growth and acid production of lactic streptococci in milk. *The Australian Journal of Dairy Technology*, 147–149.
19. Gouesbet, G., Jan, G., & Boyaval, P. (2001). *Lactobacillus delbrueckii* ssp. *bulgaricus* thermotolerance. *Lait*, *81*, 301–309.
20. Prasad, J., McJarrow, P., & Gopal, P. (2003). Heat and osmotic stress response of probiotic *Lactobacillus rhamnosus* HN001 (DR20) in relation to viability after drying. *Applied and Environmental Microbiology*, *69*, 917–925.
21. Saarela, M., Rantala, M., Hallamaa, K., et al. (2004). Stationary-phase acid and heat treatments for

improvement of the viability of probiotic lactobacilli and bifidobacteria. *Journal of Applied Microbiology, 96,* 1205–1214.

22. Wang, Y., Corrieu, G., & Beal, C. (2005). Fermentation pH and temperature influence the cryotolerance of *Lactobacillus acidophilus* RD758. *Journal of Dairy Science, 88,* 21–29.

23. Champagne, C. P., Mondou, F., Raymond, Y., & Roy, D. (1996). Effect of polymers and storage temperature on the stability of freeze-dried lactic acid bacteria. *Food Research International, 29,* 555–562.

24. Lin, W. H., Hwang, C. F., Chen, L. W., & Tsen, H. Y. (2006). Viable counts, characteristic evaluation for commercial lactic acid bacteria products. *Food Microbiology, 23,* 74–81.

25. Ishibashi, N., Tatematsu, T., Shimamura, S., et al. (1985). Effect of water activity on the viability of freeze-dried bifidobacteria and lactic acid bacteria. Fundamentals and application of freeze drying to biological materials, dyes and foodstuffs. Paris: International Institute of Refrigeration (pp. 227–232).

26. Farnworth, E. R. (2004). The beneficial effects of fermented foods—potential probiotics around the world. *Journal of Nutraceuticals Functional and Medicinal Foods, 4,* 93–117.

27. Champagne, C. P. (2009). Some technological challenges in the addition of probiotic bacteria to foods (In Press). In D. Charalampopoulos & R. Rastall (Eds.), *Prebiotics and Probiotics Science and Technology*. Springer.

28. Roy, D. (2005). Technological aspects related to the use of bifidobacteria in dairy products. *Lait, 85,* 39–56.

29. Talwalkar, A., & Kailasapathy, K. (2004). A review of oxygen toxicity in probiotic yogurts: influence on the survival of probiotic bacteria and protective techniques. *Comprehensive Reviews in Food Science and Food Safety, 3,* 117–124.

30. Champagne, C. P., Raymond, Y., & Gagnon, R. (2008). Viability of *Lactobacillus rhamnosus* R0011 in an apple-based fruit juice under simulated storage conditions at the consumer level. *Journal of Food Science, 73,* M221–M226.

31. Farnworth, E. R. (2008). The evidence to support health claims. *Journal of Nutrition, 138,* 1250S–1254S.

32. Jew, S., Vanstone, C. A., Antoine, J-M., & Jones, P. J. H. (2008). Generic and product-specific health claim processes for functional foods across global jurisdictions. *Journal of Nutrition, 138,* 1228S–1236S.

33. Reid, G. (2008). Probiotics and prebiotics: progress and challenges. *International Dairy Journal, 18,* 969–975.

34. Sanders, M. E., Walker, D. C., Walker, K. M., et al. (1996). Performance of commercial cultures in fluid milk applications. *Journal of Dairy Science, 79,* 943–955.

35. Nahaisi, M. H. (1986). *Lactobacillus acidophilus:* Therapeutic properties, production and enumeration. In

R. K. Robinson (Ed.), *Developments in Food Microbiology* (2nd edn.) (pp. 153–178). London: Elsevier Applied Science Publishing.

36. Saxelin, M., Elo, S., Salminen, S., & Vapaatalo, H. (1991). Dose response colonisation of feces after oral administration of *Lactbacillus casei* strain GG. *Microbial Ecology in Health and Disease, 4,* 209–214.

37. Saxelin, M., Ahokas, M., & Salminen, S. (1993). Dose response on the faecal colonisation of Lactobacillus strain GG administered in two different formulations. *Microbial Ecology in Health and Disease, 6,* 119–122.

38. Christensen, H. R., Larsen, C. N., Kæstel, P., et al. (2006). Immunomodulating potential of supplementation with probiotics: a dose–response study in healthy young adults. *FEMS Immunology and Medical Microbiology, 47,* 380–390.

39. Ishibashi, N., & Shimamura, S. (1993). Bifidobacteria: research and development in Japan. *Food Technology,* pp. 126, 129–130, 132–135.

40. CODEX (2003). CODEX standard for fermented milks. STAN 243–2003.

41. Marteau, P., Pochart, P., Flourié, B., et al. (1990). Effect of chronic ingestion of a fermented dairy product containing *Lactobacillus acidophilus* and *Bifidobacterium bifidum* on metabolic activities of the colonic flora in humans. *American Journal of Clinical Nutrition, 52,* 685–688.

42. Bouhnik, Y., Pochart, P., Marteau, P., et al. (1992). Fecal recovery in humans of viable *Bifidobacterium* sp ingested in fermented milk. *Gastroenterology, 102,* 875–878.

43. Bouhnik, Y., Flourie, B., Andrieux, C., et al. (1996). Effect of *Bifidobacterium* sp fermented milk ingested with or without inulin on colonic bifidobacteria and enzymatic activities in healthy humans. *European Journal of Clinical Nutrition, 50,* 269–273.

44. Kullen, M. J., Amann, M. M., O'Shaughnessy, W., et al. (1997). Differentiation of ingested and endogenous bifidobacteria by DNA fingerprinting demonstrates the survival of an unmodified strain in the gastrointestinal tract of humans. *Journal of Nutrition, 127,* 89–94.

45. Farnworth, E. R. (2006). Probiotics and Prebiotics. In R. E. C Wildman (Ed.), *Handbook of Nutracteuticals and Functional Foods* (2nd edn.) (pp. 335–352). Boca Raton, FL: CRC Press.

46. Saxelin, M., Korpela, R., & Mayra-Makinen, A. (2003). Introduction: classifying functional dairy products. In T. Mattila-Sandholm, & M. Saarela, (Eds.) *Functional Dairy Products: Vol. 1* (pp. 1–15). Boca Raton, FL: CRC Press/Woodhead Publishing Ltd.

47. Corcoran, B. M., Stanton, C., Fitzgerald, G. F., & Ross, R. P. (2005). Survival of probiotic lactobacilli in acidic environments is enhanced in the presence of metabolizable sugars. *Applied and Environmental Microbiology, 71,* 3060–3067.

48. Saarela, M., Virkajarvi, I., Alakomi, H. L., et al. (2006). Stability and functionality of freeze-dried probiotic Bifidobacterium cells during storage in juice and milk. *International Dairy Journal, 16*, 1477–1482.

49. Champagne, C. P., & Fustier, P. (2007). Microencapsulation for delivery of probiotics and other ingredients in functional dairy products. Chapter 23. In M. Saarela (Ed.), *Functional Dairy Products* (2nd edn.) (pp. 404–426). London: Woodhead Publishing.

50. Champagne, C. P. (2006). Starter cultures biotechnology: The production of concentrated lactic cultures in alginate beads and their applications in the nutraceutical and food industries. *Chemical Industry and Chemical Engineering Quarterly, 12*, 11–17.

51. Champagne, C. P., & Kailasapathy, K. (2008). Encapsulation of probiotics. Chapter 14. In N. Garti (Ed.), *Controlled release technologies for targeted nutrition* (pp. 344–369). London: Woodhead Publishing, CRC Press.

52. Goulet, J., & Wozniak, J. (2002). Probiotic stability: a multifaced reality. *Innovations in Food Technology, February*, 14–16.

53. Le-Tien, C., Millette, M., Mateescu, M. A., & Lacroix, M. (2004). Modified alginate and chitosan for lactic acid bacteria immobilization. *Biotechnology and Applied Biochemistry, 39*, 347–354.

54. Guérin, D., Vuillemard, J. C., & Subirade, M. (2003). Protection of bifidobacteria encapsulated in polysaccharide-protein gel beads against gastric juice and bile. *Journal of Food Protection, 66*, 2076–2084.

55. Iyer, C., & Kailasapathy, K. (2005). Effect of co-encapsulation of probiotics with prebiotics in increasing the viability of encapsulated bacteria under *in vitro* acidic and bile salt conditions and in yogurt. *Journal of Food Science, 70*, M18–M23.

56. Chandramouli, V., Kailasapathy, K., Peiris, P., & Jones, M. (2004). An improved method of microencapsulation and its evaluation to protect Lactobacillus sp. in simulated gastric environments. *Journal of Microbiological Methods, 56*, 27–35.

57. Mandal, S., Puniya, A. K., & Singh, K. (2006). Effect of alginate concentration on survival of microencapsulated *Lactobacillus casei* NCDC-298. *International Dairy Journal, 16*, 1190–1195.

58. Sultana, K., Godward, G., Reynolds, N., et al. (2000). Encapsulation of probiotic bacteria with alginate-starch and evaluation of survival in simulated gastrointestinal conditions and in yoghurt. *International Journal of Food Microbiology, 62*, 47–55.

59. Truelstrup-Hansen, L., Allan-Wojtas, P. M., Jin, Y. L., & Paulson, A. T. (2002). Survival of Ca-alginate microencapsulated *Bifidobacterium* spp. in milk and simulated gastrointestinal conditions. *Food Microbiology, 19*, 35–45.

60. Lee, K. Y., & Heo, T. R. (2000). Survival of *Bifidobacterium longum* immobilized in calcium alginate beads in simulated gastric juices and bile salt solution. *Applied Environmental Microbiology, 66*, 869–873.

61. Prasad, J., Gill, H., Smart, J., & Gopal, P. K. (1998). Selection and characterisation of Lactobacillus and Bifidobacterium strains for use as probiotics. *International Dairy Journal, 8*, 993–1002.

62. Olejnik, A., Lewandowska, M., Obarska, M., & Grajek, W. (2005). Tolerance of Lactobacillus and Bifidobacterium strains to low pH, bile salts and digestive enzymes [http://www.ejpau.media.pl/volume8/issue1/art-05.html]. Electronic Journal of Polish Agricultural Universities, *8*, 1–5.

63. Liu, Z., Jiang, Z., Zhou, K., et al. (2007). Screening of bifidobacteria with acquired tolerance to human gastrointestinal tract. *Anaerobe, 13*, 215–219.

64. Minekus, M., Marteau, P., Havenaar, R., & Huis in't Veld, J. H. J. (1995). A multicompartmental dynamic compute-controlled model simulating the stomach and small intestine. *Alternatives to Laboratory Animals, 23*, 197–209.

65. Hoebler, C., Lecannu, G., Belleville, C., et al. (2002). Development of an *in vitro* system simulating bucco-gastric digestion to assess the physical and chemical changes in food. *International Journal of Food Sciences and Nutrition, 53*, 389–402.

66. Mainville, I., Arcand, Y., & Farnworth, E. R. (2005). Use of a dynamic model simulating the human upper GI tract for the study of probiotics. *International Journal of Food Microbiology, 9*, 287–296.

67. Reid, A. A., Vuillemard, J. C., Britten, M., et al. (2005). Microentrapment of probiotic bacteria in a Ca + -induced whey protein gel and effects on their viability in a dynamic gastrointestinal model. *Journal of Microencapsulation, 22*, 603–619.

68. Kailasapathy, K., & Chin, J. (2000). Survival and therapeutic potential of probiotic organisms with reference to *Lactobacillus acidophilus* and *Bifidobacterium* spp. *Immunology and Cell Biology, 78*, 80–88.

69. Bansal, T., & Garg, S. (2008). Probiotics: from functional foods to pharmaceutical products. *Current Pharmaceutical Biotechnology, 9*, 267–287.

70. Gill, H. S. (1998). Stimulation of the immune system by lactic cultures. *International Dairy Journal, 8*, 535–544.

71. Farnworth, E. R. (2000). Designing a proper control for testing the efficacy of a probiotic product. *Journal of Nutraceuticals, Functional and Medical Foods, 2*, 55–63.

72. Mitsuoka, T. (2000). Significance of dietary modulation of intestinal flora and intestinal environment. *Bioscience Microflora, 19*, 15–25.

73. Farnworth, E. R. (2008). E. R. Farnworth (Ed.), *Fermented Functional Foods* (2nd edn.). Boca Raton, FL: CRC Press.

74. de Moreno de LeBlanc, A., Matar, C., LeBlanc, N., & Perdigón, G. (2005). Effects of milk fermented by *Lactobacillus helveticus* R389 on a murine breast cancer model. *Breast Cancer Research, 7*, R477–R486.

75. Vinderola, G., de Moreno de Le Blanc, A., Perdigon, G., & Matar, C. (2008). Biologically active peptides released

in fermented milk. In E. R. Farnworth (Ed.), *Handbook of Fermented Functional Foods* (2nd edn.) (pp. 209–241). Boca Raton, FL: CRC Press.

76. Tanasupawat, S., & Visessanguan, W. (2008). Thai fermented foods. In E. R. Farnworth (Ed.), *Handbook of Fermented Functional Foods* (2nd edn.) (pp. 495–511). Boca Raton, FL: CRC Press.

77. Chun, J., Kim, G. M., Lee, K. W., et al. (2007). Conversion of isoflavone glucosides to aglycones in soymilk by fermentation with lactic acid bacteria. *Journal of Food Science, 72*, M39–M44.

78. Rekha, C. R., & Vijayalakshmi, G. (2008). Biomolecules and nutritional quality of soymilk fermented with probiotic yeast and bacteria. *Applied Biochemistry and Biotechnology, 151*, 452–463.

79. Woo, A. H., Kollodge, S., & Lindsay, R. C. (1984). Quantification of major fatty acids in several cheese varieties. *Journal of Dairy Science, 67*, 874–878.

80. Bugaut, M. & Bentéjac, M. (1993). Biological effects of short-chain fatty acids in nonruminant mammals. *Annual Review of Nutrition, 13*, 217–241.

81. de Vrese, M., Stegelmann, A., Richter, B., et al. (2001). Probiotics: compensation for lactase insufficiency. *American Journal of Clinical Nutrition, 73*(suppl), 421S–429S.

82. Farnworth, E. R., Champagne, C. P., & Van Calsteren, M-R. (2008). Exopolysaccharides from lactic acid bacteria: food uses, production, chemical structures, and health benefits. In R. E. C. Wildman (Ed.), *Handbook of Nutraceuticals and Functional Foods* (2nd edn.) (pp. 353–371). Boca Raton, FL: CRC Press,.

83. Furukawa, N., Matsuoka, A., Takahashi, T., & Yamanaka, Y. (2000). Anti-metastatic effect of kefir grain components on Lewis lung carcinoma and highly metastatic B16 melanoma in mice. *Journal of the Agricultural Science Tokyo Nogyo Daigaku, 45*, 62–70.

84. Vinderola, G., Perdigón, G., Duarte, J., et al. (2006). Effects of the oral administration of the exopolysaccharide produced by *Lactobacillus kefiranofaciens* on the gut mucosal immunity. *Cytokine, 36*, 254–260.

85. Sinha, R. N., Shukla, A. K., Lal, M., & Ranganathan, B. (1982). Rehydration of freeze-dried cultures of lactic streptococci. *Journal of Food Science, 47*, 668–669.

86. De Valdez, G. F., De Giori, G. S., De Ruiz Holgado, A. P., & Oliver, G. (1985). Effect of the rehydration medium on the recovery of freeze-dried lactic acid bacteria. *Applied Environmental Microbiology, 50*, 1339–1341.

87. De Valdez, G. F., De Giori, G. S., De Ruiz Holgado, A. P., & Oliver, G. (1985). Rehydration conditions and viability of freeze-dried lactic acid bacteria. *Cryobiology, 22*, 574–577.

88. Mille, Y., Obert, J. P., Beney, L., & Gervais, P. (2004). New drying process for lactic bacteria based on their dehydration behaviour in liquid medium. *Biotechnology and Bioengineering, 88*, 71–76.

89. De Valdez, G. F., De Giori, G. S., De Ruiz Holgado, A. P., & Oliver, G. (1986). Composition of the recovery medium and its influence on the survival of freeze-dried lactic acid bacteria. *Milchwissenschaft, 41*, 286–288.

90. Reid, A. A., Champagne, C. P., Gardner, N., et al. (2007). Survival in food systems of *Lactobacillus rhamnosus* R011 microentrapped in whey protein gel particles. *Journal of Food Science, 72*, M031–M037.

91. Vinderola, C. G., Costa, G. A., Regenhardt, S., & Reinheimer, J. A. (2002). Influence of compounds associated with fermented dairy products on the growth of lactic acid starter and probiotic bacteria. *International Dairy Journal, 12*, 579–589.

92. Roy, D., Desjardins, M. L., & Mondou, F. (1995). Selection of bifidobacteria for use under cheese-making conditions. *Milchwissenschaft, 50*, 139–142.

93. Charteris, W. P., Kelly, P. M., Morelli, L., & Collins, J. K. (2002). Edible table (bio)spread containing potentially probiotic Lactobacillus and Bifidobacterium species. *International Journal of Dairy Technology, 55*, 44–56.

94. Ding, W. K., & Shah, N. P. (2007). Acid, bile, and heat tolerance of free and microencapsulated probiotic bacteria. *Journal of Food Science, 72*, M446–M450.

95. Sheu, T. Y., & Marshall, R. T. (1993). Microentrapment of lactobacilli in calcium alginate gels. *Journal of Food Science, 54*, 557–561.

96. Champagne, C. P. (2009). Development of yogurt and specialty fermented milks containing probiotics. In K. Aryana (Ed.), *Recent Advances in Probiotics and Prebiotics in Foods: Product Applications, and Wellbeing*. Lancaster PA: DEStech Publications (in press).

97. Champagne, C. P., & Gardner, N. J. (2008). Effect of storage in a fruit drink on subsequent survival of probiotic lactobacilli to gastro-intestinal stresses. *Food Research International, 41*, 539–543.

Assessment of Prebiotics and Probiotics: An Overview

Arturo Anadón, Maria Rosa Martínez-Larrañaga, Virginia Caballero, and Victor Castellano

Department of Toxicology and Pharmacology, Faculty of Veterinary Medicine, Universidad Complutense de Madrid, Madrid, Spain

1. INTRODUCTION

There is a range of new prebiotic and probiotic emerging and their market in food is growing rapidly. The prebiotics and probiotics need to be assessed for health benefits and safety, before they can be introduced in food products. The functional foods containing prebiotic compounds and probiotic bacteria have great potential for the agro-food industry, consumers and public health. For this reason, the present review intends to express the main health benefits of interest for prebiotics and probiotics as well as the main requirements for their studies and assessments.

There are certainly safety concerns for the consumer concerning the selection and dosage of non-digestive substances, mainly carbohydrates, and their ability to be tolerated and the selection of non-pathogenic bacteria strains. However, there is consensus on the prebiotic metabolic substrates (e.g. digestibility, composition,

dosage, specificity of metabolization) and on the selection of bacterial strains (e.g. counts, survival of gastrointestinal passage, growth conditions, non-pathogenicity, non-toxinogenicity, stability, identity) [1].

The current European Union legislation covers substances with a physiological effect, such as prebiotic compounds and probiotic bacteria. Any claims proposed for these substances must be based on, and substantiated by, the generally accepted scientific data. The European Union regulations will prohibit any claims referring to the prevention, treatment or cure of a human disease for a food in contrast to that proposed by other countries such as Canada and the USA [2]. One of the most difficult endeavors facing those in the prebiotic and probiotic field's substantiation of efficacy needed to support claims of health benefits.

Prebiotic and probiotic foodstuffs with identifiable functions can be rightly considered as functional following the Consensus Document

19

of the Scientific Concepts of Functional Foods in Europe [3] where the following is stated:

> A food can be regarded as 'functional' if it is satisfactorily demonstrated to affect beneficially one or more target functions in the body, beyond adequate nutritional effects, in a way that is relevant to either an improved state of health and well-being and/or reduction of risk of disease. Functional foods must remain foods and they must demonstrate their effects in amounts that can normally be expected to be consumed in the diet; they are not pills or capsules, but part of a normal food pattern.

2. PREBIOTIC CONCEPT

A prebiotic was defined by Gibson and Roberfroid [4] as: 'a non-digestive food ingredient that beneficially affects the host by selectively stimulating the growth and/or activity of one or a limited number of bacteria in the colon, and thus improves host health.' These authors revised this concept and proposed 'a new prebiotic definition as a selectively fermented ingredient that allows specific changes; both in the composition and/or activity in the gastrointestinal microbiota that confers benefits upon host well-being and health' [5, 6]. The latest definition results in an equalization of 'prebiotic' and 'bifidogenic' and includes in the definition the prebiotic index (i.e. gives the absolute increase of the fecal bifidobacteria concentration per gram of daily consumed prebiotics). According to this definition, candidate prebiotics must fulfil the following criteria which are to be proven by *in vitro* and *in vivo* tests: 1) non-digestibility (resistance to low pH gastric acid, enzymatic digestion, and intestinal absorption); 2) fermentation by the intestinal microbiotica; and 3) selective stimulation of growth and activity of intestinal bacteria [7].

Also, the prebiotics have been defined as 'a non-viable food component that confers a health benefit on the host associated with modulation of the microbiota' [8]. The definition arose from observations that particular dietary fibers bring about a specific modulation of the gut microbiota, particularly increased numbers of bifidobacteria and/or lactobacilli cell counts or a decrease in potential harmful bacteria is a sufficient criterion for health promotion. In regular terms, prebiotics are food for bacterial species, which are considered beneficial for health and well-being and it is scientifically accepted prebiotics are valuable dietary additions for modulating the growth and activity of specific bacterial species in the colon that are considered health-supporting.

3. USE OF PREBIOTICS

Although prebiotics and probiotics probably share common mechanisms of action (especially modulation of the endogenous flora), they differ in their composition and metabolism. The fate of prebiotics in the gastrointestinal tract is better known than that of probiotics. Prebiotics, like other low digestible carbohydrates, exert an osmotic effect in the gastrointestinal tract as long as they are not fermented; when they are fermented by the endogenous flora (i.e. at the place where they exhibit their prebiotic effect, they also increase intestinal gas production) [9]. The prebiotic or rather bifidogenic effects depend on the type and concentration of the prebiotic and on the bifidobacteria concentration in the intestine of the host, no simple dose-effect relationship exists. Only carbohydrates like inulin and oligofructose (OF), (*trans*-)galacto-oligosaccharides (TOS or GOS) or lactulose, which are non-digestible but can be fermented by the intestinal flora, fulfil the criteria [7]. Inulin-type fructans are the best documented oligosaccharides for their effect on intestinal bifidobacteria and are considered important prebiotic substrates.

The prebiotics usually employed and the candidate ones are indicated in Table 2.1.

With the exception of inulin (a mixture of fructo-oligo- and polysaccharides), the known prebiotics are mixtures of indigestible oligosaccharides (i.e. chains consisting of three to 10 carbohydrate monomers). Oligosaccharides are carbohydrates of low molecular weight with a degree of polymerization values (2 and 9); exhibit properties typical of dietary fibers and are found in several vegetables as fructans (i.e. asparagus, onions, garlic, and leeks), as stachyose in soybean, as well as in human breast milk and cows' milk as oligosaccharides. Oligosaccharides are readily water-soluble and exhibit some sweetness, which decreases with increasing chain length. Water-binding and gelling properties, and so the putative use as a fat substitute, increases with the number of hexose molecules and reticulation [10].

The glycosidic bonds of oligosaccharides are resistant to hydrolysis by intestinal digestive enzymes and hence are poorly degraded in the upper regions of the gastrointestinal tract, thus reaching the colon intact where oligosaccharides serve as a fermentable substrate. The colonic microbes ferment the non-digestible oligosaccharides to produce short-chain fatty acids (i.e. acetic, propionic, butyric acid), lactic acid, and gases (i.e. carbon dioxide, methane, hydrogen). Finally, it is known that the ingestion of prebiotics can elevate indigenous *bifidobacterium* and *lactobacillus* levels in the colon. Because of fermentation in the large intestine, the ingestion of higher quantities of prebiotics may lead to flatulence, abdominal disorders, and diarrhea. High levels of oligosaccharides (i.e. >10 g/day), may produce intestinal disconform and flatulence.

Oligosaccharides have been recognized as components of dietary fiber because of their interesting physiological effects, which are similar to those of well-known 'soluble' fibers [11]. The prebiotic carbohydrates are not digested by human enzymes but fermented by the flora of the large intestine. Thus, they increase biomass, feces weights, and feces frequency, have a positive effect on constipation and on the health of the mucosa of the large intestine [12, 13].

As a consequence, fermentation of oligosaccharides in the caecum-colon could contribute to the protection against colon cancer [7, 10]; a summary of mechanisms are expressed in Table 2.2.

TABLE 2.1   Common and emergent prebiotics functional food

Type of oligosaccharides

Recognized prebiotics

- Fructo-oligosaccharides (FOS), galacto-oligosaccharides (GOS), galacto-oligosaccharides (GOS)/transgalactosylated-oligosaccharides (GOS/TOS) inulin, isomalto-oligosaccharides, lactulose, pyrodextrins, soy-oligosaccharides (SOS).

Emergent prebiotics

- Genti-oligosaccharides, Gluco-oligosaccharides, isomalto-oligosaccharides (IMO), lactosucrose, levans, pectic-oligosaccharides, resistant starch, sugar alcohols, xylo-oligosaccharides (XOS).

TABLE 2.2   Mechanisms of prebiotics

- Increase in the expression or change in the composition of short-chain fatty acids to colonocytes during fermentation of prebiotics carbohydrates.
- Increased fecal weight and a mild reduction in luminal colon pH.
- A more acidic pH and modulation of the intestinal flora, especially growth stimulation of carbohydrate-fermenting bacteria.
- Decreased concentration of putrefactive, toxic, mutagenic, or genotoxic substances and bacterial metabolites, as well as of secondary bile acids and cancer-promoting enzymes.
- The bifidobacteria and lactobacilli (increased by oligosaccharides) exhibit low β-glucuronidase and nitroreductase activity.
- Decreased nitrogenous end-products and reductive enzymes.
- Production of butyric acid reinforces the regeneration of the intestinal epithelium (i.e. through its pro-apoptotic potency).
- Increased expression of the binding proteins or active carriers associated with mineral absorption.
- Enhanced immunity and modulation of mucin production.

A number of oligosaccharides have been assessed for their prebiotic potential. The dose and duration for nutrition purposes are as follows: inulin (8–40 g/day, 15–64 days), fructo-oligosaccharides (FOS) (4–12.5 g/day, 8–12 days), galacto-oligosaccharides 7.5–15 g/day, 7–21 days), soy-oligosaccharides (10 g/day, 21 days), and lactulose (3–20 g/day, 14–28 days) [14]. Overall, the dosage levels for most health benefits will range from 3 g/day for short-chain fructo-oligosaccharides to 8 g/day for mixed short- and long-chain inulin, although more may be safely consumed according to individual tolerance [15, 16]. Rao [17] reviewed the dose in relation to the extent of the elevation of bifidobacteria and indicated than even when the dose of saccharide ranged from 8 to 40 g/day, there was no correlation with the resultant elevation of bifidobacteria. In general, 10–20 g oligofructose or inulin, regardless of whether ingested in a liquid or solid meal, is considered to be without side effects. In a trial with 80 health probands the ingested quantity, after which at least one of the tested symptoms (headache, belching, flatulence, bowel contractions, or liquid stools) had been observed, was between 31 and 41 g oligofructose, corresponding to 0.04–0.06 g/kg bodyweight [7]. The consumption of 80 g/day of oligofructose in one study gave four of 12 test subjects' diarrhea [18].

Prebiotics can also be used as a supplement and special food. Supplements may provide an easy way to boost prebiotic fiber consumption giving consumers a clear, convenient, and foolproof way to obtain a particular type of prebiotic and dose level. Probiotic supplements can be found clearly labeled, and can be sprinkled directly onto food; stirred into beverages, or taken as capsules, tablets, or chewables. Because the most commonly available prebiotics are water soluble and completely clear in water, they are easily incorporated into most foods and are undetectable. Special foods such as sports drinks, weight-loss powders, ready-to-drink protein meal replacers, and nutrition bars provide a popular way for people to obtain prebiotic fiber. These food items often contain fructo-oligosaccharides, some form of inulin, or resistant starch for their fiber content and prebiotic advantages, although there may be no prebiotic-associated label claims [16].

New prebiotic compounds are emerging because of interesting physiological effects (e.g. low energy value, low carcinogenicity, prebiotic effect, improvement of mineral absorption); and support the addition of some oligosaccharides to foodstuffs that normally contain low or negligible amounts. The oligosaccharides induce an increase of bifidobacteria, especially in feces, after its consumption.

3.1. Use of Prebiotic as a Medical Purpose

Prebiotics have been used for medical purposes. Frequently, they are found in enteral nutrition products. There are used in adult and pediatric patients presenting with a wide range of medical conditions, including diabetes, cancer, renal failure, pressure ulcers, metabolic stress, trauma and immunosuppression [19]. Prebiotic enrichment of these liquid products is used as a means to provide short-chain fatty acids to colonocytes via fermentation, normalize and maintain bowel function, colon integrity, and build colonization resistance in a hospital setting. These characteristics make prebiotics appropriate for use in patients with antibiotic-associated diarrhea, various irritable bowel conditions, including colitis, and for general bowel maintenance while receiving a formulated diet for medical nutrition therapy [20]. When used in appropriate amounts, the effect of prebiotic fiber may also lead to an alteration in nitrogen excretion that is advantageous to renal patients [21, 22]. Table 2.3 expressed the use indications of prebiotics.

Wolf et al. [31] provide an information overview of the medical uses of fructo-oligosaccharides at the levels found in enteral products. The use of these products to provide total nutrition will deliver efficacious amounts of prebiotic fiber to hospitalized patients, generally in the range of

TABLE 2.3   Use indications for prebiotics

	Prebiotics to be used	Possible mechanism	Ref.
Alleviation of constipation	Lactulose, fructo-oligosaccharides, galacto-oligosaccharides	Osmotic effect and modulation of indigenous microflora.	[5]
Treatment of hepatic encephalopathy	Lactulose, Lactilol	Bacterial incorporation of nitrogen and acidification of the colonic environment which in turn reduces the breakdown of nitrogen-containing compounds to ammonia and other potential cerebral toxins.	[10, 23]
Inflammatory bowel diseases (IBD)	Inuline, fructo-oligosaccharides, galacto-oligosaccharides	Regulating immune responses to commensal and pathogenic bacteria.	[24–27]
Prevention of cholesterol gallstones	Oligosaccharides (fructo-oligosaccharides, isomalto-oligosaccharides, galacto-oligosaccharides, palatinose condensate, raffinose and soybean oligosaccharides)	Stimulating the growth of bifidobacteria *in vitro* and *in vivo*.	[28, 29]
Prevention of infections of intestinal origin	Oligosaccharides	Contributing to a greater resistance to infection. Most of *Bifidobacterium* species have scavenging function.	[29]

10 to 15g/day. For patients not receiving formulated diets, simply start with 1g/day for the first week, increasing by 1g/week until a 3g level is attained. The maximum dose that is generally recognized as safe for all persons older than age 1 year is 20g, although much higher doses have also been suggested as safe [16].

3.2. Prebiotic Sources

a) Fructans

Fructans are a group of naturally occurring oligosaccharides and fructo-oligosaccharides found in milligram quantities in onions, bananas, wheat, artichokes, garlic, and other whole foods [32]. They are also extracted from chicory or manufactured from sucrose for use in the food industry. Despite their similarities, the fructans remain distinct from each other in origin, structure, and fermentation characteristics [16]. *In vitro* testing is not sufficient for prebiotic qualification or claims of efficacy because this method cannot approach the dynamic nature of colonic metabolism. There are also method limitations that involve the metabolism of the resident microflora as well as that of the host. These factors contribute to wide variations in measurable colony-forming unit counts, short-chain fatty acid and enzyme levels, and other measurements of outcome [33]. Many factors can confound results, including the chemical composition of the proposed prebiotic, its fermentation profile, the study design, baseline distribution of a subject's colonic microbiotica, the methodologies used in observing an effect in a particular subject group, and the statistical constructs used to interpret the data [34].

b) Resistant starch

Non-fructan prebiotics are also under investigation for their fermentation characteristics, prebiotic effect, and health benefits. Resistant starch has been the subject of numerous studies that document a prebiotic effect, both as a single ingredient and in combination with fructo-oligosaccharides. Resistant starch is found in raw potatoes, cooked and cooled starchy products (retrograde starch), and in unripe fruits like bananas. Appreciable amounts of resistant starch exist in many commercial food products due to the processing effects upon starch [16]. Resistant starch is also manufactured specifically for use in the food industry. The ideal dose of resistant starch is about 20 g/day but low doses in the range of 2.5 to 5 g/day have demonstrated a prebiotic effect; the difference in dosing is due to the varying fermentation profiles of prebiotic ingredients.

The bread and cereal categories are filled with products that include meaningful amounts of resistant starch or inulin for fiber content and sometimes energy reduction. It is reported that 20 g/day of resistant starch is a minimum healthy dose [35]. Bouhnik et al. [36] found that short-chain fructo-oligosaccharides, soybean oligosaccharides, galacto-oligosaccharides, and type III resistant starch measurably raised fecal counts of *Bifidobacterium* species at reasonable dose ranges of 2.5 to 5 g/day within 7 days of administration.

It is also important to validate markers that provide predictors for efficacy on human health. This is a difficult process requiring mechanistic and epidemiological studies for validation. One large barrier to the development of biomarkers relevant to the study of probiotics and prebiotics is that the composition of the human gut flora is not fully characterized and the significance of the presence, absence or certain levels of different genera, species or strains of bacteria, is not understood.

3.3. Prebiotics and Resistance to Gastrointestinal Infections

The gut microflora and the mucosa themselves may act as barriers against invasion by potential pathogens. Bifidobacteria and lactobacilli can inhibit pathogens like *Escherichia coli*, *Campylobacter* and *Salmonella* spp. The lactic microflora of the human gastrointestinal tract is through to play a significant role in the improved colonization resistance [37]. These authors stated different mechanisms that can operate:

1. metabolic end-products, such as acids, excreted by these microorganisms may lower the gut pH, in a microniche, to levels below those at which pathogens are able to effectively compete;
2. competitive effects from occupation of normal colonization sites;
3. direct antagonism through natural antimicrobial excretion (lactic acid bacteria produce inhibitory peptides);
4. competition for nutrients and blocking of pathogen adhesion sites in the gut; and
5. enhancement of the immune system.

Moreover, many lactobacilli and bifidobacteria species are able to excrete natural antibiotics, which can have a broad spectrum of activity [38].

A potential correlation exists with reduced pathogen resistance, decreased numbers of bifidobacteria in the elderly, and the production of natural resistance factors. In essence, the natural gut flora may have been compromised through reduced bifidobacteria numbers and may have a diminished ability to deal with pathogens. If prebiotics are used to increase bifidobacteria or lactobacilli towards being the numerically predominant genus in the colon then an improved colonization resistance will result.

Several studies have been conducted using human subjects, although the dose, substrate, duration and volunteers varied. A general observation was the greater bifidogenic effect of substrates in subjects with a low initial bifidobacteria count (107/g feces) than in those with a high initial number (109.5/g feces) [39]. Also, a negative correlation between bifidobacteria and *Clostridium perfringens* was observed, suggesting that the former may inhibit growth of the latter in the intestine, supporting earlier studies [40, 41].

4. EVALUATION OF PREBIOTIC

According to the FAO Technical Meeting in 2007 on prebiotics [42] the way to evaluate and substantiate a product as a prebiotic is indicated in Figure 2.1.

Taking into account the flow-chart in Figure 2.1, the steps to be followed are:

4.1. Product Specification/Characteristics of the Prebiotic

The component, to which the claim of being prebiotic is attributed, must be characterized for any given product. This includes the source and origin, purity, chemical composition and structure, vehicle, concentration, and the amount in which it is to be delivered to the host.

4.2. Functionality

At a minimum, there needs to be evidence of a correlation between the measurable physiological outcomes and modulation of the microbiota at a specific site (primarily the gastrointestinal tract, but potentially also other sites such as vagina and skin). Also needs to correlate a specific function at a specific site with the physiological effect and its associated timeframe.

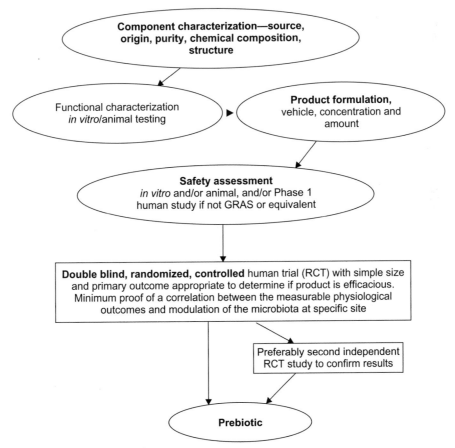

FIGURE 2.1   Guidelines for the evaluation and substantiation of prebiotics.

Within a study, the target variable should change in a statistically significant way and the change should be biologically meaningful for the target group consistent with the claim to be supported. Substantiation of a claim should be based on studies with the final product type, tested in the target host. A suitably sized randomized control trial (compared to a placebo or a standard control substance) is required, preferably with a second independent study.

Examples of physiological outcomes due to the administration of prebiotics could be:

- satiety (measured towards carbohydrates, fats, total energy intake);
- endocrine mechanisms regulating food intake and energy usage in the body;
- effects on absorption of nutrients (e.g. calcium, magnesium, trace elements, protein);
- reduced incidence or duration of infection;
- blood lipid and classic endocrine parameters;
- bowel movement and regularity;
- markers for cancer risk;
- changes in innate and acquired immunity that are evidence of a health benefit.

4.3. Qualifications

The qualifications for a prebiotic can be: *component* (chemical substance or a food grade component), *health benefit* (measurable and not due to the absorption of the component or due to the component acting alone, and over-riding any adverse effects) or *modulation* (changes in the composition or activities of the microbiota in the target host). A prebiotic can be a fiber but a fiber need not be a prebiotic.

It was stated that bifidogenic effects are not sufficient without demonstrated physiological health benefits. It is also recognized that the determining events that take place within compartments of the intestine are often difficult; specific site sampling or more sophisticated methods can reliably link

microbiota modulation with health benefits, fecal analysis will be suitable.

4.4. Safety

It is recommended that the following issues are covered in any safety assessment of a prebiotic final product formulation.

- When the product has a history of safe use in the target host, such as Generally Recognized As Safe (GRAS) or its equivalents (i.e. the Qualified Perception of Safety (QPS) in the EU, also discussed in this revision), then it is suggested that further animal and human toxicological studies may not be necessary.
- Safe consumption levels with minimal symptoms and side effects should be established.
- The product must not contain contaminants and impurities. The contaminants should be identified and measured, and the impurities should be well characterized and submitted to toxicity evaluation if needed.
- Based upon current knowledge, the prebiotic should not alter the microbiota in such a way as to have long-term detrimental effects on the host.

For functional ingredients, animal models can be used to ascertain the target organs and effects that are produced as a result of toxicity. The extent of testing necessary for a functional ingredient is increased in response to the lack of understanding of potential for toxicity because of inadequately characterized products. The following criteria must be met to derive a safe level of exposure without additional toxicology testing [43]:

1. active component(s) and related substances are well-characterized and there is adequate understanding of the lack of potential for toxicity at the human dose levels recommended based upon existing data from the literature;

2. impurities are well-characterized and there is an adequate understanding of the lack of potential for toxicity based upon existing data from the literature; and

3. the manufacturing process is standardized and reproductive.

When the active component(s) or impurities are either not fully characterized, or there is not enough data available to evaluate the potential for toxicity, the following preclinical toxicological information is needed to assess the functional ingredient: toxicity studies *in vitro* and *in vivo*, including mutagenicity studies, reproduction and teratogenicity studies, pharmacokinetics and special pharmacology studies and long-term feeding studies, following a tiered approach on a case-by-case basis. One element that must be considered in the design of animal studies for functional ingredients is the margin of safety between the no-observed-adverse-effect level (NOAEL) determined in the animal studies and the anticipated human level of intake.

5. PROBIOTICS USED IN FOOD

Probiotics are commonly defined as viable microorganisms (yeast and bacteria) that exhibit a beneficial effect on the health of the host when they are ingested. Most probiotics are marketed as foodstuffs or drugs. *Lactobacillus*, *Leuconostoc*, and *Pediococcus* species have been used extensively in food processing throughout human history, and the ingestion of foods containing live bacteria, dead bacteria, and metabolites of these microorganisms has always been around [44].

Most probiotic foods contain lactobacilli and/or bifidobacteria. Enterococci are infrequently used. Microorganisms used as probiotics are mainly bacterial strains of members of the heterogeneous group of lactic acid bacteria; lactobacilli (*L. acidophilus*, *L. casei*, *L. plantarum*, *L. reuteri*, *L. rhamnosus*, *L. salivarus*), bifidobacteria (*B. breve*,

B. longum, *B. lactis*), *Bacillus* (*B. subtilis*, *B. cereus* var. *toyoi*), *Enterococcus* (*E. faecium*) among others. The yeast *Saccharomyces boulardi* is also used as a human probiotic, although as deliverers in capsules or powders rather than in food form. It is noticed that *Bacillus* and *Lactobacillus* differ in many characteristics and that the *Bacillus* and the yeasts are not usual components of the gut microflora. While most of the species and genera are apparently safe, certain microorganisms may be problematic, particularly the enterococci (*E. faecium and E. faecalis*). These have emerged as opportunistic pathogens in hospital environments causing nosocomial infections such as endocarditis, bacteraemia, and intra-abdominal, urinary tract and central nervous system infections, and may also harbor transmissible antibiotic resistance determinants (i.e. vancomycin resistant *Enterococcus* strains) and bacilli, especially those belonging to the *B. cereus* group that are known to produce enterotoxins and an emetic toxin [45].

The selection criteria of new probiotic strains is determined by many factors such as resistance to pancreatic enzymes, acid and bile, preferably human origin (although the *S. boulardi* is not of human origin), documented health effects, known safety, and good technological properties, especially the potential probiotics [46]. It is generally assumed that probiotics are live microorganisms, generally bacteria but also yeasts which, when ingested in sufficient numbers, interact with the gut microflora and host, having a positive effect on the health of an individual.

In most cases, the safety of novel strains has been deduced mainly from the common occurrence of the species either in foods or as normal commensals in the human gut.

At present, probiotic foods are not governed under specific EU regulatory frameworks; although the Regulation (EC) No. 258/97 of the European Parliament and of the Council of 27 January 1997 concerning novel foods and novel food ingredients (OJ No. L 043, 14.02.1997, p. 1)

may cover other more novel types of probiotic species that need to be discussed and assessed in the light of the Novel Food Guidelines [47]. According to this Regulation 258/97, novel foods and food ingredients are those that have not hitherto been used for human consumption to a significant degree within the Community. Specifically, foods and food ingredients containing or consisting of, or produced from, genetically modified organisms and foods consisting of, or isolated from, microorganisms, fungi or algae belong to the category of novel foods. For GM food and feed a comprehensive, specific regulation is in force in EU [Regulation (EC) No. 1829/2003 (OJ No. L 368, 18.10.2003) and Regulation (EC) No. 1830/2003 (OJ No. L 265, 18.10.2003)]. However, it should be stated that additives and processing aids fall outside the scope of the regulation. The case of a processing aid or additive consisting of live microorganisms thus remains ambiguous. Microbial feed additives, however, are covered by Regulation (EC) No. 1831/2003 of the European Parliament and of the Council of 22 September 2003 on additives for use in animal nutrition (OJ No. L 268, 18.10.2003). And, in accordance with the guidelines of the FEEDAP Panel of EFSA, they are subjected to the detailed efficacy and safety assessment, the latter with the intention of ensuring that they are innocuous to target animals, users and consumers [45].

In the Regulation 258/97, the *nutritional information* states that nutritional consequences should be assessed at normal and maximum levels of consumption, and that the effect of anti-nutritional factors (e.g. inhibiting mineral absorption or bioavailability) on the nutritional value of the whole diet should also be assessed. The numbers involved in study groups should ensure that the study has adequate statistical power, and that all studies should comply with relevant elements and ethical principles of guidelines on good clinical practice and good laboratory practice. With respect to the *implications of Novel Food to human nutrition*, overall assessment must consider nutritional implications (expected normal intakes and at maximum levels of consumption).

Referring to the *nutritional considerations affecting toxicological testing in animals*, it is of crucial importance to carefully interpret any adverse effects seen in animal studies. It is also important to distinguish any toxic effects due to nutrition imbalance in the experimental diet and in the design animal feeding studies. The maximum level of dietary incorporation achievable without causing nutritional imbalance should be the highest dose level, while the lowest dose level should be comparable to its anticipated role in human diet. Finally, the *toxicological requirements for Novel Food* needs to be considered on a case-by-case basis. In the worst case scenario, the following elements are needed: consideration of the possible toxicity of the analytically identified individual chemical components, toxicity studies *in vitro* and *in vivo* including mutagenicity studies, reproduction and teratogenicity studies as well as long-term feeding studies and studies on potential allergenicity.

The Novel Food Regulation defines novel foods as foods and food ingredients that were not used for human consumption to a significant degree within the Community before 15 May 1997. 'Human consumption to a significant degree within the Community,' in this context, has been interpreted as being demonstrated by a food having been generally available within the Community. For example, if a food was only available in pharmacies within the Community, this would not constitute evidence of use of human consumption to a significant degree. In contrast, if a food was available in general food stores, this would constitute evidence of use for human consumption to a significant degree [48].

6. SAFETY ASPECT OF PROBIOTICS

Assessment of the safety of probiotics is not an easy task. The selection of new probiotic organisms targets new strains and even genera that are more beneficial or specific. When novel microbes and GMO are introduced, their safety and the risk-to-benefit ratio have to be carefully studied and assessed. Also, new probiotics should be of genera and strains commonly found in the healthy human intestinal microflora. The microbes could be classified as non-pathogenic (*Lactobacillus, Lactococcus, Bifidobacterium, Saccharomyces*), pathogens (*B. cereus*) and opportunistic pathogens (*Enterococcus* and other general lactic acid bacteria). Lactic acid bacteria and bifidobacteria are the most common bacterias that attach to the human intestinal mucosa and are commonly regarded as having the GRAS status. Every viable microbe able to grow under the conditions encountered in a host can cause an infection under certain circumstances, especially in immunocompromised human beings. The factors that must be addressed in the evaluation of safety of probiotics include the following: pathogenicity, infectivity, and virulence factors comprising toxicity, metabolic activity, and the intrinsic properties of the microbes. The absence of pathogenicity and infectivity is a requisite of probiotic safety. Another requisite of probiotics is that the probiotic bacteria should not produce harmful substances by metabolic activity. Platelet-aggregating activity, mucus degradation activity and antibiotic resistance should also be tested [49]. At present, it remains unknown as to whether strains with platelet aggregation properties enhance the infectious risk to a relevant extent, and whether they should be considered undesirable as probiotics.

Members of the genera *Lactococcus* and *Lactobacillus* are most commonly given GRAS status whilst members of the genera *Streptococcus* and *Enterococcus* and some other genera of lactic acid bacteria contain some opportunistic pathogens.

In terms of efficacy and adverse effects, survival of the probiotics in the gastrointestinal tract, their translocation and colonization properties, and the fate of their active components need to be recognized [50]. In the context of potential adverse effects of probiotics, four types of side effects or adverse reactions such as systemic infections, risk of deleterious metabolic activities, risk of adjuvant side effects and of immunomodulation, and risk of gene transfer have been described [51].

According to Salminen et al. [52], three approaches can be used to assess the safety of a probiotic strain: 1) studies on the intrinsic properties of the strain; 2) studies on the pharmacokinetics of the strain (survival, activity in the intestine, dose-response relationship, fecal and mucosal recovery); and 3) studies searching for interactions between the strain and the host. It is very important to identify the survival of the probiotics within the gastrointestinal tract, their translocation and colonization properties, and the fate of their active components to predict the positive effects and/or the side effects. The survival of ingested probiotics at different levels of the gastrointestinal tract differs between strains [50]. Some strains are killed in the stomach while others (e.g. bifidobacteria or *L. acidophilus*) can pass through the entire gut at very high concentrations [50]. In conclusion, the safety and stability would be an important criteria for probiotic selection.

6.1. *In Vitro* Studies

Estimation of the *in vitro* infective properties of the probiotic microorganisms using cell lines and human intestinal mucus degradation. In addition, the assessment of infectivity can be done in animal models (e.g. immunocompromised animals or lethally irradiated animals).

6.2. Animal Studies

Animal models are generally of limited value in microbiological risk assessment concerning probiotic bacteria [53]. There is a high variability in responses between animal species that makes extrapolation of results to humans hazardous. However, the maximum dose levels (tolerance study) in feed given to different animal species that have not caused any site or adverse affects are of interest. The assessment of the acute and sub-acute effects of ingestion of large amounts of the probiotic microorganisms, carried out by using an acute oral and a 90-day rodent feeding toxicity study as performed under EU or OCDE guidelines, is required especially for the new probiotics. The optimal mode of administration is by incorporation into the feed, but if this is impractical, administration in drinking water or by oral *gavage* may be used [45].

6.3. Non-invasive Tests in Animal Models and Humans

Probiotics and prebiotics can have multiple effects on a host (e.g. either directly or indirectly on the pathogenesis and progress of disease) and they require better ways to determine both their safety and toxicity. The non-invasive constitute ways to apply dynamic function testing in animal models and humans to provide reference points to which other measurements can be related (e.g. altered circulating cytokines, altered gene expression). As such, this phenotypic scaffold, alone and combined with newer molecular parameters, will improve our understanding of the interaction of luminal factors within the alimentary tract and the impact that these have on physiologically challenged mucosa and in disease both at the gastrointestinal level and in remote organs [54].

6.4. Studies in Humans

A number of short-term clinical trials on healthy volunteers attested to the safety of current probiotics. In most studies, it is only mentioned that the probiotic did not induce more adverse effects than the placebo or that its tolerance was excellent. In some studies, the presence (or absence) of gastrointestinal disorders has been especially studied, which seems

rational since the first and probably only contact between bio-products and the host occurs in the gastrointestinal tract [51].

6.5. Epidemiological and Post-marketing Surveillance

The long history of the use of probiotic microorganisms has proven their safety. As the risk, then, is very low, the best approach to assess it is probably to analyze it retrospectively in epidemiology studies and prospectively using the post-marketing pharmaco-toxicovigilance systems in populations ingesting large amounts of newly introduced probiotic microorganisms for infections in comparison to the use of traditional strains [51]. Undoubtedly, safety assessment for probiotics should always be associated with those mentioned studies.

The value of such studies depends of course on their statistical power, i.e. on the number of cases studied and the attitude of the health care system to comply with the reported tasks [55–57].

For some new probiotics additional studies could be required especially in the following:

Genotoxicity studies including mutagenicity

At least two different genotoxicity tests, a bacterial reverse mutation assay and an *in vivo* assay for clastogenicity in mammalian cells (e.g. a metaphase cytogenetic assay) should be performed. If these initial tests give an indication of mutagenicity, two additional *in vivo* studies should be carried out using two somatic tissue sites to demonstrate that *in vitro* mutagenicity is not expressed *in vivo* [45].

Toxin production and virulence factors

Under certain specific conditions, some *Bacillus* species have shown to be able to produce toxins. Knowledge of the genetic and biochemical basis for toxin production and methods for the detection of *Bacillus* toxins are reviewed and recommendations made for how best to ensure the absence of toxins (or a capacity for toxin production). The use of strains from *B. cereus* taxonomic group is strongly discouraged. The required studies start with taxonomy of the strain. In the case of organisms belonging to the *B. cereus* group, commercial test kits, laboratory bioassays and PCR-based methods are required to identify toxins and virulence factors. These latter tests are also required for bacilli [45].

Antibiotic resistance profile and transferability of resistances

Bacteria may bear transferable resistances. Lactic acid bacteria are intrinsically resistant to many antibiotics and it has been shown by antibiotic resistance screening that the spontaneous mutation rate to antibiotic resistance among lactobacilli can be quite high [58, 45] as mentioned above. Antibiotic resistance plasmids are of special interest from the safety concern aspect, because they may be conjugatively transferred to other strains, species, and even genera, including potential human and animal pathogens. Several antibiotic resistance plasmids from the lactobacilli haven were detected [59], indicated by curing experiments on the plasmid-linkage of tetracycline and erythromycin resistances in *Lactobacillus fermentum* isolated from human feces. Also, some enterococcal strains have shown a resistance to vancomycin and were able to transfer this kind of resistance to other species.

7. PREBIOTIC AND PROBIOTIC EFFICACY EVIDENCE

These compounds have been studied to varying degrees *in vitro*, in animal feeding studies, but less in human feeding studies. Available data indicate that no harmful effects have been observed in controlled clinical studies with lactobacilli and bifidobacteria. Degradation of intestinal mucus was used as the first marker of toxicity and in one study, specific commercial probiotic strains were shown to be inactive in mucosal degradation [60]. Novel compounds to be used to the human diet fall under the European Union regulatory category of 'novel foods' and will require legislated levels of safety and toxicological assessment before they can be introduced in food products. However, little legislation exists governing the use of the word 'prebiotic' itself on functional food products and there is a growing collection of commercially available products which bears the prebiotic label, but for which supportive scientific literature is sparse or lacking altogether.

7.1. *In Vitro* Evidence

It was generally agreed that *in vitro* approaches are usually too simplistic and fail to successfully mimic the conditions in the human organism, limiting their usefulness in predicting efficacy or safety in humans. Although there are limitations, many *in vitro* evaluations are quite useful and necessary as precursors to *in vivo* studies or in their own right by providing important strain characterization data. *In vitro* tests can be used as the first step of screening for probiotic safety and efficacy. Valuable *in vitro* efforts include genomic analysis, DNA-based and phenotypic strain identification and measurement of viability. These approaches are useful for the following purposes:

- quantifying the bacteria in the sample/product;
- identifying and characterizing the strain(s) being studied;
- recognizing the characterization of strain- or species-specific differences among a range of probiotic bacteria;
- insuring product quality and consistency;

- screening for survivability in the upper gastrointestinal tract;
- conducting mechanistic studies with cellular models; and
- identifying the potential safety risks [2].

7.2. Animal Models

Several animal model systems have been developed for the study of physiological effects of a number of bioactive components and diets. However, there are several important differences such as the anatomy, metabolism, and physiology between animal species and humans; therefore, the outcomes obtained from animal experiments cannot be used as proof of efficacy but only as indications, especially when doses used in animal studies are not reflective of realistic doses to be used in humans [2].

Preliminary substantiation of safety, efficacy and a plausible hypothesis of effect in animal models is important in gaining approval for human studies by institutional review boards, as only a limited range of tests can be performed in humans due to ethical issues. Furthermore, animal models allow the acquisition of tissue from a living animal host that would not be accessible from a human. These tissue samples can be of great value to advancing the understanding of the impact of probiotics and prebiotics on animal physiology [2].

7.3. Human Case Studies

Observations from a single case study are at best only suggestive of a more general effect. Most often, they only reflect peculiar effects in a specific condition and are not representative of the general population. Single case successes should be used only with caution, as they do not provide sufficient evidence of probiotic or prebiotic efficacy and it is tempting to overextend the meaning of the results. Results are likely to be biased towards a specific case and there is no

mechanism for similar reports of product failure. The sample population size is always important in proving efficacy in the general population. Although human case studies can raise public awareness, they should always be confirmed by well-designed, randomized, double blind, controlled trials. Caution should also be exercised in evaluating case studies as they relate to safety. Individual reports of rare adverse incidents can be difficult to interpret without context for evaluating the relative risk [61].

7.4. Human Trials

Well-designed, randomized, double blind, controlled trials are the core of efficacy substantiation and have been conducted with some preparations [62, 63]. However, some factors complicate this approach, especially when applied to the evaluation of functional foods [64]. It is important to define the active ingredients of a preparation to be put on the market, because many ingredients may not be stable. Effects of the functional ingredient(s) may vary when included in different food matrices, and for this reason studies should be performed on the final product. Although placebo-controlled trials are the ideal, it can be difficult to develop an appropriate placebo for some studies, especially for food delivery systems [65]. However, even if the placebo is discernible from the test product, it is still possible to blind a study (i.e. none of the participants knows which product is test and which is placebo). If a placebo-controlled trial is not possible, it is still important that the trial is randomized. Another important factor is the reproducibility of the study.

Open-label studies might provide useful information. For marketing of functional foods, the psychology of the product may be an important factor. However, although important from a marketing point of view, establishment of a psychological placebo effect would not be convincing evidence of efficacy for either scientific or regulatory scrutiny. If an open-label approach is used, randomization is still an important study design element and results must be reproducible to be considered valid [2].

Epidemiology was considered to be valuable, but the large degree of experimental 'noise' in these studies makes it difficult to detect small effects. Obtaining reliable information from consumers regarding their dietary intakes is difficult, and such studies can be costly and time consuming. Observational studies can also be valuable, but do not provide conclusive evidence.

Performing long-term intervention trials is also important, especially in order to observe the improvement of wellness. Most studies with probiotics and prebiotics are short-term (<12 week) studies. If, for example, a risk factor can be reduced with probiotic or prebiotic administration, long-term trials are necessary to investigate whether the effect will persist with time. Postmarket surveillance is important in order to monitor the long-term beneficial (or adverse) effects. It is a difficult task to perform though, since diet is not easily monitored accurately [2].

8. PREBIOTIC AND PROBIOTIC CLAIMS

8.1. European Union

The European Food Safety Authority (EFSA) has issued a scientific and technical guidance for the preparation and presentation of the application for authorization of a health claim [66] under Regulation (EC) No. 1924/2006 of the European Parliament, and The Council of 20 December 2006 on nutrition and health claims made on foods (OJ No. L 404, 30.12.2006), Corrigendum OJ L 12, 18.1.2007, pp. 3–18) requested by the European Commission.

This guidance applies to health claims related to the consumption of a food category, a food, or its constituents (including a nutrient or other substance, or a combination of nutrients/other substances); hereafter referred to as food/constituent.

The purpose of this guidance is to assist applicants in preparing and presenting their applications for authorization of health claims that fall under Article 14 of the Regulation (EC) No. 1924/2006; i.e. reduction of disease risk claims and claims referring to children's development and health. This guidance will be updated at a later stage to cover applications for authorization of the health claims which fall under Article 18 of the Regulation (EC) No. 1924/2006. In other words, applications for inclusion of health claims in the Community list of permitted claims provided for in Article 13(3) based on newly developed scientific evidence and/or include a request for the protection of proprietary data.

As specified in the Regulation (EC) No. 1924/2006, health claims should be substantiated by taking into account the totality of the available scientific data and by weighing the evidence, subject to the specific conditions of use. In particular, the evidence should demonstrate the extent to which:

- the claimed effect of the food/constituent is relevant for human health;
- a cause and effect relationship is established between the consumption of the food/constituent and the claimed effect in humans (such as: the strength, consistency, specificity, dose-response, and biological plausibility of the relationship);
- the quantity of the food/constituent and pattern of consumption required to obtain the claimed effect could reasonably be achieved as part of a balanced diet; and
- the specific study group(s) in which the evidence was obtained is representative of the target population for which the claim is intended.

In accordance with the requirements of the Regulation, the guidance imposes the layout of the submission dossier based on five parts (Table 2.4).

TABLE 2.4 Organization of the applications

Part 1	• Administrative and Technical Data
Part 2	• Food/Constituent Characteristics
Part 3	• Overall Summary of Scientific Data
Part 4	• Body of Pertinent Scientific Data Identified
Part 5	• Annexes to the Application

Organization and content of the application

Data provided in the application should be organized into five parts.

Part 1 contains the specific requirements for the **Administrative and Technical Data**:

• *Comprehensive table of contents of the application*; *application form*; *general information*. These would consist of the name and address of the company or organization, the contact person authorized to communicate with EFSA on behalf of the applicant; the nature of the application (application for authorization of a health claim pursuant to Article 14 or 13(5) of the Regulation (EC) No. 1924/2006); national and international regulatory status.
• *Health claim particulars* (specify the food/constituent for which a health claim is made; describe the relationship between the food/constituent and the claimed effect; provide a proposal for the wording of the health claim for which authorization is sought; specific conditions of use).
• *Summary of the application* and *references*.

Part 2 contains information specific to **Food/Constituent Characteristics**:

• *Food constituent* (name and characteristics; manufacturing process, stability information; bioavailability data).
• *Food or category of food* (name and composition; manufacturing process, stability information, and bioavailability data).
• *References*.

Part 3 contains:

• Tabulated summary of all pertinent studies identified.
• Tabulated summary of data from pertinent human studies.
• Written summary of data from pertinent human studies.
• Written summary of data from pertinent non-human studies.
• Overall conclusions.

Part 4 contains:

• *All pertinent scientific data that form the basis for substantiation of the health claim* (identification of pertinent scientific data). Journal abstracts and articles published in newspapers, magazines, newsletters or handouts that have not been peer-reviewed and books or chapters of books for consumers or the general public should not be cited.
• A comprehensive review of published human data (authorship, background; clearly describe the relationship between the food/constituent and the claimed effect—or surrogate markers of the claimed effect—that is being addressed in the comprehensive review; clearly define exclusion and inclusion criteria that will be applied by the applicant to select pertinent publications; literature search; identification of pertinent published human data).
• Unpublished human data.
• Identification of published non-human data.
• Unpublished non-human data.
• *Pertinent data identified* (human data and non-human data).

Part 5 comprises the **annexes to the application**:

• *Glossary abbreviations; copies/reprints of pertinent published data; full study reports of pertinent unpublished data, and other*; scientific opinion, of national/international regulatory body for health claim authorization if available.

The organization of the data identified as pertinent must be done in the order shown in Table 2.5.

TABLE 2.5   Study type of human and non-human studies

1. **HUMAN STUDIES** (dealing with the relationship between the consumption of the food/constituent and the claimed effect)
   1.1 Experimental intervention studies
   a. RCT (full randomization) (method of randomization reported as coin toss, computer generated numbers, random number tables or similar).
   b. RCT (concealed allocation).
   c. RT (non-controlled).
   1.2 Quasi-experimental intervention studies
   a. Non-randomized, controlled.
   b. Non-randomized, non-controlled.
   1.3 Observational studies
   a. Cohort studies.
   b. Case-control studies.
   c. Cross-sectional studies.
   1.4 Other [human studies dealing with the mechanisms by which the food/constituent could be responsible for the claimed effect (mechanistic studies), or studies on bioavailability].

2. **NON-HUMAN STUDIES**
   2.1 Animal studies [dealing with, e.g., the mechanisms by which the food/constituent could be responsible for the claimed effect (mechanistic studies), including studies on bioavailability].
   2.2 *Ex vivo/in vitro* studies (based on either human or animal biological samples related to the mechanisms of action by which the food/constituent could be responsible for the claimed effect).
   2.3 Other (studies reporting any combination of the above or non-classifiable among the above).

RCT = Randomized controlled trial; RT = Randomized trials.

8.2. United States

As an exemption from drug status, pursuant to amendments to the Food, Drug and Cosmetic (FDC) Act established by the Nutrition Labeling and Education (NLEA) Act of 1990 (NLEA), Food and Drug Administration (FDA) regulations allow a claim in the labeling of food that characterizes the relationship of any food substance to a disease or health-related condition if the claim is first approved by an FDA regulation, 21 of the Code of Federal Regulation (CFR) at Section 101.14. Such claims are called 'health claims.' Examples include calcium to help prevent osteoporosis, folic acid to prevent neural tube defects, and consumption of soy protein to reduce the risk of cardiovascular disease (see 21 CFR § 101.72, 101.79 and 101.82).

Statements of nutritional support, often referred to as structure/function claims, were formally authorized in the Dietary Supplement Health and Education Act of 1994 (DSHEA). Initially, such statements were regarded as being available for use only in the labeling of dietary supplements, not foods, but FDA extended the use of these claims to food in September 1997, in a Federal Register notice (www.cfsan.fda.gov/label.html).

Health claims are defined in the USA as any claims that expressly or by implication characterize the relationship of a dietary substance to a disease or health-related condition, must be pre-approved by the FDA or must be issued as authoritative statements by an agency of the US government with responsibility for dietary guidance or public health [2]. However, Section 3003 of the FDA Modernization Act (FDAMA), 1997, amends section 403(r)(3) of the FDC Act to add new sub-paragraphs (C) and (D), authorizing food labeling to include certain 'health claims' without approval by an FDA regulation.

FDA has issued new guidance to industry allowing *qualified* health claims in the labeling of conventional foods and dietary supplements. This guidance is a result of the Court of Appeals decision in the *Pearson v. Shalala* litigation (United States Court of Appeals for the District of Columbia Circuit, *Pearson v. Shalala*, 164 F.3d 650, DC Cir. 1999). In this guidance the FDA indicates that it will expand the exercise of enforcement discretion for a health claim that is not subject to an FDA approved regulation under the following circumstances [67]:

1. The claim is subject to health claim petition requirements of 21 CFR § 101.70 and has been filed for comprehensive review under 21 CFR § 101.70(J)(2).
2. The scientific evidence in support of the claim outweighs the scientific evidence against the claim, the claim is appropriately qualified, and all statements in the claim are consistent with the weight of the scientific evidence.
3. Consumer health and safety are not threatened.
4. The claim meets the general requirements for health claims at 21 CFR § 101.14 except for not meeting the significant scientific agreement requirement.

Four different health claims are allowed for dietary supplement products without an FDA approved regulation if certain legal requirements are met. Those claims are statements that:

1. claims a benefit related to a classical nutrient deficiency disease and discloses the prevalence of such disease in the United States;
2. describes the role of a nutrient or dietary ingredient intended to affect the structure or function in humans;
3. characterizes the documented mechanism by which a nutrient or dietary ingredient acts to maintain such structure or function; and
4. describes general well-being from consumption of a nutrient or dietary ingredient.

Alternatively, there are other basic rules concerning the use of 'structure/function' health claims for foods that are held to different legal requirements than the 'structure/function' type claims made for dietary supplements [67].

In proving a case for efficacy to substantiate a health or structure/function claim, a variety of sources of information may be compiled, including experience, long-standing traditional use, ethnomedical uses, animal studies, case reports, *in vitro* experiments and clinical or human volunteer trials. Animal and *in vitro* studies alone would not adequately support a health claim [2].

According to the FDA [68], the degree of qualification needed and the level of evidence supporting a health claim will be judged by the following rating system: a) significant scientific agreement exists, no qualifications are necessary; b) the evidence is not conclusive; c) the evidence is limited and not conclusive; and d) there is little scientific evidence supporting the claim.

The types of studies supporting claims will be rated: Type 1 (randomized controlled intervention trial); Type 2 (prospective observational cohort study); Type 3 (non-randomized intervention trial with concurrent or historical control); and Type 4 (cross-sectional study, case study).

The strength of the total body of scientific evidence will be rated according to:

- **Quantity** (the number of studies and number of individuals tested, weighted by study type and quality).
- **Consistency** (similarity of results from high quality studies of design Types 1 and 2.
- **Relevance** [magnitude of effect (observed in high quality studies of design Types 1 and 2) and whether the effect is physiologically meaningful and achievable].

9. QUALIFIED PRESUMPTION OF SAFETY (QPS) CONCEPT OF MICRO-ORGANISMS USED IN FOOD

Presumption being defined in the European Union as 'a belief or assumption based on reasonable evidence' and qualified to allow certain restriction to apply. The QPS approach regarding microorganisms in food and feed is a system similar to the GRAS definition, but modified to take into account the different regulatory practices in Europe. QPS provides a mechanism to recognize and give weight to prior knowledge when assessing the safety of microorganisms in food and feed production.

The QPS approach represents a possible route to harmonization of approaches for the safety assessment of microorganisms used in food/feed production without introducing unnecessary measures in areas where there has been no great concern about safety, while allowing more important safety concerns to be addressed. Therefore, QPS is suggested as an operating procedure within EFSA for risk assessment.

The traditional use of microorganisms may be placed in three categories (see Table 2.6).

QPS is not applicable to traditional, undefined microbial mixtures belonging to Categories A and B, until the mixture becomes defined, and thus regrouped in Category C. For microbes belonging to Category C, QPS is applicable and represents a useful approach to the assessment of safety. If, on this sub-division of the 'tradition use' however, the traditional undefined microbial mixture has a long history of apparent safe use, no safety assessment is needed for this particular use. However, certain issues could be addressed on a case-by-case basis, including the presence of virulence factors, toxic metabolites and antibiotic resistant determinants.

If an undefined mixture belonging to Categories A or B can be defined at a later date, QPS will then become applicable. It was suggested that for microbial mixtures with a long history of safe use, identification at species level rather than at strain level would be required in order to obtain QPS status. It should be noted that the expert consultation jointly set up by the FAO and WHO has strongly advised the use of molecular biology techniques such as 16S

TABLE 2.6   Categories of microorganisms following its traditional use

Category A	• Spontaneous fermentation processes, i.e. without any micro-organisms added intentionally and so-called back-slopping processes where an undefined mixture of micro-organisms, naturally present in a product, is recycled (e.g. olives, cream and sourdough-based bread).
Category B	• Processes based on deliberately added, but undefined microbial mixtures, which were not originally part of the natural flora in the raw material (e.g. 'Kefir', flora Danica).
Category C	• Processes using defined micro-organisms, which are identifiable at the strain level. This category includes complex microbial mixtures containing a large number of different strains, provides that each strain has been identified (i.e., known at the strain level).

rDNA sequencing or DNA/DNA hybridization and up-to-date taxonomic nomenclature for the identification of probiotic bacteria. Comparison of rDNA genes sequences is currently considered to be one of the most powerful and accurate methods for species identification.

Based on this sub-division of the 'traditional use' of microorganisms, the colloquium reached agreement as follows: for microbes belonging to Category C, QPS is applicable and represents a useful approach to the assessment of safety. It should be noted that this category included complex microbial mixtures containing a large number of different strains, provided that each strain has been identified.

In the case of novel use of a microorganism that also has a traditional use in food or feed production, the Novel Food Regulation covers the safety assessment of the products [Regulation (EC) No. 258/97 of the European Parliament and of the Council of 27 January 1997 concerning novel foods and novel food ingredients (OJ No. L 43, 14/2/1997, p. 1)]. For novel use of undefined microbial mixtures, where QPS is not possible, a full case-by-case assessment is needed. However, if the mixture can be defined, no matter how complex that mixture may be, QPS might be applicable, and necessary to optimize the safety assessment.

Taxonomic status of candidate organisms for QPS assessment

The term 'body of knowledge' should be used following the recommendation of EFSA Scientific Colloquium [69]. This term is required for the QPS safety assessment of probiotics and who should decide what defines the boundaries to that body of knowledge. Several elements will comprise the 'body of knowledge' (Figure 2.2). In addition to the peer-reviewed scientific literature, these include an understanding of the history of use of a microorganism, its industrial applications, its ecology, any clinical reports concerning the microorganisms and entries in public databases.

Purpose and advantages of QPS

Any 'generic listing' of a microorganism should be qualified, allowing the general safety of the organism/group of organisms to be concluded provided that certain specific criteria are met. QPS is a qualified generic approval system that would harmonize the safety assessment of microorganisms throughout the food chain. A case-by-case safety assessment could then be limited to only those aspects that are relevant for the organism in question (e.g. the presence of acquired antibiotic resistance determinants in a lactic acid bacterium or known virulence factors in species known to contain pathogenic strains).

Requirements of QPS

For a Notifier with a production strain falling within a taxonomic unit already granted QPS status the only requirements would be: (a) registration of a production strain with accompanying evidence of its taxonomic status and

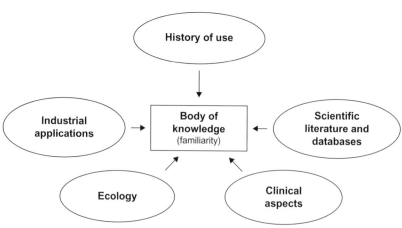

FIGURE 2.2 Components comprising the body of knowledge.

that the strain meets all of the qualifications imposed for the particular taxonomic unit; and (b) notifications of any changes in use or to production conditions.

The QPS would have to be established by those responsible for risk assessment rather than resulting from the cumulative applications of Notifiers. This might initially center on the more commonly encountered genera; in particular, those used for food application to which some form of regulation might be usefully introduced (lactic acid bacteria, bifidobacteria, *Bacillus* spp.). Thereafter, additions may be at the request of, and with the help of, Notifiers.

10. CONCLUSION

This review is focused on an overview of the assessment of prebiotics and probiotics, in respect of their safety and health benefits, before they can be introduced into food products. In the case of novel microorganisms and genetic modified organisms the question of their safety and risk-to-benefit ratio needs to be carefully established. It is recognized that there are numerous potential new applications being considered for prebiotic compounds and probiotic microorganism uses which must be assessed on the basis of the existing scientific regulatory requirements. When novel organisms and genera are selected for probiotic use, the current safety assessment procedures described in the EU Novel Foods Directive and related reviews need to be carefully followed.

There is a need for more randomized, placebo-controlled clinical trials with adequate statistical power. This requires relevant information on the dose–response effects, efficacy and safety of probiotic products. Publication in peer-reviewed journals of all clinical trials, whether the outcome is positive, negative or adverse, should be encouraged.

At present, the available information on current probiotics provides convincing safety records.

ACKNOWLEDGMENT

This work was supported by the *Comunidad de Madrid* and the *Ministerio de Educación y Ciencia*, Projects Ref. AGL2006-02031/ALI, and Consolider-Ingenio 2010 Ref. CSD/2007/00063 (FUN-C-FOOD), Madrid, Spain.

References

1. Przyrembel, H. (2001). Consideration of possible legislation within existing regulatory frameworks. *American Journal of Clinical Nutrition, 73*(Suppl.), 471S–475S.
2. Sanders, M. E, Tompkins, T., Heimbach, J., & Kolida, S. (2005). Weight of evidence needed to substantiate a health effect for probiotics and prebiotics. Regulatory considerations in Canada, EU, and US. *European Journal of Nutrition, 44*, 303–310.
3. Diplock, A. T., Aggett, P. J., Ashwell, M., et al. (1999). Scientific concepts of functional foods in Europe Consensus document. *British Journal of Nutrition, 81*(suppl), S1–S27.
4. Gibson, G. R., & Roberfroid, M. (1995). Dietary modulation of the human colonic microbiota: Introducing the concept of prebiotics. *Journal of Nutrition, 125*, 1401–1412.
5. Gibson, G. R., Probert, H. M., Van Loo, J., et al. (2004). Dietary modulation of the human colonic microbiota: updating the concept of prebiotics. *Nutrition Research Reviews, 17*, 259–275.
6. Roberfroid, M. (2007). Prebiotics: the concept revisited. *Journal of Nutrition, 137*, 830–837.
7. De Vrese, M., & Schrezenmeir, J. (2008). Probiotics, prebiotics, and synbiotics. *Advances in Biochemical Engineering/Biotechnology, 111*, 1–66.
8. FAO. (2007). FAO Technical Meeting on Prebiotics, Food Quality and Standards Service (AGNS), FAO, September 15–16.
9. Roberfoid, M., & Slavin, J. (2000). Nondigestible oligosaccharides. *Critical Review of Food Science and Nutrition, 40*, 461–480.
10. Delzenne, N. M. (2003). Oligosaccharides: state of the art. *Proceedings of the Nutrition Society, 62*, 177–182.
11. Flamm, G., Glinsmann, W., Kristchevsky, D., et al. (2001). Inulin and oligofructose as dietary fiber: A review of the evidence. *Critical Review of Food Science and Nutrition, 41*, 353–362.
12. Cherbur, C. (2002). Inulin and oligofructose in the dietary fiber concept. *British Journal of Nutrition, 87*, 159–162.
13. Nyman, M. (2002). Fermentation and bulking capacity of indigestible carbohydrates: The case of inulin and oligofructose. *British Journal of Nutrition, 87*, 163–168.

14. Conway, P. L. (2001). Prebiotics and human health: The state-of-the-art and future perspectives. *Scandinavian Journal of Nutrition, 45*, 13–21.

15. Marteau, P., & Flourie, B. (2001). Tolerance to low-digestible carbohydrates: Symptomatology and methods. *British Journal of Nutrition, 85*(Suppl. 1), S17–S21.

16. Douglas, L. C., & Sanders, M. E. (2008). Probiotics and prebiotics in dietetics practice. *Journal of the American Dietetic Association, 108*(3), 510–521.

17. Rao, A. V. (1999). Dose-response effects of inulin and oligofructose and intestinal bifidogenesis effects. *Journal of Nutrition, 129*(7S), 1442S–1445S.

18. Clausen, M. R., Jorgensen, J., & Mortensen, P. B. (1998). Comparison of diarrhea induced by ingestion of fructooligosaccharide Idolax and disaccharide lactulose: Role of osmolarity versus fermentation of malabsorbed carbohydrate. *Digestive Diseases and Sciences, 43*, 2696–2707.

19. Ross Products Division. (2005). *Ross Medical Nutrition Pocket Guide*. Columbus, OH: Abbot Laboratories.

20. Seidner, D. L., Lashner, B. A., Brzezinski, A., et al. (2005). An oral supplement enriched with fish oil, soluble fiber, and antioxidants for corticosteroid sparing in ulcerative colitis: A randomized, controlled trial. *Clinical Gastroenterology and Hepatology, 3*, 358–369.

21. Younes, H., Garleb, K., Behr, S., et al. (1995). Fermentable fibers or oligosaccharides reduce urinary nitrogen excretion by increasing urea disposal in the rat caecum. *Journal of Nutrition, 3*, 139–148.

22. Younes, H., Alphonse, J. C., Hadj-Adbelkader, M., & Remesy, C. (2001). Fermentable carbohydrates and digestive nitrogen excretion. *Journal of Renal Nutrition, 3*, 139–148.

23. Marteau, P., & Boutron-Ruault, M. C. (2002). Nutritional advantages of probiotics and prebiotics. *British Journal of Nutrition, 87*(Suppl. 2), S153–S157.

24. Cherbut, C., Michel, C., & Lecannu, G. (2003). The prebiotic characteristics of fructooligosaccharides are necessary for reduction of TNBS-induced colitis in rats. *Journal of Nutrition, 133*, 21–27.

25. Schultz, M., Munro, K., Tannock, G. W., et al. (2004). Effects of feeding a probiotic preparation (SIM) containing inulin on the severity of colitis and on the composition of the intestinal microflora in HLA-B27 transgenic rats. *Clinical and Diagnostic Laboratory Immunology, 11*, 581–587.

26. Furrie, E., Macfarlane, S., Kennedy, A., et al. (2005). Synbiotic therapy (*Bifidobacterium longum*/Synergy 1) initiates resolution of inflammation in patients with active ulcerative colitis: a randomised controlled pilot trial. *Gut, 54*, 242–249.

27. Kelly, D., Conway, S., & Aminov, R. (2005). Commensal gut bacteria: Mechanisms of immune modulation. *Trends in Immunology, 26*, 326–333.

28. Mitsuoka, T., Hidaka, H., & Eida, T. (1987). Effect of fructo-oligosaccharides on intestinal microflora. *Die Nahrung, 31*, 5–6.

29. Kohmoto, T., Fukui, F., Takaku, H., et al. (1988). Effect of isomalto-oligosaccharides on human fecal flora. *Bifidobacteria Microflora, 1*, 61–68.

30. Mitsuoka, T. (1990). Bifidobacteria and their role in human health. *Journal of Industrial Microbiology, 6*, 263–268.

31. Wolf, B. W., Chow, J. M., & Garleb, K. A. (2005). Medical foods and fructooligosaccharides. In S. Dimitriu (Ed.), *Polysaccharides: Structural Diversity and Functional Versatility* (2nd edn.) (pp. 853–866). New York: Marcel Dekker.

32. Chow, J. (2002). Probiotics and prebiotics. A brief overview. *Journal of Renal Nutrition, 12*, 76–86.

33. Blaut, M. (2002). Relationship of prebiotics and food to intestinal microflora. *European Journal of Nutrition, 41*(Suppl. 1), S11–S16.

34. Scholz-Ahrens, K. E., Schaafama, G., & van den Heuvel, E. G. (2001). Effects of prebiotics on mineral metabolism. *American Journal of Clinical Nutrition, 73*(Suppl.), 459S–464S.

35. Cassidy, A., Bingham, S. A., & Cummings, J. H. (1994). Starch intake and colorectal cancer risk. An international comparison. *British Journal of Cancer, 69*, 119–125.

36. Bounik, Y., Raskine, L., Simoneau, G., et al. (2004). The capacity of non-digestible carbohydrates to stimulate fecal bifidobacteria in health humans: A double-blind, randomized, placebo-controlled, parallel-group, dose-response relation study. *American Journal of Clinical Nutrition, 80*, 1658–1664.

37. Gibson, G. R., Saavedra, J. M., Macfarlane, S., & Macfarlane, G. T. (1997). Gastrointestinal microbial disease. In R. Fuller (Ed.), *Probiotics 2: Applications and Practical Aspects* (pp. 10–39). Andover: Chapman and Hall.

38. Gibson, G. R., McCartney, A. L., & Rastall, R. A. (2005). Prebiotics and resistance to gastrointestinal infections. *British Journal of Nutrition, 93*(Suppl. 1), S31–S34.

39. Hidaka, H., Eida, T., Takizawa, T., et al. (1986). Effects of fructooligosaccharides on intestinal flora and human health. *Bifidobacteria Microflora, 5*, 37–50.

40. Wang, X., & Gibson, G. R. (1993). Effects of the *in vitro* fermentation of oligofructose and inulin by bacteria growing in the human large intestine. *Journal of Applied Bacteriology, 75*, 373–380.

41. Gibson, G. R., & Wang, X. (1994). Bifidogenic properties of different types of fructo-oligosaccharides. *Food Microbiology, 11*, 491–498.

42. FAO Technical, Meeting Report. (2007). FAO Technical Meeting on Prebiotics, September, 15–16, 2007.

43. Kruger, C. L., & Mann, S. W. (2003). Safety evaluation of functional ingredients. *Food and Chemical Toxicology, 41*, 793–805.

44. Mäyrä-Mäkien, A., & Bigret, M. (1993). Industrial use and production of lactic acid bacteria. In S. Salminen &

A. von Wright (Eds.), *Lactic Acid Bacteria* (pp. 65–95). New York: Marcel Dekker.

45. Anadón, A., Martinez-Larrañaga, M. R., & Martinez, M. A. (2006). Probiotics for animal nutrition in the European Union. Regulation and safety assessment. *Regulatory Toxicology and Pharmacology, 45*, 91–95.

46. Ouwehand, A. C., Salminen, S., & Isolauri, E. (2002). Probiotics: an overview of beneficial effects. *Antonie van Leeuwenhoek, 82*, 279–289.

47. Jonas, D., Abtignac, E., Antoine, J. M., et al. (1996). The safety assessment of novel foods. Guidelines prepared by ILSI Europe novel foods task force. *Food and Chemical Toxicology, 34*, 931–940.

48. SANCO. (2002). Discussion Paper: Implementation of Regulation (EC) No 258/97 of the European Parliament and of the Council of 27 January 1997 concerning novel foods and novel food ingredients, July 2002 [http://ec.europa.eu/food/food/biotechnology/novelfood/discussion_en.pdf].

49. Ishibashi, N., & Yamazaki, S. (2001). Probiotics and safety. *American Journal of Clinical Nutrition, 73*(Suppl.), 465S–470S.

50. Marteau, P., Pochart, P., Bouhnik, Y., & Rambaud, J. C. (1993). Fate and effects of some transiting microorganisms in the human gastrointestinal tract. *World Review of Nutrition and Dietetics, 74*, 1–21.

51. Salminen, S., & von Wright, A. (1998). Current probiotics—safety assured? *Microbial Ecology in Health and Disease, 10*, 68–77.

52. Salminen, S., von Wright, A., Morelli, L., et al. (1998). Demonstration of safety of probiotics – a review. *International Journal of Food Microbiology, 44*, 93–106.

53. ILSI Europe. (1993). A scientific basis for regulations on pathogenic microorganisms in foods. Summary of a workshop held in May 1993 and organised by the Scientific Committee on Microbiology, ILSI Press.

54. Butler, R. N. (2008). Non-invasive tests in animal models and humans: A new paradigm for assessing efficacy of biologics including prebiotics and probiotics. *Current Pharmaceutical Design, 14*, 1341–1350.

55. Adams, M. R., & Marteau, P. (1995). On the safety of lactic acid bacteria from food. *International Journal of Food Microbiology, 27*, 263–264.

56. Aguirre, M., & Collins, M. D. (1993). Lactic acid bacteria and human clinical infection. *Journal of Applied Bacteriology, 75*, 95–107.

57. Dhodapkar, K. M., & Henry, N. K. (1996). Leuconostoc bacteriemia in an infant with short-gut syndrome: Case report and literature review. *Mayo Clinic Proceedings, 71*, 1171–1174.

58. Curragh, H. J., & Collins, M. A. (1992). High levels of spontaneous drug resistance in *Lactobacillus*. *Journal of Applied Bacteriology, 73*, 31–36.

59. Ishiwa, H., & Iwata, M. (1980). Drug resistance plasmids in *Lactobacillus fermentum*. *Journal of General and Applied Microbiology, 26*, 71–74.

60. Donohue, D., Salminen, S., & Marteau, P. (1998). Safety of probiotic bacteria. In S. Salimnen & A. von Wright (Eds.), *Lactic Acid Bacteria* (pp. 369–384). New York: Marcel Dekker.

61. Rautio, M., Jousumies-Somer, H., Kauma, H., et al. (1999). Liver abscess due to a *Lactobacillus rhamnosus* strain GG. *Clinical Infectious and Diseases, 28*, 1159–1160.

62. Kalliomaki, M., Salminen, S., Arvilommi, H., et al. (2001). Probiotics in primary prevention of atopic disease: A randomised placebo-controlled trial. *Lancet, 357*, 1076–1079.

63. Oli, M. W., Petschow, B. W., & Buddington, R. K. (1998). Evaluation of fructooligosaccharide supplementation of oral electrolyte solutions for treatment of diarrhea. Recovery of the intestinal bacteria. *Digestive Diseases and Sciences, 43*, 138–147.

64. Rafter, J. J. (2002). Scientific basis of biomarkers and benefits of functional foods for reduction of disease risk: Cancer. *British Journal of Nutrition, 88*, S219–S224.

65. Reid, G., Bruce, A. W., Fraser, N., et al. (2001). Oral probiotics can resolve urogenital infections. *FEMS Imnunology and Medical Microbiology, 30*, 49–52.

66. EFSA. (2007). Scientific and technical guidance for the preparation and presentation of the application for authorization of a health claim, Request no EFSA-Q-2007-066.

67. Noonan, W. P., & Noonan, C. (2004). Legal requirements for 'functional food' claims. *Toxicology Letters, 150*, 19–24.

68. FDA. (2003). Guidance Interim Procedures for Qualified Health Claims in the Labelling of Conventional Human Food and Human Dietary Supplements.

69. EFSA. (2005). EFSA Scientific Colloquium Summary Report. OPS Qualified Presumption of Safety of Microorganisms in Food and Feed, 13–14 December 2004, Brussels, Belgium. ISBN 92-9199-012-4 [http://www.efsa.eu.int/science/colloquium_series/no2_qps/948_en.html/].

3

Probiotics: A Historical Perspective

Julie Smolyansky

Lifeway Foods, Morton Grove, IL, USA

Microorganisms have played an essential role in food, drinks, and human health for centuries. The discovery of a symbiotic relationship between bacteria and humans led to novel ways of examining bacteria as potentially beneficial, rather than pathogenic. When mitochondria were discovered in the 1800s, scientists were struck by how much these organelles looked like bacteria. These observations led to the 'endosymbiotic' hypothesis that mitochondria descended from bacteria in a mutually beneficial relation with their human host cells. While scientists knew for a long time that bacteria could live inside animals and plants without causing disease, the symbiotic theory of bacteria and humans would take time and further research to build enough evidence to convince the scientific community [1]. In ancient times, when Eastern nomadic shepherds frequently carried pouches of fresh milk in their travels, they accidently discovered that the milk sometimes fermented into a bubbly, tasting beverage. The nomads called the drink 'kefir,' thought to originate from the Turkish word 'keif,' meaning 'good feeling.' In parts of the Caucasus Mountains, legend has it that the natives added kefir grains, with its fermenting yeasts and bacteria, to fresh milk and drank it once it soured. It is unknown how

many cultures knew about kefir, but Marco Polo is known to have spoken of kefir in his travels to the East [2].

A renewed interest in microorganisms occurred with the discovery of 'lactic acid bacteria' (LAB) in the mid-nineteenth century, and since then dairy foods fermented by these bacteria have been hypothesized to provide a wide variety of health benefits. In the past 150 years, research demonstrating that some microorganisms benefit human health led to the concept of bio-therapeutic and prophylactic uses of bacteria and the widespread use of probiotics in today's world. After Louis Pasteur demonstrated in 1857 that the fermentation process is caused by microorganisms, the first successful isolation of a LAB came shortly after. Joseph Lister isolated the strain *Bacterium lactis* in fermented milk in 1873 [3]. And so began a series of discoveries regarding microorganisms and their intimate relationship with human health. In 1885, Theodor Escherich discovered the bacterium *Escherichia coli* and later suggested a benefit of bacteria in digestion based on evidence of the early colonization of the gastrointestinal tract of infants [4]. A few years later, the discovery of bifidobacteria in the gut flora of breast-fed infants by Henri Tissier at the Institut Pasteur led

43

to the recommendation to administer bifidobacteria to infants with diarrhea. Tissier observed a lower incidence of diarrhea among breast-fed infants compared to formula-fed infants, and claimed that bifidobacteria can replace the harmful bacteria responsible for the diarrhea [5].

The works of one Nobel prize-winning scientist, Elie Metchnikoff, is often considered the birth of probiotics [6]. In Metchnikoff's book, *The Prolongation of Life*, he postulated that the lactic acid bacteria (LAB) content of fermented milk offers health benefits. Metchnikoff further suggested that ingestion of LAB can lead to increased longevity of the host, as he observed that Bulgarian peasants who consumed large amounts of sour milk lived longer than the average human [7]. He also bolstered his data with claims of his own 'feeling of general health and well-being' after ingesting the LAB. The bacteria in the sour milk were what would be later named *Lactobacillus bulgaricus* [7].

Following Metchnikoff's best-selling publication, dozens of experiments were conducted to show a beneficial association between various types of LAB and human health. Then, in the following decades, Metchnikoff's theory that LAB benefit the human gut was challenged by several scientists when they demonstrated that bifidobacteria could not survive passage through the stomach and small intestine [8, 9]. The focus then shifted to other types of LAB that could survive in the human gut but also retained the beneficial features for health. The next strains examined fitting these criteria included *Lactobacillus acidophilus*, which was discovered by Moro in 1900 and promoted by Leo Rettger, a bacteriology professor at Yale University in the 1930s. Rettger and his colleague Harry Cheplin claimed that the intestinal flora of the human gut is dependent almost entirely by the nature of the individual's diet, and that *L. acidophilus* may help certain GI ailments [10, 11].

Over the next century, much of probiotics research examined the effects of *L. acidophilus* on human health, and continues to provide evidence that other LAB strains played a significant role in human health [12]. In 1930, the first culture of *Lactobacillus casei* was isolated by Dr. Minoru Shirota at Kyoto University in Japan. Based on the hypothesis that daily ingestion of LAB promotes intestinal health and prevents disease, Dr. Shirota developed a fermented milk drink named 'Yakult,' which is still on the market today [6]. While it was not yet called a 'probiotic,' by today's standard, this was the first known commercially produced fermented milk drink. Dairy products containing LAB strains were also produced in Germany in the 1960s, and 'bio-yogurts' were first popularized here [4].

The term 'probiotics' is based on the Greek expression 'pro bios,' which means 'for life.' The first use of the word 'probiotic' was by Kollath in 1953 when he used the term to contrast favorable food complexes with antibiotics and other antimicrobial substances [4]. Lilly and Stillwell generalized the definition in 1965 when they described probiotics as 'substances secreted by one microorganism which stimulates the growth of another,' although various other definitions have been proposed and adopted since then [13]. While probiotics improve the microbial environment of the intestine, prebiotics actually stimulate growth or activity of beneficial bacteria already present in the colon. It was not until 1995 that the term 'prebiotic' was introduced by Gibson and Roberfroid as a 'non-digestible food ingredient that beneficially affects the host by selectively stimulating the growth and/or activity of one or a limited number of bacteria in the colon' [14]. In the last decade, a wealth of research on the symbiotic relationship between probiotics and prebiotics has furthered the discussion on health-enhancing foods and beverages.

CONCLUSION

More than 2000 years ago, Hippocrates advocated for the importance of food in human health when he stated 'let food be thy medicine.' This principle of healthy living is still apparent in today's world with the growing interest in foods that are functional and 'prolife.' The strength of the evidence for the benefits of microorganisms in human health has steadily increased since the start of the microbiology era in the mid-nineteenth century, and the value of probiotics has been well-established in clinical trials and other prospective studies. Furthermore, the LAB species such as *Lactobacillus* and *Bifidobacteria* that were examined more than 150 years ago remain the most commonly used probiotics even today. The drink we call kefir has high amounts of these LAB species, containing a total of 10 active microorganisms. Because kefir is such an easily digested nutritious food full of calcium, protein, and fiber, it is ideal for infants, pregnant women, nursing mothers, or the elderly. Research on the health benefits of kefir in a variety of ailments is ongoing, including intestinal tract health, immunity and the prevention of infections, infant and children's health, the management of obesity and nutritional health, and the prevention of cancer.

References

1. Zimmer, C. (2001). *Evolution: The triumph of an idea*. New York, NY: Harper-Collins Publishers Inc.
2. Novil, S. (2008). *Health Professionals, I*. Lifeway Foods, Editor.
3. Lister, J. (1873). On the lactic fermentation and its bearings on pathology. In: *Transactions of the Pathological Society of London*, pp. 425–467.
4. Goktepe, I., Vijay, K. & Juneja, M. A. (2006). *Probiotics in food safety and human health*. Boca Raton, FL: CRC Press.
5. Schrezenmeir, JaMdV. (2001). Probiotics, prebiotics, and synbiotics—approaching a definition. *American Journal of Clinical Nutrition*, 73(Suppl.), 361S–364S.
6. Mazza G. (Ed.). (2008). *Handbook of Fermented Foods*. Boca Raton, FL: CRC Press.
7. Metchnikoff, E. (1907). *The Prolongation of Life*: Optimistic Studies. London: Butterworth-Heinemann.
8. Salminen, S., von Wright, A. & Ouwehand, A. (Eds.), (2004). *Lactic acid bacteria: Microbiological and functional aspects* (3rd edn.). New York: Marcel Dekker, Inc.
9. Rettger, L. F., & Cheplin, H. A. (1921). *A treatise on the transformation of the intestinal flora with special reference to the implantation of bacillus acidophilus*. Yale University Press.
10. Cheplin, H. A., Post, C. D., & Wiseman, J. R. (1923). Bacillus acidophilus milk and its therapeutic effects. *Boston Medical and Surgical Journal*, 189, 405–411.
11. Rettger, L. (1935). *Lactobacillus acidophilus and its therapeutic application*. New Haven: Yale University Press.
12. Klaenhammer, T.e.a. (2002). *Discovering lactic acid bacteria by genomics. in seventh symposium on lactic acid bacteria: genetics, metabolism, and applications*. The Netherlands: Kluwer Academic Publishers.
13. Lilly, D. M., & Stillwell, R. H. (1965). Growth promoting factors produced by micro-organisms. *Science*, 147, 747–748.
14. Gibson, G. R., & Roberfroid, M. B. (1995). Dietary modulation of the human colonic microbiota. Introducing the concept of prebiotics. *Journal of Nutrition*, 125, 1212–1401.

Safety of Probiotic Bacteria

Federico Lara-Villoslada, Mónica Olivares and Jordi Xaus

Department of Nutrition and Health, Puleva Biotech, Granada, Spain

1. INTRODUCTION

The ingestion of lactic acid bacteria (LAB) in fermented food dates back thousands of years in the belief that they have health benefits. Elie Metchnikoff, in the early twentieth century, first related the consumption of probiotic bacteria to health effects and longevity. Since they were consumed as constituents of food, probiotic bacteria, most of them including in the genera *Lactobacillus* and *Bifodobacterium*, with some strains of *Enterococcus* and *Saccharomyces*, were generally considered as safe on the basis of a long history of use and with the assumption that they were normal commensal flora. However, health-promoting effects of probiotics, until recently poorly supported by research, has actually gained great interest, since animal models and clinical trials have demonstrated their benefits. These include: anti-infection properties [1]; beneficial effects in intestinal inflammation [2]; immunomodulatory activity [3]; or efficacy in the prevention of allergic diseases [4]. Thus, probiotics are now considered good candidates for functional foods and a high number of new bacterial strains are being identified and incorporated into food and pharmaceutical products. Not all of these strains have scientifically proven their benefits and safety, although it has been widely demonstrated that probiotic effects are strain specific, which means

that the effects of one strain cannot be extrapolated to others. Thus, it cannot be assumed that all of the probiotic strains share the historical safety of tested or traditional strains. The increasingly widespread use of probiotics, together with different reports relating probiotics with different pathological conditions, has resulted in concern about the risk of consumption of these bacteria. However, it has been reported that, in spite of the marked increase in the use of the probiotic *L. rhamnosus* GG in Finland since 1990, no significant increase in *Lactobacillus* bacteremia attributable to probiotic strains has been observed in southern Finland [5]. Thus, there is scientific evidence supporting the safety of probiotics, particularly the *Lactobacillus* strains. The objective of this chapter is to review different aspects of the safety of probiotic bacteria, such as the known risk of probiotic consumption, positioning of expert committees, and the methods actually used to demonstrate safety of these bacteria. The concept of genetic manipulation of bacteria to achieve a specific probiotic function has been suggested [6, 7]. However, the use of genetically modified organisms (GMOs) with probiotic properties is unlikely in the near future because, among other reasons, of consumer rejection. They would be considered as 'novel food' and stringent safety assessments would be required. These microorganisms are beyond the objective of this chapter, since they fall more in the area of medicine than that of food.

2. PATHOGENICITY AND INFECTIVITY OF PROBIOTIC BACTERIA

Although the absence of pathogenicity and infectivity of a microorganism is a prerequisite to considering it a probiotic, the frequent isolation of strains belonging to the same species than common probiotic bacteria from clinical infections has resulted in concerns about the possible infectivity of these bacteria. While it has been reported that lactobacilli and bifidobacteria may invade the host body by bacterial translocation and other routes [8], it seems probable that for these bacteria to cause infection, both the bacterial factors and the host factors have to be involved. In fact, the isolation of probiotic bacteria from infections is likely to be the result of opportunistic infections. All cases of probiotic sepsis have occurred in patients with an underlying immune compromise, chronic disease or debilitation and there is no report on probiotic sepsis in healthy individuals. In a review by Boyle et al. [9] the known risks of probiotic treatment are revised. These authors have reported 12 cases of bacterial sepsis temporally related to probiotic use in humans, nine cases of bacteremia, two cases of endocarditis and one case of liver abscess. All of these were associated with different risk factors such as diabetes mellitus, short gut syndrome, central nervous catheter and antibiotic diarrhea, among others. In those cases the bacteria isolated was indistinguishable from the probiotic strain consumed. *Lactobacillus rhamnosus* LGG and *Bacillus subtilis* were the most frequently isolated strains, which could be due, at least in the case of LGG, to the widespread use of these strains. No cases of infection from *Bifidobacterium* have been reported. Isolation of *Saccharomyces boulardii* from infection has been more frequent. Boyle and colleagues [9] reported 24 cases of fungal sepsis related to the consumption of this yeast

strain in individuals with different risk factors. They proposed immune comprise and prematurity as major risk factors in the treatment with probiotics and also suggested other minor risk factors such as central venous catheter, impaired intestinal barrier or concomitant treatment with antibiotics to which probiotics are resistant.

In 2008, Besselink et al. [10] reported an increased rate of mortality in patients with severe acute pancreatitis treated with a combination of six probiotics (*L. acidophilus, L. casei, L. salivarius, L. lactis, B. bifidum* and *B. lactis*) compared to patients treated with a placebo. Severe acute pancreatitis is an acute inflammatory process with high rates of mortality. In this disease, enteral nutrition helps in maintaining the integrity of the gut barrier, which is a key factor in limiting bacterial translocation. Modulation of the intestinal flora with probiotics has a rationale as a possible treatment option to limit complications. In fact, it has been demonstrated that treatment with specific probiotics could be beneficial in terms of reducing infectious complications [11]. As previously mentioned, not all probiotics have similar effects and, especially in pathological conditions, benefits and safety of probiotics have to be evaluated on a strain-by-strain basis (Table 4.1).

One theoretical concern with the safety of probiotics is the fact that most of them have been selected to have good adherence, which was initially considered important to their mechanism of action. Adherence to intestinal mucosa could also be the first step in the translocation of bacteria from gut to other tissues. This concern is supported by the fact that blood culture isolates from *Lactobacillus* spp. have greater adherence properties than do isolates from human feces or dairy products [12]. This finding could be of special interest in those cases of immaturity of the intestinal barrier such as in a newborn, especially preterm, although probiotics have been used in preterm infants with no significant adverse effects [13].

Probiotics have also been demonstrated to play an important role in immune-modulation both in animal models and clinical trials [14, 15]. The immunological effect of probiotics, while considered

TABLE 4.1 Main reports of complications associated with the consumption of probiotic bacteria[a]

Report	Age	Complication	Risk factor	Probiotic
Rautio et al. 1999 [60]	74 years	Liver abscess	Diabetes mellitus	LGG
Mackay et al. 1999 [61]	67 years	Endocarditis	Mitral regurgitation, dental extraction	*L. rhamnosus*
Kunz et al. 2004 [62]	3 months	Bacteremia	Prematurity, short gut syndrome	LGG
	10 weeks	Bacteremia	Prematurity, short gut syndrome inflammed intestine	LGG
De Groote et al. 2005 [63]	11 months	Bacteremia	Prematurity, short gut syndrome gastroctomy, CVC, parenteral nutrition rotavirus diarrhea	LGG
Land et al. 2005 [64]	4 months	Endocarditis	Cardiac surgery, antibiotic diarrhea	LGG
	6 years	Bacteremia	Cerebral palsy, jejunostomy feeding, CVC, antibiotic diarrhea	LGG
Richard et al. 1988 [65]	47 years	Bacteremia	Not stated	*B.subtilis*
	25 years	Bacteremia	Not stated	*B.subtilis*
	63 years	Bacteremia	Not stated	*B.subtilis*
	79 years	Bacteremia	Not stated	*B.subtilis*
Oggioni et al. 1998 [66]	73 years	Bacteremia	Chronic lymphocytic leukemia	*B.subtilis*
Zein et al. 2008 [67]	54 years	Bacteremia	Diabetes mellitus	*L. rhamnosus*

[a]Actualized from Boyle et al. 2006 [9]. CVC: central venous catheter. LGG: *L.rhamnosus* GG.

a beneficial property, has also raised some concerns about the use of these bacteria in specific conditions, such as pregnant mothers. Probiotics have been shown to suppress the Th2 response, which could be theoretically detrimental during pregnancy when there is a bias in T cell response to a Th2 phenotype. However, different reports have demonstrated that LGG administration to pregnant women has no adverse effects and it is effective in the reduction of early atopic disease in children at high risk [15] and in the prevention of IgE-associated allergy in cesarean-delivered children [16].

Although probiotics have been related to clinical pathologic conditions, it is unlikely that they universally possess generalized mechanisms of infectivity. Safety evaluation of short- and long-term effects of each specific strain of probiotic will be important in the selection and characterization studies, especially to those strains targeted to specific at-risk populations.

3. EXPERT COMMITTEE REPORTS AND REGULATION ON THE USE OF PROBIOTICS

3.1. Recommendations from Expert Committees

There is no international consensus on the safety of microorganisms used as probiotics. Historically, lactobacilli and bifidobacteria associated with food have been considered to be safe. A long history of consumption of these microorganisms included in human foods or in the preparation of human food has given them this presumption of safety. The ESPGHAN (European Society for Paediatric Gastroenterology, Hepatology and Nutrition) Committee of Nutrition published in 2004 a review about 'Probiotic bacteria in dietetic products for infants' considering that probiotics so far used in clinical trials can be generally considered as safe. However, surveillance for possible side effects, such as infection in high-risk groups, is lacking and is needed [17]. In 2006, a Committee of NASPGHAN (North America Society for Pediatric Gastroenterology, Hepatology and Nutrition) published a guideline of clinical practice on probiotics [18]. The committee concluded that, in general, probiotics can be considered safe even in children. However, it is recommended that caution should be used, especially when considering probiotics in patient populations with indwelling venous catheters.

With the aim of evaluating the information and scientific evidence available on the functional and safety aspects of probiotics, a joint Food and Agriculture Organization of the United Nations/World Health Organization (FAO/WHO) expert Consultation on health and nutritional properties of powder milk with live lactic acid bacteria was held in 2001 [19]. In terms of safety of probiotics, the Consultation believed that a set of general principles and practical criteria are needed to be generated to provide guidelines to test and prove to have a low risk of inducing or being associated with etiology of disease. The Consultation concluded that the evaluation of safety would require at least some studies to be performed in humans, and should address aspects of the proposed end use of the probiotic strain.

FAO/WHO convened a Working Group in 2002 to generate guidelines and recommend criteria and methodology for the evaluation of probiotics including the safety aspects [20]. In recognition of the importance of assuring safety of the probiotic bacteria, the Working Group recommended that probiotic strains be characterized at a minimum with the following tests:

1. Determination of antibiotic resistance patterns.
2. Assessment of certain metabolic activities.
3. Assessment of side effects during human studies.
4. Epidemiological surveillance of adverse incidents in consumers (post market).

5. If the strain under evaluation belongs to a specie that is known as a mammalian toxin producer, it must be tested for toxin production.
6. If the strain under evaluation belongs to a specie with known hemolytic potential, determination of hemolytic activity is required.

It is also suggested that an assessment of lack of infectivity by probiotic strains in immuno-compromised animals would add a measure of confidence in the safety of the probiotic.

3.2. Legislative Framework

However, the previously mentioned guidelines for the evaluation of probiotics in food are only recommendations, and the regulatory framework regarding the safety of human probiotics is practically non-existent. In various countries, the food microorganisms are variably classified either as additives or processing aids or as ingredients.

The United States Food and Drug Administration (FDA) does not currently regulate probiotic products. According to FDA, a microorganism used in food could be classified either as an additive, in which case it has to be approved by the FDA on the basis of safety and efficacy data, or it can be generally recognized as safe (GRAS). The GRAs status can be achieved in two ways. Either the substance or microorganism has a history of safe use in food dating before 1 January 1958, or it has been recognized by qualified experts as safe under the conditions of intended use. However, GRAS status is usually restricted to a specific application and not to a general use of the organism in another context or product. In the case of the European Union, in 2003 a document entitled 'On a generic approach to the safety assessment of microorganisms used in feed/food and feed/food production' was made available for public consultation [21]. This had been prepared by a working group consisting of members of the former Scientific Committee on Animal

Nutrition, Scientific Committee on Food and the Scientific Committee on Plants of the European Commission and is referred to as 'the QPS document.' A system was proposed for a pre-market safety assessment of selected groups of microorganisms leading to a 'Qualified Presumption of Safety (QPS).' The concept and purpose is similar to the GRAS definition used in the USA. In essence, this proposed that a safety assessment of a defined taxonomic group (e.g. genus or group of related species) could be made based on four pillars: establishing identity, body of knowledge including history of use, possible pathogenicity, and end use. If the taxonomic group did not raise safety concerns, or if safety concerns existed but could be defined and excluded (the qualification), the grouping could be granted QPS status. Thereafter, any strain of microorganism, the identity of which could be unambiguously established and assigned to a QPS group, would be free from the need for further safety assessment other than satisfying any qualifications specified. Contrary to the GRAS concept, the status QPS refers to the microorganisms and is not restricted to a specific application allowing the development of novel products. Microorganisms not considered suitable for QPS would remain subject to a full safety assessment.

The EFSA Scientific Committee recommended that a QPS system for microorganisms should be 'introduced and implemented across EFSA as an assessment tool within the framework of the current and proposed legislation for all safety considerations of microorganisms intentionally added to the food chain, regardless of purpose' [22].

Approximately 100 species of microorganisms have been referred to EFSA for a safety assessment. The majority have been the result of notifications for market authorization as sources of food and feed additives, food enzymes and plant protection products. A large majority of these 100 species were found to fall within four broad groupings:

1. Gram-positive non-sporulating bacteria (GPNS).

2. *Bacillus* species.
3. Yeasts.
4. Filamentous fungi.

The Scientific Committee elaborated a list of microorganisms considered suitable for QPS status and these were updated in 2008 [23]. The list contains 74 species of microorganisms, including 33 species of *Lactobacillus* and five of *Bifidobacterium* (Table 4.2).

Curiously the situation is more advanced for animal probiotics, where the Scientific Committee on Animal Nutrition (SCAN) adopted the 'opinion on the criteria for assessing the safety of microorganisms resistant to antibiotics of human clinical and veterinary importance' [24]. The test requirements include assessment of antibiotic resistance, genotoxicity tests and oral toxicity tests. The Panel on Additives and Products or Substances used in Animal Feed (FEEDAP) revised the SCAN opinion and adopted an opinion on the criteria used in the assessment of bacteria for resistance to

TABLE 4.2   Updated list of QPS granted lactobacilli and bifidobacteria[a]

Bifidobacteria		
B. adolescentis	B. bifidum	B. longum
B. animalis	B. breve	
Lactobacilli		
L. acidophilus	L. farciminis	L. paracasei
L. amylolyticus	L. fermentum	L. paraplantarum
L. amylovorus	L. gallinarum	L. pentosus
L. alimentarius	L. gasseri	L. plantarum
L. aviaries	L. helveticus	L. pontis
L. brevis	L. hilgardii	L. reuteri
L. bucheri	L. johnsonii	L. rhamnosus
L. casei	L. kefiranofaciens	L. sakei
L. coryniformis	L. kefiri	L. salivarius
L. crispatus	L. mucosae	L. sanfranciscensis
L. curvatus	L. panis	
L. delbrueckii		

[a]From EFSA 2008 [23].

antibiotics of human or veterinary importance that has become a technical guidance for assisting the applicants in the preparation of dossiers of Additives for Animal Feed [25].

The situation is different in the case of GMOs that would be subjected to the GMO and novel food/feed legislation.

4. EVALUATION OF THE SAFETY OF PROBIOTICS

According to the previously mentioned recommendations and guidelines, probiotics aimed to be incorporated into products for human consumption must be evaluated for safety and efficacy on a strain-by-strain basis. There are different *in vitro* and *in vivo* tests that are generally accepted to evaluate the safety of a probiotic strain, regarding both, the intrinsic properties of the individual strain as well as the effects of different doses of the strain on the host.

4.1. *In Vitro* Tests to Characterize the Safety of a Probiotic Strain

The intestinal microbiota plays an important role in many metabolic activities, including complex carbohydrate digestion, lipid metabolism and glucose homeostasis [26]. Therefore, manipulation of gut microbiota with probiotics may theoretically be associated to deleterious metabolic effects for the host. Some intrinsic properties of the probiotic strains could be detrimental, such as excessive bile salt deconjugation, degradation of mucines, production of ammonia, platelet-aggregating activity or antibiotic resistance. Analysis of those possible detrimental activities is recommended in the evaluation of the safety of probiotic strains (Table 4.3).

Determination of antibiotic resistance patterns

The emergence and the spread or resistance to antimicrobials in bacteria pose a threat to

TABLE 4.3 Main *in vitro* test used to evaluate the safety of probiotic bacteria

Antibiotic susceptibility
MIC values

Identification of the strain
Phenotypic tests
Genetic characterization (DNA/RNA hybridization, 16S sequencing)

Metabolic activities
Deconjugation of bile acids
Production of amines
Platelet-aggregating activity
Degradation of mucines
Production of D-lactic acid

human and animal health and present a major financial cost. As with any bacteria, antibiotic resistance exists among some lactic acid bacteria, including probiotic microorganisms [27]. This resistance may be related to chromosomal, transposon or plasmid located genes. Insufficient information is available on situations in which these genetic elements could be mobilized and it is not known if situations could arise where this would become a clinical problem. The enterococcal strains are normal inhabitants of the gastrointestinal tract and are present in many traditional fermented foods without any apparent risk. However, this resistance was found to be *in vitro* transferable, in addition to other enterococcal strains, and to other Gram-positive bacteria including *Listeria* [28] and *Staphylococcus aureus* [29]. Since vancomycin is one of the last antibiotics that are effective against multidrug-resistant staphylococci, Salminen et al. [27] recommend that no vancomycin-resistant enterococci should be used as either human or animal probiotics.

The joint FAO/WHO expert consultation on health and nutritional properties of powder milk with live lactic acid bacteria suggested in 2001 that further research relating to the antibiotic resistance of lactobacilli and bifidobacteria should be done [19]. The consultation recommended that probiotic bacteria should not harbor transmissible drug resistance genes encoding resistance to clinically used drugs. In the case of animal feed, where the use of antibiotics as growth promoters apparently creates selective advantages for the spread of resistance factors, this prudent precaution would be particularly important. In 2002, FAO/WHO convened a Working Group to generate guidelines and recommend criteria and methodology for the evaluation of probiotics in foods. The Working Group recommended the determination of antibiotic resistance patterns of the probiotic bacteria strains as a requirement for proof of the safety of the bacteria [20].

The extensive use of antibiotics in human and veterinary medicines and the indiscriminate use as growth promoters in animal feed have created a situation where the spread of multidrug resistances could be possible [30]. In an effort to decrease the development of resistance, various actions have been taken at Community level, including the removal of all antibiotics used for growth promotion purposes from animal feed in 2006. The Panel on Additives and Products or Substances used in Animal Feed (FEEDAP) updated the criteria used in the assessment of bacteria for resistance to antibiotics of human or veterinary importance [25]. It was proposed that the minimal inhibitory concentration (MIC) for antibiotics should be tested, as well as the MIC breakpoints *for Enterococcus faecium, E. faecalis, Pediococcus, Lactobacillus* and *Bacillus* categorizing a bacterial strain as resistant to an antibiotic. If the MIC value for a certain antibiotic resistance has been surpassed, the transferability of the resistance should be tested (if possible) by conjugation experiments. If no transfer of genes is detected, the strain should be screened for the presence of known antibiotic resistance genes. The Panel proposes one scheme for the antimicrobial resistance assessment of a bacterial strain used as feed additive (Figure 4.1). The Panel concludes that those strains of bacteria carrying an acquired resistance to antimicrobials should not be used as feed additives, unless it can be demonstrated that it is a result of chromosomal mutation.

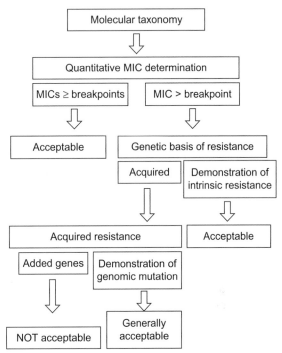

FIGURE 4.1 Scheme for the antimicrobial resistance assessment of a bacterial strain. From EFSA 2008 [25].

Identification of individual strains

Most probiotic strains mainly belong to two genera, *Lactobacillus* and *Bifidobacterium*, but other lactic acid bacteria such as *E. faecium* or *S. thermophilus*, or even non-lactic acid bacteria such as *E. coli*, are used as probiotics. The taxonomic classification of the probiotic bacteria must be accurate since this aspect can involve connotations of safety and regulation [31]. The joint FAO/WHO expert Consultation on health and nutritional properties of powder milk with live lactic acid bacteria recommended that strains should be named according to the International Code of Nomenclature, and deposited in an internationally recognized culture collection. Strain identification should be performed by phenotypic tests followed by genetic identification with methods such as DNA/RNA hybridization and 16sRNA sequencing. For the latter, the RDP (ribosomal data base project) should be used to confirm identity [19]. In the case of the Community a prerequisite for QPS status of a bacteria is the identity, unambiguously established at the taxonomic level claimed [23]. In the future, the sequencing of the completed genomes of a bacterium will allow the exact identification and classification of the bacteria and will also allow discarding of potentially harmful genes.

Metabolic activities

Probiotic bacteria could convert food components or biological secretions into secondary substances potentially harmful to the host. The production of amines during digestion of food proteins by lactobacilli and bifidobacteria has been proposed as a test to assess detrimental effects of probiotics [32]. Martín et al. [33] evaluated the production of biogenic amines by incubating six lactobacilli strains, three of which were isolated from human milk, in the presence of aminoacids in decarboxylase broth using Bover-Cid and Holzapfel's method [34]. None of the lactobacilli tested produced biogenic amines, suggesting a low deaminase activity. In previous reports, Araya-Kojima et al. [35, 36] demonstrated that *Bifidobacterium* spp. have a lower deaminase activity than other bacteria of the intestinal flora.

Deconjugation of bile acids to produce secondary bile salts is another potentially harmful activity of probiotics, since it has been reported that these salts may act as promoters of carcinogenesis [37]. Deconjugation of bile acids can be measured by the activity of the enzyme 7α-dehydroxylase. Takahashi et al. [38] reported the absence of this enzymatic activity in different strains of the genera *Lactobacillus* and *Bifidobacterium*.

Another *in vitro* safety test proposed for probiotics is the platelet-aggregating activity, which has been related to the progression of infective endocarditis [39]. Harty et al. [40] reported that five of five strains of *L. rhamnosus* isolated from infective endocarditis showed aggregating activity, whereas only eight of 16 laboratory strains

showed it. In agreement with those results, Kirjavainen et al. [41] reported that lactobacilli isolated from aortic infections have higher aggregating activity than do strains isolated from urinary or respiratory infections.

Production of D(−)-lactic acid by probiotic bacteria, especially strains of the genus *Lactobacillus*, is also a concern in the use of probiotics in children, due to D(−)-lactic acidosis, a pathologic condition characterized by neurological alterations. However, in the literature there is no cases of D(−)-lactic acidosis in healthy humans and almost all cases are related to short bowel syndrome [42, 43]. Although mammal tissues lack D-lactate dehydrogenase (DLDH) and thus they cannot use this via to metabolise D(−)-lactic acid, it has been reported that this compound is efficiently metabolized by mammals [42, 43], probably through the D-2-hydroxyacid dehydrogenase. In fact, administration of D(−)-lactic acid-producing bacteria to human infants has been shown to be safe and blood levels of D(−)-lactic acid in those infants remained under normal values [44]. In addition, lactobacilli strain producers of D(−)-lactic acid, such as *L. acidophilus*, *L. fermentum*, *L. gasseri*, *L. reuteri* or *L. plantarum*, are normally found in the fecal microbiota of healthy children and adults. Martín et al. [45] also reported the presence of strains of *L. fermentum* and *L. gasseri* in breast milk from healthy women and thus, it is supposed that those strains will be transferred to newborns through breast-feeding.

4.2. Animal Studies

Although extrapolation of results obtained from animal studies to human has limited validity, toxicity studies in experimental animals are generally accepted as a reliable tool to assess acute toxicity. However, those experiments are normally expensive and time-consuming, which makes the *in vitro* selection process of the probiotic strain to be assessed, crucial.

Acute toxicity studies, conducted by the same procedures used for testing toxicity of chemicals, have been widely used for the evaluation of probiotic safety and tolerance. These studies are carried out by oral administration of high doses of the probiotic strain to animals, usually mice, over a short period of time (usually 7 or 8 days). An important parameter to be assessed in these studies is translocation of the probiotic from gut to other tissues, since it is considered as a prerequisite for most opportunistic pathogens. However, it has been suggested that translocation of probiotics to extra-gut tissues, especially to the gut-associated lymphoid tissues (GALT), is a normal and beneficial process for the immune-modulation activity of these bacteria [46]. Zhou et al. [47] assessed the acute oral toxicity of three lactobacilli strains and found a LD_{50} higher than $50 g/kg/day$ (10^{11} cfu/mouse/day) which could be considered as 700 times the normal amount of probiotic consumed by humans. No bacteremia was detected in any of the mice and translocation of bacteria to other tissues was not different between probiotic and control mice. It is important to notice that the presence of bacteria in liver and spleen of healthy mice has been previously reported [48]. This result is in agreement with other previously published articles by Momose et al. [49] who reported a LD_{50} of $50 g/kg/day$ for *B. longum*. In a similar study, Donohue et al. [50] reported a LD_{50} of $6 g/kg/day$ for *L. rhamnosus* GG, which was considered the maximum dose that could be technically administered to mice.

In other reports, the administration of high doses of probiotics was performed during a longer period of time. Thus, daily oral administration of *L. gasseri* CECT5714 or *L. coryniformis* CECT5711 was shown to be safe for mice and the LD_{50} was reported to be higher than $5 g/kg/day$, which was the maximum dose that could be technically administered to mice [51]. Probiotic administration did not cause bacteremia and did not increase bacterial translocation to liver or spleen. In addition, no signs of infection were detected in probiotic treated mice. In a similar report, LD_{50} for oral administration of *L. salivarius* CECT5713 was higher than $5 g/kg/day$ and it was also demonstrated that intraperitoneal administration of this strain at a single dose of $50 mg/kg/day$ was safe and did not produce detrimental effects on mice [52].

Since immune compromise seems to be a risk factor for probiotic infection, animal models of immune deficiency have also been used to assess safety of different probiotic strains. Wagner et al. [53] colonized athymic mice with human isolates of *L. reuteri*, *L. acidophilus*, *B. animalis* or LGG. There were no adverse effects in adult mice but colonization with LGG or *L. reuteri* did lead to deaths in some athymic neonatal mice, thus suggesting that the immune compromise may put neonates at particular risk of probiotic infection.

An association of probiotics to germ-free animals has also been used as a criterion for safety. As an example, administration of *B. longum* to germ-free mice led to colonization of intestinal tract with this strain and translocation of *B. longum* to mesenteric lymph nodes, liver and kidney. However, the translocated bacteria did not cause either infection or any harmful effects [54].

4.3. Human Clinical Studies

An increasing interest in the manipulation of gut microbiota with probiotics has led to a large number of clinical trials or studies in human volunteers over the last two decades. Most of these were designed to analyze functional effects of a probiotic strain or food containing probiotics, but safety aspects were also implicit.

The use of probiotics in adults has been widely documented and most of the studies report that the incidence of adverse effects is no different between probiotic and placebo groups. In 2006 Olivares et al. [55] reported that oral consumption of a dairy product containing *L. coryniformis* CECT5711 (2×10^9 cfu/day) and *L. gasseri* CECT5714 (2×10^9 cfu/day) for 28 days was well tolerated by healthy adults and did not cause any adverse effects. This probiotic product enhanced the intestinal function of volunteers [55] and did cause an increment in several immunological parameters, such as the percentage of natural killer cells and plasmatic concentration of IgA [3]. In another trial, probiotic capsules containing *L. fermentum* CECT5716 (10^{10} cfu/day) consumed daily over 28 days were also well tolerated by healthy adults and enhanced the response to influenza vaccination [56].

The use of probiotics in children has been more controversial, especially in newborns. There are enough data to support the safety of probiotics in healthy children aged 6 months and older, and expert nutrition committees, such as the one from ESPGHAN [17], have found few concerns in the use of probiotics in follow-on formula (designed to feed children older than 5 months). Data from the use of probiotics in younger children are scarcer. However, acquisition of these data would be highly desirable, given the suggestion that bacteria ingested during early life are more likely to permanently colonize the intestine [57]. Finding of lactic acid bacteria in breast milk [17] could support, at least in part, the use of probiotics in dietetic products for newborns. In 2008, a breast milk strain, *L. fermentum* CECT5716 was reported to be safe in 6-month-old children [58]. Chouraqui et al. [59] assessed the safety of different probiotic strains in children of 2 weeks of age. Consumption of infant formulas containing *B. longum*, *L. rhamnosus* or *L. paracasei* did not cause any adverse effect and the growth ratio was no different between placebo and probiotic groups. It should also be noticed that different strains of probiotics have been reported to be safe in preterm infants (a specific at-risk population), with some evidence of health-promoting effects [13].

5. CONCLUSION

Although the use of probiotics is generally recognized as safe in otherwise healthy persons, in the clinical evaluation of probiotic products, apart from functional effects, safety aspects should also be addressed. Especially in at-risk populations, safety of probiotics should be analyzed on a strain-by-strain basis, taking into account that the dose and effect of one strain in a particular clinical condition cannot be extrapolated either to other strains or to other clinical conditions. Clarification of the legislative framework would be highly recommended to better elucidate the steps to be followed to state safety of a probiotic strain before being marketed.

References

1. Isolauri, E., Juntunen, M., Rautanen, T., et al. (1991). A human *Lactobacillus* strain (*Lactobacillus casei* sp strain GG) promotes recovery from acute diarrhea in children. *Pediatrics, 88*, 90–97.
2. Peran, L., Camuesco, D., Comalada, M., et al. (2005). Preventive effects of a probiotic, *Lactobacillus salivarius* ssp. *salivarius*, in the TNBS model of rat colitis. *World Journal of Gastroenterology, 11*, 5185–5192.
3. Olivares, M., Díaz-Ropero, M. P., Gómez, N., et al. (2006). The consumption of two probiotic strains, *Lactobacillus coryniformis* CECT5711 and *Lactobacillus gasseri* CECT5714, boost the immune system of healthy humans. *International Microbiology, 9*, 47–52.
4. Furrie, E. (2005). Probiotics and allergy. *Proceedings of the Nutrition Society, 64*, 465–469.
5. Saxelin, M., Chuang, N. H., Chassy, B., et al. (1996). Lactobacilli bacteremia in southern Finland, 1989–1992. *Clinical Infectious Diseases, 22*, 564–566.
6. Steidler, L., Hans, W., Schotte, L., et al. (2000). Treatment of murine colitis by *Lactococcus lactis* secreting IL-10. *Science, 289*, 1352–1355.
7. Kaur, P., Chopra, K., & Saini, A. (2002). Probiotics: potential pharmaceutical applications. *European Journal of Pharmaceutical Sciences, 15*, 1–9.
8. Berg, R. D. (1992). Translocation of indigenous gut flora. In R. Fuller (Ed.), *Probiotics, the scientific basis* (pp. 55–85). London: Chapman and Hall.
9. Boyle, R., Robins-Browne, R. M., & Tang, M. L. K. (2006). Probiotic use in clinical practice: what are the risks? *American Journal of Clinical Nutrition, 83*, 1256–1264.
10. Besselink, M., van Santvoort, H., Buskens, E., et al. (2008). Probiotic prophylaxis in predicted severe acute pancreatitis: a randomised, double-blind, placebo-controlled trial. *Lancet, 371*, 651–659.
11. Capurso, G., Marignani, M., Piciucchi, M., et al. (2008). Probiotics and severe acute pancreatitis. *Journal of Clinical Gastroenterology, 42*, S148–S153.
12. Apostolou, E., Kirjavainen, P. V., & Saxelin, M. (2001). Good adhesion properties of probiotics: a potential

risk for bacteremia? *FEMS Immunology and Medical Microbiology, 31*, 35–39.

13. Stansbridge, E. M., Walker, V., & Hall, M. A. (1993). Effects of feeding premature infants with lactobacillus GG on gut fermentation. *Archives of Disease in Childhood, 69*, 488–492.

14. Diaz-Ropero, M. P., Martin, R., Sierra, S., et al. (2006). Two *lactobacillus* strains, isolated from breast milk, differently modulate the immune response. *Journal of Applied Microbiology, 102*, 337–343.

15. Kalliomaki, M., Salminen, S., Arviolommi, H., et al. (2001). Probiotics in primary prevention of atopic disease. *Lancet, 357*, 1076–1079.

16. Kuituenen, M., Kukkonen, K., Juntunen-Backman, K., et al. (2009). Probiotics prevent IgE-associated allergy until age 5 years in cesarean delivered children but not in the total cohort (Epub ahead of print). *Journal of Allergy and Clinical Immunology.*

17. Agostoni, C., Axelsson, I., Braegger, C., et al. (2004). Probiotic bacteria in dietetic products for infants: a commentary by the ESPGHAN committee on nutrition. *Journal of Pediatric Gastroenterology and Nutrition, 38*, 365–374.

18. Michail, S., Sylvester, F., Fuchs, G., & Issenman, R. (2006). Clinical efficacy of probiotics: review of the evidence with focus on children. *Journal of Pediatric Gastroenterology and Nutrition, 43*, 550–557.

19. FAO/WHO Expert Consultation on Evaluation of Health and Nutritional Properties of Probiotics in Food Including Powder Milk with Live Lactic Acid Bacteria, October 2001. [http://www.who.int/foodsafety/publications/fs_management/en/probiotics.pdf].

20. FAO/WHO Working Group Report on Drafting Guidelines for the Evaluation of Probiotics in Food. London Ontario, Canada, April 30 and May 1, 2002. [http://www.who.int/foodsafety/publications/fs_management/en/probiotics.pdf].

21. European Commission. Working Group consisting of members of the Scientific Committee on Animal Nutrition, Scientific Committee on Food and the Scientific Committee on Plants of the European Commission. On a generic approach to the safety assessment of microorganisms used in feed/food and feed/food production. [http://ec.europa.eu/food/fs/sc/scf/out178_en.pdf].

22. EFSA. (2007). Opinion of the scientific committee on a request from EFSA on the introduction of a qualified presumption of safety (QPS) approach for assessment of selected microorganisms referred to EFSA. *The EFSA Journal, 587*, 1–16.

23. EFSA. (2008). Scientific opinion of the panel on biological hazards on a request from EFSA on the maintenance of the QPS list of microorganisms intentionally added to food or feed. *The EFSA Journal, 923*, 1–48.

24. European Commission. Opinion of the Scientific Committee on Animal Nutrition (SCAN) on the criteria for assessing the safety of micro-organisms resistant to antibiotics of human clinical and veterinary importance (Adopted in 2001, revised in 2003). [http://ec.europa.eu/food/fs/sc/scan/out108_en.pdf].

25. EFSA. (2008). Technical guidance prepared by the Panel on Additives and Products of Substances used in Animal Feed (FEEDAP) on the update of the criteria used in the assessment of bacterial resistance to antibiotics of human or veterinary importance. *The EFSA Journal, 732*, 1–15.

26. Backed, F., Ley, R. E., Sonnenburg, J. L., et al. (2005). Host-bacterial mutualism in the human intestine. *Science, 307*, 1915–1920.

27. Salminen, S., von Wright, A., Morelli, L., et al. (1998). Demonstration of safety of probiotics—A review. *International Journal of Food Microbiology, 44*, 93–106.

28. Leclercq, R., Derlot, E., Weber, M., et al. (1989). Transferable vancomycin and teicoplanin resistance in enterococcus faecium. *Antimicrobial Agents and Chemotherapy, 33*, 10.

29. Noble, W. C., Virani, Z., & Cree, R. G. (1992). Co-transfer of vancomycin and other resistance genes from *Enterococcus faecalis* NCTC 12201 to *Staphylococcus aureus*. *FEMS Microbiology Letters, 72*(2), 195–198.

30. Morelli, L., Sarra, P. G., & Bottazzi, V. (1988). *In vivo* transfer of pAM beta 1 from *Lactobacillus reuteri* to *Enterococcus faecalis*. *Journal of Applied Bacteriology, 65*(5), 371–375.

31. O'Brien, J., Crittenden, R., Ouwehand, A. C., & Salminen, S. (1999). Safety evaluation of probiotics. *Trends in Food Science & Technology, 10*, 418–424.

32. Ishibashi, N., & Yamazaki, S. (2001). Probiotics and safety. *American Journal of Clinical Nutrition, 73*, 465S–470S.

33. Martin, R., Langa, S., Reviriego, C., et al. (2003). Human milk is a source of lactic acid bacteria for the infant gut. *Journal of Pediatrics, 143*, 754–758.

34. Bover-Cid, S., & Holzapfel, W. H. (1999). Improved screening procedure for biogenic amine production by lactic acid bacteria. *International Journal of Food Microbiology, 53*, 33–41.

35. Araya-Kojima, T., Yaeshmina, T., Ishibashi, N., et al. (1995). Inhibitory effects *Bifidobacterium longum* on harmful intestinal bacteria. *Bifidobacter Microflora, 14*, 59–66.

36. Araya-Kojima, T., Yaeshmina, T., Ishibashi, N., et al. (1996). Inhibitory effects of human-derived bifidobacterium on pathogenic escherichia coli serotype O-111. *Bioscience and Microflora, 15*, 17–22.

37. Yamazaki, S., Kamimura, H., Momose, H., et al. (1982). Protective effect of bifidobacterium-monoassociation against lethal activity of *Escherichia coli*. *Bifidobacter Microflora, 1*, 55–59.

38. Takahashi, T., & Morotomi, M. (1994). Absence of cholic acid 7-dehydroxylase activity in the strains of Lactobacillus and Bifidobacterium. *Journal of Dairy Science, 77*, 3275–3286.

39. Douglas, C. W., Brown, P. R., & Preston, R. E. (1990). Platelet aggregation activity by oral streptococci. *FEMS Microbiology Letters, 72*, 63–68.

40. Harty, D. W. S., Patrikakis, M., Hume, E. B. H., et al. (1993). The aggregation of human platelets by Lactobacillus species. *Journal of General and Applied Microbiology, 139*, 2945–2951.

41. Kijavainen, P., Tuomola, E. M., Crittenden, R. G., et al. (1999). *In vitro* adhesion and platelet aggregation properties if bacteremia-associated lactobacilli. *Infection and Immunity, 67*, 2653–2655.

42. Uribarri, J., Oh, M. S., & Carroll, H. J. (1998). D-lactic acidosis. A review of clinical presentation, biochemical features and pathological mechanisms. *Medicine, 77*, 73–82.

43. Hove, H. (1998). Lactate and SCFA production in the human colon: implications for D-lactic acidosis, short bowel syndrome, antibiotic associated diarrhea, colon cancer and inflammatory bowel disease. *Danish Medical Bulletin, 45*, 15–33.

44. Connolly, E., Abrahamsson, T., & Björkesten, B. (2005). Safety of D(−)-Lactic acid producing bacteria in the human infant. *Journal of Pediatric Gastroenterology and Nutrition, 41*, 489–492.

45. Martin, R., Olivares, M., Marin, M. L., et al. (2005). Probiotic potential of three lactobacilli strains isolated from breast milk. *Human Lactation, 21*, 8–17.

46. Bengmark, S., & Jeppsson, B. (1995). Gastrointestinal surface protection and mucosa reconditioning. *Journal of Parenteral Entertainment Nutrition, 19*, 410–415.

47. Zhou, J. S., Shu, Q., Rutherfurd, K. J., et al. (2000). Acute oral toxicity and bacterial translocation studies on potentially probiotic strains of lactic acid bacteria. *Food and Chemical Toxicology, 38*, 153–161.

48. Berg, R. D. (1983). Translocation of indigenous bacteria from the intestinal tract. In R. J. Hentges (Ed.), *Human Intestinal Microflora in Health and Disease* (pp. 333–352). London: Academic Press.

49. Momose, H., Igarashi, M., Era, T., et al. (1979). Toxicological studies on *Bifidobacterium longum* BB-536. *Pharmacometrics, 17*, 881–887.

50. Donohue, D. C., & Salminen, S. (1996). Safety of Lactobacillus GG (ATCC 53103). *Asia Pacific Journal of Clinical Nutrition, 5*, 25–28.

51. Lara-Villoslada, F., Sierra, S., Martín, R., et al. (2007). Safety assessment of two probiotic strains, *Lactobacillus coryniformis* CECT5711 and *Lactobacillus gasseri* CECT5714. *Journal of Applied Microbiology, 103*, 175–184.

52. Lara-Villoslada, F., Sierra, S., Díaz-Ropero, M. P., et al. (2007). Safety assessment of the human milk-isolated probiotic *Lactobacillus salivarius* CECT5711. *Journal of Dairy Science, 90*, 3583–3589.

53. Wagner, R. D., Warner, T., Roberts, L., et al. (1997). Colonization of congenitally immunodeficient mice with probiotic bacteria. *Infection and Immunity, 65*, 3345–3351.

54. Yamazaki, S., Tsuyuki, S., & Akashiba, H. (1991). Immune response od bifidobacterium-monoassociated mice. *Bifidobacter Microflora, 10*, 19–31.

55. Olivares, M., Díaz-Ropero, M. P., Gómez, N., et al. (2006). Oral administration of two probiotic strains, *Lactobacillus coryniformis* CECT5711 and *Lactobacillus gasseri* CECT5714, enhances the intestinal function of healthy adults. *International Journal of Food Microbiology, 107*, 104–111.

56. Olivares, M., Díaz-Ropero, M. P., Sierra, S., et al. (2007). Oral intake of *Lactobacillus fermentum* CECT5716 enhances the effect of influenza vaccination. *Nutrition, 23*, 254–260.

57. Hooper, L. V., & Gordon, J. I. (2002). Commensal host-bacterial relationships in the gut. *Science, 292*, 1115–1118.

58. Maldonado, J., Narbona, E., Sempere, L., et al. (2008). Oral tolerance studies of the human milk probiotic *Lactobacillus fermentum* CECT5716. *Journal of Pediatric Gastroenterology and Nutrition, 44*, S1–S360.

59. Chouraqui, J. P., Grathwohl, D., Labaune, J. M., et al. (2008). Assessment of the safety, tolerance and protective effect against diarrhea of infant formulas containing mixtures of probiotics or probiotics and prebiotics in a randomized controlled trial. *American Journal of Clinical Nutrition, 87*, 1365–1373.

60. Rautio, M., Jousimies-Somer, H., Kauma, H., et al. (1999). Liver abscess due to a *Lactobacillus rhamnosus* strain indistinguishable from *L. rhamnosus* strain GG. *Clinical Infectious Diseases, 28*, 1159–1160.

61. Mackay, A. D., Taylor, M. B., Kibbler, C. C., & Hamilton-Miller, J. M. (1999). Lactobacillus *endocarditis* caused by a probiotic organism. *Clinical Microbiology and Infection, 5*, 292.

62. Kunz, A. N., Noel, J. M., & Fairchok, M. P. (2004). Two cases of Lactobacillus bacteremia during probiotic treatment of short gut syndrome. *Journal of Pediatric Gastroenterology and Nutrition, 38*, 457–458.

63. De Groote, M. A., Frank, D. N., Dowell, E., et al. (2005). *Lactobacillus rhamnosus* GG bacteremia associated probiotic use in a child with short gut syndrome. *The Pediatric Infectious Disease Journal, 24*, 278–280.

64. Land, M. H., Rouster-Stevens, K., Woods, C. R., et al. (2005). *Lactobacillus sepsis* associated with probiotic therapy. *Pediatrics, 115*, 178–181.

65. Richard, V., Van der Auwera, P., Snoeck, R., et al. (1988). Nosocomial bacteremia caused by *Bacillus* species. *European Journal of Clinical Microbiology & Infectious Diseases, 7*, 783–785.

66. Oggioni, M. R., Pozzi, G., Valensin, P. E., et al. (1998). Recurrent septicemia in an immunocompromised patient due to probiotic strains of *Bacillus subtilis*. *Journal of Clinical Microbiology, 36*, 325–326.

67. Zein, E. F., Karaa, S., Chemaly, A., et al. (2008). *Lactobacillus rhamnosus* septicemia in a diabetic patient associated with probiotic use: a case report. *Annales de Biologie Clinique (Paris), 66*, 195–198.

Prevention of Infections by Probiotics: An Overview

Koji Nomoto

Yakult Central Institute for Microbiological Research, Kunitachi-shi, Tokyo, Japan

1. INTRODUCTION

Infectious diseases still remain the most severe problem for humans to solve in the twenty-first century. Intestinal infectious diseases caused by pathogenic microorganisms including *Shigella, Vibrio cholera*, pathogenic *Escherichia coli, Campylobacter*, and rotavirus are the main causes of death in developing countries, where more than one billion diarrhea episodes occur every year among children younger than 5 years [1, 2]. Even in a developed country like the USA, 21–37 million cases of diarrhea occurred annually in a population of 16.5 million children [3], and *Salmonella, Campylobacter*, and enterohemorrhagic *E. coli* O157 have been problematic as etiologic bacteria of foodborne infection [4]. Moreover, overuse of antibiotics has allowed the spread of nosocomial infections with antibiotic-resistant bacteria, particularly multidrug-resistant bacteria, as adverse effects. Under these circumstances, some useful bacteria contained in yogurt, lactobacillary beverages, and other fermented foods have been medically recognized as probiotics [5, 6]. Probiotics have been identified mainly by experience of their ingestion as foods, but studies to evaluate the usefulness of probiotics based on medical criteria are underway, and many reviews of these studies have been published [7–11].

Since the concept of EBM (evidence-based medicine) was introduced in the medical field, the evidence-based evaluation of therapeutic methods has become the mainstream. The accumulation of clinical data to demonstrate the usefulness for disease control may also be important for probiotic bacterial strains. In this report, studies of the prevention of infections by probiotics in acute diarrhea, neonates and children, digestive organ surgery, and other fields are reviewed. Important points to increase the usefulness of probiotics are also discussed.

2. ACUTE DIARRHEA

2.1. Effect on Acute Infectious Diarrhea (Rotaviral Diarrhea)

Rotaviral diarrhea occurs mainly in infants aged 6 months to 2 years. Vomiting and subsequent rapid watery diarrhea continue for a short period. For treatment, fluid replacement for dehydration and nutritional management are performed. Effects of various probiotics on rotaviral diarrhea have been investigated by double blind placebo-controlled randomized studies [12–16]. There have been several reports concerning the preventive effects of *Lactobacillus* strains on acute watery diarrhea in children. For example, in a multicenter study performed in Europe [14], 291 neonatal patients aged 1–3 months admitted for diarrhea were randomly divided into two groups, and 10^{10} cfu of *L. rhamnosus* GG strain or placebo was administered after treatment of dehydration 4–6 hours after admission. The duration of diarrhea was significantly shortened in the *L. rhamnosus* GG group, compared to the placebo group. In a double blind placebo-controlled randomized study performed in patients aged 6–36 months (75% were infected with rotavirus), ingestion of *L. reuteri* SD 2222 strain (10^{10}–10^{11} cfu) for 5 days shortened the duration of watery diarrhea, compared to the placebo group [13]. In a randomized control trial (RCT) examining the effect of freeze-dried mixture of three *L. rhamnosus* strains (573L/1, 573L/2, and 573L/3) in a total dose of 10^{10} cfu showed that the *L. rhamnosus* strains shortened the duration of rotaviral diarrhea in hospitalized children in Poland [12]. There have also been several reports on the different probiotics such as *Bifidobacterium* and mixtures of several probiotic strains. In a study performed in Thailand, 175 nursery school children aged 6–36 months were divided into three test groups: the first group received powdered milk: the second group was given *Bifidobacterium* Bb12-supplemented powdered milk, and the third group was given *Bifidobacterium* Bb12- and *Streptococcus thermophilus*-supplemented powdered milk. The anti-rotavirus IgA antibody titer in saliva was measured as an index of rotaviral infection [15]. The antibody titer increased four times or more during the 8-month study period in 30.4% of the subjects in the control group that ingested powdered milk alone, but no increase in the antibody titer was noted in most subjects in the group that ingested *Bifidobacterium* Bb12 and the group that ingested *Bifidobacterium* Bb12 and *S. thermophilus*. One report of the RCT concerning the use of probiotics mixture VSL#3 (a mixture of four strains of lactobacilli: *L. acidophilus*, *L. paracasei*, *L. bulgaricus*, *L. plantarum*, three strains of bifidobacteria: *B. breve*, *B. infantis*, *B. longum*, one strain of *S. thermophilus*, including a total of 90 billion bacteria) showed that VSL#3 was effective in earlier recovery and reduced frequency of ORS administration [16]. However, there have been a couple of reports showing that LGG was not effective in the treatment of acute watery diarrhea [17, 18]. There has been a report of the meta-analysis of the effect of probiotics on acute infectious diarrhea which reviewed nine reports of the RCT including some of the above reports [19]. It concluded that *Lactobacillus* is effective as a treatment of acute infectious diarrhea. It should be noted that there was a significant positive linear association between the dose of *Lactobacillus* and the reduction of the duration of diarrhea.

On the other hand, preventive administration of probiotics for rotaviral infectious disease has been investigated. In a double blind placebo-controlled randomized study performed in 220 inpatients aged 1–18 months, the incidence of rotaviral infection was significantly lower in patients fed maternal milk than in patients fed artificial milk, but daily preventive administration of 10^{10} cfu *L. rhamnosus* GG during hospital stays did not decrease the incidence, compared to placebo administration [20]. Similarly, preventive administration of *Lactobacillus* GG reduced diarrheal symptoms, but no obvious prevention of rotaviral infection was noted in other studies [21].

2.2. Antibiotic-induced Diarrhea

Antibiotics cause diarrhea due to an imbalance of intestinal bacterial flora in 20% of patients treated. In double blind placebo-controlled randomized studies, probiotics such as *Saccharomyces boulardii* [22, 23], *Lactobacillus rhamnosus* GG strain [24], *Bifidobacterium longum* [25], and *Enterococcus faecium* SF 68 strain [26] significantly decreased the incidence of diarrhea in healthy subjects and patients treated with antibiotics. Diarrhea induced by antibiotics such as clindamycin, cephalosporin, and penicillin, due to proliferation of *Clostridium difficile* in the intestine is well-known. The above antibiotics disturb endogenous intestinal bacterial flora, and allow abnormal proliferation of endogenous *C. difficile*, which normally exists in the intestine at a low level. Diarrhea may aggravate pseudomembranous enteritis, and the recurrence rate after discontinuation of eradication treatment is high. For these problems, the preventive effect of probiotics on recurrence of *C. difficile* infection has been investigated. When *Saccharomyces boulardii* was concomitantly administered (1 g daily for 28 days) with vancomycin for eradication, recurrence was significantly prevented, compared to the placebo group (*S. boulardii* group: 16.7%, placebo group: 50%, $p = 0.05$) [23]. Digestion of toxin A or B of *C. difficile*, which are important for the pathogenicity of *C. difficile*, and receptors of these toxins on intestinal mucoepithelium by proteolytic enzyme produced by *S. boulardii* is considered to be the infection-preventive mechanism of *S. boulardii* [23]. Meta-analysis of the effects of probiotics on antibiotic-induced diarrhea in nine double blind placebo-controlled studies has been performed, and the results clarified the significance of the actions of probiotics such as *S. boulardii* and *Lactobacillus* [27].

Other meta-analyses of RCTs concluded that probiotics reduce the risk of antibiotic-associated diarrhea (AAD) in pediatric inpatients [28, 29]. However, effects of probiotics for AAD in the adults or elderly patients have not been conclusive. One RCT on 135 inpatients in the UK showed that consumption of a probiotic drink including *L. casei*, *L. bulgaricus*, and *S. thermophilus* reduced the incidence of AAD and *Clostridium difficile*-associated diarrhea (CDAD) [30]. However, *L. rhamnosus* GG

capsules had no preventive effect on AAD in US adult inpatients [31]. Moreover, bio yogurt including *L. acidophilus*, *L. delbrueckii*, *Bifidobacterium animalis*, and *S. thermophilus* had no significant effect on AAD in a placebo-controlled RCT with adult inpatients ($n = 131$) when compared with either commercial yogurt ($n = 118$) or non-treated control ($n = 120$) [32].

2.3. Traveler's Diarrhea

Traveler's diarrhea (three times or more a day) occurs in residents of developed countries after traveling to subtropical and tropical zones [33]. There have been two reports of the meta-analysis for the prevention of traveler's diarrhea by probiotics [34, 35]: McFarland reviewed 12 trials and concluded that several probiotics (mainly *S. boulardii* and a mixture of *L. acidophilus* and *B. bifidum*) had significant efficacy [34], while Takahashi et al. concluded that probiotics were not effective in TD by reviewing five RCTs [35]. The main reason for the difference may be the kinds of the probiotics used in the trials, because the former analysis included many effective trials of *S. boulardii* while the latter included only one for *S. boulardii* out of five trials. There are some factors such as trip destinations, probiotic potency during travel, medication compliance that affect the results.

3. EFFECTS OF PROBIOTICS IN NEONATES AND CHILDREN

3.1. Effects on Necrotizing Enterocolitis and Related Diseases

Necrotizing enterocolitis has been reported to occur in 10–25% of premature babies (weighing less than 1500 g) in intensive care units, or one-third to a half of neonates with extremely low birth weight [3], and surgery is necessary for most cases. The mortality is high (20–30%), and sequelae such as short-bowel syndrome and intestinal obstruction occur in about a quarter of the cases. In patients with necrotizing enterocolitis, abnormal intestinal bacterial flora with increased *Enterococcus*, *E. coli*, *Staphylococcus*, and *Clostridium perfringens* is suggested to cause aggravation of the symptoms. A decrease in the incidence of necrotizing enterocolitis by intestinal colonization by *Bifidobacterium* and *Lactobacillus* has been reported [36]. In a study performed in Colombia, 2.5×10^8 cfu *L. acidophilus* and *B. infantis* were administered to 1,237 neonates, and the incidence of necrotizing enterocolitis decreased by 60% compared to the incidence in 1,282 non-treated inpatients in the previous year [37]. In a study performed in neonates born with less than 1500 g birth weight before 32 weeks of gestation, powdered milk supplemented with 6×10^9 cfu *L. rhamnosus* GG was administered daily until discharge [38]. The incidence of necrotizing enterocolitis was slightly decreased, compared to the placebo group, but the difference was not significant. In one study in 1991 of the effect of *Lactobacillus* GG, viable cells of *Lactobacillus* GG strain were detected in feces of the patients, but no significant effect was noted [39]. Since then, several RCTs have been conducted. For example, Lin et al. have reported the results of the RCT with 367 infants: both *L. acidophilus* and *B. infantis* with breast milk were fed until discharge [40]. The incidence of death or NEC (>stage 2) was significantly lower when compared with the control group that had received breast milk alone. A report of meta-analysis of seven RCTs including the above information concluded that probiotics might reduce the risk of NEC in preterm neonates with less than 33 weeks' gestation but that the short- and long-term safety should be assessed in large trials [41]. Moreover, it suggested that more information on the dose, duration, and type of probiotic agents would be useful for more concise estimation of probiotics on NEC [41].

In Japan, Kitajima *et al.* [42] administered live *B. breve* strain Yakult (about 5×10^8 cfu/d,

4 weeks) to neonates with extremely low birth weight, and found the following: i) administered *Bifidobacterium* colonized in the intestine at a high level in a high ratio of the neonates; ii) abnormal proliferation of single intestinal bacteria such as *Enterococcus* was inhibited; and iii) intestinal gas production was inhibited. As for clinical symptoms, improvement of body weight gain, a decrease in the amount of gastric gas aspirated, and an increase in calorie intake were noted in the group colonized with *Bifidobacterium*. Kanamori et al. [43–45] reported aggravation of intestinal bacterial flora in various diseases (short bowel syndrome, Hirschsprung disease, and laryngotracheoesophageal schistasis) in consideration that aggravation of intestinal microflora caused not only by organic disorder of the digestive organs but also repeated use of antibiotics is an important issue to investigate in patients who have serious disorders in the pediatric surgery field immediately after birth. In these patients, useful anaerobes represented by *Bifidobacterium* decrease and facultative anaerobes such as *E. coli* markedly increase, and the detection rate of *Pseudomonas aeruginosa*, *Candida*, and MRSA is also high. Furthermore, the synbiotics (probiotics + prebiotics) therapy consisting of *L. casei* strain Shirota, *B. breve* strain Yakult, and galacto-oligosaccharide (enteral or intragastric administration) has been reported to improve intestinal microflora and intestinal function (peristalsis and absorption of Na^+ salt) with marked improvement of systemic symptoms.

4. PREVENTION OF INFECTIOUS COMPLICATIONS IN THE FIELD OF DIGESTIVE ORGAN SURGERY

Prevention of infectious complications after surgery for digestive organs is a major clinical task of this field. Considering that postoperative administration of antibiotics at a high dose for a long period promotes bacteremia with low sensitivity to antibiotics, such as MRSA, the basic attitude in digestive organ surgery is to refrain from the use of antibiotics. Probiotics and prebiotics have been introduced to prevent postoperative infectious complications. Rayes et al. performed a placebo-controlled randomized study in 95 patients with liver transplantation [46]. The patients were divided into the following three groups: i) the first group was treated with standard selective eradication of intestinal bacteria + postoperative early enteral nutrition; ii) the second group was treated with standard selective eradication of intestinal bacteria + postoperative early enteral nutrition (soluble and insoluble fiber and 10^9 cfu live *L. plantarum* 299 strain were supplemented); and iii) the third group was treated the same as for the second group, except that the same amount of heat-inactivated *L. plantarum* 299 were added instead of live bacteria. The incidence of postoperative infectious disease was 48% in the first group (early enteral nutrition control group), but the incidence was significantly decreased in the second group (13%). However, no significant decrease was noted in the third group, compared to the control group. The authors paid attention to recovery of immunity after surgery, and found that postoperative recovery of the CD4/CD8 ratio in peripheral blood was better in the second group than in the first group. Effects of enteral administrations of live and heat-inactivated *L. plantarum* 299 (supplemented with oat fiber) on development of sepsis after surgery in the abdominal cavity (hepatectomy, pancreatectomy, gastrectomy, resection of the large intestine, and intestinal bypass) have been compared [47]. This treatment significantly decreased the incidence of sepsis compared to standard enteral nutrition, and was particularly effective for gastrectomy and pancreatectomy.

Kanazawa et al. added probiotics (*L. casei* strain Shirota, *B. breve* strain Yakult, 5×10^9 cfu/g × 3 g each) and prebiotics (galacto-oligosaccharide 6.6 g/d) to postoperative enteral nutrition for patients with infectious complications such as wound infection, peritoneal abscess, and sepsis that occur at a high incidence after hepatectomy and extrahepatic bile duct resection and reconstruction of the biliary tract in patients with highly invasive biliary tract cancer, and investigated the protection from infections [48]. The above synbiotics therapy markedly improved intestinal microflora in the patients after surgery for bile duct cancer, and significantly decreased the incidence of infectious complications. Furthermore, patients' quality of life was also improved, with a shortening of the duration of postoperative hospital stay and the antibiotics administration period. The intestinal organic acid concentration also improved to the normal level, suggesting that the synbiotics therapy inhibited postoperative proliferation of intestinal etiologic bacteria of opportunistic infections, such as *Candida*, *Pseudomonas aeruginosa*, and *E. coli*, and their invasion into the body, by improving the intestinal environment. Considering that the preoperative oral ingestion of synbiotics, in addition to postoperative synbiotic therapy, may effectively prevent infections, a randomized controlled study was performed with a preoperative and postoperative synbiotic ingestion group and control group with the postoperative ingestion of synbiotic alone (synbiotic group: 41 patients, control group: 40 patients) [49]. *L. casei* strain Shirota-fermented drink (containing 40 billion or more live bacteria of *L. casei* strain Shirota) and *B. breve* strain Yakult-fermented drink (containing 10 billion or more live bacteria of *B. breve* strain Yakult) were selected for postoperative synbiotics, and 55% of galacto-oligosaccharides solution as a prebiotic. Preoperative synbiotic ingestion for 2 weeks (one each bottle of probiotics per day and 15 g of galacto-oligosaccharides solution per day) significantly elevated the peripheral blood NK activity and total number of lymphocytes in patients prior to surgery. Surgical stress-induced inflammatory symptoms (elevation of peripheral blood IL-6 and CRP levels) were also significantly reduced in pre- and postoperative synbiotic treatment groups, compared to the group with postoperative synbiotic treatment alone. Furthermore, the improvement of intestinal flora and conditions by postoperative synbiotics increased significantly when additionally administered synbiotic before surgery. With these findings, the incidence of postoperative infectious complications was decreased to 12.1%, and total duration of hospitalization and number of days with antibiotics treatment were also reduced, suggesting that synbiotic therapy improves the intestinal bacterial flora and prevents infectious complications in severe pathological conditions such as surgical stress.

For emergency treatment, the control of marked systemic inflammatory reactions in response to severe injuries and burns is important. A new concept of inflammatory reaction, systemic inflammatory response syndrome (SIRS), has been proposed by a joint meeting of the American College of Chest Physicians and Society of Critical Care Medicine [50]. It attempts to comprehensively define the conditions of patients described above. SIRS represents systemic inflammatory reactions to stresses, and is defined as conditions showing abnormalities in two or more of the following four body systems: body temperature, heart rate, respiratory rate, and white blood cell count. Infection-associated SIRS is defined as sepsis. Sepsis accompanied by organ disorder and abnormal perfusion in an organ is defined as severe sepsis, and severe sepsis complicated by severe hypotension, is defined as septic shock. Control of these SIRS symptoms is of major concern in emergency treatment. Shimizu et al. have investigated fecal microflora in SIRS patients considering disturbance of intestinal flora accompanied by infection of intestinal bacteria (called bacterial

translocation; BT) and found that intestinal microflora markedly disturbed in SIRS patients (25 cases, compared to healthy adults) [51]. In particular, the numbers of *Bifidobacterium* and *Lactobacillus* were 1/100 to 1/1000 of those in healthy adults, while *Staphylococcus*, which may cause BT, was increased. Moreover, aggravation of intestinal environment reflecting the above abnormality of intestinal flora resulted in reduction of intestinal organic acid levels and elevation of intestinal pH. When they administered an enteral BL seichoyaku preparation containing the *L. casei* strain Shirota, *B. breve* strain Yakult and Oligomate HP (galacto-oligosaccharides solution) to control intestinal function to SIRS patients, intestinal *Bifidobacterium* and *Lactobacillus* increased markedly, and abnormally low intestinal organic acid level also increased by synbiotics [52]. The incidences of systemic infectious diseases, such as enteritis, pneumonia, and sepsis, were also lower than the group without synbiotic treatment. The condition of patients admitted to the emergency care unit needs immediate treatment/improvement, but improvement has been observed by synbiotic therapy [52].

Bacterial translocation (BT) is defined as the passage of viable enteric bacteria from the intestinal lumen through the epithelial mucosa into the lamina propria and then into mesenteric lymph nodes (MLNs) and possibly other organs [53, 54]. Factors considered to induce BT are as follows: i) abnormal proliferation of bacteria in the intestine; ii) impairment of barrier function of the intestinal wall; and iii) failure of the biological defense system against invasive bacteria. Probiotics and prebiotics, as well as organic acids produced by their administration, may improve host resistance to some of the above three factors of BT in postoperative infectious diseases of digestive organs. As suggested by the above examples, improvement of intestinal bacterial flora by improvement of intestinal environment is particularly important.

5. OTHERS

5.1. *Helicobacter pylori*-induced Infectious Disease

Helicobacter pylori are microaerophilic Gram-negative rods, are considered to cause gastritis and peptic ulcer and suggested to be a risk factor of gastric cancer. Since various lactic acid bacterial strains and *Bifidobacterium* strains prevented infection in experimental animal models, and inhibited proliferation and urease activity of *H. pylori in vitro* [55–58], inhibition of *H. pylori* infection and its recurrence has been investigated in humans [59–62]. For example, 120 *H. pylori*-positive patients were divided into three groups, and received the following treatments: i) eradication of the bacteria with three drugs (rabeprazole, calrithromycin, and amoxicillin) for 7 days (eradication control group); ii) eradication + live *L. acidophilus* (live bacteria treatment group); or (iii) eradication + killed *L. acidophilus* (killed bacteria treatment group) [59]. *Helicobacter pylori* was eradicated in 72% of the patients in the eradication control group, and the eradication rates were increased to 88 and 87% in the live and killed bacteria treatment groups, respectively ($p = 0.03$ and $p = 0.02$, respectively), showing a significant eradication-promoting effect. Host immune system and inhibition of adsorption to glycolipid receptors are considered to be involved in the mechanism for the effect of killed bacteria, though not clarified. In another study, 53 *H. pylori*-positive patients were divided into two groups, and fermented milk containing *L. johnsonii* La1 strain was administered twice a day for 2 weeks to one group, and placebo was administered to the other group with the same schedule [60]. On endoscopy and biopsy of gastric mucosa, the density of *H. pylori* at the antrum and corpus of the stomach was significantly decreased in the *L. johnsonii* treatment group. There is no clear description with regard to improvement of clinical symptoms in this report. More clear evidence was shown

in the report by Sýkora et al., which showed the marked increase in the eradication rate by supplementation of *L. casei* DN-114-fermented milk product to the triple treatement with omeprazole, amoxicillin, and clarithromycin in a double blind controlled study with 86 *H. pylori*-positive children [63]. Probiotics were used for the eradication of residual *H. pylori* after failed triple therapy [64]: 138 patients to whom 1-week triple therapy (amoxillin, clarithromycin, and omeprazole) had failed were enrolled. One group received a 4-week pretreatment with *L. acidophilus* La5- and *B. lactis* Bb12, *L. bulgaricus*, and *S. thermophilus*-containing yogurt with the subsequent regimen of a 1-week quadruple therapy (amoxicillin, metronidazole, omeprazole, and bismuth subcitrate). The eradication rate in the group estimated by the excessive $\sigma^{13}CO_2/mL$ values of the ^{13}C-urea beath test were significantly higher than the quadruple therapy-only control [64]. In Japan, when *H. pylori*-positive healthy subjects ingested yogurt containing *L. gasseri* OLL2716 (10^9 cfu/day bacterial count, 8 weeks), the $\Delta^{13}C$ value was decreased in an urea breath test, and the serum pepsinogen I/II ratio was increased, compared to that before ingestion [62]. The effect of *B. bifidum* BF-1- and *S. thermophilus* YIT 2021-fermented milk was examined in an RCT with 79 adult volunteers who fulfilled the eligibility criteria: men and women concerned about their own stomach health, those with a UBT value at 5% and over, or those judged as positive in the PG test [65]. There was a significant difference (ΔUBT) of the UBT value from the baseline value at 8 weeks of ingestion between the *H. pylori*-positive subjects in the probiotics and placebo groups. The PG I levels in the probiotics group was also lower than the placebo group at the 12-week ingestion period [65]. The boom of yogurt sales in Japan may have been due to the study results of *H. pylori* eradication by probiotics. However, to increase the reliability of the effect, confirmation by a large-scale placebo-controlled randomized study and detailed elucidation of the action mechanism are necessary.

5.2. Prevention of Infections in the Urogenital Fields

The importance of maintenance of the healthy condition of intravaginal bacterial flora has been recognized in the gynecology field [7, 66]. From the viewpoint that maintenance of the dominant bacteria in normal vaginal microflora, *Lactobacillus*, at a high level is important for normal delivery and prevention of bacterial vaginosis, studies of introduction of probiotics into the vagina have been performed [67–71]. Most of the studies were performed by Reid's group [68–71]. They selected *Lactobacillus* strains based on adhesiveness to epithelial cells and hydrogen peroxide production [72, 73], and performed clinical studies. For example, in a study performed on 49 patients, introduction of *L. rhamnosus* GR-1 into the vagina inhibited urinary tract infection in 73% of the patients [68]. Weekly administration of 10^9 cfu *L. rhamnosus* GR-1 and *L. fermentum* B-54 as a vaginal suppository for 1 year significantly decreased the incidence of urinary tract infection, compared to the incidence in the previous year in the same subjects [69]. For the mechanism of prevention of infections, improvement of aggravation of vaginal bacterial flora consisting of more than 50 species (decrease of the dominant bacteria, endogenous *Lactobacillus*, abnormal proliferation of endogenous *Gardnerella*, *Bacteroides*, *Peptostreptococcus*, and *Prevotella*, and exogenous *E. coli* infection) is considered important. There has been a RCT concerning the supplementary use of lactobacilli with antibiotic therapy for BV [74]. Supplementary treatment with two different *Lactobacillus* strains (*L. gasseri* Lbp EB01-DSM 14869 and *L. rhamnosus* Lbp PB01-DSM 14870) does not improve the efficacy of BV therapy with clindamycin during the first month of treatment, but for women initially cured, adjunct treatment with lactobacilli during three menstrual cycles

significantly lengthens the time to relapse in the probiotic-treated group [74]. It has been shown in an animal study that activation of local immunity by *L. casei* strain Shirota played an important role in its urinary tract infection-preventing effect [75]. In contrast, there have only been a few studies of oral application. It has been reported that when 10^9–10^{10} cfu *L. rhamnosus* GR-1 and *L. fermentum* RC-14 were orally administered, these probiotics transferred from the rectum to the vagina, and harmful bacteria in the vagina, *E. coli* and fungi, decreased [76]. In 2006, an RCT was conducted to examine oral lactobacilli on bacterial vaginosis in combination with antimicrobial metronidazole therapy [71]. The 125 premenopausal women diagnosed with BV were treated with oral metronidazole twice daily for 7 days, and randomized to receive oral *L. reuteri* RC-14 or placebo twice daily for 30 days. Eighty-eight percent of the patients in the antibiotic/probiotic group were cured, while only 40% in the antibiotic/placebo group were cured. However, further clinical studies are necessary for more precise evaluation of the urogenital infection preventive effect of oral probiotics.

Bacterial vaginosis associated with disruption of vaginal microflora has been suggested to allow invasion of various pathogenic microorganisms of sexually transmitted diseases (STD) [77, 78]. Attempts to normalize vaginal bacterial flora by probiotics to inhibit the spread of STDs such as AIDS are a future task [79].

6. PROSPECTS FOR FURTHER RESEARCH

The procedure, quality (bacterial strains), and safety of clinical studies necessary for assessment of health claims of probiotics were presented in the working standard for development of probiotics presented in the expert committee of FAO/WHO in 2002 [6, 80]. Finally, the future of probiotics for prevention of infection is discussed.

6.1. Extension of Clinical Study

The first problem to be solved in the application of probiotics is insufficiency of medically reliable data, as described above. Ideally, many clinical studies that can be judged by medical criteria should be conducted. For the future of probiotics as foods, development in the direction of evidence-based probiotics is important, as evidence-based medicine is proposed in the medical field. In Japan, a system of foods specified for health use was introduced in 1991. Although preventive effects of probiotics against infectious diseases do not fall under the category of foods specified for health use, major indications may include cold, for instance, in addition to various infectious diseases described above [81].

6.2. Action Mechanism

The concepts of probiotics, prebiotics, and a combination of these, synbiotics, is still quite novel. The most common definition of probiotics in the last 10 years was 'microorganisms that provide benefits to the host by improving balance of intestinal bacterial flora' [5]. The FAO/WHO expert committee has proposed a definition, 'microorganisms that exhibit beneficial effects on host's health when ingested in a sufficient amount' [6]. This may be based on the clarification that the mechanism of probiotics is not necessarily limited to actions among intestinal microflora, and immunoregulatory action on hosts is also included. From the viewpoint of prevention of infections, basic studies focusing on the following three points may be useful: i) improvement of intestinal environment (bacterial flora, pH, and organic acid concentration); ii) activation of host defense system; and iii) elucidation of factors determining strain specificity of the effect. Regarding the first point, intestinal environment, a search for the colonization resistance system possessed by endogenous bacterial flora with regard to quorum sensing may be one approach. For the second

point, close investigation of the interactions between intestinal microorganisms and intestinal mucoepithelial cells may clarify how intestinal bacterial flora is involved in various immune and allergic diseases. For the third point, investigation of strain-specific bacterial cell structures may be important because strain-specific metabolic systems have been elucidated with regard to the signal transduction systems in bacterial cells for elucidation of bacterial factors, and immunoregulatory function has been shown to be exerted by killed probiotic cells.

6.3. Safety

Probiotics have been incorporated into eating habits and are considered generally recognized as safe (GRAS). As described above, some strains do not develop serious adverse events even if administered at a 10^9–10^{10} level to low-birthweight-born neonates, who appear to be immunologically weak, and patients after highly invasive surgery for digestive organs. However, problems have been suggested for certain bacterial *species* and strains [82–87]. The most common reports are isolation of bacteria from the inflammatory region of bacterial endocarditis [82–84]. However, the isolation frequencies of these bacteria are far lower than those of the major *Enterococcus* and *Staphylococcus* species. Probiotic strains have been isolated in severely immunocompromised patients such as those underlying diabetes [85]. However, it should be carefully considered, at least by a strain-specific manner. For example, a prospective, descriptive pilot study on 28 critically ill children was conducted in the UK for evaluation of safety of probiotic *L. casei* strain Shirota [88]. The authors concluded that the use of LcS as a probiotic in enterally fed CIC is safe [88]. On the other hand, there has been a clinical report describing an adverse event in an RCT of a probiotics mixture, Ecologic 641 (*L. acidophilus, L. casei, L. salivarius, Lactococcus lactis, B. bifidum,* and *B. lactis*) on the patients with severe acute pancreatitis [89];

although there was no significant difference in the incidence of infectious complications as the main endpoint of the study between the probiotics group and the placebo group, the probiotic treatment was associated with an increased risk of mortality. However, there have been several counter-arguments both on the appropriateness of the implementation of the study and interpretation of the results [90]. The important issue is the variation of safety among bacterial strains in the prospective effects of probiotics. Therefore, it is necessary to establish safety criteria.

7. CONCLUSION

The importance of nutritional management is advocated in the field of clinical medicine. Since many probiotics are applied as foods, establishment of standards for expression of their function in foods may also be important. From the viewpoint that nutritional management of patients has a significant influence on recovery from diseases and on prognosis, formation of a nutrition support team (NST) by hospital staff such as physicians, nurses, pharmacists, and administrative dietitians for nutritional management of patients from a comprehensive viewpoint has been introduced. It is expected that application of probiotics will spread widely as a part of nutritional management of patients in all fields.

ACKNOWLEDGMENT

I thank Mr. Hirokazu Tsuji for helpful suggestions and preparing the manuscripts.

References

1. World Health Organization. (1996). *Water and sanitation: Fact sheet 112*. Geneva: World Health Organization.
2. World Health Organization. (1994). *Programme for control of diarrheal diseases: Ninth programme report 1992–1993.* Geneva: World Health Organization.
3. Glass, R. I., Lew, J. F., Gangarosa, R. E., et al. (1991). Estimates of morbidity and mortality rates for diarrheal diseases in American children. *The Journal of Pediatrics, 118,* S27–S33.
4. Farthing, M. J. (2000). Diarrhoea: A significant worldwide problem. *International Journal of Antimicrobial Agents, 14,* 65–69.
5. Fuller, R. (1989). Probiotics in man and animals. *The Journal of Applied Bacteriology, 66,* 365–378.
6. Reid, G. (2005). The importance of guidelines in the development and application of probiotics. *Current Pharmaceutical Design, 11,* 11–16.
7. Reid, G., Jass, J., Sebulsky, M. T., & McCormick, J. K. (2003). Potential uses of probiotics in clinical practice. *Clinical Microbiology Reviews, 16,* 658–672.
8. de Vrese, M., & Marteau, P. R. (2007). Probiotics and prebiotics: Effects on diarrhea. *The Journal of Nutrition, 137*(3 Suppl. 2), 803S–811S.
9. Guandalini, S. (2008). Probiotics for children with diarrhea: An update. *Journal of Clinical Gastroenterology, 42,* S53–S57.
10. Johnston, B. C., Supina, A. L., Ospina, M., & Vohra, S. (2007). Probiotics for the prevention of pediatric antibiotic-associated diarrhea CD004827. *Cochrane Database of Systematic Reviews.*
11. Allen, S. J., Okoko, B., Martinez, E., et al. (2004). Probiotics for treating infectious diarrhoea CD003048. *Cochrane Database of Systematic Reviews.*
12. Szymański, H., Pejcz, J., Jawień, M., et al. (2006). Treatment of acute infectious diarrhoea in infants and children with a mixture of three *Lactobacillus rhamnosus* strains—a randomized, double-blind, placebo-controlled trial. *Alimentary Pharmacology & Therapeutics, 23,* 247–253.
13. Shornikova, A. V., Casas, I. A., Isolauri, E., et al. (1997). *Lactobacillus reuteri* as a therapeutic agent in acute diarrhea in young children. *Journal of Pediatric Gastroenterology and Nutrition, 24,* 399–404.
14. Guandalini, S., Pensabene, L., Zikri, M. A., et al. (2000). *Lactobacillus* GG administered in oral rehydration solution to children with acute diarrhea: A multicenter European study. *Journal of Pediatric Gastroenterology and Nutrition, 30,* 54–60.
15. Saavedra, J. M., Bauman, N. A., Oung, I., et al. (1994). Feeding of *Bifidobacterium bifidum* and *Streptococcus thermophilus* to infants in hospital for prevention of diarrhea and shedding of rotavirus. *Lancet, 344,* 1046–1049.
16. Dubey, A. P., Rajeshwari, K., Chakravarty, A., & Famularo, G. (2008). Use of VSL#3 in the treatment of rotavirus diarrhea in children: Preliminary results.

Journal of Clinical Gastroenterology, 42(Suppl. 3 Pt. 1), S126–S129.

17. Salazar-Lindo, E., Miranda-Langschwager, P., Campos-Sanchez, M., et al. (2004). *Lactobacillus casei* strain GG in the treatment of infants with acute watery diarrhea: a randomized, double-blind, placebo controlled clinical trial [ISRCTN67363048]. *BMC Pediatrics, 4*, 18–26.

18. Basu, S., Chatterjee, M., Ganguly, S., & Chandra, P. K. (2007). Efficacy of *Lactobacillus rhamnosus* GG in acute watery diarrhoea of Indian children: a randomised controlled trial. *Paediatrics & Child Health, 43*, 837–842.

19. Van Niel, C. W., Feudtner, C., Garrison, M. M., & Christakis, D. A. (2002). Lactobacillus therapy for acute infectious diarrhea in children: A meta-analysis. *Pediatrics, 109*, 678–684.

20. Mastretta, E., Longo, P., Laccisaglia, A., et al. (2002). Effect of *Lactobacillus* GG and breast-feeding in the prevention of rotavirus nosocomial infection. *Journal of Pediatric Gastroenterology and Nutrition, 35*, 527–531.

21. Szajewska, H., Kotowska, M., Mrukowicz, J. Z., et al. (2001). Efficacy of *Lactobacillus* GG in prevention of nosocomial diarrhea in infants. *The Journal of Pediatrics, 138*, 361–365.

22. Surawicz, C. M., Elmer, G. W., Speelman, P., et al. (1989). Prevention of antibiotic-associated diarrhea by *Saccharomyces boulardii*. A prospective study. *Gastroenterology, 96*, 981–988.

23. McFarland, L. V., Surawicz, C. M., Greenberg, R. N., et al. (1995). Prevention of beta lactam-associated diarrhea by *Saccharomyces boulardii* compared with placebo. *The American Journal of Gastroenterology, 90*, 439–448.

24. Pant, A. R., Graham, S. M., Allen, S. J., et al. (1996). *Lactobacillus* GG and acute diarrhoea in young children in the tropics. *Journal of Tropical Pediatrics, 42*, 16–25.

25. Colombel, J. F., Cortot, A., Neut, C., & Romond, C. (1987). Yogurt with *Bifidobacterium longum* reduces erythromycin-induced gastrointestinal effects. *Lancet, 2*, 43.

26. Buydens, P., & Debeucklaere, S. (1996). Efficacy of SF 68 in the treatment of acute diarrhea: A placebo controlled trial. *Scandinavian Journal of Gastroenterology, 31*, 887–891.

27. D'Souza, A. L., Rajkumar, C., Cooke, J., & Bulpitt, C. J. (2002). Probiotics in prevention of antibiotic-associated diarrhoea: Meta analysis. *British Medical Journal, 324*, 1361–1364.

28. Johnston, B. C., Supina, A. L., & Vohra, S. (2006). Probiotics for pediatric antibiotic-associated diarrhea: A meta-analysis of randomized placebo-controlled trials. Erratum in: CMAJ, 175, 777 (2006). *CMAJ: Canadian Medical Association journal = journal de l'Association Medicale Canadienne, 175*, 377–383.

29. Szajewska, H., Ruszczyński, M., & Radzikowski, A. (2006). Probiotics in the prevention of antibiotic-associated diarrhea in children: A meta-analysis of randomized controlled trials. *The Journal of Pediatrics, 149*, 367–372.

30. Hickson, M., D'Souza, A. L., Muthu, N., et al. (2007). Use of probiotic Lactobacillus preparation to prevent diarrhoea associated with antibiotics: randomised double-blind placebo controlled trial. *British Medical Journal, 335*, 80–84.

31. Thomas, M. R., Litin, S. C., Osmon, D. R., et al. (2001). Lack of effect of *Lactobacillus* GG on antibiotic-associated diarrhea: a randomized, placebo-controlled trial. *Mayo Clinic Proceedings, 76*, 883–889.

32. Conway, S., Hart, A., Clark, A., & Harvey, I. (2007). Does eating yogurt prevent antibiotic-associated diarrhoea? A placebo-controlled randomised controlled trial in general practice. *The British Journal of General Practice: The Journal of the Royal College of General Practitioners, 57*, 953–959.

33. DuPont, H. L., & Ericsson, C. D. (1993). Prevention and treatment of traveler's diarrhea. *The New England Journal of Medicine, 328*, 1821–1827.

34. McFarland, L. V. (2007). Meta-analysis of probiotics for the prevention of traveler's diarrhea. *Travel Medicine and Infectious Disease, 5*, 97–105.

35. Takahashi, O., Noguchi, Y., Omata, F., et al. (2007). Probiotics in the prevention of traveler's diarrhea: meta-analysis. *Journal of Clinical Gastroenterology, 41*, 336–337.

36. Lucas, A., & Cole, T. J. (1990). Breast milk and neonatal necrotizing enterocolitis. *Lancet, 336*, 1519–1523.

37. Hoyos, A. B. (1999). Reduced incidence of necrotizing enterocolitis associated with enteral administration of *Lactobacillus acidophilus* and *Bifidobacterium infantis* to neonates in an intensive care unit. *International Journal on Disability, 3*, 197–202.

38. Dani, C., Biadaioli, R., Bertini, G., et al. (2002). Probiotics feeding in prevention of urinary tract infection, bacterial sepsis, and necrotizing enterocolitis in preterm infants. A prospective double-blind study. *Biology of the Neonate, 82*, 103–108.

39. Millar, M. R., Bacon, C., Smith, S. L., et al. (1993). Enteral feeding of premature infants with Lactobacillus sp. strain GG. *Archives of Disease in Childhood, 69*, 483–487.

40. Lin, H. C., Hsu, C. H., Chen, H. L., et al. (2008). Oral probiotics prevent necrotizing enterocolitis in very low birth weight preterm infants: a multicenter, randomized, controlled trial. *Pediatrics, 122*, 693–700.

41. Deshpande, G., Rao, S., & Patole, S. (2007). Probiotics for prevention of necrotising enterocolitis in preterm neonates with very low birthweight: a systematic review of randomised controlled trials. *Lancet, 369*, 1614–1620.

42. Kitajima, H., Sumida, Y., Tanaka, R., et al. (1997). Early administration of *Bifidobacterium breve* to preterm

infants: Randomized controlled trial. *Archives of Disease in Childhood. Fetal and Neonatal Edition, 76,* F101–F107.

43. Kanamori, Y., Hashizume, K., Sugiyama, M., et al. (2001). Combination therapy with *Bifidobacterium breve, Lactobacillus casei,* and galacto-oligosaccharides dramatically improved the intestinal function in a girl with short bowel syndrome; a novel synbiotics therapy for intestinal failure. *Digestive Diseases and Sciences, 46,* 2010–2016.

44. Kanamori, Y., Hashizume, K., Sugiyama, M., et al. (2002). A novel synbiotic therapy dramatically improved the intestinal function of a pediatric patient with laryngotracheo-esophageal cleft (LTEC) in the intensive care unit. *Clinical Nutrition, 21,* 527–530.

45. Kanamori, Y., Hashizume, K., Kitano, Y., et al. (2003). Anaerobic dominant flora was reconstructed by synbiotics in an infant with MRSA enteritis. *Pediatrics International, 45,* 359–362.

46. Rayes, N., Seehofer, D., Hansen, S., et al. (2002). Early enteral supply of Lactobacillus and fiber versus selective bowel decontamination; a controlled trial in liver transplant recipients. *Transplantation, 74,* 123–127.

47. Rayes, N., Hansen, S., Seehofer, D., et al. (2002). Early enteral supply of fiber and lactobacilli versus conventional nutrition: A controlled trial in patients with major abdominal surgery. *Nutrition, 18,* 609–615.

48. Kanazawa, H., Nagino, M., Kamiya, S., et al. (2005). Synbiotics reduce postoperative infectious complications: a randomized controlled trial in biliary cancer patients undergoing hepatectomy. *Langenbeck's Archives of Surgery, 390,* 104–113.

49. Sugawara, G., Nagino, M., Nishio, H., et al. (2006). Perioperative synbiotic treatment to prevent postoperative infectious complications in biliary cancer surgery: a randomized controlled trial. *Annals of Surgery, 244,* 706–714.

50. Muckart, D. J., & Bhagwanjee, S. (1997). American College of Chest Physicians/Society of Critical Care Medicine Consensus Conference definitions of the systemic inflammatory response syndrome and allied disorders in relation to critically injured patients. *Critical Care Medicine, 25,* 1789–1795.

51. Shimizu, K., Ogura, H., Goto, M., et al. (2006). Altered gut flora and environment in patients with severe SIRS. *The Journal of Trauma, 60,* 126–133.

52. Shimizu, K., Ogura, H., Goto, M., et al. (2009). Synbiotics decrease the incidence of septic complications in patients with severe SIRS: A Preliminary Report. *Digestive Diseases and Sciences, 4,* 1071–1078.

53. Berg, R. D., & Garlington, A. W. (1979). Translocation of certain indigenous bacteria from the gastrointestinal tract to the mesenteric lymph nodes and other organs in a gnotobiotic mouse model. *Infection and Immunity, 23,* 403–411.

54. Wiest, R., & Rath, H. C. (2003). Bacterial translocation in the gut. *Best Practice & Research. Clinical Gastroenterology, 17,* 397–425.

55. Kabir, A. M., Aiba, Y., Takagi, A., et al. (1997). Prevention of *Helicobacter pylori* infection by lactobacilli in a gnotobiotic murine model. *Gut, 41,* 49–55.

56. Coconnier, M. H., Lievin, V., Hemery, E., & Servin, A. L. (1998). Antagonistic activity against Helicobacter infection *in vitro* and *in vivo* by the human *Lactobacillus acidophilus* strain LB. *Applied and Environmental Microbiology, 64,* 4573–4580.

57. Midolo, P. D., Lambert, J. R., Hull, R., et al. (1995). *In vitro* inhibition of *Helicobacter pylori* NCTC 11637 by organic acids and lactic acid bacteria. *The Journal of Applied Bacteriology, 79,* 475–479.

58. Sgouras, D., Maragkoudakis, P., Petraki, K., et al. (2004). *In vitro* and *in vivo* inhibition of *Helicobacter pylori* by Lactobacillus casei strain Shirota. *Applied and Environmental Microbiology, 70,* 518–526.

59. Canducci, F., Armuzzi, A., Cremonini, F., et al. (2000). A lyophilized and inactivated culture of *Lactobacillus acidophilus* increases *Helicobacter pylori* eradication rates. *Alimentary Pharmacology & Therapeutics, 14,* 1625–1629.

60. Felley, C. P., Corthesy-Theulaz, I., Rivero, J. L., et al. (2001). Favourable effect of an acidified milk (LC-1) on Helicobacter pylori gastritis in man. *European journal of Gastroenterology & Hepatology, 13,* 25–29.

61. Michetti, P., Dorta, G., Wiesel, P. H., et al. (1999). Effect of whey-based culture supernatant of *Lactobacillus acidophilus* (johnsonni) La1 on *Helicobacter pylori* infection in humans. *Digestion, 60,* 203–209.

62. Sakamoto, I., Igarashi, M., Kimura, K., et al. (2001). Suppressive effect of *Lactobacillus gasseri* OLL 2716 (LG21) on *Helicobacter pylori* infection in humans. *The Journal of Antimicrobial Chemotherapy, 47,* 709–710.

63. Sýkora, J., Valecková, K., Amlerová, J., et al. (2005). Effects of a specially designed fermented milk product containing probiotic *Lactobacillus casei* DN-114 001 and the eradication of *H. pylori* in children: A prospective randomized double-blind study. *Journal of Clinical Gastroenterology, 39,* 692–698.

64. Sheu, B. S., Cheng, H. C., Kao, A. W., et al. (2006). Pretreatment with Lactobacillus- and Bifidobacterium-containing yogurt can improve the efficacy of quadruple therapy in eradicating residual *Helicobacter pylori* infection after failed triple therapy. *The American Journal of Clinical Nutrition, 83,* 864–869.

65. Miki, K., Urita, Y., Ishikawa, F., et al. (2007). Effect of *Bifidobacterium bifidum* fermented milk on *Helicobacter pylori* and serum pepsinogen levels in humans. *Journal of Dairy Science, 90,* 2630–2640.

66. Reid, G. (2001). Probiotic agents to protect the urogenital tract against infection. *The American Journal of Clinical Nutrition, 73,* 437S–444S.

67. Hallen, A., Jarstrand, C., & Pahlson, C. (1992). Treatment of bacterial vaginosis with lactobacilli. *Sexually Transmitted Diseases, 19*, 146–148.

68. Reid, G., Bruce, A. W., & Taylor, M. (1995). Instillation of Lactobacillus and stimulation of indigenous organisms to prevent recurrence of urinary tract infections. *Microecology and Therapy, 23*, 32–45.

69. Reid, G., & Bruce, A. W. (1995). Low vaginal pH and urinary-tract infection. *Lancet, 346*, 1704.

70. Reid, G., Bruce, A. W., & Taylor, M. (1995). Instillation of Lactobacillus and stimulation of indigenous organisms to prevent recurrence of urinary tract infections. *Microecology and Therapy, 23*, 32–45.

71. Anukam, K., Osazuwa, E., Ahonkhai, I., et al. (2006). Augmentation of antimicrobial metronidazole therapy of bacterial vaginosis with oral probiotic *Lactobacillus rhamnosus* GR-1 and *Lactobacillus reuteri* RC-14: randomized, double-blind, placebo controlled trial. *Microbes and Infection, 8*, 1450–1454.

72. Reid, G., Cook, R. L., & Bruce, A. W. (1987). Examination of strains of lactobacilli for properties that may influence bacterial interference in the urinary tract. *The Journal of Urology, 138*, 330–335.

73. Reid, G., & Bruce, A. W. (2001). Selection of Lactobacillus strains for urogenital probiotic applications. *The Journal of Infectious Diseases, 183*, S77–S80.

74. Larsson, P. G., Stray-Pedersen, B., Ryttig, K. R., & Larsen, S. (2008). Human lactobacilli as supplementation of clindamycin to patients with bacterial vaginosis reduce the recurrence rate; a 6-month, double-blind, randomized, placebo-controlled study. *BMC Womens Health, 8*, 3–10.

75. Asahara, T., Nomoto, K., Watanuki, M., & Yokokura, T. (2001). Antimicrobial activity of intraurethrally administered probiotic *Lactobacillus casei* in a murine model of *Escherichia coli* urinary tract infection. *Antimicrobial Agents and Chemotherapy, 45*, 1751–1760.

76. Reid, G., Charbonneau, D., Erb, J., et al. (2003). Oral use of *Lactobacillus rhamnosus* GR-1 and *L. fermentum* RC-14 significantly alters vaginal flora: Randomized, placebo-controlled trial in 64 healthy women. *FEMS Immunology and Medical Microbiology, 35*, 131–134.

77. Schwebke, J. R. (2001). Role of vaginal flora as a barrier to HIV acquisition. *Current Infectious Disease Reports, 3*, 152–155.

78. Sewankambo, N., Gray, R. H., Wawer, M. J., et al. (1997). HIV-1 infection associated with abnormal vaginal flora morphology and bacterial vaginosis. Erratum in: Lancet, 350, 1036 (1997). *Lancet, 350*, 546–550.

79. Gorbach, S. L. (2002). Probiotics in the third millennium. *Digestive and Liver Disease, 34*, S2–S7.

80. Reid, G. (2005). Importance of guidelines in the development and application of probiotics. *Current Pharmaceutical Design, 11*, 11–16.

81. Turchet, P., Laurenzano, M., Auboiron, S., & Antoine, J. M. (2003). Effect of fermented milk containing probiotic *Lactobacillus casei* DN-114001 on winter infections in free-living elderly subjects: A randomized controlled pilot study. *The Journal of Nutrition Health Aging, 7*, 75–77.

82. Mackay, A. D., Taylor, M. B., Kibbler, C. C., & Hamilton-Miller, J. M. (1999). *Lactobacillus endocarditis* caused by a probiotic organism. *Clinical Microbiology and Infection, 5*, 290–292.

83. Avlami, A., Kordossis, T., Vrizidis, N., & Sipsas, N. V. (2001). *Lactobacillus rhamnosus* endocarditis complicating colonoscopy. *The Journal of Infection, 42*, 283–285.

84. Land, M. H., Rouster-Stevens, K., Woods, C. R., et al. (2005). Endocarditis by *Lactobacillus rhamnosus* due to yogurt ingestion? *Pediatrics, 115*, 178–181.

85. Rautio, M., Jousimies-Somer, H., Kauma, H., et al. (1999). Liver abscess due to a *Lactobacillus rhamnosus* strain indistinguishable from *L. rhamnosus* strain GG. *Clinical Infectious Diseases, 28*, 1159–1160.

86. Salminen, M. K., Rautelin, H., Tynkkynen, S., et al. (2004). *Lactobacillus bacteremia*, clinical significance, and patient outcome, with special focus on probiotic *L. rhamnosus* GG. *Clinical Infectious Diseases, 38*, 62–69.

87. Kunz, A. N., Noel, J. M., & Fairchok, M. P. (2004). Two cases of *Lactobacillus bacteremia* during probiotic treatment of short gut syndrome. *Journal of Pediatric Gastroenterology and Nutrition, 38*, 457–458.

88. Srinivasan, R., Meyer, R., Padmanabhan, R., & Britto, J. (2006). Clinical safety of *Lactobacillus casei shirota* as a probiotic in critically ill children. *Journal of Pediatric Gastroenterology and Nutrition, 42*, 171–173.

89. Besselink, M. G., van Santvoort, H. C., Buskens, E., et al. (2008). Probiotic prophylaxis in predicted severe acute pancreatitis: A randomised, double-blind, placebo-controlled trial. *Lancet, 371*, 651–659.

90. Reid, G., Gibson, G., Sanders, M. E., et al. (2008). International Scientific Association for Probiotics and Prebiotics. Probiotic prophylaxis in predicted severe acute pancreatitis. *Lancet, 372*, 112–113.

6

Probiotics and Prebiotics in Human Health: An Overview

Oscar Brunser and Martin Gotteland

Gastroenterology Unit and Laboratory of Microbiology and Probiotics, Institute of Nutrition and Food Technology (INTA), University of Chile, Santiago, Chile

1. PROBIOTICS: WHERE DID THEY COME FROM?

Humans have been in contact with bacteria whose properties fulfil the requisites that qualify them as probiotics for thousands of years. Under the poor conditions of hygiene prevailing during most of human history, the passage of these bacteria from one individual to another was facilitated. It is now known, that mothers transfer some of their microbiota to their offspring during breast-feeding and that the environment is another source of colonizers for the newborn, including the transfer of probiotics. Indeed, most probiotics currently studied are of human origin and have been isolated from feces.

Ilya Metchnikoff, a Russian biologist who worked at the Institut Pasteur, became interested in the aging process and the prolongation of life, and originated the concept that beneficial bacteria may be present in food and come to inhabit the colon. He studied a unique group of Bulgarians who lived much longer than the average European population and whose diet was characterized by the consumption of large amounts of a yogurt from which he isolated a *Lactobacillus*. He attributed a large part of the beneficial influence on health and aging to this microorganism. According to his hypothesis, this microorganism had the capacity to neutralize the amines, ammonia and other toxic substances generated by the chemical reactions of putrefactive bacteria in the colon. The re-establishment of a correct balance in the colonic microflora by the acidophilic bacteria in detriment of the putrefactive bacteria would prevent degenerative diseases and improve the quality of life of the consumers. Metchnikoff also postulated that this bacteria could become implanted in the colon and thus inhibit the proliferation of the undesirable microorganisms. He called this *Lactobacillus* 'Bulgarian' (*bulgaricus*) but it is not known whether the microorganism currently identified with this name corresponds to Metchnikoff's original strain, which was lost. It is possible that Metchnikoff's concept matched, to some extent, the concept currently defining probiotics. Metchnikoff wrote a book, which he published in 1908, 'The prolongation of life.

73

Optimistic studies' [1] and he launched a successful industry that produced an acidified milk and a product in tablet form containing *L. bulgaricus*; furthermore, he became a consumer of his product and lived to be 71 years, a very advanced age at that time.

Interest in the bifidobacteria started more or less contemporaneously, when Tissier described in the feces of breastfed infants the predominance of bacteria that produced lactic and acetic acid; these bacteria were bifurcated and which he named *Bacillus bifidus* [2]. This was later called *Bifidobacterium*. Tissier was the first to notice that when infants were introduced to cows' milk, their fecal flora became more varied and the bifidobacteria were no longer predominant. Since breastfed infants are more refractory to conditions such as acute diarrhea, he attributed this advantage to the growth of the bifidobacteria.

Interest in the functional capacities of lactobacilli and bifidobacteria decreased after some time, and remained low for many years as extravagant claims were made on doubtful scientific grounds about their supposed capacity to cure all kinds of diseases. In the United States, a product called 'acidophilus milk' is still available in the market and rather widely consumed by people affected by constipation and symptoms probably resulting from the irritable bowel syndrome [3].

Interest in the colonic microflora was re-established by the studies of Dubos, Savage, Savaiano and many other investigators. It became progressively evident that the microflora of the colon included large numbers of species (about 1000) and strains (numbers unknown) and that it was extremely complex. Furthermore, this ecosystem suffered changes related to age and type of feeding in infants, and during antibiotic treatments, although it returned to normality after treatments were interrupted [4]. The importance of the resident microbiota as part of the defensive mechanisms of the organism awoke the interest of specialists. They studied the genus and species whose characteristics were considered to result in the protective against some diseases,

with a shortening of the duration of their symptoms, and even in their prevention in some cases.

1.1. Characterization of Probiotics

The word 'probiotic' was coined by Parker who defined them as organisms and substances that contribute to the intestinal microbial balance [5]. Some 15 years later, Fuller expanded this concept, defining them as '... a live microbial feed supplement which beneficially affects the host animal by improving its intestinal microbial balance' [6]. This wider and more comprehensive definition emphasizes the requirement for probiotic microorganisms to be alive when ingested, that they influence the resident intestinal microbiota of the host, and that their intake brings benefit(s) to the host. However, some of the terms of this definition were considered rather vague, especially when applied to the clinical environment and, as a result, other definitions were coined. Thus, Saavedra and colleagues defined probiotics as viable microorganisms which, when ingested with food, may exert positive effects on the prevention or the treatment of specific pathologic conditions [7]. Eventually, a consensus was reached on a definition of probiotics that was expressed by a joint FAO/WHO Expert Consultation that defined them as '... live microorganisms which, when ingested in adequate numbers as part of food, benefit the health of the host' [8]. This latter definition emphasizes the concept that to obtain the desired effects probiotics must be ingested in numbers above a threshold.

It has been agreed that in order to be accepted as a probiotic, a microorganism should fulfil certain requirements: it should be of human origin (although some species have been recovered from plants or animals); and it should exhibit the capacity to withstand the effects of gastric acidity, conjugated bile salts and intestinal and pancreatic enzymes. Furthermore, the probiotic agents must be capable of adhering to enterocytes and colonocytes; they should be innocuous even when administered in large

TABLE 6.1 Species from which probiotics used in humans have been isolated

Bacteria	*Bifidobacterium*	*Leuconostoc*
Lactobacillus	*bifidus*	*Pediococcus*
acidophilus	*infantis*	*Propionibacterium*
johnsonii	*longum*	*Enterococcus*
plantarum	*thermophilus*	*Escherichia coli*
rhamnosus	*adolescentis*	*Lactococcus*
delbruecki	*catenulatus*	*Aspergillus*
reuteri	*pseudocatenulatus*	*niger*
fermentum	*lactis*	*oryzae*
brevis	*Streptococcus*	**Yeast and fungi**
lactis	*lactis*	*Saccharomyces*
cellobiosus	*cremoris*	*boulardii*
paracasei	*salivarius*	
helveticus	*intermedius*	

numbers; they should exhibit dose–response relationships and they must survive the industrial processes involved in their massive incorporation to foodstuffs [9].

A number of species and strains of bacteria, yeast and even fungi have been evaluated for their potential probiotic properties. Table 6.1 is a partial list of the microorganism species from which probiotic strains have been isolated and tested in the laboratory or have been used in the production or processing of foodstuffs [9]. Different probiotic species or even different strains from the same species may exert different, even antagonistic effects [10].

1.2. Safety of Probiotics

The main condition that probiotics have to fulfil is that they are safe to administer. Lactobacilli have been used for thousands of years in foods, mainly in dairy products, as they are present in the microbiota of animals and plants. Because of their capacity to synthesize acid, many lactobacilli have been used to produce fermented foodstuffs from meat, fish, cereals, vegetables, fruits and from the milk of almost all mammalian species. The acidified beverages were empirically administered to young children for their diarrhea-preventing potential [11]. Furthermore, the concerns about the risk of inducing D(−)-lactic acidosis during the fermentative process has been demonstrated as unfounded in some publications [12, 13]. Lactobacilli, bifidobacteria, and lactococci are all included in the category of organisms 'generally regarded as safe (GRAS)', a category in which the spore-forming bacteria, *Enterococcus*, streptococci and *Bacillus* are not included. Different probiotics have been administered to considerable numbers of individuals under controlled conditions, both infants and adults, suffering from different conditions, and have been proven to be without associated risks. In some of these trials, combinations of probiotics have been used. Furthermore, all kinds of products containing these bacteria are sold over the counter and without control to large segments of population without any undesirable affects [10]. However, concerns persist as cases of sepsis are reported periodically in the medical literature [14]. Some of the theoretical risks associated with probiotic intake include local disturbances of gastrointestinal function and metabolism, the displacement of the resident microbiota by the probiotic bacteria, adverse repercussions on the local (and systemic) immunity, the transfer of antibiotic resistance to the colonic bacteria or to potential pathogens originating from the environment. Another concern is that a probiotic may become invasive through translocation across the intestinal barrier in immunosuppressed subjects [15].

So far, there is no evidence that probiotics have the capacity to adhere to the epithelial lining of the intestine as pathogens do when invading the bloodstream. On the contrary, administration of probiotics is capable of blocking the translocation of pathogens without themselves migrating. Long-term surveillance in many countries has not demonstrated an increase of the risk of bacteremia or endocarditis due to probiotics. Even more, administration of probiotics has been shown to decrease mucosal permeability in a number of studies in humans [15, 16].

The microorganisms associated with bacteremia or endocarditis include *L. rhamnosus* GG, *L. plantarum*, *L. casei*, *L. paracasei*, *L. salivarius*, and *L. acidophilus*. Some cases have been associated with *Bifidobacterium*, *Leuconostoc* and *Pediococcus*, most of them of endogenous origin. Episodes of blood invasion associated with *Enterococcus* have been described but this microorganism is known to cause endocarditis of endogenous origin. While in some patients the associated microorganisms have been demonstrated by molecular methods to originate from the administered probiotics, this confirmation is missing in other episodes. Most of the affected patients had severe intercurrent conditions such as short bowel syndrome, intestinal feeding tubes, central venous catheters and other severe co-morbidities [14]. However, it should be emphasized again that these cases are almost anecdotic.

In 2008 the results of a multicenter, randomized, double blind, placebo-controlled study on the effects of a multispecies probiotic preparation in patients with severe acute pancreatitis were published [15, 16]. The aim was to confirm previous investigations by other groups that suggested possible beneficial effects in acute pancreatitis associated with tissue necrosis. A total of 153 patients received an experimental mixture of six different bacterial probiotics that carry the European Union label of qualified presumption of safety in two daily doses of 10^{10} by enteral tube; 144 individuals served as controls. Infectious complications occurred in more patients in the group receiving the probiotics; of the patients in the probiotic group 16% died compared with 6% in the control group. Nine patients in the probiotic group developed bowel ischemia, eight with fatal outcomes, compared to none in the control group. The authors concluded that the probiotic mixture used as a prophylactic

agent did not reduce the risk of infectious complications and, on the contrary it was associated with a considerably increased risk of mortality [17]. While eliciting considerable concern, this study raised a number of serious objections on aspects such as the model design and the randomization of patients, the use of the six different bacterial species and their high numbers, and especially, the clinical status of the patients, with a number of them already in shock or with organ failure in the experimental group when incorporated to the protocol and the microorganisms were administered to them [18–20]. The growing consensus among the specialists is that probiotics should not be administered to individuals of any age who may be at risk of organ failure or of deterioration of the intestinal barrier function [21]. Otherwise, the risk involved in the administration of probiotic bacteria is minimal as they have been administered to individuals who have suffered severe trauma, extensive surgery including cases of liver transplantation or duodenopancreatectomy, cirrhosis of the liver and mild-to-moderate hepatic encephalopathy. The need for carefully planned and controlled studies for the evaluation of the properties of probiotics results is evident if valid results are to be obtained [15, 16, 21].

1.3. Probiotics in Acute Diarrhea

Despite the multiple advances in the management of acute diarrhea, it continues to cause some three million deaths in children. Furthermore, it is one of the main causes of deterioration of their nutritional status. Even in developed countries such as the United States, diarrhea is reported as the cause of hospitalization in 13% of admitted patients and the estimated cumulative incidence is of one hospitalization due to diarrhea per 23 to 27 children under the age of 5 years. As the sanitary conditions of the environment improve through the provision of safe drinking water and adequate sewerage systems in association with the education of the population, the prevalence of diarrhea associated with bacteria such as enteropathogenic *E. coli* and *Shigella* decreases and the incidence of cases associated with rotavirus infection increases [22, 23]. The high numbers of episodes of acute diarrhea represents an economic burden for the less developed countries and for poor families who frequently cannot afford treatment. It is estimated that in the United States the combined cost of outpatient and inpatient treatment for diarrhea exceeds US$2 billion per year. Furthermore, in many cases antibiotics are unnecessarily prescribed and this represents, besides a source of disturbances of the resident microflora, the cause of antibiotic-associated diarrhea and of the appearance of resistant species and strains of bacteria.

Since 1983, a number of randomized, controlled trials using probiotics for the management of acute diarrhea have been published. These studies show that different probiotic microorganisms, *L. rhamnosus* GG (LGG), *L. reuteri*, *B. lactis* (Bb12), *B. breve* and *S. thermophilus* 065, exert protective effects or shorten the duration of this disease when induced by rotavirus [24–30]. This latter effect may be considered as modest because, while in the control children the duration of the episodes has been reported to be 2.4 ± 1.1 days, in those who received a fermented product containing LGG the episodes lasted 1.4 ± 0.8 days [26]. However, when the considerable numbers of children who may be affected are taken into consideration, a shortening of approximately 1 day in the duration of this condition represents an important decrease of the burden to the health services in terms of hospitalizations, patient loads and costs. Similar effects have been reported for the duration of febrile episodes associated with the administration of *L. reuteri* when compared to *B. lactis* Bb12. *L. reuteri* has also been associated with decreased shedding of rotavirus in feces during episodes of diarrhea and their aftermath, a finding that is important as this may decrease the rate of secondary cases [29]. This suggests that probiotics probably exhibit specificity as to their effects on acute diarrhea and its symptoms.

Probiotics do not seem to have comparable effects on the duration of bacteria-associated diarrhea; however, their administration is associated with decreases of the frequency and duration of persistent diarrhea [29].

Antibiotic-associated diarrhea (AAD) is an otherwise unexplained diarrhea that occurs in association with the administration of antibiotics [31]. The bacterial agent most commonly detected in AAD is *Clostridium difficile*, although *Klebsiella oxytoca*, multidrug resistant *Salmonella*, *C. albicans*, and *C. tropicalis* have also been implicated in some cases [32]. Almost any antibiotic is capable of inducing episodes of this disease, in particular those that decrease the resident populations of anaerobic bacteria. The incidence of this clinical entity is 5–25%, depending on the antibiotic [33]. The symptoms vary from mild episodes that end spontaneously when the antibiotic treatment is interrupted, to severe, dehydrating bloody diarrhea that may become associated with life-threatening conditions such as toxic megacolon [34]. The administration of probiotics, especially *S. boulardii* or some lactobacilli, has been demonstrated to be therapeutic options, especially the former [35, 36]. The effect of *S. boulardii* has been evaluated in only one study in infants [37]. Most studies have been carried out in adults. The effect of *S. boulardii* is associated with its capacity to neutralize the cytotoxins produced by *C. difficile*, through the release of a protease capable of degrading the toxin and its receptor in the mucosa. This yeast exerts trophic effects on the intestinal mucosa by increasing its concentrations of polyamines. It restores the levels of short-chain fatty acids, and it exerts anti-inflammatory effects by acting on the MAP kinase and NF-kB pathways and decreasing the secretion of IL-8. In addition, *S. boulardii* secretes a small peptide, the *S. boulardii* anti-inflammatory factor, that inhibits signaling pathways activated by the toxins produced by *C. difficile* [39].

1.4. Probiotics and *Helicobacter pylori* Colonization

Helicobacter pylori (*H. pylori*) is considered to be one of the most prevalent pathogens and colonizes the surface of the human gastric mucosa. Gastric colonization begins early in life, and affects a high proportion of the pediatric population, including infants in the developing countries [40]. *H. pylori* is considered as the etiological factor for gastroduodenal ulcers and a risk factor for gastric cancer, due to the early colonization process and an important factor in determining the development of gastric cancer later in life. Although all colonized individuals develop chronic gastritis, most remain asymptomatic and should not receive antibiotic treatment. This has a high cost, it is not highly effective and results in antibiotic resistance, and furthermore it induces adverse effects that affect compliance. Additionally, treated children are rapidly re-colonized.

For these reasons, it has been proposed that probiotics can be used as a tool for the dietary management of *H. pylori* colonization in at-risk populations. Some of the probiotics used in infant formulas and in child foodstuffs have been shown to interfere with *H. pylori* and/or to exert gastroprotective activities. These effects are strain specific and are related to the inhibition of *H. pylori* growth and adhesion by probiotic bacteriocins as well as to their antioxidant and anti-inflammatory properties [41]. In a randomized, double blind place to controlled trial carried out in asymptomatic colonized children, it was shown that 4-weeks administration of *L. johnsonii* NCC533 significantly decreased *H. pylori* colonization (determined by the ^{13}C-urea breath test), compared with the placebo. Interestingly, the decrease of the colonization induced by the probiotic correlated with the levels of basal colonization before treatment [42]. In another study, the same probiotic strain, alone or combined with cranberry juice, was shown to eradicate *H. pylori* in 14.9 and 22.9%, respectively, of colonized children [43].

Similar rates of eradication were observed with *S. boulardii* in another trial [44]. On the other hand, the administration of a yogurt with *L. gasseri* OLL 2716 (LG21) to *H. pylori*-positive children did not affect the density of colonization at the end of the intake period but decreased the severity of the gastric inflammation, as reflected by the lower pepsinogen I/II ratio [45].

Probiotics have also been used in combination with *H. pylori* antibiotic therapy with the aim of increasing its efficiency. In a multicenter, prospective, randomized, double blind, controlled study carried out in symptomatic children colonized by *H. pylori*, a 7-day treatment with antibiotics and omeprazole was compared with the same regimen supplemented with a fermented milk containing *L. casei* DN-114001 for 14 days [46]. The fermented product significantly increased the eradication rate from 57.5 to 84.6%. However, no differences in the rate of eradication were observed in another study carried out in 65 children, using the standard triple therapy (for 7 days) supplemented with a yogurt containing *B. animalis* and *L. casei* for 3 months [47].

These studies suggest that some probiotics may be useful to maintain low levels of *H. pylori* and to decrease the chronic inflammatory processes in the gastric antrum of colonized children. However, better designed studies with adequate sample sizes are necessary to obtain more solid conclusions.

1.5. Probiotics in Necrotizing Enterocolitis

Necrotizing enterocolitis (NEC) is a serious gastrointestinal disease observed predominantly in very low birth weight infants during their hospitalization in neonatal intensive care units in the first weeks of life. NEC is a complex, multifactorial disease probably associated with immaturity of intestinal functions and deficiencie of the local and systemic immune systems. To this must be added the effects of enteral feeding and of the microbial colonization of the gut lumen with local production of gas and of molecules that affect negatively enterocyte functions. The contribution of each of these factors to the genesis of NEC is unknown [48].

In 1999, Hoyos demonstrated that the incidence of NEC as well as its fatality rate were reduced in neonates in an intensive care unit when *Lactobacillus acidophilus* and *Bifidobacterium infantis* were administered [49]. Hoyos suggested that these results needed further investigation of bacterial gut colonization and its role in NEC. A number of other studies—including a Cochrane Database Systematic Review—which showed that enteral administration of probiotics significantly reduced the incidence of severe NEC (stage II or more) and mortality [50–55], have confirmed these studies. The mechanisms by which probiotics may prevent NEC include reduced intestinal colonization by pathogens, increased efficiency of the intestinal barrier against bacterial translocation to the bloodstream, modification of the host responses to microbial products through sensitization and immune responses, and improved efficiency of enteral nutrition.

It has not been possible to extract data regarding the outcome of the extremely low birth weight infants because of their low numbers, and in consequence, no suggestions are made for this high-risk group. The positive effects on infants weighing more than 1000 g at birth support the need for changes in their current treatment practices. Of note, no systemic infections with the probiotic microorganisms were reported in any of the studies.

1.6. Probiotics in Traveler's Diarrhea

Traveler's diarrhea (TD) is a common ailment that affects mostly people traveling from the developed to the less developed parts of the world. However, TD may also affect people going in the opposite direction, which means that for this condition there are no safe places. It is estimated that TD is the result of the ingestion of fecally contaminated food, water or any other beverages. The risk is especially high if the food is acquired from street vendors. The incubation period is 2–3 days and the duration of the symptoms is highly variable; in general, it is a self-limited condition characterized by diarrheal bowel movements, cramping abdominal pain, nausea, vomiting, and low fever. In some cases the symptoms are severe and patients may become severely dehydrated, especially children, immunocompromised individuals and the elderly. Although TD tends to affect individuals, large outbreaks have occurred affecting hundreds of passengers in settings such as cruise ships [48]. Most cases of TD are explained by the presence of pathogens such as enteropathogenic *E. coli*, enteroaggregative *E. coli*, *Salmonella* species, *Shigella* species, *Campylobacter jejuni*, *Yersinia enterocolitica*, *Plesiomonas shigelloides*, *Vibrio parahemolyticus*, *Aeromonas hydrophila*, and *Vibrio cholerae*. The diarrhea-associated types of *E. coli* are the most common cause. Other causative agents include parasites (*G. lamblia*, *E. histolytica*, *Cyclospora* and *Cryptosporidium*). Of the viruses associated with diarrhea, the most frequent findings are rotavirus and noroviruses. Affected individuals harbor more than one agent during the episode; in about one-third of patients no agent is identified [56].

The best strategy for dealing with TD is through prevention. However, in many of the cases it is necessary to institute treatment. Probiotics have been used in both capacities; this idea is conceptually sound as these microorganism are safe, compete with enteropathogens and have been shown to be effective. In placebo-controlled studies, *S. boulardii* has been demonstrated to be effective but the benefit was different depending on the geographical area to which the subjects traveled. *Lactobacillus* GG was also demonstrated to be effective [57]. On the other hand, *L. acidophilus* did not seem to be effective nor was nonviable *L. acidophilus* [58]. Mixtures of different probiotic species yielded variable results [59]. It is possible that some of the geographical differences in clinical outcomes are the result of different pathogens and different vehicles. Administration of the probiotic agents should be started 2 or 3 days before exposure and should be continued for about a week after the episode is finished.

1.7. Probiotics in the Management of Allergies

Atopic diseases such as eczema, allergic rhinitis and asthma are chronic allergic disorders whose prevalence has increased considerably over the past 20 years. According to the hygiene hypothesis, there is an inverse association between the number of infectious episodes occurring early in life and the development of atopy appearing simultaneously or a few short years later. The higher frequency of allergies may be related to other conditions such as decreases of intestinal infections, changes in food consumption patterns, industrial processing of foodstuffs resulting in the disappearance of all or some of their microbiota, and alterations of the intestinal microbiota [60]. It is estimated that food allergies affect 3.5% of adults and 8 to 10% of children; the food allergens most frequently involved are egg, peanuts, milk, fish, nuts, shellfish, wheat, kiwi and mustard.

A number of studies suggest that there exists a relationship between allergic conditions and the composition of the gut microbiota. The fecal counts of bifidobacteria in allergic infants, particularly those with atopic eczema, are significantly lower than in healthy peers [61]. *Clostridium*, *Bacteroides* and *Staphylococcus* may also be altered and their numbers may correlate with the IgE serum levels. In the population of *Bifidobacterium* of the colon of allergic infants there are higher counts of *B. adolescentis* and *B. longum* and lower counts of *B. bifidum*, in contrast to their healthy peers [62]; such a microbiota is associated with the *in vitro* synthesis of TNF-α and IL-12 by macrophage-like cells [63]. The gut microbiota participates in the establishment of immune oral tolerance by reorienting the Th2 responder

phenotype of newborns towards the Th-1 cell-mediated immune response and through the stimulation of TGF-β and IgA secretion. The microbiota also participates in the regulation of the gut barrier function, which blocks the transfer across the mucosa of food antigens and microorganisms implicated in the altered immune responses of atopic children.

It has been proposed that probiotics modulate the homeostasis of the gut microbiota and decrease the risk and the symptoms of allergies. Randomized, double blind, placebo-controlled clinical trials have been carried out to evaluate whether probiotic intake alleviates atopic eczema in children. LGG, and sometimes *Bifidobacterium* Bb12, decrease SCORAD as well as the fecal α-1 antitrypsin and TNF-α, plasmatic sCD4 and the protein X of eosinophils in urine [64]. A decrease of atopic eczema in infants from atopic families was observed when mothers were given LGG prior to delivery and during lactation (23 vs 46% in the probiotic and placebo groups, respectively) [65]; TGF-β2 levels were increased in their milk [66]. The protective effect has been shown to persist until 7 years of age [67]. This means that the administration of probiotic microorganisms prior to delivery, and 6 months afterwards, leaves an imprint in the immune system of the host that persists for years and prevents the development of atopic manifestations.

In atopic dermatitis, the daily administration of LGG for 4 weeks decreased SCORAD in the children with high IgE levels [68]. On the other hand, no improvement of SCORAD and of inflammatory parameters was observed in infants less than 5 months of age who received a hydrolyzed, whey-based formula alone or supplemented with LGG or with *L. rhamnosus* for 3 months [69].

1.8. Probiotics in the Management of the Irritable Bowel Syndrome

The irritable bowel syndrome (IBS) is a functional disorder characterized by symptoms such as abdominal pain, bloating and episodes of diarrhea or constipation. These occur in the absence of demonstrable lesions and may persist for long periods with some of the symptoms increasing or decreasing in intensity in an unpredictable manner. The affected patients represent a rather heterogeneous group in whom a variety of treatments have been assayed with variable results, mostly disappointing. With some frequency the irritable bowel syndrome becomes manifest following episodes of acute, mostly viral, diarrhea or after antibiotic treatments. For this reason, alterations of the resident microbiota have been considered to play a part in its pathogenesis. The pathophysiology of the IBS is multifactorial and may include motor and sensory dysfunction, immune responses, food sensitivity and genetic predisposition. The disease is more common in females [70, 71]. A decrease of bifidobacteria, lactobacilli and *E. coli* has been described with concomitant increases of other bacteria such as clostridia. Some patients exhibit symptoms of increased colonic fermentation including bloating and meteorism [72, 73]. Probiotics may modify the composition and metabolism of the resident flora and furthermore, exert anti-inflammatory effects, influence the adaptation of the intestinal vasculature to changing conditions in the mucosa of the colon and protect the lumen and the mucosa surface from pathogens [74]. A study in 2007 demonstrated that *Lactobacillus* strains, and especially *L. acidophilus*, induced the expression of μ-opioid and endocanabinoid receptors in cultured intestinal epithelial cells; it also mediated analgesic functions in the gut of mice, similar to the effects of morphine [75]. This suggests that the microbial flora of the gastrointestinal tract may influence visceral perception by the affected individuals.

The majority of the controlled studies on the effects of probiotic bacteria on the evolution of the irritable bowel syndrome show improvement of the symptoms experienced by patients and of their health quality of life index, with stabilization of the resident microflora but without changes in the fecal concentrations of short-chain fatty acids (SCFAs) or in the parameters indicative of inflammatory processes, such as C-reactive protein [76, 77].

1.9. Probiotics in Inflammatory Bowel Disease

Inflammatory bowel disease (IBD) is a spectrum of chronic inflammatory disorders whose etiology is unknown although genetic, immunological and psychological factors have been demonstrated to play a role in their pathogenesis.

Ulcerative colitis (UC) and Crohn's disease (CD) are the two most frequent causes of this chronic inflammation of the gastrointestinal tract; these are lifelong diseases characterized by recurrent episodes of diarrhea, frequently with blood in the feces, abdominal pain, fever, malaise and weight loss. While UC is confined to the mucosa of the colon and sometimes involves the terminal ileum (backwash ileitis), CD affects any segment of the gastrointestinal tract, it tends to affect the full thickness of the wall and generates fistulae that short circuit the affected organ to other segments of the intestinal tube or to organs close by such as the biliary tract, the urinary bladder or the skin, greatly complicating the management of these patients. Systemic compromise is more frequent in CD, affecting the eyes, joints, genitals and skin. The incidence of UC is 10 new cases per 100,000 persons/year in the United States. In the less developed countries the incidence is less, although in some countries such as Chile it has been increasing in the last 20 years; the incidence of CD is 3.4 to 14.6 per 100,000 persons/year. As with UC, the prevalence of CD is also increasing in some of the less-developed countries. For both diseases there is evidence of genetic influences [78, 79].

Medical treatment to induce remission in both conditions (UC and CD) includes the use of different types and pharmaceutical forms of corticosteroids, derivates of aminosalicylic acid, immunomodulators (azathioprine, 6-mercaptopurine, mycophenolate mofetil, tacrolimus), biological agents (infliximab, adalimumab, certolizumab, etc.), and selective adhesion molecule inhibitors (MLN02) [80]. In a proportion of cases, resection of the affected segments becomes necessary because of stricture, abscess or fistula formation or because of the risk of malignancy after many years of evolution [78, 79].

An important body of evidence has suggested that the enteric microbial flora exerts a distinct role in inducing and maintaining the activity of the intestinal inflammation processes through complex interrelations with the local immune system. It seems that some bacteria, viruses or even food antigens may act as triggers. The role of the resident microbiota in these diseases is difficult to establish; however, the fact that some antibiotics such as metronidazole and ciprofloxacin induce remissions, especially in CD, further suggests that bacteria plays a role in the causation of both diseases [81–83]. This is also the rationale for the use of probiotics. Although there have been clinical studies on the effect of probiotics in IBD, there is a scarcity of large, randomized, double blind, placebo-controlled studies. Studies have evaluated the efficacy of *E. coli* Nissle 1917 and VSL#3 for relatively short periods in patients on remission; in general, the results achieved are not different from those of 5-aminosalicylic (5-ASA) in maintaining remission [84, 85]. The main advantage of the probiotics is that they induce fewer side effects than conventional therapies. In other studies, *Lactobacillus* GG seems to be able to maintain remission for longer periods than 5-ASA does; relapse rates and clinical, endoscopic and histological scores were similar with both therapies. A study using VSL#3 showed that this combination of probiotics is beneficial as an alternative to 5-ASA in the maintenance of remission in patients with UC. Another study provided additional information on the use of the same combination as capable of maintaining remission for at least 6 weeks in 53% of patients while an

additional 24% were improved. In some patients a reduction of NFkB was observed together with an increase of anti-inflammatory cytokine release. In other studies the results are not conclusive. It seems that probiotics have strain-specific effects and that it is important to test each of these in carefully selected patients [83].

Similar results are obtained in the treatment of active UC with probiotics, administered either orally or by enema. It is possible that the administration of probiotics may magnify the effects of 5-ASA. There are suggestions that the effect of the probiotics is not the result of their direct influence on the colonic mucosa but perhaps it may be a consequence of modifications induced on the resident microflora or on the inflammatory processes [86].

The results obtained in the treatment of CD in the active stage or in remission are similar to those observed in UC. In some cases, the efficacy is not evident. It is possible to observe a certain degree of decrease of relapse rates but this is not clearcut. Another problem is the small number of patients participating in some studies. A Cochrane Review published in 2008 discourages the use of probiotics in the management of CD [87].

The situation is different in pouchitis. This is a condition characterized by mucosal inflammation occurring in an ileal reservoir following total colectomy for UC or familial adenomatous polyposis. Its incidence is higher in the former. The inflammation of the pouch mucosa occurs in continent ileostomies and in pelvic pouches. The condition is manifested clinically by increased stool frequency, urgency, diarrhea, bleeding from the mucosa and pain. Systemic symptoms such as fever are common. The treatment of this condition may be very frustrating and use has been made of metronidazole, ciprofloxacin and topical butyrate, glutamine and kaolin. Some studies in patients with pouchitis have not shown evidences of clinical or endoscopic responses with the administration of LGG; however, first episodes of this disease were delayed in another study. In two randomized, double blind, placebo-controlled studies in which participating patients were given VSL#3, relapse rates were significantly reduced after a 9-month follow-up and pouchitis development in newly operated patients was prevented. *L. acidophilus* and *B. lactis* may induce improvement of the markers of a pouch disease activity index [83, 88].

1.10. Probiotics and Cancer

Cancers of the large intestine are the third most prevalent form of the disease in men (after lung and prostate cancers) and in women (after breast and lung cancers). In non-disseminated disease the 5-year survival rate may be 63% although if metastatic spread has already occurred at the time of discovery, the 5-year survival rate is close to 10%. Most cancers arise from adenomatous polyps after a long evolution through the accumulation of a succession of mutations to genes such as *TP53*, *APC*, and *K-ras*. A number of epidemiological studies suggest that there is a relationship between the appearance of colonic cancers and the quality of the diet [89]. Because of this, and due to the fact that most sporadic colon cancers appear in areas with high counts of bacteria and fecal stagnation (the cecum, the ascending and descending colon and the rectum), the role of the resident microflora in carcinogenesis has awakened considerable interest. As probiotics modulate the colonic microbiota and stimulate local and systemic immunity, a natural interest was also awakened to further explore these aspects [90]. It is possible that some bacteria from the resident microbiota may release carcinogenic compounds into the colonic lumen as a result of their metabolism of unabsorbed molecules. There is evidence suggesting that the consumption of fermented milk products containing lactobacilli and bifidobacteria may play a role in preventing cancer of the colon and rectum but the mechanisms responsible for this effect are not fully understood and may be linked to different factors. Part of this

effect is attributed to the decline of fecal beta-glucuronidase, nitroreductase and azoreductase activities induced in healthy individuals by two strains of *Lactobacillus acidophilus* (NCFM and N-2) after 10 days of intake. When the intake of these agents is interrupted, the activity of these enzymes returns to their previous levels in 3 to 4 weeks [89]. Not every probiotic shares this property as some (*L. rhamnosus* DR20, *L. plantarum* 299v and *L. acidophilus*) do not decrease these enzymes in feces, compared with *L. casei* Shirota which is highly effective [89].

Probiotics may also play a protective role through the binding and/or degradation of carcinogens, many of them originating from the western type diet, rich in red meats processed by broiling. Studies in mice indicate that the use of some lactobacilli reduce the uptake of mutagens by different tissues. Observations in human volunteers have disclosed that consumption of preparations containing lactobacilli reduces the urinary and fecal excretion of mutagenic compounds [91]. The presence of probiotics in the colon is associated with changes in the physico-chemical environment of the lumen (changes in the pH and redox potential). Additionally, SCFAs are produced by the bacterial fermentation of indigestible polysaccharides and butyrate has been shown to induce apoptosis of damaged cultured cells of colonic origin. Butyrate also reduces the number of aberrant crypt foci in rats treated with the carcinogen azoxymethane [92].

Other mechanisms by which probiotics may act as anti-tumorigenic factors are the enhancement of the local and systemic immune responses and the production of molecules that neutralize or block mutagens; another possibility is that these molecules may be directly anti-tumorigenic [89].

Although the evidence for beneficial effects of probiotics in human tumorigenesis is indirect, there is an accumulating body of information from experimental models that suggests that they exert anti-neoplastic effects. The need for carefully planned, long-term studies in humans is evident as probiotics may be useful agents in the prevention of the earliest stages in the onset of the evolution of cancer.

1.11. Effects of Probiotics on Distant Organs

Probiotics induce changes in organs distant from the gastrointestinal tract, besides modifying the quality of its mucosal barrier and the patterns of response of its immune system. Two studies have evaluated the effects of the oral intake of mixtures of probiotics in individuals affected by episodes of common cold or upper respiratory tract infections. Individuals in the probiotics group experienced shorter episodes of common cold with reduced intensity of symptoms and with enhancement of cytotoxic and T suppressor (CD8+) and T helper (CD4+) cells [93]. In the second study the number of episodes of common cold and influenza decreased considerably as well as the overall severity of symptoms; in this latter study the subjects in the experimental group received prebiotics or lactoferrin in addition to the probiotics [94]. As the experimental design and mixtures of bacteria tested in both studies are not identical, it is difficult to establish comparisons between these mixtures and their effects. The roles played by the prebiotics and the lactoferrin are not evident. Anyway, these studies show that probiotics have effects beyond the digestive tract.

Another example of this type of effect is the decrease in the severity of atopy in infants whose mothers had received *L. rhamnosus* GG before delivery and then for 6 months if the infants were breastfed. Alternatively, *L. rhamnosus* was added to the formula for the same length of time if the infant was not breastfed [66, 67]. The interesting finding of these studies is that the protective effect of this single probiotic extended for at least 7 years, which means that intake of these microorganisms leaves an imprint in the immune system that persists for long periods of time.

It has been shown that the oral administration of *L. casei* together with the intravesical administration of epirubicin to patients operated on for bladder cancer was associated with a higher percentage of patients with a 3-year symptom-free survival rate although the overall survival and the progression-free period were not influenced. Again this shows that probiotics exert effects in distant organs. These effects are probably mediated by changes in the local and systemic immune responses, the patterns of cytokine synthesis, the stimulation of natural killer and cytotoxic cells, the stimulation of macrophages, the changes in the quality of the intestinal barrier, and many other functions which have not been evaluated in depth [95].

2. THE PREBIOTIC CONCEPT

The original definition of prebiotics, proposed by Gibson and Roberfroid in 1995, defined them as indigestible dietary carbohydrates which beneficially affect the health of the host by selectively stimulating the growth or the activity of one or more bacterial populations in the colon, mainly lactobacilli and bifidobacteria [96]. Then, in 2007, the FAO Technical Meeting on Prebiotics proposed a broader definition to encompass new prebiotics and to reflect more accurately the current understanding of the microbial ecology of the human microbiota: 'A prebiotic is a non-viable food component that confers a health benefit on the host, associated with modulation of the microbiota' [97]. It is interesting to note that according to this new definition, dietary components other than non-digestible carbohydrates could also be considered as prebiotics. This is the case, for example, of the nucleotides and the casein-derived glycomacropeptide of human milk, which are capable of modulating the colonic microbiota of the newborn [98, 99]. The FAO report states that prebiotics must be food-grade components (not drugs) well-characterized from the chemical point of view. They can be a form of dietary fiber, although not all dietary fiber is necessarily a prebiotic. Another important point is that the measurable health-promoting effects of the prebiotics must not be due to their absorption into the bloodstream or the component acting alone; the metabolic activities or the composition of the microbiota of the target host must be modulated by the sole presence of this dietary component or of the formulation in which it is being delivered. This is accomplished through fermentation, as a result of receptor blockage or other mechanisms.

2.1. Prebiotics in Human Milk

Oligosaccharides are present in human milk in concentrations ranging from 7 to 12 g/L, much higher than those found in bovine milk which only contains traces of these molecules [100]. They are synthesized in the mammary gland through the binding of galactose (Gal) and N-acetylglucosamine (GlcNAc) to lactose and the incorporation of fucose and sialic acid which determines their classification into neutral and acidic oligosaccharides and explains the great variety of their chemical structures (more than 130 described) [101]. The presence of N-acetylglucosamine and fucose differentiates human milk oligosaccharides from galacto-oligosaccharides (GOS). The human milk oligosaccharides may be considered as prebiotic components as they are neither digested nor absorbed in the small intestine, reaching the infant's colon where they are fermented. The neutral oligosaccharidic fraction is a relevant factor in this process and it contributes to the development of the *Bifidobacterium*-rich microbiota characteristic of breastfed infants [102]. On the other hand, the acidic fraction could prevent the adhesion of pathogenic bacteria to the intestinal epithelium [103]. This latter property is due to the fact that they display specific moieties that act as analogues of host cell surface receptors to which enteropathogens may bind; this

blockage of the enteropathogen binding results in their subsequent elimination in the feces and in the prevention of infectious episodes. In consequence, the great structural diversity of these oligosaccharides may be considered as an adaptive response on the part of the mother to the diversity of pathogens present in the environment.

2.2. Sources of Prebiotics

Poly- and oligosaccharides are widely available in the diet [104]. They are mainly found in traditionally consumed vegetables, where they constitute a reserve of energy to be used during germination. Some oligosaccharides with prebiotic activity are also found in the milk of other mammals. Chitin, which is used to produce chitosan (by desacetylation), is considered the most abundant polysaccharide in nature after cellulose; it is found in the exoskeleton of crustaceans, insects and in some fungi.

The prebiotics most commonly used in the elaboration of foodstuffs, including baby foods, are fructans (inulin and fructo-oligosaccharides, FOS) and galacto-oligosaccharides (GOS) [105, 106]. They are considered as GRAS and their health-promoting effects have been widely studied. Inulin, for example, is a mixture of polymers composed by fructose units forming lineal chains with variable degrees of polymerization, bound to a single glucose moiety. Inulin is isolated and purified from chicory after extraction with hot water. It may be used as a fat substitute in some foodstuffs, improving their texture and mouthfeel and decreasing their energy density [107].

On the other hand, many new prebiotics, either of natural (soy oligosaccharides, resistant starch, etc.) or synthetic origin (xylo-oligosaccharides, pyrodextrin, isomalte-oligosaccharides, lactosucrose, polydextrose, lactulose) are emerging in the world markets. Many of these new products have been developed in Japan where some are currently commercialized. However, it is important to note that many of these new compounds have been studied mainly in *in vitro* and animal models. In consequence, it is necessary to carry out more clinical trials to confirm their safety as well as their healthy effects in humans.

2.3. Health-promoting Effects Associated with Prebiotic Intake

Inhibition of enteropathogens

Many enteropathogens use oligosaccharide moieties in the enterocyte glycocalix as receptors: receptor binding is the first step in the colonization process that results in the subsequent appearance of functional derangements and digestive symptoms. It has been proposed that the improved understanding of the characteristics of these binding sites could result in the design of a new generation of 'optimized' prebiotics capable of interfering with enteropathogen binding, as illustrated by those present in human milk [103].

Prebiotics may also exert antibacterial effects through the short-chain fatty acids (SCFAs) released during the fermentation processes, which decreases the intra-colonic pH and inhibits pathogen growth. The bacterial populations whose growth has been stimulated by prebiotics may also inhibit the growth of pathogens, as it has been observed *in vitro* with *E. coli*, *Campylobacter*, *Shigella* y *Salmonella* spp., and reduce their adhesion to epithelial cells [108]. Based on these observations it has been proposed that prebiotic intake could decrease the risk of infectious diarrhea. However, few studies have confirmed these results in humans [109]. Prebiotics may also contribute to the restoration of the homeostasis of the intestinal microbiota when this is altered, for example, by antibiotic administration [4].

2.4. Prebiotics and the Risk of Colorectal Cancer

Dietary fiber has been considered to participate in the protection against the development of colorectal cancer [110]. In animal models of colonic tumorogenesis induced in rats by azoxymethane, the dietary administration of oligofructose (10%) decreased the number of aberrant crypts in the colonic epithelium and their evolution to malignant tumours [111]. On the other hand, fructo- and galacto-oligosaccharides have been shown to affect the expression of fecal procarcinogenic enzymatic activities of bacterial origin such as β-glucuronidase, nitroreductase and azoreductase [112]. It has not been clearly determined if those effects are due to the direct inhibition of these activities by the prebiotics, or whether this occurs through the higher counts of bifidobacteria and lactobacilli and/or the decrease of other populations such as members of the genus *Clostridium*. Another important aspect contributing to the decrease of the risk of colorectal cancer is the cecal concentration of butyrate. In fact, this SCFA is important to maintain a healthy colonic epithelium because it is the main source of energy for the colonocytes and favors their differentiation and apoptosis, resulting in the elimination of potentially cancerous cells.

2.5. Prebiotics and Minerals Bioavailability

The adequate intake of calcium and magnesium is crucial for bone health and the prevention of osteoporosis in at-risk populations. The addition of GOS to the diet of rats has been shown to increase the absorption of these minerals while this effect was reduced in animals treated with neomycin, suggesting a role for the colonic microbiota in this effect [113]. The administration of FOS to gastrectomized animals, which normally present a decreased absorption of calcium, stimulates the expression of calbindin in the colonic mucosa and increases the retention of calcium in the skeleton in comparison with controls receiving sucrose [114].

Contradictory results have been observed in studies in humans; this could be due to differences between the doses of prebiotics, the timing of their administration, the calcium content of the diet, the segment of the skeleton evaluated, and the age of the subjects [115]. This phenomenon could be explained by the fact that prebiotics fermentation decreases intracolonic pH and this improves the solubility of calcium and magnesium as well as their bioavailability. For example, the daily intake of oligofructose and long-chain inulin from chicory enhanced in postmenopausal women the fractional absorption of Ca and Mg compared with placebo. Bone formation, evaluated by serum osteocalcin, was improved after 6 weeks of treatment [116]. Even though this process was not quantitatively considerable, it contributes to reverse the negative calcium balance existing in postmenopausal women and in men >65 years of age, decreasing the risk of osteoporosis in the absence of an adequate calcium intake. Interestingly, a similar protective effect has been observed in teenagers [117]; this could be associated with a decrease of body mass index [118].

2.6. Prebiotics and the Regulation of Blood Lipids

High levels of plasmatic triglycerides and cholesterol, in addition to abdominal obesity, arterial hypertension and insulin resistance, are important components of the metabolic syndrome, a pathological condition associated with an increased risk of cardiovascular diseases. Studies in animal models and in humans indicate that prebiotic intake could decrease blood triglyceride and cholesterol levels [119]. Various mechanisms have been proposed to explain such effects. Some prebiotics, like the β-glucans in barley, are known to form viscous gels when in aqueous solution; it has been proposed that in the intestinal lumen such gels decrease pancreatic lipase activity and interfere with the

incorporation of cholesterol into micelles [120]. This effect, however, may not be considered as prebiotic as it does not occur through the modulation of the colonic microbiota.

As previously stated, the fermentation of prebiotics in the colon produces high amounts of SCFAs, mainly acetate, propionate and butyrate. Once absorbed by the colonic mucosa, acetate and propionate reach the systemic circulation and arrive in the liver. In this organ, acetate may be used as a substrate for the *de novo* synthesis of triglycerides and cholesterol while propionate tends to exert an antagonist effect by inhibiting the genic expression of lipogenic enzymes involved in the synthesis of these molecules [121, 122]. In consequence, the propionate/acetate ratio produced by the fermentation of prebiotics is an important factor in determining their capacity to decrease circulating lipids.

The majority of studies that evaluated the effects of prebiotics on blood lipids have been done with inulin and oligofructose. Although convincing lipid-lowering effects have been observed in animals, high doses had to be used. Few studies have been carried out in humans and their results are contradictory. While some do not report any effects of inulin or oligofructose on serum lipids in normolipidemic subjects, others have shown reductions in serum triglycerides, with moderate changes in serum total and LDL cholesterol; in hyperlipidemic subjects the primary effect is the lowering of cholesterol levels [119].

2.7. Prebiotics and the Regulation of Food Intake

Obesity is an important public health problem worldwide as it constitutes a risk factor for the development of chronic diseases such as type 2 diabetes and cardiovascular diseases. One of the most interesting aspects of prebiotic use is their capacity for modulating food intake. Studies in animal models have demonstrated that the administration of oligofructose in rats stimulates in the epithelium of the distal ileon the differentiation of enteroendocrine L cells and their subsequent release of the incretin Glucagon Like Peptide-1 (GLP-1) [123, 124]. In addition to its insulin-like effects, GLP-1 exerts anorexigenic effects in the central nervous system, resulting in lower food intake and decreased weight gain. Some studies in humans seem to confirm these observations, suggesting that the incorporation of FOS in foodstuffs may be an interesting tool for appetite regulation [118, 125].

2.8. Prebiotics and Intestinal Transit and Constipation

Constipation is a common ailment in children and adults and its prevalence tends to be even higher in the elderly. The composition of the intestinal microbiota changes with age, with a marked decrease of the *Bifidobacterium* population [126]; it has been proposed that this phenomenon is implicated in the genesis of the constipation. In fact, it is known that alterations of the intestinal microbiota can affect intestinal motility, and that the SCFAs produced by the fermentative processes (involving bifidobacteria) have an important effect on transit time. In consequence, it has been proposed that probiotics and/or prebiotics could be useful tools in the dietary management of constipation, by increasing the numbers of bifidobacteria. It is interesting to note that lactulose, a widely used laxative, is also a prebiotic as it is not digestible in the small intestine and can be used as a substrate to stimulate *Bifidobacterium* growth in the colon [127]. Other prebiotics such as lactitol, GOS and FOS have also proven effective in treating chronic constipation in the elderly [128–130]. Mixtures of GOS/FOS incorporated to infant milk formulae have also been shown to soften stool consistency in constipated children [131, 132].

3. CONCLUSION

The information reviewed indicates that there is a growing understanding of the role played by the resident microbiota on human health, including the prevention or amelioration of a number of conditions and symptoms. While probiotics are foreign microbial agents that act as enzymatic systems and stimulate the local and systemic immune system, prebiotics act by stimulating colonic fermentative processes and enhancing the proliferation of endogenous species and strains of bacteria. It has been shown that prebiotics may exert additional systemic effects through the stimulation of endocrine mechanisms that regulate satiety and weight gain.

References

1. Metchnikoff, Y. (1908). *The prolongation of life*. Optimistic studies. London: William Heinemann.
2. Mitsuoka, T. (1990). Bifidobacteria and their role in human health. *Journal of Industrial Microbiology & Biotechnology, 6*, 263–268.
3. Tannock, G. W. (2003). Probiotics: Time for a dose of realism. *Current Issues in Intestinal Microbiology, 4*, 33–42.
4. Brunser, O., Gotteland, M., Cruchet, S., et al. (2006). Effect of a milk formula with prebiotics on the intestinal microbiota of infants after an antibiotic treatment. *Pediatric Research, 59*, 451–456.
5. Parker, R. B. (1974). Probiotics, the other half of the antibiotic story. *Animal Nutrition Health, 29*, 4–8.
6. Fuller, R. (1989). Probiotics in man and animals. *The Journal of Applied Bacteriology, 66*, 365–378.
7. Saavedra, J. M., Abi-Hanna, A., Moore, N., & Yolken, R. H. (2004). Long-term consumption of infant formulas containing live probiotic bacteria: Tolerance and safety. *The American Journal of Clinical Nutrition, 79*, 261–267.
8. Joint FAO/WHO. (2001). *Expert Consultation on Evaluation of Health and Nutritional Properties of Probiotics in Foods*. Geneva: WHO.
9. Wilson, M. (2005). Manipulation of the indigenous microbiota. In M. Wilson (Ed.), *Microbial inhabitants of humans. Their ecology and role in health and disease* (pp. 395–419). Cambridge: Cambridge University Press.
10. Sanders, M. E. (2008). Probiotics: Definition, sources, selection, and uses. *Clinical Infectious Diseases, 46*(Suppl. 2), S58–S61.
11. Brunser, O., Gotteland, M., & Cruchet, S. (2007). Functional fermented milk products. In C. Agostoni, &

O. Brunser (Eds.), *Issues in complementary feeding. Nestlé Nutrition Workshop Series: Vol. 60* (pp. 215–250). Basel: Nestec Ltd, Vevey; S. Karger AG.

12. Connoly, E. (2005). Abrahamsson Th, Björkstén B. Safety of D(-) lactic acid producing bacteria in the human infant. *Journal of Pediatric Gastroenterology and Nutrition, 41*, 489–492.

13. Haschke-Becher, E., Brunser, O., Cruchet, S., et al. (2008). Urinary D-lactate excretion in infants receiving *Lactobacillus johnsonii* (La1) with formula. *Annals of Nutrition & Metabolism, 53*, 240–244.

14. Land, M. H., Rouster-Stevens, K., Woods, C. R., et al. (2005). *Lactobacillus* sepsis associated with probiotic therapy. *Pediatrics, 115*, 178–181.

15. Snydman, D. R. (2008). The safety of probiotics. *Clinical Infectious Diseases, 46*, S11–S104.

16. Hord, N. G. (2008). Eukariotic-microbiotic crosstalk: Potential mechanisms for health benefits of prebiotics and probiotics. *Annual Review of Nutrition, 28*, 215–231.

17. Besselink, M. G., van Santvoort, H. C., Buskens, E., et al. (2008). Dutch Acute Pancreatitis Study Group. Probiotic prophylaxis in predicted severe acute pancreatitis: A randomised, double-blind, placebo-controlled trial. *Lancet, 371*, 651–659.

18. Reid, G., Gibson, G., Guarner, F., & Versalovic, J. (2008). Probiotic prophylaxis in predicted severe acute pancreatitis. *Lancet, 372*, 112–113.

19. Reddy, B. S., & McFie, J. (2008). Probiotic prophylaxis in predicted severe acute pancreatitis. *Lancet, 372*, 113.

20. Marteau, Ph. (2008). Probiotic prophylaxis in predicted severe acute pancreatitis. *Lancet, 372*, 114–115.

21. Bengmark, S. (2008). Is probiotic prophylaxis worthwhile in patients with predicted severe acute pancreatitis? *Nature Clinical Practice. Gastroenterology & Hepatology, 5*, 602–603.

22. Araya, M., Figueroa, G., Espinoza, J., et al. (1985). Acute diarrhoeal disease in children under 7 years of age living in a periurban slum in Santiago, Chile. *The Journal of Hygiene (Cambridge), 95*, 457–467.

23. Espinoza, J., Araya, M., Figueroa, G., et al. (1989). Diarrea aguda en población infantil marginal de Santiago. In A. E. Lattes, M. Farren, & J. MacDonald (Eds.), *Salud, mortalidad infantil y perinatal en América Latina* (pp. 207–223). Ottawa: La Técnica Impresora, Buenos Aires. International Development Research Centre.

24. Clements, M. L., Levine, M. M., Ristaino, P. A., et al. (1983). Exogenous lactobacilli fed to man—their fate and ability to prevent diarrheal disease. *Progress in Food & Nutrition Science, 7*, 29–37.

25. Brunser, O., Araya, M., Espinoza, J., et al. (1989). Effect of an acidified milk on diarrhoea and the carrier state in infants of low socio-economic stratum. *Acta Paediatrica Scandinavica, 78*, 259–264.

26. Isolauri, E., Juntunen, M., Rautanen, T., et al. (1991). A human *Lactobacillus* strain (*Lactobacillus casei* sp strain GG) promotes recovery from acute diarrhea in children. *Pediatrics, 88*, 90–97.

27. Majamaa, H., Isolauri, E., Saxelin, M., & Vesikari, T. (1995). Lactic acid bacteria in the treatment of acute rotavirus gastroenteritis. *Journal of Pediatric Gastroenterology and Nutrition, 20*, 333–338.

28. Shornikova, A. V., Isolauri, E., Burkanova, L., et al. (1997). A trial in the Karelian Republic of oral rehydration and *Lactobacillus* GG for treatment of diarrhea. *Acta Paediatrica, 86*, 460–465.

29. Weizman, Z., Asli, G., & Alsheikh, A. (2005). Effect of a probiotic infant formula on infections in child care centers: Comparison of two probiotic agents. *Pediatrics, 115*, 5–9.

30. Szajewska, H., Setty, M., Mrukowicz, J., & Guandalini, S. (2006). Probiotics in gastrointestinal diseases in children: Hard and not-so-hard evidence of efficacy. *Journal of Pediatric Gastroenterology and Nutrition, 42*, 454–475.

31. Bartlett, J. G. (2002). Antibiotic-associated diarrhea. *The New England Journal of Medicine, 346*, 334–339.

32. Zollner-Schwetz, I., Högenauer, C., Joainig, M., et al. (2008). Role of *Klebsiella oxytoca* in antibiotic-associated diarrhea. *Clinical Infectious Diseases, 47*, 74–78.

33. Wiström, J., Norrby, S. R., Myhre, E. B., et al. (2001). Frequency of antibiotic-associated diarrhoea in 2462 antibiotic-treated patients: A prospective study. *The Journal of Antimicrobial Chemotherapy, 47*, 43–50.

34. Jaber, M. R., Olafsson, S., Fung, W. L., & Reeves, M. E. (2008). Clinical review of the management of fulminant *Clostridium difficile* infection. *The American Journal of Gastroenterology, 103*, 195–203.

35. Arvola, T., Laiho, K., Torkkeli, S., et al. (1999). Prophylactic *Lactobacillus* GG reduces antibiotic-associated diarrhea in children with respiratory infections: A randomized study. *Pediatric Research, 104*, e-64.

36. Szymański, H., Armańska, M., Kowalska-Duplaga, K., & Szajewska, H. (2008). *Bifidobacterium longum* PL03, *Lactobacillus rhamnosus* KL53A, and *Lactobacillus plantarum* PL02 in the prevention of antibiotic-associated diarrhea in children: A randomized controlled pilot trial. *Digestion, 78*, 13–17.

37. Buts, J. P., Corthier, G., & Delmee, M. (1993). *Saccharomyces boulardii* for *Clostridium difficile*-associated enteropathies in infants. *Journal of Pediatric Gastroenterology and Nutrition, 16*, 419–425.

38. Eng, S., & Surawicz, C. (2004). Colitis pseudomembranous. In L. R. Johnson (Ed.), *Encyclopedia of gastroenterology* (pp. 379–381). San Diego: Academic Press.

39. Vandenplas, Y., Brunser, O., & Szajewska, H. (2009). *Saccharomyces boulardii* in childhood. *European Journal of Pediatrics, 168*, 253–265.

A. INTRODUCTION AND OVERVIEW

40. Langat, A. C., Ogutu, E., Kamenwa, R., & Simiyu, D. E. (2006). Prevalence of *Helicobacter pylori* in children less than three years of age in health facilities in Nairobi Province. *East African Medical Journal, 83,* 471–477.

41. Gotteland, M., Brunser, O., & Cruchet, S. (2006). Systematic review: Are probiotics useful in controlling gastric colonization by *Helicobacter pylori*? *Alimentary Pharmacology & Therapeutics, 23,* 1077–1086.

42. Cruchet, S., Obregon, M. C., Salazar, G., et al. (2003). Effect of the ingestion of a dietary product containing *Lactobacillus johnsonii* La1 on *Helicobacter pylori* colonization in children. *Nutrition, 19,* 716–721.

43. Gotteland, M., Andrews, M., Toledo, M., et al. (2008). Modulation of *Helicobacter pylori* colonization with cranberry juice and *Lactobacillus johnsonii* La1 in children. *Nutrition, 24,* 421–426.

44. Gotteland, M., Poliak, L., Cruchet, S., & Brunser, O. (2005). Effect of regular ingestion of *Saccharomyces boulardii* plus inulin or *Lactobacillus acidophilus* LB in children colonized by *Helicobacter pylori*. *Acta Paediatrica, 94,* 1747–1751.

45. Sakamoto, I., Igarashi, M., Kimura, K., et al. (2001). Suppressive effect of *Lactobacillus gasseri* OLL 2716 (LG21) on *Helicobacter pylori* infection in humans. *The Journal of Antimicrobial Chemotherapy, 47,* 709–710.

46. Sýkora, J., Valecková, K., Amlerová, J., et al. (2005). Effects of a specially designed fermented milk product containing probiotic *Lactobacillus casei* DN-114 001 and the eradication of *H. pylori* in children: A prospective randomized double-blind study. *Journal of Clinical Gastroenterology, 39,* 692–698.

47. Goldman, C. G., Barrado, D. A., Balcarce, N., et al. (2006). Effect of a probiotic food as an adjuvant to triple therapy for eradication of *Helicobacter pylori* infection in children. *Nutrition, 22,* 984–988.

48. Martin, C. R., & Walker, W. A. (2008). Probiotics: Role in pathophysiology and prevention in necrotizing enterocolitis. *Seminars in Perinatology, 32,* 127–137.

49. Hoyos, A. B. (1999). Reduced incidence of necrotizing enterocolitis associated with enteral administration of *Lactobacillus acidophilus* and *Bifidobacterium infantis* to neonates in an intensive care unit. *International Journal of Infectious Diseases, 3,* 197–202.

50. Dani, C., Biadaioli, R., Bertini, G., et al. (2002). Probiotics feeding in prevention of urinary tract infection, bacterial sepsis and necrotizing enterocolitis in preterm infants. A prospective double-blind study. *Biology of the Neonate, 82,* 103–108.

51. Bin-Nun, A., Bromiker, R., Wilschanski, M., et al. (2005). Oral probiotics prevent necrotizing enterocolitis in very low birth weight neonates. *The Journal of Pediatrics, 147,* 192–196.

52. Deshpande, G., Rao, S., & Patole, S. (2007). Probiotics for prevention of necrotising enterocolitis in preterm neonates with very low birthweight: A systematic review of randomised controlled trials. *Lancet, 369,* 1614–1620.

53. Lin, H. C., Su, B. H., Chen, A. C., et al. (2005). Oral probiotics reduce the incidence and severity of necrotizing enterocolitis in very low birth weight infants. *Pediatrics, 115,* 1–4.

54. Lin, H. C., Hsu, C. H., Chen, H. L., et al. (2008). Oral probiotics prevent necrotizing enterocolitis in very low birth weight preterm infants: A multicenter, randomized, controlled trial. *Pediatrics, 122,* 693–700.

55. Alfaleh, K., & Bassler, D. (2008). Probiotics for prevention of necrotizing enterocolitis in preterm infants CD005496. *Cochrane Database of Systematic Reviews, 23*(1).

56. McFarland, L. V. (2007). Meta-analysis of probiotics for the prevention of traveler's diarrhea. *Travel Medicine and Infectious Disease, 5,* 97–105.

57. Marteau, P. R., de Vrese, M., Cellier, C. J., & Schrezenmeir, J. (2001). Protection from gastrointestinal diseases with the use of probiotics. *The American Journal of Clinical Nutrition, 73*(Suppl. 2), 430S–436S.

58. Briand, V., Buffet, P., Genty, S., et al. (2006). Absence of efficacy of nonviable *Lactobacillus acidophilus* for the prevention of traveler's diarrhea: A randomized, double-blind, controlled study. *Clinical Infectious Diseases, 43,* 1170–1175.

59. Ericsson, C. D. (2005). Nonantimicrobial agents in the prevention and treatment of traveler's diarrhea. *Clinical Infectious Diseases, 41*(Suppl. 8), S557–S563.

60. Grüber, C., Wendt, M., Sulser, C., et al. (2007). Randomized, placebo-controlled trial of *Lactobacillus rhamnosus* GG as treatment of atopic dermatitis in infancy. *Allergy, 62,* 1270–1276.

61. Sepp, E., Julge, K., Mikelsaar, M., & Bjorksten, B. (2005). Intestinal microbiota and immunoglobulin E responses in 5-year-old Estonian children. *Clinical and Experimental Allergy, 35,* 1141–1146.

62. He, F., Ouwehand, A. C., Isolauri, E., et al. (2001). Comparison of mucosal adhesion and species identification of bifidobacteria isolated from healthy and allergic infants. *FEMS Immunology and Medical Microbiology, 30,* 43–47.

63. He, F., Morita, H., Ouwehand, A. C., et al. (2002). Stimulation of the secretion of pro-inflammatory cytokines by *Bifidobacterium* strains. *Microbiology and Immunology, 46,* 781–785.

64. Isolauri, E., Arvola, T., Sutas, Y., et al. (2000). Probiotics in the management of atopic eczema. *Clinical and Experimental Allergy, 30,* 1604–1610.

65. Kalliomaki, M., Salminen, S., Arvilommi, H., et al. (2001). Probiotics in primary prevention of atopic

disease: A randomized placebo-controlled trial. *Lancet, 357,* 1076–1079.

66. Rautava, S., Kalliomaki, M., & Isolauri, E. (2002). Probiotics during pregnancy and breast-feeding might confer immunomodulatory protection against atopic disease in the infant. *The Journal of Allergy and Clinical Immunology, 109,* 119–121.

67. Kalliomaki, M., Salminen, S., Poussa, T., & Isolauri, E. (2007). Probiotics during the first 7 years of life: A cumulative risk reduction of eczema in a randomized, placebo-controlled trial. *The Journal of Allergy and Clinical Immunology, 119,* 1019–1021.

68. Viljanen, M., Kuitunen, M., Haahtela, T., et al. (2005). Probiotic effects on faecal inflammatory markers and on faecal IgA in food allergic atopic eczema/dermatitis syndrome infants. *Pediatric Allergy and Immunology, 16,* 65–71.

69. Brouwer, M. L., Wolt-Plompen, S. A., Dubois, A. E., et al. (2006). No effects of probiotics on atopic dermatitis in infancy: A randomized placebo-controlled trial. *Clinical and Experimental Allergy, 36,* 899–906.

70. Cremonini, F., & Talley, N. J. (2005). Irritable bowel syndrome: Epidemiology, natural history, health care seeking and emerging risk factors. *Gastroenterology clinics of North America, 34,* 189–204.

71. Saito, Y. A., Cremonini, F., & Talley, N. J. (2004). Association of the 1438G/A and 102T/C polymorphism of the 5-HT2A receptor gene with irritable bowel syndrome 5-HT2A gene polymorphism in irritable bowel syndrome. *Journal of Clinical Gastroenterology, 38,* 561–566.

72. Spiller, R. C. (2007). Role of infection in irritable bowel syndrome. *Journal of Gastroenterology, 42*(Suppl. 17), 41–47.

73. O'Mahony, L., McCarthy, J., Kelly, P., et al. (2005). *Lactobacillus* and *Bifidobacterium* in irritable bowel syndrome: Symptom responses and relationship to cytokine profiles. *Gastroenterology, 128,* 541–551.

74. Hanson, L.Å., & Yolken, R. H. (1997). Probiotics, other nutritional factors, and intestinal microflora. *Nestlé Nutrition Workshop Series* (Vol. 42). Philadelphia: Nestec Ltd, Vevey/ Lippincot-Raven Publishers.

75. Rousseaux, C., Thuru, X., Gelot, A., et al. (2007). *Lactobacillus acidophilus* modulates intestinal pain and induces opioid and cannabinoid receptors. *Nature Medicine, 13,* 35–37.

76. Kajander, K., Krogius-Kurikka, L., Rinttilä, T., et al. (2007). Effects of multispecies probiotic supplementation on intestinal microbiota in irritable bowel syndrome. *Alimentary Pharmacology & Therapeutics, 26,* 463–473.

77. Kajander, K., Myllyluoma, E., Rajili -Stojanovi , M., et al. (2008). Clinical trial: Multispecies probiotic supplementation alleviates the symptoms of irritable bowel syndrome and stabilizes intestinal microbiota. *Alimentary Pharmacology & Therapeutics, 27,* 48–57.

78. Mow, W. S., & Abreu, M. T. (2004). Crohn's disease. In L. R. Johnson (Ed.), *Encyclopedia of gastroenterology: Vol. I* (pp. 509–520). San Diego: Academic Press.

79. Langmead, L., & Rampton, D. S. (2004). Colitis, ulcerative. In L. R. Johnson (Ed.), *Encyclopedia of gastroenterology: Vol. I* (pp. 385–399). San Diego: Elsevier/Academic Press.

80. Kozuch, P. L., & Hanauer, S. B. (2008). Treatment of inflammatory bowel disease: A review of medical therapy. *World Journal of Gastroenterology, 14,* 354–377.

81. Damaskos, D., & Kolios, G. (2008). Probiotics and prebiotics in inflammatory bowel disease: Microflora 'on the scope'. *British Journal of Clinical Pharmacology, 65,* 453–467.

82. Fedorak, R. N. (2008). Understanding why probiotic therapies can be effective in treating IBD. *Journal of Clinical Gastroenterology, 42*(Suppl 3 Pt 1), S111–S115.

83. Geier, M. S., Butler, R. N., & Howarth, G. S. (2007). Inflammatory bowel disease: Current insights into pathogenesis and new therapeutic options; probiotics, prebiotics and synbiotics. *International Journal of Food Microbiology, 115,* 1–11.

84. Rembacken, B. J., Snelling, A. M., Hawkey, P. M, et al. (1999). Non-pathogenic *Escherichia coli* versus mesalazine for the treatment of ulcerative colitis: A randomised trial. *Lancet, 354,* 635–639.

85. Henker, J., Müller, S., Laass, M. W., et al. (2008). Probiotic *Escherichia coli* Nissle 1917 (EcN) for successful remission maintenance of ulcerative colitis in children and adolescents: An open-label pilot study. *Zeitschrift Fur Gastroenterologie, 46,* 874–875.

86. Ewaschuk, J. B., Tejpar, Q. Z., Soo, I., et al. (2006). The role of antibiotic and probiotic therapies in current and future management of inflammatory bowel disease. *Current Gastroenterology Reports, 8,* 486–498.

87. Butterworth, A. D., Thomas, A. G., & Akobeng, A. K. (2008). Probiotics for induction of remission in Crohn's disease CD006634. *Cochrane Database of Systematic Reviews.*

88. Jonkers, D., & Stockbrügger, R. (2007). Probiotics in gastrointestinal and liver diseases. *Alimentary Pharmacology & Therapeutics, 26*(Suppl. 2), 133–148.

89. Geier, M. S., Butler, R. N., & Howarth, G. S. (2006). Probiotics, prebiotics and synbiotics: A role in chemoprevention for colorectal cancer? *Cancer Biology & Therapy, 5,* 1265–1269.

90. Fotiadis, C. I., Stoidis, C. N., Spyropoulos, B. G., & Zografos, E. D. (2008). Role of probiotics, prebiotics and synbiotics in chemoprevention for colorectal cancer. *World Journal of Gastroenterology, 14,* 6453–6457.

91. Capurso, G., Marignani, M., & Delle Fave, G. (2006). Probiotics and the incidence of colorectal cancer: When evidence is not evident. *Digestive and Liver Disease, 38*(Suppl. 2), S277–S282.

92. Lan, A., Lagadic-Gossmann, D., Lemaire, C., et al. (2007). Acidic extracellular pH shifts colorectal cancer cell death from apoptosis to necrosis upon exposure to propionate and acetate, major end-products of the human probiotic propionibacteria. *Apoptosis, 12,* 573–591.

93. de Vrese, M., Winkler, P., Rautenberg, P., et al. (2005). Effect of *Lactobacillus gasseri* PA 16/8, *Bifidobacterium longum* SP 07/3, *B. bifidum* MF 20/5 on common cold episodes: A double blind, randomized, controlled trial. *Clinical Nutrition, 24,* 481–491.

94. Pregliasco, F., Anselmi, G., Fonte, L., et al. (2008). A new chance of preventing winter diseases by the administration of symbiotic formulations. *Journal of Clinical Gastroenterology, 42*(Suppl. 3 Pt 2), S224–S233.

95. Naito, S., Koga, H., Yamaguchi, A., et al. (2008). Prevention of recurrence with epirubicin and *Lactobacillus casei* after transurethral resection of bladder cancer. *Journal D'urologie, 179,* 485–490.

96. Gibson, G. R., & Roberfroid, M. B. (1995). Dietary modulation of the human colonic microbiota: Introducing the concept of prebiotics. *The Journal of Nutrition, 125,* 1401–1412.

97. Piñeiro, M., Asp, N. G., Reid, G., et al. (2008). FAO Technical meeting on prebiotics. *Journal of Clinical Gastroenterology, 42*(Suppl. 3 Pt 2), S156–S159.

98. Singhal, A., Macfarlane, G., Macfarlane, S., et al. (2008). Dietary nucleotides and fecal microbiota in formula-fed infants: A randomized controlled trial. *The American Journal of Clinical Nutrition, 87,* 1785–1792.

99. Brück, W. M., Redgrave, M., Tuohy, K. M., et al. (2006). Effects of bovine alpha-lactalbumin and casein glycomacropeptide-enriched infant formulae on faecal microbiota in healthy term infants. *Journal of Pediatric Gastroenterology and Nutrition, 43,* 673–679.

100. Kunz, C., Rudloff, S., Baier, W., et al. (2000). Oligosaccharides in human milk: Structural, functional, and metabolic aspects. *Annual Review of Nutrition, 20,* 699–722.

101. Miller, J. B. (1999). Human milk oligosaccharides: 130 reasons to breast feed. *The British Journal of Nutrition, 82,* 333–335.

102. German, J. B., Freeman, S. L., Lebrilla, C. B., & Mills, D. A. (2008). Human milk oligosaccharides: Evolution, structures and bioselectivity as substrates for intestinal bacteria. *Nestle Nutrition Workshop Series. Paediatric Programme, 62,* 205–218.

103. Morrow, A. L., Ruiz-Palacios, G. M., Jiang, X., & Newburg, D. S. (2005). Human-milk glycans that inhibit pathogen binding protect breast-feeding infants against infectious diarrhea. *The Journal of Nutrition, 135,* 1304–1307.

104. Vijn, I., & Smeekens, S. (1999). Fructan: More than a reserve carbohydrate? *Plant Physiology, 120,* 351–360.

105. Kolida, S., & Gibson, G. R. (2007). Prebiotic capacity of inulin-type fructans. *The Journal of Nutrition, 137,* 2503S–2506S.

106. Fanaro, S., Boehm, G., Garssen, J., et al. (2005). Galacto-oligosaccharides and long-chain fructo-oligosaccharides as prebiotics in infant formulas: A review. *Acta Paediatrica Supplement, 94,* 22–26.

107. Archer, B. J., Johnson, S. K., Devereux, H. M., & Baxter, A. L. (2004). Effect of fat replacement by inulin or lupin-kernel fibre on sausage patty acceptability, post-meal perceptions of satiety and food intake in men. *The British Journal of Nutrition, 91,* 591–599.

108. Servin, A. L. (2004). Antagonistic activities of lactobacilli and bifidobacteria against microbial pathogens. *FEMS Microbiology Reviews, 28,* 405–440.

109. Duggan, C., Penny, M. E., Hibberd, P., et al. (2003). Oligofructose-supplemented infant cereal: Two randomized, blinded, community-based trials in Peruvian infants. *The American Journal of Clinical Nutrition, 77,* 937–942.

110. Mason, J. B., & Kim, Y. (1999). Nutritional strategies in the prevention of colorectal cancer. *Current Gastroenterology Reports, 1,* 341–353.

111. Reddy, B. S., Hamid, R., & Rao, C. V. (1997). Effect of dietary oligofructose and inulin on colonic preneoplastic aberrant crypt foci inhibition. *Carcinogenesis, 18,* 1371–1374.

112. McBain, A. J., & MacFarlane, G. T. (2001). Modulation of genotoxic enzyme activities by non-digestible oligosaccharide metabolism in *in-vitro* human gut bacterial ecosystems. *Journal of Medical Microbiology, 50,* 833–842.

113. Chonan, O., Takahashi, R., & Watanuki, M. (2001). Role of activity of gastrointestinal microflora in absorption of calcium and magnesium in rats fed beta1-4 linked galactooligosaccharides. *Bioscience, Biotechnology, and Biochemistry, 65,* 1872–1875.

114. Ohta, A., Motohashi, Y., Sakai, K., et al. (1998). Dietary fructooligosaccharides increase calcium absorption and levels of mucosal calbindin-D9k in the large intestine of gastrectomized rats. *Scandinavian Journal of Gastroenterology, 33,* 1062–1068.

115. Scholz-Ahrens, K. E., Schaafsma, G., van den Heuvel, E. G., & Schrezenmeir, J. (2001). Effects of prebiotics on mineral metabolism. *The American Journal of Clinical Nutrition, 73*(Suppl. 2), 459S–464S.

116. Holloway, L., Moynihan, S., Abrams, S. A., et al. (2007). Effects of oligofructose-enriched inulin on intestinal absorption of calcium and magnesium and bone turnover markers in postmenopausal women. *The British Journal of Nutrition, 97,* 365–372.

117. Griffin, I. J., Davila, P. M., & Abrams, S. A. (2002). Non-digestible oligosaccharides and calcium absorption in girls with adequate calcium intakes. *The British Journal of Nutrition, 87*(Suppl. 2), S187–S191.

118. Abrams, S. A., Griffin, I. J., Hawthorne, K. M., & Ellis, K. J. (2007). Effect of prebiotic supplementation and calcium intake on body mass index. *The Journal of Pediatrics, 151,* 293–298.

119. Pereira, I., & Gibson, G. R. (2002). Effects of consumption of probiotics and prebiotics on serum lipid levels in humans. *Critical Reviews in Biochemistry and Molecular Biology, 37,* 259–281.

120. Almirall, M., Francesch, M., Perez-Vendrell, A. M, et al. (1995). The differences in intestinal viscosity produced by barley and beta-glucanase alter digesta enzyme activities and ileal nutrient digestibilities more in broiler chicks than in cocks. *The Journal of Nutrition, 125,* 947–955.

121. Delzenne, N. M., Daubioul, C., Neyrinck, A., et al. (2002). Inulin and oligofructose modulate lipid metabolism in animals: Review of biochemical events and future prospects. *The British Journal of Nutrition, 87*(Suppl. 2), S255–S259.

122. Demigné, C., Morand, C., Levrat, M. A., et al. (1995). Effect of propionate on fatty acid and cholesterol synthesis and on acetate metabolism in isolated rat hepatocytes. *The British Journal of Nutrition, 74,* 209–219.

123. Cani, P. D., Dewever, C., & Delzenne, N. M. (2004). Inulin-type fructans modulate gastrointestinal peptides involved in appetite regulation (glucagon-like peptide-1 and ghrelin) in rats. *The British Journal of Nutrition, 92,* 521–526.

124. Cani, P. D., Hoste, S., Guiot, Y., & Delzenne, N. M. (2007). Dietary non-digestible carbohydrates promote L-cell differentiation in the proximal colon of rats. *The British Journal of Nutrition, 98,* 32–37.

125. Cani, P. D., Neyrinck, A. M., Maton, N., & Delzenne, N. M. (2005). Oligofructose promotes satiety in rats fed a high-fat diet: Involvement of glucagon-like Peptide-1. *Obesity Research, 13,* 1000–1007.

126. Woodmansey, E. J., McMurdo, M. E., Macfarlane, G. T., & Macfarlane, S. (2004). Comparison of compositions and metabolic activities of fecal microbiotas in young adults and in antibiotic-treated and non-antibiotic-treated elderly subjects. *Applied and Environmental Microbiology, 70,* 6113–6122.

127. Bouhnik, Y., Attar, A., Joly, F. A., et al. (2004). Lactulose ingestion increases faecal bifidobacterial counts: A randomised double-blind study in healthy humans. *European Journal of Clinical Nutrition, 58,* 462–466.

128. Rajala, S. A., Salminen, S. J., Seppänen, J. H., & Vapaatalo, H. (1988). Treatment of chronic constipation with lactitol sweetened yoghurt supplemented with guar gum and wheat bran in elderly hospital patients. *Comprehensive Gerontology A, 2,* 83–86.

129. Teuri, U., & Korpela, R. (1998). Galacto-oligosaccharides relieve constipation in elderly people. *Annals of Nutrition & Metabolism, 42,* 319–327.

130. Kleesen, B., Sykura, B., Zunft, H.-J., & Blaut, M. (1997). Effects of inulin and lactose on fecal microflora, microbial activity and bowel habit in elderly constipated persons. *The American Journal of Clinical Nutrition, 65,* 1397–1402.

131. Mihatsch, W. A., Hoegel, J., & Pohlandt, F. (2006). Prebiotic oligosaccharides reduce stool viscosity and accelerate gastrointestinal transport in preterm infants. *Acta Paediatrica, 95,* 843–848.

132. Bongers, M. E., de Lorijn, F., Reitsma, J. B., et al. (2007). The clinical effect of a new infant formula in term infants with constipation: A double-blind, randomized cross-over trial. *Nutrition Journal, 11*(6), 8.

A. INTRODUCTION AND OVERVIEW

PREBIOTICS IN HEALTH PROMOTION

7

Pre- and Probiotics in Liver Health and Function

Mirjam Looijer-van Langen and Karen Madsen

Division of Gastroenterology, Department of Medicine, University of Alberta, Edmonton, AB, Canada

1. STRUCTURE AND FUNCTION OF THE LIVER

The liver is the largest solid organ in the body and is located in the right upper quadrant of the abdomen, just below the diaphragm. The weight ranges from approximately 1300 grams in females to 1800 grams in males, and constitutes approximately 1.8–3.1% of total bodyweight. The liver has a typical wedge-shape, with its tip pointing to the spleen and the base against the right abdominal wall. The liver reaches from the fifth intercostal space in the midclavicular line down to the right costal margin. Two lobes form the liver, a large right lobe and smaller left lobe. The two lobes are separated by the falciform ligament, which also connects the liver to the diaphragm and anterior abdominal wall. In the centre of the inferior liver surface the hilus is located, which consists of the portal vein, hepatic artery, common hepatic duct, lymph vessels and hepatic nerve plexus. The porta hepatica is where veins and arteries enter the liver and bile canaliculi leave the liver. These structures are all held together by the perivascular fibrous capsule. Twenty-five percent of the blood supply to the liver comes from the hepatic artery and 75% comes from the portal vein system. The oxygen supply comes for 50% from the arterial blood supply and for 50% from the relatively oxygen deprived portal vein system.

The liver has numerous roles, including the removal and excretion of drugs, body wastes, and hormones; synthesis of plasma proteins; production of bile; removal of bilirubin; storage of vitamins, minerals, and sugars; processing of nutrients absorbed from the digestive tract; production of immune factors; and removal of bacteria (Table 7.1). Hepatocytes make up the bulk of the organ and are arranged in plates that radiate from each portal triad towards adjacent central veins. All hepatocytes appear to perform the same physiological and metabolic functions, although there is some functional heterogeneity within the various lobes due to the presence of nutrient and hormonal gradients within the liver. Sinusoidal lining cells comprise at least four distinct cellular populations: endothelial cells, Kupffer cells, stellate (perisinusoidal) cells,

TABLE 7.1   Functions of the liver

Function	Compound
Hemostasis	Vitamins (fat-soluble: A, D, E, K) Proteins Fat and cholesterol Hormones
Synthesis	Proteins including the clotting factors Bile acids Heparin Somatomedins Estrogen Angiotensinogen Cholesterol Acute phase proteins
Storage	Vitamins Glycogen Cholesterol Iron, copper Fats
Excretion	Cholesterol, bile acids, phospholipids Bilirubin Drugs Poisons including heavy metals Hormones
Filtration	Toxins Nutrients including amino acids, sugars, and fats Bilirubin, bile acids IgA Drugs Dead or damaged cells in circulatory system
Immune	Excretes IgA into lumen of intestinal tract Kupffer cells

and pit cells. Endothelial cells are flattened elongated sinusoidal cells. Numerous cytoplasmic projections and clustered fenestrae are present, and function as a filtration barrier. A main function of the endothelial cell is filtration of various macromolecules from the sinusoidal blood, thus enabling substances such as glycoproteins and polysaccharides direct contact with hepatocytes, but excluding and protecting the liver from larger cellular components. Kupffer cells are tissue macrophages that form an important part of the body's reticuloendothelial system. The major functions of Kupffer cells include phagocytosis of foreign particles, removal of endotoxins and other toxic substances, and modulation of the immune response through the release of mediators. Stellate cells (also called perisinusoidal fat-storing or Ito cells) store vitamin A, and transform into fibroblasts in response to hepatic injury, thus contributing to hepatic fibrosis. Pit cells (also called liver-associated lymphocytes and large granulae lymphocytes) are nonparenchymal T cells distributed within the sinusoidal lumen in loose contact with the endothelial or Kupffer cells. These cells function as natural killer cells.

2. GUT-LIVER AXIS

The ability of the intestinal tract to act as a barrier between the massive load of microbes in the gut lumen and the closely regulated internal milieu is absolutely essential for human health. In our evolution as vertebrates we have developed elegant mechanisms to co-exist with bacteria. Colonization of the intestine with bacteria begins during the birth process, and within several months, a relatively stable bacterial population resides in our intestines. Intestinal microflora produce numerous compounds (i.e. ammonia, ethanol, acetaldehyde, phenols, benzodiazepines) which affect and are metabolized by the liver. In addition, microbial cellular structures (lipopolysaccharide, DNA, lipoteichoic acid) and secreted bioactive factors influence the host physiology and immune system through interactions with both the innate and the adaptive immune system. A failure of the intestinal tract to maintain gut microbes within the lumen appears to have a key role in the pathogenesis of various liver diseases and sepsis. There is some evidence that bacterial translocation and resultant endotoxemia induce an inflammatory response that triggers the cachexia syndrome in liver disease. In addition, endoscopy studies have demonstrated mucosal inflammation and altered gut microflora in patients with liver disease and portal hypertension, which in and of themselves would then contribute to systemic inflammation in the liver. Several strains of probiotics have demonstrated effectiveness in modulating gut permeability and cytokine secretion, thus the rationale for using these strains to potentially treat or prevent liver disease is an attractive prospect. Altering gut microflora with non-invasive and immunomodulatory probiotic organisms has been proposed as adjunctive therapy to reduce the level of bacterial translocation and prevent the onset of sepsis and liver disease. This chapter focuses on the latest evidence on the use of pre- and probiotics in liver disease, including non-alcoholic fatty liver disease, alcoholic liver disease, cirrhosis, spontaneous bacterial peritonitis, hepatic encephalopathy, and liver transplantation and resection.

3. PROBIOTIC EFFECTS IN EXPERIMENTAL ANIMAL MODELS OF LIVER INJURY

Different experimental animal liver disease models have been used to study the efficacy of pro- and prebiotics. These models are especially useful to identify and provide insight into possible mechanisms of pro- and prebiotics in the treatment and/or prevention of liver disease.

3.1. Animal Models of Acute Liver Injury

Numerous studies have shown probiotic treatment to reduce bacterial translocation and decrease hepatocellular damage in acute liver injury animal models (Table 7.2). One of the most commonly used models of acute liver injury involves the injection of D-galactosamine (D-GalN) with or without lipopolysaccharide (LPS) as D-galactosamine (D-GalN) increases the susceptibility of mice to LPS-induced injury by impairing liver metabolism [1]. Rectal administration of probiotic bacteria (*L. reuteri*, *L. rhamnosus*, *L. plantarum*, *L. fermentum*) in combination with arginine in the D-GalN model resulted in decreased hepatic inflammatory cell infiltration and hepatocellular necrosis. This was associated with decreased bacterial translocation in the probiotic treated animals. In this study, *L. plantarum* clearly showed superior results compared to the other probiotic strains [2].

In a second study in this model, the beneficial effects of *L. plantarum* with arginine were confirmed in that liver enzymes and bilirubin levels were decreased [3]. In another study, pre-treatment with oral VSL#3 (*Bifidobacterium longum*, *Bifidobacterium breve*, *Bifidobacterium infantis*, *Lactobacillus casei*, *Lactobacillus plantarum*, *Lactobacillus acidophilus*, *Lactobacillus delbrueckii* subsp. *Bulgaricus*, *Streptococcus salivarius* subsp. *Thermophilus*) prevented the breakdown in intestinal barrier function, reduced bacterial translocation, and significantly attenuated liver injury in an LPS/GalN liver injury model through a PPAR?-dependent mechanism [4]. Lactulose, a prebiotic, and *L. plantarum* prevented liver injury and bacterial translocation in a study by Kasravi et al. [5]. In addition, a remarkable decrease in enterobacteriaceae counts in the intestine was observed in lactobacilli treated rats [5].

A difference in effect of bifidobacteria strains compared to lactobacilli has been described. One study using the strains *B. animalis*, *L. acidophilus*, *L. rhamnosus* and *L. plantarum* demonstrated that while the lactobacilli strains reduced bacterial translocation and hepatocellular damage, *B. animalis* treatment actually increased bacterial translocation to the mesenteric lymph nodes and did not prevent hepatocellular damage [6]. A similar failure of a *Bifidobacterium* strain was seen in a study

TABLE 7.2   Pre- and probiotics in experimental animal models of liver disease

Study reference	Animal model	Pro/prebiotics and dose	Treatment duration (days) (prior or following)	Study outcome
Adawi 1997 [2]	D-galactosamine	L. reuteri, L. rhamnosus, L. plantarum, L. fermentum (± 2% arginine); 3×10^9 cfu/day	8 prior	↓ BT and translocated bacteria. ↓ liver enzymes, bilirubin, necrosis and inflammatory cell infiltration with L. plantarum.
Adawi 1998 [3]	D-galactosamine	L. plantarum+ arginine; 3×10^9 cfu/day	8 prior	↓ liver enzymes and bilirubin.
Adawi 2001 [6]	D-galactosamine	B. animalis, L. acidophilus, L. rhamnosus, L. rhamnosus, L. plantarum; 3×10^9 cfu/day	8 prior	Lactobacilli reduced BT and hepatocellular damage; B. animalis increased BT to MLN.
Kasravi 1997 [5]	D-galactosamine	L. reuteri, L. plantarum, lactulose; $2.5–5 \times 10^9$ cfu/day	8 prior	Lactulose decreased liver injury and BT; Lactobacillus (+ neomycin) moderately decreased liver injury and BT.
Osman 2007 [7]	D-galactosamine	L. plantarum, B. infantis (6×10^8 cfu/day) ± blueberry powder	8 prior	Decreased ALT, bilirubin, TNF-α, MPO and acetic acid, increased glutathione values; decreased liver IL-1β, BT (except B. infantis group).
Ewaschuk 2007 [4]	D-galactosamine + LPS sepsis	VSL#3; 2.8×10^8 cfu/day	7 prior	Prevention of breakdown in intestinal barrier function, reduced BT and attenuated liver injury.
Neyrinck 2004 [10]	Liver injury after endotoxic shock and sepsis	FOS (10 g/100 g)	21 prior	Decreased ALT, histologic liver damage, increased numbers of large phagocytic Kupffer cells, improved LPS clearance.
Wiest 2003 [8]	Portal hypertension	Lactobacillus; 8×10^9 cfu/day	9 prior	No changes in BT or bacterial flora compared to placebo.
Marotta 2005 [9]	Alcohol pancreatitis related liver damage	L. acidophilus, L. helveticus, Bifidobacterium	21 following	Decreased ALT, AST, endotoxin levels, improved histological steatosis score.
Xing 2005 [11]	Ischemia reperfusion liver injury	B. catenulatum, L. fermentum or both (1.2×10^9 cfu/day)	8 prior	Decreased endotoxemia, ALT, TNF-α, MDA; ameliorated liver histology and intestinal mucosal ultrastructure, reduced BT, increased lactobacilli and bifidobacteria.

BT, bacterial translocation; MLN, mesenteric lymph nodes; ALT, alanine transaminase; MPO, myeloperoxidase; LPS, lipopolysaccharide; AST, aspartate aminotransferase; MDA, malondialdehyde; TNF, tumor necrosis factor; FOS, fructo-oligosaccharide.

by Osman et al. [7]. In this study, *Lactobacillus plantarum* and *Bifidobacterium infantis* administration with or without added blueberry powder were investigated. While a significant decrease was seen in all treated groups for bilirubin, liver TNF-α, myeloperoxidase activity, and caecal acetic acid content, only *L. plantarum* decreased liver IL-1β secretion and bacterial translocation to the liver and lymph nodes [7]. However, *Lactobacillus acidophilus* or *Lactobacillus* GG containing yogurt did not influence bacterial translocation or intestinal flora in portal vein ligated rats, which is a model of prehepatic portal hypertension [8].

A mixture of *Lactobacillus acidophilus*, *Lactobacillus helveticus* and bifidobacteria decreased ALT, AST, endotoxin levels and histological steatosis score in an experimental acute alcohol pancreatitis-related rat model [9]. Prebiotic treatment has also shown some benefit in acute injury models. Rats treated with fructo-oligosaccharides showed decreased ALT levels compared to controls, less histological liver damage, and increased numbers of large phagocytic Kupffer cells with improved capability of TNF-α clearance [10]. The effects of *Lactobacillus and Bifidobacterium* on ischemia-reperfusion liver injury have also been investigated. Treatment with either *B. catenulatum* or *L. fermentum* resulted in decreased endotoxemia and improved liver function and structure. Again, this was associated with reduced bacterial translocation [11].

3.2. Summary

Despite some contradictory results, animal studies predominantly show a positive effect of pro- and prebiotic treatment in acute liver injury models. Improvement of bacterial translocation, decreased liver enzymes and pro-inflammatory cytokines and decreased hepatocellular damage have been observed in several studies of acute liver injury. There is a clear strain-dependence to the beneficial effects. Although results from animal studies cannot be directly translated to the human condition, they do help to unravel the possible mechanisms of pro- and prebiotics, and clearly point to an effect on gut barrier function to be important in the ability of probiotics and prebiotics to ameliorate liver injury.

4. NON-ALCOHOLIC AND ALCOHOLIC FATTY LIVER DISEASE AND CIRRHOSIS

Non-alcoholic fatty liver disease (NAFLD) represents a spectrum of alterations in liver histology characterized by predominantly macrovesicular steatosis that by definition are not caused by the over-consumption of alcohol [12, 13]. NAFLD comprises a group of liver diseases including simple fatty liver (steatosis), non-alcoholic steatohepatitis (NASH) and cirrhosis (end-stage irreversible liver disease with scarring) [12, 14]. All of these refer to a state of accumulation of fat in the liver cells. Liver steatosis is often associated with a number of conditions including obesity, malnutrition, intestinal malabsorption, insulin resistance, metabolic syndrome and endocrine disease. It can also develop in response to hepatotoxic drugs, alcohol, accumulation of transition metals and hepatitis C infection [15, 16]. NASH represents an advanced stage of fatty liver disease and is associated with different degrees of inflammation and scarring of the liver. A clear link between bacterial overgrowth and liver damage in NAFLD and NASH has been established [17]. These conditions may progress to cirrhosis. No established treatment exists for this potentially serious disorder. Current management of NAFLD and NASH is largely conservative and includes diet regimen, aerobic exercise, and interventions towards the associated metabolic abnormalities. The primary concern is to prevent progression to end-stage liver cirrhosis and liver failure. Among the most promising medications are weight reducing drugs (sibutramin, orlistat), insulin sensitizers (metformin, rosiglitazone), lipid lowering agents (clofibrate, probucol, gemfibrozil), antioxidants, and cytoprotective agents (acetylcysteine, vitamin E, ursodeoxycholate). However, to date no definitive therapy or treatment has been established [18].

Alcoholic liver disease (ALD) is the major cause of liver disease in western countries. Histopathologically, ALD is very similar to NAFLD. Pathogenic mechanisms are also similar (i.e. increased endogenous production of ethanol, direct activation of inflammatory cytokines in luminal cells and non-parenchymal liver cells). Causes and most important treatment (abstinence) are obviously different.

Liver cirrhosis is a frequent phenomenon and final consequence of various chronic liver diseases such as alcohol abuse, autoimmune hepatitis, hepatitis B and C virus and hemochromatosis. Liver cirrhosis is characterized by replacement of liver tissue by fibrous scar tissue and regenerative nodules, which leads to progressive loss of liver function [19–22].

4.1. Probiotic Effects in Animal Models of Chronic Liver Disease

The intestinal microflora is an important factor in the pathogenesis of fatty liver disease. Treatments aimed at reducing bacterial overgrowth inhibit the development of steatohepatitis [23–25]. Several studies have examined the ability of probiotics to attenuate liver disease in various chronic models (Table 7.3). A high fat diet has been shown to deplete hepatic natural killer T cell (NKT) function leading to the development of insulin resistance and hepatic steatosis. Probiotics (VSL#3) were shown to improve hepatic steatosis in mice on a high fat diet by preventing hepatic natural killer cell depletion [26]. In a controlled study in Ob/ob mice, a model of NAFLD, treatment with VSL#3 improved liver histology,

reduced hepatic total fatty acid content, and decreased serum ALT levels. Furthermore, TNF-α activity was significantly reduced in VSL#3 treated mice, as well as insulin resistance [27]. The hypothesis that probiotic VSL#3 ameliorates the methionin-choline-deficient (MCD) diet-induced mouse model of NASH was tested by Velayudham et al. [28]. Although VSL#3 failed to prevent MCD-induced liver steatosis or inflammation, VSL#3 did reduce MCD diet-induced liver fibrosis resulting in diminished accumulation of collage and α-smooth muscle actin [28]. In an alcohol-induced injury model, Nanji et al. [24] demonstrated that rats fed *Lactobacillus* GG in addition to ethanol had a lower pathology score and reduced plasma endotoxin levels. In models using carbon tetrachloride (CCl4) to induce hepatic fibrosis, studies have shown strains of *Lactobacillus* (*L. brevis*, *L. acidophilus*) and *Bifidobacterium* (*B. longum*) to have a hepatoprotective effect by inhibiting β-glucoronidase productivity [29, 30]. β-glucuronidase is an enzyme that transforms endogenous and exogenous compounds, such as benzopyrene glucuronides to toxic compounds. *Lactobacillus* GG, however, failed to prevent bacterial translocation [31]. A combination of antioxidants with *Lactobacillus johnsonii* also showed beneficial effects in this model in that the treatment suppressed bacterial translocation to mesenteric lymph nodes, reduced ileal and cecal counts of enterobacteria and enterococci, and reduced intestinal malondialdehyde levels and endotoxemia [32].

Nicaise et al. [33] studied the effects of a wild-type *L. plantarum* strain and a genetically engineered ammonia hyperconsuming strain of *L. plantarum* on hyperammonia in two different rodent models of liver disease (CCl4 model of chronic liver insufficiency, and TCA-induced acute liver injury). Ammonia levels were decreased in the chronic liver insufficiency model by *Lactobacillus* administration. In the TCA model, probiotics significantly increased survival and decreased blood and fecal ammonia levels. The genetically engineered *Lactobacillus* strain showed a

TABLE 7.3 Pre- and probiotics in animal models of cirrhosis

Reference	Animal model	Pro/prebiotics and dose	Treatment duration	Study outcome
Ma 2008 [26]	High fat induced hepatic steatosis rat model	VSL#3, 1.5×10^9 cfu/day	4 weeks	Protection against NKT cell depletion, insulin resistance and hepatic steatosis, reduced inflammatory signaling.
Liu 2003 [27]	Ob/ob mice NAFLD model	VSL#3, 1.5×10^9 cfu/day	4 weeks	Slightly improved liver histology, reduced hepatic total fatty acid content, decreased ALT.
Velayudham 2009 [28]	MCD diet induced NASH mouse model	VSL#3	10 weeks	Improvement of liver fibrosis; no protection against inflammation and steatosis formation.
Nanji 1994 [24]	Alcoholic induced liver injury	*L.* GG (10^{10} cfu/day)	4 weeks	Reduced pathology score and lower endotoxin levels.
Han 2004 [29]	CCl4	*L. brevis, L. acidophilus, B. longum* (0.5–2 gram/kg bwt)	4 weeks	Inhibition of B-glucuronidase production, reduced AST and ALT.
Bauer 2002 [31]	CCl4	*L.* GG ($1–2 \times 10^9$ cfu/day) ± norfloxacin	8–10 days	Failure to prevent BT and ascitic fluid infection, in spite of successful intestinal colonization.
Nicaise 2008 [33]	TCA & CCl4	*L. plantarum*, wildtype or hyperammonia consuming genetically engineered strain $10^{7–9}$ cfu/day (TCA) and 10^{10} cfu/day (CCl4)	3–4 days	Increased survival, reduced astrocyte swelling, decreased blood and fecal ammonia levels in both models with probiotics.
Chiva 2002 [32]	CCl4 cirrhosis	*L. johnsonii*, 10^9 cfu/day	10 days	Decreased enterobacteria and enterococci, BT, MDA levels and endotoxemia.

NKT, natural killer T cell; ALT, alanine transaminase; AST, aspartate transaminase; BT, bacterial translocation; MDA, malondialdehyde; NAFLD, non-alcoholic fatty liver disease; MCD, methionine choline deficient; CCL4, carbon tetrachloride; TCA, tricarboxylic acid.

beneficial effect at a lower dose than the wild-type strain [33].

4.2. Probiotic Effects in Human Studies

The effects of VSL#3 on hepatic steatosis were evaluated in an open-labeled pilot trial in four adult patients [34]. Patients received VSL#3 for 4 months at which time liver fat was measured by proton magnetic resonance spectroscopy. Unexpectedly, all four subjects experienced a significant increase in liver fat at the end of 4 months, which failed to support the hypothesis that probiotics would reduce hepatic steatosis in humans [34]. In another study, 66 adult males admitted to a psychiatric hospital with a diagnosis of alcoholic psychosis were enrolled in a prospective RCT to study the effects of probiotics on bowel flora and alcohol-induced liver injury [35]. Patients were randomized to receive 5 days of *B. bifidum* and *L. plantarum* versus standard therapy (abstinence plus vitamins). After 5 days of probiotic therapy alcoholic patients had significantly increased numbers of both bifidobacteria and lactobacilli compared to the standard treated group along with lower AST and ALT scores [35]. A study performed by Liu et al. [36] with Synbiotic 2000 or prebiotics alone showed that after 1 month of therapy the Child-Pugh classification improved in 47% of synbiotic treated patients compared to 8% of patients receiving placebo and 29% of patients receiving prebiotics. Improved outcome measures were serum albumin, bilirubin and prothrombin time [36] (Table 7.4).

Another randomized controlled study administered *Escherichia coli* Nissle bacteria to cirrhotic patients for 42 days [37]. A control group received a sucrose placebo capsule. An improvement of Child-Pugh score (resulting from decrease in bilirubin level and improvement of ascites and endotoxemia) and a trend toward lower endotoxin levels was observed, although the results were not statistically significant. In the *E. coli* Nissle treated group an increase of colonization with *Lactobacillus* spp. and *Bifidobacterium* spp. from 33 to 50% occurred, whereas in the placebo treated group no important changes in the microbiological composition were found [37]. The effect of probiotic treatment on neutrophil function and cytokine responses in patients with compensated alcoholic cirrhosis was investigated by Stadlbauer et al. [38]. Twelve patients received *Lactobacillus casei* three times daily for 4 weeks. Data were compared to healthy patients and cirrhotic patients not receiving probiotics. Baseline neutrophil phagocytic capacity in patients was significantly lower compared to healthy controls, but normalized at the end of the study, whereas non-treated patients didn't improve.

IL-10 secretion, endotoxin-stimulated levels of sTNFR1 and 2 were significantly lower at the end of the study as was TLR4 expression [38]. A third study investigated the effect of a combination of probiotics (*L. acidophilus*, *B. bifidus*, *L. rhamnosus*, *L. plantarum*, *L. salivarius*, *L. bulgaricus*, *L. lactis*, *L. casei*, *B. breve*) and a prebiotic (fructo-oligosaccharide) in HCV-related chronic hepatitis, alcoholic cirrhosis and NASH patients [39]. Liver transaminases, total proteins, albumin, λ-globulins, cytokines, malondialdehyde and 4-hydroxinonenal were measured. Three months of treatment did not affect any of the parameters in HCV-related chronic hepatitis patients. NASH patients showed a decrease in ALT and λ-GT at the end of treatment. In alcoholic cirrhosis patients a significant improvement of liver damage and liver function tests was observed [39]. Another study investigated the effects of VSL#3 in NAFLD and alcoholic cirrhotic patients compared to HCV positive patients with chronic hepatitis with or without liver cirrhosis. A significant improvement in plasma levels of MDA and 4-HNE were found in both NAFLD and alcoholic liver cirrhosis patients. Cytokine levels (IL-6, IL-10 and TNF-α) only improved in the alcoholic liver cirrhosis patients. No such improvements were seen in the HCV patients. However, routine liver damage tests and plasma S-NO levels were improved in all patients at the end of treatment [40]. A small study studied the effects of VSL#3 treatment in compensated or early decompensated cirrhosis patients [41]. Decreased plasma endotoxin levels, increased TNF-α serum levels, and a significant reduction in plasma aldosterone was observed. No changes in the hepatic venous pressure gradient or intestinal permeability were found.

Summary

In both animal and human studies pro- and prebiotic treatment ameliorated and prevented liver damage in NAFLD. Only one small study

TABLE 7.4 Pre- and probiotics in human studies of cirrhosis

Study reference	Study design	Pro/prebiotics and dose	Treatment duration	Study outcome
Solga 2008 [34]	Steatosis pts ($n = 4$)	VSL#3	4 months	↑ in liver fat.
Kirpich 2008 [35]	ALD, open-labeled, randomized prospective trial ($n = 66$)	*B. bifidum* (0.9×10^8 cfu/day and *L. plantarum* (0.9×10^9 cfu/day)	5 days	↑ fecal bifidobacteria and lactobacilli, ↓ AST and ALT.
Liu 2004 [36]	Cirrhosis with MHE ($n = 97$)	2.5 g each of beta glucan, inulin, pectin, resistant starch ± freeze-dried *P. pentosaceus, L. mesenteroides, L. paracasei, L. plantarum* (10^{10} cfu/day each)	30 days	↑ fecal content of lactobacilli, ↓ ammonia levels, reversal of MHE, ↓ in endotoxemia, improved Child-Pugh score; synbiotics more beneficial.
Lata 2007 [37]	Cirrhosis ($n = 39$)	*E. coli* Nissle 2.5–25×10^9 cfu/day	42 days	↓ endotoxemia, improvement of Child-Pugh score.
Stadlbauer 2008 [38]	Compensated alcoholic cirrhosis ($n = 32$)	*Lactobacillus casei* shirota (2×10^{10}/day)	4 weeks	Normalization of neutrophil phagocytic capacity, endotoxin stimulated levels of sTNFR1,2 and IL-10 decreased. TLR4 expression normalized.
Loguercio 2002 [39]	HCV-related chronic hepatitis, alcoholic cirrhosis, NASH ($n = 32$)	*L. acidophilus, bifidus, rhamnosus, plantarum, salivarius, bulgaricus, lactis, casei, breve*, FOS	3 months	NASH: improvement ALT and γ-GT; alcoholic cirrhosis: improvement of liver damage, function tests; HCV pts no improvements.
Loguercio 2005 [40]	NAFLD, alcoholic liver cirrhosis, chronic hepatitis, HCV related cirrhosis ($n = 78$)	VSL#3, 450 billion (2×2/die)	3 months	↓ ALT, AST, S-NO levels; NAFLD and AC improved levels of MDA and 4-HNE; TNF-α, IL-6 and IL-10 reduction in AC group.
Tandon 2009 [41]	Compensated or very early decompensated cirrhosis ($n = 8$)	VSL#3 (1.8×10^{10}) twice daily	2 months	↓ plasma endotoxin levels, ↑TNF-α serum levels, ↓ in plasma aldosteron. No change in HVPG or intestinal permeability.

AST, aspartate transaminase; ALT, alanine transaminase; MHE, minimal hepatic encephalopathy; TLR, toll-like receptor; NASH, non-alcoholic steato-hepatitis; γ-GT, gamma-glutamyl transaminase; HCV, hepatitis C virus; S-NO, S-nitrosothiols; NAFLD, non-alcoholic fatty liver disease; AC, alcoholic cirrhosis; MDA, malondialdehyde; 4-HNE, 4-hydroxynonenal; ALD, alcoholic liver disease; FOS, fructo-oligosaccharide; HVPG, hepatic venous pressure gradient.

showed an increase in liver fat. The majority of studies observed reduced hepatic steatosis formation, reduced pathology scores, lowered endotoxin levels, decreased liver enzymes, decreased ammonia levels and improved Child-Pugh score. Interestingly there was no improvement in hepatitis C patients after probiotic treatment and in more advanced disease pro- and prebiotics were not able to ameliorate disease. This indicates that administration will probably be mostly useful in preventing progression of disease more than improving end-stage liver disease.

4.3. Hepatic Encephalopathy

Hepatic encephalopathy (HE) is a common and serious complication of chronic liver disease which may substantially impair daily functioning and quality of life in patients [42–44]. Minimal HE (MHE) is a term that describes patients with chronic liver disease who have no clinical symptoms of brain dysfunction, but do perform worse on psychometric tests compared to healthy controls [44–47]. MHE affects as much as 60% of cirrhotic patients. The exact pathogenesis of HE still remains uncertain and is probably multifactorial. Gut flora metabolism products, such as ammonia, endotoxin, mercaptans and benzodiazepine-like substances, have been recognized as important factors in recent years [43, 48, 49]. Treatment of HE aims at the reduction of the production and absorption of these toxins by modulating the type and quantity of protein intake, reducing intestinal transit time and modifying microbial flora by reducing proteolytic and increasing saccharolytic flora [50–53]. Present treatment strategies include lactulose (a prebiotic) and poorly absorbable antibiotics (neomycin) [54]. Lactulose remains undigested until it reaches the colon where it functions to inhibit bacterial ammonia production and trap ammonia as non-diffusable ammonium in the intestinal lumen [55]. This may not be the optimal therapy for all HE patients, however, due to side effects and patients' poor compliance with therapy. Some patients find lactulose unpalatable and lactulose use is associated with increased flatulence, diarrhea and abdominal pain. Therefore other safe and better tolerated treatment options, like probiotics and other prebiotics are being evaluated [56] (Table 7.5).

Probiotics may have multiple beneficial effects in the treatment of minimal HE by modulating the microflora which can lead to decreased ammonia levels. This can be achieved by decreasing intestinal permeability and bacterial urease secretion, increasing ammonia excretion and improving nutritional status of gut epithelial cells. Furthermore, probiotics can decrease oxidative stress and inflammation in hepatocytes which leads to increased function and capacity to clear and decrease uptake of toxins and ammonia [17, 57, 58].

In a study by Jia et al. [56], the effects of Golden Bifid (a highly concentrated combination of probiotic containing lactobacilli, bifidobacteria and a mixture of *Streptococcus thermophilus* strains) were compared with lactulose in a rat experimental MHE model induced by thioacetamide. In this study both probiotics and lactulose lowered the levels of hyperammonemia and hyperendotoxemia, thereby decreasing the incidence of MHE and inflammatory reaction in the liver [57]. One of the earliest human studies using probiotic therapy in hepatic encephalopathy was reported by Macbeth et al. in 1965 [59]. Two HE patients were treated with *Lactobacillus acidophilus* and both patients showed a reduction in blood ammonia levels and improvement of neurological status [59].

A second small study at that time conducted by Read et al. [60] compared freeze-dried *Lactobacillus acidophilus* (Enpac) with and without neomycin treatment to normal diet in 10 hepatic encephalopathy patients. Sixty percent of patients treated with both Enpac and neomycin showed a decrease in arterial ammonia level. EEG improvements were found in five patients [60].

A pilot, placebo-controlled study of 55 cirrhotic patients with MHE performed by Liu et al. [36] compared the effects of oral supplementation of synbiotics (consisting of four freeze-dried bacteria: *P. pentosaceus, L. mesenteroides, L. paracasei and L. plantarum*) along with 10 grams of fermentable fiber (beta glucan, inulin, pectin and resistant starch (cocktail 2000)). Treatment lasted for 30 days and was compared to fermentable fiber alone or placebo. Prevention of cecal overgrowth with *Escherichia coli* and *Staphylococcus* spp. was observed in the synbiotic group. *Lactobacillus* species were significantly increased. Prebiotic treated patients had decreased *E. coli* bacteria and showed a significant increase in bifidobacteria.

TABLE 7.5 Pre- and probiotics in hepatic encephalopathy

Study reference	Study design	Pro/prebiotics and dose	Treatment duration	Study outcome	Adverse effects
Jia 2005 [56]	TAA animal study ($n = 36$)	Golden bifid (1.5 g/kg), lactulose 8 mL/kg	8 days prior to disease induction	↓ MHE; ↓ blood ammonia; ↓ endotoxemia; ↓ liver inflammation. No difference between lactulose and probiotics.	
Macbeth 1965 [59]	Case report ($n = 2$)	*L. acidophilus* 3–6 × 10^{12} cfu/day	3 days	↓ gram-negative flora, ↓ ammonia, ↑ fecal lactobacilli; improved EEG.	Not mentioned
Read 1966 [60]	($n = 10$)	Freeze-dried *L. acidophilus* (Enpac) ($2 \times 10^8 - 4 \times 10^8$ or 9×10^8 cfu/day)	1–4 weeks	↑ fecal lactobacilli; improvement in EEG; ↓ blood ammonia.	High dose produced stupor (probably due to high protein level in Enpac)
Liu 2004 [36]	Cirrhosis with MHE; ($n = 97$)	2.5 g each of beta glucan, inulin, pectin, resistant starch ± freeze-dried *P. pentosaceus*, *L. mesenteroides*, *L. paracasei*, *L. plantarum* (10^{10} cfu/day each); 30 days	30 days	↑ fecal lactobacilli; ↓ blood ammonia; reversal of MHE; ↓ endotoxemia; improved Child-Pugh score; synbiotics more beneficial.	Well tolerated
Loguercio 1987 [61]	RCT ($n = 40$)	E. SF68 6 capsules/day or 120 mL lactulose	20 days	Probiotics as effective as lactulose in ↓ blood ammonia, improving mental state and psychometric performance.	Diarrhea and abdominal pain reported with lactulose
Loguercio 1995 [62]	($n = 40$)	*E. faecium* (SF68), 4.5×10^8 cfu/day, lactulose 90 mL/day	3×4 weeks	↓ blood ammonia and enhanced Reitan's test times; beneficial effects maintained in washout period.	No
Bajaj 2008 [50]	RCT ($n = 25$)	*L. bulgaricus*, *S. thermophilus*	60 days	Improved MHE reversal, improved neuropsychological tests, protection against OHE development.	No
Malaguarnera 2006 [63]	RCT ($n = 60$)	*B. longum* and FOS (2.5 g)	90 days	↓ blood ammonia levels and ↑ performance on neuropsychological tests.	Well tolerated

TAA, thioacetamide; MHE, minimal hepatic encephalopathy; EEG, electroencephalography; RCT, randomized controlled trial; OHE, overt hepatic encephalopathy; FOS, fructo-oligosaccharide.

B. PREBIOTICS IN HEALTH PROMOTION

Placebo treated patients had no change in micro-flora composition. Furthermore, supply of the synbiotic composition or just prebiotics led to a significant decrease of venous ammonia, serum endotoxin levels, reversal of MHE and improvement of liver function (Child-Pugh score) in approximately half of the patients. Interestingly, fermentable fibers alone were also effective in a substantial proportion of patients. All treatments were well-tolerated and there were no reports of adverse side effects [36]. *Enterococcus* SF68 improved neurological symptoms, lowered ammonia levels and enhanced tolerance to protein load in a controlled study in 40 compensated cirrhotic HE patients [61]. Moreover, the effects of *Enterococcus* persisted 2 weeks after treatment withdrawal. This was in contrast to a second group receiving 30 mL of lactulose four times daily, which improved as well, but effects were lost after treatment stopped. Diarrhea and abdominal pain were reported with lactulose treatment. No adverse effects were reported with *Enterococcus* treatment [61]. Loguercio et al. [61] compared lactulose treatment with *Enterococcus faecium* SF68 treatment in cirrhotic patients with hepatic encephalopathy. Patients received one of the two treatments for three periods of 4 weeks, each interrupted by a 2-week drug free interval. After the complete treatment period, *Enterococcus* treated patients showed decreased blood ammonia levels and improved neurological status. These improvements were more significant than patients receiving lactulose treatment. Furthermore, *Enterococcus* treated patients maintained improvement after the 2-week drug free interval, whereas lactulose treated patients returned to basal values during these 2 weeks. No adverse effects of *Enterococcus* treatment were reported [62]. In a study by Bajaj et al. [50], 25 non-alcoholic MHE cirrhotics were randomized to receive probiotic yogurt or no treatment for 60 days. A significantly higher percentage of patients receiving yogurt reversed MHE compared to no treatment patients (71 vs 0% $p = 0.003$). Twenty-five percent of control patients versus

0% of yogurt patients developed overt hepatic encephalopathy during the trial. No adverse effects of yogurt treatment were observed [50]. A randomized double blind, placebo-controlled study performed with *Bifidobacterium longum* and fructo-oligosaccharides (FOS) was conducted in 60 cirrhotic patients with MHE [63]. Neurophysiological, liver function and neuropsychological assessments were investigated. After 90 days of treatment ammonia levels were significantly decreased, neurological testing and MMSE were significantly improved in the *Bifidobacterium longum* and FOS group compared to the control [63].

Summary

The use of prebiotics in hepatic encephalopathy is not new. The effectiveness of lactulose in this condition has long been proven and therefore lactulose has been the standard therapy. However, lactulose can cause many intolerable side effects, leading to an increased level of research into alternative prebiotic and probiotic therapies. Probiotics were shown to be at least as effective as lactulose in improving neurophysiological scoring and reducing ammonia blood levels. Probiotics were also better tolerated than lactulose.

4.4. Spontaneous Bacterial Peritonitis and Bacterial Translocation in Liver Disease

Spontaneous bacterial peritonitis (SBP) is a common complication in patients with cirrhosis. SBP is an infection of the ascetic fluid, mostly caused by a single bacterial species in the absence of any other intra-abdominal source. It is the most characteristic and serious infection occurring in patients with cirrhosis. SBP results from bacterial translocation which is the migration of bacteria from the intestinal lumen to mesenteric lymph nodes or other extra-intestinal sides [64, 65]. Cirrhotic patients are predisposed to develop SBP and other bacterial infections due to increased potential for bacterial overgrowth and bacterial translocation. This is caused by increased permeability of the small intestinal wall combined with impaired antibacterial defense mechanisms [66]. Various studies have recorded that patients with liver cirrhosis have varying degrees of imbalance of the intestinal flora which can predispose for bacterial overgrowth and subsequent problems of bacterial infection. Functional studies have demonstrated that increased intestinal permeability occurs in animal cirrhosis models and patients with cirrhosis, especially in those with advanced liver disease [67–72].

The inpatient mortality rate associated with SBP remains high, in the order of 20–30% [73–76]. In response to BT the gut immune system produces and releases TNF-α, especially in the presence of bacterial overgrowth. The complications of bacterial infections may have severe adverse clinical consequences, since this associated increase in pro-inflammatory cytokines and endotoxins exacerbates hepatic dysfunction, encephalopathy and the hemodynamic disturbances that underlie the development of portal hypertension and hepatorenal syndrome [66, 77–79]. In severe cases bacterial infection can lead to sepsis, which is a common cause of death in patients with cirrhosis [80, 81]. The mortality rate associated with bacterial infection in cirrhotic patients is more than 20 times higher than that in the general population [82].

Prophylactic antibiotic treatment has been shown to be of benefit in high risk patients. However, long-term use of antibiotics increases the risk of infection with antibiotic-resistant bacteria as shown in several studies [83–85]. Use of nephrotoxic antibiotics also adds to the risk of renal failure in this setting [86]. Since bacterial infection is such a severe complication and threat in cirrhotic patients and current therapy is inadequate, this highlights the need for investigation into non-antibiotic based strategies, such as pre-, pro- and synbiotics. Preliminary data of pre- and probiotic treatment in both *in vitro* and *in vivo* settings of bacterial translocation and its infective complications such as SBP are emerging. The hypothesis is that probiotics can have beneficial effects on the underlying causes of SBP, such as intestinal bacterial overgrowth, intestinal flora imbalance, impaired barrier function and bacterial translocation [36, 52, 87–90]. An additional advantage of probiotic treatment could be the decrease in circulating endotoxin levels [52, 88].

Summary

To date the only data on the effects of pro- and prebiotics and BT are coming from experimental animal studies. These current data are somewhat conflicting. Most lactobacilli strains induce a decrease in bacterial translocation, but some bifidobacteria strains increase bacterial translocation. Unfortunately, there are no data from clinical studies on the effects of pre- and probiotics in the prevention of bacterial translocation and spontaneous bacterial peritonitis in liver disease patients. More rigorous studies with different probiotic strains are needed to investigate which strains are beneficial and which may be harmful in this aspect before we can use probiotics as a means for prevention of bacterial translocation.

4.5. Liver Transplantation

Liver transplantation is a highly successful treatment for patients with end-stage liver disease and acute liver failure. However, serious postoperative complications can significantly compromise patient survival. Despite advanced surgical techniques and broad-spectrum antibiotic prophylaxis and treatment, bacterial infection is still the most common cause of morbidity within the first 3 postoperative months [91–93]. Therefore prevention of nosocomial infections is a major issue in post-transplant patients. Liver transplant patients are particularly susceptible to bacterial infections, with reported rates as high as 30 to 86% [91–93]. Furthermore, postoperative infections with subsequent need for antibacterial and antiviral treatments are associated with a significantly higher incidence of graft loss [93] (Table 7.6).

A new concept in the prevention of post-transplant complications is the administration of pre- and probiotics. Studies in liver transplant patients using early enteral nutrition with oat fiber and live or heat-killed *L. plantarum* 299 decreased infection rates significantly from 48% in the control group (which received conventional selective bowel decontamination with tobramycin, amphotericin B and colistin sulfate) to 13% with live bacteria and 34% with heat-killed bacteria. The mean duration of antibiotic therapy, total hospital stay and stay on the intensive care unit were also shorter for the group receiving live probiotics compared to the other two groups. No adverse effects of synbiotics were reported and intake was well tolerated [95]. A second randomized controlled study investigated the effects of a composition of four lactobacilli and fibers compared to fiber only ($n = 66$). Treatment started the day before surgery and continued for 14 days. Thirty-day infection rate, length of hospital stay, duration of antibiotic therapy, non-infectious complications and side effects of enteral nutrition were recorded. In this study the incidence of postoperative bacterial infection was significantly reduced from 48% with only prebiotics to 3% with synbiotics. In addition, the use of antibiotics was significantly shorter in the latter group. In both groups mainly mild or moderate infections occurred. Interestingly, non-infectious complication rates were higher in synbiotic treated patients compared to prebiotic treated patients (36 vs 12%). These complications included: biliary tract stenosis or fistulas, lienalis steal syndrome, abdominal hemorrhage, acute renal failure and non-function of the liver followed by re-transplantation [96].

4.6. Liver Resection

Liver resection is conducted in patients suffering from liver carcinoma or metastases or when part of the liver is donated. After liver resection, approximately 30% of patients develop infections and 10% develop intra-abdominal sepsis [97]. If the resection is more extensive the incidence of infection can even be as high as 45% [98]. If liver resection is complicated by infection, the risk of liver failure is 50% and the mortality rate is over 40% [97]. Most common causes for the development of infection after liver resection are the limited hepatic clearance of LPS, excessive cytokine production in the liver, reduction of the function of the reticulo-endothelial system, and reduced intestinal blood flow [99–102].

One experimental study investigated the effect of pre- and probiotics on bacterial translocation in rats after liver resection, with or without simultaneous colon anastomosis. Rats were fed a combination of four probiotics (*P. pentosaceus*, *Lactococcus raffinlocatis*, *L. paracasei*, *L. plantarum*) and four fibers (betaglucan, inulin, pectin and resistant starch). Application of the pre- and probiotics significantly decreased bacterial concentration in lymph nodes, but not liver and spleen [103]. These findings are compatible with a report in rats with liver failure following 90% hepatectomy. In this study, treatment with *Lactobacillus reuteri* in combination with fermentable oatmeal was associated with a significant reduction in bacterial translocation [104]. Kanazawa et al. investigated the impact of synbiotics on the clinical course of hepatectomy in bile duct carcinoma patients [105]. Twenty-one patients received enteral nutrition plus a synbiotic combination of *B. breve* and *L. casei* as well as galacto-oligosaccharides (12 g/day) postoperatively for 14 days. Results were compared to 23 patients only receiving enteral nutrition. In the synbiotics group, 19% had bacterial infections compared to 52% in the control group. Furthermore, beneficial bacteria (lactobacilli and bifidobacteria) in feces were increased in the

TABLE 7.6 Pre- and probiotics in liver transplantation and liver resection (animal and human studies)

Study reference	Study design	Pro/prebiotics and dose	Treatment duration	Study outcome	Adverse effects
Rayes 2002 [95]	RCT ($n = 95$) (liver transplantation pts)	*L. plantarum* live (2×10^9 cfu/day) of heat-killed + oat fibers; started on day of OK	12 days	↓ bacterial infection, (most prominent with live bacteria); ↓duration of antibiotic therapy and mean total hospital stay, and ICU stay in live group.	Well tolerated
Rayes 2005 [96]	Double-blind ($n = 66$) (liver transplantation pts)	5 g/day each of betaglucan, inulin, pectin, resistant starch ± *P. pentosaceus, Leuconostoc mesenteroides, L. paracasei, L. plantarum* (2×10^{10} cfu/day) treatment added to enteral nutrition	14 days	Synbiotics shorter antibiotic therapy. Synbiotics group 36% of non-infectious complications, prebiotics group 12%. Synbiotics group showed lower nosocomial infection rates than prebiotics (3 vs 48%).	Reports of diarrhea and abdominal cramps 10–20% pts
Seehofer 2004 [103]	($n = 68$) (animal study liver resection)	*P. pentosaceus, Lactococcus raffinolactis, L. paracasei, L. plantarum* (10^9 cfu/day), 0.4 g betaglucan, inulin, pectin, resistant starch	5 days	↓ BT in the lymph nodes.	n/a
Wang 1995 [104]	(Animal study liver resection)	*L. reuteri* and oatmeal	8–10 days	↓ BT.	n/a
Kanazawa 2005 [105]	RCT ($n = 44$) (liver resection pts)	*B. breve* (10^8 cfu/day) *L. casei* (10^8 cfu/day) 12 g GOS	14 days	↓ infection; ↑ beneficial bacteria; ↓ pathogenic bacteria in feces.	Not mentioned
Sugawara 2006 [106]	RCT ($n = 81$); (liver resection pts)	Pre-OK: 4×10^{10} *L. casei* strain shirota (Yakult). 1×10^{10} *B. breve* and 15 g GOS; Post-OK: 1×10^8 *L. casei* and *B. breve*	2 or 4 weeks	Pre-OK effect: ↑ NK activity, and lymphocyte counts; ↓ IL-6; Post-OK: ↓ Il-6; ↓ WBC counts; ↓ CRP; ↑ bifidobacteria; incidence of postoperative infections decreased.	No

RCT, randomized controlled trial; ICU, intensive care unit; BT, bacterial translocation; GOS, galacto-oligosaccharide; NK, natural killer cell; WBC, white blood cells; CRP, C-reactive protein.

probiotics group, whereas a decrease was seen in the control group. Harmful bacteria (enterobacteriaceae, pseudomonas and candida) were decreased in the probiotics group and increased in the control group. In addition, a significant reduction of pathogenic bacteria and an increase of organic acids in the feces were observed [105].

In a second study with 81 patients undergoing hepatobiliary resection for bile duct carcinoma, the same synbiotics were given in a higher concentration. Pre- and postoperative treatment with synbiotics resulted in significantly lower bacterial infection rates compared to only postoperative treatment (12.1 vs 30%). Moreover, in this group, an increased activity of natural killer cells and a lower concentration of IL-6 levels in the blood were observed [106].

Summary

The few animal and human studies of pro- and prebiotic effects in liver transplantation and resection show a beneficial effect of this treatment. Decreased bacterial infection rates and duration of antibiotic therapy were observed. The effect seems to be more prominent if treatment is started before the operation and if pro- and prebiotics are administered together.

5. CONCLUSION

Pre- and probiotics are a safe, convenient and easy to administer treatment. To date, no serious side effects have been observed in studies with liver disease patients. From the current studies, there is some evidence to suggest that pro- and prebiotics may have a role in the treatment and/or prevention of liver disease by maintaining gut barrier function, modulating innate and adaptive immune function, and reducing concentrations of harmful intestinal microbes. Unfortunately, a lack of carefully designed randomized controlled trials and differences in use of bacterial strains, doses, length of administration, outcome measurements and moment of initiation of treatment make it hard to draw any final conclusions at this point. There seems to be a promising role for pro- and prebiotics in prevention of steatosis, improvement of liver function in cirrhosis, improvement of hepatic encephalopathy and prevention of infectious complications in post-transplant and hepatectomy patients. However, further studies will be necessary to investigate what probiotic strains and what dosage is most effective and safe for treatment of different liver conditions.

References

1. Lehmann, V., Freudenberg, M. A., & Galanos, C. (1987). Lethal toxicity of lipopolysaccharide and tumor necrosis factor in normal and D-galactosamine-treated mice. *The Journal of Experimental Medicine, 165*, 657–663.
2. Adawi, D., Kasravi, F. B., Molin, G., & Jeppsson, B. (1997). Effect of Lactobacillus supplementation with and without arginine on liver damage and bacterial translocation in an acute liver injury model in the rat. *Hepatology, 25*, 642–647.
3. Adawi, D., Molin, G., & Jeppsson, B. (1998). Inhibition of nitric oxide production and the effects of arginine and Lactobacillus administration in an acute liver injury model. *Annals of Surgery, 228*, 748–755.
4. Ewaschuk, J., Endersby, R., Thiel, D., et al. (2007). Probiotic bacteria prevent hepatic damage and maintain colonic barrier function in a mouse model of sepsis. *Hepatology, 46*, 841–850.
5. Kasravi, F. B., Adawi, D., Molin, G., et al. (1997). Effect of oral supplementation of lactobacilli on bacterial translocation in acute liver injury induced by D-galactosamine. *Journal of Hepatology, 26*, 417–424.
6. Adawi, D., Ahrne, S., & Molin, G. (2001). Effects of different probiotic strains of Lactobacillus and Bifidobacterium on bacterial translocation and liver injury in an acute liver injury model. *International Journal of Food Microbiology, 70*, 213–220.
7. Osman, N., Adawi, D., Ahrne, S., et al. (2007). Endotoxin- and D-galactosamine-induced liver injury improved by the administration of Lactobacillus, Bifidobacterium and blueberry. *Digestive and Liver Disease, 39*, 849–856.
8. Wiest, R., Chen, F., Cadelina, G., et al. (2003). Effect of Lactobacillus-fermented diets on bacterial translocation and intestinal flora in experimental prehepatic portal hypertension. *Digestive Diseases and Sciences, 48*, 1136–1141.
9. Marotta, F., Barreto, R., Wu, C. C., et al. (2005). Experimental acute alcohol pancreatitis-related liver damage and endotoxemia: synbiotics but not metronidazole have a protective effect. *Chinese Journal of Digestive Diseases, 6*, 193–197.
10. Neyrinck, A. M., Alexiou, H., & Delzenne, N. M. (2004). Kupffer cell activity is involved in the hepatoprotective effect of dietary oligofructose in rats with endotoxic shock. *The Journal of Nutrition, 134*, 1124–1129.
11. Xing, H. C., Li, L. J., Xu, K. J., et al. (2005). Intestinal microflora in rats with ischemia/reperfusion liver injury. *Journal of Zhejiang University Science, B 6*, 14–21.
12. Vuppalanchi, R., & Chalasani, N. (2009). Nonalcoholic fatty liver disease and nonalcoholic steatohepatitis: Selected practical issues in their evaluation and management. *Hepatology, 49*, 306–317.

13. Gan, S. K., Adams, L. A., & Watts, G. F. (2008). The trials and tribulations of the treatment of nonalcoholic fatty-liver disease. *Current Opinion in Lipidology, 19*, 592–599.

14. Shifflet, A., & Wu, G. Y. (2009). Non-alcoholic steato-hepatitis: An overview. *Journal of the Formosan Medical Association, 108*, 4–12.

15. Sokol, R. J., Devereaux, M., Dahl, R., & Gumpricht, E. (2006). 'Let there be bile'—understanding hepatic injury in cholestasis. *Journal of Pediatric Gastroenterology and Nutrition, 43*(Suppl. 1), S4–S9.

16. Rubbia-Brandt, L., Leandro, G., Spahr, L., et al. (2001). Liver steatosis in chronic hepatitis C: A morphological sign suggesting infection with HCV genotype 3. *Histopathology, 39*, 119–124.

17. Solga, S. F., & Diehl, A. M. (2003). Non-alcoholic fatty liver disease: Lumen-liver interactions and possible role for probiotics. *Journal of Hepatology, 38*, 681–687.

18. Portincasa, P., Grattagliano, I., Palmieri, V. O., & Palasciano, G. (2006). Current pharmacological treatment of nonalcoholic fatty liver. *Current Medicinal Chemistry, 13*, 2889–2900.

19. Purohit, V., Gao, B., & Song, B. J. (2009). Molecular mechanisms of alcoholic fatty liver. *Alcoholism, Clinical and Experimental Research, 33*, 191–205.

20. Albano, E. (2008). New concepts in the pathogenesis of alcoholic liver disease. *Expert Review of Gastroenterology and Hepatology, 2*, 749–759.

21. Zeng, M. D., Li, Y. M., Chen, C. W., et al. (2008). Guidelines for the diagnosis and treatment of alcoholic liver disease. *Journal of Digestive Diseases, 9*, 113–116.

22. Reuben, A. (2008). Alcohol and the liver. *Current Opinion in Gastroenterology, 24*, 328–338.

23. Yin, M., Wheeler, M. D., Kono, H., et al. (1999). Essential role of tumor necrosis factor alpha in alcohol-induced liver injury in mice. *Gastroenterology, 117*, 942–952.

24. Nanji, A. A., Khettry, U., & Sadrzadeh, S. M. (1994). Lactobacillus feeding reduces endotoxemia and severity of experimental alcoholic liver (disease). *Proceedings of the Society for Experimental Biology and Medicine, 205*, 243–247.

25. Iimuro, Y., Gallucci, R. M., Luster, M. I., et al. (1997). Antibodies to tumor necrosis factor alfa attenuate hepatic necrosis and inflammation caused by chronic exposure to ethanol in the rat. *Hepatology, 26*, 1530–1537.

26. Ma, X., Hua, J., & Li, Z. (2008). Probiotics improve high fat diet-induced hepatic steatosis and insulin resistance by increasing hepatic NKT cells. *Journal of Hepatology, 49*, 821–830.

27. Li, Z., Yang, S., Lin, H., et al. (2003). Probiotics and antibodies to TNF inhibit inflammatory activity and improve nonalcoholic fatty liver disease. *Hepatology, 37*, 343–350.

28. Velayudham, A., Dolganiuc, A., Ellis, M., et al. (2009). VSL#3 probiotic treatment attenuates fibrosis without changes in steatohepatitis in a diet-induced nonalcoholic steatohepatitis model in mice. *Hepatology, 49*, 989–997.

29. Han, S. Y., Huh, C. S., Ahn, Y. T., et al. (2005). Hepatoprotective effect of lactic acid bacteria, inhibitors of beta-glucuronidase production against intestinal microflora. *Archives of Pharmacal Research, 28*, 325–329.

30. Chen, L., Pan, D. D., Zhou, J., & Jiang, Y. Z. (2005). Protective effect of selenium-enriched Lactobacillus on CCl4-induced liver injury in mice and its possible mechanisms. *World Journal of Gastroenterology, 11*, 5795–5800.

31. Bauer, T. M., Fernandez, J., Navasa, M., et al. (2002). Failure of Lactobacillus spp. to prevent bacterial translocation in a rat model of experimental cirrhosis. *Journal of Hepatology, 36*, 501–506.

32. Chiva, M., Soriano, G., Rochat, I., et al. (2002). Effect of *Lactobacillus johnsonii* La1 and antioxidants on intestinal flora and bacterial translocation in rats with experimental cirrhosis. *Journal of Hepatology, 37*, 456–462.

33. Nicaise, C., Prozzi, D., Viaene, E., et al. (2008). Control of acute, chronic, and constitutive hyperammonemia by wild-type and genetically engineered Lactobacillus plantarum in rodents. *Hepatology, 48*, 1184–1192.

34. Solga, S. F., Buckley, G., Clark, J. M., et al. (2008). The effect of a probiotic on hepatic steatosis. *Journal of Clinical Gastroenterology, 42*, 1117–1119.

35. Kirpich, I. A., Solovieva, N. V., Leikhter, S. N., et al. (2008). Probiotics restore bowel flora and improve liver enzymes in human alcohol-induced liver injury: A pilot study. *Alcohol, 42*, 675–682.

36. Liu, Q., Duan, Z. P., Ha, D. K., et al. (2004). Synbiotic modulation of gut flora: Effect on minimal hepatic encephalopathy in patients with cirrhosis. *Hepatology, 39*, 1441–1449.

37. Lata, J., Novotny, I., Pribramska, V., et al. (2007). The effect of probiotics on gut flora, level of endotoxin and Child-Pugh score in cirrhotic patients: Results of a double-blind randomized study. *European Journal of Gastroenterology & Hepatology, 19*, 1111–1113.

38. Stadlbauer, V., Mookerjee, R. P., Hodges, S., et al. (2008). Effect of probiotic treatment on deranged neutrophil function and cytokine responses in patients with compensated alcoholic cirrhosis. *Journal of Hepatology, 48*, 945–951.

39. Loguercio, C., De, S. T., Federico, A., et al. (2002). Gut-liver axis: a new point of attack to treat chronic liver damage? *The American Journal of Gastroenterology, 97*, 2144–2146.

40. Loguercio, C., Federico, A., Tuccillo, C., et al. (2005). Beneficial effects of a probiotic VSL#3 on parameters of liver dysfunction in chronic liver diseases. *Journal of Clinical Gastroenterology, 39*, 540–543.

41. Tandon, P., Moncrief, K., Madsen, K., et al. (2009). Effects of probiotic therapy on portal pressure in patients with cirrhosis: A pilot study. *Liver International, 29*(7), 1110–1115.

B. PREBIOTICS IN HEALTH PROMOTION

42. Ferenci, P., Lockwood, A., Mullen, K., et al. (2002). Hepatic encephalopathy – definition, nomenclature, diagnosis, and quantification: Final report of the working party at the 11th World Congresses of Gastroenterology, Vienna, 1998. *Hepatology, 35*, 716–721.

43. Ferenci, P. (1991). Pathophysiology of hepatic encephalopathy. *Hepatogastroenterology, 38*, 371–376.

44. Blei, A. T., & Cordoba, J. (2001). Hepatic encephalopathy. *The American Journal of Gastroenterology, 96*, 1968–1976.

45. Romero-Gomez, M., Ramos-Guerrero, R., Grande, L., et al. (2004). Intestinal glutaminase activity is increased in liver cirrhosis and correlates with minimal hepatic encephalopathy. *Journal of Hepatology, 41*, 49–54.

46. Kharbanda, P. S., Saraswat, V. A., & Dhiman, R. K. (2003). Minimal hepatic encephalopathy: Diagnosis by neuropsychological and neurophysiologic methods. *Indian Journal of Gastroenterology, 22*(Suppl. 2), S37–S41.

47. Weissenborn, K., Ennen, J. C., Schomerus, H., et al. (2001). Neuropsychological characterization of hepatic encephalopathy. *Journal of Hepatology, 34*, 768–773.

48. Nomura, F., & Takekoshi, K. (1994). Zinc and selenium metabolism in liver cirrhosis. *Nippon Rinsho, 52*, 165–169.

49. Yurdaydin, C., Walsh, T. J., Engler, H. D., et al. (1995). Gut bacteria provide precursors of benzodiazepine receptor ligands in a rat model of hepatic encephalopathy. *Brain Research, 679*, 42–48.

50. Bajaj, J. S., Saeian, K., Christensen, K. M., et al. (2008). Probiotic yogurt for the treatment of minimal hepatic encephalopathy. *The American Journal of Gastroenterology, 103*, 1707–1715.

51. Bajaj, J. S. (2008). Minimal hepatic encephalopathy matters in daily life. *World Journal of Gastroenterology, 14*, 3609–3615.

52. Garcia-Tsao, G., & Wiest, R. (2004). Gut microflora in the pathogenesis of the complications of cirrhosis. *Best Practice & Research. Clinical Gastroenterology, 18*, 353–372.

53. Weber, F. L., Jr. (1996). Lactulose and combination therapy of hepatic encephalopathy: The role of the intestinal microflora. *Digestive Diseases, 14*(Suppl. 1), 53–63.

54. Dbouk, N., & McGuire, B. M. (2006). Hepatic encephalopathy: A review of its pathophysiology and treatment. *Current Treatment Options in Gastroenterology, 9*, 464–474.

55. Riordan, S. M., & Williams, R. (1997). Treatment of hepatic encephalopathy. *The New England Journal of Medicine, 337*, 473–479.

56. Jia, L., & Zhang, M. H. (2005). Comparison of probiotics and lactulose in the treatment of minimal hepatic encephalopathy in rats. *World Journal of Gastroenterology, 11*, 908–911.

57. Sheth, A. A., & Garcia-Tsao, G. (2008). Probiotics and liver disease. *Journal of Clinical Gastroenterology, 42*(Suppl. 2), S80–S84.

58. Sharma, P., Sharma, B. C., Puri, V., & Sarin, S. K. (2008). An open-label randomized controlled trial of lactulose and probiotics in the treatment of minimal hepatic encephalopathy. *European Journal of Gastroenterology & Hepatology, 20*, 506–511.

59. Macbeth, W. A., Kass, E. H., & McDermott, W. V., Jr. (1965). Treatment of hepatic encephalopathy by alteration of intestinal flora with *Lactobacillus acidophilus*. *Lancet, 1*, 399–403.

60. Read, A. E., McCarthy, C. F., Heaton, K. W., & Laidlaw, J. (1966). *Lactobacillus acidophilus* (enpac) in treatment of hepatic encephalopathy. *British Medical Journal, 1*, 1267–1269.

61. Loguercio, C., Del Vecchio, B. C., & Coltorti, M. (1987). Enterococcus lactic acid bacteria strain SF68 and lactulose in hepatic encephalopathy: A controlled study. *The Journal of International Medical Research, 15*, 335–343.

62. Loguercio, C., Abbiati, R., Rinaldi, M., Romano, A., et al. (1995). Long-term effects of *Enterococcus faecium* SF68 versus lactulose in the treatment of patients with cirrhosis and grade 1-2 hepatic encephalopathy. *Journal of Hepatology, 23*, 39–46.

63. Malaguarnera, M., Greco, F., Barone, G., et al. (2007). *Bifidobacterium longum* with fructo-oligosaccharide (FOS) treatment in minimal hepatic encephalopathy: A randomized, double-blind, placebo-controlled study. *Digestive Diseases and Sciences, 52*, 3259–3265.

64. Koulaouzidis, A., Bhat, S., & Saeed, A. A. (2009). Spontaneous bacterial peritonitis. *World Journal of Gastroenterology, 15*, 1042–1049.

65. Guarner, C., & Soriano, G. (1997). Spontaneous bacterial peritonitis. *Seminars in Liver Disease, 17*, 203–217.

66. Wiest, R., & Garcia-Tsao, G. (2005). Bacterial translocation (BT) in cirrhosis. *Hepatology, 41*, 422–433.

67. Llovet, J. M., Bartoli, R., March, F., et al. (1998). Translocated intestinal bacteria cause spontaneous bacterial peritonitis in cirrhotic rats: Molecular epidemiologic evidence. *Journal of Hepatology, 28*, 307–313.

68. Zuckerman, M. J., Menzies, I. S., Ho, H., et al. (2004). Assessment of intestinal permeability and absorption in cirrhotic patients with ascites using combined sugar probes. *Digestive Diseases and Sciences, 49*, 621–626.

69. Pascual, S., Such, J., Esteban, A., et al. (2003). Intestinal permeability is increased in patients with advanced cirrhosis. *Hepatogastroenterology, 50*, 1482–1486.

70. Di, L. V., Venturi, C., Baragiotta, A., et al. (2003). Gastroduodenal and intestinal permeability in primary biliary cirrhosis. *European Journal of Gastroenterology & Hepatology, 15*, 967–973.

71. Campillo, B., Pernet, P., Bories, P. N., et al. (1999). Intestinal permeability in liver cirrhosis: Relationship with severe septic complications. *European Journal of Gastroenterology & Hepatology, 11*, 755–759.

72. Ersoz, G., Aydin, A., Erdem, S., et al. (1999). Intestinal permeability in liver cirrhosis. *European Journal of Gastroenterology & Hepatology, 11*, 409–412.

73. Rimola, A., Navasa, M., & Arroyo, V. (1995). Experience with cefotaxime in the treatment of spontaneous bacterial peritonitis in cirrhosis. *Diagnostic Microbiology and Infectious Disease, 22*, 141–145.

74. Rimola, A., Salmeron, J. M., Clemente, G., et al. (1995). Two different dosages of cefotaxime in the treatment of spontaneous bacterial peritonitis in cirrhosis: Results of a prospective, randomized, multicenter study. *Hepatology, 21*, 674–679.

75. Ricart, E., Soriano, G., Novella, M. T., et al. (2000). Amoxicillin-clavulanic acid versus cefotaxime in the therapy of bacterial infections in cirrhotic patients. *Journal of Hepatology, 32*, 596–602.

76. Sort, P., Navasa, M., Arroyo, V., et al. (1999). Effect of intravenous albumin on renal impairment and mortality in patients with cirrhosis and spontaneous bacterial peritonitis. *The New England Journal of Medicine, 341*, 403–409.

77. Strauss, E., Gomes de Sa Ribeiro, Mde. (2003). Bacterial infections associated with hepatic encephalopathy: Prevalence and outcome. *Annals of Hepatology, 2*, 41–45.

78. Strauss, E., & Caly, W. R. (2003). Spontaneous bacterial peritonitis. *Revista da Sociedade Brasileira de Medicina Tropical, 36*, 711–717.

79. Riordan, S. M., & Williams, R. (2003). Mechanisms of hepatocyte injury, multiorgan failure, and prognostic criteria in acute liver failure. *Seminars in Liver Disease, 23*, 203–215.

80. Brann, O. S. (2001). Infectious complications of cirrhosis. *Current Gastroenterology Reports, 3*, 285–292.

81. Borzio, M., Salerno, F., Piantoni, L., et al. (2001). Bacterial infection in patients with advanced cirrhosis: A multicentre prospective study. *Digestive and Liver Disease, 33*, 41–48.

82. Vilstrup, H. (2003). Cirrhosis and bacterial infections. *Romanian Journal of Gastroenterology, 12*, 297–302.

83. Cereto, F., Molina, I., Gonzalez, A., et al. (2003). Role of immunosuppression in the development of quinolone-resistant *Escherichia coli* spontaneous bacterial peritonitis and in the mortality of *E. coli* spontaneous bacterial peritonitis. *Alimentary Pharmacology & Therapeutics, 17*, 695–701.

84. Campillo, B., Dupeyron, C., Richardet, J. P., et al. (1998). Epidemiology of severe hospital-acquired infections in patients with liver cirrhosis: Effect of long-term administration of norfloxacin. *Clinical Infectious Diseases, 26*, 1066–1070.

85. Campillo, B., Dupeyron, C., & Richardet, J. P. (2001). Epidemiology of hospital-acquired infections in cirrhotic patients: Effect of carriage of methicillin-resistant *Staphylococcus aureus* and influence of previous antibiotic therapy and norfloxacin prophylaxis. *Epidemiology and Infection, 127*, 443–450.

86. Hampel, H., Bynum, G. D., Zamora, E., & El-Serag, H. B. (2001). Risk factors for the development of renal dysfunction in hospitalized patients with cirrhosis. *The American Journal of Gastroenterology, 96*, 2206–2210.

87. Zhao, H. Y., Wang, H. J., Lu, Z., & Xu, S. Z. (2004). Intestinal microflora in patients with liver cirrhosis. *Chinese Journal of Digestive Diseases, 5*, 64–67.

88. Garcia-Tsao, G. (2004). Bacterial infections in cirrhosis. *Canadian Journal of Gastroenterology, 18*, 405–406.

89. Laudanno, O. M., Cesolari, J. A., Godoy, A., et al. (2008). Bioflora probiotic in immunomodulation and prophylaxis of intestinal bacterial translocation in rats. *Digestive Diseases and Sciences, 53*, 2667–2670.

90. Paturi, G., Phillips, M., Jones, M., & Kailasapathy, K. (2007). Immune enhancing effects of *Lactobacillus acidophilus* LAFTI L10 and *Lactobacillus paracasei* LAFTI L26 in mice. *International Journal of Food Microbiology, 115*, 115–118.

91. Wade, J. J., Rolando, N., Hayllar, K., et al. (1995). Bacterial and fungal infections after liver transplantation: an analysis of 284 patients. *Hepatology, 21*, 1328–1336.

92. Dominguez, E. A. (1995). Long-term infectious complications of liver transplantation. *Seminars in Liver Disease, 15*, 133–138.

93. Mazariegos, G. V., Molmenti, E. P., & Kramer, D. J. (1999). Early complications after orthotopic liver transplantation. *The Surgical Clinics of North America, 79*, 109–129.

94. Cainelli, F., & Vento, S. (2002). Infections and solid organ transplant rejection: A cause-and-effect relationship? *The Lancet Infectious Diseases, 2*, 539–549.

95. Rayes, N., Seehofer, D., Hansen, S., et al. (2002). Early enteral supply of lactobacillus and fiber versus selective bowel decontamination: A controlled trial in liver transplant recipients. *Transplantation, 74*, 123–127.

96. Rayes, N., Seehofer, D., Theruvath, T., et al. (2005). Supply of pre- and probiotics reduces bacterial infection rates after liver transplantation—a randomized, double-blind trial. *American Journal of Transplantation, 5*, 125–130.

97. Shigeta, H., Nagino, M., Kamiya, J., et al. (2002). Bacteremia after hepatectomy: An analysis of a single-center, 10-year experience with 407 patients. *Langenbeck's Archives of Surgery, 387*, 117–124.

98. Togo, S., Matsuo, K., Tanaka, K., et al. (2007). Perioperative infection control and its effectiveness in hepatectomy patients. *Journal of Gastroenterology and Hepatology, 22*, 1942–1948.

99. Wang, X., Andersson, R., Ding, J., et al. (1993). Reticuloendothelial system function following acute

liver failure induced by 90% hepatectomy in the rat. *HPB Surgery, 6,* 151–162.

100. Wang, X. D., Soltesz, V., Andersson, R., & Bengmark, S. (1993). Bacterial translocation in acute liver failure induced by 90 per cent hepatectomy in the rat. *The British Journal of Surgery, 80,* 66–71.

101. Wang, X. D., Parsson, H., Andersson, R., et al. (1994). Bacterial translocation, intestinal ultrastructure and cell membrane permeability early after major liver resection in the rat. *The British Journal of Surgery, 81,* 579–584.

102. Wang, X. D., Guo, W. D., Wang, Q., et al. (1994). The association between enteric bacterial overgrowth and gastrointestinal motility after subtotal liver resection or portal vein obstruction in rats. *The European Journal of Surgery, 160,* 153–160.

103. Seehofer, D., Rayes, N., Schiller, R., et al. (2004). Probiotics partly reverse increased bacterial translocation after simultaneous liver resection and colonic anastomosis in rats. *The Journal of Surgical Research, 117,* 262–271.

104. Wang, X. D., Soltesz, V., Molin, G., & Andersson, R. (1995). The role of oral administration of oatmeal fermented by Lactobacillus reuteri R2LC on bacterial translocation after acute liver failure induced by subtotal liver resection in the rat. *Scandinavian Journal of Gastroenterology, 30,* 180–185.

105. Kanazawa, H., Nagino, M., Kamiya, S., et al. (2005). Synbiotics reduce postoperative infectious complications: A randomized controlled trial in biliary cancer patients undergoing hepatectomy. *Langenbeck's Archives of Surgery, 390,* 104–113.

106. Sugawara, G., Nagino, M., Nishio, H., et al. (2006). Perioperative synbiotic treatment to prevent postoperative infectious complications in biliary cancer surgery: A randomized controlled trial. *Annals of Surgery, 244,* 706–714.

Prebiotics in Infant Formulas: Risks and Benefits

Jose M. Moreno Villares

Nutrition Unit, Department of Pediatrics, Hospital Universitario 12 de Octubre, Madrid, Spain

1. INTRODUCTION

The human intestinal microbiota is composed of 10^{13} to 10^{14} microorganisms whose collective genome (microbiome) contains at least 100 times as many genes as our own genome. In a way we can say that humans are superorganisms whose metabolism represents an amalgamation of microbial and human attributes. Evidence is accumulating that the interaction of the intestinal microflora with the intestinal mucosa cells plays a significant role in subsequent health, including autoimmune diseases, allergies and gastrointestinal diseases. A deeper knowledge in the close relationship between host and microflora will help us to better understand the health status, to develop new ways for optimizing our personal nutrition and how to forecast our individual and societal predispositions to some diseases [1]. Consideration should be given to the role of microbes in the gut through the lens of the evolutionary history of prokaryotic-eukaryotic relations, as Neish affirms [2]. Neish recommends a departure from the usual paradigm of microbes as presumptive pathogens, assuming that prokaryotic–eukaryotic interactions in the gut are generally mutually beneficial. Newborn babies and infants possess a functional but immature immune system which protects against infections. The maturation of this immune system is closely related to the acquisition of an appropriate gut microflora. Breast milk contains a number of biological, active compounds that can improve the infant's immune system directly or through components that help to establish a determined intestinal flora. Whilst it is not possible to produce infant formulas that have identical compositions and properties to breast milk, potential health benefits could arise from the supplementation of these products with one or a combination of functional food ingredients. There is increasing evidence that such dietary modulations could be beneficial for the host by effecting a health-promoting modification in the composition and the activities of gut microflora. This chapter reviews the strength of evidence regarding the immune-stimulating effects of one of these components, prebiotics, and how they are used in current infant formulas. The risks associated to its use and what is the regulatory status of prebiotics in infant formulas will be also reviewed.

2. DEVELOPMENT OF THE INFANT IMMUNE SYSTEM

At birth the gastrointestinal tract is essentially germ-free, with intestinal colonization occurring during birth or shortly afterwards. Within the first days of life, mucosal surfaces of the gastrointestinal as well as the respiratory tract become colonized with bacteria. The first colonization of the intestine is one of the most critical immunologic exposures faced by the newborn infant because microbial niches become established, allowing long-term colonization as part of the biofilm located in the glycocalyx of the epithelial layer [3].

The lymphoid system is not yet mature, although it is developed. The fetal immune system develops at least partial functional competence before birth but lacks full capacity to generate sustained immune responses. Lymphocytes T and B are naïve. Activation of T lymphocytes results in a type Th2 response, that is production of cytokines IL-4 and IL-5 and very low Th1 cytokine γ-interferon [4].

Although after birth there is an immense exposition to a wide spectrum of commensal and pathogenic microorganisms, the immune system does not respond to every stimulus. The corresponding pathogen-associated molecular patterns are recognized by receptors of the immune system, and this shapes the direction of the immune system's development through childhood to adulthood.

During pregnancy, the immune system of the fetus co-exists with the mother's immune system. After birth, the immune system must switch in order to protect the infant against pathogens and to develop tolerance to harmless non-self antigens, such as food antigens. At birth, T lymphocytes exhibit a Th2-profile, characterized by a limited ability to produce cytokines. Until this immune defense is set, infants are at risk for serious infection. Throughout the first months after birth these Th2-skewed responses are modified towards a low-level immunity, predominantly Th1-cytokines and IgG antibodies, particularly IgG1 [5]. On the other side, the immune system is tightly controlled by its own regulatory network to prevent inappropriate immune reactions from resulting in pathologic conditions. If this system fails, the result can be allergy or autoimmune disease. An interesting review can be found in Refs [2] and [6].

The close relationship between colonic microflora and host cells has a central role in health and disease. Dietary modulation is important for improved gut health, especially during the highly-sensitive stage of infancy [7–9].

Marked differences in the composition of gut flora have been recognized in response to the infant feeding regimen. Differences in gut microflora composition and incidences of infections exist between breast-fed and formula-fed infants, with the former thought to have improved protection.

Although there are different elements in infant feeding that can play a role in modifying gut microflora we will only discuss the role of prebiotics, especially when added to infant formulas.

3. BREAST MILK AND DEFENSE AGAINST INFECTIONS AND ALLERGIC MANIFESTATIONS

Breast-feeding is the ideal mode of feeding for the newborn infant. Breast milk confers passive immunity to the newborn. Clearly, the effect of human milk on the postnatal development of the intestinal flora cannot be attributed to a single ingredient. Breast milk contains 0.4 to 1.0 g/L

TABLE 8.1   Immunological active ingredients of human milk

Class	Ingredient
Immunoglobulins	sIgA, sIgG, sIgM
Antimicrobial proteins	Lactoferrin
	Lysozyme
	Lactoperoxidase
Leukocytes, macrophages	
Cytokines	IL-1, IL-6, TNF-α, γ-TNF, IL-12, IL-10, IL-8, chemokines
Hormones and growth factors	Granulocyte-macrophage colony stimulating factor, erythropoietin, cortisol
Long-chain polyunsaturated fatty acids	Docosahexaenoic acid (DHA)
	Arachidonic acid
Oligosaccharides	Galacto-oligosaccharides
Minerals	Zn, Se, Cu, Fe, Mn, Ca
Vitamins	Vitamin A, E, D3, C, B12
Nucleotides	AMP, CMP, GMP, IMP, UMP
Sialic acid	
Gangliosides	
Nucleotide-hydrolyzing antibodies	
Complement and complement receptors	
Toll-like receptors	
Milk peptides	

secretory IgA, antimicrobial protein (lactoferrin, lysozyme), leukocytes, cytokines and chemokines, hormones, fatty acids, oligosaccharides, as well as minerals, vitamins and other components that may contribute to the defense against infections (Table 8.1) [10, 11]. Breast-feeding protects against atopy [12] and infections [13]. In classical long-term epidemiological studies, it has been demonstrated that breast-fed infants are better protected against infections of the gut, respiratory and urinary tract when compared to those who are formula-fed [14, 15].

We focus on human milk oligosaccharides (HMO) later in the chapter. Breast milk contains at least 80 different oligosaccharides. Many of them act as receptor analogous that inhibit the binding of bacterial and viral pathogens or toxins to gut epithelial cells. Oligosaccharides also promote the proliferation of commensal *Bifidobacterium* spp. and lactobacilli in the intestinal tract [16].

4. PREBIOTICS: BENEFICIAL ACTIONS

Two different approaches towards modifying the development and balance of intestinal microflora can be taken: one is the addition of live bacteria and bifidobacteria (probiotics) and the other is the addition of oligosaccharides that survive passage through the small intestine and reach the colon where they are used by colonic bacteria, involving the manipulation of its energy sources (prebiotics) [17]. A prebiotic is a non-digestible food ingredient that beneficially affects the host by selectively stimulating the growth and/or activity of one or a limited number of bacterial species already resident in the colon [18]. The characteristics of a prebiotic are that they:

1. are neither hydrolyzed nor absorbed in the upper part of the gastrointestinal tract;
2. can be a selective substrate for one or a few beneficial bacteria in the colon;
3. are able to alter the colonic microflora towards a healthier composition.

Although any dietary component that reaches the colon intact is a potential prebiotic, most of the interest is aimed at non-digestible oligosaccharides [19]. Fructo-oligosaccharides (FOS) and galacto-oligosaccharides (GOS) have demonstrated beneficial effects on the intestinal microflora. Oligosaccharides are sugars containing between two and twenty units. They can occur naturally in fruits and vegetables or be produced by the hydrolysis of polysaccharides.

As prebiotics are not digestible, they are fully available to the bacteria that reside in the intestinal tract and interact with the intestinal microbiota. Prebiotic consumption shifts the composition of the intestinal microbiota towards those associated with a healthy condition in the host [20]. As the composition of the microbiota is modified, the types of bacterial metabolites into which prebiotics are converted are also modified, e.g. producing a greater amount of short-chain fatty acids (SCFAs). The SCFAs have important effects in the intestinal tract. Butyrate has an essential role in maintaining the metabolism, proliferation and differentiation of the various epithelial cell types. Many of these metabolites are absorbed into the blood and enter the systemic circulation interacting with many physiologic processes.

In this way prebiotics act: a) at improving intestinal transit time [21]; b) increasing the absorption of minerals, mainly calcium and manganese [22]; c) with anticancer effects, mainly in the prevention or progression of colon cancer [23, 24]; d) modifying lipid metabolism [25]; and e) modulating various systemic immune markers [26]. The possible therapeutic application of some prebiotics in specific clinical conditions such as inflammatory bowel diseases [27–29], and others [30] will be further analyzed in other chapters in this book.

5. PREBIOTICS AND HUMAN MILK

Shortly after birth, the previously sterile infant gut begins to be colonized by bacteria, facultative anaerobes and strict anaerobes, from the birth canal and its surroundings. Microbial flora of the female genital tract, sanitary conditions, and the type of delivery, all have an effect on the level and frequency of various species colonizing the infant gut. But the main factor contributing to the establishment of a particular microflora is the type of feeding. In the gastrointestinal system of breast-fed babies (Figure 8.1), bifidobacteria are soon selected and become predominant. Formula-fed babies harbor a varied flora consisting of bifidobacteria, *Escherichia coli*, and *Bacteriodes* [31]. When complementary feeding is introduced, a diversification of the flora occurs (Figure 8.2).

The bifidogenic effect of human milk has been ascribed to oligosaccharides, lactoferrin, and nucleotides [32]. But the two last components seem to have more an inhibitory effect of the pathogenic flora rather than a direct stimulus to the development of bifidobacteria. Then, we can say that human milk stimulates the growth of bifidobacteria because of its high oligosaccharide content. Human milk oligosaccharides (HMOs) are a combination of five monosaccharides: glucose, galactose, sialic acid, fructose, and N-acetyl-glucosamine. They are synthesized in the mammalian gland by specific enzymes,

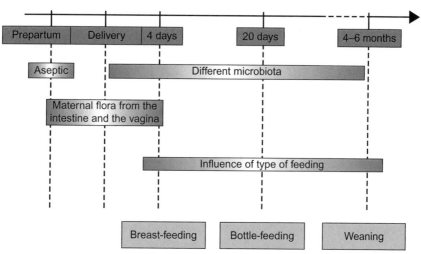

FIGURE 8.1   Factors influencing intestinal colonization.

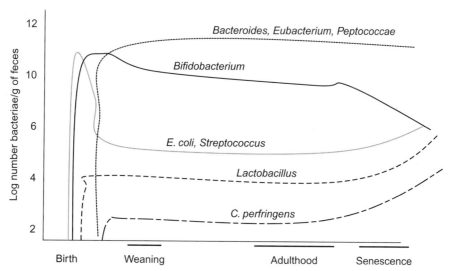

FIGURE 8.2   Development of intestinal microbiota according to age.

the glycosyltransferases, in sequences of five to 10 monosaccharides [33]. Human milk contains at least 21 different kinds of oligosaccharides composed of many different molecules. These oligosaccharides are predominantly neutral, low molecular weight molecules, and depending on the Lewis blood group of the mother. HMOs represent the third largest components (after lactose and lipids) in breast milk, occurring at a concentration of 12–14g/L in mature milk and 20–23g/L in colostrum [34]. On the contrary, cows' milk, commonly used to prepare infant formulas, contains less than 1g/L oligosaccharides. HMOs are very resistant to enzymatic hydrolysis. Beside their role into the intestinal lumen, they can be absorbed and cross the brush border membrane of the intestine [35]. In this case, they may have a systemic effect and their properties not restricted to the mucosal environment. Experimental studies have shown that the human milk-derived acidic oligosaccharide fraction is able to enhance the production of certain cytokines as well as γ-interferon [36]. The same authors also demonstrated that some plant-derived oligosaccharides have a similar effect.

There are substantial differences in quality and quantity of HMOs among different nursing mothers, but it has not been determined whether there is a relationship between quantity and quality of HMOs and the presence of different bacterial species in the composition of intestinal microflora [33].

It has since been reported that human milk already has a probiotic effect as it also contains lactic acid bacteria. In this sense we could more properly talk of the synbiotic effect of human milk [37, 38].

6. PREBIOTICS IN INFANT FEEDS

Due to their complexity, oligosaccharides with an identical structure to HMOs are not available as dietary ingredients. Searching for alternatives, several mixtures of GOS and FOS have been tested. Inuline and oligofructose are safe inducers of a *Bifidus* flora, so it appears clear its use in infant feedings [39–41]. The most extensive experience is available for long-chain fructo-oligosaccharides obtained from chicory extract and galacto-oligosaccharides gained from enzymatic synthesis of lactose [42]. While in Europe these are the most common prebiotics added to infant formulas (10% inulin with 5–60 fructose monomers and 90% galacto-oligosaccharides 2–7 monomers), in Japan they use isomalto-oligosaccharides and xylo-oligosaccharides. Also, acidic oligosaccharides such as pectin hydrolysate are under investigation [43]. Structurally, the acidic

oligosaccharides of human milk are characterized by their content in sialic acid.

The formulas supplemented with a prebiotic mixture are reported to have multiple effects mediated through changes in the flora, the immune system and other mechanisms [44, 45].

It has been demonstrated an increase in the bifidobacteria and lactobacilli content in feces of term infants after 28 days of supplementation with a mixture FOS/GOS, in a dose-related mode (with 0.4 and 0.8 g/dL), compare to the levels seen in breast-fed infants (Figure 8.3) [20, 46].

In preterm infants of about 31 weeks' gestational age and about 1 week old, a double blind, randomized controlled study was performed comparing standard formula with a formula containing 1 g/dL of a prebiotic mixture. During the 28 days study period the number of fecal bifidobacteria and lactobacilli increased in the prebiotic formula group to levels seen in the breast-fed group, used as a control. The difference in composition of the fecal flora between the standard formula and the prebiotic formula group was highly significant. At the same time, a significant reduction in the total number of relevant pathogens in the fecal flora was found [47]. Moreover, stool consistency and stool frequency were similar in the breast-fed and the supplemented group [48, 49]. Stool characteristics in the group fed the supplemented formula were close to those found in the human milk. The authors postulate that prebiotic mixtures may help in improving intestinal tolerance to enteral feeding in preterm infants [50]. The prebiotic mixture might also have improved calcium absorption as indicated by a similar urinary Ca/P ratio in prebiotic-fed and breast-fed babies [51].

This change in flora was correlated with an increase in the metabolic activity (pH, lactate and short-chain fatty acid, (SCFA) production) [52]. Nineteen infants who received a prebiotic mixture of (GOS/FOS) 6 g/L, presented in the feces a higher fecal acetate ratio and lactate concentration and lower pH after 16 weeks than did the group receiving a standard formula or a formula

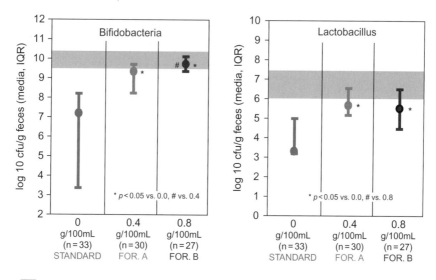

Reference range (IQR) in breast-fed infants (n = 15)

FIGURE 8.3   Modification in the amount of bifidobacteria and lactobacilli according to the amount of GOS+FOS in the formula (g/100 mL). Formula A: 0.4g/100mL. Formula B: 0.8g/100mL. Standard: non-supplements.

supplemented with *Bifidobacterium anima-lis* (6.0×10^{10} viable cells per liter) [53]. Using molecular biology techniques it was observed that the species of bifidobacteria present in infant-fed FOS/GOS supplemented formula corresponded with the patterns seen in breast-feeding. That is, *B. infantis*, *B. breve*, and *B. longum* as predominant in breast-fed and supplemented infants, while the infants receiving a standard formula have lower levels of *B. breve* and higher levels of *B. catenulatum* and *B. adolescentis* [54]. This shift in microflora was accompanied by a reduction in potential pathogens.

Early evidence led to the publication of a statement by the Scientific Committee on Food of the European Commission on 13 December 2001 in which the addition of the prebiotic mixture (10% FOS, 90% GOS) at a concentration of 0.8g/dL to infant formula was considered safe [55].

A few other studies have been done using only fructo-oligosaccharides (FOS). When used in infant formula at a concentration of 1.5g/L or 3.0g/L for 5 weeks FOS alone did not show

significant differences in fecal *Lactobacillus* or *Bifidobacterium* counts [56]. Furthermore, there were an increased number of adverse events (flatulence, spit-ups, and loose stools).

In 2004, the Committee on Nutrition of the European Society of Pediatric Gastroenterology, Hepatology and Nutrition pointed out that at that moment no conclusive recommendation could be done on the benefits of the addition of a prebiotic mixture to an infant formula. They suggested performing prospective clinical trials designed to show the clinical benefits of such an approach [57].

Since then, several new trials have been published (Table 8.2). The putative effect of prebiotic formulae on the immune system has been demonstrated by studies on the incidence of infections during the first year of life and on atopic dermatitis. In a prospective, randomized, placebo-controlled open trial, infants receiving the prebiotics mixture over a 12 month period have significantly fewer episodes of GI and respiratory tract infections [58, 59]. In another study in infants at risk for atopy, the use of the prebiotic formula

TABLE 8.2 Clinical trial on prebiotic supplementation in infant formulae

Authors (year)	Number of infants	Sub-groups	Prebiotic mixture	Length of the study	Results
Brunser (2006)	110 (12–24 m)	SF: 66 PF: 64	Oligofructose + inulin 0.45/dL	3 weeks	↑ bifidobacteria in feces after amoxicillin treatment
Moro (2006)	259	SF: 104 PF: 102	GOS + FOS 0.8 g/dL	6 months	↑ bifidobacteria in feces ↓ atopic dermatitis (9.8 vs 23.1%)
Bruzzese (2006)	281	SF: 145 PF: 136	GOS + FOS 0.8 g/dL	12 months	↓ acute diarrhea episodes (0.15 vs 0.28 episodes/infant) ↓ infants with diarrhea (17 vs 34%) ↓ respiratory tract infections (19 vs 35% infant with ≥ 3 infections) ↓ infants needing antibiotics (30 vs 49%)
Arslanoglu (2007)	206	SF: 130 PF: 129	GOS + FOS 0.8 g/dL	6 months	↓ number of infectious episodes ↓ respiratory tract infections ↓ infants needing antibiotics
Arslanoglu (2008)	134	SF: 68 PF: 66	GOS + FOS 0.8 g/dL	24 months	↓ number of allergic manifestations ↓ respiratory tract infections ↓ infants needing antibiotics
Mihatsch (2006)	20 prematures (GE: 24–31 weeks)	SF: 10 PF: 10	GOS + FOS 1 g/dL	14 days	Laxative effect. Decreased transit time

SF: Standard formula. PF: Prebiotic supplemented formula.

demonstrated a protective effect at 6 months [60]. In a follow-up at 2 years, there was still a lower incidence of allergic manifestations in the group of infants who received a prebiotic supplemented formula when compared with a standard one [61]. Potential mechanisms of the prebiotic effect may be by improving the gut barrier and enhancing fecal secretory IgA levels.

Beside the preventive effects on infections and allergic disorders, there may be other potential beneficial effects [62]. Mihatsch demonstrated in 20 preterm infants that the addition of 1 g/100 mL of GOS/FOS significantly reduced stool viscosity and accelerated gastrointestinal transport when compared with a placebo (maltodextrin) [63]. This may be an advantage if we could prove whether GOS/FOS facilitates enteral feeding advancement in these preterm infants. Further trials are required.

Inulin and oligofructose have also been studied in special infant formulae as well as in weaning foods for toddlers. Tolerance to increased fiber intake in the form of FOS as part of a weaning food has been well-documented. Its consumption led to more regular and softer stools as well as decreased frequency of symptoms associated with constipation [64].

A double blind study comparing a formula containing partially hydrolyzed protein, a high β-palmitic acid level, and non-digestible oligosaccharides demonstrated that, when compared with standard infant formula, it led to higher counts of bifidobacteria in the feces and was well-tolerated while supporting satisfactory growth [65]. Combinations of prebiotic oligosaccharides with pectin-derived acidic oligosaccharides also appear to be clinically safe and effective on modifying infant microbiota [66].

In 2008, Fanaro and colleagues published a paper giving the results on the supplementation with GOS (5 g/L) on follow-on formula for 18 weeks. The data indicate that this supplementation positively influences the bifidobacteria flora and the stool consistency during the supplementation period [67].

Although these were initially promising results, additional studies are needed in order to confirm the evidence of clinical benefits [68].

As more studies support the hypothesis that human milk has a synbiotic effect than exclusively a prebiotic one, there is an increased interest in demonstrating the safety and efficacy of combination or prebiotics plus probiotics both in the prevention of gastrointestinal infections and diarrhea, prevention of the onset of allergy, and usefulness in the treatment of atopic disease. Initial studies are on the way [69].

7. SIDE EFFECTS

Because the neonatal period is a critical period of development when microbes become established in the gastrointestinal tract, the long-term effects of manipulation of gut microbiota during this time are more amplified than effects of later manipulations. That is a reason for caution regarding perinatal and neonatal manipulation of the intestinal microflora [70].

Oligosaccharides are, in general, considered as very safe. Infants fed a prebiotic inulin/GOS mixture in an infant formula grew well, had a stable water balance, and did not show undesirable effects. Prebiotics are mostly not absorbed in the small bowel, exerting an osmotic effect in the intestinal lumen, and are fermented in the colon in short-chain fatty acids and gas. Prebiotics are usually well-tolerated, but if supplied in excessive amounts may have undesirable effects consisting of excessive flatus, borborygmi, abdominal pain, and diarrhea [71]. A worsening of the symptoms after the administration of up to 20 grams per day of FOS in adult patients with gastroesophageal reflux have been reported [72].

It seems clear that the tolerance is related to their nature, dose, individual sensitivity factors, and adaptation to chronic consumption. Total doses of less than 20 grams per day are well-tolerated [73].

8. REGULATION OF THE ADDITION OF PREBIOTICS TO INFANT FORMULAS

The Scientific Committee on Food of the European Union considered the addition of this oligosaccharide mixture (GOS 90% + FOS 10%) at 0.8 g/dL, when added to an infant formula, as safe [55]. This was confirmed in the last European Union Directives of December 2006 (Commission directive 2006/141/EC on infant formulae and follow-up formulae) [74]. The Scientific Panel on Dietetic Products, Nutrition and Allergies of the European Commission considered in 2004 that there is no evidence of benefits to infants from the addition of FOS (1.5 to 3.0 g/L) to infant formula, while reasons for safety concerns remain (prevalence of adverse events, including loose stools) [75].

9. CONCLUSIONS

One of the most challenging current research areas is the potential beneficial effect of prebiotics on the immune system of young infants [76, 77]. Prebiotics in early nutrition may have profound effects on the intestinal barrier, internal milieu and defense mechanisms. It has been well-established that a prebiotic mixture in infant formula has a bifidogenic effect. Are there long-term health benefits related to an early intervention? A few clinical studies report encouraging data on immune-mediated effects of prebiotic supplementation: less gastrointestinal and respiratory infections, less atopic dermatitis in the first years of life. It is probable that both effects are related. Clearly, additional research is needed on the optimal composition, dosage, and combinations of different oligosaccharides [78]. Moreover, should prebiotics be used in case of illness? Which are the effects of adding prebiotics to special infants' formulas? The functional effects of prebiotics on infant health and the long-term effects of different dietary prebiotics on adult health and gastrointestinal diseases need to be further studied in controlled intervention trials [79].

SUMMARY

- Based on experimental data there is evidence that prebiotic oligosaccharides can modulate the natural defense system against infection during infancy.
- It has been demonstrated that a mixture of fructo-oligosaccharides and galacto-oligosaccharides added to an infant formula (0.88 g/dL) significantly increases the number of bifidobacteria in feces in a dose-related way and reduces the number of pathogens when compared with unsupplemented formula.
- Clinical studies report encouraging data on immune-mediated effects of prebiotic supplementation: less gastrointestinal and respiratory infections, less atopic dermatitis at an early age.

References

1. Gill, S. R., Pop, M., DeBoy, R. T., et al. (2006). Metagenomic analysis of the human distal gut microbiome. *Science, 312*, 1355–1359.
2. Neish, A. S. (2009). Microbes in gastrointestinal health and disease. *Gastroenterology, 136*, 65–80.
3. Sonnenburg, J. L., Angenent, L. T., & Gordon, G. I. (2004). Getting a grip on things: How do communities of bacterial symbionts become established in our intestine? *Nature Immunology, 5*, 569–573.
4. Szépfalusi, Z. (2008). The maturation of the fetal and neonatal immune system. *The Journal of Nutrition, 138*, 1773S–1781S.
5. Holt, P. G., & Jones, C. A. (2000). The development of the immune system during pregnancy and early life. *Allergy, 55*, 688–697.
6. Calder, P. C., Krauss-Etschmann, S., de Jong, E. C., et al. (2006). Early nutrition and immunity. Progress and perspectives. *The British Journal of Nutrition, 96*, 774–790.
7. Hooper, L. V., Midtvedt, T., & Gordon, J. I. (2002). How host-microbial interations shape the nutrient environment of the mammalian intestine. *Annual Review of Nutrition, 22*, 283–307.

8. Bach, J. F. (2002). The effect of infections on susceptibility to autoimmune and allergic disease. *The New England Journal of Medicine, 347*, 911–920.

9. Renz, H., Blumer, N., Virna, S., et al. (2006). The immunological basis of the hygiene hypothesis. *Chemical Immunology and Allergy, 91*, 30–48.

10. Garofalo, R. P., & Goldman, A. S. (1999). Expression of functional immunomodulatory and anti-inflammatory factors in human milk. *Clinics in Perinatology, 26*, 361–367.

11. Goldman, A. S., Chheda, S., & Garoffalo, R. (1997). Spectrum of immunomodulating agents in human milk. *International Journal of Pediatric Hematology/Oncology, 4*, 491–497.

12. Gdalevich, M., Mimouni, D., David, M., & Mimouni, M. (2001). Breast-feeding and the onset of atopic dermatitis in childhood: A systematic review and meta-analysis of prospective studies. *Journal of the American Academy of Dermatology, 45*, 520–527.

13. Pettigrew, M., Khodaee, M., Gillespie, B., et al. (2003). Duration of breastfeeding, daycare and physician visits among infants 6 months and younger. *Annals of Epidemiology, 13*, 431–435.

14. Levy, J. (1998). Immunonutrition: The pediatric experience. *Nutrition, 14*, 641–647.

15. López Alarcón, M., Villalpando, S., & Fajardo, A. (1997). Breast-feeding lowers the frequency and duration of acute respiratory infection and diarrhea in infants under six months of age. *The Journal of Nutrition, 127*, 436–443.

16. Niers, L., Stasse-Wolthius, M., Rombouts, F. M., & Rijkers, G. T. (2007). Nutritional support for the infant's immune system. *Nutrition Reviews, 65*, 347–360.

17. Hord, H. G. (2007). Eukaryotic-microbiota crosstalk: Mechanisms for health benefits of prebiotics and probiotics. *Annual Review, 28*, 1–17.

18. Gibson, G. R., & Roberfroid, M. B. (1995). Dietary modulation of the human colonic microbiota: Introducing the concept of prebiotics. *The Journal of Nutrition, 125*, 1401–1412.

19. Delzenne, N. M. (2003). Oligosaccharides: State of the art. *The Proceedings of the Nutrition Society, 62*, 177–182.

20. Gibson, G. R., Beatty, E. R., Wang, X., & Cummings, J. H. (1995). Selective stimulation of Bifidobacteria in the human colon by oligofructose and inulin. *Gastroenterology, 108*, 975–982.

21. Cherbut, C. (2003). Motor effects of short-chain fatty acids and lactate in the gastrointestinal tract. *The Proceedings of the Nutrition Society, 62*, 95–99.

22. Tahiri, M., Tressol, J. C., Arnaud, J., et al. (2003). Effect of short-chain fructo-oligosaccharides on intestinal calcium absorption and calcium status in postmenopausal women: A stable-isotope study. *The American Journal of Clinical Nutrition, 77*, 449–457.

23. Pool-Zobel, B., Van Loo, J., Rowland, I., & Roberfroid, M. (2002). Experimental evidences on the potential of prebiotics fructans to reduce the risk of colon cancer. *The British Journal of Nutrition, 87*(Suppl. 2), S273–S281.

24. Wollowski, I., Rechkemmer, G., & Pool-Zobel, B. (2002). Protective role of probiotics and prebiotics in colon cancer. *The American Journal of Clinical Nutrition, 73*, 451S–455S.

25. López, H. W., Levrat-Verny, M. A., Coudray, C., et al. (2001). Class 2 resistant starches lower plasma and liver lipids and improve mineral retention in rats. *The Journal of Nutrition, 131*, 1283–1289.

26. Van Loo, J. A. E. (2004). The basis, the potential, and the emerging evidence. *Journal of Clinical Gastroenterology, 38*, S70–S75.

27. Guarner, F. (2007). Prebiotics in inflammatory bowel disease. *The British Journal of Nutrition, 98*(Suppl. 1), S85–S89.

28. Leenen, C. H. M., & Dieleman, L. A. (2007). Inulin and oligofructose in chronic inflammatory bowel disease. *The Journal of Nutrition, 137*, 2572S–2575S.

29. Duggan, C., Gannon, J., & Walker, W. A. (2002). Protective nutrients and functional foods for the gastrointestinal tract. *The American Journal of Clinical Nutrition, 75*, 789–808.

30. Lenoir-Wijnkoop, I., Sanders, M. E., Cabana, M. D., et al. (2007). Probiotic and prebiotic influence beyond the intestinal tract. *Nutrition Reviews, 65*, 469–489.

31. Harmsen, H. J., Wildeboer-Veloo, A. C., Raangs, G. C., et al. (2000). Analysis of intestinal flora development in breast-fed infants by using molecular identification and detection methods. *Journal of Pediatric Gastroenterology and Nutrition, 30*, 61–67.

32. Mountzouris, K. C., McCartney, A. L., & Gibson, G. R. (2002). Intestinal microflora of human infants and current trends for its nutritional modulation. *The British Journal of Nutrition, 87*, 405–420.

33. Coppa, G. V., Bruni, S., Morelli, L., et al. (2004). The first prebiotics in humans. Human milk oligosaccharides. *Journal of Clinical Gastroenterology, 38*, S80–S83.

34. Coppa, G. V., Pierani, P., Zampini, L., et al. (1999). Oligosaccharides in human milk during different phases of lactation. *Acta Paediatrica Supplement, 88*, 89–94.

35. Kunz, C., Rudloff, S., Baier, W., et al. (2000). Oligosaccharides in human milk: Structural, functional, and metabolic aspects. *Annual Review of Nutrition, 20*, 699–722.

36. Eiwegger, T., Schmitt, J., Boehm, G., et al. (2004). Human milk-derived oligosaccharides and plant-derived oligosaccharides stimulate cytokine production of cord blood T-cells *in vitro*. *Pediatric Research, 56*, 536–540.

37. Martín, R., Langa, S., Reviriego, C., et al. (2003). Human milk is a source of lactic acid bacteria for the infant gut. *The Journal of Pediatrics, 143*, 754–758.

38. Martín, R., Jiménez, E., Olivares, M., et al. (2006). *Lactobacillus salivarius* CECT 5713, a potential probiotic

strain isolated from infant feces and breast milk of a mother-child pair. *International Journal of Food Microbiology*, 112, 35–43.

39. Vandenplas, Y. (2002). Oligosaccharides in infant formula. *The British Journal of Nutrition*, 87, S293–S296.

40. Fanaro, S., Boehm, G., Garssen, J., et al. (2005). Galacto-oligosaccharides and long-chain fructo-oligosaccharides as prebiotics in infant formulas: A review. *Acta Paediatrica Supplement*, 94, 22–26.

41. Vitoria Miñana, I. (2007). Oligosacáridos en nutrición infantil: fórmula infantil, alimentación complementaria y del adolescente. *Acta Pediatrica Espanola*, 65, 175–179.

42. Boehm, G., Stahl, B., Garssen, J., et al. (2005). Prebiotics in infant formulas. Immune modulators during infancy. *Nutrafoods*, 4, 51–57.

43. Fanaro, S., Jelinek, J., Stahl, B., et al. (2005). Acidic oligosaccharides from pectin hydrolysate as new component for infant formulae: Effect on intestinal flora, stool characteristics, and pH. *Journal of Pediatric Gastroenterology and Nutrition*, 41, 186–190.

44. Veereman, G. (2007). Pediatric applications of inuline and oligofructose. *The Journal of Nutrition*, 137, 2585S–2589S.

45. Boehm, G., Jelinek, J., Stahl, B., et al. (2004). Prebiotics in infant formula. *Journal of Clinical Gastroenterology*, 38, S76–S79.

46. Moro, G., Minoli, I., Mosca, M., et al. (2002). Dosage-related bifidogenic effects of galacto- and fructo-oligosaccharides in formula-fed term infants. *Journal of Pediatric Gastroenterology and Nutrition*, 34, 291–295.

47. Knol, J., Boehm, G., Lidestri, M., et al. (2005). Increase of faecal bifidobacteria due to dietary oligosaccharides induces a reduction of clinically relevant pathogen germs in the faeces of formula-fed preterm infants. *Acta Paediatr*, 94(Suppl. 449), 31–33.

48. Boehm, G., Marini, A., & Jelinek, J. (2000). Bifidogenic oligosaccarides in a preterm formula. *Journal of Pediatric Gastroenterology and Nutrition*, 31(Suppl. 2), S26.

49. Boehm, G., Lidestri, M., Casetta, P., et al. (2002). Supplementation of a bovine milk formula with an oligosaccharide mixture increases counts of faecal bifidobacteria in preterm infants. *Archives of Disease in Childhood. Fetal and Neonatal Edition*, 86, F178–F181.

50. Boehm, G., Fanaro, S., Jelinek, J., et al. (2003). Prebiotic concept for infant nutrition. *Acta Paediatrica Supplement*, 441, 64–67.

51. Marini, A., Negretti, F., Boehm, G., et al. (2003). Pro- and prebiotics administration in preterm infants: Colonization and influence on faecal flora. *Acta Paediatrica Supplement*, 441, 80–81.

52. Knol, J., Scholtens, P., Kafka, C., et al. (2005). Colon microflora in infants fed formula with galacto- and fructo-oligosaccharides: More like breast-fed infants. *Journal of Pediatric Gastroenterology and Nutrition*, 40, 36–42.

53. Bakker-Zierikzee, A. M., Alles, M. S., Knol, J., et al. (2005). Effects of infant formula containing a mixture of galacto- and fructo-oligosaccharides or viable *Bifidobacterium animalis* on the intestinal microflora during the first 4 months of life. *The British Journal of Nutrition*, 94, 783–790.

54. Haarman, M., & Knol, J. (2005). Quantitative real-time PCR assays to identify and quantify fecal *Bifidobacterium* species in infants receiving a prebiotic infant formula. *Applied and Environmental Microbiology*, 71, 2318–2324.

55. EC Scientific Committee on Food. Additional statement on the use of resistant short chain carbohydrates (oligofructosyl-saccharose and oligogalactosyl-lactose) in infant formulae and in follow-on formulae. Brussels, 13 December 2001.

56. Euler, A. R., Mitchell, D. K., Kline, R., & Pickering, L. K. (2005). Prebiotic effect of fructo-oligosaccharide supplemented term infant formula at two concentrations compared with unsupplemented formula and human milk. *Journal of Pediatric Gastroenterology and Nutrition*, 40, 157–164.

57. Agostoni, C., Axelsson, I., Goulet, O., et al. (2004). ESPGHAN Committee on Nutrition. Prebiotic oligosaccharides in dietetic products for infants: A commentary by the ESPGHAN Committee on Nutrition. *Journal of Pediatric Gastroenterology and Nutrition*, 39, 465–473.

58. Bruzzese, E., Volpicelli, M., Salvini, F., et al. (2006). Effect of early administration of GOS/FOS on the prevention of intestinal and extra-intestinal infections in healthy infants. *Journal of Pediatric Gastroenterology and Nutrition*, 42, e95.

59. Arslanoglu, S., Moro, G. E., & Boehm, G. (2007). Early supplementation of prebiotics oligosaccharides protects formula-fed infants against infections during the first 6 months of life. *The Journal of Nutrition*, 137, 2420–2424.

60. Moro, G., Arslanoglu, S., Stahl, B., et al. (2006). A mixture of prebiotic oligosaccharides reduces the incidence of atopic dermatitis during the first six months of age. *Archives of Disease in Childhood*, 91, 814–819.

61. Arslanoglu, S., Moro, G. E., Schmitt, J., et al. (2008). Early dietary intervention with a mixture of prebiotics oligosaccharides reduces incidence of allergic manifestations and infections during the first two years of life. *The Journal of Nutrition*, 138, 1091–1095.

62. Brunser, O., Gotteland, M., Cruchet, S., et al. (2006). Effect of milk formula with prebiotics on the intestinal microbiota of infants after an antibiotic treatment. *Pediatric Research*, 59, 451–456.

63. Mihatsch, W. A., Hoegel, J., & Pohlandt, F. (2006). Prebiotic oligosaccharides reduce stool viscosity and accelerate gastrointestinal transport in preterm infants. *Acta Paediatrica*, 95, 843–848.

64. Moore, N., Chao, C., Yang, L. P., et al. (2003). Effects of fructo-oligosaccharide-supplemented infant

cereal: A double-blind, randomized trial. *The British Journal of Nutrition, 90,* 581–587.

65. Schmelzle, H., Wirth, S., Skopnik, H., et al. (2003). Randomized double-blind study of the nutritional efficacy and bifidogenicity of a new infant formula containing partially hydrolyzed protein, a high β-palmitic acid level, and nondigestible oligosaccharides. *Journal of Pediatric Gastroenterology and Nutrition, 36,* 343–351.

66. Magne, F., Wahiba, H., Suau, A., et al. (2008). Effects on faecal microbiota of dietary and acidic ologosaccharides in children during partial formula feeding. *Journal of Pediatric Gastroenterology and Nutrition, 46,* 580–588.

67. Fanaro, S., Marten, B., Bagna, R., et al. (2008). Galacto-oligosaccharides are bifidogenic and safe at weaning: A double-blind randomized multicenter study. *Journal of Pediatric Gastroenterology and Nutrition, 48,* 82–88.

68. Osborn, D. A., & Sinn, J. K. (2008). Prebióticos en neonatos para la prevención de la enfermedad alérgica y la hipersensibilidad alimentaria. La Biblioteca Cochrane Plus 2008 número 2 (available in http://www.update-software.com).

69. Chouraqui, J. P., Grathwohl, D., Labaune, J. M., et al. (2008). Assessment of the safety, tolerance, and protective effect against diarrhea of infant formulas containing mixtures of probiotics or probiotics and prebiotics in a randomized controlled trial. *The American Journal of Clinical Nutrition, 87,* 1365–1373.

70. Neu, J. (2007). Perinatal and neonatal manipulation of the intestinal microbiome: A note of caution. *Nutrition Reviews, 65,* 282–285.

71. Marteau, P., & Flourié, B. (2001). Tolerance to low-digestible carbohydrates: Symptomatology and methods. *The British Journal of Nutrition, 85*(Suppl.), S17–S21.

72. Piche, T., des Varannes, S. B., Sacher-Huvelin, S., et al. (2003). Colonic fermentation influences lower esophageal sphincter in gastroesophageal reflux disease. *Gastroenterology, 124,* 894–902.

73. Marteau, P., & Seksik, P. (2004). Tolerance of probiotics and prebiotics. *Journal of Clinical Gastroenterology, 38,* S67–S69.

74. Commission directive 2006/141/EC on infant formulae and follow-up formulae. Available from: http://ec.europa.eu/food.

75. Opinion of the Scientific Panel on Dietetc Products, Nutrition and Allergies on a request from the Commission relating to the safety and suitability for particular nutritional use by infants of fructooligosaccharides in infant formulae and follow-on formulae. Request No EFSA-Q-2003-020. Adopted on 19 February 2004. http://www.efsa.eu.int/p_diet_en.html.

76. Veereman-Wauters, G. (2005). Application of prebiotics in infant foods. *The British Journal of Nutrition, 93*(Suppl. 1), S57–S60.

77. Parracho, H., McCartney, A. L., & Gibson, G. R. (2007). Probiotics and prebiotics in infant nutrition. *The Proceedings of the Nutrition Society, 66,* 405–411.

78. Niers, L., Stasse-Wolthuis, M., Rombouts, F. M., & Rijkers, G. T. (2007). Nutritional support for the infant's immune system. *Nutrition Reviews, 65,* 347–360.

79. Aggett, P. J., Agostoni, C., Axelsson, I., et al. (2003). Nondigestible carbohydrates in the diets of infants and young children: A commentary by the ESPGHAN Committee on Nutrition. *Journal of Pediatric Gastroenterology and Nutrition, 36,* 329–337.

Prebiotics as Infant Foods

Gigi Veereman-Wauters

Pediatric Gastroenterology and Nutrition, Queen Paola Children's Hospital—ZNA,
Antwerp, Belgium

1. INTRODUCTION

Prebiotic fibers have been added to infant milk formulas in Japan for the last 20 years. In Europe, prebiotics were introduced into infant foods around the year 2000, with initially very little published scientific evidence to support their use. Since then, the body of scientific data suggesting positive health benefits for infants, and the scarcity of adverse events with the dosages consumed, have encouraged infant food manufacturers to offer prebiotic supplements. In this chapter, we will discuss the various forms of infant foods and the prebiotics used to supplement these foods. Emphasis will be placed on the available clinical studies in this age group.

2. HOW ARE INFANTS FED?

The natural alimentation of the newborn infant is breast milk. International recommendations are to breast-feed whenever possible. Specific programs have been implemented in many countries to encourage breast-feeding in hospital settings [1]. The best alternative for human milk is humanized formula milk, mostly based on cows' milk. Infant milk formula (IMF) is subject to stringent regulations for composition and hygiene [2]. Manufacturers seek to improve formulae to bring them closer to the gold standard: human milk. Numerous IMF are on the market: they vary in protein source (cows' milk, soy), degree of hydrolysis, types of carbohydrates and lipids. Some formulations are adapted to specific conditions such as prematurity, allergy, cholestasis, etc. Babies who are unable to feed orally need tube feeding. During the first year of life, IMF is mostly used for enteral feeding, later replaced by specially packaged enteral formulae for tube feeding.

The development of intestinal digestive capacity and oral-motor skills allows weaning around 4 months of age. However, since the increase in allergic diseases, the so-called 'allergic march' weaning to solid food is recommended around 6 months in babies with a family history of atopy [3]. Vegetables, fruit and complex carbohydrates are introduced gradually. Breast milk or IMF remain the sole protein source until the introduction of meat or fish around 8 months. A toddler should drink around 500 mL of milk-based products and be offered a variety of fresh fruit, vegetables and slow carbohydrates. In practice, the products consumed are IMF, full milk, milk products such as yogurt, cheeses, vegetables and fruit, pasta, bread, cereals, rice, cookies, etc. Some commercial products are suitable candidates for enrichment with prebiotics.

3. PREBIOTICS IN HUMAN BREAST MILK

Human breast milk contains both nutritive and non-nutritive factors. Its composition is highly adapted to the infant's needs: it varies with gestational age at birth, with the duration of lactation and individually. Breast milk fulfils all of the nutritional needs during the first weeks of life. In addition, the non-nutritive bioactive components have protective and stimulatory functions that are only partially elucidated. Breast milk contains a wide range of specific and non-specific anti-microbial factors, cytokines, anti-inflammatory substances, hormones, growth modulators and digestive enzymes. Protection from infections is secured by secretory IgA, IgM and IgG, lactoferrin, lysozyme, complement C3, leukocytes, lipids and fatty acids, antiviral mucins and GAG peptides [4]. It has been known for over a century that human milk contains a 'bifidus factor', meaning that human milk favors the development of a bifidus predominant flora. The non-digestible oligosaccharides in human milk (HMO) are considered to be the 'bifidus factor' [5, 6]; in other words and according to current definitions: the non-digestible HMO are the first prebiotics. Human milk is protective against infections [7] and also against atopy [8]. Both these characteristics might thus be at least attributed to the 'bifidus factor' or the HMO.

Human milk stimulates the growth of bifidobacteria because of this high oligosaccharide content [9]. In contrast, bovine milk, and thus formula, contains very little oligosaccharides.

Oligosaccharides are the third largest component of human milk: lactose content being 53–61 g/L, fat 30–50 g/L, oligosaccharides (with DP 3–50) 10–12 g/L and protein 810 g/L [10]. There are thousands of different HMO components. The HMO are predominantly neutral (90%) and low molecular weight molecules. Negatively charged acidic structures are 10%: acidic oligosaccharides (AOS) [9]. Their production depends on enzymes encoded by the genes associated with expression of the Lewis blood group system of the mother [11]. They inspired the addition of non-digestible oligosaccharides and inulin to infant food in order to foster a comparable bifidogenic effect. However, there is much more to the HMO than their prebiotic (bifidogenic) effect. Their anti-infective properties are mainly due to the demonstrated inhibition of pathogen binding to host cell ligands. Due to the similarity of HMO to epithelial cell surface carbohydrates, an inhibitory effect on the adhesion of pathogens to the cell surface is most likely but yet unproven in humans. Thus many functions of the HMO remain to be unveiled: their possible suppressive effect on pathogens, anti-inflammatory effects and direct immune regulatory effects in the gut. Since absorption is possible, putative systemic effects need consideration [12].

So far, the literature has mainly focused on the bifidogenic effects of prebiotics in infant foods and not on the other direct effects they may have.

4. THE RATIONALE FOR USING PREBIOTICS IN INFANT FOODS

The hypothesis behind initially supplementing infant foods with prebiotics was mostly to obtain a bifidogenic effect. Bifidobacteria were first described in 1899 as an essential part of the gut flora of breast-fed infants [13]. Fortunately the introduction of 90% galacto-oligosaccharides

(GOS)/10% inulin mixtures in formula in Europe did not lead to any noticeable side effects and was considered a successful innovation. The scientific rationale for recommending supplementation of prebiotics to infant foods is based on the effects on the flora and the consequences on the development of the immune system, although many effects of these are still insufficiently documented. Furthermore, it is probable that prebiotic supplementation has important direct effects, influences nutrient absorption and metabolic regulation.

Establishment of the intestinal flora soon after birth plays a crucial role in the development of the innate and adaptive immune system [14]. In normal circumstances, the newborn baby is inoculated by the mother's flora when passing through the birth canal. A diverse flora residing in the mother's vagina and intestine colonizes her baby. In the case of a cesarean section, this step obviously does not take place. Babies born through cesarean section harbor lower numbers of bifidobacteria and bacteroides and are more often colonized with *C. difficile* [15]. This may be the mechanism leading to a higher incidence of allergy as children born by cesarean section have a higher risk of asthma than those born by vaginal delivery, particularly children of allergic parents [16].

In the gastrointestinal (GI) system of breast-fed babies bifidobacteria are soon selected and become predominant. This situation remains until weaning. The introduction of formula or solid food immediately leads to diversification of the flora, which is reflected by alterations of stool color, consistency and odor. Formula fed babies harbor a varied flora consisting of bifidobacteria, *E. coli* and bacteroides [17–19]. Thus, infants are a unique age group in which the change is made from bifidus predominant to diverse flora.

The age when the change occurs is determined by the duration of exclusive breast-feeding and by the intake of prebiotic supplements. The aim of conserving a bifidogenic effect on the infant's intestinal flora is to counteract the current rise of allergic diseases [20] and to protect from GI infections [21]. The immune system of newborns is characterized by a Th2 profile, meaning that type 2 helper cells and their cytokines predominate. These generate IgE producing cells and eosinophilic stimulation leading to allergic inflammation [14]. A normal assemblage of intestinal bacteria promotes a Th1 response, restoring the balance towards tolerance [22]. Bifidobacteria induce a Th1 response [23]. Lack of adequate bacterial stimulation has been incriminated as the culprit for the increased incidence of allergic disease, also called the 'allergic march' [24]. However, the hygiene hypothesis does not account for changes related to the earlier, far more significant drop in infectious diseases. Therefore, it is now suggested to rather focus on differences in microbial exposure [24, 25].

Allergic and non-allergic children harbor different types of flora: non-allergic children having higher counts of aerobic bacteria, lactobacilli and bifidobacteria [26]. It appears that *Bifidobacterium bifidus* has stronger adhesive properties and may be specifically protective against allergy as opposed to *Bifidobacterium adolescentis* [27].

In addition to the favorable bifidogenic effects, prebiotics may have direct effects such as binding of pathogens [12], but the molecular structure will be determinant.

Inulin has been shown to improve calcium availability *in vitro* [28]. Oligofructose and inulin improve calcium absorption and bone mineralization in adolescents [29–31]. Although calcium absorption in infancy deserves attention, clinical studies are not yet available on this subject.

In adolescents it has also been shown that 8 g/d of a mixed short and long degree of polymerization inulin-type fructans have a favorable effect on body mass index (BMI) [32]. It has been claimed that breast-feeding protects against obesity in later life. However, the causative factor may be the lower protein content of human milk [33] and some epidemiological studies do not confirm an association between breastfeeding and overweight [34]. It is unclear at present whether early administration of the right prebiotics may protect against obesity.

Chains of mainly ↓(1–4) and ↓(1–6) linked galactose with terminal glucose DP = 2 to 7

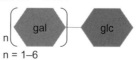

n = 1–6

FIGURE 9.1   Structure GOS.

5. TYPES OF PREBIOTICS STUDIED IN INFANTS

It has been impossible to reproduce the HMO contained in breast milk. The prebiotics that have been used in clinical studies in infants belong to the categories of inulin-type fructans (β-(2-1) linear fructans) and galacto-oligosaccharides 2–7 monomers, called GOS. GOS are supposed to mimic HMO. HMO contains galactose, glucose, N-acetylglucosamine, fucose or sialic acid as monosaccharide components. GOS are side products of lactose hydrolysis in fermented milk and milk products, containing β(1-4) and β(1-6) linked galactose with terminal glucose (Figure 9.1). The inulin type fructans are short chain (DP ≤ 4) oligofructose or long chain (DP = 5–60) inulin (HP), called FOS in commercial products. They are manufactured from chicory but are also present in many other plants such as artichokes, leeks, wheat and bananas (Figure 9.2). Mixtures have been used such as inulin/GOS: a combination of 10% inulin and 90% galacto-oligosaccharides and Synergy 1®: a combination of 30% oligofructose and 70% inulin HP, otherwise named oligofructose-enriched inulin.

Various other ingredients have been used (Table 9.1), and their effects are described in the following sections on clinical studies.

In France, a fermented milk formula was studied (fermentation with *Bifidobacterium breve* c50 and *Streptococcus thermophilus* 065) and it was argued that the (unidentified) metabolites resulting from the fermentation process are prebiotics [35].

Chains of ↓-1,2-glycosidic linked fructose with/without glucose

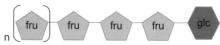

n = 1–4   : Oligofructose or fructo-oligosaccharides
n = 1–56 : Inulin (FOS)

FIGURE 9.2   Structure inulin/FOS.

TABLE 9.1   Prebiotics studied in infant

Prebiotic	Reference
Infant Milk Formula	
GOS	Japan since 1980
Fermented milk	[42]
Oligofructose	[39, 58]
AOS (no effect!)	[31]
Inulin/GOS (10:90)	[43–45]
Oligofructose/Inulin (50:50)	[49]
DX/GOS (50:50)	[33, 34]
PDX/GOS/Lactulose(50:33:17)	[33, 34]
Acidic/Neutral OS (20:80)	[32]
AOS/Inulin/GOS	[31]
ORS Solution	
Oligofructose (no effect!)	[62]
Cereals	
Oligofructose	[65–67]
Inulin/GOS (10:90)	[63]
Oligofructose/Inulin (70:30)	[69, 70]

AOS, acidic oligosaccharides; GOS, galacto-oligosaccharides; OS, oligosaccharides; PDX, polydextrose.

Since human milk contains 15 to 25% acidic oligosaccharides (AOS), a study was conducted comparing standard formula supplemented with either maltodextrin as control, 2 g/L AOS (obtained from pectin) or AOS plus 6 g/L inulin/GOS [36]. A prospective study on the immune effects of neutral and AOS in preterm infants is being conducted in the Netherlands [37].

Ziegler et al. conducted a randomized, double blind study to evaluate the tolerability and effect on infant growth of term newborns with a prebiotic blend of polydextrose (PDX) and GOS (50:50 ratio, 4 g/L), or formula supplemented with a prebiotic blend of PDX, GOS and lactulose in a 50:33:17 ratio (8 g/L) [38]. PDX, GOS and lactulose in various combinations and dosages (4 and 8 g/L) were also studied by Nakamura et al. [39].

6. CLINICAL STUDIES PERFORMED IN PRETERM INFANTS

Preterm infants are a particularly vulnerable group because many barrier functions and the immune system are still in a developmental phase. A few studies have been performed using prebiotics (Figure 9.3).

It was shown in preterm infants that the prebiotic mixture of inulin/GOS (10% inulin and 90% galacto-oligosaccharides) at a concentration of 1 g/L increases fecal bifidobacteria counts to the level of breast-fed infants [40, 41] and that their feces contain fewer colony-forming units/g of potential enteric pathogens [42].

Enrichment of formula for premature infants at 1 g/dL with the inulin/GOS mixture over 2 weeks lowers stool viscosity and shortens intestinal transit time measured with carmine red dye [43]. This finding is encouraging as it may facilitate the advancement of enteral feedings.

Kapiki et al. compared the effect of formula supplemented only with FOS (4 g/L) with a control formula. In the prebiotic-treated group, numbers of bifidobacteria in stool and the proportion of infants colonized with bifidobacteria were higher after 7 days compared with the control group; there was also a significantly higher number of *Bacteroides* spp. in the FOS group, daily stool frequency increased. Of note, weight gain during the study was significantly greater in the control group. The greater weight gain in the control group may well have been due to added maltodextrin, but this will require experimental confirmation by calculating the net caloric intakes [44].

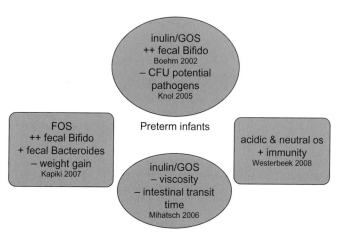

FIGURE 9.3   Clinical studies applying prebiotics in food for preterm infants.

At the time of writing, a large prospective study is being conducted in the Netherlands aiming at understanding the role of neutral and AOS in postnatal modulation of the immune response and postnatal adaptation of the gut [37]. Necrotizing enterocolitis (NEC) is a subject of interest in the premature infant. Probiotics may have a protective effect [45] but prebiotics have not yet been studied in preterm infants. In an animal model (quails) oligofructose supplementation enhanced the level of bifidobacteria, provided they were present, and decreased the number of clostridia, thereby protecting against NEC [46].

7. CLINICAL STUDIES PERFORMED IN TERM INFANTS

In Japan, IMF has been supplemented with GOS for over 20 years but no literature on the subject appears to be available. Local reports from a specific brand demonstrate increased counts of fecal bifidobacteria and lactobacilli with galactosyl-lactose supplements [35].

Many well-documented studies are available on the effect of IMF supplemented with the mixture of inulin/GOS (10% inulin and 90% galacto-oligosaccharides). After 28 days of supplementation, bifidus counts show a dose related increase (4 g/L and 8 g/L) and lactobacilli also significantly increase from baseline to levels seen in breast-fed babies. Moreover, the types of bifidobacteria and lactobacilli correspond with the patterns seen with breast-feeding [47–51].

The lower dosage of 4 g/L fails to always significantly increase the number of bifidobacteria [52].

A formula enriched with a mixture of FOS/inulin (50:50) at 8 g/L (Synergy 1®) from birth has comparable bifidogenic effects as inulin/GOS, demonstrated by fluorescence in situ hybridization (FISH) analysis of the stools, softens stools, is well-tolerated and allows normal growth [53]. A study in newborns with formula supplemented

with PDX and GOS (4 g/L) or PDX, GOS, lactulose at 4 and 8 g/L using various stool analysis techniques (culture-based selective enumeration, quantitative real-time PCR and FISH) showed only few significant changes in bacterial subpopulations at any time point. However, bacterial communities were less stable at a younger age, indicating that early administration is crucial in order to influence flora [39].

The shift towards breast-fed type flora is accompanied by a reduction in potential pathogens [51, 52, 54]. These changes in the bacterial populations and their metabolic activities lead to lower stool pH 8 and production of short-chain fatty acid (SCFA) profiles comparable to breast-fed infants, with higher acetate and lower propionate levels [42] or higher acetate and lactate levels [55]. This last report, however, fails to demonstrate a superior bifidogenic effect compared to standard formula [55].

A consistent clinical effect obtained by prebiotic formula is softer stools [48]. It's unclear whether this is due to the flora shift, to an osmotic effect, to SCFA or to all of the above. The putative effect of prebiotic formula on the immune system has been demonstrated by studies on the incidence of infections and on atopic dermatitis during the first 2 years of life. In a prospective, randomized, placebo controlled open trial, infants receiving the inulin/GOS mixture over a 12-month period had significantly less episodes of GI and respiratory tract infections [21]. A partial hydrolysate enriched with the same prebiotic mixture taken for 6 months also decreased the number of infections at 1 [56] and even 2 years [57].

A prospective, double blind, randomized placebo controlled study in infants at risk for atopy brilliantly demonstrated a protective effect of the inulin/GOS enriched hydrolyzed formula at 6 months when compared with a maltodextrine containing formula [58]. After 6 months, fewer infants in the prebiotic treated group had atopic dermatitis compared to the controls based on a validated clinical quantitative index. However, there was a relatively high dropout rate of 20.5%. Arslanoglu et al. reported the results of a follow-up of this study until 2 years of life. The cumulative incidence of atopic dermatitis, recurrent wheezing and allergic urticaria were higher in the maltodextrin group than in the prebiotic group [57]. However, in another study, supplementation with PDX/GOS led to significant eczema [58]. Therefore, a Cochrane analysis concluded in 2007 that the evidence does not confirm that prebiotics protect against allergic disease [59].

Potential mechanisms of the prebiotic effect may be improved gut barrier, as was shown to be the case [60]. The prebiotic mixture also enhances fecal secretory IgA levels [51, 61].

A short prospective, randomized, crossover intervention with 1.5 grams and 3 grams oligofructose/L formula showed a laxative effect of the higher dose but failed to document alterations in fecal flora. However, 1 week intervention may have been too short to permit changes in the species composition and metabolic activities of the GI bacteria [62].

Infants fed the prebiotic inulin/GOS mixture [41] or oligofructose alone [63] in formula grow well, have a stable water balance and no noted undesirable side effects.

Studies using formula milk fermented with *Bifidobacterium breve* c50 and *Streptococcus thermophilus* 065 demonstrated a bifidogenic effect [64] and decreased severity of acute gastroenteritis but no effect on incidence [65].

Studies with PDX/GOS/lactulose showed normal weight gain and growth. Stools were looser in the supplemented groups compared with the control formula days. Diarrhea was higher in the PDX/GOS group, eczema was significantly higher in the PDX/GOS group (see earlier) and irritability was significantly higher in the PDX/GOS/lactulose group. The most frequent reason given for withdrawal from the study was gas, particularly in the PDX/GOS/lactulose group [38].

The combination of AOS/inulin/GOS has the same effects on intestinal flora, fecal pH and stool consistency as the classical inulin/GOS mixture. AOS alone is well tolerated but has no clinical effect. Infants grew well with all supplements [36].

In conclusion, prebiotic formulas for term infants are reported to have multiple positive effects mediated through changes in the flora, the immune system and other mechanisms (Figure 9.4).

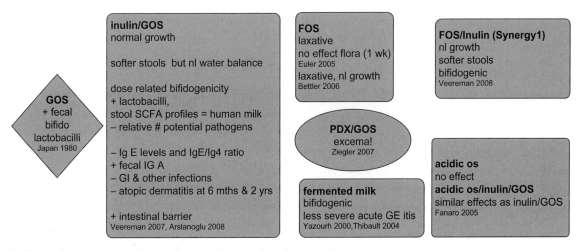

FIGURE 9.4 Clinical studies applying prebiotics in food for term infants.

Another approach has been the addition of prebiotics to oral rehydration solution (ORS) for acute diarrhea. However, a mixture of FOS and inulin added to ORS in the treatment of acute infectious diarrhea with mild or moderate dehydration failed to show any significant benefit [66].

8. CLINICAL STUDIES PERFORMED IN TODDLERS

Toddlers take a variety of solid foods which allows the addition of prebiotics to cereals or other prepared food or beverages (Figure 9.5).

The addition of the inulin/GOS mixture in weaning foods of 4- to 6-month-old infants in a daily dose of 4.5 grams over 6 weeks succeeds in increasing the bifidus population from 43 to 57% of the fecal flora. This change was significantly different from the non-supplemented group [67]. The inulin/GOS mixture administered to healthy toddlers in daily amounts of 4.5 grams results in SCFA patterns with higher acetate and lower butyrate [68].

The combination of inulin and oligofructose has been studied more often in weaning food

after the first year of life. Clinical effects suggest improved immune response, as indicated by a lower incidence of febrile episodes. Inulin and oligofructose are bifidogenic and decrease the number of some pathogens. A study by Saavedra and Tschernia performed in 1999 first reported the effect of oligofructose (up to 3 grams daily) in weaning foods consumed by toddlers attending day care. These otherwise healthy toddlers had softer stools, less emesis, regurgitation and perceived discomfort and interestingly fewer fever episodes [69]. A similar set-up in toddlers attending day care and taking 2 grams oligofructose daily for 3 weeks confirmed a protective effect against fever. These toddlers also had fewer infectious episodes requiring antibiotic treatment, fewer episodes of diarrhea and emesis, less flatulence. Fecal microbial analysis confirmed the suspected bifidogenic effect during supplementation. Simultaneously clostridia counts dropped and both shifts subsided after a 2-week washout period [70]. Moore showed that an average daily consumption of 0.74 grams oligofructose (max 3 g) succeeds in softening stools but observed no alterations in other GI symptoms [71].

Prebiotics have been tested in disease states such as diarrhea. In breast-fed Peruvian children

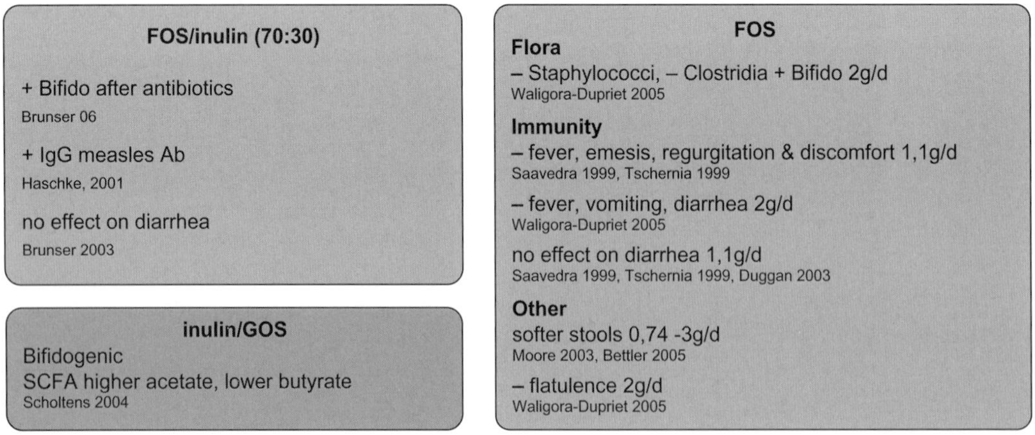

FIGURE 9.5   Clinical studies applying prebiotics in food for toddlers.

no effect was seen on the incidence of diarrhea by adding oligofructose to cereals, with or without Zn [72].

A mixture of oligofructose and inulin (70/30 Prebio 1®) at 2.25 g/d for 3 weeks is protective of the bifidus flora during amoxicillin treatment. Prebiotic treatment did not cause any GI symptoms but also did not alter stool frequency or consistency [73]. The same Prebio 1® mixture was shown to enhance antibody response to measles vaccination when given 4 weeks before. No effect was seen on GI tolerance [74].

9. PREBIOTICS IN DIFFERENT TYPES OF INFANT FOODS

More than 400 general prebiotic food products are on the market. Currently, infant foods with prebiotics are marketed mostly in Asia and Europe. IMF has been enriched with prebiotics in Japan since the 1980s [75]. More than 400 general prebiotic food products are on the market. Regulations regarding food ingredients vary by country. Overall, health claims need to be validated.

The addition of a mixture of 10% inulin and 90% galacto-oligosaccharides in a concentration of 0.8 g/dL to infant formula was recognized safe by the European Commission in December 2001. This was confirmed in the last EU Directives of December 2006 (Commission Directive 2006/141/EC on infant formulae and follow-up formulae [76]) with the following wording in Annex 1: 'fructo-oligosaccharides and galacto-oligosaccharides may be added to infant formula ... their content shall not exceed 0.8 g/% in a combination of 90% oligogalactosyl-lactose and 10% high molecular weight fructosyl-saccharose ... other combinations may be used.' The document further mentions in article 5: 'the formula is manufactured from protein sources ... and other food ingredients ... whose suitability for particular nutritional use by infants from

birth has been established by generally accepted scientific data.'

In the USA, the FDA's Center for Food Safety and Applied Nutrition (CFSAN) regulates probiotics and prebiotics marketed as dietary supplement or food ingredients. The product Vivinal GOS (Friesland Foods Domo) received GRAS status (generally recognized as safe) from the US Food and Drug Administration (FDA) in September 2008 [77]. As a result, Vivinal GOS could be used in infant formula and other food categories. Vivinal GOS contains GOS, lactose, glucose, and a small amount of galactose [78].

The demand and interest for prebiotics in general, and in infant foods in particular, is growing rapidly from a small base and is a potentially high revenue market. For young infants, prebiotics could be incorporated in IMF of different types, in enteral feeding formulae, in ORS or other fluids. After weaning, potential vehicles are breakfast cereals, baked goods and any type of prepared fruit or vegetable meal.

A key benefit of prebiotics is that they are easier to include in formula and transitions food than probiotics. This is why they perhaps have a greater market potential for infant and toddler foods that must be sterilized.

10. SAFETY

At the reported dosages (under 1 g/L) most prebiotics have a laxative effect in infant and toddlers but have not caused dehydration. Fermentation causes gas production and generates SCFA. Flatulence was reported to be an inconvenience in only one study [38]. Overall, prebiotic supplementation is very well tolerated by infants and toddlers. The effect of increased luminal SCFA has not been well addressed so far. An animal model (rats) was used to explore the effect of high luminal concentration of organic acids, based on the hypothesis that intestinal barrier function may be compromised. Neonatal rats were fed a mixture of inulin/GOS/Inulin, 12:88 at 5.6 g/L from the seventh day of life until weaning. Luminal concentrations of acetate and lactate increased but intestinal flora, permeability and tight junctions remained unaltered. However, GOS/inulin supplementation was associated with increased bacterial translocation towards the spleen [79]. These findings prompt a cautious approach especially in patients with immature gut.

11. CONCLUSIONS

The addition of prebiotics to infant foods has generated enthusiasm because 'the bifidus factor' from breast milk can be reproduced. Enriched IMF offers practical solutions in daily clinical practice for the treatment of hard stools. However, the effects of prebiotic supplementation may be far more profound by modulating the immune system in a beneficial way, thereby reducing the incidence of infections and atopy. At this time, the longest follow-up is 2 years and limited to a single study [57]. All reported intervention studies are short-term.

Particular attention should be paid to the specific type of prebiotic used, as it is clear from the current data that results of clinical studies with a particular ingredient may not be extrapolated. The desired 'bifidogenic effect' of prebiotics is probably only the top of the iceberg as each structure may have direct effects (e.g. binding of pathogens). Therefore, prebiotics cannot be viewed merely as a 'pro-drug' for probiotics. Our considerations of these food supplements for infants should not be any different than our considerations of bioactive drugs, especially since important health claims, such as immune modulation, are put forward. Dosages, clarity about composition and possible side effects need careful attention.

References

1. de Boer, A. S., & Darnton-Hill, I. (1994). A good start in life: Breast-feeding in hospital. *World Health Forum, 15,* 66–68.

2. Koletzko, B., Baker, S., Cleghorn, G., et al. (2005). Global standard for the composition of infant formula: recommendations of an ESPGHAN coordinated international expert group. *Journal of Pediatric Gastroenterology and Nutrition, 41,* 584–599.

3. Fiocchi, A., Assa'ad, A., & Bahna, S. (2006). Food allergy and the introduction of solid foods to infants: A consensus document. Adverse Reactions to Foods Committee, American College of Allergy, Asthma and Immunology *Ann Allergy Asthma Immunol, 97,* 10–20; quiz 21, 77.

4. Prentice, A. (1996). The constituents of human milk. In T. U. N. U. Press (Ed.), *Food and Nutrition Bulletin.* Tokyo, Boston: United Nations University.

5. Mata, L. J., & Wyatt, R. G. (1971). The uniqueness of human milk. Host resistance to infection. *The American Journal of Clinical Nutrition, 24,* 976–986.

6. Kunz, C., Rudloff, S., Baier, W., et al. (2000). Oligosaccharides in human milk: Structural, functional, and metabolic aspects. *Annual Review of Nutrition, 20,* 699–722.

7. Howie, P. W., Forsyth, J. S., Ogston, S. A., et al. (1990). Protective effect of breast feeding against infection. *BMJ (Clinical Research edn.), 300,* 11–16.

8. Rothenbacher, D., Weyermann, M., Beermann, C., & Brenner, H. (2005). Breastfeeding, soluble CD14 concentration in breast milk and risk of atopic dermatitis and asthma in early childhood: birth cohort study. *Clinical and Experimental Allergy, 35,* 1014–1021.

9. Stahl, B., Thurl, S., Zeng, J., et al. (1994). Oligosaccharides from human milk as revealed by matrix-assisted laser desorption/ionization mass spectrometry. *Analytical Biochemistry, 223,* 218–226.

10. Newburg, D. S., & Neubauer, S. H. (1995). Handbook of milk composition. Academic Press.

11. Newburg, D. S., Ruiz-Palacios, G. M., & Morrow, A. L. (2005). Human milk glycans protect infants against enteric pathogens. *Annual Review of Nutrition, 25,* 37–58.

12. Kunz, C., & Rudloff, S. (2008). Potential anti-inflammatory and anti-infectious effects of human milk oligosaccharides. *Advances In Experimental Medicine and Biology, 606,* 455–465.

13. Tissier, H. (1899). *Societe De Biologie, 51,* 943–945.

14. Kirjavainen, P., & Gibson, G. R. (1999). Healthy gut microflora and allergy: Factors influencing development of the microbiota. *Annales Medicinae, 31,* 288–292.

15. Penders, J., Thijs, C., Vink, C., et al. (2006). Factors influencing the composition of the intestinal microbiota in early infancy. *Pediatrics, 118,* 511–521.

16. Roduit, C., Scholtens, S., de Jongste, J. C., et al. (2009). Asthma at 8 years of age in children born by caesarean section. *Thorax, 64,* 107–113.

17. Harmsen, H. J. M., Wildeboer-Veloo, A. C. M., Raangs, G. C., et al. (2000). Analysis of intestinal flora development in breast-fed and formula-fed infants by using

molecular identification and detection methods. *Journal of Pediatric Gastroenterology and Nutrition, 30,* 61–67.

18. Langhendries, J., Paquay, T., Hannon, M., & Darimont, J. (1998). Acquisition de la flore intestinale néonatale: rôle sur la morbidité et perspectives thérapeutiques. *Archives de Pédiatrie, 5,* 644–653.

19. Storla, P., & Lee, A. (1982). The microbial ecology of the large bowel of breast-fed and formula-fed infants during the first year of life. *Journal of Medical Microbiology, 15,* 189–203.

20. Asher, M. I., Montefort, S., Bjorksten, B., et al. (2006). Worldwide time trends in the prevalence of symptoms of asthma, allergic rhinoconjunctivitis, and eczema in childhood: ISAAC Phases One and Three repeat multi-country cross-sectional surveys. *Lancet, 368,* 733–743.

21. Bruzzese, E., Volpicelli, M., Squeglia, V., et al. (2009). A formula containing galacto- and fructo-oligosaccharides prevents intestinal and extra-intestinal infections: An observational study. *Clinical Nutrition, 28,* 156–161.

22. Sudo, N., Sawamura, S., Tanaka, K., et al. (1997). The requirement of intestinal bacterial flora for the development of an IgE production system fully susceptible to oral tolerance induction. *Journal of Immunology, 159,* 1739–1745.

23. Hessle, C., Andersson, B., & Wold, A. E. (2000). Gram-positive bacteria are potent inducers of monocytic interleukin-12 (IL-12) while gram-negative bacteria preferentially stimulate IL-10 production. *Infection and Immunity, 68,* 3581–3586.

24. Strachan, D. P. (2000). Family size, infection and atopy: The first decade of the 'hygiene hypothesis'. *Thorax, 55*(Suppl. 1), S2–S10.

25. Bloomfield, S. F., Stanwell-Smith, R., Crevel, R. W., & Pickup, J. (2006). Too clean, or not too clean: The hygiene hypothesis and home hygiene. *Clinical and Experimental Allergy, 36,* 402–425.

26. Bjorksten, B., Sepp, E., Julge, K., et al. (2001). Allergy development and the intestinal microflora during the first year of life. *The Journal of Allergy and Clinical Immunology, 108,* 516–520.

27. He, F., Ouwehand, A., Isolauri, E., et al. (2001). Comparison of mucosal adhesion and species identification of bifidobacteria isolated from healthy and allergic infants. *FEMS Immunology and Medical Microbiology, 30,* 43–47.

28. Bosscher, D., Van Caillie-Bertrand, M., Van Cauwenbergh, R., & Deelstra, H. (2003). Availabilities of Calcium, Iron, and Zinc from dairy infant formulas is affected by soluble dietary fibers and modified starch fractions. *Nutrition, 19,* 641–645.

29. van den Heuvel, E., Muys, T., van Dokkum, W., & Schaafsma, G. (1999). Oligofructose stimulates calcium absorption in adolescents. *The American Journal of Clinical Nutrition, 69,* 544–548.

30. Griffin, I. J., Davila, P. M., & Abrams, S. A. (2002). Non-digestible oligosaccharides and calcium absorption in girls with adequate calcium intakes. *The British Journal of Nutrition, 87*(Suppl. 2), S187–S191.

31. Abrams, S. A., Griffin, I. J., Hawthorne, K. M., et al. (2005). A combination of prebiotic short- and long-chain inulin-type fructans enhances calcium absorption and bone mineralization in young adolescents. *The American Journal of Clinical Nutrition, 82,* 471–476.

32. Abrams, S. A., Griffin, I. J., Hawthorne, K. M., & Ellis, K. J. (2007). Effect of prebiotic supplementation and calcium intake on body mass index. *Journal of Pediatric, 151,* 293–298.

33. Koletzko, B., von Kries, R., Monasterolo, R. C., et al. (2009). Can infant feeding choices modulate later obesity risk? *The American Journal of Clinical Nutrition, 89,* 1530S–1532S.

34. Neutzling, M. B., Hallal, P. R., Araujo, C. L., et al. (2009). Infant feeding and obesity at 11 years: Prospective birth cohort study. *International Journal of Pediatric Obesity,* 1–7.

35. Ghisoefi, J. (2003). Dietary fibre and prebiotics in infant formulas. *Proceedings of the Nutrition Society, 62,* 183–185.

36. Fanaro, S., Jelinek, J., Stahl, B., et al. (2005). Acidic oligosaccharides from pectin hydrolysate as new component for infant formulae: Effect on intestinal flora, stool characteristics, and pH. *Journal of Pediatric Gastroenterology and Nutrition, 41,* 186–190.

37. Westerbeek, E. A., van Elburg, R. M., van den Berg, A., et al. (2008). Design of a randomised controlled trial on immune effects of acidic and neutral oligosaccharides in the nutrition of preterm infants: Carrot study. *BMC Pediatrics, 8,* 46.

38. Ziegler, E., Vanderhoof, J. A., Petschow, B., et al. (2007). Term infants fed formula supplemented with selected blends of prebiotics grow normally and have soft stools similar to those reported for breast-fed infants. *Journal of Pediatric Gastroenterology and Nutrition, 44,* 359–364.

39. Nakamura, N., Gaskins, H. R., Collier, C. T., et al. (2009). Molecular ecological analysis of fecal bacterial populations from term infants fed formula supplemented with selected blends of prebiotics. *Applied and Environmental Microbiology, 75,* 1121–1128.

40. Boehm, G., Lidestri, M., Casetta, P., et al. (2002). Supplementation of a bovine milk formula with an oligosaccharide mixture increases counts of faecal bifidobacteria in preterm infants. *Archives of Disease in Childhood. Fetal and Neonatal Edition, 86,* F178–F181.

41. Schmelzle, H., Wirth, S., Skopnik, H., et al. (2003). Randomized double-blind study of the nutritional efficacy and bifidogenicity of a new infant formula containing partially hydrolyzed protein, a high beta-palmitic acid level, and non-digestible oligosaccharides. *Journal of Pediatric Gastroenterology and Nutrition, 36,* 343–351.

B. PREBIOTICS IN HEALTH PROMOTION

42. Knol, J., Boehm, G., Lidestri, M., et al. (2005). Increase of faecal bifidobacteria due to dietary oligosaccharides induces a reduction of clinically relevant pathogen germs in the faeces of formula-fed preterm infants. *Acta Paediatrica (Oslo, Norway: 1992). Supplement, 94*, 31–33.

43. Mihatsch, W. A., Hoegel, J., & Pohlandt, F. (2006). Prebiotic oligosaccharides reduce stool viscosity and accelerate gastrointestinal transport in preterm infants. *Acta Paediatrica, 95*, 843–848.

44. Kapiki, A., Costalos, C., Oikonomidou, C., et al. (2007). The effect of a fructo-oligosaccharide supplemented formula on gut flora of preterm infants. *Early Human Development, 83*, 335–339.

45. Alfaleh, K., & Bassler, D. (2008). Probiotics for prevention of necrotizing enterocolitis in preterm infants. Cochrane Database Syst Rev: CD005496.

46. Butel, M. J., Waligora-Dupriet, A. J., & Szylit, O. (2002). Oligofructose and experimental model of neonatal necrotising enterocolitis. *The British Journal of Nutrition, 87*(Suppl. 2), S213–S219.

47. Haarman, M., & Knol, J. (2006). Quantitative real-time PCR analysis of fecal Lactobacillus species in infants receiving a prebiotic infant formula. *Applied and Environmental Microbiology, 72*, 2359–2365.

48. Moro, G., Minoli, I., Mosca, M., et al. (2002). Dosage-related bifidogenic effects of galacto- and fructooligosaccharides in formula-fed term infants. *Journal of Pediatric Gastroenterology and Nutrition, 34*, 291–295.

49. Haarman, M., & Knol, J. (2005). Quantitative real-time PCR assays to identify and quantify fecal Bifidobacterium species in infants receiving a prebiotic infant formula. *Applied and Environmental Microbiology, 71*, 2318–2324.

50. Knol, J., Scholtens, P., Kafka, C., et al. (2005). Colon microflora in infants fed formula with galacto- and fructo-oligosaccharides: More like breast-fed infants. *Journal of Pediatric Gastroenterology and Nutrition, 40*, 36–42.

51. Scholtens, P. A., Alliet, P., Raes, M., et al. (2008). Fecal secretory immunoglobulin A is increased in healthy infants who receive a formula with short-chain galacto-oligosaccharides and long-chain fructo-oligosaccharides. *Journal of Nutrition, 138*, 1141–1147.

52. Costalos, C., Kapiki, A., Apostolou, M., & Papathoma, E. (2008). The effect of a prebiotic supplemented formula on growth and stool microbiology of term infants. *Early Human Development, 84*, 45–49.

53. Veereman, G., Staelens, S., Van de Broek, H., et al. (2008). *Physiological and bifidogenic effects of prebiotic supplements in infant formula.* Iguassu, Brasil: World Congres Of Pediatric Gastroenterology Hepatology and Nutrition.

54. Knol, J., Boehm, G., Lidestri, M., et al. (2005). Increase of faecal bifidobacteria due to dietary oligosaccharides induces a reduction of clinically relevant pathogen germs in the faeces of formula-fed preterm infants. *Acta Paediatr, 94*(Suppl. 449), 31–33.

55. Bakker-Zierikzee, A. M., Alles, M. S., Knol, J., et al. (2005). Effects of infant formula containing a mixture of galacto- and fructo-oligosaccharides or viable *Bifidobacterium animalis* on the intestinal microflora during the first 4 months of life. *The British Journal of Nutrition, 94*, 783–790.

56. Arslanoglu, S., Moro, G. E., & Boehm, G. (2007). Early supplementation of prebiotic oligosaccharides protects formula-fed infants against infections during the first 6 months of life. *Journal of Nutrition, 137*, 2420–2424.

57. Arslanoglu, S., Moro, G. E., Schmitt, J., et al. (2008). Early dietary intervention with a mixture of prebiotic oligosaccharides reduces the incidence of allergic manifestations and infections during the first two years of life. *Journal of Nutrition, 138*, 1091–1095.

58. Moro, G., Arslanoglu, S., Stahl, B., et al. (2006). A mixture of prebiotic oligosaccharides reduces the incidence of atopic dermatitis during the first six months of age. *Archives of Disease in Childhood, 91*, 814–819.

59. Osborn, D. A., & Sinn, J. K. (2007). Prebiotics in infants for prevention of allergic disease and food hypersensitivity. Cochrane Database Syst Rev: CD006474.

60. Francavilla, R., Castellaneta, S., Masciale, A., et al. (2006). Intestinal permeability and faecal flora of infants fed with prebiotic supplemented formula: A double blind placebo controlled study. *Journal of Pediatric Gastroenterology and Nutrition, 42*, PN2–PN21.

61. Bakker-Zierikzee, A. M., Tol, E. A., Kroes, H., et al. (2006). Faecal SIgA secretion in infants fed on pre- or probiotic infant formula. *Pediatric Allergy and Immunology, 17*, 134–140.

62. Euler, A., Mitchell, D., Kline, R., & Pickering, L. (2005). Prebiotic effect of fructo-oligosaccharide supplemented term infant formula at two concentrations compared with unsupplemented formula and human milk. *Journal of Pediatric Gastroenterology and Nutrition, 40*, 157–164.

63. Bettler, J., & Euler, A. (2006). An evaluation of the growth of term infants fed formula supplemented with fructo-oligosaccharide. *International Journal of Probiotics and Prebiotics, 1*, 19–26.

64. Yazourh, A., Mullie, C., Leroux, B., Romond, C., & Romond, M. B. (2000). [Probiotic effect on reproduction of intestinal flora of the infant]. *Arch Pediatr, 7*(Suppl. 2), 244s–246s.

65. Thibault, H., Aubert-Jacquin, C., & Goulet, O. (2004). Effects of long-term consumption of a fermented infant formula (with *Bifidobacterium breve* c50 and *Streptococcus thermophilus* 065) on acute diarrhea in healthy infants. *Journal of Pediatric Gastroenterology and Nutrition, 39*, 147–152.

66. Hoekstra, J. H., Szajewska, H., Zikri, M. A., et al. (2004). Oral rehydration solution containing a mixture of

non-digestible carbohydrates in the treatment of acute diarrhea: A multicenter randomized placebo controlled study on behalf of the ESPGHAN working group on intestinal infections. *Journal of Pediatric Gastroenterology and Nutrition, 39,* 239–245.

67. Scholtens, P. A., Alles, M. S., Bindels, J. G., et al. (2006). Bifidogenic effects of solid weaning foods with added prebiotic oligosaccharides: a randomised controlled clinical trial. *Journal of Pediatric Gastroenterology and Nutrition, 42,* 553–559.

68. Scholtens, P., Alles, M., Van der Linde, E. G. M., et al. (2004). Addition of prebiotic oligosaccharides to solid weaning foods affects the metabolic activity of the intestinal micoflora. *Journal of Pediatric Gastroenterology and Nutrition, 39,* S12–S13.

69. Saavedra, J. M., & Tschernia, A. (2002). Human studies with probiotics and prebiotics: clinical implications. *British Journal of Nutrition, 87,* S241–S246.

70. Waligora-Dupriet, A. J., Campeotto, F., Nicolis, I., et al. (2007). Effect of oligofructose supplementation on gut microflora and well-being in young children attending a day care centre. *International Journal of Food Microbiology, 113,* 108–113.

71. Moore, N., Chao, C., Yang, L.-P., et al. (2003). Effects of fructo-oligosaccharide-supplemented infant cereal: A double-blind, randomized trial. *British Journal of Nutrition, 90,* 581–587.

72. Duggan, C., Penny, M., Hibberd, P., et al. (2003). Oligofructose-supplemented infant cereal: 2 randomized, blinded, community-based trials in Peruvian infants. *The American Journal of Clinical Nutrition, 77,* 937–942.

73. Brunser, O., Gotteland, M., Cruchet, S., et al. (2006). Effect of a milk formula with prebiotics on the intestinal microbiota of infants after an antibiotic treatment. *Pediatric Research, 59,* 451–456.

74. Firmansyah, A., Pramita, G., Carrie Fassler, A., et al. (2001). Improved humoral response to measles vaccine in infants receiving infant cereal with fructo-oligosaccharides. *Journal of Pediatric Gastroenterology and Nutrition, 31,* A521.

75. Consulting, U. The World Prebiotic Market. <http://www.ubic-consulting.com/food/ingredient/chemical-industries/world-prebiotics-market.html >

76. Commission directive (2006) 2006/141/EC on infant formulae and follow-up formulae.

77. Starling, S. (2008). Prebiotic wins GRAS approval, <http://www.nutraingredients-usa.com/Regulation/Prebiotic-wins-GRAS-approval >

78. Product portfolio. <http://www.vivinalgos.com/index.php?id = 20 >

79. Barrat, E., Michel, C., Poupeau, G., et al. (2008). Supplementation with galactooligosaccharides and inulin increases bacterial translocation in artificially reared newborn rats. *Pediatric Research, 64,* 34–39.

Prebiotics in the Gastrointestinal Tract

Sandra Macfarlane

University of Dundee, Microbiology and Gut Biology Group,
Ninewells Hospital Medical School, Dundee, UK

1. INTRODUCTION

Many hundreds of different species and strains of bacteria have been identified in the human gastrointestinal tract, with numbers increasing progressively from the proximal colon to the distal large bowel. Viable cell counts in fecal material range from about 10^{11} to 10^{12} per gram [1, 2], and the vast majority of these organisms are strict anaerobes [3, 4] which play an important role in host digestive physiology, metabolism and development of the immune system [5]. The composition of the intestinal microbiota is determined by a variety of host, microbiological, dietary and environmental factors, which can vary markedly between individuals at the level of species and strains. When the microbiota is perturbed due to changes in diet, disease, age, or the use of drugs or antibiotics [6–8], then dysbiosis can occur, which can result in a decreased ability to resist invading pathogens, or increases in potentially pathogenic indigenous bacteria with the concomitant loss of beneficial species. Most of our knowledge of bacterial communities in the large intestine was initially derived using viable

counting techniques [1, 2]. However, this has been largely superseded by a range of molecular methods for microbiota analysis [9, 10], which has improved our ability to study the effects of therapeutic manipulation on the structure and composition of the gut ecosystem.

Prebiotics are non-digestible oligosaccharides (NDO) which selectively stimulate the growth of intestinal bacteria, such as lactobacilli and bifidobacteria that have health promoting properties for the host [11, 12]. These bacteria are generally regarded as safe because they mainly ferment carbohydrates, are not pathogenic and are non-toxigenic, while they have a role in colonization resistance and frequently manifest immunomodulatory properties in the host. Prebiotics have been shown to reduce colonic transit times due to their laxative effects, enhance colonization resistance to enteral pathogens [13], increase production of short-chain fatty acids (SCFA) [14], and aid in preventing bacterial translocation [15]. They have also been shown to reduce numbers of certain bacteria in the gut, such as clostridia, bacteroides, enterococci and enterobacteria, some species of which may be detrimental to health, and have the ability to produce more toxic metabolites as waste products of metabolism, such as indoles, phenols, ammonia, thiols, H_2S and amines, that may be involved in the etiology of colorectal cancer (see later).

The most widely studied NDO are inulins and their associated fructo-oligosaccharides (FOS), which are fructose-containing polymers of 2 to 60 chain length with a terminal glucose residue [12]. These are found naturally occurring in plants such as Jerusalem artichokes (up to 20% inulin), onions (up to 6% inulin), bananas (<1% inulin) and chicory roots (up to 20% inulin) [16, 17]. Other potential NDO prebiotics include galacto-oligosaccharides (GOS) [17], soya-oligosaccharides [18], xylo-oligosaccharides [19], pyrodextrins, isomalto-oligosaccharides [20], and the disaccharide lactulose [21]. There are believed to be few safety issues in the use of prebiotics and several European studies have indicated that GOS is safe to add to infant feeds [22]. The addition of up to 0.8 grams $100 mL^{-1}$ of the prebiotic mixture comprising 90% GOS and 10% FOS in infant formula feeds has been approved by the EU Scientific Committee on Food (SCF) for use in infant feeds [23]. However, one constraint on the use of prebiotics is that consumption of high levels can lead to undesirable side effects such as abdominal discomfort, cramping, flatulence and diarrhea [24–26].

This chapter will focus on modulation of the gastrointestinal microbiota by prebiotics, and their abilities to impact on colonic diseases by restoring more beneficial bacterial populations and in the aging gut.

2. MODULATING THE INTESTINAL MICROBIOTA

The gastrointestinal tract contains diverse communities of bacteria which are present not only in the gut lumen, but also on mucosal surfaces. Until comparatively recently, selective and non-selective culture methods were the standard techniques used to quantitate bacterial populations in feces, and the total number of species was thought to be in the range of 400–500 [27]. However, these methods have been shown to result in an underestimation of bacterial population sizes and microbial diversity [28, 29], and may lead to an overestimation of some groups such as bacteroides and bifidobacteria [30, 31]. Several studies using fecal material have indicated that only about 40–60% of total bacteria counted under the microscope are able to be detected using culture techniques [27, 32].

Thus the desire to have more high-throughput methods of analysis, and to detect the components of the microbiota that are more difficult to culture, has led to the development of many new molecular techniques for analysis of the intestinal microbiota, many of which are based on nucleic acid hybridization technologies, and usually involve analyses of 16S rRNA [27, 28, 30, 33, 34]. These include non-quantitative molecular fingerprinting techniques such as denaturing gradient electrophoresis (DGGE) [35] and clone library analysis, as well as more quantitative techniques such as fluorescent *in situ* hybridization (FISH) [36] or quantitative PCR (7, 9, 10, 37). The use of molecular methodologies has been shown in several studies to be useful in increasing our understanding of the effects of prebiotics on the gastrointestinal microbiota [9, 10].

Doses of 4–15 g/d of inulin or oligofructose have been shown in several feeding studies to be able to modulate the composition of the intestinal microbiota, and increase levels of bifidobacteria [38, 39]. A few studies have shown that prebiotics can also stimulate the growth of some lactobacilli [40], and even small amounts of NDO added to the diet have been shown to significantly affect bacterial populations in the gut [41]. Unlike probiotics, which are live microbial supplements that can be added to the diet, prebiotics affect the growth of indigenous organisms already present in the gut. However, in certain groups of individuals such as in patients with inflammatory bowel disease (IBD) [42] or the elderly [43], where there is a loss of beneficial bacteria (see later), it may be more useful to use a synbiotic combination of a prebiotic with a probiotic [16] to obtain maximum health benefits.

By modulating the composition of the intestinal microbiota, prebiotics can also increase levels of SCFA, resulting in lower intestinal pH, and the inhibition of a number of pathogenic species. SCFA formation is one of the most important physiological processes mediated by intestinal bacteria [44]. These fermentation products are absorbed from the gut, and can provide up to 10% of the host's daily energy requirements [45]. SCFA also affect intestinal epithelial cell transport processes, energy transduction in colonocytes, growth and cellular differentiation, hepatic control of lipid and carbohydrate metabolism, and provide energy to muscle, kidney, heart and brain [46]. The main SCFA produced are acetate, propionate and butyrate. Butyrate is important in that it is the principal fuel for colonocytes, and has been linked with the prevention of colon cancer and IBD (see later). Since greater than 95% of SCFA are absorbed in the gut, the amount that is produced with different prebiotics cannot be readily measured in fecal material. This has led to the use of *in vitro* models, such as various forms of batch culture, single or multistage continuous culture models of the gastrointestinal tract, to compare the fermentability of different prebiotics [47, 48]. In one study using pH controlled fermentors, 10 g/L, FOS and GOS were shown to increase acetate and butyrate formation, with transient accumulations of lactate and succinate [49]. Interestingly, bifidobacteria and lactobacilli produce acetate and lactate but not butyrate. However, several studies have indicated that prebiotics can increase levels of butyrate *in vivo* and *in vitro* [50, 51]. In a study by Langlands and coworkers, feeding 7.5 grams of inulin and 7.5 grams of FOS per day was shown to increase levels of butyrate,

and increase numbers of bifidobacteria and eubacteria on the colonic mucosa [51]. This suggested that the eubacteria might be using lactate formed during bifidobacterial fermentation to produce butyrate. In 2006, butyrate-producing species such as *Anaerostipes caccae* and *Eubacterium halli* were shown to be able to cross-feed on lactate produced by *B. adolescentis* growing on FOS, while a non-lactate utilizing, butyrate-forming *Roseburia* sp. could assimilate carbohydrate fragments formed when the *Bifidobacterium* hydrolyzed complex polymeric substrates [52]. While the main populations of bacteria stimulated by prebiotics are thought to be bifidobacteria and lactobacilli, due to this cross-feeding, the final outcome of fermentation may be affecting a larger number of bacterial groups than was initially thought. Increased numbers of eubacteria and roseburia have been found in studies with inulin, and clostridia have also been shown to utilize FOS [53] and bacteroides and clostridia to ferment GOS [54, 55].

While many studies on prebiotics have principally concentrated on SCFA formation, and increases in bifidobacterial numbers in feces, *in vitro* studies have shown that they may also inhibit the adherence of intestinal pathogens, which could be due to the prebiotic mimicking pathogen receptors on epithelial cells. The attachment of enteropathogenic *Escherichia coli* (EPEC) to HEp-2 and Caco-2 cell lines was shown to be inhibited by GOS, which was more effective than either inulin or FOS in this respect [56] and transgalacto-oligosaccharides (TOS) were reported to increase the protective abilities of *B. breve* in mice infected with *Salmonella enterica* serovar Typhimurium [57].

3. PREBIOTICS AND IBD

The two main forms of idiopathic IBD are ulcerative colitis (UC) and Crohn's disease (CD).

Germ-free animals do not get colitis unless repopulated with bacteria, and this suggests that bacterial species belonging to the normal intestinal microbiota play a key role in the pathogenesis of UC [58]. UC is confined to the colon and the symptoms include rectal bleeding, diarrhea and abdominal pain, whereas CD is a more heterogeneous condition that can occur along the entire length of the gastrointestinal tract [58]. The etiology of IBD is unclear, but is thought to be multifactorial, involving not only the colonic microbiota, but also genetic and environmental factors, as well as dysregulation of the immune system leading to an imbalance of pro-inflammatory cytokine formation, and the Th1 and Th2 responses modulated through NF-κB [58]. Treatment for UC usually involves suppression or modulation of the host inflammatory response using corticosteroids, aminosalicylates or immunomodulatory agents, depending on the severity and localization of the disease. However, some individuals cannot tolerate these treatments, which can have various debilitating side effects [59]. Surprisingly, given the degree of microbial involvement in IBD, the few studies that have been done using antibiotics to treat UC have suggested that they are of limited use. Antibiotic resistance can also develop, and unless specifically targeted, antibiotics can cause severe disturbances in the microbiota. Moreover, bacteria involved in inflammatory processes in UC probably grow in biofilms on the mucosa [42, 60], which have been shown to be resistant to antibiotics [61].

Dysbiosis in the colonic microbiota is thought to occur in IBD, and several studies have shown that lower levels of bifidobacteria and increased concentrations of putatively pathogenic bacteria, enterococci, enterobacteria and other Gram-positive cocci [42, 62, 63] occur in both UC and CD.

Evidence suggests that prebiotics such as FOS, GOS and inulin are useful in animal studies with induced colitis. In rat and murine models, they have been shown to reduce mucosal inflammation, reduce inflammatory markers [64], increase butyrate concentrations, increase numbers of lactobacilli and bifidobacteria, and attenuate NF-κB activation [65].

However, at the time of writing, there have been few human clinical trials of the effects of prebiotics in IBD [58]. Welters and colleagues [66] demonstrated an improvement in 20 patients with pouchitis, which is a clinical condition in patients who have had an ileal pouch-anal anastomosis after total colectomy, using 24 grams of inulin over a relatively short experimental period of 3 weeks. Although the study was not placebo controlled, improvements were found in endoscopic and histological scores, together with a reduction in bacteroides, and increases in fecal butyrate. Two small open label studies have been done looking at FOS and inulin in children and adults. The first was a crossover trial in which 10 children with active CD were randomized to a combination of inulin and FOS for 3 weeks, or were given a placebo. Significant improvements were seen in weight gain, and a decrease in the pediatric Crohn's disease activity index was found in the prebiotic group [67]. In the second study, 15 patients with active Crohn's were given 15 grams of FOS daily, which resulted in significantly increased levels of fecal bifidobacteria, and reductions in the Harvey Bradshaw clinical index [68]. Increased numbers of IL-10 positive dendritic cells were detected in the prebiotic group, as well as in dendritic cells expressing the pattern recognition receptors, TLR2 and TLR4.

FOS and inulin have been shown to modify not only the bacterial compositions of feces, but also of mucosa-associated microbiotas in the upper and lower gut [51]. This may be of clinical relevance, since UC primarily affects the mucosa, and in several studies, a reduction in bifidobacteria has been detected on the colonic mucosa [42]. Furrie and coworkers [10] reported a double blind randomized controlled trial in which a synbiotic was fed to UC patients for 4 weeks. Eighteen individuals were involved in the study, and those receiving the synbiotic were given 12 grams of Synergy 1® (oligofructose-enriched inulin) and 2×10^{11} live *Bifidobacterium longum* per day. Levels of mucosal bifidobacteria increased 42-fold in patients receiving the synbiotic, compared to 4.6-fold in those receiving the placebo. At the end of the study, the prebiotic group had significant reductions in mucosal pro-inflammatory cytokines (TNF-α, IL-1α) and inducible human β-defensins (hBD). hBD are anti-microbial peptides only formed by epithelial cells in inflamed tissues, but unlike the pro-inflammatory cytokines, they are not produced by inflammatory infiltrates, making them good markers of epithelial healing. In the most severely ill patients, C-reactive protein fell to normal levels. Regeneration of the epithelium and a decrease in inflammation occurred in the synbiotic patients at the end of the trial, with reductions in both histology and sigmoidoscopy scores.

4. CANCER

Diets low in fruits and vegetables, and high levels of animal fats and proteins, along with lifestyle and genetics factors have been implicated in the pathogenesis of colorectal cancer (CRC), which is now the third most common cancer worldwide. There is good evidence for the involvement of intestinal bacteria in the etiology of this disease, since they are able to produce a range of mutagenic and genotoxic compounds. Several bacterial enzymes such as β-glucosidase, β-glucuronidase, nitroreductase and azoreductase are thought to be involved in the production of genotoxic substances from dietary or environmental precursors, and increased proteolysis can lead to more toxic substances such as indoles, phenols and amines being formed. The use of prebiotics is a promising method of supplementing the diet to protect against bowel cancer, by increasing the availability of fermentable carbohydrate, reducing putrefactive processes, and modulating bacterial physiology and ecology to decrease the production of toxic metabolites. However, results from studies on the ability of prebiotics to reduce these enzyme activities have been mixed, and in several studies, prebiotics have had no effect on these genotoxic enzymes. In one investigation, no differences were detected in fecal β-glucosidase or β-glucuronidase activities after feeding inulin to constipated elderly volunteers [69]. Other work showed that consumption of 12.5 grams of FOS per day had no effect on either azoreductase, nitroreductase or β-glucuronidase [70]. However, in one human feeding study involving 12 volunteers, while 4 grams of FOS per day had no effect on nitroreductase activity, reduced levels of fecal β-glucosidase were detected [71], and feeding 12 healthy young volunteers 15 grams of GOS or inulin per day was shown to significantly increase levels of acetate and reduced β-glucuronidase [72]. Then in 2008, in a larger 4-week randomized crossover study involving 53 healthy subjects, lactulose and inulin combined was shown to significantly reduce fecal β-glucuronidase activity [73].

Production of SCFA such as butyrate by intestinal bacteria may play a role in reducing cancer risk, and the survival of tumor cells [74]. Butyrate has been shown to induce apoptosis (programmed cell death) [75] and to be able to modulate genes involved in regulating oxidative and metabolic stress in human colon cell lines [76]. It has also been shown to induce glutathione S-transferases in tumor cell lines, which may be linked to detoxification of dietary carcinogens [77], and to suppress both cytokine-induced and constitutive expression of the transcription factor NF-κB in HT-29 cell lines [78]. In one study, intravenous administration of acetate was shown to increase peripheral blood antibody production and NK activity in cancer patients, compared to controls [79].

The majority of the work done so far on prebiotics and colon cancer has been done in animals, where the cancer has been chemically induced, and in most of these, prebiotics were shown to reduce the numbers of pre-cancerous aberrant crypt foci [17, 80]. In one study, reduced levels of fecal and cecal genotoxins were found after feeding azoxymethane treated rats a synbiotic combination of inulin/FOS, and two probiotic bacteria (*Lactobacillus rhamnosus* and *Bifidobacterium lactis*), or the prebiotic alone, which correlated with a reduction in tumor incidences [81]. Rafter and colleagues carried out a human cancer study that was a randomized, double blind, placebo controlled trial using a combination of 12 g/day inulin/FOS, and two probiotic bacteria *Lactobacillus rhamnosus* GG and *Bifidobacterium lactis* Bb12 [82]. The investigation involved 37 colon cancer patients, and 43 polypectomized patients, who were at high risk for colon cancer, for 12 weeks. Increased numbers of lactobacilli and bifidobacteria were detected in stools, and levels of *C. perfringens* decreased. The synbiotic also significantly reduced the ability of fecal water to induce necrosis in colonic cell lines, reduced colorectal cell proliferation, and enhanced epithelial function in the polypectomized subjects. Several immune markers were also measured in the study, and although the synbiotic was found to have no effect on the systemic immune system, its consumption was shown to increase production of INF-γ in the cancer patients, and to prevent an increase of IL-2 by peripheral blood mononuclear cells [83].

5. THE AGING GUT

There is an increasing elderly population worldwide. As people get older their health often deteriorates, and they have a greater susceptibility to chronic diseases and gastrointestinal infections, which results in increased morbidity and mortality. Several human gut functions are affected with age, including reductions in intestinal immunity associated with age-related T cell changes, and reductions in antibody production, as well as a decline in cell-mediated immunity [84, 85] which increases their susceptibility to gastrointestinal infections [86]. The elderly often suffer from loss of taste and the ability to chew, which may lead to malnutrition, which has been linked to a decline in immune responses [87]. They also have decreased intestinal transit times, which can lead to constipation, and results in increased proteolysis and the formation of toxic putrifactive metabolites such as phenols, amines, sulfide, ammonia and indoles.

Increased numbers of proteolytic bacteria such as fusobacteria and clostridia have been detected in elderly people, with a greater increase in clostridia occurring after antibiotic treatment [43]. Early studies on fecal material demonstrated that lower numbers of colonic anaerobes, particularly bifidobacteria and higher numbers of yeasts, enterobacteria, streptococci and *Clostridium perfringens,* occurred in the elderly gut [88–90]. In a cultural study by Woodmansey and colleagues [43], along with the increase in potentially more harmful bacteria such as clostridia, enterococci and enterobacteria in older people, a concomitant decrease in numbers and species diversity of beneficial bacteria such as bifidobacteria was detected. Other studies have also detected a reduction in bifidobacterial species diversity in older people, with the fecal microbiota reported to be comprised of only one or two dominant bifidobacteria, in particular *B. adolescentis* and *B. longum* [91, 92]. Changes in bifidobacteria are of particular interest because of their association with gut health. It has been suggested that reduced abilities of bifidobacteria to adhere to the colonic mucosa may be a factor in the decline of these organisms in older people [92, 93].

These findings would suggest that this is a particularly good target group for prebiotic usage in the human population, in that there is considerable scope for improving the composition of their gut microbiotas. These individuals would benefit from the immunomodulatory and bifidogenic properties of prebiotics in improving intestinal health. The majority of prebiotic studies on the elderly so far have been designed to determine their effects on constipation. While the results of these investigations are mixed, prebiotics have been shown to be of benefit in several studies involving elderly constipated volunteers. In one double blinded feeding study, Kleesen and coworkers fed 25 healthy elderly constipated volunteers 20 g/d of lactose or inulin for 8 days, and then increased the amount to 40 g/day for a further 10 days [94]. With lactose, the numbers of enterococci increased while clostridia and lactobacilli decreased. With inulin, the numbers of bifidobacteria detected in feces increased, and the numbers of enterobacteria and enterococci went down, with nine of the 10 volunteers showing a reduction in the symptoms of constipation. Although these were very high doses, this study demonstrates the beneficial effects of inulin in older people. In two other studies by the same group, involving constipated elderly men, feeding 10 g/d oligofructose was reported to increase stool weight from 32 to 69 grams per day [95], while isomalto-oligosaccharides were able to increase stool weights by 70% [96].

Bartosch and colleagues [9] carried out a placebo controlled randomized, double blind controlled trial to determine whether feeding a synbiotic comprising 6 grams of the prebiotic Synergy 1® (a mixture of oligofructose and long-chain inulin) in combination with a capsule containing 10^{10} colony forming units (CFU) each of B. bifidum and B. lactis could elicit significant changes in microbiota composition in fecal samples of healthy elderly people (mean age 73). The study lasted 4 weeks and a combination of molecular and cultural techniques was used. The synbiotic was given to nine elderly volunteers twice per day, and was compared to those given a placebo containing malto-oligosaccharides and potato starch. Increased numbers and diversity of bifidobacteria were detected during the feeding period in the test group compared to the placebo group, which could not be accounted for by the probiotics alone, and in some individuals given the synbiotic, bifidobacterial numbers

remained high for several weeks after cessation of synbiotic administration. Indigenous bifidobacterial species, particularly B. adolescentis and B. angulatum, and some lactobacilli (e.g. L. cateneforme) also increased greatly during synbiotic feeding, compared to the placebo group. This demonstrates that the prebiotic may be beneficial in elderly people to restore levels of beneficial immuno-stimulatory bacteria.

In one double blind placebo controlled trial, the effects of xylo-oligosaccharides (XOS) in the elderly has also been studied [97]. XOS can be found in bamboo shoots, fruit, vegetables and honey. Four sources of XOS were given per day to 22 elderly subjects (mean age 78.6 years) for 3 weeks. A significant increase in the number of fecal bifidobacteria was detected in the XOS group, while no significant increases were found in the placebos. The authors also indicated that fecal moisture content went up in the prebiotic group, and that there was a reduction in fecal pH, which was probably due to increased SCFA production by intestinal bacteria. The supplement did not affect nutrient intakes or the hematologic or biochemical parameters of the volunteers.

In order to assess the effects of nutritional supplementation with prebiotics on not only bifidobacteria, but also inflammatory parameters, Shiffrin and colleagues carried out a randomized placebo controlled double blinded study involving 74 elderly patients (mean age 70), living in either nursing homes or in the community [98]. The subjects were given 1.3 grams of oligosaccharide daily for 12 weeks. While no significant difference was found in fecal microbiota or in nutritional parameters, a reduction in pro-inflammatory gene activation was detected in the prebiotic group, particularly with respect to TNF-α and IL-6 specific mRNA in blood leukocytes. This suggests that prebiotics may improve low level inflammatory responses in the elderly.

Clostridium difficile associated diarrhea (CDAD) is one of the most common nosocomial infections in the elderly, particularly following antibiotic treatment. Several studies have shown that probiotics can be beneficial in preventing CDAD; however, there have been few studies on the effects of prebiotics in these patients. Two large investigations were done by Lewis and coworkers [99, 100]. In the first study, prebiotics were used with the aim of preventing the incidence of infection, and in the second, in preventing relapse. While no reduction was found in the incidence of *C. difficile*, levels of fecal bifidobacteria were increased, and a significant reduction was detected in the rate of relapse in the prebiotic group compared to the placebos. *In vitro* fermentation studies with mixed cultures of fecal bacteria growing on inulin and GOS (oligomate 55) have demonstrated that the oligosaccharides, especially GOS, inhibited growth and toxin production by *Clostridium difficile* [49]. However, while the GOS preparation in particular was shown to be bifidogenic, stimulating growth of *B. adolescentis*, *B. angulatum* and *B. bifidum*, these organisms were not responsible for suppressing the pathogen, indicating that other species in the microbiota were protective. These studies indicate that prebiotics alone, or in combination as a synbiotic, can be beneficial in CDAD.

6. CONCLUSIONS—FUTURE CHALLENGES FOR PREBIOTICS IN THE GASTROINTESTINAL TRACT

It is now well-recognized that an imbalance in bacterial populations occurs in several gastrointestinal disorders and in the elderly. Evidence from studies undertaken to date has indicated that prebiotics and synbiotics can beneficially modulate the intestinal microbiota, and that they have promising therapeutic potential for treating IBD and colon cancer, and in maintaining a healthy microbial balance in the aging gut. However, there are still great deficiencies in our knowledge of the mechanisms of prebiotic action

and their involvement in disease processes. This will be enhanced in the future by the use of new more sensitive molecular techniques for microbiological analysis, as well as in measurements of immunological and cellular markers.

References

1. Moore, W. E. C., & Holdeman, L. V. (1974). Human fecal flora: The normal flora of 20 Japanese-Hawaiians. *Applied Microbiology, 27*, 961–979.
2. Finegold, S. M., Sutter, V. L., & Mathisen, G. E. (1983). Normal indigenous intestinal flora. In D. J. Hentges (Ed.), *Human intestinal microflora in health and disease* (pp. 3–31). New York: Academic Press.
3. Finegold, S. M., Attebery, H. R., & Sutter, V. L. (1974). Effect of diet on human fecal flora: Comparison of Japanese and American diets. *American Journal of Clinical Nutrition, 27*, 1456–1469.
4. Hentges, D. J. (1993). The anaerobic microflora of the human body. *Clinical Infectious Diseases, 16*, S175–S180.
5. Cummings, J. H., & Macfarlane, G. T. (1997). Colonic microflora: Nutrition and health. *Nutrition, 13*, 476–479.
6. Simon, G. L., & Gorbach, S. L. (1984). Intestinal flora in health and disease. *Gastroenterology, 86*, 174–193.
7. Bartosch, S., Woodmansey, E. J., Patterson, J. C., et al. (2004). Characterization of bacterial communities in feces from healthy elderly volunteers and hospitalized elderly patients by using real-time PCR and effects of antibiotic treatment on the fecal microbiota. *Applied and Environmental Microbiology, 70*, 3575–3581.
8. Moore, W. E., & Moore, L. H. (1995). Intestinal floras of populations that have a high risk of colon cancer. *Applied and Environmental Microbiology, 61*, 3202–3207.
9. Bartosch, S., Woodmansey, E. J., Paterson, J. C., et al. (2005). Microbiological effects of consuming a synbiotic containing *Bifidobacterium bifidum*, *Bifidobacterium lactis* and oligofructose in elderly patients, determined by real-time polymerase chain reaction and counting of viable bacteria. *Clinical Infectious Diseases, 40*, 28–37.
10. Furrie, E., Macfarlane, S., Kennedy, A., et al. (2004). Synbiotic therapy (*Bifidobacterium longum*/Synergy 1™) initiates resolution of inflammation in patients with active ulcerative colitis: A randomised controlled pilot trial. *Gut, 54*, 242–249.
11. Gibson, G. R., & Roberfroid, M. B. (1995). Dietary modulation of the human colonic microbiota: Introducing the concept of prebiotics. *Journal of Nutrition, 125*, 1401–1412.
12. Macfarlane, S., Macfarlane, G. T., & Cummings, J. H. (2006). Prebiotics in the gastrointestinal tract. *Alimentary Pharmacology & Therapeutics, 24*, 701–714.

13. Gibson, G. R., & Wang, X. (1994). Regulatory effects of bifidobacteria on the growth of other colonic bacteria. *Journal of Applied Bacteriology, 77*, 412–420.

14. Cherbut, C., Michel, C., & Lecannu, G. (2003). The prebiotic characteristics of fructooligosaccharides are necessary for reduction of TNBS-induced colitis in rats. *Journal of Nutrition, 133*, 21–27.

15. Bosscher, D., Loo, J. V., & Franck, A. (2006). Inulin and oligofructose as prebiotics in the prevention of intestinal infections and diseases. *Nutrition Research Reviews, 19*, 216–226.

16. Macfarlane, S. (2006). Therapeutic use of synbiotics: The use of synbiotics as therapies for maintaining health of the digestive tract. *AGRO Fd Indust High Technology, 17*(2), 21–23.

17. Macfarlane, G. T., Steed, H., & Macfarlane, S. (2008). Bacterial metabolism and health-related effects of galacto-oligosaccharides and other prebiotics. *Journal of Applied Microbiology, 104*, 305–344.

18. Saito, Y., Tanaka, T., & Rowland, I. R. (1992). Effects of soybean oligosaccharides on the human gut microflora *in vitro* culture. *Microbial Ecology in Health and Disease, 5*, 105–110.

19. Campbell, J. M., Fahy, G. C., & Wolf, B. W. (1997). Selected indigestible oligosaccharides affect large bowel mass and fecal short-chain fatty acids, pH and microflora in rats. *Journal of Nutrition, 127*, 130–136.

20. Gostner, A., Blaut, M., Schaffer, V., et al. (2006). Effect of isomalt consumption on faecal microflora and colonic metabolism in healthy volunteers. *British Journal of Nutrition, 95*, 40–50.

21. Tuohy, K. M., Ziemer, C. J., Klinder, A., et al. (2002). A human volunteer study to determine the prebiotic effects of lactulose powder on human colonic microbiota. *Microbial Ecology in Health and Disease, 14*, 165–173.

22. Moro, G. E., Arslanoglu, S., Stahl, B., et al. (2006). A mixture of prebiotic oligosaccharides reduces the incidence of atopic dermatitis during the first six months of age. *Archives of Disease in Childhood, 91*, 814–819.

23. Scientific Committee on Food (SCF) (2003). Report of the Committee on Food on the revision of essential requirements of infant formulae and follow-on formulae. In *EU Commission Report SCF/CS/NUT/IF/65, Final 18 May*. Brussels: European Commission, Health and consumer Protection Directorate-General.

24. Deguchi, Y. (1997). Effects of beta 1-4-galacto-oligosaccharide administration on defecation of healthy volunteers with a tendency to constipation. *Japan Journal of Nutrition, 55*, 13–22.

25. Teuri, U., Korpela, R., Saxelin, M., et al. (1998). Increased fecal frequency and gastrointestinal symptoms following ingestion of galacto-oligosaccharide containing yoghurt. *Journal of Nutritional Science and Vitaminology, 44*, 465–471.

26. Saavedra, J. M., & Tschernia, A. (2002). Human studies with probiotics and prebiotics: Clinical implications. *British Journal of Nutrition, 87*, S241–S246.

27. Macfarlane, S., & Macfarlane, G. T. (2004). Bacterial diversity in the large intestine. *Advances in Applied Microbiology, 54*, 261–289.

28. Wilson, K. H., & Blitchington, R. B. (1996). Human colonic biota studied by ribosomal DNA sequence analysis. *Applied and Environmental Microbiology, 62*, 2273–2278.

29. O'Sullivan, D. J. (1999). Methods for the analysis of the intestinal flora. In G. W. Tannock (Ed.), *Probiotics: A critical review* (pp. 23–44). Wymondham, UK: Horizon Scientific Press.

30. Dore, J., Sghir, A., Hannequart-Gramet, G., et al. (1998). Design and evaluation of a 16S rRNA-targeted oligonucleotide probe for specific detection and quantitation of human faecal *Bacteroides* populations. *Systematic and Applied Microbiology, 21*, 65–71.

31. Sghir, A., Gramet, G., Suau, A., et al. (2000). Quantification of bacterial groups within human fecal flora by oligonucleotide probe hybridization. *Applied and Environmental Microbiology, 66*, 2263–2266.

32. Tannock, G. W., Munro, K., Harmsen, H. J. M., et al. (2000). Analysis of the fecal microflora of human subjects consuming a probiotic containing *Lactobacillus rhamnosus* DR20. *Applied and Environmental Microbiology, 66*, 2578–2588.

33. Woese, C. R. (1987). Bacterial evolution. *Microbiology Reviews, 51*, 221–227.

34. Amann, R. I., Ludwig, W., & Schleifer, K. H. (1995). Phylogenetic identification and *in situ* detection of individual microbial cells without cultivation. *Microbiology Reviews, 59*, 143–169.

35. Ahmed, S., Macfarlane, G. T., Fite, A., et al. (2007). Mucosa-associated bacterial diversity in relation to human terminal ileum and colonic biopsy samples. *Applied and Environmental Microbiology, 73*, 7435–7442.

36. Harmsen, H. J., Gibson, G. R., Elfferich, P., et al. (2000). Comparison of viable cell counts and fluorescence in situ hybridization using specific rRNA-based probes for the quantification of human fecal bacteria. *FEMS Microbiology Letters, 183*, 125–129.

37. Fite, A., Macfarlane, G. T., Cummings, J. H., et al. (2004). Identification and quantitation of mucosal and faecal desulfovibrios using real-time PCR. *Gut, 53*, 523–529.

38. Ito, M., Deuguchi, Y., Miyamori, A., et al. (1990). Effects of administration of galacto-oligosaccharides on the human faecal microflora, stool weight and abdominal sensation. *Microbial Ecology in Health and Disease, 3*, 285–292.

39. Gibson, G. R., & Roberfroid, M. B. (1995). Dietary modulation of the human colonic microbiota: Introducing the concept of prebiotics. *Journal of Nutrition, 125*, 1401–1412.

B. PREBIOTICS IN HEALTH PROMOTION

40. Smiricky-Tjardes, M. R., Grieshop, C. M., Flickinger, E. A., et al. (2003). Dietary galacto-oligosaccharides affect ileal and total-tract nutrient digestibility, ileal and fecal bacterial concentrations, and ileal fermentative characteristics of growing pigs. *Journal of Animal Sciences*, 81, 2535–2545.

41. Macfarlane, S., & Macfarlane, G. T. (2003). Food and the large intestine. In R. Fuller & G. Perdigon (Eds.), *Gut flora, nutrition, immunity and health* (pp. 24–51). Oxford: Blackwell Publishing.

42. Macfarlane, S., Furrie, E., Cummings, J. H., & Macfarlane, G. T. (2004). Chemotaxonomic analysis of bacterial populations colonizing the rectal mucosa in patients with ulcerative colitis. *Clinical Infectious Diseases*, 38, 1690–1699.

43. Woodmansey, E. J., McMurdo, M. E. T., Macfarlane, G. T., & Macfarlane, S. (2004). Comparison of compositions and metabolic activities of fecal microbiotas in young adults and in antibiotic-treated and non-antibiotic-treated elderly subjects. *Applied and Environmental Microbiology*, 70, 6113–6122.

44. Macfarlane, S., & Macfarlane, G. T. (2002). Regulation of short chain fatty acid production. *PNS*, 62, 67–72.

45. Macfarlane, G. T., & Cummings, J. H. (1991). The colonic flora, fermentation and large bowel digestive function. In S. F. Phillips, J. H. Pemberton, & R. G. Shorter (Eds.), *The large intestine: Physiology, pathophysiology and disease* (pp. 51–92). New York: Raven Press.

46. Cummings, J. H. (1995). Short chain fatty acids. In G. R. Gibson & G. T. Macfarlane (Eds.), *Human colonic bacteria: Role in nutrition, physiology and health* (pp. 101–130). Boca Raton: CRC Press.

47. Macfarlane, G. T., & Macfarlane, S. (2007). Models for intestinal fermentation: Association between food components, delivery systems, bioavailability and functional interactions in the gut. *Current Opinion in Biotechnology*, 18, 156–162.

48. Tzortzis, G., Goulas, A. K., Gee, J. M., & Gibson, G. R. (2005). A novel galacto-oligosacccharide mixture increases the bifidobacterial population numbers in a continuous *in vitro* fermentation system and in the proximal colonic contents of pigs *in vivo*. *Journal of Nutrition*, 135, 1726–1731.

49. Hopkins, M. J., & Macfarlane, G. T. (2003). Nondigestible oligosaccharides enhance bacterial colonization resistance against *Clostridium difficile in vitro*. *Applied and Environmental Microbiology*, 69, 1920–1927.

50. Topping, D. L., & Clifton, P. M. (2001). Short chain fatty acids and human colonic function: Roles of resistant starch and nonstarch polysaccharides. *Physiological Reviews*, 81, 1031–1064.

51. Langlands, S. J., Hopkins, M. J., Coleman, N., & Cummings, J. H. (2004). Prebiotic carbohydrates modify the mucosa associated microflora of the human large bowel. *Gut*, 53, 1610–1616.

52. Belenguer, A., Duncan, S. F., Calder, A. G., et al. (2006). Two routes of metabolic cross-feeding between *Bifidobacterium adolescentis* and butyrate producing anaerobes from the human gut. *Applied and Environmental Microbiology*, 72, 3593–3599.

53. Duncan, S. H., Scott, K. P., Ramsay, A. G., et al. (2003). Effects of alternative dietary substrates on competition between human colonic bacteria in an anerobic fermentor system. *Applied and Environmental Microbiology*, 69, 1136–1142.

54. Ohtsuka, K., Benno, Y., Endo, A., et al. (1989). Effects of 4′-galactosyl-lactose on human intestinal microflora. *Bifidus*, 2, 143–149.

55. Sako, T., Matsumoto, K., & Tanaka, R. (1999). Recent progress on research and applications of non-digestable galacto-oligosaccharides. *International of Dairy Journal*, 9, 69–80.

56. Shoaf, K., Mulvey, G. L., Armstrong, G. D., & Hutkins, R. W. (2006). Prebiotic galacto-oligosaccharides reduce adherence of enteropathogenic *Escherichia coli* to tissue culture cells. *Infection and Immunity*, 74, 6920–6928.

57. Asahara, T., Nomoto, K., Shimizu, K., et al. (2001). Increased resistance of mice to *Salmonella enterica* serovar Typhimurium infection by synbiotic administration of Bifidobacteria and transgalactosylated oligosaccharides. *Journal of Applied Microbiology*, 91, 985–996.

58. Macfarlane, S., Steed, H., & Macfarlane, G. T. (2009). Intestinal bacteria in IBD. *Critical Reviews in Clinical Laboratory Sciences*, 46, 25–54.

59. Navarro, F., & Hanauer, S. B. (2003). Treatment of inflammatory bowel disease: safety and tolerability issues. *American Journal of Gastroenterology*, 98, S18–S23.

60. Macfarlane, S., Furrie, E., Kennedy, A., et al. (2005). Mucosal bacteria in ulcerative colitis. *The British Journal of Nutrition*, 93, 67–72.

61. Anwar, H., Dasgupta, M. K., & Costerton, J. W. (1990). Testing the susceptibility of bacteria in biofilms to antibacterial agents. *Antimicrobial Agents and Chemotherapy*, 34, 2043–2046.

62. Favier, C., Neut, C., Mizon, C., et al. (1997). Fecal beta-D-galactosidase production and bifidobacteria are decreased in Crohn's disease. *Digestive Diseases and Sciences*, 42, 817–822.

63. Cummings, J. H., Macfarlane, G. T., & Macfarlane, S. (2003). Intestinal bacteria and ulcerative colitis. *Current Issues in Intestinal Microbiology*, 4, 9–20.

64. Videla, S., Vilaseca, J., Antolin, M., et al. (2001). Dietary inulin improves distal colitis induced by dextran sodium sulphate in the rat. *The American Journal of Gastroenterology*, 96, 1486–1493.

65. Kanauchi, O., Mitsuyama, K., Araki, Y., & Andoh, A. (2003). Modification of intestinal flora in the treatment

of inflammatory bowel disease. *Current Pharmaceutical Design, 9*(4), 333–346.

66. Welters, C. F., Heineman, E., Thunnissen, F. B., et al. (2002). Effect of dietary inulin supplementation on inflammation of pouch mucosa in patients with ileal pouch-anal anastomosis. *Diseases of the Colon and Rectum, 45,* 621–627.

67. Hussey, T. A., Issenman, R. M., Persad, R., et al. (2003). Nutrition therapy in pediatric Crohn's disease patients improves nutrition status and decreases inflammation. *Journal of Pediatric Gastroenterology, 37,* A341.

68. Lindsay, J. O., Whelan, K., Stagg, A. J., et al. (2006). Clinical, microbiological, and immunological effects of fructo-oligosaccharide in patients with Crohn's disease. *Gut, 55,* 348–355.

69. Kleessen, B., Sykura, B., Zunft, H. J., & Blaut, M. (1997). Effects of inulin and lactose on fecal microflora, microbial activity and bowel habit in elderly constipated persons. *American Journal of Clinical Nutrition, 65,* 1397–1402.

70. Bouhnik, Y., Flourie, B., Riottot, M., et al. (1996). Effects of fructo-oligosaccharides ingestion on fecal bifidobacteria and selected metabolic indexes of colon carcinogenesis in healthy humans. *Nutrition and Cancer, 26,* 21–29.

71. Buddington, R. K., Williams, C. H., Chen, S. C., & Witherly, S. A. (1996). Dietary supplement of neosugar alters the fecal flora and decreases activities of some reductive enzymes in human subjects. *The American Journal of Clinical Nutrition, 63,* 709–716.

72. Van Dokkum, W., Wezendonk, B., Srikumar, T. S., & Van den Heuvel, E. G. (1999). Effect of nondigestible oligosaccharides on large-bowel functions, blood lipid concentrations and glucose absorption in young healthy male subjects. *European Journal of Clinical Nutrition, 53,* 1–7.

73. De Preter, V., Raemen, Y. H., Cloetens, L., et al. (2008). Effect of dietary intervention with different pre- and probiotics on intestinal bacterial enzyme activities. *European Journal of Clinical Nutrition, 62,* 225–231.

74. Scheppach, W., & Weiler, F. (2004). The butyrate story: Old wine in new bottles?. *Current Opinion in Clinical Nutrition and Metabolic Care, 7,* 563–567.

75. Hague, A., Manning, A. M., Hanlon, K. A., et al. (1993). Sodium butyrate induces apoptosis in human colonic tumour cell lines in a p53-independent pathway: Implications for the possible role of dietary fibre in the prevention of large bowel cancer. *International Journal of Cancer, 55,* 498–505.

76. Sauer, J., Richter, K. K., & Pool-Zobel, B. L. (2007). Physiological concentrations of butyrate favourably modulate genes of oxidative and metabolic stress in primary human colon cells. *Journal of Nutritional Biochemistry, 18,* 736–745.

77. Pool-Zobel, B. L., Selvaraju, V., Sauer, J., et al. (2005). Butyrate may enhance toxological defense in primary, adenoma and tumor human colon cells by favourably modulating expression of glutathione S-transferases genes, an approach in nutrigenomics. *Carcinogenesis, 26,* 1064–1076.

78. Inan, M. S., Rasoulpour, R. J., Yin, L., et al. (2000). The luminal short-chain fatty acid butyrate modulates NF-κB activity in a human colonic epithelial cell line. *Gastroenterology, 118,* 724–734.

79. Ishizaka, S., Kikuchi, E., & Tsujii, T. (1993). Effects of acetate on human immune system. *Immunopharmacology Immunotoxicology, 15,* 151–162.

80. Rowland, I. R., Rumney, C. J., Coutts, J. T., & Lievense, L. C. (1998). Effect of *Bifidobacterium longum* and inulin on gut bacterial metabolism and carcinogen-induced aberrant crypt foci in rats. *Carcinogenesis, 19,* 281–285.

81. Klinder, A., Forster, A., & Caderni, G. (2004). Fecal water genotoxicity is predictive of tumour-preventative activities by inulin-like oligofructoses, probiotics (*Lactobacillus rhamnosus* and *Bifidobacterium lactis*) and their symbiotic combination. *Nutrition Cancer, 49,* 144–155.

82. Rafter, J., Bennett, M., Caderni, G., et al. (2007). Dietary synbiotics reduce cancer risk factors in polypectomized and colon cancer patients. *American Journal of Clinical Nutrition, 85,* 488–496.

83. Roller, M., Clune, Y., Collins, K., et al. (2007). Consumption of prebiotic inulin enriched with oligofructose in combination with the probiotics *Lactobacillus rhamnosus* and *Bifidobacterium lactis* has minor effects on selected immune parameters in polypectomised and colon cancer patients. *British Journal of Nutrition, 97,* 676–684.

84. Ginaldi, L., Martinis, M. D., D'Ostilio, A., et al. (1999). Immunological changes in the elderly. *Ageing Clinical and Experimental Researchs, 11,* 281–286.

85. Effros, R. B. (2001). Ageing and immune system. *Novartis Foundation Symposium, 235,* 130–145.

86. Lovat, L. B. (1996). Age related changes in gut physiology and nutritional status. *Gut, 38,* 306–309.

87. Lesourd, B. M., Laisney, C., Slavatore, R., et al. (1994). Decreased maturation of T-cell populations in the healthy elderly: Influence of nutritional factors on the appearance of double negative CD4-CD8-CD2+ cells. *Archives of Gerontology and Geriatrics, 4,* S149–S154.

88. Gorbach, S. L., Nahas, L., Lerner, P. I., & Weinstein, L. (1967). Studies of intestinal microbiota. I. Effects of diet, age, and periodic sampling on numbers of fecal microorganisms in man. *Gastroenterology, 53,* 845–855.

89. Mitsuoka, T. (1973). Intestinal flora and aging. *Nutrition Reviews, 223,* 333–342.

90. Hopkins, M. J., Sharp, R., & Macfarlane, G. T. (2001). Age and disease related changes in intestinal bacterial populations assessed by cell culture, 16S rRNA abundance, and community cellular fatty acid profiles. *Gut, 48,* 198–205.

91. Gavini, F., Cayuela, C., Antoine, J. M., et al. (2001). Differences in distrubution of bifidobacterial and enterobacterial species in human faecal microflora of three different (children, adults, elderly) age groups. *Microbial Ecology in Health and Disease, 13,* 40–45.

92. He, F., Ouwehand, A. C., Isolauri, E., et al. (2001). Differences in composition and mucosal adhesion of bifidobacteria isolated from healthy adults and healthy seniors. *Current Microbiology, 43,* 351–354.

93. Ouwehand, A. C., Isolauri, E., Kirjavainan, P. V., & Salminen, S. J. (1999). Adhesion of four *Bifidobacterium* strains to human intestinal mucus from subjects in different age groups. *FEMS Microbiology Letters, 172,* 61–64.

94. Kleesen, B., Sykura, B., Zunft, H. J., & Blaut, M. (1997). Effects of inulin and lactose on fecal microflora, microbial activity, and bowel habit in elderly constipated persons. *The American Journal of Clinical Nutrition, 65,* 1397–1402.

95. Chen, H. L., Lu, Y. H., Lin, J. J., & Ko, L. Y. (2000). Effects of fructooligosaccharide on bowel function and indicators of nutritional status in constipated elderly men. *Nutritional Research, 20,* 1725–1733.

96. Chen, H. L., Lu, Y. H., Lin, J. J., & Ko, L. Y. (2001). Effects of isomalto-oligosaccharides on bowel functions and indicators of nutritional status in constipated elderly men. *Journal of the American College of Nutrition, 20,* 44–49.

97. Chung, Y. C., Hsu, C. K., Ko, C. Y., & Chan, Y. C. (2007). Dietary intake of xylooligosaccharides improves the intestinal microbiota, fecal moisture, and pH value in the elderly. *Nutritional Research, 27,* 756–761.

98. Schiffrin, E. J., Thomas, D. R., Kumar, V. B., et al. (2007). Systemic inflammatory markers in older persons: The effect of oral nutritional supplementation with prebiotics. *Journal of Nutrition Health Aging, 11,* 475–479.

99. Lewis, S., Burmeister, S., & Brazier, J. (2005). Effect of the prebiotic oligofructose on relapse of *Clostridium difficile*-associated diarrhoea: A randomized, controlled study. *Clinical Gastroenterology Hepatologie, 3,* 442–448.

100. Lewis, S., Burmeister, S., Cohen, S., et al. (2005). Failure of dietary oligofructose to prevent antibiotic-associated diarrhoea. *Alimentary Pharmacology & Therapeutics, 21,* 469–477.

PREBIOTICS AND PROBIOTICS AS THERAPIES

Prebiotics and Probiotics for the Prevention or Treatment of Allergic Asthma

Wojciech Feleszko and Joanna Jaworska

Department of Pediatric Pneumology and Allergy, The Medical University of Warsaw,
The Medical University Children's Hospital, Warszawa, Poland

1. INTRODUCTION

An obvious decrease of microbial exposure in early childhood is believed to be one of the most probable causes of the worldwide increase in morbidity in allergic diseases. This hypothesis is consequently supported by accumulating evidence from epidemiologic observations, suggesting crucial effects of microbial factors on early immune development. It has been previously shown that neonates, that go on to develop allergic disease, demonstrate a distinct pattern of early microbial gut colonization [1]. Therefore, it seems clear that these microbiota are essential to normal immune development and oral tolerance. Altogether, these studies gave rise to the experimental investigations on the potential application of microbial products to reduce allergic immune responses. As a consequence, several strains have already been identified to display documented health benefits in human beings. The rationale for potential probiotic application in allergic disease has been summarized as:

1. Epidemiological data suggesting a causative effect of high microbial exposure and protective, anti-allergic effects.
2. Neonates and infants demonstrate a certain level of immune 'deviation' resulting in subsequent allergic disease, suggesting a need for early protective intervention.
3. A 'critical time window' of immune development in early infancy includes exposure to large amount of gut-colonizing bacteria.
4. A 'western life style' stands for changing pattern of gut microflora and increase in allergic diseases.
5. Application of microbiota in experimental models augments immunoregulatory mechanisms.
6. Gut microflora is believed to induce oral tolerance.

Concurrently, studies demonstrate that infants with allergies demonstrate a certain level of immune dysregulation before onset of the disease, and further that gut microbiota possess immune regulatory activity. Together, these findings provide an interesting concept of therapeutic use of live intestinal strains in order to influence the development of an allergic disease. This attractive option appeared initially to be supported by both preventive [2] and therapeutic [3] studies on probiotics in allergic disease.

2. PROBIOTICS: MECHANISMS OF ACTION

According to our current understanding of immune phenomena, the immune system requires systematic environmental pressure in order to develop properly. Strong and direct evidence for the concept that contact with microorganisms through their constant pressure have an impact on the maturation of the immune system, comes from studies in animals grown in a germ-free environment (gnotobiotic animals). These animals develop only weak immunoregulatory mechanisms, and are at risk of acquiring diseases associated with immune dysfunction. These animals have been shown not only to be deficient in effective immune response to pathogens [4], but also to lack immune tolerance, thus over-expressing 'pro-allergic' T helper type 2 (Th2)-biased immune responses to an orally delivered antigen [5]. Interestingly, in these animals oral application of non-pathogenic lactic acid bacteria led to re-establishing oral tolerance mechanisms [6], suggesting an outstanding role of continuous oral microbial exposure for full immune competence.

The gut microbiota is the major source of microbial exposure, composed of more than 10^{14} microorganisms, or 10 times the number of cells in the entire body with a total weight of 1 kg. Microbial colonization of the gastrointestinal tract seems to depend upon lifestyle and geographic factors. Various studies have suggested a potential link between differences in the composition of the gut microbiota in infants living in various countries with a high and a low prevalence of allergies. Similarly, intestinal microflora differs significantly between healthy infants and infants with allergies [7, 8].

Probiotics are defined as living microorganisms which, on ingestion in certain numbers, exert health benefits beyond inherent general nutrition. Meanwhile, evidence is accumulating that probiotic bacterial strains—limited mainly to lactobacilli and bifidobacteria—can influence the immune system through a number of different ways. There have been multiple different effects of probiotics on the immune system described (summarized in Table 11.1). However, their clinical consequences remain to be elucidated. Probiotic bacteria have already been shown to act through circulating monocytes, local dendritic cells, and effector T and B cells, predominantly by reducing local inflammation. Interestingly, at least some of the anti-inflammatory effects of probiotic bacteria are attributed to their direct action on enterocytes, and mediated through TLR (mainly TLR9 and possibly TLR2 and TLR4) expressed on enterocytes [9]. They have also been demonstrated to control the systemic limiting antigen load by increasing the integrity of the intestinal barrier.

Of note, probiotic bacteria induce systemic immune regulatory mechanisms and therefore might regulate immune responses in distant organs by driving T cell regulatory network [10–12]. They preferentially elicit two substantial T cell lineages, which counterbalance the predominance of the pro-allergic, T helper 2 directed immune response: the T helper 1 cells and the T helper 3/T regulatory 1 cells, respectively [2, 3, 13, 14]. These cell types comprise the most immunosuppressive lineage of lymphocytes locally in the gut, and their activity suppresses the predisposition towards allergic reactions.

The crucial role in this network is attributed to dendritic cells. When primed with probiotic

TABLE 11.1 Probiotics and the immune system—evidence

Pathway	Activity in experimental models and clinical settings	Immunomodulatory effects
Local effects		
• Toll-like receptors	TLR9-mediated anti-inflammatory effects	Decreased Th2 responses
• Enterocytes	Decreased cell signaling Augmented production of TGF-β	Local immunosuppression Local tolerance mechanisms
• DCs	Increased activity of DCs in the gut	Tolerogenic DCs
• Tregs	Local TGF-β and IL-10 producing cells	Increased local TGF-β—induces IgA, Treg activity, tolerogenic DCs
• B cells	Increased IgA production	Reduced systemic antigen load
• T cells	Th1 skewing	Reduced Th2 responses
• Mucosal barrier	Increased regeneration and integrity of intestinal barrier Enhanced mucus production	Reduced gut permeability for allergens/antigens
Systemic effects		
• T cells	See above	
• B cells	Increased IgA production in distal sites	Increased antimicrobial immunity
• Monocytes	Improved circulation of monocytes	Increased antimicrobial immunity?

bacteria DCs have been shown to produce IL-10 and by these means induce tolerogenic milieu for surrounding T cells [12, 15, 16]. Preliminary animal studies show unequivocally that probiotic feeding promotes immunoregulatory activity in the gut, by inducing regulatory T cell populations that act in distal mucosal sites [17, 18]. In these experiments local increased T regulatory responses are associated with systemic activation of regulatory mechanisms and inhibition of systemic allergic inflammation. Logically, probiotic microorganisms were shown in human beings to indirectly influence the newborns' immunity by activating tolerance mechanisms, even if given to lactating mothers via an increase in breast milk TGF-β concentration [19].

The impact of probiotic treatment on systemic IgE concentrations reveals conflicting results. In the majority of studies, which showed beneficial effects of probiotic treatment on atopic eczema and dermatitis, IgE responses stayed unaffected [2, 20–23]. However, application of probiotics along with prebiotics was observed to increase serum IgE concentrations [24], but this effect paradoxically was associated with protection from IgE-mediated allergy. It is also well-recognized that intestinal microbiota positively affects IgA production, both locally (in the gut) as well as in distal sites (respiratory tract). The gut-associated lymphoid tissue (GALT) supplements in part the integrated common mucosal immune system, which consists of various mucosae across the body, and provides sufficient numbers of IgA-producing lymphoblasts, that are generated and maturate in the GALT. This phenomenon has also been shown for the T cells that are committed to Treg lineage in the gut before seeding to distal mucosal sites in the respiratory tract. These observations provide a possible explanation for how the gut micobiota seem to enhance systemic regulatory mechanisms and enhance IgA production in distal organs [25–27].

A previously described enhanced effect of probiotic supplementation on monocyte maturations remains less clear and further studies are needed to verify systemic effects of gut microbiota on bone marrow-derived cell populations [8]. It is worth stressing that all these effects seem to be related to particular bacterial species, as indicated by previous studies. Among others *L. casei* and *L. reuteri* and, but not *L. plantarum*, were shown to modulate dendritic cell function to induce the commitment of IL-10-producing regulatory T cells [15].

3. CLINICAL EFFECTS OF PROBIOTICS AND PREBIOTICS IN THE TREATMENT OF ALLERGIC ASTHMA

The vast majority of studies to investigate the beneficial role of probiotics in the treatment of allergies have analyzed their efficacy in early allergic diseases like food allergy and atopic dermatitis. In this line of investigation research focused on the use of probiotics in children with atopic dermatitis demonstrating mild but promising effects (this subject will be extensively discussed in the other chapters). These studies allowed for the selection of some probiotic strains demonstrating the most efficacious effects in clinical settings. In the second line of investigations, clinical studies were addressed to demonstrate potential therapeutic effects of probiotics in the treatment and prevention of allergic airway diseases (Tables 11.2 and 11.3).

The first study to address this (Table 11.2) demonstrated no clinical improvement in young adults with moderate asthma when treated with probiotic-fortified yogurt (*n* = 15) during the 56-week treatment period compared with a placebo group [28]. The second study again included young adults, in which the severity of the disease was not known and documented no significant difference in symptoms in all participants after 28 weeks; however, a slight (non-significant) decrease in the challenge symptoms was noted in the group receiving probiotics

(*Lactobacillus rhamnosus*) [29]. These were both very small studies and only included young adults who are less likely to be susceptible for successful immune modulation. One further study in a larger cohort (*n* = 187) [30] found no beneficial effect after 12 months of treatment in toddlers with allergic asthma (age 2–5 years) receiving *L. casei*. The second study in children with asthma (*n* = 17) did not demonstrate any improvement in patients receiving *Enterococcus faecalis* strain while also receiving acupuncture for 22 weeks [31].

In summary, there are no studies proving any favorable effects of probiotics on allergic asthma either in children or in older individuals. The lack of effect of these products in established asthmatic phenotype suggests that if any beneficial effect exists, it should be limited to a hypothetical 'time window of opportunity' before allergic disease is established. This 'window of opportunity' has been postulated to be located in early infancy, since the first onset of allergy frequently occurs within the first months of life and this time is crucial for the maturation of the immune system including the gut defense mechanisms [9, 32].

4. ROLE OF PROBIOTICS AND PREBIOTICS IN PREVENTION OF ALLERGIC ASTHMA

Clinical studies in individuals with established allergic disease have failed to demonstrate any beneficial effect. On the other hand, previous reports from animal studies suggested an existence of a critical 'time window of opportunity' for successful immune modulation with probiotics [9, 32]. Therefore, it appeared logical, from an immunological point of view, to investigate the benefits of probiotics in very early infancy, when the immune system is under development. There are now a number

TABLE 11.2 Characteristics and summary of four RCTs that evaluated the therapeutic effects of probiotics on asthma

Trial	No. of patients (age)	Severity of asthma	Study duration	Treatment	Probiotic strain	Type of outcomes	Outcomes	Conclusion
Wheeler, 1997 [28]	15 (13–45 years)	moderate	56 weeks	yogurt containing probiotics vs placebo for 4 weeks	*Lactobacillus acidophilus* (7.6×10^8 CFU)	Clinical and laboratory	no differences in quality of life no difference in FEV1 no difference in blood eosinophils no difference in cytokine levels no difference in total IgE levels	No effect
Helin, 2002 [29]	38 (young adults)	not reported	28 weeks	capsules twice daily for 22 weeks	*Lactobacillus rhamnosus* (10^{10} CFU)	Clinical	no differences in symptoms score during season no differences in symptoms prevalence no decrease in symptoms score during pollen season	No effect
Giovannini, 2007 [30]	187 (2–5 years)	intermittent to moderate persistent	12 months	fermented milk containing probiotic vs placebo	*Lactobacillus casei* (10^{10} CFU)	Clinical and laboratory	longer mean time free of episodes of asthma no differences in cumulative number of episodes of asthma no differences in mean duration of an episode of asthma	No effect
Stockert, 2007 [31]	17 (6–12 years)	>1 year intermittent or mild persistent	22 weeks	drops of suspension for 7 weeks	*Enterococcus faecalis* (18×10^7 CFU)	Clinical and laboratory	no differences in quality of life no differences in cortisone use no differences in number of days missed from school due to infections/bigger amount of patients without a single day of a febrile infection no difference in FEV1 no difference in blood eosinophils no difference in cytokine levels no difference in total IgE levels	No effect

TABLE 11.3   Characteristics and summary of the 13 RCTs that evaluated the preventive effects of probiotics on asthma

Trial	No. of patients (age)	Participant characteristic	Study duration	Type of intervention	Probiotic strain	Outcomes	Conclusion
Kalliomaki, 2001 [2]	132 (of initial 159); (36 Hbd–6 months)	term infants with family history of allergic disease	2 years	PREVENTION: probiotic was given prenatally to pregnant woman for 2–4 weeks before delivery and after birth to breast-feeding mothers or to children for 6 months	LGG	reduced frequency of atopic eczema no significant difference in asthma prevalence in childhood	No effect
Taylor, 2006 [33]	226; (0–6 months)	term infants of atopic women	12 months	PREVENTION: probiotic freeze-dried powder dissolved in water and given orally from birth to 6 months vs placebo	Lactobacillus acidophilus LAVRI-A1	no significant difference in asthma incidence in infancy	No effect
Abrahamsson, 2007 [20]	188 (of initial 232); (36 Hbd–6 months)	term infants with family history of allergic disease	2 years	PREVENTION: probiotic freeze-dried, suspended in coconut and peanut oil given to mother for 4 weeks before delivery and baby for 12 months after delivery vs placebo	Lactobacillus reuteri	Non-significant lower cumulative incidence of asthma no significant difference in asthma incidence in infancy higher cumulative incidence of wheeze including asthma no difference in the cumulative incidence of eczema no difference in circulating IgE no difference in infections rate	No effect
Kukkonen, 2007 [35]	925 (of initial 1223); (36 Hbd–6 months)	term infants with family history of allergy	2 years	PREVENTION: probiotic mixture was given prenatally to pregnant woman daily for 2–4 weeks before delivery and after birth to infants for 6 months (together with prebiotic) vs placebo	LGG, L. rhamnosus LC705, Bifidobacterium breve Bb99, Propionibacterium freudenreichii ssp. Schermani	no effect of all allergic disease reduced frequency of atopic eczema	No effect
Kopp, 2008 [22]	94 (of initial 102); (34 Hbd–6 months)	term infants with family history of allergic disease	2 years	PREVENTION: probiotic vs placebo was given prenatally to pregnant woman daily for 4–6 weeks before delivery and after birth for 6 months	LGG	no difference in severity of atopic dermatitis more frequent episodes of recurrent wheezing bronchitis ($P = 0.03$)	LGG not recommended for primary prevention

Reference	Number; (age)	Population	Duration	Intervention	Strains	Results	Effect
Soh, 2008 [38]	253; (0–6 months)	term infants with family history of allergic disease	1 year	PREVENTION: cows' milk formula with or without probiotic daily for 6 months	Bifidobacterium longum BL999 and Lactobacillus rhamnosus	no difference in incidence of eczema	No effect
Wickens, 2008 [21]	474; (36 Hbd–6 months)	term infants with family history of allergic disease	2 years	PREVENTION: probiotic (2 strains) vs placebo was given prenatally to pregnant woman for 4 weeks before delivery and after birth to breast-feeding mothers and to children for 6 months	L. rhamnosus, HN001 and Bifidobacterium animalis subsp. lactis	reduced risk of atopic eczema no significant impact on atopy	No effect
Kuitunen, 2009 [34]	891 (of initial 1223); (26 Hbd–6 months)	term infants with family history of allergic disease	5 years	PREVENTION: probiotic mixture was given prenatally to pregnant woman daily for 2–4 weeks before delivery and after birth to infants for 6 months (together with prebiotic) vs placebo	LGG, L. rhamnosus LC705, Bifidobacterium breve Bb99, Propionibacterium freudenreichii ssp. Schermani	no difference in frequencies of eczema, allergic rhinitis or asthma less IgE-associated eczema and less IgE sensitization in cesarean-delivered children	No effect
Thornton, Morgan et al., Swansea, United Kingdom	600; (36 Hbd–6 months)	term infants with family history of allergic disease	5 years	PREVENTION: probiotic mixture was given prenatally to pregnant woman daily for 2–4 weeks before delivery and after birth to infants for 6 months vs placebo	Lactobacillus salivaris, Lactobacillus paracasei, Bifidobacterium infantis, Bifidobacterium bifidum	study not complete	
Niers, Rijkers, Hoekstra et al., Utrecht, The Netherlands	120; 36 Hbd–12 months	term infants with family history of allergic disease	12 months	PREVENTION: probiotic mixture (3 strains) was given prenatally to pregnant woman daily for 4 weeks before delivery and after birth to infants for 12 months vs placebo	Lactococcus lactis, Bifidobacterium infantis, Bifidobacterium bifidum	study not complete	
Lau, Wahn, and Hamelmann, Berlin, Germany	650; (0–6 months)	term infants with family history of allergic disease	3 years	PREVENTION: probiotic mixture (2 strains) directly to a child daily for 6 months	Streptococcus faecalis DSM 16440, Escherichia coli, DSM 17252	Study not complete	

of reports taking up the role of probiotics in primary prevention of allergic asthma (as detailed in Table 11.3). The pioneer study to investigate the role of probiotics in this context undertook to administer *L. rhamnosus* to mothers (starting 2–4 weeks before delivery) and to infants in the first 6 months of life [2]. Although this report revealed an apparent reduction in the incidence of eczema at 2 years, no significant decrease in respiratory allergy, IgE levels, or allergic sensitization anti-asthmatic was observed. A number of subsequent research papers with other strains of lactobacilli also did not find any favorable effects on allergic asthma prevention.

1. In one of the studies [33] in which *Lactobacillus acidophilus* was given probiotic supplementation for the first 6 months of life did not alter early immune responses and no significant difference in asthma incidence was found.

2. In two other studies [20, 34], probiotic administration (three different strains) was associated with reduced incidence of IgE-associated eczema, indicating potential positive effect on asthma incidence. However, this effect (non-significant lower cumulative incidence of asthma) was observed only in the first study by Abrahamsson ($n = 188$) and was not reproduced in the other reports [20]. Of note, in the second study a combination of strains and prebiotic galacto-oligosaccharides was used.

3. There are now four other published studies (recapitulated in Table 11.3) and at least three other studies in progress at the time of writing to investigate the efficacy of a range of probiotic species for allergy prevention, most using pre- and postnatal infant supplementation. The four published reports failed to show any reduction in allergic airway disease despite changes in intestinal colonization. Rather, there was a disconcerting increase in the frequency of wheezy bronchitis in one study and, astonishingly, the authors concluded that probiotic supplementation cannot generally be recommended for the primary prevention of allergy.

The vast majority of presented studies used probiotics and one [34, 35] tested a combination of pro- and prebiotics. Despite promising immunomodulatory effects, as tested in animal models, none of these studies demonstrated any clear effect on asthma prevention. Basing on this, at this stage it is not reasonable to recommend probiotics and/or prebiotics for respiratory allergy prevention. However, prospective analysis of these populations may allow for an assessment on long-term outcomes, particularly in respect to possible effects on allergic asthma. The outcomes of the other studies (Table 11.3) are expected with great anticipation, especially in respect to the prevention of atopic eczema.

5. FINAL REMARKS

5.1. Prebiotics

There is an interesting discrepancy between promising results from the animal studies, suggesting the therapeutic potential of probiotic strains in airway allergy and the results from clinical studies. Moreover, a number of studies demonstrate some beneficial effects on the suppression of the Th2-directed immune responses and potential therapeutic application in atopic eczema and allergic rhinitis [8, 36]. Therefore, one may speculate that supplementation with a single probiotic strain might be insufficient to have a major impact on the very diverse intestinal flora and the multidirectional interactions between the gut microbiota and the host. This notion has led to a transfer in interest to dietary supplements that could promote more massive effect on gut microbiota—namely, prebiotics. These compounds, which include non-digestible but fermentable oligosaccharides, accelerate the growth of beneficial microbial species like *Bifidobacterium* and *Lactobacillus*. Therefore, it appeared logical from a microbiological standpoint that increasing the consumption of foods containing these products can positively affect the composition and activity of intestinal microbiota. This is a possible mechanism by which the increased consumption of grains and cereals has some protective effects, as it has been seen in epidemiologic studies. As there is only one study showing no protection from allergic asthma when pre- and probiotics were used [34, 35], we believe that, at this stage, there is still too little data to confirm or exclude directly the immunologic or therapeutic effects of prebiotic supplements.

5.2. Different Strains

Possible explanations for the various results among trials in atopic eczema, allergic rhinitis and allergic asthma may include differences in the bacterial strains used and individual factors that could affect microbial responsiveness and allergic susceptibility. Taking into consideration good experimental evidence from animals to suggest its effectiveness in allergy prevention and a limited number of strains used in the presented studies, one cannot dismiss the notion that this approach may still be useful when a more potent probiotic strain will be found and applied successfully.

5.3. Adverse Effects

Despite the fact that probiotic food supplements are believed to be relatively harmless, it might happen that some commercially available products might enclose some milk contaminants and therefore cause side effects in anaphylactic individuals. The significance of this should be thoroughly explored in further studies, since there are prevention studies reporting adverse

outcomes [22, 37]. These reports arouse caution in the middle of the growing public enthusiasm for probiotics.

6. CONCLUSION

It is clear from the review of the presented literature that this issue cannot be definitively resolved at this time, and there is currently not enough data to recommend or reject this as a part of routine management in any allergic disease or for prevention. Even though there have been great expectations, currently there is general agreement that more trials are warranted to confirm this, and that any benefits are not likely to be impressive.

References

1. Bjorksten, B., Sepp, E., Julge, K., et al. (2001). Allergy development and the intestinal microflora during the first year of life. *The Journal of Allergy and Clinical Immunology, 108*, 516–520.
2. Kalliomaki, M., Salminen, S., Arvilommi, H., et al. (2001). Probiotics in primary prevention of atopic disease: a randomised placebo-controlled trial. *Lancet, 357*, 1076–1079.
3. Isolauri, E., Arvola, T., Sutas, Y., et al. (2000). Probiotics in the management of atopic eczema. *Clinical and Experimental Allergy, 30*, 1604–1610.
4. Cross, M. L., & Gill, H. S. (2001). Can immunoregulatory lactic acid bacteria be used as dietary supplements to limit allergies? *Int Arch Allergy Immunol, 125*, 112–119.
5. Sudo, N., Sawamura, S., Tanaka, K., et al. (1997). The requirement of intestinal bacterial flora for the development of an IgE production system fully susceptible to oral tolerance induction. *Journal of Immunology (Baltimore, Md.: 1950), 159*, 1739–1745.
6. Sudo, N., Yu, X. N., Aiba, Y., et al. (2002). An oral introduction of intestinal bacteria prevents the development of a long-term Th2-skewed immunological memory induced by neonatal antibiotic treatment in mice. *Clinical and Experimental Allergy, 32*, 1112–1116.
7. Bjorksten, B. (2005). Genetic and environmental risk factors for the development of food allergy. *Curr Opin Allergy Clin Immunol, 5*, 249–253.

8. Prescott, S. L., & Bjorksten, B. (2007). Probiotics for the prevention or treatment of allergic diseases. *The Journal of Allergy and Clinical Immunology, 120*, 255–262.

9. Feleszko, W., Jaworska, J., & Hamelmann, E. (2006). Toll-like receptors—novel targets in allergic airway disease (probiotics, friends and relatives)., *533*, 308–318.

10. Noverr, M. C., & Huffnagle, G. B. (2004). Does the microbiota regulate immune responses outside the gut? *Trends in Microbiology, 12*, 562–568.

11. Shida, K., & Nanno, M. (2008). Probiotics and immunology: separating the wheat from the chaff. *Trends in Immunology, 29*, 565–573.

12. Borchers, A. T., Selmi, C., Meyers, F. J., et al. (2009). Probiotics and immunity. *Journal of Gastroenterology, 44*, 26–46.

13. Rautava, S., Kalliomaki, M., & Isolauri, E. (2005). New therapeutic strategy for combating the increasing burden of allergic disease: Probiotics—A Nutrition, Allergy, Mucosal Immunology and Intestinal Microbiota (NAMI) Research Group report. *The Journal of Allergy and Clinical Immunology, 116*, 31–37.

14. Vanderhoof, J. A., & Young, R. J. (2004). Current and potential uses of probiotics. *Ann Allergy Asthma Immunol, 93*, S33–S37.

15. Smits, H. H., Engering, A., van der Kleij, D., et al. (2005). Selective probiotic bacteria induce IL-10-producing regulatory T cells *in vitro* by modulating dendritic cell function through dendritic cell-specific intercellular adhesion molecule 3-grabbing nonintegrin. *The Journal of Allergy and Clinical Immunology, 115*, 1260–1267.

16. Kopp, M. V., Goldstein, M., Dietschek, A., et al. (2008). *Lactobacillus* GG has *in vitro* effects on enhanced interleukin-10 and interferon-gamma release of mononuclear cells but no *in vivo* effects in supplemented mothers and their neonates. *Clinical and Experimental Allergy, 38*, 602–610.

17. Feleszko, W., Jaworska, J., Rha, R. D., et al. (2007). Probiotic-induced suppression of allergic sensitization and airway inflammation is associated with an increase of T regulatory-dependent mechanisms in a murine model of asthma. *Clinical and Experimental Allergy, 37*, 498–505.

18. Yoo, J., Tcheurekdjian, H., Lynch, S. V., et al. (2007). Microbial manipulation of immune function for asthma prevention: inferences from clinical trials. *Proceedings of the American Thoracic Society, 4*, 277–282.

19. Prescott, S. L., Wickens, K., Westcott, L., et al. (2008). Supplementation with *Lactobacillus rhamnosus* or *Bifidobacterium lactis* probiotics in pregnancy increases cord blood interferon-gamma and breast milk transforming growth factor-β and immunoglobin A detection. *Clinical and Experimental Allergy, 38*, 1606–1614.

20. Abrahamsson, T. R., Jakobsson, T., Bottcher, M. F., et al. (2007). Probiotics in prevention of IgE-associated eczema: a double-blind, randomized, placebo-controlled trial. *The Journal of Allergy and Clinical Immunology, 119*, 1174–1180.

21. Wickens, K., Black, P. N., Stanley, T. V., et al. (2008). A differential effect of 2 probiotics in the prevention of eczema and atopy: a double-blind, randomized, placebo-controlled trial. *The Journal of Allergy and Clinical Immunology, 122*, 788–794.

22. Kopp, M. V., Hennemuth, I., Heinzmann, A., & Urbanek, R. (2008). Randomized, double-blind, placebo-controlled trial of probiotics for primary prevention: no clinical effects of Lactobacillus GG supplementation. *Pediatrics, 121*, e850–e856.

23. Viljanen, M., Savilahti, E., Haahtela, T., et al. (2005). Probiotics in the treatment of atopic eczema/dermatitis syndrome in infants: a double-blind placebo-controlled trial. *Allergy, 60*, 494–500.

24. Marschan, E., Kuitunen, M., Kukkonen, K., et al. (2008). Probiotics in infancy induce protective immune profiles that are characteristic for chronic low-grade inflammation. *Pulmonary Pharmacology & Therapeutics, 38*, 611–618.

25. Prescott, S. L., & Dunstan, J. A. (2005). Immune dysregulation in allergic respiratory disease: the role of T regulatory cells. *Pulmonary Pharmacology & Therapeutics, 18*, 217–228.

26. Macdonald, T. T., & Monteleone, G. (2005). Immunity, inflammation, and allergy in the gut. *Science, 307*, 1920–1925.

27. Suzuki, K., & Fagarasan, S. (2008). How host-bacterial interactions lead to IgA synthesis in the gut. *Trends in Immunology, 29*, 523–531.

28. Wheeler, J. G., Shema, S. J., Bogle, M. L., et al. (1997). Immune and clinical impact of *Lactobacillus acidophilus* on asthma. *Ann Allergy Asthma Immunol, 79*, 229–233.

29. Helin, T., Haahtela, S., & Haahtela, T. (2002). No effect of oral treatment with an intestinal bacterial strain, *Lactobacillus rhamnosus* (ATCC 53103), on birch-pollen allergy: a placebo-controlled double-blind study. *Allergy, 57*, 243–246.

30. Giovannini, M., Agostoni, C., Riva, E., et al. (2007). A randomized prospective double-blind controlled trial on effects of long-term consumption of fermented milk containing *Lactobacillus casei* in pre-school children with allergic asthma and/or rhinitis. *Pediatric Research, 62*, 215–220.

31. Stockert, K., Schneider, B., Porenta, G., et al. (2007). Laser acupuncture and probiotics in school age children with asthma: a randomized, placebo-controlled pilot study of therapy guided by principles of Traditional Chinese Medicine. *Pediatric Allergy and Immunology, 18*, 160–166.

32. Hamelmann, E., & Wahn, U. (2002). Immune responses to allergens early in life: when and why do allergies arise? *Clinical and Experimental Allergy, 32*, 1679–1681.

33. Taylor, A., Hale, J., Wiltschut, J., et al. (2006). Evaluation of the effects of probiotic supplementation from the neonatal period on innate immune development in infancy. *Clinical and Experimental Allergy, 36*, 1218–1226.

34. Kuitunen, M., Kukkonen, K., Juntunen-Backman, K., et al. (2009). Probiotics prevent IgE-associated allergy until age 5 years in cesarean-delivered children but not in the total cohort. *The Journal of Allergy and Clinical Immunology, 123*, 335–341.

35. Kukkonen, K., Savilahti, E., Haahtela, T., et al. (2007). Probiotics and prebiotic galacto-oligosaccharides in the prevention of allergic diseases: a randomized, double-blind, placebo-controlled trial. *The Journal of Allergy and Clinical Immunology, 119*, 192–198.

36. Vliagoftis, H., Kouranos, V. D., Betsi, G. I., & Falagas, M. E. (2008). Probiotics for the treatment of allergic rhinitis and asthma: systematic review of randomized controlled trials. *Annals of Allergy, Asthma & Immunology, 101*, 570–579.

37. Taylor, A. L., Dunstan, J. A., & Prescott, S. L. (2007). Probiotic supplementation for the first 6 months of life fails to reduce the risk of atopic dermatitis and increases the risk of allergen sensitization in high-risk children: a randomized controlled trial. *The Journal of Allergy and Clinical Immunology, 119*, 184–191.

38. Soh, S. E., Aw, M., Gerez, I., et al. (2009). Probiotic supplementation in the first 6 months of life in at risk Asian infants—effects on eczema and atopic sensitization at the age of 1 year. *Clinical and Experimental Allergy, 32*, 571–578.

Probiotics and Prebiotics:
Role in Surgery Recuperation?

José Eduardo de Aguilar-Nascimento

**Department of Surgery, Medical Sciences School,
The Federal University of Mato Grosso, Cuiaba, Brazil**

1. INTRODUCTION

The prevalence of postoperative infections is still alarming and continues to represent a major problem in surgical units. Sepsis is still a main cause of postoperative morbidity and mortality after abdominal surgery [1]. Sepsis, as defined by the American College of Chest Physicians/Society of Critical Care Medicine consensus definition, is the systemic inflammatory response syndrome due to an infection [2], and is currently the tenth overall leading cause of deaths in the United States, with fatality rates between 20 and 50% [3].

The gastrointestinal tract of healthy individuals contains approximately 10-fold more microbes than the total of eukaryotic body cells [4]. This huge amount of indigenous flora is constrained in the intestinal intraluminal space especially due to the properties of the gut barrier. The disruption of the gut barrier can result in an invasion of either microbes or endotoxin to the organism, resulting in systemic inflammation and septic complications. Bacterial translocation is a well-known phenomenon defined as the passage of viable indigenous bacteria from the intestinal tract through the epithelial mucosa to the mesenteric lymph nodes, and then to the systemic circulation [5]. In surgical patients bacterial translocation is a source of inflammation, sepsis, and is directly associated to postoperative infections [6, 7]. In agreement, gut origin bacteria predominates in postoperative infections. The most frequent aerobic bacteria are *Escherichia coli* and *Enterococci* sp., and the main anaerobic bacteria are the *Bacteroides fragilis* group, *Peptostreptococcus* spp. and *Clostridium* spp. [8] (Table 12.1).

2. RATIONALE FOR THE USE OF PROBIOTICS IN SURGERY

Regardless of the correct use of prophylactic antibiotics and accurate surgical technique, postoperative infections remain a serious concern, an important cause of morbidity and mortality, and an enormous source of costs in surgical practice [1]. Therefore, new strategies should be developed to minimize this problem.

171

TABLE 12.1 The most frequent bacteria in abdominal infections [8]

Anaerobic bacteria	Aerobic bacteria
α-Haemolytic streptococci	*Peptostreptococcus* spp.
β-Haemolytic streptococci	*Microaerophilic streptococci*
Enterococcus spp.	*Propionibacterium acnes*
Staphylococcus aureus	*Veillonella parvulla*
Escherichia coli	*Clostridium* spp.
Klebsiella pneumoniae	*Fusobacterium* spp.
Proteus mirabilis	*Bacteroides fragilis* group
Serratia marcescens	*Prevotella* spp.
Pseudomonas aeruginosa	

TABLE 12.2 Level of interaction between microbes and host

Level of interaction	Quality of interaction
1. Intraluminal	Microbe–microbe
2. Intraluminal	Microbe–gut epithelium
3. Gut wall, lymphonodes	Microbe–immune system

The normal microbiota protects the organism from colonization of pathogenic species, produces short-chain fatty acids (SCFA) to nourish the epithelium, induces local and systemic immunity, and helps gut motility [9]. As it is possible to manipulate the composition of the gastrointestinal microflora by administration of pre- and probiotics it seems logical that this therapy may have a role in preventing infections in surgical patients. Probiotics are defined as preparations containing adequate numbers of viable, defined microorganisms, which confer to the host health benefits [10, 11]. Prebiotics are non-digestible sugars that selectively stimulate the growth of certain colonic bacteria (bifidobacteria and lactobacilli), thereby increasing the body's natural resistance to invading pathogens [12]. In addition, there is increasing evidence that fermentable dietary fibers and the newly described prebiotics can modulate various properties of the immune system, including those of the gut-associated lymphoid tissues (GALT), secondary lymphoid tissues and peripheral circulation [13].

The interaction between bacteria and host plays an important role in the understanding of mechanisms of bacterial translocation, systemic inflammatory response syndrome (SIRS), and the development of postoperative infections. This interaction take place in three levels as described in Table 12.2. At the gut lumen, interaction between microbiota may prevent colonization and enhance the digestion and absorption of various nutrients. In surgical patients, the interaction balance between these three levels is modified due to either the initial insult (chronic disease, trauma, burn, etc.) or the use of antibiotics.

Specific probiotic strains prevent bacterial overgrowth of potential pathogens by direct antimicrobial effects (such as lactic acid production) and competitive growth. The physical property of the gut barrier is fundamental in protecting the organism from the invasion of pathogenic bacteria. Various conditions during the operation, such as gut manipulation, resection, and the placement of sutures, can disrupt the continuity of the mucosal barrier. The inflammatory response to trauma increases the gut permeability enhancing bacterial translocation [6, 7]. The immune system plays a crucial role in preventing infections. Continuous cross-talking between the gut microbiota and the immune system induces a suitable immune response to the invasion of bacteria [9, 11]. In this context, probiotics may confer protection against all mechanisms involved in bacterial translocation. All at once probiotics can generate SCFA and consequently enhance mucosal trophism, increase intestinal motility, and enhance the innate immune system, i.e. they could promote beneficial effects to the patients by acting on the three levels of the host-microbial interaction [9, 12]. For these reasons, it is thought that probiotics may prevent bacterial translocation and consequently may diminish postoperative infections (Table 12.2).

3. RATIONALE FOR THE USE OF PREBIOTICS IN SURGERY

Prebiotics are selectively fermented ingredients which allow specific changes, both in the composition and/or activity in the gastrointestinal microflora that confers benefits upon host well-being and health [14]. They are dietary fibers including inulin or pectin with a well-established positive impact on the intestinal microflora. A number of poorly digested carbohydrates fall into the category of prebiotics, including certain fibers and resistant starches, but the most widely described prebiotics are non-digestible oligosaccharides. Prebiotics may promote various beneficial effects into the gastrointestinal tract. However, most of the health effects of prebiotics are indirect, i.e. mediated by the intestinal microflora, and therefore less well-proven [15]. The combination of pre- and probiotics is called 'synbiotics'. Gibson and Roberfroid defined synbiotics as a mixture of prebiotics and probiotics that beneficially affects the host by improving the survival and implantation of live microbial dietary supplements in the gastrointestinal tract, by selectively stimulating the growth and activating the metabolism of one or a limited number of health-promoting bacteria, and thus improving host welfare [9, 14].

In the surgical field, the association of probiotics and prebiotics seems reasonable due to their synergic effect at the mucosal barrier setting. A number of both experimental and clinical studies aiming at investigating this hypothesis have been conducted with interesting results.

4. ANIMAL STUDIES

Experimental studies have shown that the use of probiotics may prevent sepsis, reduce mortality or decrease the rate of bacterial translocation in various animal models [16–18]. Tsunoda et al.

reported that the pretreatment with *Lactobacillus casei* reduced mortality in rats submitted to fecal peritonitis [19]. Mangell et al. demonstrates that pretreatment with *Lactobacillus plantarum* protects against an *E. coli*-induced increase in intestinal permeability [20].

Qin et al. performed an excellent study in a rat model of peritonitis induced by cecal ligation and perforation. Rats receiving parenteral nutrition were randomized after creation of experimental peritonitis to be either treated or not treated with probiotics via a jejunostomy tube for 5 days. The occludin expression, the integrality of the gut epithelial tight junction and microvilli, the bacterial translocation rate and endotoxin in blood in probiotics group, all improved as compared with the control group [21]. Aguilar-Nascimento et al. showed that a diet supplemented with probiotics (*Streptococcus thermophilus* e *Lactobacillus helveticus*) during the pre- and postoperative periods in rats submitted to colonic resection and anastomosis enhanced colonic weight and anastomotic bursting strength postoperatively. IgA levels increased from intra- to postoperative periods only in animals receiving probiotics supplementation [22].

5. CLINICAL TRIALS

Some controlled clinical trials have investigated the benefits of probiotics in various surgical conditions. The potential effects of prebiotics in the gastrointestinal tract are:

- increased production of SCFA;
- increased energy uptake;
- selectively increases the population of bifidobacteria and lactobacilli;
- increased colonization resistance;
- prevention of bacterial translocation;
- prevention of diarrhea;
- prevention of constipation;
- stimulation of mineral absorption;
- prevention of colorectal cancer.

5.1. Trauma

Few randomized trials have looked into the effects of either probiotics or synbiotics in the trauma setting. In the three trial diets studied here all patients were administered by tube feeding. In a double blind, placebo controlled trial, Kotzampassi et al. randomized 65 patients to receive a synbiotic formula containing synbiotics (Synbiotic 2000 Forte, Medipharm, Sweden) or maltodextrin as placebo once daily for 15 days. The formula contained 10^{11} cfu/g of each of the four bacteria: *Pediococcus pentosaceus, Leuconostoc mesenteroides, L. paracasei* ssp. *paracasei*; and *L. plantarum*, in association with inulin, oat bran, pectin, and resistant starch as prebiotics. All patients were critically ill due to severe multiple trauma. Infection rate (63 vs 90%; $p = 0.01$), days of mechanical ventilation (16.7 ± 9.5 vs 29.7 ± 16.5 days; $p = 0.001$), and length of intensive care stay (27.7 ± 15.2 vs 41.3 ± 20.5; $p = 0.01$) was significantly decreased in the synbiotic group [23].

Another randomized controlled trial included 113 multiple injured patients into four groups to receive enteral nutrition supplemented with glutamine or fermentable fiber; peptide diet; or fibers combined with the same Synbiotic 2000 formula (Synbiotic 2000 Forte, Medipharm, Sweden), a mixture containing live lactobacilli and specific bioactive fibers. There were no differences in the days of mechanical ventilation, intensive care unit stay, or multiple-organ failure scores between the patient groups. However, patients receiving the synbiotic formula had less lung infections and reduced intestinal permeability than others [24].

Twenty subjects in an intensive care setting due to traumatic brain injury were randomized by Falcão de Arruda and Aguilar-Nascimento to receive early enteral feeding with a standard formula that was associated or not associated with both glutamine (30 g) and probiotics (*Lactobacillus johnsonii* La 1 (LC1®; Nestlé, São Paulo, Brazil) for at least 5 days. The infection rate was higher in controls (100%) when compared with the study group (50%; $p = 0.03$) and the median (range) number of infections per patient was significantly greater ($p < 0.01$) in the control group [3 (1–5) days] compared with the study group [1 (0–3) days]. Both the critical care unit stay [22 (7–57) compared with 10 (5–20) days; $p < 0.01$; median (range)] and days of mechanical ventilation [14 (3–53) compared with 7 (1–15) days; $p = 0.04$; median (range)] were higher in the patients in the control group than in the study group. The central hypothesis of this study was that the association of glutamine with probiotics might promote a synergistic and favorable action in trauma patients. Glutamine would improve both the enterocyte and immune cell nutrition, whereas the presence of probiotic bacteria would beneficially alter the intraluminal environment [25].

In summary, all of these studies in trauma patients attested to the potential benefits of probiotics/synbiotics in the postoperative outcome.

5.2. Major Abdominal Operation (Mainly Colorectal)

In elective abdominal operations the benefits of probiotics/synbiotics are less palpable. Four controlled randomized trials have investigated the postoperative outcome of patients submitted to elective abdominal operations, mainly colorectal surgeries, and in three studies no significant advantage of the probiotics/synbiotics was found [26–29].

McNaught et al. included 129 patients undergoing elective major abdominal surgery to receive perioperatively either an oral preparation containing *Lactobacillus plantarum* 299v or a control diet. There was no significant difference between the two groups regarding bacterial translocation rate (12 vs 12%; $p = 0.82$), gastric colonization with enteric organisms (11 vs 17%; $p = 0.42$), or septic morbidity (13 vs 15%; $p = 0.74$) [26]. The same group performed another randomized trial [27], this time enrolling 72 patients to receive an oral synbiotic formula (*Lactobacillus acidophilus* La5, *Bifidobacterium lactis* Bb-12, *Streptococcus thermophilus*, and *Lactobacillus bulgaricus*, in association to oligofructose). Sixty-five other patients made up the placebo group. Again, the findings showed no significant differences between the synbiotic and control groups in bacterial translocation (12.1 vs 10.7%; $p = 0.81$), gastric colonization (41 vs 44%; $p = 0.72$), various surrogates of systemic inflammation, or septic complications (32 vs 31%; $p = 0.88$). A third study performed by the same group, this time in patients undergoing elective colorectal resection, failed to find any beneficial effect of synbiotics in the postoperative outcome [28].

In a non-homogeneous population of patient candidates to major abdominal operations, Rayes et al. randomized [29] 90 subjects to receive either parenteral nutrition and fiber-free enteral nutrition (group A), enteral fiber-containing nutrition with living *Lactobacillus* (group B), or heat-killed *Lactobacillus* (group C) for 7 days. The incidence of infections was significantly lower ($p = 0.01$) in groups B and C, with enteral nutrition containing fibers (10% each), than in group A (30%). Patients receiving living *Lactobacillus* had antibiotics for a significantly shorter time ($p = 0.04$) than patients in groups A and C. However, the length of hospital stay and the incidence of non-infectious complications did not differ significantly.

It is reasonable to assume that the findings in trauma patients are most appreciable when compared to elective major abdominal operations. Although the reasons for this lack of effectiveness are not clear at present, it is interesting to notice that all elective studies that failed used the oral route while the enteral route for administration of probiotics/synbiotics was used in studies performed in the trauma care. This particular point in the methodology of the study may play a role to explain the differences seen in postoperative outcome because some probiotic strains may not survive the acidic environment of the stomach. Other possible explanations are the short period of treatment (a median of 4 days in the trials associated with no beneficial effect), and the distinct clinical condition of the enrolled patients.

5.3. Pancreas Resection

Resection of the pancreas alone or associated with the duodenum is a major operation and is associated with high morbidity and mortality, mainly due to postoperative infections. Fathy et al. have reviewed the outcome of 216 periampullary tumors treated by Whipple pancreaticoduodenectomy from 2000 to 2006. Pancreaticogastrostomy was done in 183 patients and pancreaticojejunostomy in 33 patients. Operative mortality was 3.2%, but 33% patients developed one or more complications, mainly infections [30]. A systematic review involving 578 randomized patients and six randomized trials showed that mortality ranged from 0 to 7.1% and morbidity from 20.8 to 59% [31].

In this context, two randomized trials have tested probiotics/synbiotics in patients undergoing pancreatic resections [32, 33]. Nomura et al. allocated 64 patients into two groups before pancreaticoduodenectomy (30 receiving probiotics and 34 controls). The probiotics group received a mixture of *Enterococcus faecalis* T-110, *Clostridium butyricum* TO-A, and *Bacillus mesentericus* TO-A (BIO-THREE, Toa Pharmaceutical, Japan) 3 to 15 days before the operation, and then reintroduced on the second postoperative day. There was no statistical difference in mortality rate, though the incidence of infectious complications in the probiotics group (23%) was significantly lower ($p = 0.02$) than in the controls (53%) [32].

Another randomized trial performed by Rayes et al. showed the similar beneficial effect of symbiotic in this subset of surgical patients. They randomized 80 patients following pylorus-preserving pancreatoduodenectomy to receive enteral nutrition containing either a composition of prebiotics and probiotics (Synbiotic 2000, Medipharm, Kågerod, Sweden and Des Moines, USA) or only prebiotics. The synbiotic group received—via the jejunum—a combination containing four different lactic acid bacteria: 1010 *Pediacoccus pentosaceus* 5–33:3 (dep.nr LMG P-20608), *Leuconostoc mesenteroides* 77:1 (dep. nr LMG P-20607), *Lactobacillus paracasei* subspecies paracasei F19 (dep.nr LMG P-17806), and *Lactobacillus plantarum* 2362 (dep.nr LMG P-20606). They also received four bioactive fibers: 2.5 g of each betaglucan, inulin, pectin, and resistant starch, totaling 10 g per dose, or 20 g per day. The findings showed that the incidence of postoperative bacterial infections was significantly lower with symbiotic therapy (12.5%) than with fibers only (40%). In addition, the duration of antibiotic therapy was significantly shorter in the latter group [33].

5.4. Biliary Tree and Liver

Septic complications after liver resection remain a difficult problem and a major, well-recognized complication after hepatectomy [34]. The morbidity rate in liver resection can reach as high as 81.0% [35]. Given that synbiotics can improve the intestinal microbial environment and activate host immune function, leading to prevention of bacterial translocation, some randomized trials have investigated whether this beneficial effect might reduce infectious complications after hepatectomy or liver transplantation.

A randomized controlled trial investigated the effect of synbiotics on intestinal integrity and microflora, as well as on surgical outcome, in patients undergoing high-risk hepatectomy. Forty-four patients undergoing hepatectomy for biliary malignancies were randomized to receive postoperatively enteral nutrition that included or did not include synbiotics (a combination of 10^8 *Bifidobacterium breve* Yakult and *L. casei* Shiroti, and galacto-oligosaccharides). The incidence of infectious complications was 19% (4/21) in the synbiotics group and 52% (12/23) in controls ($p < 0.05$) [36].

In an excellent controlled trial, Sugawara et al. randomized 101 patients with biliary cancer

involving the hepatic hilus before hepatectomy to receive either postoperative enteral feeding with synbiotics (postoperative group) or the same composition in the preoperative plus postoperative periods (perioperative group). Postoperative synbiotics used in both groups were Yakult BL Seichoyaku (Yakult Honsha, Japan) containing 1×10^8 of the living *Lactobacillus casei* strain Shirota, and 1×10^8 of the living *Bifidobacterium breve* strain Yakult, per gram; as well as galacto-oligosaccharides (Oligomate 55, Yakult Honsha, Japan). As a preoperative synbiotic treatment, patients received orally one 80 mL bottle of Yakult 400 (Yakult Honsha, Japan) containing at least 4×10^{10} of the living *Lactobacillus casei* strain Shirota; one 100-mL bottle of Bifiel (Yakult Honsha) containing at least 1×10^{10} of the living *Bifidobacterium breve* strain Yakult; and the same prebiotics for 2 weeks before hepatectomy. In 81 patients who completed the trial postoperative serum IL-6, white blood cell counts, and C-reactive protein were significantly lower in the perioperative group than in the postoperative group ($p < 0.05$). Moreover, the incidence of postoperative infectious complications was approximately two-fold greater (30.0%) in the postoperative group than in the perioperative group (12.1%) ($p < 0.05$). The authors concluded that preoperative oral administration of synbiotics enhances immune responses, attenuates systemic postoperative inflammatory responses, improves intestinal microbial environment, and reduces postoperative infectious complications after hepatobiliary resection for biliary tract cancer [37].

These two randomized trials clearly show that the use of synbiotics impact the outcome of patients submitted to liver resection. In addition to these important findings, the administration of synbiotics for liver transplant recipients has also decreased the infectious morbidity in two other randomized trials published by Rayes et al. [38, 39]. These results are especially significant because sepsis is the most important cause of death in liver transplant recipients. In the second study, they allocated 66 patients to

TABLE 12.3 Summary of randomized trials in current literature

Author	Type of patients	Time of administration	Composition	Route	Infection outcome
Kotzampassi et al. [23]	Trauma	15 days post-op	*Pediococcus pentosaceus, Leuconostoc mesenteroides, L. paracasei ssp. paracasei*, and *L. plantarum*, and inulin, oat bran, pectin, and resistant starch.	Enteral	63 vs 90% ($p = 0.01$)
McNaught et al. [26]	Major abdominal operations	± 9 days pre-op; ± 5 days post-op	*Lactobacillus plantarum* 299v.	Oral	NS
Spindler-Vesel et al. [24]	Trauma	Not stated	Lactobacilli and specific bioactive fibers.	Enteral	Reduction of infection ($p = 0.02$)
Falcão de Arruda et al. [25]	Head trauma	At least 5 days	*Lactobacillus johnsonii* La 1 and glutamine.	Enteral	50 vs 100% ($p = 0.03$)
Anderson et al. [27]	Major abdominal operations	± 12 days pre-op; ± 5 days post-op	*Lactobacillus acidophilus* La5, *Bifidobacterium lactis* Bb-12, *Streptococcus thermophilus*, and *Lactobacillus bulgaricus*, in association to oligofructose.	Oral	NS
Reddy et al. [28]	Colorectal	Preoperative; not stated	*Lactobacillus acidophilus* La5, *Bifidobacterium lactis* Bb-12, *Streptococcus thermophilus*, and *Lactobacillus bulgaricus*, in association to oligofructose.	Oral	NS
Rayes et al. [29]	Major abdominal operations	7 days post-op	*Lactobacillus*.	Enteral	10 vs 30% ($p = 0.01$)
Nomura et al. [32]	Pancreas resection	3–15 days pre-op	*Enterococcus faecalis* T-110, *Clostridium butyricum* TO-A, and *Bacillus mesentericus* TO-A.	Enteral	23 vs 53% ($p = 0.02$)
Rayes et al. [33]	Pancreas resection	1 day pre-op; 8 days post-op	*Pediacoccus pentosaceus, Leuconostoc mesenteroides, Lactobacillus paracasei* subspecies *paracasei* F19, and *Lactobacillus plantarum* 2362 plus betaglucan, inulin, pectin, and resistant starch.	Enteral	12.5 vs 40% ($p < 0.01$)
Kanazawa et al. [36]	Liver resection	14 days post-op	*Bifidobacterium breve* Yakult and *L. casei* Shirota, and galacto-oligosaccharides.	Enteral	19 vs 52% ($p < 0.05$)
Sugawara et al. [37]	Liver resection	14 days pre- and 14 days post-op	*Bifidobacterium breve* Yakult and *L. casei* Shirota, and galacto-oligosaccharides.	Oral/Enteral	12.1 vs 30% ($p < 0.049$)
Rayes et al. [38]	Liver transplantation	7 days post-op	*Lactobacillus plantarum* 299 and oat fiber.	Enteral	13 vs 34 vs 48% ($p = 0.01$)
Rayes et al. [39]	Liver transplantation	14 days post-op	*Pediacoccus pentosaceus, Leuconostoc mesenteroides, Lactobacillus paracasei* subspecies *paracasei* F19, and *Lactobacillus plantarum* 2362 plus betaglucan, inulin, pectin, and resistant starch.	Enteral	3 vs 48% ($p < 0.05$)

receive either a mixture of four probiotic bacteria and four fibers or the fibers only for a period of 14 days by early postoperative enteral nutrition. They reported a significant decrease in the incidence of postoperative bacterial infections; being 48% with only fibers and 3% with probiotics and fibers.

6. CONCLUSION

This review has shown that there is good evidence coming out of controlled randomized trials to prescribe synbiotics to surgical patients, mainly those in the trauma setting, and those candidates to elective biliary and liver resection, liver transplantation, and pancreatic resection. However, in colorectal operations, the usefulness of probiotics/synbiotics are less appreciable. Randomized trials using synbiotics by enteral route versus controls seems to be associated with a more significant decrease in infectious morbidity rate than trials in which synbiotics were administered orally. However, the available studies (Table 12.3) have used diverse methodology and tested different probiotic strains and synbiotics [40, 41]. As the effect of probiotics/synbiotics depends on the strains, the concentration of probiotics and on the duration of the therapy, further studies are necessary.

References

1. Emmanuel, K., Weighardt, H., Bartels, H., et al. (2005). Current and future concepts of abdominal sepsis. *World Journal of Surgery*, 29(1), 3–9.
2. Bone, R. C, Balk, R. A., Cerra, F. B., et al. (1992). Definitions for sepsis and organ failure and guidelines for the use of innovative therapies in sepsis. The ACCP/SCCM Consensus Conference Committee. American College of Chest Physicians/Society of Critical Care Medicine. *Chest*, 101, 1644–1655.
3. Angus, D. C., Linde-Zwirble, W. T., Lidicker, J., et al. (2001). Epidemiology of severe sepsis in the United States: Analysis of incidence, outcome, and associated costs of care. *Critical Care Medicine*, 29, 1303–1310.
4. Farthing, M. J. G. (2004). Bugs and the gut: An unstable marriage. *Best Practice & Research. Clinical Gastroenterology*, 18, 233–239.
5. MacFie, J., O'Boyle, C., Mitchell, C. J., et al. (1999). Gut origin of sepsis: A prospective study investigating associations between bacterial translocation, gastric microflora, and septic morbidity. *Gut*, 45, 223–228.
6. Schietroma, M., Carlei, F., Cappelli, S., & Amicucci, G. (2006). Intestinal permeability and systemic endotoxemia after laparotomic or laparoscopic cholecystectomy. *Annals of Surgery*, 243(3), 359–363.
7. MacFie, J., Reddy, B. S., Gatt, M., et al. (2006). Bacterial translocation studied in 927 patients over 13 years. *The British Journal of Surgery*, 93(1), 87–93.
8. Brook, I. (2008). Microbiology and management of abdominal infections. *Digestive Diseases and Sciences*, 53(10), 2585–2591.
9. Hooper, L. V., & Gordon, J. L. (2001). Commensal host-bacterial relationships in the gut. *Science*, 292, 1115–1118.
10. Food and Agricultural Organization of the United Nations and World Health Organization Working Group. (2002). *Working group report: guidelines for the evaluation of probiotics*. London, Ontario, Canada: World Health Organization.
11. Macfarlane, G. T., & Cummings, J. H. (2002). Probiotics, infection and immunity. *Current Opinion in Infectious Diseases*, 15, 501–506.
12. Cummings, J. H., & Macfarlane, G. T. (2002). Gastrointestinal effects of prebiotics. *The British Journal of Nutrition*, 87(2), S145–S151.
13. Schley, P. D., & Field, C. J. (2002). The immune-enhancing effects of dietary fibres and prebiotics. *The British Journal of Nutrition*, 87(Suppl 2), S221–S230.
14. Gibson, G. R., & Roberfroid, M. B. (1995). Dietary modulation of the human colonic microbiota: Introducing the concept of prebiotics. *The Journal of Nutrition*, 125, 1401–1412.
15. de Vrese, M., & Schrezenmeir, J. (2008). Probiotics, prebiotics, and synbiotics. *Advances in Biochemical Engineering/Biotechnology*, 111, 1–66.
16. Adawi, D., Ahrné, S., & Molin, G. (2001). Effects of different probiotic strains of Lactobacillus and Bifidobacterium on bacterial translocation and liver injury in an acute liver injury model. *International Journal of Food Microbiology*, 70(3), 213–220.
17. Gun, F., Salman, T., Gurler, N., & Olgac, V. (2005). Effect of probiotic supplementation on bacterial translocation in thermal injury. *Surgery Today*, 35(9), 760–764.
18. Luyer, M. D., Buurman, W. A., Hadfoune, M., et al. (2005). Strain-specific effects of probiotics on gut barrier integrity following hemorrhagic shock. *Infection and Immunity*, 73(6), 3686–3692.
19. Tsunoda, A., Shibusawa, M., Tsunoda, Y., et al. (2002). Effect of *Lactobacillus casei* on a novel murine model of

abdominal sepsis. *The Journal of Surgical Research*, 107(1), 37–43.

20. Mangell, P., Nejdfors, P., Wang, M., et al. (2002). *Lactobacillus plantarum* 299v inhibits *Escherichia coli*-induced intestinal permeability. *Digestive Diseases and Sciences*, 47(3), 511–516.

21. Qin, H. L., Shen, T. Y., Gao, Z. G., et al. (2005). Effect of lactobacillus on the gut microflora and barrier function of the rats with abdominal infection. *World Journal of Gastroenterology : WJG*, 11(17), 2591–2596.

22. Aguilar-Nascimento, J. E., Prado, S., Zaffani, G., et al. (2006). Perioperative administration of probiotics: Effects on immune response, anastomotic resistance and colonic mucosal trophism. *Acta Cirurgica Brasileira*, 21(Suppl 4), 80–83.

23. Kotzampassi, K., Giamarellos-Bourboulis, E. J., Voudouris, A., et al. (2006). Benefits of a synbiotic formula (Synbiotic 2000 Forte) in critically ill trauma patients: Early results of a randomized controlled trial. *World Journal of Surgery*, 30(10), 1848–1855.

24. Spindler-Vesel, A., Bengmark, S., Vovk, I., et al. (2007). Synbiotics, prebiotics, glutamine, or peptide in early enteral nutrition: a randomized study in trauma patients. *JPEN. Journal of Parenteral and Enteral Nutrition*, 31(2), 119–126.

25. Falcão de Arruda, I. S., & de Aguilar-Nascimento, J. E. (2004). Benefits of early enteral nutrition with glutamine and probiotics in brain injury patients. *Clinical Science (London, England: 1979)*, 106(3), 287–292.

26. McNaught, C. E., Woodcock, N. P., et al. (2002). A prospective randomised study of the probiotic *Lactobacillus plantarum* 299v on indices of gut barrier function in elective surgical patients. *Gut*, 51, 827–831.

27. Anderson, A. D. G., McNaught, C. E., Jain, P. K., & MacFie, J. (2004). Randomised clinical trial of synbiotic therapy in elective surgical patients. *Gut*, 53, 241–245.

28. Reddy, B. S., MacFie, J., Gatt, M., et al. (2007). Randomized clinical trial of effect of synbiotics, neomycin and mechanical bowel preparation on intestinal barrier function in patients undergoing colectomy. *The British Journal of Surgery*, 94, 546–554.

29. Rayes, N., Hansen, S., Seehofer, D., et al. (2002). Early enteral supply of fiber and lactobacilli versus conventional nutrition: a controlled trial in patients with major abdominal surgery. *Nutrition*, 18, 609–615.

30. Fathy, O., Wahab, M. A., Elghwalby, N., et al. (2008). 216 cases of pancreaticoduodenectomy: Risk factors for postoperative complications. *Hepatogastroenterology*, 55(84), 1093–1098.

31. Diener, M. K., Knaebel, H. P., Heukaufer, C., et al. (2007). A systematic review and meta-analysis of pylorus-preserving versus classical pancreaticoduodenectomy for surgical treatment of periampullary and pancreatic carcinoma. *Annals of Surgery*, 245(2), 187–200.

32. Nomura, T., Tsuchiya, Y., Nashimoto, A., et al. (2007). Probiotics reduce infectious complications after pancreaticoduodenectomy. *Hepatogastroenterology*, 54(75), 661–663.

33. Rayes, N., Seehofer, D., Theruvath, T., et al. (2007). Effect of enteral nutrition and synbiotics on bacterial infection rates after pylorus-preserving pancreatoduodenectomy: A randomized, double-blind trial. *Annals of Surgery*, 246(1), 36–41.

34. Matsumata, T., Yanaga, K., Shimada, M., et al. (1995). Occurrence of intra-abdominal septic complications after hepatic resections between 1985 and 1990. *Surgery Today*, 25, 49–54.

35. Nagino, M., Kamiya, J., Uesaka, K., et al. (2001). Complications of hepatectomy for hilar cholangiocarcinoma. *World Journal of Surgery*, 25, 1277–1283.

36. Kanazawa, H., Nagino, M., Kamiya, S., et al. (2005). Synbiotics reduce postoperative infectious complications: A randomized controlled trial in biliary cancer patients undergoing hepatectomy. *Langenbeck's Archives of Surgery*, 390(2), 104–113.

37. Sugawara, G., Nagino, M., Nishio, H., et al. (2006). Perioperative synbiotic treatment to prevent postoperative infectious complications in biliary cancer surgery: A randomized controlled trial. *Annals of Surgery*, 244(5), 706–714.

38. Rayes, N., Seehofer, D., Hansen, S., et al. (2002). Early enteral supply of Lactobacillus and fiber versus selective bowel decontamination: A controlled trial in liver transplant recipients. *Transplantation*, 74(1), 123–128.

39. Rayes, N., Seehofer, D., Theruvath, T., et al. (2005). Supply of pre- and probiotics reduces bacterial infection rates after liver transplantation—a randomized, double-blind trial. *American Journal of Transplantation*, 5, 125–130.

40. van Santvoort, H. C., Besselink, M. G., Timmerman, H. M., et al. (2008). Probiotics in surgery. *Surgery*, 143(1), 1–7.

41. Rayes, N., Seehofer, D., & Neuhaus, P. (2008). Prebiotics, probiotics, synbiotics in surgery—are they only trendy, truly effective or even dangerous? [Epub ahead of print]. *Langenbecks Archives of Surgery*, Dec 16.

13

Prebiotics and Probiotics in Therapy and Prevention of Gastrointestinal Diseases in Children

Silvia Salvatore[1] and Yvan Vandenplas[2]

[1]Clinica Pediatrica, Università dell'Insubria, Ospedale 'F. Del Ponte,' Varese, Italy
[2]Department of Pediatrics, Universitair Ziekenhuis Kinderen Brussel,
Vrije Universiteit Brussel, Brussels, Belgium

1. INTRODUCTION

The knowledge of the beneficial effect of some microorganisms on health is not new. It is already more than 2000 years ago since the Roman author Plinius The Old recommended fermented milk in the treatment of acute gastroenteritis. The modern concept of using microorganisms in the treatment of disease dates from more than a century ago [1]. As early as in 1906, Tissier noted that significant stool colonization with bifidobacteria was protective against the likelihood of the development of diarrhea in children [2]. However, the term 'probiotic' (meaning 'for life') was not used until the 1960s. During the past two decades or so the number of publications on gastrointestinal flora in different gastrointestinal disorders has literally exploded, especially in the area of acute infectious gastroenteritis, although only a limited number of strains have been tested in children.

Simultaneously, the demonstration of the benefit of prebiotics, such as galacto-oligosaccharide (GOS), fructo-oligosaccharide (FOS) and inulin have been investigated. This chapter will focus on the gastrointestinal effects of prebiotics and probiotics in children.

2. PREBIOTICS AND THE GUT

Breast milk is the golden standard for infant nutrition. Its composition is complex and not reproducible, whereas its functional properties represent the model for modern formulas. More than 130 different oligosaccharides have been recognized in human milk and their bifidogenic and anti-infective properties have been demonstrated [3–5].

Supplementing infant formulas with oligosaccharides similar to those present in human milk

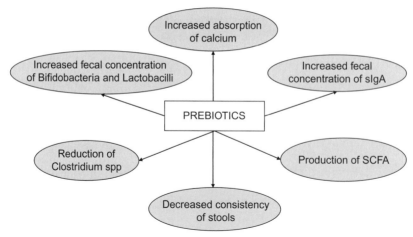

FIGURE 13.1 Prebiotics and the gut: proven effects in children.

and mimicking the microflora of breast-fed infants may have clinical potential benefits in infants' health specifically in terms of prevention of infections and allergy, and mineral absorption. Research has focused on the role of inulin, FOS, GOS and their fermentation derivatives represented by short-chain fatty acids (SCFA) such as butyric, acetic and propionic acid [6]. The SCFA are an important source of energy for gut cells, decrease the luminal pH and participate in electrolyte and water absorption. The effects and clinical importance of SCFA will not be discussed in this chapter.

3. THE GASTROINTESTINAL EFFECTS OF PREBIOTICS IN ASYMPTOMATIC INFANTS

3.1. Prebiotic Supplementation in Infant Formula and Intestinal Flora

The first study on the effect of a formula containing GOS (2%) in infants dates back to 1982 and showed fecal characteristics (stool consistency, colour and pH) similar to that obtained with human milk. The percentages of bifidobacteria in the fecal flora were 93% in the breast-fed group, 69% in the GOS group and 61% in the commercial control formula group [7].

Infant formulae containing GOS (0.24g/100mL) or a mixture of GOS and FOS (at doses of 0.4 to 0.8g/100mL, with a ratio of 9:1) significantly increased, both in term and preterm infants, the number of intestinal bifidobacteria (with a dosage-related effect [5]) and lactobacilli when compared to infants fed a control formula [5, 8–12]. No significant difference was present between infants fed supplemented formulae and human milk in terms of strains and concentration of bifidobacteria and lactobacilli [12]. Higher frequencies and softer stools were reported with the GOS and FOS supplementation (with a ratio of 9:1) at dosages of 0.4g/100mL [5, 13], 0.8g/100mL [5, 14, 15] and 1g/100mL [8]; or with only GOS (0.24g/100mL) [9] or FOS (3.0g/L [16] to 4.0g/L [17]) compared to standard formulae. A different combination of prebiotics (polydextrose, GOS, and lactulose), at two different intake levels (4g/L and 8g/L) confirmed the significant decrease of stool consistency but resulted in increased stool frequency only at 30 days of life and in the group with 8g/L of supplementation [18].

In addition, a reduction in the absolute number of possible harmful bacteria was seen to indicate that prebiotic substances might have the capacity to protect against enteral infections [10, 13, 17].

A double blind, placebo controlled, randomized intervention trial (DBRCT) in 82 healthy, full-term, partially breast-fed children from 1 week to 3 months old, evaluated the effect of the addition of a mixture of GOS (0.54 g/100 mL) and FOS (0.06 g/100 mL) alone or in combination with pectin-derived acidic oligosaccharides (0.2 g/100 mL) in whey-based formula. An increase of the *Bifidobacterium genus* ($p = 0.0001$), and a decrease of proportions for the bacteroides ($p = 0.02$) and the *Clostridium coccoides* group ($p = 0.01$) in both oligosaccharide groups were demonstrated using quantitative fluorescent *in situ* hybridization (FISH) coupled to flow cytometry. The intervention was protracted up to 2 months after cessation of breast-feeding and the increase of bifidobacteria persisted with a stronger affect when acidic oligosaccharides were present ($p < 0.01$) [19].

The beneficial effects of an infant milk formula with GOS/FOS (6 g/L, ratio 9:1) on improving the percentages of bifidobacteria (60 vs 53%, $p = 0.04$) and reducing the *Clostridium* spp. (0.0 vs 3.27%, $p = 0.006$) was confirmed, with FISH analysis of stool samples, in another DBRCT on 187 healthy infants with an intervention period in the first 26 weeks of life [20].

However, in the studies with formulae supplemented with only FOS, the results are less homogeneous. A dosage of FOS of 0.15 or 0.3 g/L significantly increased the concentration of *Enterococcus* and *Clostridium* compared to breast-fed infants ($p < 0.05$) and had a significant transitory bifidogenic affect only in the group with 0.15 g/L ($p = 0.045$ vs standard formula) disappearing 7 days after the conclusion of supplementation [16]. In another infant trial 0.4/100 mL of FOS a significant higher number of bacteroides and bifidobacteria, and proportion of infants colonized with bifidobacteria, and lower concentration of *Escherichia coli* and enterococci were noted compared to a maltodextrine-enriched formula ($p = 0.03$) [17].

Supplementation with 0.24 g/100 mL GOS [9] or a mixture of GOS and FOS (6 g/L or 8 g/L, ratio 9:1) [10, 21] also mimicked, in formula-fed infants, the metabolic activity of the intestinal microflora from breast-fed infants with a reduction of the pH and a similar fecal fatty acid pattern. There was a significant increase of acetate and lactate and decrease of propionate levels compared to infants fed unsupplemented formula.

3.2. Prebiotic Supplementation in Solids

The effects of an addition of prebiotic oligosaccharides in solids such as cereals and weaning foods have been less studied.

In one DBRCT, 56 healthy infants were randomly assigned to receive either 0.75 g FOS per serving of cereal or placebo for 28 days. Average FOS consumption was 0.74 g/d and as high as 3.00 g/d. There was no difference between the groups in the stool pH, tolerance and in crying, spitting-up or colic. FOS consumption led to more regular (1.99 mean number of stools per infant per day vs 1.58 in the control group, $p = 0.02$) and softer stools [22].

In a DBRCT with an intervention period of 6 weeks in 35 infants (aged 4 to 6 months), the addition of GOS/FOS (ratio 9:1, 4.5 g/d) to weaning products (Vivinal GOS, Borculo Domo Ingredients, Zwolle, the Netherlands; Raftiline HP, Orafti active food ingredients, Tienen, Belgium) determined a significant increase in the fecal percentage of bifidobacteria compared to enrollment ($p = 0.03$) and control group ($p = 0.03$) [23].

A mean intake of $0.74 + 0.39$ g FOS/day in cereals consumed by toddlers attending daycare reduced the chance of having 'hard' stools in favor of stools of 'soft' or 'loose' consistency [24]. A mean intake of 1.2 g/day oligofructose over 6 months resulted in adequate growth and a reduction of vomiting, regurgitation, pain at defecation, febrile events, respiratory symptoms, antibiotic use and day-care absenteeism, but without any difference in diarrhea.

Significantly less flatulence, vomiting, fever and diarrhea occurred in 7–19 months healthy children observed for 15 days and supplemented for 3 weeks with 2 g/day FOS [25].

3.3. Prebiotic Supplementation and Mineral Absorption

Oligofructose and inulin (0.4 g/dL) increased the availability of calcium to 16.7 and 17.2%, respectively [26]. A formula containing GOS and FOS (0.8 g/dL, ratio 9:1) stimulated calcium absorption in preterm infants [27]. Oligofructose did not change the availability of zinc, but inulin (0.4 g/dL) increased zinc availability to 12.2% [26].

Calcium absorption was significantly higher (38.2 ± 9.8% vs 32.3 ± 9.8%; $p = 0.01$), in a group of 59 girls receiving a mixture of 8 g/d inulin and oligofructose (ratio of 70:30, Synergy) over a 3-week period in comparison to groups receiving the same amount of FOS alone or placebo [28]. After 1 year of supplementation, the same treatment also significantly improved bone mineral density [28]. In a randomized controlled feeding study (9-day periods) in 12 adolescent boys, FOS at 15 g/d significantly improved fractional Ca absorption [29]. In 100 children (9–13 years) a 1-year supplement of mixed long- and short-chain inulin (8 g/d) increased calcium absorption and bone mineral density [30].

4. GUT IMMUNE EFFECTS

4.1. Prebiotics

In a trial comparing standard infant formulae, one formula with 0.6 g/100 mL GOS/FOS (ratio 9:1) and one with probiotics (6×10^9 cfu *Bifidobacterium animalis* Bb12/100 mL) showed a trend towards an increased fecal secretory IgA level with only the prebiotic formula compared to a standard formula reaching statistical significance at the age of 16 weeks [31]. A significant increased production of fecal secretory immunoglobulin A (sIgA) (719 μg/g vs 263 μg/g, $p < 0.001$) was demonstrated after 26 weeks of intervention, investigating the effect of an infant milk formula with 0.6 g/100 mL GOS/FOS (ratio 9:1) in 187 healthy infants [20].

In a prospective DBRCT, healthy term infants with a parental history of atopy were fed either prebiotic-supplemented (8 g/L GOS/FOS, ratio 9:1) or placebo-supplemented (8 g/L maltodextrin) hypoallergenic formula during the first 6 months of life. Infants in the prebiotic group had significantly fewer episodes of all types of infections combined ($p = 0.01$) and lower cumulative incidences of any respiratory recurring infections (3.9 and 2.9% vs 13.5 and 9.6% in the placebo group, $p < 0.05$) [32].

Oligofructose (Orafti Group, Tienen, Belgium) added to infant cereal (0.55 g/15 g cereal, average consumed 0.67 g prebiotic/d, or 0.11 g/kg/d) for 6 months failed to show a significant benefit in response to Haemophilus Influenza type B vaccinations, weight gain, visits to the clinic, hospitalizations and use of antibiotics. However, infants were partially breast-fed for more than 85% of the observational period [33].

4.2. Probiotics

Many different strain-specific mechanisms of action have been demonstrated for probiotics (Figure 13.2) [34]. The protective affects of probiotics involve [35–39]:

- direct antagonism against pathogens through competitive inhibition of adhesion to the epithelium and of specific bacterial toxins;
- production of intestinal mucin;
- bacteriocins or other antimicrobic molecules;
- restoration of tight junction protein structure;
- secretion of defensins;

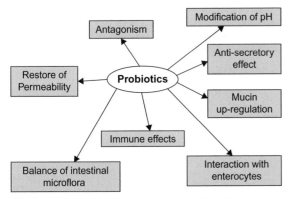

FIGURE 13.2 Mechanism of action of probiotics in the gut.

- interaction with dendritic cells;
- toll-like receptors and intracellular pathways;
- activation of macrophages and NK cells;
- stimulaton of gut lymphoid tissue (GALT) immunoglobulins and specific cytokines; and
- modulation of innate and adaptive immunity.

A formula with viable bifidobacteria significantly increased total and anti-poliovirus fecal IgA in seven children after 21 days of intake [40]. Kaila et al. demonstrated that LGG (1×10^{10} cfu bd for 5 days) significantly increased humoral immune response in Rotavirus enteritis [41], more relevant with viable than inactivated probiotic [42].

Timing of supplementation and efficacy on colonization may well be critical. Adherence of B.Bb12 improves in the presence of *L. casei* GG, both in healthy infants and during episodes of diarrhea, suggesting that synergism may well occur [43].

Saccharomyces boulardii exerts specific anti-inflammatory and antimicrobial properties. It counteracts bacterial toxins, induces host immune response, influences inflammatory pathways (NF-κB, MAPK), improves the maturation of brush border enzymes (lactase, sucrase, maltase and aminopeptidase) and of glucose carriers in the enterocyte-membrane through a 54-KDa protease and the release of prolamine and soluble factors [44–46].

No data have been reported so far combining *Saccharomyces boulardii* with bifidobacteria or lactobacilli.

Reduced Paneth cell defensin expression and related decreased antimicrobial peptides and change in the colonizing microbiota have been reported in ileal Crohn's disease and in necrotizing enterocolitis (NEC) [47].

Stress, at any age, may also produce different effects on the gastrointestinal system, such as a reduction of the number of lactobacilli, an up-regulation of virulence factors and an increased growth, epithelial adherence and mucosal uptake of Gram-negative pathogens, e.g. *E. coli* and *Pseudomonas* [48]. Probiotics can counteract stress-induced changes in intestinal barrier function, visceral sensitivity and gut motility [48].

5. ACUTE INFECTIOUS GASTROENTERITIS

5.1. Prevention

The best protection from infectious diseases such as gastroenteritis is achieved by breast milk. Promotion of (exclusive) breast-feeding should be maximally endorsed in infants. Among protective components of human milk, different oligosaccharides play an important role. The presence of probiotic bacteria has also been demonstrated [49]. To recreate these benefits, probiotics and prebiotic oligosaccharides have been added to infant formula.

Prebiotics

Saran et al. showed that feeding fermented milk to Indian infants over a period of 6 months resulted in a significantly better weight gain and a 50% reduction of infectious diarrhea [50]. The addition of *Bifidobacterium lactis* HN019 and GOS in milk improved the iron status and produced a 10% reduction of diarrhea and a significant effect in morbidity and bloody diarrhea [51]. Data on the prevention of infectious gastroenteritis with prebiotic oligosaccharides are only limited to one prospective Italian multicenter open-label RCT in 342 healthy term infants (aged between 15 and 120 days, mean age 53.7 ± 32.1 days) fed with a prebiotic-enriched (0.4 g/100 mL of a mixture of GOS and FOS with a ratio of 9:1) formula for 12 months [52]. The incidence of gastroenteritis was lower in the supplemented group than in the controls (0.12 ± 0.04 vs 0.29 ± 0.05 episodes/child/12 months; CI 95% mean difference -0.3–0.03; $p = 0.015$) (10.4 vs 23.8% numbers of children with ≥ 1 episode of diarrhea; $p = 0.01$, RR 0.44; CI 95%, RR 0.22–0.86). A transient increase in body weight was observed in children on prebiotics compared to controls during the first 6 months of follow-up ($p < 0.01$) [52].

Oligofructose (Orafti Group, Tienen, Belgium) added to infant cereal (0.55 g/15 g cereal, average consumed 0.67 g prebiotic/d, or 0.11 g/kg/d) for 6 months did not show any protective effect in terms of episodes, days, or severity of diarrhea or Rotavirus infection rate. However, infants were partially breast-fed for more than 85% of the observational period [33].

Probiotics

Saavedra et al. showed that *Streptococcus* (*Str.*) *thermophilus* and *Bifidobacterium* (*B.*) *bifidum* (later renamed *B. lactis*) prevented nosocomial-acquired diarrhea in a small group of children admitted for long stays to a chronic care institution [53].

A formula supplemented with the viable *B. lactis* strain Bb12 failed to demonstrate a significant benefit compared to placebo in the prevalence of diarrhea in 90 healthy infants living in residential nurseries or foster care centers (28.3 vs 38.7%) despite a 30% reduction of the risk (RR 0.7, 95% confidence interval 0.4–1.3) [54]. A formula fermented with *B. breve* c50 and *Str. thermophilus* 065 was well accepted, resulted in normal growth of infants and reduced

the severity of diarrhea episodes but did not significantly reduce incidence, duration of diarrhea episodes or number of hospital admissions [55].

LGG was shown to reduce nosocomial infection, especially for Rotavirus gastroenteritis, in one study [56], but did not produce a statistically significant protective effect in a large double blind randomized study in 220 children [57].

Seven children would need to be treated with a probiotic to prevent one patient from developing nosocomial rotaviral gastroenteritis [58] but the effect is far less significant if the incidence of diarrhea (episodes per patient/month) rather than the percentage of patients with diarrhea is taken into account [58]. According to the current literature and cost:benefit ratio, there is not enough evidence to recommend the routine use of probiotics to prevent nosocomial diarrhea [59].

Three large RCT provide evidence of a very modest effect (statistically significant, but of questionable clinical importance) of three probiotic strains (LGG, *L. reuteri*, *B. lactis*) on the prevention of community-acquired diarrhea [59].

A large Finnish study included 571 children attending day-care centers and supplemented with LGG did not show a significant difference in the number of days with diarrhea but a 16% reduction in the number of days of absence due to gastrointestinal and respiratory illnesses [60]. Another study involving 210 healthy children in child health care centers showed a lower frequency and shorter duration of diarrhea during a follow-up of 3 months when *Lactobacillus reuteri* (better) or *B. lactis* (Bb12) were given to the children [61]. The protective effect of BB12 on diarrhea was not confirmed in another trial [62].

One RCT from Pakistan involving 100 children with acute watery diarrhea reported a significant difference in the incidence of episodes of diarrhea in the group receiving *S. boulardii* compared with the control group during a 2-month follow-up (0.32 vs 0.56, $p = 0.04$) [63].

5.2. Treatment

Prebiotics

In Bangladesh, green banana (250 g/L) and pectin (4 g/kg), in addition to a rice-based diet, significantly reduced fecal stool, rehydration needed, vomiting and the duration of diarrhea [64]. Supplementation of ORS with a prebiotic such as hydrolized guar gum significantly reduced diarrhea (from 90 to 74 hours) without modification of fecal volume [65].

In a multicenter European DBRCT in 144 boys (1–36 months) with acute diarrhea and mild to moderate dehydration, the addition of a mixture of non-digestible carbohydrates (soya polysaccharide 25%, a-cellulose 9%, arabic gum 19%, FOS 18.5%, inulin 21.5%, resistant starch 7%) to oral rehydration solution (ORS), did not determine a significant difference in terms of fecal volume, duration of diarrhea (82 ± 39 hours vs 97 ± 76 hours, $p = 0.2$), hospitalization or parenteral rehydration [66].

Probiotics

In the treatment of acute infectious gastroenteritis, probiotics have shown the best evidence of efficacy. Conversely, there have been almost no studies performed on chronic diarrhea of infectious origin.

Lactobacillus rhamnosus GG is the most extensively studied. LGG (2×10^{11} bd for 5 days), compared to placebo, significantly reduced the duration of hospitalization in Rotavirus diarrhea (1.4 vs 2.4 days) in 71 children treated with ORS [67]. The efficacy of LGG (1×10^{11} cfu/g bd for 2 days) in reducing the duration of non-bloody diarrhea (31 vs 75% of the controls at 48 hours) was confirmed in a study in 40 Pakistani children admitted for severe diarrhea and malnutrition [68]. Shornikova et al. showed, in a trial in 123 hospitalized children (33% with Rotavirus

and 21% with bacterial diarrhea), similar results with LGG (5×10^9 cfu/g bd for 5 days and ORS) in reducing the duration of viral diarrhea (2.7 vs 3.7 days) [69]. The same group assessed the efficacy of *L. reuteri* at two different doses (10^7 and 10^{10} cfu/g once a day for 5 days) in 66 hospitalized children with Rotavirus diarrhea. The probiotic reduced the duration of diarrhea with a dose-dependent effect (2.5 days in the placebo group vs 1.9 and 1.5 in the *L. reuteri* groups, respectively) [70]. In out patient children *L. casei* GG (3×10^9 cfu/g bd for a maximum of 6 days) halved the duration of diarrhea and also significantly reduced Rotavirus shedding [71]. A multicenter European prospective, RCT with LGG (10^{10} cfu/250 mL) as add-on to ORS in 287 children with acute diarrhea, showed a significant decrease of the duration of diarrhea with about 10% (a mean duration of diarrhea of 123 hours in the placebo group versus 110 hours in the intervention group) [72]. A more detailed analysis showed that the difference was greatest in the Rota-positive group (115 vs 136 hours) and that there was no difference in the subgroup with invasive pathogens (about 1/5th of all inclusions) (124 vs 121 hours' duration of diarrhea) [72]. *Lactobacillus acidophilus* LB (Lacteol Fort®, a product containing heat-killed lactobacilli, 10^{10} for five doses) was tested in 73 children with acute diarrhea (50% Rotavirus positive) resulting in a similar reduction of duration (43 vs 57 hours) [73]. However, at least three RCTs in developing countries negated the beneficial effect of LGG and *L. acidophilus* in acute diarrhea, likely related to the distinct etiological profile [74–76]. In children with more severe diarrhea, there was no demonstrable benefit of *L. casei* GG [75, 77]. Absence of shortening of the duration of diarrhea was also reported for a mixture of *L. acidophilus*, *B. bifidum* (later renamed *B. lactis*) and *L. bulgaricus* [77]. The *L. paracasei* strain ST11 did not reduce the volume of stool output in Rotavirus infection but improved the outcome of non-Rotavirus diarrhea in children from Bangladesh [78]. Three meta-analyses concluded that the majority of the studies had been performed in the developed world, and that *L. rhamnosus* GG is the probiotic bacteria with the best evidence of efficacy, especially for viral diarrhea [79–81]. In particular, the duration of (viral) diarrhea was significantly reduced (about 17 hours or 0.7 days) (relative risk (RR) 0.40 and four children treated (NNT) to protect one subject from diarrhea) compared to controls [80]. The efficacy of LGG appeared to be related to the logarithm of the dose ($>10^{11}$ as the most efficient dose) [81]. A Cochrane review examined 23 RCT and 1,917 participants (1,449 children) and highlighted the beneficial effect of probiotics (especially LGG) as add-on treatment to ORS in reducing the risk of diarrhea at 3 days (RR 0.66; 95% CI, 0.55–0.77; random effects model, 15 studies), and the mean duration of diarrhea (of about 30 hours with a RR 0.7), without significant side effects in immune-competent subjects [82]. More data are needed for strains less studied such as *Streptococcus thermophilus*, *L. acidophilus* and *bulgaricus* [82]. Shamir and coworkers showed a reduction in the duration of acute gastroenteritis from $1.96 + 1.24$ to $1.43 + 0.71$ days ($p = 0.017$) with an addition of 10^9 cfu *Streptococcus thermophilus*, *B. lactis*, *L. acidophilus*, 10 mg zinc and 0.3 g FOS per day [83].

Other studies have recently been published using bacterial probiotics on acute diarrhea.

An Italian open RCT compared the efficacy of five probiotic preparations (*L. rhamnosus* strain GG; *S. boulardii*; *Bacillus clausii*; a mix of *L. delbrueckii var bulgaricus*, *Streptococcus thermophilus*, *L. acidophilus*, and *Bifidobacterium bifidum*; or *Enterococcus faecium* SF68) in 571 outpatient children aged 3–36 months, with acute diarrhea. A significant effect ($p < 0.001$) (-32 and -37 hours compared to 115 hours of ORS alone) was demonstrated only for LGG and the mixed product [84].

In one DBRCT, 87 Polish children (age range: 2 months to 6 years) with infectious diarrhea were administered a mixture of three *L. rhamnosus* strains (573L/1; 573L/2; 573L/3) at a dose 1.2×10^{10} cfu or placebo, twice daily, for 5 days. In an intention to treat analysis, the mean duration of Rotaviral diarrhea (76 ± 5 vs 115 ± 67 h, $p = 0.03$) but not of diarrhea of other aetiology, and the duration of parenteral rehydration (15 ± 14 vs 38 ± 33 h, $p = 0.006$) were significantly shortened [85].

A DBRCT on acute Rotavirus diarrhea in 224 Indian children showed that VSL #3 probiotic mixture significantly reduced stool frequency and ORS requirement and improved recovery rates and stool consistency from day 2 up to 8 hours of day 4 [86].

In the same country, LGG administered once or twice daily confirmed its significant efficacy in reducing the frequency and duration of diarrhea, requirement for intravenous therapy, and hospital stay in a DBRCT enrolling 559 hospitalized children with acute diarrhea [87].

Saccharomyces boulardii is a non-pathogenic yeast isolated from the lychee fruit in Indonesia and introduced into France since 1950 for the treatment of diarrhea. The first DBRCT of *S. boulardii* was performed more than 15 years ago: diarrhea persisted for more than 7 days in 12% in the placebo group and in 3% in the experimental group [88]. Since then, several DBRCTs performed with *S. boulardii* in children with acute gastroenteritis have systematically shown a significant improvement in comparison to a placebo. A consecutive series of 130 Mexican children, 3 months to 3 years old, with acute infectious diarrhea, were treated with ORS and placebo or *S. boulardii* (600 mg/d) for 5 days [89]. A significant decrease in the number of stools was apparent from day 2 onwards [89]. After 48 hours, the percentage of children considered cured was almost 50% in the *S. boulardii* group compared to 8% in the placebo group; on day 4, resolution was up to 95% in the intervention group compared to just 50% in the placebo group [89]. Kurugol treated 200 children with acute diarrhea with 250 mg *S. boulardii* or a placebo for 5 days: duration of both diarrhea and hospital stay decreased within approximately 24 hours [90]. Villaruel and co-workers showed similar results in ambulatory care in Argentina: diarrhea persisted for more than 7 days in 27% of a placebo group compared to 7% in a group treated with *S. boulardii* for 6 days, with a greater affect if treatment was started within the first 2 days of the disease [91]. *Saccharomyces boulardii* also improved tolerance of feeding in children with chronic *Giardia lamblia* infection [92]. Furthermore, *S. boulardii* demonstrated efficacy in amebiasis and HIV-diarrhea [93, 94]. An open RCT in Pakistani children with acute infectious gastroenteritis showed that administration of 500 mg *S. boulardii* for 5 days significantly reduced the frequency of stools and duration of diarrhea (3.5 days vs 4.8 days, $p = 0.001$) and resulted 2 months later in a 50% decrease in re-infection rates and 30% better weight gain [63]. One meta-analysis was aimed at evaluating the effectiveness of *S. boulardii* in treating acute infectious diarrhea in children (94). Data from five RCTs [63, 89–91, 96] and 619 participants were included. Combined data from four RCTs showed that *S. boulardii* significantly reduced the duration of diarrhea compared with the control. The pooled weighted mean difference was −1.1 days (95% CI −1.3 to −0.8) with a fixed model and remained significant in a random affect model. *S. boulardii* significantly reduced the risk of diarrhea on days 3, 6, and 7. In addition, the risk of diarrhea lasting >7 days was significantly reduced in the *S. boulardii* group versus control group (1 RCT, $n = 88$, RR 0.25, 95% CI 0.08–0.83, NNT 5, 95% CI 3–20). This meta-analysis concluded that, in otherwise healthy infants and children with acute infectious gastroenteritis, the use of *S. boulardii* compared with a control treatment is associated with a moderate therapeutic benefit that is reproducible regardless of the outcome measure studied. In other words, duration of diarrhea, chance of cure or risk of diarrhea at certain point intervals, number of stools, and length of hospital stay [95]. Another RCT was carried out in Myanmar and involved 100 children with acute diarrhea. *Saccharomyces boulardii* reduced the duration

of diarrhea compared with placebo (3.08 ± 0.95 vs 4.68 ± 1.23 days, respectively) [97].

Given these new data, the previous mentioned meta-analysis was updated. Based on the pooled results of six RCTs involving 756 children, *S. boulardii*, compared to placebo or no intervention, reduced the duration of diarrhea by 22 hours (WMD −22, CI −26 to −18) [37].

A shortening of the duration of diarrhea, as well as a reduced hospital stay, suggests a relevant social and economic benefit of biotherapeutic treatment in adjunction to ORS in acute infectious gastroenteritis in children.

While numerous clinical trials have been published evaluating different probiotics in the treatment of acute gastroenteritis, trials vary in relation to strains tested, dosage, methodological quality, diarrhea definitions and outcomes. Most studies show a statistically significant effect that is of only moderate clinical benefit, with a greatest effect in viral and watery diarrhea [59]. Greater efficacy has been shown if the probiotic is administered early in the disease. Probiotics in acute diarrhea of diverse causes reduced the duration in children of about 57% (35–71%) [98]. In general, there is a lack of data from community-based trials and from developing countries, although there is now an increasing body of evidence with *S. boulardii* in these populations.

6. ANTIBIOTIC ASSOCIATED DIARRHEA (AAD)

Antibiotic treatment is known to disturb gastrointestinal microflora, which results in a range of clinical symptoms, especially diarrhea. While *Clostridium difficile* is the most common infectious agent isolated, in most cases of AAD a causative organism is not found. The incidence of AAD in children in first line medicine is about 10%, independent of the reason for antibiotic administration [99]. The risk for

AAD is increased in young children (18% in children younger than 2 years) and with some oral antibiotics such as amoxicillin-clavulanate (23% with this antibiotic) [100].

6.1. Prebiotics

Only one RCT of prebiotics on the prevention of pediatric AAD has been reported. In children aged 1–2 years a mixture of 70:30 inulin:oligofructose (0.45 g/100 mL, ratio 70:30, Prebio 1) at 2.25 g/d for 3 weeks after 1 week of amoxicillin therapy significantly increased fecal bifidobacteria but did not change diarrheal symptoms [100].

6.2. Probiotics

According to two meta-analyses, selected probiotics (LGG, *B. lactis*, *Str. thermophilus* and *S. boulardii*) reduce the risk of AAD [101, 102] by approximately 60%, from 28.5% to 11.9% (RR 0.44, 95% CI 0.25–0.77) in children [101].

Preplanned subgroup analysis showed that a reduction of the risk of AAD was associated with the use of LGG (two RCTs, 307 participants, RR 0.3, 95% CI 0.15–0.6), *S. boulardii* (one RCT, 246 participants, RR 0.2, 95% CI 0.07–0.6), or *B. lactis* and *Str. thermophilus* (one RCT, 157 participants, RR 0.5, 95% CI 0.3–0.95) [101]. The NNT with probiotics to avoid AAD in one patient would be seven patients according to one meta-analysis [101] or 10 patients if only considered in a study on *Saccharomyces boulardii* [103].

As is the case with all yeasts, *S. boulardii* is naturally resistant to antibiotics. Simultaneous oral intake of amoxicillin and *S. boulardii* doubles the number of *S. boulardii* surviving in the gastrointestinal tract [104].

According to a randomized controlled trial, the dose of LGG to prevent AAD should be of at least 10–20 billion cfu daily [105].

A combination of *L. acidophilus* and *L. bulgaricus* was ineffective in preventing diarrhea in children receiving amoxicillin therapy during a DBRCT [106].

Ten studies met the inclusion criteria in the recent Cochrane review [107]. Trials included treatment with either *Lactobacilli* spp., *Bifidobacterium* spp., *Streptococcus* spp., or *Saccharomyces boulardii* alone or in combination. Six studies used a single strain probiotic agent and four combined two probiotic strains. The per protocol analysis for 9/10 trials reporting on the incidence of diarrhea show statistically significant results favoring probiotics over active/non-active controls (RR 0.49; 95% CI 0.32 to 0.74). However, an intention to treat analysis showed non-significant results overall (RR 0.90; 95% CI 0.50 to 1.63). Five of 10 trials monitored for adverse events ($n = 647$); none reported a serious adverse event [107].

A combination of 10^8 colony-forming units of *Bifidobacterium longum* PL03, *Lactobacillus rhamnosus* KL53A and *Lactobacillus plantarum* PL02 administered orally twice daily for the duration of antibiotic treatment did not significantly alter the rate of AAD (relative risk 0.5, 95% CI 0.06–3.5) in 78 children (ages: 5 months to 16 years), although it reduced the frequency of stools (mean difference -0.3 stool/day, 95% CI -0.5 to -0.07) [108].

Another trial in 240 children (aged 3 months to 14 years) in the same group showed efficacy of administration of *Lactobacillus rhamnosus* (strains E/N, Oxy and Pen) (2×10^{10} colony-forming units orally twice daily throughout antibiotic treatment) in the prevention of AAD in an intention to treat analysis. Any diarrhea (> or = 3 loose or watery stools/day for > or = 48 hours occurring during or up to 2 weeks after the antibiotic therapy) occurred in nine (7.5%) patients in the probiotic group and in 20 (17%) patients in the placebo group (RR 0.45, 95% CI 0.2–0.9) [109].

From the above data, probiotics show promise in the prevention of pediatric AAD but do not withstand intention to treat analysis. Before routine use is recommended, further studies (with limited losses of subjects to follow-up) are merited. Trials should involve those probiotic strains and doses with the most promising evidence (i.e., LGG at 5–40×10^9 cfu daily, or *S. boulardii* at 250–500 mg daily). More data are needed in children who develop a severe AAD.

7. CLOSTRIDIUM DIFFICILE INFECTION

There is little evidence to support the routine use of probiotics in preventing the recurrence of *Clostridium difficile* infection or to treat existing *C. difficile* diarrhea [59, 110]. In the meta-analysis, only *S. boulardii* was reported to be effective in *C. difficile* disease [102]. LGG showed some benefit in the prevention of relapsing *C. difficile* only in a small open-label trial in children [111].

8. TRAVELERS' DIARRHEA

Travelers' diarrhea is a frequent condition (rates can range from 5 to 50%, depending on the destination) of great socio-economic impact.

8.1. Prebiotics

There appear to be no study assessments on the affects of prebiotics to prevent travelers' diarrhea in children.

8.2. Probiotics

The use of probiotics for this disease remains controversial and no data on children are available.

9. IRRITABLE BOWEL SYNDROME (IBS)

9.1. Prebiotics

There are currently no published RCT concerning the use of prebiotics alone in IBS. Prebiotics may increase gas production in the gut because of their fermentation [112, 113]. This might preclude prebiotic use in diarrhea-predominant IBS, or where bloating or gas are prominent symptoms, but might allow their mild laxative properties [113] to be useful in constipation-predominant IBS. No trials have been performed in children.

9.2. Probiotics

A different intestinal microflora (reduced number of bifidobacteria and lactobacilli) [114] and mucosal inflammation [115] have been reported in adult IBS and may be suggestive of probiotic efficacy.

Data in children are limited. A randomized trial of 6 weeks with LGG versus placebo showed overall negative results in 50 children and young adults (6–20 years), although there was a lower incidence of perceived abdominal distension in the LGG group ($p = 0.02$) [116]. In another report, LGG was more effective than a placebo (33 vs 5%, RB 6.3, 95% CI 1.2–38, NNT 4, 95% CI 2–36) and reduced frequency of pain ($p = 0.02$) (but not pain severity) only in the children classified as IBS compared to the group with functional dyspepsia or functional abdominal pain [117].

In a Cochrane review [118] only these two trials [116, 117], both testing LGG in 168 children, provided analyzable data. The pooled odds ratio for improvement of symptoms was 1.17 (95% CI 0.62, 2.21) showing no evidence of benefit from *Lactobacillus* supplementation.

A meta-analysis of probiotics for IBS included overall 20 (adult and pediatric) trials (1,404 subjects) with 23 probiotic treatment arms and 20 different strains (used alone or in combination, in different concentration). A high degree of heterogeneity of the trials (generally small and of short duration) was highlighted. Overall, probiotic use was associated with less likelihood of global IBS symptoms compared to placebo (RR = 0.77, 95% CI 0.62–0.94) and abdominal pain (RR = 0.78, 95% CI 0.69–0.88) by the end of the follow-up. Data were not sufficient to examine the efficacy of individual probiotic strains [119]. A strong placebo affect (reported in a range of 5–72%) [119] and a lack of uniformity of the IBS population may have hindered a clearer demonstration of the affect of probiotics in this disorder.

10. CONSTIPATION

10.1. Prebiotics

This paragraph will not consider lactulose as a possible prebiotic and will focus only on GOS, FOS and inulin effects.

In healthy infants, different GOS and FOS supplementations alone (0.24 g/100 mL of GOS [9] and 0.3 g/100 mL [16] to 0.4 g/100 mL [17] of FOS) or in combinations (0.4 g/100 mL to 1 g/100 mL) [5, 8, 13–15] resulted in decreased consistency and increased frequency of stools compared to standard formulas.

The laxative properties of inulin have also long been known [120] with a better benefit compared to other oligosaccharides probably due to its higher molecular weight and lower solubility resulting in slower fermentation.

However, a clear benefit in constipated patients still needed to be demonstrated in children.

10.2. Probiotics

The absence of an intestinal flora in germ-free animals resulted in an abnormal intestinal morphology and immune response and in decreased gastrointestinal motility [121]. Bifidobacteria and lactobacilli produce lactic, acetic and other acids resulting in a lowering of pH in the colon that may enhance peristalsis and subsequently decreases colonic transit time [122, 123].

A DBRCT in 45 children with constipation showed that both the strain *L. rhamnosus* Lcr35 (8×10^8 cfu/day) and magnesium oxide produced a similar significant increase in defecation frequency ($p = 0.03$), less use of an enema ($p = 0.04$), and less hard stools ($p = 0.01$) compared to the placebo group. Also, although only in the probiotic group, there was a significant decrease in abdominal pain ($p = 0.03$) [124]. Conversely, the addition of LGG (10^9 cfu/day) to lactulose as standard treatment did not offer any additional benefit in another DBRCT including 84 children with constipation (<3 bowel movements per week) [125].

A pilot study in 20 children showed that a daily intake of a probiotic mixture (Ecologic®Relief, 4×10^9 cfu) containing three bifidobacteria (*bifidum*, *longum* and *infantis*) and three lactobacilli (*casei*, *plantarum* and *rhamnosus*) determined a significant decrease in abdominal pain ($p = 0.04$ after 2 weeks and $p = 0.006$ after 4 weeks). There was also a significant decrease in the number of faecal incontinence episodes ($p = 0.01$). The increase in stool frequency was significant only in the subgroup of patients presenting with <3 bowel movements per week ($p = 0.01$) [126].

One 7-month prospective DBRCT enrolling 134 infants reported fewer incidences of constipation and hard stools in the group fed an experimental formula containing 2×10^7 cfu of *Bifidobacterium longum* BL999 and 4 g/L of a prebiotic mixture (90% GOS and 10% FOS) [127].

11. INFLAMMATORY BOWEL DISEASE (IBD)

The concept of dysbiosis, a breakdown of tolerance to autologous flora and of balance between 'protective' and 'harmful' intestinal bacteria, is gaining credibility in the multiple etiologic factors of IBD. The concept that the enteric flora is of profound importance in the development of CD is supported by the absence of disease in germ-free conditions. Equally important is the recognition that a specific disease-associated gene, such as Nod-2, encodes an intracellular molecule essential in the inflammatory response to bacterial peptidoglycans, and the induced production of IFN-γ by extracts of proper commensal flora [128].

11.1. Prebiotics

There are very limited results on prebiotics alone in either UC or CD, although some data on anti-inflammatory properties of prebiotics (lactulose, inulin, FOS, or a combination of them) on animal models of intestinal inflammation do exist [6].

An open pilot study evaluated the effect of a daily dose of 3–6 g of N-acetyl-glucosamine (a bifidogenic oligosaccharide also present in human milk) administered orally as adjunct therapy in 12 children with severe treatment-resistant IBD or rectally as sole therapy in nine children with distal ulcerative colitis or resistant proctitis. Eight of the 12 children treated orally and five out of nine treated rectally showed clear improvement. In all cases biopsied there was evidence of histological improvement, and a significant increase in epithelial and lamina propria glycosaminoglycans [129].

11.2. Probiotics

At the time of writing, only one RCT has been performed in children with IBD [130]. A 2-year follow-up study with LGG in children with Crohn's disease in remission resulted in a non-significant difference in relapse rate (31 vs 17% in the placebo group) and in the time lapse before the relapse [130].

It is noteworthy that, despite any current evidence of benefit of probiotics, almost 80% of the children with an IBD have a regular intake of probiotics [131].

12. HELICOBACTER PYLORI

The use of probiotics and food with bioactive components in *H. pylori*-colonized subjects with gastric inflammation is supported by many observations [132]. Specific strains of *Lactobacillus* and *Bifidobacterium* exert *in vitro* bactericidal affects against *H. pylori* through the release of bacteriocins or the production of organic acids, and/or the inhibition of adhesion to epithelial cells [132]. In addition, the antioxidant and anti-inflammatory properties exerted by specific probiotics may stabilize the gastric barrier function and decrease mucosal inflammation [132].

The single or combined treatment with only *Lactobacillus johnsonii* La1 and cranberry juice, given daily for 3 weeks, reached an eradication rate of 15 and 23% in 271 randomized children compared to 1.5% in the control group (placebo/heat-killed La1)($p < 0.01$) [133]. In 141 Chilean children, Hp was eradicated in 66%, 12% and 6.5% of the children by the standard eradication treatment, *Saccharomyces boulardii* plus inulin or *Lactobacillus acidophilus* LB groups while no spontaneous clearance was observed in the children without treatment [134].

In a multicenter, prospective, DBRCT supplementation with fermented milk, containing live special probiotic *L. casei* DN-114 001 (Actimel), conferred an enhanced therapeutic benefit on Hp eradication in 86 children with gastritis on triple therapy in both ITT ($p = 0.0045$) and PP analysis ($p = 0.0019$) [135].

Conversely, probiotic food consisting of 250 mL of a commercial yogurt containing *Bifidobacterium animalis* and *Lactobacillus casei* (10^7 cfu/mL) did not improve the eradication rates when added to treatment in 65 Argentinian children [136].

A prospective open study performed in 90 symptomatic children showed that the addition of *S. boulardii* to the standard eradication treatment confers a 12% non-significant enhanced therapeutic benefit on *H. pylori* eradication (93 vs 81%, $p = 0.75$) and reduces significantly the incidence of side effects (8 vs 31%, $p = 0.047$) [137].

In 40 chidren, *L. reuteri* ATCC 55730 (10^8 cfu) significantly reduced frequency and intensity of antibiotic-associated side effects during eradication therapy [138].

A review showed an improvement of Hp and decrease in Hp density after administration of probiotics in seven out of nine human studies considered. The addition of probiotics to standard antibiotic treatment significantly improved Hp eradication rates (81 vs 71%, $p = 0.03$) and reduced Hp therapy-associated side effects (23 vs 46%, $p = 0.04$) [139].

One systematic review and meta-analysis including 10 RCT (two in children) [135, 136] and nearly 500 patients (72 children) in the treated group demonstrated that fermented milk-based probiotic preparations improve Hp eradication rates by approximately 5–15%, whereas the affect on adverse effects was heterogeneous [140].

13. COLICS AND REGURGITATION

13.1. Prebiotics

A formula containing partially hydrolyzed whey protein, modified vegetable oil with a high beta-palmitic acid content, prebiotic oligosaccharides 0.8 g/dL GOS/FOS (ratio 9:1) significantly increased stool frequency and reduced the frequency of colic and the number of regurgitation episodes after 1 and 2 weeks in 200 full-term healthy infants [15]. The same formula induced a significant reduction in crying episodes in infants with colic after 7 and 14 days when compared with a standard formula or simethicone [141].

13.2. Probiotics

In a prospective trial 90 breast-fed colicky infants were assigned randomly to receive either the probiotic *L. reuteri* (10^8 live bacteria per day) or simethicone (60 mg/day) for 28 days. The mothers avoided cows' milk in their diet. Infants receiving *L. reuteri* showed a significant reduction in daily crying time ($p < 0.005$ by day 7, and $p < 0.001$ on days 14, 21, and 28). At the end of the study, a significantly higher proportion of responders were present in the probiotic group (95 vs 7%, $p < 0.001$) compared to the simethicone group [142].

14. PRETERM NEWBORNS

Feeding tolerance, regurgitation, mean daily crying, and stool frequency significantly improved in 10 preterm newborns receiving *Lactobacillus reuteri* ATCC 55730 (10^8 cfu a day) for 30 days. In addition, the gastric emptying rate was significantly increased and fasting antral area was significantly reduced compared to a placebo group [143].

Candida species increasingly cause morbidity and mortality in the premature infant in neonatal intensive care units. A pilot DBRCT in preterm neonates has demonstrated that LGG administered in the first month of life significantly reduces enteric Candida colonization [144].

15. NECROTIZING ENTEROCOLITIS

Necrotizing enterocolitis (NEC) is a severe condition occurring especially in preterm babies.

Abnormal gastrointestinal flora development has been hypothesized as one of the possible etiologic factors. In addition, through prevention of bacterial migration across the mucosa, competitive exclusion of pathogenic bacteria, and enhancing the immune responses in the host, prophylactic enteral probiotics may play a role in reducing NEC [145].

At least three RCTs with different lactobacilli and bifidobacteria showed a significant reduction in the development of NEC [146–148]. A supplementation of preterm infants with *S. boulardii* did not protect from NEC [149]. Nine eligible trials randomizing 1,425 infants were included in one Cochrane meta-analysis [145] and showed that enteral probiotic supplementation significantly reduced the incidences of severe NEC (stage II or more) [typical RR 0.32 (95% CI 0.17, 0.60)] and mortality [typical RR 0.43 (95% CI 0.25, 0.75)] in preterm infants. There was no evidence of a significant reduction of nosocomial sepsis [typical RR 0.93 (95% CI 0.73, 1.19)] or days on total parenteral nutrition (TPN) [WMD −1.9 (95% CI −4.6, 0.77)]. The included trials reported no systemic infection with the probiotics supplemental organism. Data regarding outcome of ELBW (<1000 g) infants could not be extracted from the available studies considered [145].

Another prospective multicenter RCT, conducted in Taiwan, enrolled 434 very low birth weights infants (<1500 g). *Bifidobacterium bifidum* and *Lactobacillus acidophilus* added to breast milk or mixed feeding (breast milk and formula) were given twice daily for 6 weeks in the study group. The incidences of death or NEC (Bell's stage > or = 2) was significantly lower in the study group. No adverse effect was reported [150].

Because cases of bacteremia and sepsis have been related to probiotic administration, further large RCTs are required in this high-risk age group before the routine use of probiotics to reduce the risk for NEC can be recommended in preterm babies.

16. SAFETY AND SIDE EFFECTS

16.1. Prebiotics

Prebiotics are considered safe and without side effects. Flatulence, bloating and osmotic diarrhea may occur if inulin-derived oligosaccharides and GOS are taken in large amounts [6] but the threshold of the recommended dose still needs to be clarified because of the different individual prebiotic intake in common diet. Doses as high as 30 g/d (roughly 0.5 g/kg) have been associated with gastrointestinal side effects in adults [151]. In infants fed a FOS supplemented formula (1.5 or 3.0 g/L), gastrointestinal side effects were significantly higher ($p = 0.03$) compared to human milk and dose-dependent with flatulence occurring in 21 and 31%, looser stools in 15 and 31%, and spitting-up in 12 and 28% in the two FOS groups, respectively [16]. When a different combination of prebiotics (polydextrose, GOS, and lactulose) was considered, increased irritability appeared in the group fed 8 g/L of prebiotics (16 vs 4% of controls, $p = 0.03$), whereas in a significantly higher proportion of infants taking the formula supplemented with 4 g/L, diarrhea (18 vs 4% of controls, $p = 0.008$) and eczema (18 vs 7% of controls and 4% of 8 g/L groups, $p = 0.046$ and $p = 0.008$, respectively) occurred [18].

16.2. Probiotics

Probiotics are 'generally regarded as safe', with no reported drug interactions and side effects such as septicemia and fungemia have only been very rarely reported in high-risk situations, such as in patients with immunodeficiency, short gut, central venous catheter [152]. Two cases of bacteriemia attributable to *Lactobacillus* supplementation, with identical molecular clinical and supplement isolates, were reported in an infant and a child without underlying gastrointestinal disease or immunocompromised status [153]. Fungemia has even been reported in an adult patient with deep central venous lines hospitalized in a bed next to a patient treated with the yeast [154]. Probiotic enterococci and even lactobacilli, may act as reservoirs for antibiotic resistance genes and might transfer their resistance genes to pathogenic bacteria through their plasmids [155, 156]. Antibiotic sensitivity is currently required to commercialize a bacterial probiotic product. The absence of transfer of genetic material between microorganisms is relevant, especially in antibiotic-associated diarrhea and immunocompromised patients.

17. KEY POINTS

- Different supplementation of GOS and FOS positively affects the intestinal microflora and may improve immune status and calcium absorption.
- Prebiotics are considered safe and without side effects. Flatulence, irritability and looser diarrhea may occur especially if taken at high dosage.
- Probiotics are a heterogeneous group of microorganisms with differences in mechanisms of action, biological activity and dose.
- Proven efficacy of selected probiotics (mostly LGG, S. boulardii, L. reuteri) have been demonstrated in different gastrointestinal disorders such as acute infectious and antibiotic diarrhea, H. pylori infection and NEC.
- Probiotics have no reported drug interactions and side effects such as septicemia and fungemia have only been very rarely reported in high-risk situations. Strain specificity and concentration are of utmost importance.

18. CONCLUSIONS

18.1. Prebiotics

The evidence for supplemented prebiotics such as GOS, FOS and inulin is currently limited

to changes in stool consistency and increased concentration of bifidobacteria and lactobacilli after different supplementation. In pediatric age, there is an increasing body of evidence suggesting a reduced incidence of frequent occurring infections and an improved calcium absorption.

18.2. Probiotics

The spectrum of application of probiotics is continuously expanding despite little evidence to support this broad use (Figure 13.3).

Current recommendations for probiotic use in gastrointestinal disorders in children include a grade A for treatment of acute diarrhea, reduction of side effects eradication treatment in Hp infection, prevention of antibiotic-associated diarrhea, and NEC. More studies are needed to prove efficacy in IBD, IBS, infantile colic and constipation (Table 13.2).

Because of strain-affect specificity, only those organisms that have been clinically tested can be recommended. *L. casei* GG and *S. boulardii* were the best studied but different probiotics

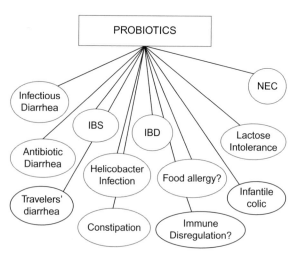

FIGURE 13.3   Spectrum of clinical application of probiotics in gastrointestinal disorders in children.

TABLE 13.1 Evidence of efficacy of probiotics in pediatric gastrointestinal disorders

Gastrointestinal disorder	Level of evidence	Strain with the best efficacy	Notes
Acute infectious diarrhea	A	LGG Saccharomyces boulardii Lactobacillus reuteri	Better effect if: – Early administration – High dose – Mild-to moderate diarrhea
Antibiotic associated diarrhea	A	LGG Saccharomyces boulardii	Risk reduced by 52%; better benefit if assumed within 72 hrs of starting antibiotics
Colic	A	Lactobacillus reuteri ATCC 55730	Efficacy in term and preterms. Imroved gastric emptying
Constipaton	B	Lactobacilli (L. rhamnosus Lcr35) and Bifidobacteria	Insufficient data
Crohn's	B	–	Only 1 study with LGG with negative results
Helicobacter pylori infection	A	L. casei DN-114 001, L. johnsonii LA1, L. reuteri ATCC 55730, Saccharmyces boulardii	Enhanced eradication rate (5–15%) and reduced antibiotic side-effects
Irritable Bowel Syndrome	B	LGG	Lower abdominal distension and pain frequency. Only 2 trials
NEC	A	Lactobacillli (acidophilus) and Bifidobacteria (bifidum)	Insufficient data on ELBW

(such as bifidobacteria and *L. reuteri*) showed beneficial effects in specific conditions. Since some commercialized products are combinations of different strains, and synergism as well as antagonism may occur, laboratory and clinical testing is mandatory before preferring them to a single-strain product.

References

1. Lilly, D. M., & Stillwell, R. H. (1965). Probiotic growth promoting factors produced by microorganisms. *Science*, 147, 747–748.
2. Tissier, H. (1906). Traitement des infections intestinales par la méthode de la transformation de la flore bactérienne de l'intestin. *Comptes Rendus Social Biology*, 60, 359–361.
3. McVeagh, P., & Miller, J. B. (1997). Human milk oligosaccharides: Only the breast. *Journal of Paediatrics and Child Health*, 33, 281–286.
4. Agostoni, C., Axelsson, I., Goulet, O., et al. (2004). Prebiotic oligosaccharides in dietetic products for infants: a commentary by the ESPGHAN Committee on nutrition. *Journal of Pediatric Gastroenterology and Nutrition*, 39, 465–473.
5. Moro, G., Minoli, I., Mosca, M., et al. (2002). Dosage-related bifidogenic effects of galacto- and fructo-oligosaccharides in formula-fed term infants. *Journal of Pediatric Gastroenterology and Nutrition*, 34, 291–295.
6. Macfarlane, S., Macfarlane, G. T., & Cummings, J. H. (2006). Review articles: Prebiotics in the gastrointestinal tract. *Alimentary Pharmacology & Therapeutics*, 24, 701–714.
7. Yahiro, M., Nishikawa, I., Murakami, Y., et al. (1982). Studies on application of galactosyllactose for infant formula. *Reports of Research Laboratories, Snow Brand Milk Products Co*, 78, 27–32.
8. Boehm, G., Lidestri, M., Casetta, P., et al. (2002). Supplementation of a bovine milk formula with an oligosaccharide mixture increases counts of fecal bifidobacteria in preterm infants. *Archives of Disease in Childhood. Fetal and Neonatal Edition*, 86, F178–F181.

9. Ben, X. M., Zhou, X. Y., Zhao, W. H., et al. (2004). Supplementation of milk formula with galacto-oligosaccharides improves intestinal micro-flora and fermentation in term infants. *Chinese Medical Journal (Engl)*, *117*, 927–931.

10. Knol, J., Scholtens, P., Kafka, C., et al. (2005). Colon microflora in infants fed formula with galacto- and fructo-oligosaccharides: More like breast-fed infants. *Journal of Pediatric Gastroenterology and Nutrition*, *40*(1), 36–42.

11. Haarman, M., & Knol, J. (2005). Quantitative real-time PCR assays to identify and quantify fecal Bifidobacterium species in infants receiving a prebiotic infant formula. *Applied and Environmental Microbiology*, *71*, 2318–2324.

12. Haarman, M., & Knol, J. (2006). Quantitative real-time PCR analysis of fecal Lactobacillus species in infants receiving a prebiotic infant formula. *Applied and Environmental Microbiology*, *72*, 2359–2365.

13. Costalos, C., Kapiki, A., Apostolou, M., & Papathoma, E. (2008). The effect of a prebiotic supplemented formula on growth and stool microbiology of term infants. *Early Human Development*, *84*(1), 45–49.

14. Schmelzle, H., Wirth, S., Skopnik, H., et al. (2003). Randomized double-blind study of the nutritional efficacy and bifidogenicity of a new infant formula containing partially hydrolyzed protein, a high betapalmitic acid level, and non-digestible oligosaccharides. *Journal of Pediatric Gastroenterology and Nutrition*, *36*, 343–351.

15. Savino, F., Cresi, F., Maccario, S., et al. (2003). 'Minor' feeding problems during the first months of life: Effect of a partially hydrolysed milk formula containing fructo- and galacto-oligosaccharides.. *Acta Paediatrica Supplement*, *441*, 86–90.

16. Euler, A. R., Mitchell, D. K., Kline, R., & Pickering, L. K. (2005). Prebiotic effect of fructo-oligosaccharide supplemented term infant formula at two concentrations compared with unsupplemented formula and human milk. *Journal of Pediatric Gastroenterology and Nutrition*, *40*, 157–164.

17. Kapiki, A., Costalos, C., Oikonomidou, C., et al. (2007). The effect of a fructo-oligosaccharide supplemented formula on gut flora of preterm infants. *Early Human Development*, *83*(5), 335–339.

18. Ziegler, E., Vanderhoof, J. A., Petschow, B., et al. (2007). Term infants fed formula supplemented with selected blends of prebiotics grow normally and have soft stools similar to those reported for breast-fed infants. *Journal of Pediatric Gastroenterology and Nutrition*, *44*(3), 359–364.

19. Magne, F., Hachelaf, W., Suau, A., et al. (2008). Effects on faecal microbiota of dietary and acidic oligosaccharides in children during partial formula feeding. *Journal of Pediatric Gastroenterology and Nutrition*, *46*(5), 580–588.

20. Scholtens, P. A., Alliet, P., Raes, M., et al. (2008). Fecal secretory immunoglobulin A is increased in healthy infants who receive a formula with short-chain galacto-oligosaccharides and long-chain fructo-oligosaccharides. *The Journal of Nutrition*, *138*(6), 1141–1147.

21. Bakker-Zierikzee, A. M., Alles, M. S., Knol, J., et al. (2005). Effects of infant formula containing a mixture of galacto- and fructo-oligosaccharides or viable *Bifidobacterium animalis* on the intestinal microflora during the first 4 months of life. *The British Journal of Nutrition*, *94*, 783–790.

22. Moore, N., Chao, C., Yang, L. P., et al. (2003). Effects of fructo-oligosaccharide-supplemented infant cereal: a double-blind, randomized trial. *The British Journal of Nutrition*, *90*(3), 581–587.

23. Scholtens, P. A., Alles, M. S., Bindels, J. G., et al. (2006). Bifidogenic effects of solid weaning foods with added prebiotic oligosaccharides: A randomised controlled clinical trial. *Journal of Pediatric Gastroenterology and Nutrition*, *42*, 553–559.

24. Saavedra, J. M., & Tschernia, A. (2004). Human studies with probiotics and prebiotics: Clinical implications. *The British Journal of Nutrition*, *87*(S2), S241–S246.

25. Waligora-Dupriet, A. J., Campeotto, F., Nicolis, I., et al. (2007). Effect of oligofructose supplementation on gut microflora and well-being in young children attending day care centre. *International Journal of Food Microbiology*, *113*(1), 108–113.

26. Bosscher, D., Van Caillie-Bertrand, M., Van Cauwenbergh, R., & Deelstra, H. (2003). Availabilities of calcium, iron, and zinc from dairy infant formulas is affected by soluble dietary fibers and modified starch fractions. *Nutrition*, *19*, 641–645.

27. Lidestri, M., Agosti, M., Marini, A., & Boehm, G. (2003). Oligosaccharides might stimulate calcium absorption in formula-fed preterm infants. *Acta Paediatrica Supplement*, *91*, 91–92.

28. Griffin, I. J., Davila, P. M., & Abrams, S. A. (2002). Non-digestible oligosaccharides and calcium absorption in girls with adequate calcium intakes. *The British Journal of Nutrition*, *87*(S2), S187–S191.

29. van den Heuvel, E., Muys, T., van Dokkum, W., & Schaafsma, G. (1999). Oligofructose stimulates calcium absorption in adolescents. *The American Journal of Clinical Nutrition*, *69*, 544–548.

30. Abrams, S. A., Griffin, I. J., Hawthorne, K. M., et al. (2005). A combination of prebiotic short and long-chain inulin-type fructans enhances calcium absorption and bone mineralization in young adolescents. *The American Journal of Clinical Nutrition*, *82*, 471–476.

31. Bakker-Zierikzee, A. M., Tol, E. A., Kroes, H., et al. (2006). Faecal SIgA secretion in infants fed on pre- or probiotic infant formula. *Pediatric Allergy and Immunology*, *17*, 134–140.

32. Arslanoglu, S., Moro, G. E., & Boehm, G. (2007). Early supplementation of prebiotic oligosaccharides protects formula-fed infants against infections during the

first 6 months of life. *The Journal of Nutrition, 137*(11), 2420–2424.

33. Duggan, C., Penny, M. E., Hibberd, P., et al. (2003). Oligofructose-supplemented infant cereal: 2 randomized, blinded, community-based trials in Peruvian infants. *The American Journal of Clinical Nutrition, 77,* 937–942.

34. Michail, S., Sylvester, F., Fuchs, G., & Issenman, R. (2006). Clinical efficacy of probiotics: Review of the evidence with focus on children. *Journal of Pediatric Gastroenterology and Nutrition, 43,* 550–557.

35. Salvatore, S., Hauser, B., Devreker, T., et al. (2007). Probiotics and zinc in acute infectious gastroenteritis in children: Are they effective?. *Nutrition, 23*(6), 498–506.

36. Canny, G. O., & McCormick, B. A. (2008). Bacteria in the intestine, helpful residents or enemies from within? *Infection and Immunity, 76*(8), 3360–3373.

37. Vandenplas, Y., Brunser, O., & Szajewska, H. (2008). Saccharomyces boulardii in childhood. *Journal of Medicinal Food.*

38. Doron, S., Snydman, D. R., & Gorbach, S. L. (2005). LGG: Bacteriology and clinical applications. *Gastroenterology Clinics of North America, 34,* 483–498.

39. Szajewska, H., & Mrukowicz, J. Z. (2005). Use of probiotics in children with acute diarrea.. *Pediatrica Drugs, 7,* 111–122.

40. Fukushima, Y., Kawata, Y., Hara, H., et al. (1998). Effect of a probiotic formula on intestinal IgA production in healthy children. *International Journal of Food Microbiology, 42,* 39–44.

41. Kaila, M., Isolauri, E., Soppi, E., et al. (1992). Enhancement of the circulating antibody secreting cell response in human diarrhea by a human Lactobacillus strain. *Pediatric Research, 32,* 141–144.

42. Kaila, M., Isolauri, E., Saxelin, M., et al. (1995). Viable versus inactivated *Lactobacillus* strain GG in acute Rotavirus diarrhoea. *Archives of Disease in Childhood, 72,* 51–53.

43. Juntunen, M., Kirjavainen, P. V., Ouwehand, A. C., et al. (2001). Adherence of probiotic bacteria to human intestinal mucus in healthy infants and during ROTAvirus infection. *Clinical and Diagnostic Laboratory Immunology, 8,* 293–296.

44. Billoo, A. G., Memon, M. A., Khaskheli, S. A., et al. (2006). Role of a probiotics (*Saccharomyces boulardii*) in the management and prevention of diarrhea. *World Journal of Gastroenterology, 12,* 4557–4560.

45. Buts, J. P., & De Keyser, N. (2006). Effects of *Saccharomyces boulardii* on intestinal mucosa. *Digestive Diseases and Sciences, 51,* 1485–1492.

46. Dahan, S., Dalmasso, G., Imbert, V., et al. (2003). *Saccharomyces boulardii* interferes with enterohemorrhagic *Escherichia coli*-induced signaling pathways in T84 cells. *Infection and Immunity, 71,* 766–773.

47. Salzman, N. H., Underwood, M. A., & Bevins, C. L. (2007). Paneth cells, defensins, and the commensal microbiota: a hypothesis on intimate interplay at the intestinal mucosa. *Seminars in Immunology, 19*(2), 70–83.

48. Lutgendorff, F., Akkermans, L. M., & Söderholm, J. D. (2008). The role of microbiota and probiotics in stress-induced gastro-intestinal damage. *Current Molecular Medicine, 8*(4), 282–298.

49. Lara-Villoslada, F., Olivares, M., Sierra, S., et al. (2007). Beneficial effects of probiotic bacteria isolated from breast milk. *The British Journal of Nutrition, 98*(S1), S96–S100.

50. Saran, S., Gopalan, S., & Krishna, T. P. (2002). Use of fermented foods to combat stunting and failure to thrive. *Nutrition, 18,* 393–396.

51. Sazawal, S., Dhingra, U., Sarkar, A., et al. (2004). Efficacy of milk fortified with a probiotic *Bifidobacterium lactis* (DR-10TM) and prebiotic galacto-oligosaccharides in prevention of morbidity and on nutritional status. *Asia Pacific Journal of Clinical Nutrition, 13*(S), S28.

52. Bruzzese, E., Volpicelli, M., Squeglia, V., et al. (2009). A formula containing galacto- and fructo-oligosaccharides prevents intestinal and extra-intestinal infections: An observational study. *Clinical Nutrition, 28,* 156–161.

53. Saavedra, J. M., Bauman, N. A., Oung, I., et al. (1994). Feeding of *Bifidobacterium bifidum* and *Streptococcus thermophilus* to infants in hospital for prevention of diarrhoea and shedding of rotavirus. *Lancet, 344,* 1046–1049.

54. Chouraqui, J. P., Van Egroo, L. D., & Fichot, M. C. (2004). Acidified milk formula supplemented with *Bifidobacterium lactis*: Impact on infant diarrhea in residual care settings. *Journal of Pediatric Gastroenterology and Nutrition, 38,* 288–292.

55. Thibault, H., Aubert-Jacquin, C., & Goulet, O. (2004). Effects of long-term consumption of a fermented infant formula (with *Bifidoacterium Breve* c50 and *Streptococcus thermophilus* 065) on acute diarrhea in healthy infants. *Journal of Pediatric Gastroenterology and Nutrition, 39,* 147–152.

56. Szajewska, H., Kotowska, M., Mrukowicz, J. Z., et al. (2001). Efficacy of LGG in prevention of nosocomial diarrhea in infants. *The Journal of Pediatrics, 138,* 361–365.

57. Mastretta, E., Longo, P., Laccisaglia, A., et al. (2002). Effect of a LGG and breast-feeding in the prevention of rotavirus nosocomial infection. *Journal of Pediatric Gastroenterology and Nutrition, 35,* 527–531.

58. Szajewska, H., & Mrukowicz, J. Z. (2005). Use of probiotics in children with acute diarrhea. *Paediatrica Drugs, 7,* 111–122.

59. Szajewska, H., Setty, M., Mrukowicz, J., & Guandalini, S. (2006). Probiotics in gastrointestinal disease in

children: Hard and not-so-hard evidence of efficacy. *Journal of Pediatric Gastroenterology and Nutrition, 42,* 454–475.

60. Hatakka, K., Savilahti, E., Pönkä, A., et al. (2001). Effect of long-term consumption of probiotic milk on infections in children attending day care centres: Double blind, randomised trial. *BMJ, 322,* 1327.

61. Weizman, Z., Asli, G., & Alsheikh, A. (2005). Effect of a probiotic infant formula on infections in childcare centers: Comparison of two probiotic agents. *Pediatrics, 115,* 5–9.

62. Chouraqui, J. P., Van Egroo, L. D., & Fichot, M. C. (2004). Acidified milk formula supplemented with *Bifodobacterium lactis*: impact on infant diarrhea in residential care settings. *Journal of Pediatric Gastroenterology and Nutrition, 38,* 288–292.

63. Billoo, A. G., Memon, M. A., Khaskheli, S. A., et al. (2006). Role of a probiotics (*Saccharomyces boulardii*) in the management and prevention of diarrhea. *World Journal of Gastroenterology, 12,* 4557–4560.

64. Rabbani, G. H., Teka, T., Zaman, B., et al. (2001). Clinical studies in persistent diarrhea: dietary management with green banana or pectin in Bangladeshi children. *Gastroenterology, 121*(3), 554–560.

65. Alam, N. H., Meier, R., Schneider, H., et al. (2000). Partially hydrolyzed guar gum-supplemented oral rehydration solution in the treatment of acute diarrhea in children. *Journal of Pediatric Gastroenterology and Nutrition, 31,* 503–507.

66. Hoekstra, J. H., Szajewska, H., Zikri, M. A., et al. (2004). Oral rehydration solution containing a mixture of nondigestible carbohydrates in the treatment of acute diarrhea: A multicenter randomized placebo controlled study on behalf of the ESPGHAN working group on intestinal infections. *Journal of Pediatric Gastroenterology and Nutrition, 39,* 239–245.

67. Isolauri, E., Juntunen, M., Rautanen, T., et al. (1991). A human Lactobacillus strain (*Lactobacillus casei* sp. strain GG) promotes recovery from acute diarrhea in children. *Pediatrics, 88,* 90–97.

68. Raza, S., Graham, S. M., & Allen, S. J. (1995). LGG promotes recovery from acute non-bloody diarrhea in Pakistan. *The Pediatric Infectious Disease Journal, 14,* 107–111.

69. Shornikova, A. V., Isolauri, E., Burkanova, L., et al. (1997). A trial in the Karelian Republic of oral rehydration and LGG for treatment of acute diarrhoea. *Acta Paediatrica, 86,* 460–465.

70. Shornikova, A. V., Casas, I. A., Mykkanen, H., et al. (1997). Bacteriotherapy with *Lactobacillus reuteri* in Rotavirus gastroenteritis. *The Pediatric Infectious Disease Journal, 16,* 1103–1107.

71. Guarino, A., Berni Canani, R., Spagnuolo, M. I., et al. (1997). Oral bacterial therapy reduces the duration of symptoms and viral excretion in children with mild diarrhea. *Journal of Pediatric Gastroenterology and Nutrition, 25,* 516–519.

72. Guandalini, S., Pensabene, L., Zikri, M. A., et al. (2000). LGG administered in oral rehydration solution in children with acute diarrhea: A multicenter European trial. *Journal of Pediatric Gastroenterology and Nutrition, 30,* 214–216.

73. Simakachorn, N., Pichaipat, V., Rithipornpaisarn, P., et al. (2000). Clinical evaluation of the addition of lyophilized, heat-killed *Lactobacillus acidophilus* LB to oral rehydration therapy in the treatment of acute diarrhea in children. *Journal of Pediatric Gastroenterology and Nutrition, 30,* 68–72.

74. Costa-Ribeiro, H., Ribeiro, T. C., Mattos, A. P., et al. (2003). Limitations of probiotic therapy in acute, severe dehydrating diarrhea. *Journal of Pediatric Gastroenterology and Nutrition, 36,* 112–115.

75. Khanna, V., Alam, S., & Malik, A. (2005). Efficacy of tyndalized *Lactobacillus acidophilus* in acute diarrhea. *Indian Journal of Pediatrics, 72,* 935–938.

76. Salazar-Lindo, E., Miranda-Langschwager, P., Campos-Sanchez, M., et al. (2004). Lactobacillus casei strain GG in the treatment of infants with acute watery diarrhea: A randomized, double-blind, placebo controlled clinical trial [ISRCTN67363048]. *BMC Pediatrics, 4,* 18.

77. Kowalska-Duplaga, K., Fyderek, K., Szajewska, H., & Janiak, R. (2004). Efficacy of Trilac® in the treatment of acute diarrhoea in infants and young children—a multicentre, randomized, double-blind placebo-controlled study. *Pediatria Współczesna, 3,* 295–299.

78. Sarker, S. A., Sultana, S., Fuchs, G. J., et al. (2005). Lactobacillus paracasei strain ST11 has no effect on rotavirus but ameliorates the outcome of nonrotavirus diarrhea in children from Bangladesh. *Pediatrics, 116,* e221–e228.

79. Huang, J. S., Bousvaros, A., Lee, J. W., et al. (2002). Efficacy of probiotic use in acute diarrhea in children: a meta-analysis. *Digestive Diseases and Sciences, 47,* 2625–2634.

80. Szajewska, H., & Mrukowicz, J. Z. (2001). Probiotics in the treatment and prevention of acute infectious diarrhea in infants and children: A systematic review of published randomized, double-blind, placebo-controlled trials. *Journal of Pediatric Gastroenterology and Nutrition, 33,* S17–S25.

81. Van Niel, C. W., Feudtner, C., Garrison, M. M., & Christakis, D. A. (2002). Lactobacillus therapy for acute infectious diarrhea in children: a meta-analysis. *Pediatrics, 109,* 678–684.

82. Allen, S. J., Okoko, B., Martinez, E., et al. (2004). Probiotics for treating infectious diarrhea CD003048. *Cochrane Database of Systematic Reviews* (2).

83. Shamir, R., Makhoul, I. R., Etzioni, A., & Shehadeh, N. (2005). Evaluation of a diet containing probiotics

and zinc for the treatment of mild diarrheal illness in children younger than one year of age. *Journal of the American College of Nutrition, 24*, 370–375.

84. Canani, R. B., Cirillo, P., Terrin, G., et al. (2007). Probiotics for treatment of acute diarrhoea in children: randomised clinical trial of five different preparations. *BMJ, 335*(7615), 340–343.

85. Szymanski, H., Pejcz, J., Jawien, M., et al. (2006). Treatment of acute infectious diarrhoea in infants and children with a mixture of three *Lactobacillus rhamnosus* strains—a randomized, double-blind, placebo-controlled trial. *Alimentary Pharmacology & Therapeutics, 23*, 247–253.

86. Dubey, A. P., Rajeshwari, K., Chakravarty, A., & Famularo, G. (2008). Use of VSL#3 in the treatment of rotavirus diarrhea in children: Preliminary results. *Journal of Clinical Gastroenterology, 42*(S3), S126–S129.

87. Basu, S., Paul, D. K., Ganguly, S., et al. (2008). Efficacy of high-dose *Lactobacillus rhamnosus* GG in controlling acute watery diarrhea in indian children: a randomized controlled trial. *Journal of Clinical Gastroenterology, 43*(3), 208–213.

88. Höchter, W., & Chase, D. (1990). Hagenhoff G. Saccharomyces boulardii bei akuter Erwachsenendiarrhoe. *Munchener Medizinische Wochenschrift, 132*, 188–192.

89. Cetina-Sauri, G., & Sierra Basto, G. (1994). Therapeutic evaluation of *Saccharomyces boulardii* in children with acute diarrhea. *Annales de Pediatrie, 41*, 397–400.

90. Kurugol, Z., & Koturoglu, G. (2005). Effects of *Saccharomyces boulardii* in children with acute diarrhoea. *Acta Paediatrica, 94*, 44–47.

91. Villarruel, G., Rubio, D. M., Lopez, F., et al. (2007). *Saccharomyces boulardii* in acute childhood diarrhea: A randomized, placebo-controlled study. *Acta Paediatrica, 96*, 538–541.

92. Castañeda, C., Garcia, E., Santa Cruz, M., et al. (1995). Effects of *Saccharomyces boulardii* in children with chronic diarrhea, especially cases due to giardiasis. *Revista Mexicana de Puericultura y Pediatria, 2*, 12–16.

93. Mansour-Ghanaei, F., Dehbashi, N., Yazdanparast, K., & Shafaghi, A. (2003). Efficacy of *Saccharomyces boulardii* with antibiotics in acute amoebiasis. *World Journal of Gastroenterology, 9*, 1832–1833.

94. Saint-Marc, T., Rossello-Prats, L., & Touraine, J. L. (1991). Efficacy of *Saccharomyces boulardii* in the treatment of diarrhea in AIDS. *Annales de Medecine Interne (Paris), 142*, 64–65.

95. Szajewska, H., Skórka, A., & Dylag, M. (2007). Meta-analysis: *Saccharomyces boulardii* for treating acute diarrhoea in children. *Alimentary Pharmacology & Therapeutics, 25*, 257–264.

96. Hafeez, A., Tariq, P., Ali, S., et al. (2002). The efficacy of *Saccharomyces boulardii* in the treatment of acute watery diarrhea in children: A multicentre randomized controlled trial. *Journal of College of Physicians Surgery Pakistan, 12*, 432–434.

97. Htwe, K., Yee, K. S., Tin, M., & Vandenplas, Y. (2008). Effect of *Saccharomyces boulardii* in the treatment of acute watery diarrhea in Myanmar children: A randomized controlled study. *The American Journal of Tropical Medicine and Hygiene, 78*, 214–216.

98. Sazawal, S., Hiremath, G., Dhingra, U., et al. (2006). Efficacy of probiotics in prevention of acute diarrhoea: a meta-analysis of masked, randomised, placebo-controlled trials. *The Lancet Infectious Diseases, 6*, 374–382.

99. Turck, D., Bernet, J. P., Marx, J., et al. (2003). Incidence and risk factors of oral antibiotic associated diarrhea in an outpatient pediatric population. *Journal of Pediatric Gastroenterology and Nutrition, 37*, 22–26.

100. Brunser, O., Gotteland, M., Cruchet, S., et al. (2006). Effect of a milk formula with prebiotics on the intestinal microbiota of infants after an antibiotic treatment. *Pediatric Research, 59*, 451–456.

101. Szajewska, H., Ruszczynski, M., & Radzikowski, A. (2006). Probiotics in the prevention of antibiotic-associated diarrhea in children: A meta-analysis of randomized controlled trials. *The Journal of Pediatrics, 149*, 367–372.

102. McFarland, L. V. (2006). Meta-analysis of probiotics for prevention of antibiotic associated diarrhea and the treatment of *Clostridium difficile* disease. *The American Journal of Gastroenterology, 101*, 812–822.

103. Szajewska, H., & Mrukowicz, J. (2005). Meta-analysis: non-pathogenic yeast *Saccharomyces boulardii* in the prevention of antibiotic-associated diarrhoea. *Alimentary Pharmacology & Therapeutics, 22*, 365–372.

104. Klein, S. M., Elmer, G. W., McFarland, L. V., et al. (1993). Recovery and elimination of the biotherapeutic agent, *Saccharomyces boulardii*, in healthy human volunteers. *Pharmaceutical Research, 10*, 1615–1619.

105. Vanderhoof, J. A., Whitney, D. B., Antonson, D. L., et al. (1999). LGG in the prevention of antibiotic-associated diarrhea in children. *The Journal of Pediatrics, 135*, 564–568.

106. Tankanow, R. M., Ross, M. B., Ertel, I. J., et al. (1990). A double-blind, placebo-controlled study of the efficacy of Lactinex in the prophylaxis of amoxicillin induced diarrhea. *DICP, 24*, 382–384.

107. Johnston, B. C., Supina, A. L., Ospina, M., & Vohra, S. (2007). Probiotics for the prevention of pediatric antibiotic-associated diarrhea CD004827. *Cochrane Database of Systematic Reviews* (2).

108. Szymański, H., Armańska, M., Kowalska-Duplaga, K., & Szajewska, H. (2008). *Bifidobacterium longum* PL03, *Lactobacillus rhamnosus* KL53A, and *Lactobacillus plantarum* PL02 in the prevention of antibiotic-associated

diarrhea in children: a randomized controlled pilot trial. *Digestion*, 78(1), 13–17.

109. Ruszczyński, M., Radzikowski, A., & Szajewska, H. (2008). Clinical trial: effectiveness of *Lactobacillus rhamnosus* (strains E/N, Oxy and Pen) in the prevention of antibiotic-associated diarrhoea in children. *Alimentary Pharmacology & Therapeutics*, 28(1), 154–161.

110. Segarra-Newnham, M. (2007). Probiotics for Clostridium difficile-associated diarrhea: focus on Lactobacillus rhamnosus GG and Saccharomyces boulardii. *The Annals of Pharmacotherapy*, 41, 1212–1221.

111. Biller, J. A., Katz, A. J., Flores, A. F., et al. (1995). Treatment of recurrent *Clostridium difficile* colitis with LGG. *Journal of Pediatric Gastroenterology and Nutrition*, 21, 224–226.

112. Stone-Dorshow, T., & Levitt, M. D. (1987). Gaseous response to ingestion of a poorly absorbed fructo-oligosaccharide sweetener. *The American Journal of Clinical Nutrition*, 46, 61–65.

113. Cummings, J. H., & Macfarlane, G. T. (2002). Gastrointestinal effects of prebiotics. *The British Journal of Nutrition*, 87, S145–S151.

114. Malinen, E., Rinttila, T., & Kajander, K. (2005). Analysis of the fecal microbiota of irritable bowel syndrome patients and healthy controls with real-time PCR. *The American Journal of Gastroenterology*, 100, 373–382.

115. Aerssens, J., Camilleri, M., & Coulie, B. (2008). Alterations in mucosal immunity identified in colon of patients with irritable bowel syndrome. *Clinical Gastroenterology and Hepatology*, 6, 194–205.

116. Bausserman, M., & Michail, S. (2005). The use of LGG in irritable bowel syndrome in children: a double-blind randomized control trial. *The Journal of Pediatrics*, 147, 197–201.

117. Gawrońska, A., Dziechciarz, P., Horvath, A., & Szajewska, H. (2007). A randomized double-blind placebo-controlled trial of LGG for abdominal pain disorders in children. *Alimentary Pharmacology & Therapeutics*, 25(2), 177–184.

118. Huertas-Ceballos, A. A., Logan, S., Bennett, C., & Macarthur, C. (2009). Dietary interventions for recurrent abdominal pain (RAP) and irritable bowel syndrome (IBS) in childhood CD003019. *Cochrane Database of Systematic Reviews* (1).

119. McFarland, L. V., & Dublin, S. (2008). Meta-analysis of probiotics for the treatment of irritable bowel syndrome. *World Journal of Gastroenterology*, 14(17), 2650–2661.

120. Lewis, H. B. (1912). The value of inulin as a food-stuff. *Journal of the American Medical Association, LVIII*, 1176–1177.

121. Vandenplas, Y., & Benninga, M. (2009). Probiotics and functional gastrointestinal disorders in children. *Journal of Pediatric Gastroenterology and Nutrition, 48*, S107–S109.

122. Picard, C., Fioramonti, J., Francois, A., et al. (2005). Review article: bifidobacteria as probiotic agents—physiological effects and clinical benefits. *Alimentary Pharmacology & Therapeutics*, 22, 495–512.

123. Marteau, P., Cuillerier, E., Meance, S., et al. (2002). *Bifidobacterium animalis* strain DN-173 010 shortens the colonic transit time in healthy women: a double-blind, randomized, controlled study. *Alimentary Pharmacology & Therapeutics*, 16, 587–593.

124. Bu, L. N., Chang, M. H., Ni, Y. H., et al. (2007). *Lactobacillus casei rhamnosus* Lcr35 in children with chronic constipation. *Pediatrics International*, 49, 485–490.

125. Banaszkiewicz, A., & Szajewska, H. (2005). Ineffectiveness of LGG as an adjunct to lactulose for the treatment of constipation in children: a double-blind, placebo-controlled randomized trial. *The Journal of Pediatrics*, 146, 364–369.

126. Bekkali, N. L. H., Bongers, M. E. J., et al. (2007). The role of a probiotics mixture in the treatment of childhood constipation: a pilot study. *Nutrition Journal*, 6, 17.

127. Puccio, G., Cajozzo, C., & Meli, F. (2007). Clinical evaluation of a new starter formula for infants containing live *Bifidobacterium longum* BL999 and prebiotics. *Nutrition*, 23(1), 1–8.

128. MacDonald, T. T., & Monteleone, G. (2005). Immunity, inflammation, and allergy in the gut. *Science, 307*, 1920–1925.

129. Salvatore, S., Heuschkel, R., Tomlin, S., et al. (2000). A pilot study of N-acetyl glucosamine, a nutritional substrate for glycosaminoglycan synthesis, in paediatric chronic inflammatory bowel disease. *Alimentary Pharmacology & Therapeutics*, 14, 1567–1579.

130. Bousvaros, A., Guandalini, S., Baldassano, R. N., et al. (2005). A randomized, double-blind trial of LGG versus placebo in addition to standard maintenance therapy for children with Crohn's disease. *Inflammatory Bowel Diseases*, 11, 833–839.

131. Day, A. S. (2004). Use of complementary and alternative medicines by children and adolescents with inflammatory bowel disease. *Journal of Paediatrics and Child Health*, 40, 681–684.

132. Gotteland, M., Brunser, O., & Cruchet, S. (2006). Systematic review: are probiotics useful in controlling gastric colonization by *Helicobacter pylori*? *Alimentary Pharmacology & Therapeutics*, 23, 1077–1086.

133. Gotteland, M., Andrews, M., Toledo, M., et al. (2008). Modulation of *Helicobacter pylori* colonization with cranberry juice and *Lactobacillus johnsonii* La1 in children. *Nutrition*, 24(5), 421–426.

134. Gotteland, M., Poliak, L., Cruchet, S., & Brunser, O. (2005). Effect of regular ingestion of *Saccharomyces boulardii* plus inulin or *Lactobacillus acidophilus* LB

in children colonized by *Helicobacter pylori*. *Acta Paediatrica*, *94*(12), 1747–1751.

135. Sýkora, J., Valecková, K., Amlerová, J., et al. (2005). Effects of a specially designed fermented milk product containing probiotic *Lactobacillus casei* DN-114 001 and the eradication of *H. pylori* in children: A prospective randomized double-blind study. *Journal of Clinical Gastroenterology*, *39*(8), 692–698.

136. Goldman, C. G., Barrado, D. A., Balcarce, N., et al. (2006). Effect of a probiotic food as an adjuvant to triple therapy for eradication of *Helicobacter pylori* infection in children. *Nutrition*, *22*(10), 984–988.

137. Hurduc, V., Plesca, D., Dragomir, D., et al. (2009). A randomized, open trial evaluating the effect of *Saccharomyces boulardii* on the eradication rate of *Helicobacter pylori* infection in children. *Acta Paediatrica*, *98*(1), 127–131.

138. Lionetti, E., Miniello, V. L., Castellaneta, S. P., et al. (2006). *Lactobacillus reuteri* therapy to reduce side-effects during anti-*Helicobacter pylori* treatment in children: A randomized placebo controlled trial. *Alimentary Pharmacology & Therapeutics*, *24*(10), 1461–1468.

139. Lesbros-Pantoflickova, D., Corthésy-Theulaz, I., & Blum, A. L. (2007). Helicobacter pylori and probiotics. *The Journal of Nutrition*, *137*(3S2), 812S–818S.

140. Sachdeva, A., & Nagpal, J. (2009). Effect of fermented milk-based probiotic preparations on *Helicobacter pylori* eradication: a systematic review and meta-analysis of randomized-controlled trials. *European Journal of Gastroenterology & Hepatology*, *21*(1), 45–53.

141. Savino, F., Palumeri, E., Castagno, E., et al. (2006). Reduction of crying episodes owing to infantile colic: a randomized controlled study on the efficacy of a new infant formula. *European Journal of Clinical Nutrition*, *60*, 1304–1310.

142. Savino, F., Pelle, E., Palumeri, E., et al. (2007). Lactobacillus reuteri (American type culture collection strain 55730) versus simethicone in the treatment of infantile colic: A prospective randomized study. *Pediatrics*, *119*, e124–e130.

143. Indrio, F., Riezzo, G., Raimondi, F., et al. (2008). The effects of probiotics on feeling tolerance, bowel habitus, and gastrointestinal motility in reterm newborns. *The Journal of Pediatrics*, *152*(6), 801–806.

144. Manzoni, P. (2007). Use of *Lactobacillus casei* subspecies *Rhamnosus* GG and gastrointestinal colonization by Candida species in preterm neonates. *Journal*

of Pediatric Gastroenterology and Nutrition, 45(S3), S190–S194.

145. Alfaleh, K., & Bassler, D. (2008). Probiotics for prevention of necrotizing enterocolitis in preterm infants CD005496. *Cochrane Database of Systematic Reviews* (1).

146. Lin, H. C., Su, B. H., & Oh, W. (2006). Oral probiotics prevent necrotizing enterocolitis. *The Journal of Pediatrics*, *148*, 849.

147. Bin-Nun, A., Bromiker, R., Wilschanski, M., et al. (2005). Oral probiotics prevent necrotizing enterocolitis in very low birth weight neonates. *The Journal of Pediatrics*, *147*, 192–196.

148. Dani, C., Biadaioli, R., Bertini, G., et al. (2002). Probiotics feeding in prevention of urinary tract infection, bacterial sepsis and necrotizing enterocolitis in preterm infants. A prospective double-blind study. *Biologia Neonatorum*, *82*, 103–108.

149. Costalos, C., Skouteri, V., Gounaris, A., et al. (2003). Enteral feeding of premature infants with *Saccharomyces boulardii*. *Early Human Development*, *74*, 89–96.

150. Lin, H. C., Hsu, C. H., Chen, H. L., et al. (2008). Oral probiotics prevent necrotizing enterocolitis in very low birth weight preterm infants: a multicenter, randomized, controlled trial. *Pediatrics*, *122*(4), 693–700.

151. Rumessen, J. J., & Gudmand-Hoyer, E. (1998). Fructans of chicory: intestinal transport and fermentation of different chain lengths and relation to fructose and sorbitol malabsorption. *The American Journal of Clinical Nutrition*, *68*, 357–364.

152. Borriello, S. P., Hammes, W. P., Holzapfel, W., et al. (2003). Safety of probiotics that contain Lactobacilli or Bifidobacteria. *Clinical Infectious Diseases*, *36*, 775–780.

153. Cabana, M. D., Shane, A. L., Chao, C., & Oliva-Henker, M. (2006). Probiotics in primary care pediatrics. *Clinical Pediatrics*, *45*, 405–410.

154. Cassone, M., Serra, P., Mondello, F., et al. (2003). Outbreak of *Saccharomyces cerevisiae* subtype *boulardii fungemia* in patients neighboring those treated with a probiotic preparation of the organism. *Clinical Microbiology*, *41*, 5340–5343.

155. Mathur, S., & Singh, R. (2005). Antibiotic resistance in food lactic acid bacteria—review. *International Journal of Food Microbiology*, *105*, 281–295.

156. Temmerman, R., Pot, B., Huys, G., & Swings, J. (2003). Identification and antibiotic susceptibility of bacterial isolates from probiotic products. *International Journal of Food Microbiology*, *81*, 1–10.

Probiotics and Prebiotics: Effects on Diarrhea

Michael de Vrese and B. Offick

Institute of Physiology and Biochemistry of Nutrition,
Federal Dairy Research Center, Kiel, Germany

1. INTRODUCTION

Fermented milk products have been consumed throughout the world for thousands of years, as evidenced by their depiction in Sumerian wall paintings dating back to 2500 BC.[1] Consumption in those days were already considered to be beneficial to health, partly due to a reduced risk related to hygiene. At 76 BC, the Roman historian Plinius recommended the administration of fermented milk products for treating gastroenteritis (reference cited in Bottazzi [1]).

At the beginning of the twentieth century, Carre [2], Tissier [3] and Metchnikoff [4] had the idea to suppress and displace harmful bacteria in the intestine by orally administered 'beneficial' ones and by this improve microbial balance, health and longevity. To be more precise, Tissier recommended the administration of bifidobacteria to infants suffering from diarrhea,

claiming that bifidobacteria supersede the putrefactive bacteria causing the disease. Nobel Prize winner (1908) Elie Metchnikoff from the Pasteur Institut in Paris claimed that the intake of lactobacilli-containing yogurt results in a reduction of toxin-producing bacteria in the gut and this is associated with increased longevity of the host. Based on the work of Metchnikoff, in 1919 Isaac Carasso developed the first industrially produced yogurt the way we know it today, as a therapy to treat life-threatening diarrhea in children, which was sold in pharmacies.

The term 'probiotics' itself was created in the 1950s by W. Kollath [5]. In 1965, Lilly and Stillwell used this term for live bacteria and spores as animal feed supplements that should help limiting the use of antibiotics in animal husbandry [6]. According to the definition of the FAO/WHO, probiotics are 'live microorganisms, which, when administered in adequate

---

[1]At the time fermented milk products already played an important role in dairy farming, possibly because of the climatic conditions according to a Persian version of the Old Testament (Genesis 18:8), which states that Abraham owed his longevity to the consumption of sour milk.

205

amounts, confer a health benefit on the host.' Other definitions emphasize the importance of the intestinal and non-intestinal microflora[2]: 'a probiotic is a preparation or product containing viable, defined microorganisms in sufficient numbers, which alter the microflora in a compartment of the host and by that exert health effects in this host' [7]. Numerous probiotic microorganisms (e.g. *Lactobacillus rhamnosus* GG, *L. reuteri*, bifidobacteria and certain strains of *L. casei* or the *L. acidophilus* group) are used in probiotic food, particularly fermented milk products, or have been investigated—as well as *Escherichia coli* strain Nissle 1917, certain enterococci (*Enterococcus faecium* SF68) and the probiotic yeast *Saccharomyces boulardii*—with regard to their medicinal use.

The similar-sounding term 'prebiotic,' which was introduced into the scientific literature by Gibson and Roberfroid in 1995 [8], characterizes a special type of dietary fiber with specific bifidogenic properties, but without nutrient character.

Both probiotics and prebiotics are food components that almost fulfil the definition of a functional food (defined as 'foods and food components that provide a health benefit beyond basic nutrition' [9]); particularly the term 'beyond nutrition,' since bacteria have no nutrient character. Fermented milk with health-promoting 'probiotic' properties is one of the oldest functional foods.

Most health effects attributed to pro- and prebiotics are related, directly or indirectly (i.e. mediated by the immune system) to the gastrointestinal tract. This is not only because prebiotic carbohydrates, food probiotics or therapeutically used microorganisms are applied normally via the oral route. The mechanisms and the efficacy of a probiotic effect often depends on interactions with the specific microflora of the host, on inhibition of intestinal pathogens, on the reduction of harmful metabolites in the gut, and on effects on the gut-associated lymphoid system (GALT).

According to this, the effect of probiotics to prevent diarrhea or inflammatory bowel disease has been particularly studied [10, 11]. A published meta-analysis of 34 randomized placebo-controlled human studies concluded that probiotics do significantly reduce diarrhea, amongst others antibiotics-associated diarrhea incidences by 35 to 65%, traveler's diarrhea incidences by 6 to 21% and diarrhea incidences due to other reasons by 8 to 53%. Overall, the risk of acute diarrhea was reduced by 57% in children and by 26% in adults [12].

2. THE USE OF PROBIOTICS IN DIARRHEA

Most people experience frequent, loose, and watery bowel movements once or twice a year. This change from the usual pattern of stools is recognized as diarrhea. According to the WHO, diarrhea is defined as 'the passage of three or more loose or liquid stools per day, or more frequently than is normal for the individual' [13]. Diarrhea occurs when fluid absorption by the colon is insufficient, e.g. if the colon is damaged or inflamed.

There are several types of diarrhea:

1. Osmotic diarrhea, due to the maldigestion and malabsorption of osmotic active nutrients, which pull water into the bowels (e.g. lactose intolerance).
2. Motility-related diarrhea, due to rapid movement of food through the intestines and increased colon peristalsis.

---

[2]The term 'microbiota' is often used instead, because the 'microflora' comprise organisms of various *phyla* (bacteria, fungi, unicellular eukaryotes).

3. Secretory diarrhea, characterized by an increase in the active secretion and/or an inhibition of the absorption of ions, commonly due to the release of toxins in bacterial or viral infections or alterations of the autochthonal (originating in the place where found) microflora.

4. Inflammatory diarrhea, due to damage to the mucosal lining or brush border, which leads to a passive loss of protein-rich fluids (exudation), and a decreased ability to absorb these lost fluids.

Therefore, causes of diarrhea can be due to viral or bacterial infections, foodborne illnesses, allergies, food and particularly lactose intolerance, or the ingestion of laxatives or foods with laxative properties and may be accompanied by abdominal pain, nausea and vomiting. Diarrhea can also be a symptom of more serious diseases, such as Montezuma's Revenge (traveler's diarrhea), dysentery, cholera, or botulism. It can also be indicative of severe radiation sickness or a chronic syndrome such as the irritable bowel syndrome or Crohn's disease.

In all types of diarrhea, probiotic bacteria show a more or less preventive or therapeutic effect, dependent on the bacterial strain and its antimicrobial, immunomodulatory and anti-inflammatory properties. They support the intestinal defense against viruses, potentially harmful bacteria or toxins at all levels (autochthonal microbiota in the gut, the mucosal barrier and the gut-associated lymphoid tissue or GALT), stabilize a balanced composition of the intestinal microbiota and prevent an excessive overgrowth of commensals and/or potential harmful bacteria of the autochthonal microbiota.

3. THE INTESTINAL MICROBIOTA

The intestinal microbiota is characterized by its high quantitative mass and its high qualitative diversity. Although most of the microbiota is autochthonous, allochthonous microbiota is also found (e.g. most pathogens). At birth, the gut is sterile and is colonized in the first 5 days after birth with aerobics (*E. coli*, lactobacilli and enterococci) and anaerobics (bacteroides and bifidobacteria), which originate from the maternal intestinal and vaginal flora and the 'hospital flora.' The intestinal microbiota is vulnerable up to 3–5 years of age and stable afterwards, although there are marked differences in microbial composition between individuals [14].

The commensal intestinal microbiota is characterized by a predominantly saccharolytic metabolism, i.e. it covers its energy requirements in large part through the fermentation of intestinal secreta, particularly complex carbohydrates from intestinal mucus, and from undigested dietary carbohydrates. In comparison with this, proteolytic metabolism and the digestion of other dietary residues plays only a minor role. The fermentation of complex carbohydrates results in the production of short-chain fatty acids (SCFA) such as acetate, propionate and butyrate, as well as of other terminal products such as lactate, ethanol, succinate, carbon dioxide, hydrogen, and methane [15, 16]. SCFA decrease gut pH [17], help increase gut motility [18], help absorption of nutrients such as calcium, magnesium, and iron [19], and provide energy for the colonic epithelium and the host [20]. Furthermore, luminal instillation of butyrate has been shown to be effective in the treatment of human ulcerative colitis and related inflammatory disorders [21, 22].

Even if the intestinal microbiota is relatively stable in adults, it can be negatively affected by poor diet, lifestyle habits, stress, illness, antibiotics treatment, other medications and aging; in the elderly, bifidobacteria counts drop and enterobacteria and clostridia increase (Fig. 14.1).

It is generally accepted that a so-called 'healthy' and balanced intestinal microbiota is a prerequisite for health, particularly for gastrointestinal well-being, regular development and function of the immune system and the

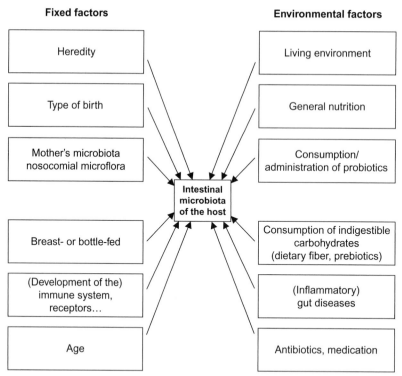

FIGURE 14.1   Factors affecting the intestinal microbiota.

prevention of pathogen infection and diarrhea. However, there is no consensus of which constituents an 'ideal' microbiota should be composed, but there is thought to be one, which is predominantly saccharolytic and SCFA and lactic acid-releasing, and which contains high numbers of lactobacilli and bifidobacteria at the expense of the disadvantage of more proteolytic or even potentially harmful bacteria.

4. THE MUCOSAL BARRIER

The gastrointestinal mucosa forms a barrier between the body and a lumenal environment. The mucosa allows the transport of nutrients across the epithelium while it prevents the passage of harmful molecules and organisms into the organism. The exclusionary properties of the

gastrointestinal mucosa are referred to as the 'mucosal barrier.' This comprises the intrinsic barrier (epithelial cell line) and the extrinsic barrier (digestive secretions, such as gastric and pancreatic juice, deconjugated bile acids and antimicrobial peptides).

Various *in vitro* and animal studies have investigated the influence of probiotics on epithelial homeostasis. Yan et al. showed that two soluble proteins produced by *L. rhamnosus* GG significantly reduced TNF-induced intestinal epithelial damage and inhibited apoptosis of intestinal epithelial cells [23]. Furthermore, *E. coli* Nissle 1917 improved intestinal barrier function in a colitis mouse model [24]. In another study, pre-treatment of rats with *L. helveticus* R0052 or *L. rhamnosus* R0011 reduced the stress-induced impairment of the intestinal barrier by the reduction of bacterial adhesion in the gut and bacterial translocation to the mesenteric lymph nodes [25].

5. THE GUT-ASSOCIATED LYMPHOID TISSUE

The GALT includes both organized lymphoid compartments, consisting of Peyer's patches, regional lymphatics, and mesenteric lymph nodes; and dispersed lymphoid cells in the intraepithelial leukocyte spaces and the gut lamina propria.

The lumen of the gastrointestinal tract represents the environment outside of the body, comprising nutrients on the one hand and many harmful microorganisms and molecules on the other. The immune system distinguishes between what is harmful and what is not. Thus, various immune cells comprise in the digestive tube, such as M cells and dendritic cells (DCs). M cells, which occur in the intestinal epithelium, endocytose protein and peptide antigens, and transport them into the underlying tissue. The antigens are taken up by local DCs and macrophages, which present them to T and B lymphocytes in the lymph nodes, leading via a signal cascade to the secretion of chemokines, cytokines, IgA and the appearance of other immune cells. The secretory IgA is transported through the epithelial cells into the lumen, where, for example, it interferes with adhesion and invasion of bacteria. The insufficient stimulation or differentiation of DCs leads to the deletion of effector T cells and the secretion of anti-inflammatory cytokines such as IL-10 and TGF-β. This generates regulatory T cells that regulate the immune response against commensal bacteria [26].

The immune system is adversely affected by age, certain bacterial strains, certain diseases, poor diet, obesity, stress, and intense exercise [27–30]. In this respect, the often asked question on how probiotics beneficially affect the immune system of healthy subjects is generally answered with the note that probiotics can be conductive to reduce the risk and/or the duration of transient disruptions of the balance between immune system and intestinal microbiota and thus reduce the risk of diseases.

However, it is not possible to characterize the effect of probiotics on the immune system as generally positive or negative, as the effects were usually described as 'modulation,' 'balancing' or 'normalization.' This comprises, as shown in various *in vitro* studies and clinical studies, an enhanced immune defense against pathogen bacteria and viruses due to an increase of pro-inflammatory cytokine release (IFN-γ, IL-2, IL-6, TNF-α) and decreased (and thus normalized) release of pro-inflammatory cytokines in chronic inflammatory diseases (Table 14.1).

6. INFECTIOUS DIARRHEA CAUSED BY VIRUSES OR BACTERIA

Gastrointestinal infections due to viruses (typically rotavirus), bacteria (*Salmonella*, *Shigella*, *Listeria*, or pathogenic strains of *E. coli*), but also by eukaryotic protozoa (*Giardia*, *Entamoeba*, *Microsporidium*) or parasitic metazoa (e.g. the nematode *Strongyloides stercoralis*) are the most common and severe causes of diarrhea. However, in most cases, the lack of hygiene and/or clean drinking water and food are responsible.

Infectious diarrhea is classified as acute diarrhea (less than 14 days from infection to onset of diarrhea) and persistent diarrhea (more than 14 days from infection to onset of diarrhea). In both cases, clinical studies investigated the effect of probiotics on prevention, therapy, or alleviation of adverse effects of an antibiotic therapy.

Since in the 1990s probiotic bacteria and the yeast *Saccharomyces boulardii* have been recognized to prevent diarrhea, alleviate gastrointestinal complaints or shorten acute infections, these effects have been investigated extensively. Most studies have been performed in infants, hospitalized children and in children from day care centers, as a beneficial effect of probiotics was expected in children due to a modifiable immune system and/or a severe infection.

TABLE 14.1   Examples of immunomodulatory effects of probiotics

Immunological function	Parameter/target group	Result
Innate (non-specific) immunity		IL-12 ↑, NK cells ↑, phagocytosis ↑, neutophils ↑, monocytes ↑
Adaptive/acquired (specific) immunity	Immunoglobulins, Food allergy associated Ig	IgA ↑, sIgA ↑, IgG ↑, virus-neutralizing antibodies ↑, IgE ↓
Mucosal integrity	Intestinal epithelium Intestinal barrier	Cell damage, apoptosis ↓, β-defensin-2 ↑, barrier function ↑, bacterial translocation ↓
Recognition of bacteria*	Toll-like receptors (TLRs) Mannose receptor	TLR-2 ↑, CD-206 ↑
Release of pro-inflammatory (TH1-) cytokines	Healthy subjects Chronically inflamed subjects	IFN-γ, IL-6 ↑, TNF-α ↑, IFN-γ ↓, IL-2 ↑, IL-6 ↓, TNF-α ↓
Release of anti-inflammatory cytokines	Healthy subjects	IL-10 ↑
	Chronically inflamed subjects	IL-10 ↓
Release of pro-allergic cytokines	Allergic subjects	IL-5 ↓

*Triggering pro-inflammatory reactions.

Therefore, this effect is perhaps the best documented beneficial probiotic effect [31–36].

In most studies a single lactobacillus strain or the yeast *S. boulardii* were used, less trials were performed with bifidobacteria or mixtures of several strains of probiotic bacteria [37]. Particularly, the effects of probiotic microorganisms on the incidence (preventive effect) as well as the severity and/or duration of acute infectious diarrhea (therapeutic effect) were investigated in these studies, and a reduction of the incidence of diarrhea (RR 0.66) or the duration of diarrheal episodes by about 1 day were the most often observed beneficial effects [38–41]. Altogether, controlled clinical studies and meta-analyses [41] showed that there is evidence to suggest beneficial effects on infectious diarrhea of several strains of probiotic microorganisms (Table 14.2), particularly of the lactobacilli *L. rhamnosus* GG and *L. reuteri*, as well as the yeast *Saccharomyces boulardii*; whereas less studies have been performed showing anti-diarrheal effects of other lactobacilli (*L. acidophilus*, *L. plantarum*), bifidobacteria, *E. coli* 'Nissle 1917', or mixed-strain probiotics (e.g. VSL#3[3] or *L. acidophilus* LA5 plus *Bifidobacterium lactis* BB12[4]).

L. rhamnosus strain Goldin and Gorbach (LGG; ATCC 53103) is named after two American scientists who had performed a successful systematic search for a probiotic bacterial strain for use in humans. LGG was the first bacterial strain used in foods, in particular in fermented milk products. No other probiotic bacterial strain was more often used (predominantly successfully) in clinical trials investigating the effect on diarrhea and other diseases [42].

[3]VSL#3: *Streptococcus thermophilus* + *Bifidobacterium breve* + *B. longum* + *B. infantis* + *L. acidophilus* + *L. plantarum* + *L. paracasei* + *L. delbrueckii* ssp. *bulgaricus*.
[4]LA5 and/or BB12: mostly used for the production of probiotic fermented milk products (frequently together with *S. thermophilus*).

TABLE 14.2 Probiotic bacteria with clinically proven beneficial effects in diarrheal disorders

Lactobacilli

L. acidophilus	L. fermentum	L. johnsonii
L. brevis	L. helveticus	L. plantarum
L. casei	L. paracasei	L. rhamnosus

Bifidobacteria

B. adolescentis	B. breve	B. longum
B. animalis	B. infantis	
B. bifidum	B. lactis	

Others

Enterococcus faecium	Saccharomyces boulardii
Lactococcus lactis ssp. lactis	

Multistrain probiotics

La5 + Bb12
(+ S. thermophilus)
VSL#3

The strain *L. reuteri* produces a very active bacteriocin[5] (Reuterin). This explains the usefulness of this probiotic in factory farming (turkeys) and beneficial effects particularly on bacterial infectious diarrhea [34].

E. coli strain Nissle 1917 is predominantly effective in infectious diseases. However, a study investigating its effects on acute diarrhea in infants and toddlers showed a significantly decreased duration of diarrhea [43, 44].

The tropical yeast *S. boulardii* (which has now been re-identified as a strain of *Saccharomyces cerevisiae* or baker's (brewer's) yeast) was first isolated from the lychee and mangosteen fruit in 1923 by Henri Boulard. This French scientist had observed that South East Asian natives chewed these fruits as a medication against cholera. Mannose residues on the surface of *S. boulardii* bind adhesin-mediated to (pathogenic) bacteria preventing them from adhering to intestinal brush border and facilitating their elimination from the body via defecation [45]. Furthermore, *S. boulardii* proteolytically degrades *Clostridium difficile* toxin A and B [46] and has anti-inflammatory effects [47, 48]. *S. boulardii* is used as preventive and therapeutic efficacy in infectious diarrhea and other intestinal disorders and has been proven in numerous randomized controlled (small-scale) clinical trials in children [49–51] and adults [52], which have been summarized in several reviews and meta-analyses [53, 54].

However, in other studies, lactobacilli [55, 56], bifidobacteria or *S. boulardii* had no effect on the duration or incidence of infectious diarrhea, or they were effective in persistent diarrhea [57] but ineffective in severe acute diarrhea [58]. In another trial using five different commercial probiotic preparations ($\sim 10^8$–10^{10} cfu/day), only LGG and a probiotic mix of four bacterial strains (*L. acidophilus*, *Bifidobacterium bifidum*, *S. thermophilus* and *L. delbrueckii* ssp. *bulgaricus*) were effective in decreasing the duration of diarrhea and the daily stool output, whereas the other strains tested (strains of *S. boulardii*, *Bacillus clausiii* and *Enterococcus faecium*) were not [59].

Altogether, an actual literature search[6] retrieved 35 randomized controlled (mostly small-scale) clinical trials in which beneficial effects of probiotics on acute diarrhea were demonstrated, whereas eight studies showed no effect. In 60% of the studies with a positive outcome, lactobacilli were given. The others used bifidobacteria (6%), yogurt, *E. coli* Nissle 1917 or *E. faecium* SF 68 (3% each), *S. boulardii* or a mixed strain probiotic (11% each). In most studies, therapeutic

---

[5]Bacteriocins are peptides or proteins that kill other bacteria by disturbing synthesis, function and structure of the bacterial cell wall. The advantage over antibiotics is the minimal risk for the host microflora and the absence of a risk of developing resistance because of the narrow spectrum of killing activity, which is directed against a limited number of other bacterial strains of the same or a closely related species.

[6]de Vrese and Offick, unpublished data.

effects of probiotics on acute (predominantly rotavirus-induced) diarrhea were investigated, and most frequently a reduction of the duration of diarrheal episodes by between 0.8 and 1.2 days was observed (according to a mean relative risk, RR = 0.43). Only four studies were available investigating the effect of probiotics on the prevention of acute diarrhea. A decreased incidence of diarrhea was found in only two of these studies. The other two studies showed a reduced length and/or severity of diarrhea in the probiotic groups. A combined analysis of probiotic effects on prevention of acute diarrhea and antibiotics-associated diarrhea showed significantly less days with diarrhea in the probiotic groups compared with the controls (mean values 2 vs 8 days per trial period; RR = 0.13–0.65).

7. DIARRHEA IN NEWBORNS

Early inoculation of a plasmid-free human *E. coli* into human newborns did not affect early colonization of the gut but reduced the frequency of acute diarrhea during the first year of life [60].

8. ROTAVIRUS-INDUCED DIARRHEA IN (HOSPITALIZED) CHILDREN

Virus- (mainly rotavirus-) induced diarrhea is still a major problem and frequent cause of death, especially in hospitalized children and in developing countries. Due to their cost-effectiveness and the absence of adverse side effects, probiotics have been used to treat such diarrheas for some time.

One of the first studies, which was performed in 71 Finnish children, demonstrated that the mean duration of diarrhea was significantly shorter after treatment with *L. casei* sp. strain GG (1.4 ± 0.8 days) than after placebo

treatment (2.4 ± 1.1 days) [61]. In another Finnish study performed in 49 infants (6–35 months old) three different freeze-dried lactic acid bacteria preparations were given. The mean (SD) duration of diarrhea was 1.8 (0.8) days in infants who received LGG, 2.8 (1.2) days in those receiving *L. casei* subsp. *rhamnosus*, and 2.6 (1.4) days in those receiving yogurt bacteria (33). In a recent randomized, double blind, placebo-controlled study treatment of 230 subjects suffering from rotavirus diarrhea with the probiotic product VSL#3, increased the stool consistency and decreased the stool frequency [37], whereas other trials used lactobacilli strains, which also decreased the duration and incidence of diarrhea [62].

Altogether, in an actual analysis[7] of nine randomized, controlled trials on the effect of probiotics (8 × lactobacilli, 1 × VSL#3) specifically on rotavirus-induced diarrhea, all studies showed that probiotics are effective in treating rotavirus-induced diarrhea. Thereby the use of probiotics, as compared with a placebo, was associated with a significantly reduced risk particularly of longer-lasting diarrhea (>3 days) in hospitalized children (RR 0.43 (95% CI, 0.34–0.53; fixed-effect model).

9. GASTROINTESTINAL COMPLAINTS AND DIARRHEA IN CHILDREN FROM DAY CARE CENTERS

Four studies were performed in young healthy children from day care centers, without the examination of the nature of the causative pathogens, probably mainly viral [63–66].

A French study group examined 287 children (aged 18.9 ± 6.0 months) in day care nurseries administered daily with either unfermented jellied milk, conventional yogurt or a probiotic yogurt product containing 10^8 cfu/mL *L. casei*. Products were given for 1 month each, interrupted by 1 month without supplementation.

[7]de Vrese and Offick, unpublished data.

The conventional yogurt shortened the mean duration of diarrhea from 8 days down to 5 days; the probiotic product was even better at 4.3 days ($p < 0.01$), while the incidence of diarrhea was not different between groups [63]. The study was expanded to a randomized, controlled multicenter clinical trial in a total of 928 children (aged 6–24 months). The daily administration of *L. casei*-containing fermented milk for 2 months decreased the frequency of diarrhea compared with the administration of conventional yogurt (15.9 vs 22%, $p < 0.05$) [64]. In another study, Finnish children from day care centers, who consumed milk containing a probiotic *L. rhamnosus* strain during the winter, had 16% less days of absence from day care due to diarrhea and gastrointestinal and respiratory tract infections than the control group [65]. Similarly, infants from Israeli child care centers consuming *B. lactis* Bb12 or *L. reuteri* SD2112 had less infectious diseases (diarrhea, cold), a reduced incidence of diarrhea (from 0.31 ± 0.09 to 0.13 ± 0.08 or 0.02 ± 0.01, respectively), and a shorter duration of episodes (from 0.59 ± 0.25 days to 0.37 ± 0.29 or 0.15 ± 0.03 days, respectively) [66].

Another study group showed that the administration of acidified milk formula supplemented with *B. lactis* Bb12 significantly decreased the days with diarrhea in infants in residential care settings (probiotic group: 1.15 ± 2.5 days; placebo group: 2.3 ± 4.5 days), but was not different from the placebo (conventional formula without probiotics) in the incidence of diarrhea (probiotic group: 28.3%; placebo group: 38.7%) and the duration of diarrhea episodes (probiotic group: 5.1 ± 3.3 days; placebo group: 7 ± 5.5 days) [67].

10. DIARRHEA IN UNDERNOURISHED CHILDREN

A study performed in 204 undernourished Peruvian children (6–24 months) showed that

LGG reduced the frequency of diarrhea from 6.0 to 5.2 episodes per child and year ($p < 0.05$) [68].

11. STUDIES IN ADULTS

Only a few studies investigating the effect of probiotics on infectious diarrhea have been performed in adults. In a study by Pereg et al., 529 Israeli soldiers consumed yogurt with or without probiotic *L. casei* cultures. In the probiotic group, 12% had diarrhea compared to 16% in the control group. The duration of the diarrhea was 2.6 days in the probiotic group versus 3 days in the control group. These differences were not significant [69]. Another study performed in 211 adults showed that the administration of *Enterococcus* SF 68 for 5 days significantly reduced the duration of diarrhea [35]. And a meta-analysis showed that probiotics reduced the risk of acute diarrhea of diverse causes by 26% (7–49%) among adults compared with 57% (35–71%) among children [12, 70].

12. TRAVELER'S DIARRHEA

Investigations on the effect of probiotic bacteria on traveler's diarrhea showed inconsistent results, possibly due to differences between probiotic strains, the traveled countries, the local microflora, specific (eating) habits of the travelers or the way of administration of the probiotic (before or during travel, as a capsule or a fermented milk product). Whereas some studies revealed less or shortened episodes of diarrhea in subjects consuming the probiotic [71–74], others found no such effect [75, 76].

Two meta-analyses investigated the effect of probiotics on traveler's diarrhea. The meta-analysis of McFarland showed that probiotics significantly prevent the incidence of traveler's diarrhea (RR = 0.85, 95% CI 0.79, 0.91, $p < 0.001$) [77] and Sazawal and colleagues showed that the risk of traveler's diarrhea was reduced by 8% (−6 to 21%) [12].

13. ANTIBIOTIC-ASSOCIATED DIARRHEA

Administration of certain probiotic strains before and during antibiotic treatment reduced the frequency and/or duration of episodes of antibiotic-associated diarrhea and the severity of symptoms in most clinical studies [78–86].

In these trials, both probiotic preparations and probiotic fermented milk products were applied, in part with considerable success. For example, a fermented multistrain probiotic (LA-5 plus Bb12) milk drink prevented 80% of AAD in adult hospitalized patients [87]. On average, in randomized, controlled clinical studies in the probiotic group, a duration of diarrhea of 2 days was observed compared with 8 days in the control group.

The administration of a fermented milk product containing *B. animalis* ssp. *lactis* and *L. acidophilus* (2×10^7–2×10^9 cfu/day) for 4 weeks before and during an *H. pylori* eradication therapy led to significantly less episodes of diarrhea (7 vs 22% of the subjects) compared with the placebo group [88]. Furthermore, in this study the applied probiotica *per se* (i.e. already before the antibiotic therapy) and/or the milk acids contained in the product, reduced the activity of *H. pylori* in the gut, albeit without completely eradicating this bacterium [88]. Similarly, the administration of *S. boulardii* during a triple anti-*H. pylori* therapy in 124 Turkish adults significantly reduced the number of subjects suffering from diarrhea (probiotic group: 14.5%, placebo group: 30.6%) [89].

On the other hand, a study using a mix of probiotics (*B. longum, L. rhamnosus, L. plantarum*) in 78 Polish children, treated by antibiotics because of otitis media, respiratory tract infections and/or urinary tract infections, showed a similar rate of diarrhea in the probiotic and the placebo group [90]. Several other papers did not report any positive effects either [91–97]. Of the 10 studies that did not show any beneficial effect of probiotics on antibiotic-associated diarrhea or only a reduced frequency of stools but not of diarrhea, most studies were performed on adults or elderly and only one study was performed on infants or children.

In some cases, antibiotic treatment and particularly the use of modern broad-spectrum antibiotics, which may eradicate members of the 'normal' protective gut flora, can result in life-threatening pseudomembranous colitis (also called *Clostridium difficile* associated diarrhea (CDAD) or antibiotic-associated colitis). CDAD is associated with the abundance of anaerobic toxigenic bacteria (particularly strains of *Clostridium difficile*), characterized by diarrhea, abdominal pain and fever, and has emerged as a major healthcare problem. Routine treatment includes metronidazole or vancomycin. Fecal bacteriotherapy, i.e. infusion of fecal bacteria from a healthy donor, has been used with high success to restore the imbalanced intestinal flora of CDAD patients, whereas probiotic bacteria (e.g. *L. casei, L. bulgaricus,* and *S. thermophilus* [98]) or *Saccharomyces boulardii* [99] reduced the incidence or recurrence of CDAD in some studies but were ineffective in others.

Altogether, several meta-analyses investigating the efficacy of probiotics in the prevention of antibiotic-associated diarrhea showed that administration of LGG, *L. acidophilus* spec., *L. reuteri* spec., *L. plantarum* spec., yogurt, several strains of bifidobacteria or *S. boulardii* is associated with a significantly reduced incidence of diarrhea by up to 52%, according to a relative risk (RR = 0.44) [12, 82, 84, 100]. In one meta-analysis four out of six trials showed that LGG is effective in preventing antibiotic-associated diarrhea and one trial reduced the number of days with diarrhea [82], whereas only two out of four studies included in a systematic review [101] showed a significant reduction of CDAD.

14. DIARRHEA IN IMMUNOCOMPROMISED SUBJECTS

Chemo- and radiotherapy frequently cause severe disturbances of the immune system and the indigenous intestinal microflora, accompanied by diarrhea and/or increased cell counts of fungi (*Candida albicans*) in the gastrointestinal tract and other organs. Both side effects were ameliorated by the administration of probiotic bacteria before and during chemo- [102] or radiotherapy [103–105]. On the other hand, one randomized, placebo-controlled, multicenter study performed in 85 patients receiving *L. casei* or placebo during radiotherapy showed that diarrhea or the use of loperamide was not different between the two groups (30 out of 44 patients in the probiotic group and 24 out of 41 in the placebo group) [106].

It was shown that probiotic products are well-tolerated by HIV patients [107], but in most investigations, they do not exert antidiarrheal effects in these patients [108,109] with the exception of *S. boulardii*, which significantly increased the recovery rate and weight gain of AIDS patients suffering from diarrhea in one study [110].

15. BACTERIAL OVERGROWTH

Small bowel bacterial overgrowth is a disorder of excessive bacterial growth in the small intestine, defined as $= 10^5$ total cfu/mL jejunal secretions. Unlike the colon, the small bowel is usually not rich with bacteria. It occurs in the absence of muscular activity in the small bowel, which allows the bacteria to stay longer, and multiply in the small bowel and spread backwards from the colon into the small bowel. Typical symptoms of small bowel bacteria overgrowth are diarrhea, nausea, bloating and vomiting.

Only a few studies have examined the effect of probiotic bacteria on small bowel bacterial overgrowth. Successful studies showed the normalization of the small bowel microflora [111], decreased frequency of diarrhea [112], decreased release of toxic N-metabolites [113], whereas two further studies did not show any beneficial effect of *S. boulardii* [114] or *L. fermentum* KLD [115] compared to conventional antibiotics treatment or a placebo, respectively.

16. LACTOSE INTOLERANCE

Lactose intolerance is the inability to digest significant amounts of lactose, because the required enzyme β-galactosidase (also called lactase) is absent or its availability is lowered. The consumption of milk or other products containing lactose results in gastrointestinal symptoms such as nausea, cramps, bloating, flatulence, abdominal pain, and diarrhea. It is estimated that 75% of adults worldwide show some decrease in lactase activity during adulthood.

It is well-known that fermented milk products improve the tolerance of milk products and thus avoid intolerance symptoms. This effect is attributable to the microbial β-galactosidase of the bacteria, which survives the passage through the stomach and is released in the small intestine [116]. It was shown that, beside probiotic bacteria [117], yogurt is very effective or even more effective in improving lactose digestion, thus the effect does not depend on the survival of the bacteria in the small intestine [118, 119]. The effect of the β-galactosidase of many probiotic bacteria might be lower compared to the effect of yogurt, because of a low activity of the enzyme or an incomplete release of the enzyme due to high resistance against acid and bile salts of the bacteria [120].

Yogurt cultures improve the digestion of lactose and reduce or prevent lactose-induced diarrhea in lactose intolerant subjects. Thus, in a cross-over study with nurses from Africa or Korea, acute gastrointestinal complaints after ingestion of 12.5/25 mg lactose (yogurt) was reduced by >75% compared to a watery lactose suspension; furthermore, no diarrhea was observed [116]. Other probiotic cultures, which improve lactose digestion to a lesser extent, might reduce the lactose-induced gastrointestinal complaints due to modulation of the microbiotia and/or a reduced complaint perception [121].

17. INFLAMMATORY INTESTINAL DISEASES

Crohn's disease (CD) and colitis ulcerosa (ulcerative colitis, UC) are known as inflammatory bowel diseases (IBD). The precise pathogenesis is not yet fully understood. Nowadays, it is postulated that the cause is an aggressive, cell-mediated answer of the immune system to a combination of specific endogenous and environmental factors (e.g. infections) in subjects with a specific genetic background. It is assumed that the inflammation of the mucosa is the result of the disturbance of the autochthonous intestinal microflora and the stimulation of pro-inflammatory immunological processes. Thus, probiotic bacteria with anti-inflammatory properties might improve the health and well-being of affected patients and positively influence the intestinal microbiota.

Although IBD is not a diarrheal disease in the strict sense of the word, and although diarrhea occurs only in a part of the cases of Crohn's disease and colitis ulcerosa, inflammatory intestinal diseases are listed here. In the corresponding clinical studies, beneficial effects of probiotics on diarrhea are not always mentioned, but it can be concluded that alleviation or the prevention of IBD and IBD symptoms may potentially include diarrhea.

Studies in rats or mice showed that the application of lactobacilli, bifidobacteria, *Lactococcus lactis* or non-food probiotics, particularly non-pathogenic strains of *E. coli* (e.g. strain Nissle 1917) prevents or treats colitis [122–125].

Similarly, patients with inflammatory bowel diseases [126–132], diverticulitis [133] or inflammation of an ileal pouch [134] showed an improvement of the symptoms and a higher quality of life [135]. The beneficial effects of probiotics were demonstrated mainly in the prevention and treatment of pouchitis and in maintaining remission of mild to moderate ulcerative colitis. Probiotics appear to be less effective in patients with Crohn's disease.

However, in most of these studies only a small number of patients were investigated, and the probiotic agent, dosage and duration of treatment varied widely between them. Therefore, more randomized clinical trials are still required to further define the role of probiotics as preventive and therapeutic agents [136].

17.1. Colitis Ulcerosa

Colitis ulcerosa usually affects the lining of the rectum and lower part of the colon, but can also spread throughout the entire colon. Many theories exist about what causes UC. It is assumed that it might be caused by an overreaction of the immune system to normal bacteria in the digestive tract. The inflammation in the colon causes the colon to empty frequently, causing cramps and diarrhea mixed with blood and mucus.

Probiotics were used both to induce remission (resolution of inflammation) initially and to prevent a relapse of the disease. Several studies showed that *E. coli* Nissle was as effective as Mesalazin, the standard treatment drug, in preventing a relapse [130, 137–139]. Studies investigating the effect of other probiotics (LGG, bifidobacteria, lactobacilli, VSL#3) to prevent a relapse of the disease compared to a placebo also showed that the probiotics were more effective [140–143]. On the other hand, the induction of a remission of UC by fecal bacteriotherapy or administration of accepted probiotics did reverse UC only in some selected patients [144] or was the same in the verum and placebo group, respectively [145, 146].

17.2. Crohn's Disease

Crohn's disease primarily affects the lining of the small and large intestines, but can affect the digestive system anywhere from the mouth to the anus. The disease is named after Dr. Burrill B. Crohn. The inflammation affects all layers of the gut and causes abdominal pain, diarrhea, vomiting, and weight loss.

The study by Plein and Hotz was one of the first randomized, controlled studies, investigating the effect of probiotics on Crohn's disease. They showed that S. boulardii significantly reduced the incidence of diarrhea in Crohn's disease patients [147]. Further studies showed that probiotics prevent relapses of the disease [148–150]. However, again the results of a meta-analysis showed that the evidence of a beneficial effect of probiotics is low because of the low number of subjects included in the respective studies [151].

17.3. Pouchitis

Pouchitis is an inflammation of the lining of the pouch (small bowel pocket), which is created to hold bowel movements in patients with UC who have had all of their large intestine or colon removed. The pouch is a considerably smaller reservoir than the colon; thus, patients tend to have more frequent bowel movements (6–8 times a day), and the reduced absorption of water in the pouch leads to diarrhea.

Antibiotic and anti-inflammatory therapy is the most common treatment for pouchitis. The use of probiotics, in particular VSL#3, for the prevention and treatment of pouchitis has been investigated in double blind, controlled or open clinical studies. Probiotics were effective in the prevention of primary pouchitis [152, 153] and the prevention of relapse of pouchitis [134, 154], whereas probiotics did not induce remission in all patients with acute pouchitis [155]. In two other studies, milk fermented with La-5 and Bb12 [156] or LGG [157] did not induce remission in any patient and only a slight improvement of the composition of the pouch flora and symptoms was observed.

17.4. Collagenous Colitis and Lymphocytic Colitis

Collagenous colitis and lymphocytic colitis are inflammatory conditions of the colon, also called microscopic colitis, because the inflammation is not visible and a biopsy is necessary to make a diagnosis. Symptoms are chronic, non-bloody, watery diarrhea and cramps. At the time of writing, two studies investigating the effects of probiotics on this condition are available. In an open trial, the probiotic E. coli Nissle significantly decreased the frequency of stools per day from 7.6 ± 4.8 to 3.7 ± 5.8 ($p = 0.034$) [158], and a randomized, placebo-controlled, double blind, multicenter study showed that a mix of probiotic bacteria (L. acidophilus LA-5, B. animalis ssp. lactis Bb12) decreased the number of liquid stools per week in collagenous colitis [159].

17.5. Irritable Bowel Syndrome

Irritable bowel syndrome (IBS) is the name for a variety of functional bowel disorders without (known) organic cause. Characteristic symptoms are chronic abdominal pain, cramping and discomfort, flatulence, meteorisms and a change in bowel habits (either diarrhea or obstipation, or both). IBS is a common disorder and women are more likely to contract IBS and to suffer from more severe symptoms. The cause of IBS is currently unknown. It is probably a combination of different factors, including abnormal gastrointestinal tract movements and psychological disorders. Furthermore, alterations of the intestinal microflora (low numbers of lactobacilli and bifidobacteria) may be involved in the initiation and/or chronicity of the symptoms [160, 161].

Nevertheless, little attention has been paid to the potential advantages of correcting this imbalance by using probiotics. Some studies have shown (dose-dependent) improvements in bloating, flatulence, bowel dysfunction, incomplete evacuation, abdominal pain or the overall quality of life in response to probiotics [161–165], whereas others failed to show any significant positive effect [166, 167], at least with respect to the primary outcome parameter [168].

Hamilton-Miller reviewed the results of 12 clinical trials, involving a total of 1371 patients treated with probiotics (169). Although in 10 trials (of which five were randomized, double blind and placebo controlled) the use of probiotics was beneficial, the probiotic agents, dosages and duration of treatment varied too widely between the studies. Furthermore, the number of patients included was too small to allow any definite conclusions other than the assumption that probiotics might be more effective in preventing IBS than in its treatment [169].

Extending the literature search to 2008 and that limitation to randomized, controlled clinical studies in adults yielded one, five or two studies, in which none, at least one, or all IBS symptoms tested (pain, flatulence, meteorism and diarrhea/obstipation) were improved by L. acidophilus, L. plantarum, L. salivarius, B. infantis, LGG or VSL#3.[8]

as their synbiotic combination with probiotic bacteria (strains of L. plantarum, L. paracasei or B. bifidum), increased bifidobacteria and lactobacilli or inhibited various human and animal pathogenic bacteria strains (Clostridium spez., E. coli, Campylobacter jejuni, Enterobacterium spez., Salmonella enteritidis or S. typhimurium) in vitro [172] or in mice [173], piglets [174] or humans [175, 176].

Only relatively few studies observed or examined result in preventive or therapeutic health effects. At least there are some experimental indications on beneficial effects of inulin, oligofructose or galacto-oligosaccharides, given alone or as a synbiotic, in the case of experimental colitis in rats [177], of rotavirus-induced, C. difficile-associated and other diarrheal diseases [176, 178] and of refractory enterocolitis [179]. The administration of 12 g oligofructose per day for the prevention of traveler's diarrhea showed moderate success [180], while the frequency of antibiotics-associated diarrhea in children [181] or the elderly [182], infectious diarrhea in children [183] as well as diarrhea associated with an irritable colon [184] could not be reduced significantly. There do not appear to be any findings concerning the potential application of prebiotics in the case of obstipation.

18. IMPACT OF PREBIOTICS ON THE INTESTINAL FLORA

Positive effects of pre- and synbiotics on the intestinal flora [170, 171] (i.e. growth-promotion of potentially protective bacteria—bifidobacteria and in part lactobacilli) and/or the inhibition of potentially pathogenic microorganisms, as well as stabilization of the intestinal environment by lowering the pH and release of short-chain organic acids, have been investigated and confirmed frequently by in vitro and in vivo trials. Inulin, oligofructose or oligosaccharides as well

19. PREBIOTIC INFANT FORMULAE—EFFECTIVE AGAINST INFANTILE DIARRHEAS?

Formulas for bottle-fed infants have been developed which soften and acidify (pH 5–6) stools and induce an intestinal flora with high bifidus content similar to that of 2–3-month-old breast-fed infants [185, 186]. For this purpose, milk-based infant formulae were enriched with either probiotic bifidobacteria and lactobacilli or

[8]de Vrese and Offick, unpublished data.

bifidogenic fructo- and galacto-oligosaccharides [185–188].

The human breast milk contains more than 130 different oligosaccharides and glycoconjugates at a concentration of 12–14 g/L (compared to cows' milk: <1 g/L). These include short- or longer-chain, linear or branched chain, neutral or acidic, and apart from simple sugars like galactose, glucose and fructose they are also sugar derivatives like amino sugars or uronic acids. The oligosaccharides and glycoconjugates play a major role in the bifidogenic, protective and immunomodulating properties of human breast milk [185, 186]. However, the complexity of the composition excludes the possibility to develop a comparable formula.

One further property of human breast milk that still cannot be simulated with commercially available prebiotics, is namely the inhibition of the adhesion of (pathogenic) bacteria on endothelic cells. This inhibition is caused by certain, more complex oligosaccharides in human breast milk, which are receptor-analogues to the adhesion molecules of the intestinal mucosa [185, 186].

Several published studies show a beneficial effect of prebiotics on health, although the quantity, structure and composition of the added prebiotics need to be optimized and further studies are needed to confirm the current results. It was shown that the administration of conventional infant formulae supplemented with 0.4 to 1 g/100 mL oligofructose and/or (more frequently) galacto-oligosaccharides for 3 to 12 weeks significantly increased the bifidobacteria in the fecal flora from 20 to approximately 60% (breast-fed infants: ~80%), and to stool characteristics similar to that of breast-fed infants [189–193].

In addition, animal studies as well as studies in infants and children, show other possible advantages of supplementing infant food with prebiotics, probiotics or synbiotics, such as less necrotizing enterocolitides [194, 195] or less rotavirus- and otherwise induced diarrhea in children [196–198]. Furthermore, administration of prebiotics to children in Thailand, Brazil, Mexico, Spain and Portugal suffering partly from malnutrition, increased calcium adsorption, supported immunogenicity as well as relief of atopic and allergic problems, and improved all in growth and health [185, 199–201].

20. CONCLUSIONS: CONTRADICTORY OR NEGATIVE STUDY RESULTS—LACK OF EFFICACY?

Despite the unquestionable market success of pro- and prebiotic foods; the increasingly exponential published clinical studies, meta-analyses and reviews on probiotics; and an increasing understanding of the underlying mechanisms of anti-diarrheal effects of pro- and prebiotics and their interactions with the intestinal flora and the immune system, it is frequently argued that pro- and prebiotics have no health effects—mostly with reference to negative or contradictive study outcomes and/or the low number of study participants. These objections, however, disregard the fact that clinical studies yield statistical results, and can have, due to strain, matrix, and target group specificity of pro- and prebiotic effects, variable effects in different individuals and/or (age) groups. This means that each consumer and each physician needs to test whether, and to what extent, healthy consumers as well as patients may profit from pro- and prebiotics.

Nevertheless prevention, abatement or shortening of rotavirus-induced or antibiotic-associated (acute) diarrhea are considered to be well-established probiotic effects, as well as an aid in the alleviation of complaints due to lactose intolerance. For others with intestinal inflammation and/or disordered intestinal microbiota-associated diarrheal diseases, the tentative use/application of probiotics (rather than prebiotics) is considered an option. Overall, a general recommendation to consume probiotics cannot yet be given as further clinical studies with a larger number of participants are still needed.

References

1. Bottazzi, V. (1983). Food and feed production with microorganisms. *Biotechnology, 5,* 315–363.
2. Carre, C. (1887). Ueber Antagonisten unter den Bacterien. *Correspondenz-Blatt fuer Schweizer Aerzte, 17,* 385–392.
3. Tissier, H. (1906). Traitement des infections intestinales par la méthode de la flore bactérienne de l'intestin. *Comptes Rendus Des Seances De La Societe De Biologie Et De Ses Filiales, 60,* 359–361.
4. Metchnikoff, E. (1907). Lactic acid as inhibiting intestinal putrefaction. In: *The prolongation of life: optimistic studies.* London: W. Heinemann (pp. 161–183). 4.
5. Kollath, W. (1953). The increase of the diseases of civilization and their prevention. *Munchener Medizinische Wochenschrift, 95,* 1260–1262.
6. Lilly, D. M., & Stillwell, R. H. (1965). Probiotics. Growth promoting factors produced by micro-organisms. *Science, 147,* 747–748.
7. Schrezenmeir, J., & de Vrese, M. (2001). Probiotics, prebiotics, and synbiotics: approaching a definition. *American Journal of Clinical Nutrition, 73,* 361–364.
8. Gibson, G. R., & Roberfroid, M. B. (1995). Dietary modulation of the colonic microbiota: introducing the concept of prebiotics. *Journal of Nutrition, 125,* 1401–1412.
9. Institute of Food Technologists, Functional Foods: Opportunities and Challenges (2005). Available at http://members.ift.org/IFT/Research/IFTExpertReports/functionalfoods_report.htm (Accessed and printed on April 1, 2009).
10. Marteau, P., de Vrese, M., Cellier, C., & Schrezenmeir, J. (2001). Protection from gastrointestinal diseases using probiotics. *American Journal of Clinical Nutrition, 73,* 430S–436S.
11. de Vrese, M., & Marteau, P. R. (2007). Probiotics and prebiotics: effects on diarrhea. *Journal of Nutrition, 137,* 803S–811S.
12. Sazawal, S., Hiremath, G., Dhingra, U., et al. (2006). Efficacy of probiotics in prevention of acute diarrhoea: a meta-analysis of masked, randomised, placebo-controlled trials. *Lancet Infectious Diseases, 6,* 374–382.
13. WHO. Available at http://www.who.int/topics/diarrhoea/en/ (Accessed and printed on April 1, 2009).
14. Eckburg, P. B., Bik, E. M., Bernstein, C. N., et al. (2005). Diversity of the human intestinal microbial flora. *Science, 308,* 1635–1638.
15. Mcfarlane, S., & Macfarlane, G. T. (2003). Regulation of short-chain fatty acid production. *Proceedings of the Nutrition Society, 62,* 67–72.
16. Wong, J. M., de Souza, R., Kendall, C. W., et al. (2006). Colonic health: fermentation and short chain fatty acids. *Journal of Clinical Gastroenterology, 40,* 235–243.
17. Hijova, E., & Chmelarova, A. (2007). Short chain fatty acids and colonic health. *Bratisl Lek Listy, 108,* 354–358.
18. Cherbut, C., Ferrier, L., Rozé, C., et al. (1998). Short-chain fatty acids modify colonic motility through nerves and polypeptide YY release in the rat. *American Journal of Physiology, 275,* 1415–1422.
19. Guarner, F., & Malagelada, J. R. (2003). Gut flora in health and disease. *Lancet, 361,* 512–519.
20. Bergman, E. (1990). Energy contribution of volatile fatty acids from the gastrointestinal tract in various species. *Physiological Reviews, 70,* 567–590.
21. Wachtershauser, A., & Stein, J. (2000). Rationale for the luminal provision of butyrate in intestinal diseases. *European Journal of Nutrition, 39,* 164–171.
22. Vernia, P., Annese, V., Bresci, G., et al. (2003). Topical butyrate improves efficacy of 5-ASA in refractory distal ulcerative colitis: results of a multicentre trial. *European Journal of Clinical Investigation, 33,* 244–248.
23. Yan, F., Cao, H., Cover, T. L., et al. (2007). Soluble proteins produced by probiotic bacteria regulate intestinal epithelial cell survival and growth. *Gastroenterology, 132,* 562–575.
24. Ukena, S. N., Singh, A., Dringenberg, U., et al. (2007). Probiotic *Escherichia coli* Nissle 1917 inhibits leaky gut by enhancing mucosal integrity. *PloS ONE, 2,* e1308.
25. Zareie, M., Johnson-Henry, K., Jury, J., et al. (2006). Probiotics prevent bacterial translocation and improve intestinal barrier function in rats following chronic psychological stress. *Gut, 55,* 1553–1560.
26. Steinman, R. M. (2003). Some interfaces of dendritic cell biology. *APMIS, 111,* 675–697.
27. Yang, E. V., & Glaser, R. (2000). Stress-induced immunomodulation: impact on immune defenses against infectious disease. *Biomedicine & Pharmacotherapy, 54,* 245–250.
28. Ginaldi, L., De Martinis, M., Monti, D., & Franceschi, C. (2004). The immune system in the elderly: activation-induced and damage-induced apoptosis. *Immunologic Research, 30,* 81–94.
29. Gleeson, M. (2007). Immune function in sport and exercise. *Journal of Applied Physiology, 103,* 693–699.
30. Wolowczuk, I., Verwaerde, C., Viltart, O., et al. (2008). Feeding our immune system: impact on metabolism. *Clin Dev Immunol,* Article 639803.
31. Saavedra, J. M., Baumann, N. A., Oung, I., et al. (1994). Feeding of *Bifidobacterium bifidum* and *Streptococcus thermophilus* to infants in hospital for prevention of diarrhea and shedding of rotavirus. *Lancet, 34,* 1046–1049.

32. Isolauri, E., Joensuu, J., Suolamalainen, H., et al. (1995). Improved immunogenecity of oral DxRRV reassortant rotavirus vaccine by *Lactobacillus casei* GG. *Vaccine, 13*, 310–312.

33. Majamaa, H., Isolauri, E., Saxelin, M., & Vesikari, T. (1995). Lactic acid bacteria in the treatment of acute rotavirus gastroenteritis. *Journal of Pediatric Gastroenterology Nutrition, 20*, 333–338.

34. Shornikova, A. V., Casas, I. A., Isolauri, E., & Vesikari, T. (1997). *Lactobacillus reuteri* as a therapeutic agent in acute diarrhea in young children. *Journal of Pediatric Gastroenterology Nutrition, 24*, 399–404.

35. Buydens, P., & Debeuckelaere, S. (1996). Efficacy of SF68 in the treatment of acute diarrhea. A placebo controlled trial. *Scandinavian Journal of Gastroenterology, 31*, 887–891.

36. Guandalini, S., Pensabene, L., Zikri, M. A., et al. (2000). *Lactobacillus* GG administered in oral rehydration solution to children with acute diarrhea: a multicenter European trial. *Journal of Pediatric Gastroenterology Nutrition, 30*, 54–60.

37. Dubey, A. P., Rajeshwari, K., Chakravarty, A., & Famularo, G. (2008). Use of VSL#3 in the treatment of rotavirus diarrhea in children: preliminary results. *Journal of Clinical Gastroenterology, 42*(Suppl. 3 Pt. 1), S126–S129.

38. Allan, S. J., Okoko, B., Martinez, E., et al. (2004). Probiotics for treating infectious diarrhoea CD003048. *Cochrane Database Syst Rev*(2).

39. Huang, J. S., Bousvaros, A., Lee, J. W., et al. (2002). Efficacy of probiotic use in acute diarrhea in children: a meta-analysis. *Digestive Diseases and Sciences, 47*, 2625–2634.

40. Guandalini, S. (2008). Probiotics for children with diarrhea: an update. *Journal of Clinical Gastroenterology, 42*(Suppl. 2), S53–S57.

41. Van Niel, C. W., Feudtner, C., Garrison, M. M., & Christakis, D. A. (2002). Lactobacillus therapy for acute infectious diarrhea in children: a meta-analysis. *Pediatrics, 109*, 678–684.

42. Szajewska, H., Skórka, A., Ruszczyński, M., & Gieruszczak-Białek, D. (2007). Meta-analysis: *Lactobacillus* GG for treating acute diarrhoea in children. *Alimentary Pharmacology & Therapeutic, 25*(8), 871–881.

43. Krammer, H. J., Kamper, H., von Bunau, R., et al. (2006). Probiotic drug therapy with *E. coli* strain Nissle 1917 (EcN): results of a prospective study of the records of 3807 Patients. *Zeitschrift Fur Gastroenterologie, 44*, 651–656.

44. Henker, J., Laass, M., Blokhin, B. M., et al. (2007). The probiotic *Escherichia coli* strain Nissle 1917 (EcN) stops acute diarrhea in infants and toddlers. *European Journal of Pediatrics, 166*, 311–318.

45. Gedek, B. R. (1999). Adherence of *Escherichia coli* serogroup O 157 and the Salmonella typhimurium mutant DT 104 to the surface of *Saccharomyces boulardii. Mycoses, 42*(4), 261–264.

46. Castagliuolo, I., Riegler, M. F., Valenick, L., et al. (1999). *Saccharomyces boulardii* protease inhibits the effects of *Clostridium difficile* toxins A and B in human colonic mucosa. *Infection and Immunity, 67*(1), 302–307.

47. Dahan, S., Dalmasso, G., Imbert, V., et al. (2003). *Saccharomyces boulardii* interferes with enterohemorrhagic *Escherichia coli*-induced signaling pathways in T84 cells. *Infection and Immunity, 71*(2), 766–773.

48. Thomas, S., Przesdzing, I., Metzke, D., et al. (2009). *Saccharomyces boulardii* inhibits lipopolysaccharide-induced activation of human dendritic cells and T cell proliferation. *Clinical and Experimental Immunology, 155*, 78.

49. Kurugöl, Z., & Koturoglu, G. (2005). Effects of *Saccharomyces boulardii* in children with acute diarrhea. *Acta Peadiatrica, 94*, 44–47.

50. Villarruel, G., Rubio, D. M., Lopez, F., et al. (2007). *Saccharomyces boulardii* in acute childhood diarrhoea: a randomized, placebo-controlled study. *Acta Paediatrica, 96*, 538–541.

51. Htwe, K., Yee, K. S., Tin, M., & Vandenplas, Y. (2008). Effect of *Saccharomyces boulardii* in the treatment of acute watery diarrhea in Myanmar children: a randomized controlled study. *American Journal of Tropical Medicine and Hygiene, 78*, 214–216.

52. Billoo, A. G., Memon, M. A., Khaskheli, S. A., et al. (2006). Role of a probiotic (*Saccharomyces boulardii*) in management and prevention of diarrhoea. *World Journal of Gastroenterology, 12*, 4557–4560.

53. McFarland, L., & Bernasconi, P. (1993). *Saccharomyces boulardii*: a review of an innovative biotherapeutic agent. *Microbial Ecology in Health and Disease, 6*, 157–171.

54. Szajewska, H., Skórka, A., & Dylag, M. (2007). Meta-analysis: *Saccharomyces boulardii* for treating acute diarrhoea in children. *Alimentary Pharmacology & Therapeutic, 25*(3), 257–264.

55. Salazar-Lindo, E., Miranda-Langschwager, P., Campos-Sanchez, M., et al. (2004). *Lactobacillus casei* strain GG in the treatment of infants with acute watery diarrhea: a randomized, double-blind, placebo controlled clinical trial. *BMC Pediatrics, 4*, 18.

56. Costa-Ribeiro, H., Ribeiro, T. C., Mattos, A. P., et al. (2003). Limitations of probiotic therapy in acute, severe dehydrating diarrhea. *Journal of Pediatric Gastroenterology Nutrition, 36*, 112–115.

57. Basu, S., Chatterjee, M., Ganguly, S., & Chandra, P. K. (2007). Efficacy of *Lactobacillus rhamnosus* GG in persistent diarrhoea in Indian children: a randomised controlled trial. *Journal of Clinical Gastroenterology, 41*(8), 756–760.

58. Basu, S., Chatterjee, M., Ganguly, S., & Chandra, P. K. (2007). Efficacy of *Lactobacillus rhamnosus* GG in acute

watery diarrhoea of Indian children: a randomised controlled trial. *Journal of Paediatric Child Health*, 43, 837–842.

59. Canani, B. R., Cirillo, P., Terrin, G., et al. (2007). Probiotics for treatment of acute diarrhoea in children: randomised clinical trial of five different preparations. *BMJ*, 335, 340.

60. Figueiredo, P. P., Vieira, E. C., Nicoli, J. R., et al. (2001). Influence of oral inoculation with plasmid-free human *Escherichia coli* on the frequency of diarrhea during the first year of life in human newborns. *Journal of Pediatric Gastroenterology Nutrition*, 33(1), 70–74.

61. Isolauri, E., Juntunen, M., Rautanen, T., et al. (1991). A human Lactobacillus strain (*Lactobacillus casei* sp strain GG) promotes recovery from acute diarrhea in children. *Pediatrics*, 88(1), 90–97.

62. Rosenfeldt, V., Michaelsen, K. F., Jakobsen, M., et al. (2002). Effect of probiotic Lactobacillus strains in young children hospitalized with acute diarrhea. *Pediatric Infectious Disease Journal*, 21, 411–416.

63. Pedone, C. A., Bernabeu, A. O., Postaire, E. R., et al. (1999). The effect of supplementation with milk fermented by *Lactobacillus casei* DN-114 001, on acute diarrhoea in children attending day care centres. *International Journal of Clinical Practice*, 53, 179–184.

64. Pedone, C. A., Arnaud, C. C., Postaire, E. R., et al. (2000). Multicenter study on 928 children attending day care centers to evaluate the effect of milk fermented by *Lactobacillus casei* DN-114 001 on the incidence of diarrhoea. *International Journal of Clinical Practice*, 54, 568–571.

65. Hatakka, K., Savilahti, E., Ponka, A., et al. (2001). Effect of long term consumption of probiotic milk on infections in children attending day care centres: double blind, randomised trial. *BMJ*, 322, 1327.

66. Weizman, Z., Asli, G., & Alsheikh, A. (2005). Effect of a probiotic infant formula on infections in child care centers: comparison of two probiotic agents. *Pediatrics*, 115, 5–9.

67. Chouraqui, J. P., Van Egroo, L. D., & Fichot, M. C. (2004). Acidified milk fromula supplemented with bifidobacterium lactis: impact on infant diarrhea in residential care settings. *Journal of Pediatric Gastroenterology Nutrition*, 38(3), 288–292.

68. Oberhelman, R. A., Gilman, R. H., Sheen, P., et al. (1999). A placebo-controlled trial of Lactobacillus GG to prevent diarrhea in undernourished Peruvian children. *Journal of Pediatrics*, 134, 15–20.

69. Pereg, D., Kimhi, O., Tirosh, A., et al. (2005). The effect of fermented yogurt on the prevention of diarrhea in a healthy adult population. *American Journal of Infection Control*, 33, 122–125.

70. Szajewska, H., & Mrukowicz, J. Z. (2005). Probiotics in the treatment and prevention of acute infectious diarrhea in infants and children: a systematic review of published randomized, double-blind, placebo-controlled trials. *Journal of Pediatric Gastroenterology Nutrition*, 33, S17–S25.

71. Black, F. T., Andersen, P. L., Orskov, J. et al. (1989). Prophylactic efficacy of lactobacilli on travelers' diarrhea. In: Steffen, R. (ed.) Travel medicine. Conference on international travel medicine 1, Zurich, Switzerland. Berlin: Springer, 333–335.

72. Hilton, E., Kolakowski, P., Smith, M., & Singer, C. (1997). Efficacy of *Lactobacillus* GG as a diarrhoea preventive. *Journal of Travel Medicine*, 4, 3–7.

73. Oksanen, P. J., Salminen, S., Saxelin, M., et al. (1990). Prevention of travelers' diarrhoea by *Lactobacillus* GG. *Annals of Medicine*, 22, 53–56.

74. Kollaritsch, H., Holst, H., Grobara, P., & Wiedermann, G. (1993). Prevention of travelers' diarrhea with *Saccharomyces boulardii*. Results of a placebo controlled double-blind study. *Fortschritte Der Medizin*, 111(9), 152–156.

75. de dios Pozo-Olano, J., Warram, J. H., Gomez, R. G. & Cavazos, M. G. (1978). Effect of a lactobacilli preparation on travelers' diarrhea. A randomized, double blind clinical trial. 74, 829–830.

76. Katelaris, P. H., Salam, I., & Farthing, M. J. G. (1995). Lactobacilli to prevent travelers' diarrhea? *New England Journal of Medicine*, 333, 1360–1361.

77. McFarland, L. V. (2007). Meta-analysis of probiotics for the prevention of travelers' diarrhea. *Travel Medicine Infectious Disease*, 5, 97–105.

78. Armuzzi, A., Cremonini, F., Bartolozzi, F., et al. (2001). The effects of oral administration of Lactobacillus GG on antibiotic-associated gastrointestinal side-effects during *Helicobacter pylori* eradication therapy. *Alimentary Pharmacology & Therapeutic*, 15, 163–169.

79. Arvola, T., Laiho, K., Torkkeli, S., et al. (1999). Prophylactic *Lactobacillus* GG reduces antibiotic-associated diarrhea in children with respiratory infections: a randomised study. *Pediatrics*, 104, E64.

80. Cremonini, F., Di Caro, S., Nista, E. C., et al. (2002). Meta-analysis: the effect of probiotic administration on antibiotic-associated diarrhea. *Alimentary Pharmacology & Therapeutic*, 16, 1461–1467.

81. Kotowska, M., Albrecht, P., & Szajewska, H. (2005). *Saccharomyces boulardii* in the prevention of antibiotic-associated diarrhoea in children: a randomized double-blind placebo-controlled trial. *Alimentary Pharmacology & Therapeutic*, 21, 583–590.

82. McFarland, L. V. (2006). Meta-analysis of probiotics for the prevention of antibiotic-associated diarrhea and the treatment of *Clostridium difficile* disease. *American Journal of Gastroenterology*, 101, 812–822.

83. Katz, J. A. (2006). Probiotics for the prevention of antibiotic-associated diarrhea and *Clostridium difficile* diarrhea. *Journal of Clinical Gastroenterology*, 40, 249–255.

84. Szajewska, H., Ruszczynski, M., & Radzikowski, A. (2006). Probiotics in the prevention of antibiotic-associated diarrhea in children: A meta-analysis of randomized controlled trials. *Journal of Pediatrics, 149*, 367–372.

85. Hawrelak, J. A., Whitten, D. L., & Myers, S. P. (2005). Is *Lactobacillus rhamnosus* GG effective in preventing the onset of antibiotic-associated diarrhoea: a systematic review. *Digestion, 72*, 51–56.

86. Duman, D. G., Bor, S., Ozutemiz, O., et al. (2005). Efficacy and safety of *Saccharomyces boulardii* in prevention of antibiotic-associated diarrhoea due to *Helicobacter pylori* eradication. *European Journal of Gastroenterol Hepatology, 17*, 1357–1361.

87. Wenus, C., Goll, R., Loken, E. B., et al. (2008). Prevention of antibiotic-associated diarrhoea by a fermented probiotic milk drink. *European Journal of Clinical Nutrition, 62*, 299–301.

88. de Vrese, M. (2003). Effects of probiotic bacteria on gastrointestinal symptoms, *Helicobacter pylori* activity and antibiotics-induced diarrhoea. *Gastroenterology, 124*, A560.

89. Cindoruk, M., Erkan, G., Karakan, T., et al. (2007). Efficacy and safety of *Saccharomyces boulardii* in the 14-day triple anti-*Helicobacter pylori* therapy: a prospective randomized placebo-controlled double-blind study. *Helicobacter, 12*, 309–316.

90. Szymanski, H., Armanska, M., Kowalska-Duplaga, K., & Szajewska, H. (2008). *Bifidobacteria longum* PL03, *Lactobacillus rhamnosus* KL53A, and *Lactobacillus plantarum* PL02 in the prevention of antibiotic-associated diarrhea in children: a randomized controlled pilot trial. *Digestion, 78*, 13–17.

91. Thomas, M. R., Litin, S. C., Osmon, D. R., et al. (2001). Lack of effect of *Lactobacillus* GG on antibiotic-associated diarrhea: a randomized, placebo-controlled trial. *Mayo Clinic Proceedings, 76*, 883–889.

92. Kim, M. N., Kim, N., Lee, S. H., et al. (2008). The effects of probiotics on PPI-triple therapy for *Helicobacter pylori* eradication. *Helicobacter, 13*, 261–268.

93. Plummer, S., Weaver, M. A., Harris, J. C., et al. (2004). *Clostridium difficile* pilot study: effects of probiotic supplementation on the incidence of *C. difficile* diarrhoea. *International Microbiology, 7*, 59–62.

94. Safdar, N., Barigala, R., Said, A., & McKinley, L. (2008). Feasibility and tolerability of probiotics for prevention of antibiotic-associated diarrhoea in hospitalized US military veterans. *Journal of Clinical Pharmacy and Therapeutics, 33*, 663–668.

95. Stein, G. Y., Nanim, R., Karniel, E., et al. (2007). Probiotics as prophylactic agents against antibiotic-associated diarrhea in hospitalized patients. *Harefuah, 146*(7), 520–522.

96. Sullivan, A., Johansson, A., Svenungsson, B., & Nord, C. E. (2004). Effect of *Lactobacillus* F19 on the emergence of antibiotic-resistant microorganisms in the intestinal microflora. *Journal of Antimicrobial Chemotherapy, 54*, 791–797.

97. Tankanow, R. M., Ross, M. B., Ertel, I. J., et al. (1990). A double-blind, placebo-controlled study of the efficacy of Lactinex in the prophylaxis of amoxicillin-induced diarrhea. *DICP, 24*(4), 382–384.

98. Hickson, M., D'Souza, A. L., Muthu, N., et al. (2007). Use of probiotic Lactobacillus preparation to prevent diarrhoea associated with antibiotics: randomised double blind placebo controlled trial. *BMJ, 335*(7610).

99. McFarland, L. V., Surawicz, C. M., Greenberg, R. N., et al. (1994). A randomized placebo-controlled trial of *Saccharomyces boulardii* in combination with standard antibiotics for *Clostridium difficile* disease. *JAMA, 271*(24), 1913–1918.

100. Johnston, B. C., Supina, A. L., & Vohra, S. (2006). Probiotics for pediatric antibiotic-associated diarrhea: a meta-analysis of randomized placebo-controlled trials. *CMAJ, 175*, 377–383.

101. Dendukuri, N., Costa, V., McGegor, M., & Brophy, J. M. (2005). Probiotic therapy for the prevention and treatment of *Clostridium difficile*-associated diarrhea: a systematic review. *CMAJ, 173*, 167–170.

102. Tomoda, T., Nakano, Y., & Kageyama, T. (1988). Intestinal Candida overgrowth and Candida infection in patients with leukemia: effect of Bifidobacterium administration. *Bifidobact, 7*, 71–74.

103. Delia, P., Sansotta, G., Donato, V., et al. (2002). Prevention of radiation-induced diarrhea with the use of VSL#3, a new high-potency probiotic preparation. *American Journal of Gastroenterology, 97*, 2150–2152.

104. Urbancsek, H., Kazar, T., Mezes, I., & Neumann, K. (2001). Results of a double-blind, randomized study to evaluate the efficacy and safety of Antibiophilus in patients with radiation-induced diarrhoea. *European Journal of Gastroenterology Hepatology, 13*, 391–396.

105. Delia, P., Sansotta, G., Donato, V., et al. (2007). Famularo G. Use of probiotics for prevention of radiation-induced diarrhea. *World Journal of Gastroenterology, 13*, 912–915.

106. Giralt, J., Regadera, J. P., Verges, R., et al. (2008). Effects of probiotic Lactobacillus casei DN-114 001 in prevention of radiation-induced diarrhea: results from multicenter, randomized, placebo-controlled nutritional trial. *Int J Radiat Oncol Biol Phys, 71*, 1213–1219.

107. Wolf, B. W., Wheeler, K. B., Ataya, D. G., & Garleb, K. A. (1998). Safety and tolerance of *Lactobacillus reuteri* supplementation to a population infected with the human immunodeficiency virus. *Food and Chemical Toxicology, 36*, 1085–1094.

108. Salminen, M. K., Tynkkynen, S., Rautelin, H., et al. (2004). The efficacy and safety of probiotic *Lactobacillus rhamnosus* GG on prolonged, non-infectious diarrhea in HIV patients on antiviral therapy: a randomized,

placebo-controlled, crossover study. *HIV Clinical Trials*, 5(4), 183–191.

109. Trois, L., Cardoso, E. M., & Miura, E. (2008). Use of probiotics in HIV-infected children: a randomized double-blind controlled study. *Journal of Tropical Pediatrics*, 54(1), 19–24.

110. Saint-Marc, T., Blehaut, H., Musial, C., & Touraine, J. (1995). AIDS related diarrhea: a double-blind trial of *Saccharomyces boulardii*. *Sem Hôsp Paris*, 71, 735–741.

111. Vanderhoof, J. A., Young, R. J., Murray, N., & Kaufman, S. S. (1998). Treatment strategies for small bowel bacterial overgrowth in short bowel syndrome. *Journal of Pediatric Gastroenterology Nutrition*, 27, 155–160.

112. Gaon, D., Garmendia, C., Murrielo, N. O., et al. (2002). Effect of Lactobacillus strains (*L. casei* and *L. acidophilus* strains cerela) on bacterial overgrowth-related chronic diarrhea. *Medicina (B Aires).*, 62, 159–163.

113. Siemenhoff, M. L., Dunn, S. R., Zollner, G. P., et al. (1996). Biomodulation of the toxic and nutritional effects of small bowel bacterial overgrowth in endstage kidney disease using freeze-dried *Lactobacillus acidophilus*. *Mineral and Electrolyte Metabolism*, 22, 92–96.

114. Attar, A., Flourie, B., Rambaud, J. C., et al. (1999). Antibiotic efficacy in small intestinal bacterial overgrowth-related chronic diarrhea: a crossover, randomized trial. *Gastroenterology*, 117(4), 794–797.

115. Stotzer, P. O., Blomberg, L., Conway, P. L., et al. (1996). Probiotic treatment of small intestinal bacterial overgrowth by Lactobacillus fermentum KLD. *Scandinavian Journal of Infectious Diseases*, 28, 615–619.

116. de Vrese, M., Kuhn, C., Titze, A., et al. (1997). Einfluß von Art und Viabilität von Laktobazillen in Sauermilchprodukten auf die Laktoseverdauung.. *Akt Ernähr*, 22, 44.

117. Gaon, D., Doweck, Y., Gomez Zavaglia, A., et al. (1995). Lactose digestion by milk fermented with *Lactobacillus acidophilus* and *Lactobacillus casei* of human origin. *Medicina (B Aires)*, 55, 237–242.

118. de Vrese, M., Stegelmann, A., Richter, B., et al. (2001). Probiotics—compensation for lactase insufficiency. *American Journal of Clinical Nutrition*, 73, 361–364.

119. Labayen, I., & Martinez, J. A. (2003). Probiotic bacteria and lactase deficiencies. *Gastroenterol Hepatology*, 26, S64–S72.

120. Suhr, M., de Vrese, M., & Barth, C. A. (1995). Differenzierende Untersuchung der β-galactosidaseaktivität von Wirts- und Mikroflora nach Joghurtverzehr. *Milchwissenschaft*, 50, 629–633.

121. Shaw, A. D., & Davies, G. J. (1999). Lactose Intolerance: Problems in Diagnosis and Treatment. *Journal of Clinical Gastroenterology*, 28, 208–216.

122. Caplan, M. S., Miller-Catchpole, R., Kaup, S., et al. (1999). Bifidobacterial supplementation reduces the incidence of necrotising enterocolitis in a neonatal rat model. *Gastroenterology*, 117, 577–583.

123. Dieleman, L. A., Goerres, M. S., Arends, A., et al. (2003). Lactobacillus GG prevents recurrence of colitis in HLA-B27 transgenic rats after antibiotic treatment. *Gut*, 52, 370–376.

124. Li, Z., Yang, S., Lin, H., et al. (2003). Probiotics and antibodies to TNF inhibit inflammatory activity and improve non-alcoholic fatty liver disease. *Hepatology*, 37, 343–350.

125. Madsen, K. L., Doyle, J. S., Jewell, L. D., et al. (1999). Lactobacillus species prevents colitis in interleukin 10 gene-deficient mice. *Gastroenterology*, 116, 1107–1114.

126. Gionchetti, P., Rizello, F., Venturi, A., & Campieri, M. (2000). Probiotics in infective diarrhea and inflammatory diseases. *Journal of Gastroenterol Hepatology*, 15, 489–493.

127. Faubion, W. A., & Sandborn, W. J. (2000). Probiotic therapy with *E. coli* for ulcerative colitis: take the good with the bad. *Gastroenterology*, 18, 630–635.

128. Guandalini, S. (2002). Use of Lactobacillus-GG in paediatric Crohn's disease. *Digestive and Liver Disease*, 34, S63–S65.

129. Malin, M., Suomalainen, H., Saxelin, M., & Isolauri, E. (1996). Promotion of IgA immune response in patients with Crohn's disease by oral bacteriotherapy with Lactobacillus GG. *Annals of Nutrition and Metabolism*, 40, 137–145.

130. Rembecken, B. J., Snelling, A. M., Hawkey, P. M., et al. (1999). Non-pathogenic *Escherichia coli* versus mesalazine for the treatment of ulcerative colitis: a randomised trial. *Lancet*, 354, 635–639.

131. Shanahan, F. (2000). Probiotics and inflammatory disease: is there a scientific rational? *Inflammatory Bowel Diseases*, 6, 107–115.

132. Chapman, T. M., Plosker, G. L., & Figgitt, D. P. (2007). Spotlight on VSL#3 probiotic mixture in chronic inflammatory bowel diseases. *Bio Drugs*, 21(1), 61–63.

133. Fricu, P., & Zavoral, M. (2003). The effect of non-pathogenic *Escherichia coli* in symptomatic uncomplicated diverticular disease of the colon. *European Journal of Gastroenterology Hepatology*, 15, 313–315.

134. Gionchetti, P., Rizzello, F., Venturi, A., et al. (2000). Oral bacteriotherapy as maintenance treatment in patients with chronic pouchitis: a double-blind, placebo-controlled trial. *Gastroenterology*, 119, 305–309.

135. Gupta, P., Andrew, H., Kirschner, B. S., & Guandalini, S. (2000). Is *Lactobacillus* GG helpful in children with Crohn's disease? Results of a preliminary, open-label study. *Journal of Pediatric Gastroenterology Nutrition*, 31, 453–457.

136. Mach, T. (2006). Clinical usefulness of probiotics in inflammatory bowel diseases. *J Physiol Pharmacol*, 57(Suppl. 9), 23–33.

137. Kruis, W., Schütz, E., Fric, P., et al. (1997). Double-blind comparison of an oral *Escherichia coli* preparation and

mesalazine in maintaining remission of ulcerative colitis. *Alimentary Pharmacology & Therapeutic, 11*, 853–858.

138. Kruis, W., Fric, P., Pokrotnieks, J., et al. (2004). Maintaining remission of ulcerative colitis with the probiotic *Escherichia coli* Nissle 1917 is as effective as with standard mesalazine. *Gut, 53*, 1617–1623.

139. Henker, J., Müller, S., Laass, M. W., et al. (2008). Probiotic *Escherichia coli* Nissle 1917 (EcN) for successful remission maintenance of ulcerative colitis in children and adolescents: an open-label pilot study Epub 2008 Sep 22. *Zeitschrift Fur Gastroenterologie, 46*(9), 874–875.

140. Venturi, A., Gionchetti, P., Rizzello, F., et al. (1999). Impact on the composition of the faecal flora by a new probiotic preparation: preliminary data on maintenance treatment of patients with ulcerative colitis. *Alimentary Pharmacology & Therapeutic, 13*(8), 1103–1108.

141. Ishikawa, H., Akedo, I., Umesaki, Y., et al. (2003). Randomized controlled trial of the effect of bifidobacteria-fermented milk on ulcerative colitis. *Journal of the American College of Nutrition, 22*(1), 56–63.

142. Cui, H. H., Chen, C. L., Wang, J. D., et al. (2004). Effects of probiotic on intestinal mucosa of patients with ulcerative colitis. *World Journal of Gastroenterology, 10*(10), 1521–1525.

143. Zocco, M. A., dal Verme, L. Z., Cremonini, F., et al. (2006). Efficacy of *Lactobacillus* GG in maintaining remission of ulcerative colitis. *Alimentary Pharmacology & Therapeutic, 23*(11), 1567–1574.

144. Borody, T. J., Warren, E. F., Leis, S., et al. (2003). Treatment of ulcerative colitis using fecal bacteriotherapy. *Journal of Clinical Gastroenterology, 37*(1), 42–47.

145. Kato, K., Mizuno, S., Umesaki, Y., et al. (2004). Randomized placebo-controlled trial assessing the effect of bifidobacteria-fermented milk on active ulcerative colitis. *Alimentary Pharmacology & Therapeutic, 20*(10), 1133–1141.

146. Bibiloni, R., Fedorak, R. N., Tannock, G. W., et al. (2005). VSL#3 probiotic-mixture induces remission in patients with active ulcerative colitis. *American Journal of Gastroenterology, 100*(7), 1539–1546.

147. Plein, K., & Hotz, J. (1993). Therapeutic effects of *Saccharomyces boulardii* on mild residual symptoms in a stable phase of Crohn's disease with specific respect to chronic diarrhea—a pilot study. *Zeitschrift Fur Gastroenterologie, 31*, 129–134.

148. Guslandi, M., Mezzi, G., Sorghi, M., & Testoni, P. A. (2000). *Saccharomyces boulardii* in maintenance treatment of Crohn's disease. *Digestive Diseases and Sciences, 45*(7), 1462–1464.

149. Malchow, H. A. (1997). Crohn's disease and *Escherichia coli*. A new approach in therapy to maintain remission of colonic Crohn's disease? *Journal of Clinical Gastroenterology, 25*(4), 653–658.

150. Schultz, M., Timmer, A., Herfarth, H. H., et al. (2004). *Lactobacillus* GG in inducing and maintaining remission of Crohn's disease. *BMC Gastroenterology, 15*(4), 5.

151. Rolfe, V. E., Fortun, P. J., Hawkey, C. J., & Bath-Hextall, F. (2006). Probiotics for maintenance of remission in Crohn's disease Cd004826. *Cochrane Database Syst. Review, 4*.

152. Gosselink, M. P., Schouten, W. R., van Lieshout, L. M., et al. (2004). Delay of the first onset of pouchitis by oral intake of the probiotic strain *Lactobacillus rhamnosus* GG. *Diseases of the Colon & Rectum, 47*(6), 876–884.

153. Gionchetti, P., Rizzello, F., Helwig, U., et al. (2003). Prophylaxis of pouchitis onset with probiotic therapy: a double-blind, placebo-controlled trial. *Gastroenterology, 124*(5), 1202–1209.

154. Mimura, T., Rizzello, F., Helwig, U., et al. (2004). Once daily high dose probiotic therapy (VSL#3) for maintaining remission in recurrent or refractory pouchitis. *Gut, 53*, 108–114.

155. Kuzela, L., Kascak, M., & Vavrecka, A. (2001). Induction and maintenance of remission with nonpathogenic *Escherichia coli* in patients with pouchitis. *American Journal of Gastroenterology, 96*(11), 3218–3219.

156. Laake, K. O., Bjørneklett, A., Aamodt, G., et al. (2005). Outcome of four weeks' intervention with probiotics on symptoms and endoscopic appearance after surgical reconstruction with a J-configurated ileal-pouch-anal-anastomosis in ulcerative colitis. *Scandinavian Journal of Gastroenterology, 40*(1), 43–51.

157. Kuisma, J., Mentula, S., Jarvinen, H., et al. (2003). Effect of *Lactobacillus rhamnosus* GG on ileal pouch inflammation and microbial flora. *Alimentary Pharmacology & Therapeutic, 17*(4), 509–515.

158. Tromm, A., Niewerth, U., Khoury, M., et al. (2004). The probiotic *E. coli* strain Nissle 1917 for treatment of collagenous colitis: first results of an open-label trial. *Zeitschrift Fur Gastroenterologie, 42*, 365–369.

159. Wildt, S., Munck, L. K., Vinter-Jensen, L., et al. (2006). Probiotic treatment of collagenous colitis: a randomized, double-blind, placebo-controlled trial with *Lactobacillus acidophilus* and *Bifidobacterium animalis* subsp lactis. *Inflammatory Bowel Diseases, 12*, 395–401.

160. Fanigliulo, L., Comparato, G., Aragona, G., et al. (2006). Role of gut microflora and probiotic effects in the irritable bowel syndrome. *Acta Biomedicine, 77*, 85–89.

161. Nobaek, S., Johansson, M. L., Molin, G., et al. (2000). Alteration of intestinal microflora is associated with reduction in abdominal bloating and pain in patients with irritable bowel syndrome. *American Journal of Gastroenterology, 95*(5), 1231–1238.

162. Halpern, G. M., Prindiville, T., Blankenburg, M., et al. (1996). Treatment of irritable bowel syndrome with Lacteol Fort: a randomized, double-blind, cross-over trial. *American Journal of Gastroenterology, 91*(8), 1579–1585.

C. PREBIOTICS AND PROBIOTICS AS THERAPIES

163. Niedzielin, K., Kordecki, H., & Birkenfeld, B. (2001). A controlled, double-blind, randomized study on the efficacy of *Lactobacillus plantarum* 299 V in patients with irritable bowel syndrome. *European Journal of Gastroenterology Hepatology, 13*(10), 1143–1147.

164. O'Mahony, L., McCarthy, J., Kelly, P., et al. (2005). Lactobacillus and bifidobacterium in irritable bowel syndrome: symptom responses and relationship to cytokine profiles. *Gastroenterology, 128*(3), 541–551.

165. Whorwell, P. J., Altringer, L., Morel, J., et al. (2006). Efficacy of an encapsulated probiotic *Bifidobacterium infantis* 35624 in women with irritable bowel syndrome. *American Journal of Gastroenterology, 101*, 1581–1590.

166. Sen, S., Mullan, M. M., Parker, T. J., et al. (2002). Effect of *Lactobacillus plantarum* 299v on colonic fermentation and symptoms of irritable bowel syndrome. *Digestive Diseases and Sciences, 47*(11), 2615–2620.

167. O'Sullivan, M. A., & O'Morain, C. A. (2000). Bacterial supplementation in the irritable bowel syndrome. A randomised double-blind placebo-controlled crossover study. *Digestive and Liver Disease, 32*, 294–301.

168. Kim, H. J., Camilleri, M., McKinzie, S., et al. (2003). A randomized controlled trial of a probiotic, VSL#3, on gut transit and symptoms in diarrhoea-predominant irritable bowel syndrome. *Alimentary Pharmacology & Therapeutic, 17*(7), 895–904.

169. Hamilton-Miller, J. M. T. (2001). Probiotics in the management of irritable bowel syndrome: a review of clinical trials 212–216(5). *Microbial Ecology in Health and Disease, 13*(4).

170. Kolida, S., Tuohy, K., & Gibson, G. R. (2002). Prebiotic effects of inulin and oligofructose. *British Journal of Nutrition, 87*, S193–S197.

171. Bielecka, M., Biedrzycka, E., & Majkowska, A. (2002). Selection of probiotics and prebiotics for synbiotics and confirmation of their *in vivo* effectiveness. *Food Research International, 35*, 139–144.

172. Fooks, L. J., & Gibson, G. R. (2002). *In vitro* investigations of the effect of probiotics and prebiotics on selected human intestinal pathogens. *FEMS Microbiology Ecology, 39*, 67–75.

173. Asahara, T., Nomoto, K., Shimizu, K., et al. (2001). Increased resistance of mice to *Salmonella enterica* serovar Typhimurium infection by synbiotic administration of Bifidobacteria and transgalactosylated oligosaccharides. *Journal of Applied Microbiology, 91*, 985–996.

174. Bomba, A., Nemcova, R., Gancarcikova, S., et al. (2002). Improvement of the probiotic effect of microorganisms by their combination with maltodextrins, fructo-oligosaccharides and polyunsaturated fatty acids. *British Journal of Nutrition, 88*, S95–S99.

175. Langlands, S. J., Hopkins, M. J., Coleman, N., & Cummings, J. H. (2004). Prebiotic carbohydrates modify the mucosa associated microflora of the human large bowel. *Gut, 53*(11), 1610–1616.

176. Cummings, J. H., & Macfarlane, G. (2002). Gastrointestinal effects of prebiotics. *British Journal of Nutrition, 87*, S145–S151.

177. Videla, S., Vilaseca, J., Antolin, M., et al. (2001). Dietary inulin improves distal colitis induced by dextran sodium sulfate in the rat. *American Journal of Gastroenterology, 96*, 1486–1493.

178. Lewis, S., Burmeister, S., & Brazier, J. (2005). Effect of the prebiotic oligofructose on relapse of *Clostridium difficile*-associated diarrhea. A randomized, controlled study. *Clinical Gastroenterol Hepatology, 3*(5), 442–448.

179. Kanamori, Y., Sugiyama, M., Hashizume, K., et al. (2004). Experience of long-term synbiotic therapy in seven short bowel patients with refractory enterocolitis. *Journal of Pediatric Surgery, 39*(11), 1686–1692.

180. Cummings, J. H., Christie, S., & Cole, T. J. (2001). A study of fructo oligosaccharides in the prevention of travelers' diarrhoea. *Alimentary Pharmacology & Therapeutic, 15*, 1139–1145.

181. Brunser, O., Gotteland, M., Cruchet, S., et al. (2006). Effect of a milk formula with prebiotics on the intestinal microbiota of infants after an antibiotic treatment. *Pediatric Research, 59*, 451–456.

182. Lewis, S., Burmeister, S., Cohen, S., et al. (2005). Failure of dietary oligofructose to prevent antibiotic-associated diarrhoea. *Alimentary Pharmacology & Therapeutic, 21*, 469–477.

183. Duggan, C., Penny, M. E., Hibberd, P., et al. (2003). Oligofructose-supplemented infant cereal: 2 randomized, blinded, community-based trials in Peruvian infants. *American Journal of Clinical Nutrition, 77*, 937–942.

184. Hunter, J. O., Tuffnell, Q., & Lee, A. J. (1999). Controlled trial of oligofructose in the management of irritable bowel syndrome. *Journal of Nutrition, 129*, 1451S–1453S.

185. Mountzouris, K. C., McCartney, A. L., & Gibson, G. R. (2002). Intestinal microflora of human infants and current trends for its nutritional modulation. *British Journal of Nutrition, 87*, 405–420.

186. Vandenplas, Y. (2002). Oligosaccharides in infant formula. *British Journal of Nutrition, 87*, S293–S296.

187. Agarwal, R., Sharma, N., Chaudhry, R., et al. (2003). Effects of oral *Lactobacillus* GG on enteric microflora in low-birth-weight neonates. *Journal of Pediatric Gastroenterology Nutrition, 36*, 397–402.

188. Millar, M. R., Bacon, C., Smith, S. L., et al. (1993). Enteral feeding of premature infants with *Lactobacillus* GG. *Archives of Disease in Childhood, 69*, 483–487.

189. Boehm, G., Casetta, P., Lidestri, M., et al. (2001). Effect of dietary oligosaccharides (OS) on faecal bifidobacteria in formula-fed preterm infants. *Journal of Pediatric Gastroenterology Nutrition, 32*, 393.

190. Moro, G., Minoli, I., Mosca, F., et al. (2002). Dosage-related bifidogenic effects of galacto- and fructo-oligosaccharides in formula-fed term infants. *Journal of Pediatric Gastroenterology Nutrition, 34*, 291–295.

191. Knol, J., Boehm, G., Lidestri, M., et al. (2005). Increase of faecal bifidobacteria due to dietary oligosaccharides induces a reduction of clinically relevant pathogen germs in the faeces of formula-fed preterm infants. *Acta Paediatrica Suppl, 94*(449), 31–33.

192. Knol, J., Scholtens, P., Kafka, C., et al. (2005). Colon microflora in infants fed formula with galacto- and fructo-oligosaccharides: more like breast-fed infants. *Journal of Pediatric Gastroenterology Nutrition, 40*(1), 36–42.

193. Fanaro, S., Boehm, G., Garssen, J. et al. Galacto-oligosaccharides and long-chain fructo-oligosaccharides as prebiotics in infant formulas: a review. Acta Paediatr Suppl, 94 (449), 22–26.

194. Danan, C., Huret, Y., Tessèdre, A-C., et al. (2000). Could oligosaccharide supplementation promote gut colonization with a beneficial flora in preterm infants? *Journal of Pediatric Gastroenterology Nutrition, 30*, 217–219.

195. Butel, M-J., Waligora-Dupriet, A-J., & Szylit, O. (2002). Prebiotics and experimental model of neonatal necrotising enterocolitis. *British Journal of Nutrition, 87*, S213–S219.

196. Juffrie, M. (2002). Fructo-oligosaccharides and diarrhea. *Bioscience Microflora, 21*, 31–34.

197. Saavedra, J., & Tschernia, A. (2002). Human studies with probiotics and prebiotics: clinical implications. *British Journal of Nutrition, 87*, S241–S246.

198. Waligora-Dupriet, A. J., Campeotto, F., Nicolis, I., et al. (2007). Effect of oligofructose supplementation on gut microflora and well-being in young children attending day care centre. *International Journal of Food Microbiology, 113*, 108–113.

199. Fisberg, M., Maulen, I., Vasquez, E., et al. (2000). Effect of oral supplementation with and without synbiotics on catch-up growth in preschool children Abstract 987. *Journal of Pediatric Gastroenterology Nutrition, 31*.

200. Firmansyah, A., Pramita, G. D., Carrié Fässler, A. L., et al. (2000). Improved humoral immune response to measles vaccine in infants receiving infant cereals with fructo-oligosaccharides Abstract 521. *Journal of Pediatric Gastroenterology Nutrition, 31*.

201. Nopchinda, S., Varavithya, W., Phuapradit, P., et al. (2002). Effect of *Bifidobacterium* Bb12 with or without *Streptococcus thermophilus* supplemented formula on nutritional status. *Journal of the Medical Association of Thailand, 85*, S1225–S1231.

15

Probiotics and AIDS Treatment

Livia Trois

Ottawa, Ontario, Canada

1. INTRODUCTION

Even with the development in HIV medical treatment research, many social and clinical factors can affect functional status and quality of life for HIV-infected children. Due to the immune cell dysfunction and subsequent immunodeficiency, there are many clinical manifestations, as gastrointestinal dysfunction, leading to electrolyte imbalance, malnutrition and severe weight loss. HIV is recognized to alter the structure and the function of human small intestines. As a result, there is dysregulation of the gut immunity followed by frequent and complicated diarrhea, disruption of bowel structure and function, and malnutrition. Malabsorption in HIV has been frequently shown in the literature and it might contribute directly to CD4 count decrease, malnutrition, wasting and reduced body-mass index, and increased viral load [1–3]. Because intestinal dysfunction is frequent in pediatric HIV infection—which includes carbohydrate malabsorption, steatorrhea, increased intestinal permeability, and intestinal iron malabsorption—it is extremely important to restore intestinal digestive-absorptive function at an early stage of HIV in order to reverse immune derangement [4]. The disordered immune system itself contributes to mucosal injury, which can exacerbate even more the immunodeficiency and enhance the HIV replication [5, 6].

It is quite common among HIV-infected children to have a depression of immune function caused by malnutrition, which is potentially reversible by restoring gut microflora and nutritional rehabilitation [3]. A study by Brantley et al. [7] found a strong association between severe diarrhea and wasting in AIDS-infected humans and both protozoal pathogens and subtherapeutic levels of antiretroviral medications. Since intestinal dysfunction is common in HIV infection—that is, carbohydrate malabsorption, frequent diarrhea, steatorrhea—the intestinal permeability is increased, and might cause enteric pathogens translocation, propitiated by bacterial gastrointestinal overgrowth [8–10]. Probably the whole intestinal dysfunction is fundamentally reflected by the immune status, due to the fact that nearly 70% of the immune system response is localized in the digestive tract, as the gut flora can interact with the innate immunity and influence the adaptive immune response in an important relation between the immune system and the environment. Among this population, we

229

can also have the situation aggravated by the poor absorption and metabolism of antiretroviral drugs [11–13].

As the probiotics, defined as live microbial feed supplements, can improve intestinal microbial balance and promote health benefits, we can give them a goal of enhanced mucosal immune defense. This mechanism can happen through enhancing macrophage activity, elevating the numbers of killer cells, T cells, and interferon; and their action against pathogenic microbial colonization and translocation. Consequently, probiotic therapy may help the immune system and restore intestinal digestive-absorptive function [14–18].

Immune responses, placed in the intestinal epithelium, associated with probiotics and epithelial cells, might be sufficient to trigger signaling cascades that activate underlying immune cells in the lamina propria [19]. The immunostimulatory properties of probiotics were discussed in a preview study, and how they might be helpful in the treatment of AIDS improving quality of life, since low CD4 count has been shown to be predictive of disease progression and the development of opportunistic infections [20].

2. THE THERAPY OF PROBIOTIC'S IMMUNE STIMULATION IN HIV PATIENTS

Probiotics have been administered both prophylactically and therapeutically in an attempt to modify the mucosal, epithelial, intestinal and systemic immune activity in ways that may benefit human health. They are reported to improve microbial balance in the intestinal tract and display both antibacterial and immune regulatory effects in humans [21]. Due to these characteristics, acute infectious diarrhea is the most investigated field in the area of probiotic use in children, followed by the immune stimulation. The literature demonstrated that probiotics has

a good safety profile. The rationale for using probiotics for the above-mentioned purposes is based on the assumption that they modify the composition of the intestinal microflora and act against enteric pathogens [22, 23].

The HIV children have no chance, as a healthy child does, to develop a balanced microfloral, for the most important gut first colonization happens through breast-feeding, followed by exposure to the environment, maternal flora, delivery characteristics, and use of antibiotics. After 2 years of age, the gastrointestinal microbiota has implications on the functional ability of gut flora to optimize its activities in nutrition, food and drugs absorption and metabolism, vitamin synthesis, defense and education of the local immune system. More than 500 species of bacteria interact with the innate immune system and play a critical role there [13].

Probiotics, a commensal bacteria, interact with the host immune system, acting as an important antigenic stimulus for the improvement of gut-associated lymphoid tissue (GALT), starting the local immune responses [19]. The protection role of the microflora is mediated by a number of mechanisms, such as competitive exclusion, increasing normal intestinal barrier function, stimulating immunoglobulin (Ig)A production. Among the explanations known to date, there is a reasonable one for the probiotic stimulation of the immune response. The gut-associated lymphoid tissue can affect immune responses at other mucosal surfaces, through the production of IgA, crossing Peyer's patches and stimulation of T lymphocyte helpers, inducing phenotype and B cell response, resulting in modulation of the indigenous microbiota composition in HIV-infected patients [4, 24]. It has been proven that the microbiota has a positive impact on immune regulation. There are some studies relating probiotics and immune-response, as shown by Meyer et al., through an increase in CD8+ and CD4+ in healthy women. However, the proof of probiotics' direct involvement needs to be studied further [25].

The GALT has enormous functions, since almost 70% of the human immune system is localized in the digestive tract, as mentioned before. Therefore, the probiotic therapy plays an important role in the HIV child's health. Moreover, because most of the probiotics do not permanently colonize the intestine as they just pass through the intestine, they must be taken regularly and in sufficient quantities; at least 5 billion colony-forming units (cfu) or more, to maintain adequate amounts in the colon and to promote periodic immune stimulation [17, 18]. In addition, there can also be a huge difference of persistence among probiotic strains, reflecting their capacity to modulate immunity. Different bacteria elicit different cytokine responses from epithelial cells, inducing the GALT in many ways [13, 19].

From an analysis of the literature, we can see why probiotics should be used for the immune response. Most of the studies clearly demonstrated increased phagocytosis, a response by IgA and IgM, B cell responses, and other cytokines, such as alpha IFN and IL-10. The authors conclude that to induce optimal immunologic modulation it may be wise to use multiple organisms, thereby stimulating a broad immune benefit [26].

Another topic that must be considered is the duration of the probiotic therapy. The literature suggests at least 1 month's supplement period in order to achieve immunostimulatory effects. Less than that could not be enough to stimulate the immune system. However, the continuous administration of probiotics may not be the best method of administration. The immune enhancement properties of probiotics may require periodic pulse dosing [18, 27].

3. DOSAGE

There is no consensus on the dosage number of bacteria that has to be consumed to produce a beneficial health effect. The daily dosage of probiotic(s) varies greatly, from 2 to 40 billion bacteria/day. Each application for a health claim will be different, but apparently there is a minimum number of 5 million probiotic bacteria to be taken as a therapy to have significant results, and it could range to 3 trillion cfu in specific cases, as used for the remission of ulcerative colitis. Most clinical studies in children use 5 to 10 billion cfu/day or a little higher depending on the purpose and bacterial strain properties [13, 28].

4. SECURITY

There is no published evidence that the consumption of probiotics, containing lactobacilli or bifidobacteria—lactic acid bacteria (LAB) type, increases the risk of opportunistic infection among immunocompromised patients. In the literature there are two studies showing the safety of probiotics consumption by HIV patients. Probiotics are even being used to prevent diarrhea in AIDS patients [24, 29–31].

A review of available clinical trials made by the ESPGHAN Committee on Nutrition confirms that cases of infection with *Bifidobacterium* during supplementation have not been reported. Also, the increased consumption of *Lactobacillus* GG in food products has not resulted in an increased incidence of bacteremia, except in a rare case of a severely ill immunocompromised host [32]. The only adverse effects that could occur are mild abdominal discomfort and flatulence. Consequently, probiotics so far used in clinical trials can be generally considered as safe in healthy children and even in immunocompromised children [25].

5. A PREVIOUS STUDY

In a previous study, a randomized double blind controlled trial, we tried to determine whether the use of probiotics could improve the immune response marked by CD4 cells/mm^3 counts and reduce liquid stool episodes of HIV-infected children. We studied 77 HIV-infected children (2–12 years old), divided into two groups. In one, 38 children received probiotics (formula containing *Bifidobacterium bifidum* with *Streptococcus thermophilus*—2.5×10^{10} cfu) and in the other, 39 children received a standard formula (control group), for 2 months [20].

The results of the study, in immunoresponse markers, showed an increase in the mean CD4 count in the probiotics group ($p = 0.049$), and on the intestinal dysfunction we could see a positive response. A similar reduction in liquid stool consistency happened in both groups ($p < 0.06$), with a slight enhancement in the probiotics group ($p < 0.522$), and there was an increase in the incidence of normal stool consistency ($p < 0.01$) [20].

6. CONCLUSION

In conclusion, this study showed that probiotics might have immunostimulatory properties and can be helpful in the treatment of HIV-infected children, since the antiretroviral therapy had not changed during the study. It must be emphasized that not all probiotics have immunomodulatory properties capable of increasing the CD4 count. This is shown in this study by *Bifidobacterium bifidum* and *Streptococcus thermophilus*, a 3-week draw-study performed by Schifrin et al. which presented an increase in global phagocytic activity of blood phagocytes (granulocytes and monocytes) and in a further study by Meyer et al., with healthy women, which showed a stimulator effect of LAB in activating T cells [33, 34, 20].

Hirose et al. showed a positive result of daily intake of probiotics, as a heat-killed *Lactobacillus plantarum* strain, for 12 weeks. This randomized, double blind, placebo-controlled study, placed with healthy adults, suggests that the probiotic therapy augments acquired immunity, especially T cell helpers (CD4+), thereby improving

the health-related quality of life, reinforcing our interest in using probiotics in patients with AIDS, looking for their quality of life [35].

References

1. Yolken, R. H., Hart, W., Oung, I., et al. (1991). Gastrointestinal dysfunction and disaccharide intolerance in children infected with human immunodeficiency virus. *The Journal of Pediatrics, 118*, 359–363.
2. Missmer, S. A., Spiegelman, D., Gorbach, S. L., & Miller, T. L. (2000). Predictors of change in the functional status of children with human immunodeficiency virus infection. *Pediatrics, 106*(2), 1–7.
3. Wittenberg, D., Benítz, C. V., Canani, R. B., et al. (2004). HIV infection: Working group report of the second world congress of pediatric gastroenterology, hepatology, and nutrition. *Journal of Pediatric Gastroenterology and Nutrition, 39*(2), S640–S646.
4. Guarino, A., Spangnuolo, M. I., Giacomet, V., et al. (2002). Effects of nutritional rehabilitation on intestinal function and on CD4 cell number in children with HIV. *Journal of Pediatric Gastroenterology and Nutrition, 34*, 366–371.
5. Yolken, R. H., Hart, W., Oung, I., et al. (1991). Gastrointestinal dysfunction and disaccharide intolerance in children infected with human immunodeficiency virus. *The Journal of Pediatrics, 118*(3), 359–363.
6. Ansari, N. A., Kombe, A. H., Kenyon, T. A., et al. (2003). Pathology and causes of death in a series of human immunodeficiency virus-positive and negative pediatric referral hospital admissions in Botswana. *The Pediatric Infectious Disease Journal, 22*, 43–47.
7. Brantley, R. K., Williams, K. R., Silva, T. M. J., et al. (2003). AIDS-associated diarrhea and wasting in Northeast Brazil is associated with subtherapeutic plasma levels of antiretroviral medications and with both bovine and human subtypes of *Cryptosporidium parvum*. *BJID, 7*(1), 16–22.
8. Miller, T. L., McQuinn, L., & Orav, E. J. (1997). Upper gastrointestinal endoscopy as a diagnostic tool for children with human immunodeficiency virus infection. *The Journal of Pediatrics, 130*, 766–773.
9. Miller, T. L. (2002). Nutritional interventions in pediatric HIV: It's hard to hit a moving target. *JPGN, 34*(4), 353–356.
10. Johnson, S., Hendson, W., Crewe-Brown, H., et al. (2000). Effect of human immunodeficiency virus infection on episodes of diarrhea among children in South Africa. *The Pediatric Infectious Disease Journal, 19*, 972–979.
11. Ball, C. S. (1998). Global issues in pediatric nutrition: AIDS. *Nutrition, 14*(10), 767–770.
12. Jirapinyo, P., Brewster, D., Succi, R. C. M., et al. (2002). HIV disease: Working group report of the first world congress of pediatric gastroenterology, hepatology,

and nutrition. *Journal of Pediatric Gastroenterology and Nutrition, 35*(2), S134–S142.

13. Kligler, B., Hanaway, P., & Cohrssen, A. (2007). Probiotics in children. *Pediatric Clinics of North America, 54,* 949–967.

14. Fuller, R., & Gibson, G. R. (1997). Modification of the intestinal microflora using probiotics and prebiotics. *Scandinavian Journal of Gastroenterology, 32*(Suppl.) 222, 28–31.

15. Vanderhoof, J. A. (2001). Probiotics: Future directions. *The American Journal of Clinical Nutrition, 73*(Suppl.), 1152S–1155S.

16. Tuomola, E., Crittenden, R., Playne, M., et al. (2001). Quality assurance criteria for probiotic bacteria. *The American Journal of Clinical Nutrition, 73*(Suppl.), 393S–398S.

17. Duggan, C., Gannon, J., & Walker, W. A. (2002). Protective nutrients and functional foods for the gastrointestinal tract. *The American Journal of Clinical Nutrition, 75,* 789–808.

18. Kalliomäki, M., & Isolauri, E. (2003). Role of intestinal flora in development of allergy. *Current Opinion in Allergy and Clinical Immunology, 3,* 15–20.

19. Corthésy, B., Rex Gaskins, H., & Mercenier, A. (2007). Cross-talk between probiotic bacteria and the host immune system1, 2. *Journal of Nutrition, 137,* 3S–781S.

20. Trois, L., Cardoso, E. M., & Miura, E. (2008). Use of probiotics in HIV-infected children: A randomized double-blind controlled study (Epub 2007 Sep 17). *Journal of Tropical Pediatrics, 54*(1), 19–24.

21. Johnston, B. C., Supina, A. L., Ospina, M., & Vohra, S. (2007). Probiotics for the prevention of pediatric antibiotic-associated diarrhea. *Cochrane Database of Systematic Reviews* Issue 2. Art. No: CD004827. DOI: 10.1002/14651858.CD004827.pub2.

22. Vandenplas, Y. (1999). Bacteria and yeasts in the treatment of acute and chronic infectious diarrhea. Bacteria. *Clinical Microbiology and Infection, 5*(6), 299–307.

23. Bernaola Aponte, G., Bada Mancilla, C. A., Carreazo Pariasca, N. Y., & Rojas Galarza, R. A. (2008). Probiotics for treating persistent diarrhoea in children (Protocol). *Cochrane Database of Systematic Reviews.*

24. Wolf, B. W., Wheeler, K. B., Ataya, D. G., & Garleb, K. A. (1998). Safety and tolerance of *Lactobacillus reuteri* supplementation to a population infected with the human immunodeficiency virus. *Food and Chemical Toxicology, 36,* 1085–1094.

25. Kligler, B., & Cohrssen, A. (2008). Probiotics. *American Family Physician, 78*(9), 1073–1078.

26. Flock, M. H., & Montrose, D. C. (2005). Use of probiotics in humans: an analysis of the literature. *Gastroenterology Clinics of North America, 34,* 547–570.

27. Saavedra, J. M., Bauman, N. A., Oung, I., et al. (1994). Feeding of *Bifidocterium bifidum* and *Streptococcus thermophilus* to infants in hospital for prevention of diarrhea and shedding of rotavirus. *Lancet, 344,* 1046–1049.

28. Farnworth, E. R. (2008). The evidence to support health claims for probiotics 1, 2. *Journal of Nutrition, 138*(6), 1250S–1254S.

29. Cunningham-Rundles, S., Ahrné, A., & Bengmark, S., et al. (2000). Probiotics and immune response. *The American Journal of Gastroenterology, 95,* S22–S25.

30. Borriello, S. P., Hammes, W. P., & Holzapfel, W. et al. (2003). Safety of probiotics that contain Lactobacilli or Bifidobacteria. *Clin Inf Dis, 36,* 775–780.

31. Penna, F. J., Filho, L. A. P., Calçado, A. C., et al. (2000). Up-to-date clinical and experimental basis for the use of probiotics. *The Journal of Pediatrics (Rio J), 76*(Suppl. 2), 209S–217S.

32. Agostini, C., Axelsson, I., Braegger, C., et al. (2004). ESPGHAN Committee on Nutrition: Probiotic bacteria in dietetic products for infants: Commentary by the ESPGHAN Committee on Nutrition. *Journal of Pediatric Gastroenterology and Nutrition, 38,* 365–374.

33. Schifrin, E. J., Brassart, D., & Servin, A. L., et al. (1997). Immune modulation of blood leukocytes in humans by lactic acid bacteria: Criteria for strain selection. *The American Journal of Clinical Nutrition, 66,* 515S–520S.

34. Meyer, A., Micksche, M., Herbacek, I., & Elmadfa, I. (2006). Daily intake of probiotic as well as conventional yogurt has a stimulating effect on cellular immunity in young healthy women. *Annals of Nutrition & Metabolism, 50,* 282–289.

35. Hirose, Y., Murosaki, S., & Yamamoto, Y., et al. (2006). Daily intake of heat-killed *Lacrobacillus plantarum* L-137 augments acquired immunity in healthy adults. *Journal of Nutrition, 136,* 3069–3073.

PROBIOTICS AND HEALTH

16

Probiotics and Prebiotics in Metabolic Disorders and Obesity

Yolanda Sanz and Arlette Santacruz

Microbial Ecophysiology and Nutrition Group, Institute of Agrochemistry and
Food Technology (CSIC), Burjassot, Valencia, Spain

1. INTRODUCTION

Obesity is viewed as one of the major current public-health issues due to its high prevalence and associated co-morbidities worldwide. Obesity constitutes a risk factor for a number of related disorders including type-2 diabetes mellitus, cardiovascular diseases and nonalcoholic fatty liver disease. Obesity results from a long-term positive imbalance between energy intake and expenditure. Multiple pathways interact to regulate energy balance and appetite, which are integrated in the central nervous system and finally determine lipid accumulation and body weight. Hormones synthesized in enteroendocrine cells of the gastrointestinal tract and peripheral tissues, where signals are integrated by the peripheral and central nervous system (gut–brain axis), are critical in regulation of appetite and body weight. These are produced in response to nutrients and energy status and, therefore, they could partially be modulated by dietary strategies. The long-term control of ingestion seems to be primarily mediated by signals

emanating from the adipose tissue (leptin) and pancreas (insulin), which are released in response to food ingestion and fat storage [1]. The short-term control of ingestion is primarily controlled by signaling pathways emanating from the gastrointestinal tract, including orexigenic peptides (ghrelin), which trigger hunger signals, and anorexigenic peptides (cholecystokinin, glucagon-like peptide-1 [GLP-1] and peptide tyrosine-tyrosine [PYY]), which drive satiety signals.

Obesity is also associated with a state of chronic low-grade inflammation and increased susceptibility to infection due to malfunction of the immune system. Obese individuals show increased macrophage infiltration in the adipose tissue along with production of inflammatory adipokines, cytokines and associated immune factors. Inflammatory immune mediators (e.g. C-reactive protein, tumor-necrosis factor [TNF]-α, interleukin [IL]-6, and monocyte chemotactic protein 1 [MCP-1]) and adipokines (leptin and resistin) are elevated in obese mice and human subjects, whereas production of the anti-inflammatory and insulin-sensitizing

237

adipokine adiponectin is reduced [2]. In fact, chronic activation of the innate immune system is regarded as a risk factor for the development of obesity and associated disorders, which might be under the immunomodulatory effects of the dietary compounds.

The increased prevalence of obesity and metabolic-associated disorders is thought to be the result of societal changes associated with regular intake of energy-dense foods and low physical activity worldwide [3]. Interventions based on dietary energy restrictions and increased physical activity have partially contributed to bodyweight control, but they have usually yielded limited and temporal weight loss. Pharmacological therapies have not fully succeeded in effectively treating obesity for long-term periods and have side effects [4]. In this context, the understanding of the contribution of interactions between environmental factors and predisposing genes to metabolic conditions is critical to progress on the development of more effective preventive and therapeutic strategies.

The human gut is populated by a vast number of bacterial species that reach concentrations ranging from 10^7 to 10^{12} cells per gram of intestinal content from the small intestine to the colon. This microbial community evolves with its host throughout life by establishing symbiotic and mutualistic relationships, which favor their co-existence [5]. The collective genome (microbiome) of the gut microbiota contains at least 100 times as many genes as the human genome, providing additional features and contributing to human physiological diversity [6, 7]. The gut microbiota serves a number of relevant functions to the metabolism, immunity and defense of the host against external aggressions. The metabolism of the gut microbiota contributes to energy salvage, improvement of complex polysaccharide digestion and production of vitamins and other essential nutrients [8]. The gut microbiota also regulates epithelial permeability as well as many aspects of innate and acquired immunity, protecting the host form pathogen invasion and

chronic inflammation [9, 10]. The concept that a balanced gut microbiota is required for maintaining a good nutritional and health status, has led to the design of dietary strategies to favor the prevalence of beneficial bacteria. These include the administration of prebiotic oligosaccharides, probiotics and synbiotics (a combination of pro- and prebiotics) in the form of functional foods and supplements. Probiotics are defined as live microbes that, when administered in adequate amounts, confer a health benefit to the host [11]. The genus *Bifidobacterium* is the predominant in the intestinal tract of infants, especially when they are breast-fed; this bacterial group also represents about 3–7% of the total microbiota in the intestine of healthy adults and it is associated with beneficial effects [9]. The genus *Lactobacillus* also inhabits the human gastrointestinal tract and some species are widely used in diverse food fermentations. These features have made these two bacterial genera the most attractive as probiotics for human consumption. Prebiotics are non-digestible dietary ingredients that allow changes, both in the composition and/or activity of the gastrointestinal microbiota, which confer benefits to the host's health [12]. Galactosyl-oligosaccharides (GOS) and inulin-type fructans (long-chain inulin and short-chain derivatives, e.g. oligofructose (OFS)) are the prebiotics most commonly commercialized [13]. In this chapter, the knowledge on the contribution of the gut microbiota to obesity and associated-metabolic disorders and the evidence on the possible benefits of interventions with probiotic, prebiotics and synbiotics are reviewed.

2. GUT MICROBIOTA COMPOSITION ASSOCIATED WITH OBESITY AND METABOLIC DISORDERS

Obesity has been associated with phylum and group-specific changes in the microbiota, reduced bacterial diversity and altered representation of bacterial genes corresponding to diverse metabolic pathways, which suggest a functional relationship between the microbiota and the host involved in bodyweight regulation [14, 15].

Increases in the relative abundance of *Firmicutes* and proportional reductions in *Bacteroidetes* have been associated with obesity by comparisons between the distal gut microbiota of genetically obese *ob/ob* mice (leptin deficient) and their lean (*ob/+* or *+/+*) littermates by DNA sequencing [16]. A higher proportion of *Archaea* was also found on the cecal microbiota of these genetically obese mice in comparison with their lean littermates and, therefore, linked to obesity [17]. Diet-induced obesity in animal models has also been associated with increased representation of *Eubacterium dolichum* from the *Firmicutes* division, which was also diminished by subsequent dietary manipulations to limit weight gain [18]. Obese Zucker rats (*fa/fa*) also showed reduced *Bifidobacterium* counts quantified by fluorescence *in situ* hybridization (FISH) and increased abundance of *Halomonas* and *Sphingomonas* detected by PCR and denaturing gradient gel electrophoresis (DGGE), compared to lean rats. These changes were associated with different metabolic phenotypes, including lower levels of urinary hippurate and creatinine, higher levels of urinary isoleucine, leucine and acetate and higher plasma levels of LDL and VLDL in obese than in lean rats [15].

Similar deviations in the relative fecal proportions of *Firmicutes* and *Bacteroidetes* have been associated with human obesity [19]. In addition, obese human adults submitted to a hypocaloric diet (either low carbohydrate- or low fat-containing diet) showed significant increases in fecal proportions of *Bacteroidetes* parallel to weight loss over a 1-year-long intervention [19]. Furthermore, a lower proportion of *Bacteroidetes* and a higher proportion of *Actinobacteria* have been associated with obesity by comparisons between the fecal microbiota of obese and lean

twin human subjects [14]. An increased abundance of *Bacteroidetes* was also related to increased genome functional diversity by DNA sequencing [14]. A larger-scale intervention study has demonstrated that both a calorie-restricted diet and increased physical activity induce changes in the gut microbiota structure of obese adolescents, correlated with weight loss and body mass index (BMI) Z-score reductions [20, 21]. *C. histolyticum, C. lituseburense* and *E. rectale-C. coccoides* proportions dropped significantly, while those of the *Bacteroides-Prevotella* group increased after the intervention in those adolescents who experienced significant weight reductions (> 4kg representing 8.1% of their body weight) as determined by FISH (20). In agreement, *Bacteroides fragilis* group and *Lactobacillus* group numbers increased while *Clostridium coccoides* group and *B. longum* numbers dropped significantly in those adolescents that experience important weight loss as determined by quantitative real-time PCR [21]. Moreover, the effectiveness of the lifestyle intervention on bodyweight loss seemed to be influenced by the composition of the individual's microbiota [21]. Other reports indicated that a dietary intervention, based on reducing carbohydrate intake, led to reductions in populations of *Bifidobacterium* and *Roseburia* spp. and *Eubacterium rectale* sub-groups of clostridial cluster XIVa in obese human subjects, while no differences were detected in *Bacteroides* or other clostridial clusters [22]; however, relationships to body weight were not established. Studies on the evolution of mammals and their gut microbes by DNA sequencing also pointed out that the diet is a fundamental driver for changes in gut bacterial diversity, which increases from carnivore to omnivore to herbivore [23].

Differences in fecal microbiota composition were shown to precede overweight in children early in life. While children maintaining normal weights showed a greater number of bifidobacteria, children becoming overweight showed a greater number of *Staphylococcus aureus* in feces during infancy [24].

The imbalanced gut microbiota composition associated with genetic or diet-induced obesity has also been shown to be reversible by oral transfer of the gut microbiota from lean mice to a germ-free recipient [18, 25] or by administration of prebiotic substrates to animal models at least over short-term periods [26]. On the light of this evidence, the intentional manipulation of the composition of gut microbiota via dietary strategies has been considered a possible tool to revert or prevent overweight and particularly metabolic-associated disorders [18, 25, 26], although direct evidence on such hypothesis is still limited.

3. GUT MICROBIOTA, NUTRIENT METABOLISM AND ENERGY STORAGE

Comparisons between germ-free mice and colonized mice by the conventional distal gut microbiota have demonstrated that the microbiota increases the host's ability to both harvest energy from the diet and store this energy in adipocytes, contributing to bodyweight gain [27]. The intestinal microbiota develops an important biochemical activity within the human body by both providing additional metabolic capacities to the host [6] and regulating diverse aspects of cellular differentiation and gene expression via host-microbe interactions [28]. The intestinal microbiota provides enzymes involved in the utilization of non-digestible carbohydrates and host-derived glycoconjugates (e.g. chondroitin sulphate, mucin, hyaluronate and heparin), deconjugation and dehydroxylation of bile acids, cholesterol reduction and biosynthesis of vitamins (K and B group), isoprenoids and amino acids (e.g. lysine and threonine) [6, 28]. In particular, the ability of the commensal microbiota to utilize complex dietary polysaccharides, which would otherwise be inaccessible to humans, seems to contribute to the ability of the host to harvest energy from the diet. This may represent 10% of the daily energy supply in omnivores and up to 70% in herbivores [29]. This metabolic activity leads to the generation of short-chain fatty acids (SCFAs) (mainly butyrate, acetate and propionate), which are almost completely absorbed along the gastrointestinal tract. Increased production of SCFAs indicates activation of the metabolic activity of the colonic microbiota that could contribute to energy supply. However, the contribution of each SCFA to body weight remains unclear. Butyrate is extensively utilized by enterocytes and generally regarded as a healthy metabolite, since it exerts anti-inflammatory effects and contributes to glucagon-like peptide 1 (GLP-1) secretion involved in satiety [30]. However, the production of butyrate has also been associated with increased prevalence of *C. perfringens*, which could explain its association and that of the *Firmicutes* phylum with obesity in animal and human studies [31]. Acetate and propionate could access the portal circulation and oppositely impact lipid metabolism. Acetate seems to contribute to lipid and cholesterol synthesis in the liver by activating the cytosolic acetyl S CoA synthetase 2, while propionate may inhibit lipid synthesis from acetate [32]. Several clostridial clusters of *Firmicutes* are also involved in acetogenesis [33], which could partly explain the inverse relationship between *Firmicutes* and bodyweight reductions in human studies. The removal of the hydrogen generated in the last stages of polysaccharide fermentation by the action of methanogenic microorganisms also activates the metabolism and growth of polysaccharide degrading bacteria, which could explain the association between the methanogenic *Archaea* and obesity [34].

The commensal microbiota has also been shown to induce expression of genes involved in the processing and absorption of dietary carbohydrates and complex lipids in the host, favoring fat storage [27, 35]. For instance, ileal expression of a monosaccharide transporter (Na + /glucose co-transporter) was induced in *B. thetaiotaomicron* mono-colonized mice, which would lead to increasing the absorption of dietary monosaccharides and SCFA and, thereby, promoting *de novo* synthesis of lipids in the liver [35]. *Eubacterium dolichum* was also shown to favor import and processing of simple sugars in subjects under a western-style diet, explaining the mechanistic basis of its association with obesity [18]. The colonization of germ-free mice by conventional microbiota also increased liver expression of key enzymes (acetyl-CoA carboxylase and fatty acid synthase) involved in the *de novo* fatty acid biosynthetic pathways, and transcriptional factors (ChREBP and SREBP-1) involved in hepatocyte lipogenic responses to insulin and glucose [27]. In addition, the colonization reduced the levels of circulating fasting-induced adipose factor (Fiaf) and the skeletal muscle and liver levels of phosphorylated AMP-activated protein kinase, which altogether contribute to fat storage [36]. The colonization of germ-free mice by *B. thetaiotaomicron* also increased the expression of other components involved in the host's lipid absorption machinery, including a pancreatic-lipase related protein that hydrolyzes triacylglycerols, a cytosolic fatty acid binding protein (L-FABP) involved in intracellular trafficking of fatty acids, and the apolipoprotein A-IV that mediates export of triacylglycerols re-synthesized in the enterocyte [35].

Components of the commensal gut microbiota could also regulate serum lipids and cholesterol by taking part in the bile acid metabolism. Bacterial enzymes mainly catalyze the deconjugation and dehydroxylation of bile acids, which alter the solubilization and absorption of dietary lipids throughout the intestine [37]. Fecal commensal bacteria were also shown to reduce cholesterol to coprostanol and, thus, increase its excretion in feces [38].

4. GUT MICROBIOTA AND NEUROENDOCRINE FUNCTION

Neuroendocrine secretions synthesized in the enteric nervous system and enteroendocrine cells of the gastrointestinal tract mucosa, peripheral organs and tissues (adipose tissue, pancreas, and liver) contribute to regulation of energy balance (or deregulation in obesity) in communication with the central nervous system.

Comparisons between germ-free and conventionalized mice indicated that the gut microbiota, as a whole, stimulates the synthesis of leptin, with a proportional increase in body fat and insulin resistance [27]. Leptin is the dominant long-term signal informing the brain of energy stores that inhibits food intake. However, leptin deficiency is not a common cause of obesity but leptin resistance, associated with increased serum levels, hunger and reduced energy expenditure. Some of the receptors of neuropeptides involved in regulation of satiety and hunger (NPY and alpha-melanocortin-stimulating hormone) are also regulated by leptin. Increased leptin levels usually associated with obesity could also promote a Th1-type cytokine secretion and contribute to the inflammatory tone [39]. Short-chain fatty acids, which mainly derived from the fermentative activity of the gut microbiota, have been shown to be ligands for G protein-coupled receptors, such as Gpr41, expressed in the distal small intestine, colon, and adipocytes, which upon activation stimulate the expression of peptide hormones (e.g. leptin and PYY) involved in appetite and energy metabolism [40]. The results have revealed that Gpr41 plays a pivotal role in regulating the flow of calories between the diet and the host in a microbiota-dependent manner. In particular, a Gpr41-deficiency was associated with reduced expression of PYY, which is an enteroendocrine peptide that modulates gut motility, transit rate, and reduced harvest of energy from the diet. Autoantibodies against key appetite-regulating neuropeptides and peptide hormones (e.g. alpha-melanocyte-stimulating hormone, NPY, agouti-related protein, ghrelin and leptin) have also been detected in sera of human subjects and rats [41]. The sequence homology found between these neuropeptides and proteins from some members of the intestinal microbiota has suggested that the microbiota could influence their production and, therefore, eating behavior.

Gut microbiota composition also seems to be affected by stress and hormone production, which could affect energy balance. Stress during the late stages of pregnancy, associated with elevated plasma cortisol levels, led to reductions in fecal bifidobacterial counts [42]. Gut colonization by the commensal microbiota has also been shown to affect the development of neural systems that govern the endocrine response to stress and, in particular, the hypothalamic-pituitary-adrenal (HPA) reaction to stress. In germ-free mice higher plasma adrenocorticotropic hormone (ACTH) and corticosterone elevation in response to restraint stress, was detected as well as reduced brain-derived neurotrophic factor (BDNF) expression levels in the cortex and hippocampus relative to conventional mice [43]. Moreover, the exaggerated HPA stress response in germ-free mice was reversed by inoculation with *Bifidobacterium infantis*, while inoculation with enteropathogenic *Escherichia coli* enhanced the response to stress. Out of these secretions, BDNF deficiency has been associated with eating disorders and glucocorticoids also well-known for their critical role in metabolism. In particular, alterations in tissue-specific cortisol levels may influence lipogenic and gluconeogenetic pathways in fat and liver, associated with obesity and development of insulin resistance [44]. Germ-free rats showed increased amounts of gastrin and serotonin-gastric immunoreactive cells in the gastric mucosa, serotonin and motilin immunoreactive cells in the ileum and serotonin-immunoreactive cells in the colonic mucosa than conventional raised rats [45]. In the obesity field, it is well-known that the serotoninergic system

plays an important role in eating behavior in humans and has been considered a target for the development of obesity and type-2 diabetes drugs [46].

5. GUT MICROBIOTA AND IMMUNE DYSFUNCTION ASSOCIATED WITH OBESITY

The innate immune system is able to differentiate between harmful and harmless antigens mainly by their detection through pattern-recognition receptors (PRRs) of epithelial and innate immune cells (dendritic cells [DCs] and macrophages), such as Toll-like receptors (TLRs) [9]. In response to danger, TLR stimulation leads to activating the transcription of different down-stream effector systems (e.g. NFκB system and mitogen-activated kinases) with production of pro-inflammatory cytokines (e.g. TNF-α, IL-1β, and IL-6) [47]. In contrast, commensal bacteria maintain immune homeostasis by producing a transient activation of the NFκB cascade or its suppression by diverse mechanisms, including induction of anti-inflammatory cytokines (e.g. IL-10) [9]. Toll-like receptors and derived cytokines also play a pivotal role in linking innate and adaptive immunity through exerting action on dendritic cells (DCs) and their interaction with T cells. These interactions influence the differentiation of T cells in different subpopulations (Th1, Th2, IL-10-secreting T regulatory type 1 [Tr1] or Th17), which are required to ensure appropriate protective responses to infections and harmful antigens, without leading to overreactions and chronic inflammation [48].

Scientific evidence has demonstrated that both the lipopolysaccharide (LPS) of Gram-negative bacteria and dietary saturated fatty acids can activate TLR4 inducing up-regulation of common intracellular inflammatory pathways, such as the c-Jun N-terminal kinase and NFκB with secretion of pro-inflammatory cytokines and chemokines in adipocytes and macrophages, related to the induction of insulin resistance and increased adiposity [49]. Metabolic endotoxemia, characterized by an increase in serum LPS levels, has been demonstrated to be an inflammatory factor, causative of bodyweight gain, insulin resistance and diabetes in high fat fed animal models [26, 50]. In contrast, the inhibition of the gut microbiota by antibiotic administration (norfloxacin and ampicillin) in two different mouse models of insulin resistance resulted in reduced serum LPS levels, low grade inflammation, obesity and type-2 diabetes, demonstrating the link between the gut microbiota and certain metabolic disorders [24]. In humans, increased LPS serum levels of *Chlamydia pneumoniae* have also been associated with an elevated BMI [51].

Infiltration of macrophages with a pro-inflammatory phenotype (M1 cells) into the adipose tissue is also associated with obesity, and their abundance is related to the level of insulin resistance in obese patients. In this context, microbial stimuli involved in Th1 cytokine production are also thought to be able to divert macrophages into M1 cells that, unlike Th2 cytokine-polarized M2 cells, are a source of inflammatory signals.

Malfunction of DCs is also characteristic of obesity. In obese mice (*ob/ob*), DCs are less potent in stimulation of allogenic T cells *in vitro* and this is associated with secretion of immunosuppressive cytokines such as transforming growth factor beta (TGF-β). The *in vivo* steady-state number of epidermal DCs was also increased and related to the absence of functional leptin [52]. In mice, transgenic for a T cell receptor specifically recognizing a peptide of ovalbumin, the specific T cell immune response was impaired under a high fat diet and the expression of this defect was different depending on whether T cells were naïve or antigen experienced [53]. Spleen T cells from naïve high fat diet fed transgenic mice exhibited a strong inflammatory profile after *in vitro* ovalbumin stimulation, as shown by the markedly increased interferon

(IFN)-gamma/IL-4 ratio as compared to cells from standard diet fed mice. Inversely, spleen T cells from ovalbumin-immunized high fat diet mice were impaired in their antigen-dependent proliferation compared to cells from standard diet fed mice. Therefore, the findings indicated that naïve T cells could participate actively in the low-grade systemic inflammation observed in overweight patients. Moreover, the impaired activity of antigen experienced T cells could have major consequences in the defense against infection and vaccination [53]. Therefore, DCs and T cells may be sensitive to metabolic alterations, explaining the immunodeficiency associated with obesity [54]. In the light of this evidence, it has been suggested that probiotics and prebiotics with immunomodulatory properties could regulate the immune responses to control the low-grade inflammatory status and malfunction of the immune system associated with obesity and related metabolic disorders, reported in some *in vivo* studies discussed in the following sections.

6. PROBIOTIC EFFECTS ON METABOLIC AND OBESITY BIOMARKERS *IN VIVO*

6.1. Probiotic Effects on Metabolic and Obesity Biomarkers in Animal Models

The pre-clinical studies carried out to evaluate the affects of classical probiotic strains (*Lactobacillus* and *Bifidobacterium*), combined or not with prebiotics (synbiotics), on diverse metabolic parameters of conventional animals and animal models of obesity, insulin resistance and hypercholesterolemia are summarized in Table 16.1.

Feeding rats with skim milk fermented by *L. gasseri* SBT2055 led to reductions in adipocyte size in mesenteric white adipose tissue, increased numbers of small adipocytes in mesenteric and retroperitoneal adipose tissues, and reduced serum leptin concentrations when compared with control fed rats [55]. These results suggested a role of the probiotic in the regulation of adipose tissue growth and probably in obesity [55]. *L. acidophilus* ATCC 4356 and 43121 supernatants administrated into rat central nervous system led to a decrease in body weight of rats and an increase in the expression of leptin in specific areas of the brain and retroperitoneal adipose tissue [56]. A synbiotic treatment consisting of a mixture of *L. rhamnosus* GG, *B. lactis* Bb12, and inulin exerted an effect on plasma concentrations of two neuropeptides involved in gut physiology and satiety in conventional rats of different age [57]. This synbiotic treatment increased the portal plasma concentrations of NPY (orexigenic) and PYY (anorexigenic) in adult rats; while in elderly animals, it decreased the NPY concentration. Although this study was focused on the effects of this dietary supplement on the gastrointestinal tract functions (gastric emptying, acid secretion and gut motility), a role of neuropeptide modulation in eating behavior could not be disregarded.

Dietary supplementation of high fructose-induced diabetic rats with a probiotic product (dahi) containing *L. acidophilus* NCDC14 and *L. casei* NCDC19 delayed the onset of glucose intolerance, hyperglycemia, hyperinsulinemia, dyslipidemia, and oxidative stress [58]. The probiotic fed group showed lower increases in several metabolic biomarkers of diabetes risk (Table 16.1), suggesting positive effects of the product on the evolution of this disorder and its complications [58]. In addition, the same probiotics were shown to increase the efficacy of the dahi product to suppress the progression of streptozotocin-induced diabetes in rats by inhibiting depletion of insulin, diabetic dyslipidemia, lipid peroxidation and nitrite formation (Table 16.1) [59].

The effect of the probiotic product VSL#3, which consists of several *Lactobacillus*, *Bifidobacterium* and *Streptococcus* strains, and its mechanisms of action on diet-induced obesity, steatosis and insulin resistance were evaluated in wild-type male C57BL6 mice, which were fed either normal or high fat diets [60]. Oral probiotic treatment significantly improved the insulin resistance, hepatic NKT cell depletion and hepatic steatosis induced by the high fat diet. This effect was NKT cell-dependent, resulted from the attenuation of the TNF-α and IκB kinase inflammatory signaling, and led to an improved sensitivity in insulin signaling [60].

L. acidophilus ATCC 43121 exerted positive effects on serum cholesterol and lipoprotein levels in hypercholesterolemia-induced rats (Table 16.1). In particular, the increase in the insoluble bile acid lithocholic acid was associated with reduced blood cholesterol levels in rats fed hypercholesterol diets supplemented with the probiotic. Overall, the positive affects of *L. acidophilus* ATCC 43121 on cholesterol levels seemed to be due to its activity in the deconjugation and dehydroxylation of bile acids [47]. The administration of the probiotic *L. paracasei* NCC2461 to germ-free mice colonized with human baby microbiota was shown to alter the host systemic lipid metabolism [61]. The probiotic supplementation resulted in decreased plasma concentrations of VLDL and LDL lipoproteins and increased concentrations of hepatic triglycerides. These affects were related to changes in the enterohepatic recirculation of bile acids, characterized by increases in taurocholic and tauro-β-muricholic acid recycling, possibly due to the relative inability of the human microbiota to deconjugate murine bile acids. It was suggested that the increased recycling of bile acids was associated with increased intestinal absorption of dietary lipids, reduced secretion of VLDL-associated triglycerides and consequently accumulation of lipids in the liver [61]. Similarly, the administration of either *L. paracasei* NCC2461 or *L. rhamnosus* NCC4007 to the same mice model led to comparable changes in lipid metabolism and, apparently, stimulated glycolysis [62]. This probiotic supplementation was also associated with significant reduction of acetate and butyrate in the cecal content and with reduced

TABLE 16.1   Effects of probiotics on body weight and metabolic biomarkers in animals

Probiotic/symbiotic/dose	Animal model	Duration	Outcome	Reference
L. gasseri SBT2055 Fermented milk with 6×10^7 cfu/g.	Male Sprague-Dawley rats.	28 days	↓Adipocyte size in mesenteric white adipose tissue ↑Numbers of small adipocytes in mesenteric and retroperitoneal adipose tissues ↓Serum leptin concentrations	[55]
L. acidophilus ATCC 4356 and 43121 supernatants.	Male Sprague-Dawley rats.	1 injection in the central nervous system	↓Body weight ↑Leptin expression in brain and retroperitoneal adipose tissue	[56]
L. rhamnosus GG and *B. lactis* Bb12 (2.2×10^9 cfu each/g diet) and inulin (8%).	Male Sprague-Dawley rats.	21 days	↑Portal plasma NPY and PYY concentration in adult rats ↓Portal plasma NPY concentrations in elderly rats	[57]
L. acidophilus NCDC14 and *L. casei* NCDC19 in dahi product (10^8 cfu/g).	High fructose-induced diabetic male Wistar rats.	8 weeks	↓Blood glucose, glycosylated hemoglobin, plasma insulin, liver glycogen, plasma total cholesterol, TAG[1], LDL cholesterol, VLDL cholesterol, blood free fatty acids ↓Thiobarbituric acid-reactive substances ↑Reduced glutathione in liver and pancreatic tissues	[58]
L. acidophilus NCDC14 and *L. casei* NCDC19 in dahi product (7.3×10^9 cfu/g).	Streptozotocin (STZ)-induced diabetes in Wistar rats.	28 days	↓Incremental peaks and delayed reduction of insulin secretion during oral glucose tolerance test ↓Oxidative damage in pancreatic tissues by inhibiting the lipid peroxidation and formation of nitric oxide ↑Glutathione content and activities of superoxide dismutase, catalase and glutathione peroxidase	[59]
VSL#3 (*B. breve, B. lactis*[2], *L. acidophilus, L. plantarum, L. paracasei, L. bulgaricus* and *S. thermophilus*) (1.5×10^9 cfu/day).	Male C57BL6 mice with steatosis and insulin resistance induced by a high-fat diet.	28 days	↑Hepatic NKT cell numbers ↓Inflammatory signaling improving steatosis and insulin resistance	[60]

(Continued)

TABLE 16.1 (Continued)

Probiotic/symbiotic/dose	Animal model	Duration	Outcome	Reference
L. acidophilus ATCC 43121 (2×10^6 cfu/day).	Hypercholesterolemia-induced in Sprague-Dawley rats.	21 days	↓Total serum cholesterol and VLDL + IDL + LDL cholesterol ↑Total fecal acid sterols excretion and ↓Primary bile acids ↑Secondary bile acids	[47]
L. paracasei NCC2461 (10^8 cfu/day).	Female germ-free mice C3H colonized with human baby flora.	14 days	↓Plasma VLDL and LDL ↑Hepatic TAG ↓Glutathione	[61]
L. paracasei NCC2461 and *L. rhamnosus* NCC4007 (10^8 cfu/day).	Female germ-free mice C3H colonized with human baby flora.	14 days	↓Plasma VLDL and LDL ↑TAG ↓Fecal excretion of bile acids ↓Acetate and butyrate in the cecum ↓Acetate/propionate in the liver	[62]
L. paracasei NCC2461 or *L. rhamnosus* NCC4007 (10^8 cfu/day) with GOS[3] (3%).	Female germ-free mice C3H colonized with human baby flora.	14 days	↑Propionate and butyrate in cecum with *L. rhamnosus* ↓Isobutyrate in cecum with *L. paracasei* ↓Liver TAG ↑Glycogen with *L. paracasei*	[63]
L. rhamnosus GG (10^8 cfu/day) with GOS[2] (3%).	Female germ-free mice C3H colonized with human baby flora.	14 days	↓Hepatic lipids and serum lipoproteins ↑*Bifidobacterium* and *B. longum*	[31]

[1]TAG, triacylglycerol.
[2]Previously labeled as *B. longum* and *B. infantis*.
[3]GOS, galactosyl-oligosaccharides.

hepatic acetate:propionate ratio, related with the serum lipid lowering effects [62]. Furthermore, the combined administration of these probiotics with GOS in comparison with their individual administration to the same mice model indicated that the prebiotic positively influenced hepatic lipids and exerted a stronger affect on the gut microbiota composition than the probiotics [63]. In particular, *L. paracasei* NCC2461 in combination with GOS led to the highest reductions in hepatic triglycerides and increases in hepatic amino acids and glycogen, suggesting increased gluconeogenesis and glycogenesis. *L. rhamnosus* NCC4007 in combination with GOS increased urinary taurine and creatine, suggesting a higher muscular activity and possible changes in energy expenditure [63]. Similarly, studies focused on the effects of GOS combined or not with *L. rhamnosus* NCC4007 on a humanized flora mice model have showed that synbiotic administration reduced the levels of plasma lipoproteins, hepatic triglycerides and kidney lipids [31]. The prebiotic seemed to be the main ingredient responsible for the reduction of triglycerides in the liver, whereas the probiotic *L. rhamnosus* was the main one responsible for the decrease in plasma lipoproteins. The synbiotic also induced a remarkable stimulation of both growth and activity of bifidobacteria and, in particular, of *B. longum* [31]. Probiotic supplementation also reduced ascorbate in the adrenal gland, which is an essential co-factor of catecholamine biosynthesis, anti-oxidation and adrenal steroidogenesis and could be related to changes in lipoproteins and gluconeogenesis.

6.2. Probiotic Effects on Biomarkers of Metabolic Disorders in Humans

The human clinical trials carried out to investigate the possible benefits of probiotic intake on serum lipids and cholesterol levels and, more recently, on blood pressure and glucose regulation are summarized in Table 16.2.

Supplementation of hypercholesterolemic patients with the probiotic bacteria *L. plantarum* 299v significantly lowered the serum concentrations of LDL cholesterol and fibrinogen [64]. A functional food product containing the same strain, *L. plantarum* 299v, was also shown to decrease different biomarkers of cardiovascular disease risk shown in Table 16.2 of heavy smokers. Monocytes isolated from the subjects treated with *L. plantarum* 299v also showed significantly reduced adhesion to native and stimulated human umbilical vein endothelial cells. Therefore, the probiotic product seemed to reduce cardiovascular disease risk factors [65]. The possible hypocholesterolemic affect of yogurt supplemented with *L. acidophilus* 145, *B. longum* 913 and OFS in comparison with control yogurt was evaluated through a cross-over trial in women [66]. This trial included three periods (7 weeks each): in the first period, control yogurt was administered to all 29 women; in the second period, synbiotic yogurt was administered to 18 women and control yogurt to 11 women; and in the third period, the reverse of that in the second period was administered. Although serum concentrations of total cholesterol and the LDL cholesterol were not influenced by the synbiotic, the HDL cholesterol concentration increased significantly and the ratio of LDL/HDL cholesterol decreased [66]. In contrast, the administration of capsules containing *L. fermentum* to subjects with elevated serum cholesterol did not lead to significant changes in total cholesterol, HDL cholesterol, triglyceride or liver enzyme activities over time. Only LDL cholesterol levels showed a modest downward trend on both probiotic and placebo groups [67]. Similarly, the effect of the intake of capsules containing *L. acidophilus* DDS-1 and *B. longum* UABL-14 and 10–15 mg OFS on plasma lipids of normocholesterolemic young women and men was evaluated [68]. In this study, plasma concentrations of total cholesterol, HDL cholesterol, LDL cholesterol and triglyceride were not altered by consumption of synbiotic or placebo

TABLE 16.2　Effects of probiotics on biomarkers of metabolic disorders in humans

Probiotic/symbiotic (dose/day)	Administration pattern/duration	Study-design[1]	Outcome	Reference
L plantarum 299 v (5.0 × 10⁷ cfu/day fermented milk).	Hypercholesterolemic patients; heavy smokers/6 weeks.	CRDB CRDB	↓Plasma LDL cholesterol and fibrinogen	[64]
			↓Systolic blood pressure, leptin and fibrinogen, F(2)-isoprostanes and interleukin 6 and cardiovascular risk	[65]
L. acidophilus 145 (10⁶⁻⁸ cfu/g), *B. longum* 913 (at least 10⁵ cfu/g) and 1% OFS[4] in yogurt containing the starter cultures *S. thermophilus* and *Lactococcus lactis* (300 g/ daily).	Healthy women, 15 normocholesterolemic and 14 hypercholesterolemic; three periods of 7 weeks: (1) control for all/(2) and (3) control-symbiotic exchange.	CO	↑Plasma HDL cholesterol ↓LDL/HDL cholesterol ratio Total cholesterol and LDL cholesterol NS[2]	[66]
L. fermentum PCC (2 × 10⁹ cfu/capsule; 2 cap/ day).	Hypercholesterolemic patients/10 weeks.	CDB	Plasma total cholesterol, HDL cholesterol, and TAG[3] or liver enzymes NS	[67]
L. acidophilus DDS-1 *B. longum* UABL-14 (10⁹ cfu) plus OFS[4] (10–15 mg) per capsule; 3 cap/day.	55 normocholesterolemic subjects; 2 months or 2 menstrual cycles.	CRSB	Plasma concentrations of total cholesterol, HDL cholesterol, LDL cholesterol and TAG NS	[68]
L. rhamnosus GG and *B. lactis* Bb12 (10⁹ cfu each/day) plus dietary recommendations.	Intake by women from first trimester of pregnancy onwards.	CRDB/SB	Highest and lowest intakes of specific nutrients associated with higher blood pressure in children of 6 months	[69]
L. rhamnosus GG and *B. lactis* Bb12 (10⁹ cfu each/day) plus dietary counseling.	Intake by women from first trimester of pregnancy onwards.	CRDB/SB	↓Blood glucose concentrations ↑Glucose tolerance during pregnancy and over the 12-month postpartum period	[70]

[1]C, placebo-controlled; R, randomized; DB, double blind; SB, single blind trial; CO, cross-over.
[2]NS, no significant effects.
[3]TAG, triacylglycerol.
[4]OFS, oligofructose (short-chain inulin-type fructan).

capsules [68]. Probiotic supplementation to pregnant mothers is also thought to influence the mother and infant metabolism and later health. Thus, the impact of maternal nutrition together with probiotic supplementation (*L. rhamnosus* GG and *B. lactis* Bb12) during pregnancy on infant blood pressure was determined in a clinical trial, which included three pregnant women groups: the first followed a modified dietary intake according to current recommendations and probiotics (diet/probiotic), the second followed dietary recommendations and received placebo (diet/placebo), and the third received placebo (control/placebo) from the first trimester of pregnancy onwards [69]. The highest and lowest intakes of specific nutrients, such as carbohydrates and monounsaturated fatty acids, were associated with higher blood pressure in children at the age 6 months compared with the middle ones, suggesting that dietary counseling can promote child health by programming blood pressure. A similar intervention study on the effects of probiotic supplementation together with dietary counseling on glucose metabolism in pregnant women was conducted recently, leading to more conclusive results [70]. Blood glucose concentrations were the lowest in the diet/probiotic group during pregnancy and over the 12-month postpartum period. Glucose tolerance was also better in the diet/probiotic group compared with the control/placebo group during the last trimester of pregnancy and over the 12-month postpartum period. The study suggests that dietary counseling with probiotics can improve blood glucose control in a normoglycemic population and, thus, may provide potential novel means for the prophylactic and therapeutic management of glucose disorders [70].

7. PREBIOTIC EFFECTS ON METABOLIC AND OBESITY BIOMARKERS *IN VIVO*

7.1. Prebiotic Effects on Metabolic and Obesity Biomarkers in Animal Models

A number of reports have shown that some prebiotics play beneficial roles in weight management and biomarkers of metabolic disorders in conventional and several animal models (Table 16.3). Most studies have focused on the evaluation of inulin-type fructans (inulin and OFS) and, lately, of GOS. The beneficial effects of prebiotics have been mainly explained by their ability to regulate lipid metabolism, glycemia, low-grade inflammation, and peptide hormones controlling hunger and satiety. These beneficial roles are partly due to the ability of prebiotics to modify the gut microbiota composition and its associated functions in immunity and metabolism.

Overall, the administration of inulin-type fructans has been shown to decrease serum lipids, liver lipids (steatosis), fat mass development and food intake in normal and in obese rats, mice and hamsters; and to exert antidiabetic and anti-inflammatory affects in streptozotocin-treated rats and high fat fed mice [71]. Doses of 10% inulin-type fructans on a weight basis have generally been effective on animal studies, although the effect varied depending on the prebiotic type, diet and animal model (Table 16.3).

In diverse animal models (fat fed rats/hamsters, apolipoprotein E-deficient mice and obese [*cp/cp*] corpulent rats, lacking a functional leptin receptor), inulin-type fructans primarily regulate serum lipids by decreasing triglyceridemia, in the fasted and/or the postprandial state, together or not with cholesterolemia [72–74]. The hypotriglyceridemic effects of inulin-type fructans seem to be due to a reduction in *de novo* fatty acid synthesis in the liver by a reduced gene expression and activity of lipogenic enzymes and lower hepatic secretion rate of VLDL-triacylglycerol, while repression of lipogenesis is not observed in adipose tissue [75]. The decrease in plasma cholesterol has been attributed either to the ability of the propionic acid generated by the gut microbiota to inhibit cholesterol synthesis, to bacterial modifications in the bile acid metabolism leading to impaired re-absorption of circulating bile acids, or to the steroid-biding properties of the prebiotics, leading its fecal excretion [76]. In other models, such as in obese *fa/fa* Zucker rats, having a leptin receptor defect, administration of inulin-type fructans reduced hepatic steatosis, without affecting postprandial triglyceridemia, probably due to a reduced availability of non-esterified fatty acids coming from adipose

TABLE 16.3　Prebiotic effects on metabolic and obesity biomarkers in animal models

Prebiotic	Animal model	Dose/duration	Outcome	Reference
Inulin	Male golden Syrian hamsters fed a high fat and cholesterol diet.	8, 12 or 16/100 g diet for 5 weeks	↓Plasma cholesterol all dose ↓VLDL-cholesterol at 16% ↓Plasma TAG[1] at 12–16% ↓Hepatic cholesterol at 8%	[72]
Inulin/OFS[2]/inulin plus OFS	Male apo E-deficient mice.	10 g/100 g diet for 16 weeks	↓Plasma cholesterol with inulin ↓Plasma TAG with all fructans ↓Hepatic cholesterol with inulin and inulin-OFS ↓Hepatic TAG with all	[73]
Inulin/inulin plus high protein	Obese (cp/cp) male James C. Russell corpulent (JCR: LA-cp) rats.	9 g/100 g diet for 3 weeks	↑GLP-1 secretion ↓Plasma glucose ↓Plasma TAG ↓Plasma cholesterol	[74]
OFS	Obese (fa/fa) Zucker rats.	10 g/100 g diet for 7 weeks	↓Hepatic TAG Fat mass development measured as epididymal fat mass ↓Body weight slightly	[77]
OFS	Obese (fa/fa) Zucker rats.	10 g/100 g diet for 8 weeks	↓Hepatic TAG ↓Energy intake and body weight	[78]
OFS	Male Wistar-Han rats fed a high fructose diet.	10 g/100 g diet for 4 weeks	↓Plasma leptin ↓Hepatic TAG	[79]
Inulin	Male Wistar rats fed a high fat/high sucrose diet.	5 g/100 g diet for 8 weeks	↓Plasma TAG and fatty acids ↓Plasma glucose ↓Hepatic TAG and fatty acids	[80]

Prebiotic	Model	Dose/duration	Effects	Ref.
Inulin/OFS[1]/inulin plus OFS	Wistar rats.	10 g/100 g diet for 16 weeks	↓Elevated blood pressure; ↓Heart peroxidation and renal damages; ↓Plasma TAG	[81]
OFS	Streptozotocin-treated diabetic male Wistar rats.	10 g/100 g diet for 6 weeks	↓Food intake; ↑Glucose tolerance and insulin secretion; ↑Portal and colonic GLP-1(7-36)	[82]
OFS	High fat diet fed male C57bl6/J mice.	10 g/100 g diet for 4 weeks	↓Energy intake, epididymal fat mass and body weight gain; ↓Glycemia; ↑Colonic proglucagon expression; ↑Insulin secretion	[83]
OFS	High fat fed male C57bl6/J mice.	10 g/100 g diet for 14 weeks	↓Endotoxemia, plasma and adipose tissue pro-inflammatory cytokines; ↑Glucose tolerance and glucose-induced insulin secretion	[26]
OFS	*ob/ob* mice C57BL/6.	10 g/100 g diet for 4 weeks	↓Intestinal permeability; ↓Inflammatory markers (LPS, cyokines, etc.); ↑Portal plasma GLP-2 levels and the jejunum and colon precursor proglucagon mRNA	[84]
GOS[3]	Germ-free mice plus human baby microbiota.	3 g/100 g diet for 2 weeks	↓Hepatic and kidney TAG	[31]

[1]TAG triacylglycerol.
[2]OFS, oligofructose (short-chain inulin-type fructan).
[3]GOS, galactosyl-oligosaccharides.

tissue, since fatty mass and body weight were reduced [77, 78]. In addition, positive effects on liver triglycerides (steatosis) have been reported, for instance, in conventional rats fed a high-fructose diet and a high fat/high sucrose diet [79, 80]. The affects of inulin-type fructans on hepatic lipids were related to their fermentation products derived from the metabolic activity of the gut microbiota, which led to increased cecal and portal vein concentrations of propionate in rats fed fructans compared with controls. In hepatocytes isolated from liver of Zucker rats, it was shown that propionate, at the concentrations measured in the portal vein of rats treated with fructans, selectively decreased the incorporation of acetate into total lipids, a phenomenon that could contribute, along with the lower energy intake, to less triglyceride accumulation in the liver [78]. In some studies, administration of inulin has also led to both reductions in total serum cholesterol and hepatic cholesterol content, for instance in apoE-deficient animals [73] and fat and cholesterol fed hamsters [72]. In general, the effects of long-chain inulin on lipid metabolism and associated disorders (e.g. atherosclerosis risk) seem to be more potent than those of OFS [73]. In diverse animal models, fructan feeding also led to reductions in fat mass development and body weight for long treatments [77].

Inulin-type fructans also show beneficial effects against common features of metabolic syndrome and type-2 diabetes [81]. In fructose-fed rats, which constitute a model of metabolic syndrome, inulin supplementation and the combination of OFS and inulin supplementation prevented fructose-induced elevated blood pressure, susceptibility to heart peroxidation and renal damages. Moreover, inulin, OFS and the combination of OFS and inulin prevented fructose-induced hypertriglyceridemia. Therefore, dietary supplementation with inulin-type fructans was efficient against fructose-induced hypertension and the effects were most pronounced for long-chain inulin and its combination. The anti-hypertensive effect of inulin could be explained by the reduction of the high fructose-induced oxidative stress [81]. In the streptozotocin-treated rat, OFS intake also lowered postprandial glycemia and partially restored insulin secretion [82]. In high fat diet fed mice, supplementation with OFS also reduced body weight, epididymal fat mass and glycemia [83]. Improvements in glucose tolerance resulting from OFS consumption have been explained by the roles of fructans in lipogenesis and its relation to glucose and insulin levels, as well as by their effects on expression of anorexigenic peptides, such as GLP-1 [82]. In particular, the fermentation products of OFS promoted L cell differentiation in the proximal colon leading to an increase of GLP-1 level in the portal vein and its precursor, proglucagon mRNA, in the proximal colon, which promotes satiety [71]. OFS was also able to modulate other gastrointestinal peptides (such as PYY and ghrelin) that could be involved in the control of food intake in rats. Moreover, the administration of OFS to high fat fed mice increased the intestinal *Bifidobacterium* numbers and normalized the endotoxemia associated with the high fat diet [26]. *Bifidobacterium* numbers significantly and positively correlated with improved glucose tolerance, glucose-induced insulin secretion and normalized inflammatory tone (decreased endotoxemia, and plasma and adipose tissue pro-inflammatory cytokines). Furthermore, the administration of OFS to genetically obese mice (*ob/ob*) has been shown to induce specific changes in the gut microbiota characterized by increases in *Lactobacillus*, *Bifidobacterium*, and *C. coccoides-E. rectale* groups, which led to reductions in intestinal permeability and to an improvement in tight-junction integrity and inflammatory markers (plasma LPS and cytokines and decreased hepatic expression of inflammatory and oxidative stress markers [84]. These effects were associated with increases in portal plasma GLP-2 levels and its precursor (the proglucagon mRNA), in the jejunum and colon. Thus, the results demonstrated that gut microbiota participates to the inflammatory phenotype of *ob/ob* mice and that

TABLE 16.4 Prebiotic effects on metabolic disorders and obesity biomarkers in humans

Prebiotic	Subjects/dose and duration	Study-design[1]	Outcome	Reference
Inulin	Healthy subjects, non-obese, 10 g/day for 3 weeks.	CRDB CO	↓Plasma TAG ↓Hepatic lipogenesis Plasma cholesterol NS[2]	[85]
OFS[3]	Subjects with hypercholesterolemia, 10.6 g/day for 2 months.	CRDB CO	↓Postprandial insulin response Lipids NS	[86]
OFS	Patients with non-alcoholic steatohepatitis, 16 g/day for 8 weeks.	CRDB CO	↓Serum aminotransferases and aspartate aminotransferase Plasma lipids NS	[87]
Lactulose and rhamnose	Healthy men, 25 g/d for 4 weeks.	CR CO	↓Plasma TAG Plasma cholesterol NS	[88]
GOS[4] and lcOFS[5] (9/1)	Infants till 6 months of age, 0.6 g/100 mL.	CRDB	Plasma cholesterol and LDL-cholesterol NS	[89]
OFS	Healthy, 20 g/day for 4 weeks.	DB CO	↓Basal hepatic glucose production Insulin-stimulated glucose metabolism NS	[90]
OFS	Type 2 diabetics, 20 g/day for 4 weeks.	DB	Glucose and lipids NS	[91]
OFS	Healthy, non-obese subjects 21–39 years, 16 g/day for 2 weeks.	CRSB	↑Satiety following breakfast and dinner ↓Reduces hunger and prospective food consumption following dinner	[92]
OFS	Healthy, non-obese subjects , 9–3 years, 8 g/day for 12 months.		↓Increase in body mass index (BMI), BMI Z-score and total fat mass	[93]

[1]C, placebo-controlled; R, randomized; DB, double blind; SB, single blind trial; CO, cross-over.
[2]NS, no significant effects.
[3]OFS, oligofructose (short-chain inulin-type fructans).
[4]GOS, galactosyl-oligosaccharides.
[5]lcFOS, long-chain inulin-type fructans.

prebiotic-induced changes in the gut microbiota contribute to the improvement of the gut barrier function during obesity and diabetes [84].

More recently, the effects of another classical prebiotic, GOS, on lipids and glucose metabolism have been evaluated in animals. In germ-free mice colonized by human baby microbiota, the administration of GOS for 2 weeks also led to increases in *B. longum*, *B. breve* and *B. distasonis* in the jejunum and feces, while *E. coli* and *C. perfringens* counts were reduced in feces. Prebiotic supplementation also led to reductions of lipids in the liver and kidney, but not in blood plasma lipoproteins. The effects on hepatic lipids were related to the ability of prebiotics to reduce the hepatic lipogenic enzyme activity and incorporation of triacylglycerol into nascent lipoproteins as well as to reduce postprandial insulinemia and glycemia [31]. Prebiotic supplementation also led to increases of pancreatic (phosphocholine, betaine, dimethylglycine and sarcosine), and liver (choline and betaine) metabolites, which suggest higher betaine synthesis from choline and stimulated transmethylation in the methionine cycle, evidenced by reduced levels of cysteine in the pancreas. This alteration of transmethylation metabolic pathways (homocysteine-betaine) could be of interest to the control of metabolic disorders due the role of homocysteine in insulin release and pancreatic β cell function in diabetes [31].

7.2. Prebiotic Effects on Metabolic and Obesity Biomarkers in Humans

In humans, inulin-type fructans have been generally found to be effective on normalization of metabolic disorder biomarkers at doses of 10–20 g/day, although the results have not been as consistent as those reported in animals [74].

In general, human studies demonstrate that prebiotics can reduce triglyceridemia and to a lesser extent cholesterolemia. The effects of inulin seemed to be more consistent than those of OFS and, specially, in a situation of increased liver-lipogenesis (high carbohydrate diet) and hyperlipidemia. Supplementation with inulin to subjects under a moderately high carbohydrate, low fat diet has been shown to exert a beneficial affect on plasma lipids. In particular, healthy subjects submitted to this intervention showed decreased hepatic lipogenesis and plasma triacylglycerol concentrations, suggesting an effect on the reduction of atherosclerosis risk factors [85]. OFS intake also led to slight significant effects on postprandial insulin response, but not on lipid metabolism in individuals with mild hypercholesterolemia [86]. Ingestion of OFS decreased serum aminotransferases and aspartate aminotransferase in seven patients with non-alcoholic steatohepatitis, suggesting a putative interest in the management of liver diseases; however, this intervention only caused a slight decrease in plasma triacylglycerol concentrations [87]. Lactulose, which increases colonic acetate production, and L-rhamnose, which increases propionate, have been shown to decrease serum triacylglycerols, but did not affect serum cholesterol concentrations in healthy men [88]. An infant formula containing GOS and long-chain fructo-oligosaccharides in a ratio of 9:1, did not exert significant effects on total cholesterol and LDL cholesterol in infants compared with those receiving a control infant formula [89].

Prebiotic effects on glucose metabolism, satiety and body weight have also been evaluated in humans, showing moderate positive results that seem to depend on the metabolic status of the human subjects (health or diabetic). For instance, a daily consumption of 20 g fructo-oligosaccharides decreased basal hepatic glucose production in healthy subjects, without any affect on insulin-stimulated glucose metabolism [90]. However, this prebiotic had no affect on glucose and lipid metabolism in type 2 diabetics [91]. In a pilot study with 10 human subjects, OFS treatment also increased satiety following breakfast and dinner, reduced hunger and prospective food consumption following dinner

[92]. A long-term study (12 months) including 100 subjects, showed that subjects who received the prebiotic supplement had a smaller increase in BMI, BMI Z-score and total fat mass, compared with the control group [93].

8. CONCLUSION

Scientific evidence has demonstrated an association between the composition of the gut microbiota and body weight, which is under the influence of the diet and the lifestyle. The use of systems biology, together with metagenomic and metabolomic approaches, have also revealed a large number of roles possibly played by the gut microbiota in the metabolic and immune dysfunction associated with obesity. On this basis, the use of dietary strategies targeting the gut ecosystem has emerged as an additional tool to control metabolic disorders. So far only a few trials have demonstrated that the administration of probiotics, prebiotics and their combination (synbiotics) exerts moderate positive effects *in vivo*. Nevertheless, the findings indicate that advances in this field could be of value in improving the intervention strategies to treat and prevent obesity and its associated metabolic disorders. The future success of these strategies will entirely depend on a better understanding of the complex interactions taking place between the human genome, the microbiome and the diet.

ACKNOWLEDGMENTS

This work was supported by grants AGL2008-01440/ALI and Consolider Fun-C-Food CSD2007-00063 from the Spanish Ministry of Science and Innovation and AP 124/09 from Consejería de Sanidad (Valencia, Spain). The scholarship to A. Santacruz from CONACYT (Mexico) is fully acknowledged.

References

1. Konturek, S. J., Konturek, J. W., Pawlik, T., & Brzozowski, T. (2004). Brain-gut axis and its role in the control of food intake. *Journal of Physiology and Pharmacology, 55*, 137–154.
2. Zeyda, M., & Stulnig, T. M. (2007). Adipose tissue macrophages. *Immunology Letters, 112*, 61–67.
3. Bellisari, A. (2008). Evolutionary origins of obesity. *Obesity Reviews, 9*, 165–180.
4. Hays, N. P., Galassetti, P. R., & Coker, R. H. (2008). Prevention and treatment of type 2 diabetes: Current role of lifestyle, natural product, and pharmacological interventions. *Pharmacology and Therapeutics, 118*, 181–191.
5. Xu, J., Mahowald, M. A., Ley, R. E., et al. (2007). Evolution of symbiotic bacteria in the distal human intestine. *PLoS Biology, 19*, e156.
6. Gill, S. R., Pop, M., Deboy, R. T., et al. (2006). Metagenomic analysis of the human distal gut microbiome. *Science, 312*, 1355–1359.
7. Turnbaugh, P. J., Ley, R. E., Hamady, M., et al. (2007). The human microbiome project. *Nature, 449*, 804–810.
8. Reid, G., Sanders, M. E., Gaskins, H. R., et al. (2003). New scientific paradigms for probiotics and prebiotics. *Journal of Clinical Gastroenterology, 37*, 105–118.
9. Sanz, Y., Nadal, I., & Sánchez, E. (2007). Probiotics as drugs against human gastrointestinal infections. *Rec Pat Anti-Infect Drug Disc, 2*, 148–156.
10. Medina, M., Izquierdo, E., Ennahar, S., & Sanz, Y. (2007). Differential immunomodulatory properties of *Bifidobacterium logum* strains: relevance to probiotic selection and clinical applications. *Clinical and Experimental Immunology, 150*, 531–538.
11. FAO/WHO working group Guidelines for the Evaluation of Probiotics in Food. 2002. http://ftp.fao.org/es/esn/food/wgreport2.pdf.
12. Roberfroid, M. (2007). Prebiotics: the concept revisited. *Journal of Nutrition, 137*, 830–837.
13. Haarman, M., & Knol, J. (2005). Quantitative real-time PCR assays to identify and quantify fecal *Bifidobacterium* species in infants receiving a prebiotic infant formula. *Applied and Environmental Microbiology, 71*, 2318–2324.
14. Turnbaugh, P. J., Hamady, M., Yatsunenko, T., et al. (2009). A core gut microbiome in obese and lean twins. *Nature, 457*, 480–484.
15. Waldram, A., Holmes, E., Wang, Y., et al. (2009). Top-down systems biology modelling of host metabotype-microbiome associations in obese rodents [Epub ahead of print]. *Journal of Proteome Research, 10*.
16. Ley, R. E., Bäckhed, F., Turnbaugh, P., et al. (2005). Obesity alters gut microbial ecology. *Proceedings of the National Academy of Sciences of the United States of America, 102*, 11070–11075.

17. Samuel, B. S., Hansen, E. E., Manchester, J. K., et al. (2007). Genomic and metabolic adaptations of *Methanobrevibacter smithii* to the human gut. *Proceedings of the National Academy of Sciences of the United States of America, 104,* 10643–10648.

18. Turnbaugh, P. J., Bäckhed, F., Fulton, L., & Gordon, J. I. (2008). Diet-induced obesity is linked to marked but reversible alterations in the mouse distal gut microbiome. *Cell Host Microbe, 17,* 213–223.

19. Ley, R. E., Turnbaugh, P. J., Klein, S., & Gordon, J. I. (2006). Microbial ecology: human gut microbes associated with obesity. *Nature, 444,* 1022–1023.

20. Nadal, I., Santacruz, A., Marcos, A., et al. (2008). Shifts in clostridia, bacteroides and immunoglobulin-coating fecal bacteria associated with weight loss in obese adolescents [Epub ahead of print]. *International Journal of Obesity, 9.*

21. Santacruz, A., Marcos, A., Wärnberg, J., et al. (2009). Interplay between weight loss and gut microbiata composition in overweight adolescents [Epub ahead of print]. *Obesity, 2.*

22. Duncan, S. H., Belenguer, A., Holtrop, G., et al. (2007). Reduced dietary intake of carbohydrates by obese subjects results in decreased concentrations of butyrate and butyrate-producing bacteria in feces. *Applied and Environmental Microbiology, 73,* 1073–1078.

23. Ley, R. E., Lozupone, C. A., Hamady, M., et al. (2008). Worlds within worlds: evolution of the vertebrate gut microbiota. *Nature Reviews Microbiology, 6,* 776–788.

24. Kalliomäki, M., Collado, M. C., Salminen, S., & Isolauri, E. (2008). Early differences in fecal microbiota composition in children may predict overweight. *The American Journal of Clinical Nutrition, 87,* 534–538.

25. Turnbaugh, P. J., Ley, R. E., Mahowald, M. A., et al. (2006). An obesity-associated gut microbiome with increased capacity for energy harvest. *Nature, 444,* 1027–1031.

26. Cani, P. D., Neyrinck, A. M., Fava, F., et al. (2007). Selective increases of bifidobacteria in gut microflora improve high-fat-diet-induced diabetes in mice through a mechanism associated with endotoxemia. *Diabetologia, 50,* 2374–2383.

27. Bäckhed, F., Ding, H., Wang, T., et al. (2004). The gut microbiota as an environmental factor that regulates fat storage. *Proceedings of the National Academy of Sciences of the United States of America, 101,* 15718–15723.

28. Hooper, L. V., Midtvedt, T., & Gordon, J. I. (2002). How host-microbial interactions shape the nutrient environment of the mammalian intestine. *Annual Review of Nutrition, 22,* 283–307.

29. Flint, H. J., Bayer, E. A., Rincon, M. T., et al. (2008). Polysaccharide utilization by gut bacteria: potential for new insights from genomic analysis. *Nature Reviews Microbiology, 6,* 121–131.

30. Hamer, H. M., Jonkers, D., & Venema, K. (2008). The role of butyrate on colonic function. *Alimentary Pharmacology & Therapeutics, 27,* 104–119.

31. Martin, F. P., Sprenger, N., Yap, I. K., et al. (2009). Pan-organismal gut microbiome-host metabolic crosstalk [Epub ahead of print]. *Journal of Proteome Research, 13.*

32. Wolever, T. M., Spadafora, P. J., Cunnane, S. C., & Pencharz, P. B. (1995). Propionate inhibits incorporation of colonic [1,2–13C] acetate into plasma lipids in humans. *The American Journal of Clinical Nutrition, 61,* 1241–1247.

33. Leitch, E. C., Walker, A. W., Duncan, S. H., et al. (2007). Selective colonization of insoluble substrates by human faecal bacteria. *Environmental Microbiology, 9,* 667–679.

34. Samuel, B. S., & Gordon, J. I. (2006). A humanized gnotobiotic mouse model of host-archaeal-bacterial mutualism. *Proceedings of the National Academy of Sciences of the United States of America, 103,* 10011–10016.

35. Hooper, L. V., Wong, M. H., Thelin, A., et al. (2001). Molecular analysis of commensal host-microbial relationships in the intestine. *Science, 291,* 881–884.

36. Bäckhed, F., Manchester, J. K., Semenkovich, C. F., & Gordon, J. I. (2007). Mechanisms underlying the resistance to diet-induced obesity in germ-free mice. *Proceedings of the National Academy of Sciences of the United States of America, 104,* 979–984.

37. Ridlon, J. M., Kang, D. J., & Hylemon, P. B. (2006). Bile salt biotransformations by human intestinal bacteria. *Journal of Lipid Research, 47,* 241–259.

38. Norin, E. (2008). Intestinal cholesterol conversion in adults and elderly from four different European countries. *Annals of Nutrition & Metabolism, 52,* 12–14.

39. Matarese, G., & La Cava, A. (2004). The intricate interface between immune system and metabolism. *Trends in Immunology, 25,* 193–200.

40. Samuel, B. S., Shaito, A., Motoike, T., et al. (2008). Effects of the gut microbiota on host adiposity are modulated by the short-chain fatty-acid binding G protein-coupled receptor, Gpr41. *Proceedings of the National Academy of Sciences of the United States of America, 105,* 16767–16772.

41. Fetissov, S. O., Hamze-Sinno, M., Coëffier, M., et al. (2008). Autoantibodies against appetite-regulating peptide hormones and neuropeptides: putative modulation by gut microflora. *Nutrition, 24,* 348–359.

42. Bailey, M. T., Lubach, G. R., & Coe, C. L. (2004). Prenatal stress alters bacterial colonization of the gut in infant monkeys. *Journal of Pediatric Gastroenterology and Nutrition, 38,* 414–421.

43. Sudo, N., Chida, Y., Aiba, Y., et al. (2004). Postnatal microbial colonization programs the hypothalamic-pituitary-adrenal system for stress response in mice. *The Journal of Physiology, 558,* 263–275.

44. Simonyte, K., Rask, E., Näslund, I., et al. (2009). Obesity is accompanied by disturbances in peripheral

glucocorticoid metabolism and changes in FA recycling [Epub ahead of print]. *Obesity, 9.*

45. Uribe, A., Alam, M., Johansson, O., et al. (1994). Microflora modulates endocrine cells in the gastrointestinal mucosa of the rat. *Gastroenterology, 107,* 1259–1269.

46. Marston, O. J., & Heisler, L. K. (2009). Targeting the serotonin 2C receptor for the treatment of obesity and type 2 diabetes. *Neuropsychopharmacology, 34,* 252–253.

47. Park, Y. H., Kim, J. G., Shin, Y. W., et al. (2007). Effect of dietary inclusion of *Lactobacillus acidophilus* ATCC 43121 on cholesterol metabolism in rats. *J Microb Biotech, 17,* 655–662.

48. Baba, N., Samson, S., Bourdet-Sicard, R., et al. (2008). Commensal bacteria trigger a full dendritic cell maturation program that promotes the expansion of non-Tr1 suppressor T cells. *Journal of Leukocyte Biology, 84,* 468–476.

49. Tsukumo, D. M., Carvalho-Filho, M. A., Carvalheira, J. B., et al. (2007). Loss-of-function mutation in Toll-like receptor 4 prevents diet-induced obesity and insulin resistance. *Diabetes, 56,* 1986–1998.

50. Siebler, J., Galle, P. R., & Weber, M. M. (2008). The gut-liver-axis: Endotoxemia, inflammation, insulin resistance and NASH. *Journal of Hepatology, 48,* 1032–1034.

51. Lajunen, T., Vikatmaa, P., Bloigu, A., et al. (2008). Chlamydial LPS and high-sensitivity CRP levels in serum are associated with an elevated body mass index in patients with cardiovascular disease. *Innate Immunity, 14,* 375–382.

52. Macia, L., Delacre, M., & Abboud, G., et al. (2006). Impairment of dendritic cell functionality and steady-state number in obese mice. *Journal of Immunology, 177,* 5997–6006.

53. Verwaerde, C., Delanoye, A., Macia, L., et al. (2006). Influence of high-fat feeding on both naive and antigen-experienced T cell immune response in DO10.11 mice. *Scandinavian Journal of Immunology, 64,* 457–466.

54. Abdullahi, M., Annibale, B., Capoccia, D., et al. (2008). The eradication of *Helicobacter pylori* is affected by body mass index (BMI). *Obesity Surgery, 18,* 1450–1454.

55. Sato, M., Uzu, K., Yoshida, T., et al. (2008). Effects of milk fermented by *Lactobacillus gasseri* SBT2055 on adipocyte size in rats. *The British Journal of Nutrition, 99,* 1013–1017.

56. Sousa, R., Halper, J., Zhang, J., et al. (2008). Effect of *Lactobacillus acidophilus* supernatants on body weight and leptin expression in rats. *BMC Complementary and Alternative Medicine, 8,* 5.

57. Lesniewska, V., Rowland, I., Cani, P. D., et al. (2006). Effect on components of the intestinal microflora and plasma neuropeptide levels of feeding *Lactobacillus delbrueckii, Bifidobacterium lactis,* and inulin to adult and elderly rats. *Applied and Environmental Microbiology, 72,* 6533–6538.

58. Yadav, H., Jain, S., & Sinhá, P. R. (2007). Antidiabetic effect of probiotic dahi containing *Lactobacillus acidophilus* and *Lactobacillus casei* in high fructose fed rats. *Nutrition, 23,* 62–68.

59. Yadav, H., Jain, S., & Sinha, P. R. (2008). Oral administration of dahi containing probiotic *Lactobacillus acidophilus* and *Lactobacillus casei* delayed the progression of streptozotocin-induced diabetes in rats. *The Journal of dairy research, 75,* 189–195.

60. Ma, X., Hua, J., & Li, Z. (2008). Probiotics improve high fat diet-induced hepatic steatosis and insulin resistance by increasing hepatic NKT cells. *Journal of Hepatology, 49,* 821–830.

61. Martin, F. P., Dumas, M. E., Wang, Y., et al. (2007). A top-down systems biology view of microbiome-mammalian metabolic interactions in a mouse model. *Molecular Systems Biology, 3,* 112.

62. Martin, F. P., Wang, Y., Sprenger, N., et al. (2008). Probiotic modulation of symbiotic gut microbial-host metabolic interactions in a humanized microbiome mouse model. *Molecular Systems Biology, 4,* 157.

63. Martin, F. P., Wang, Y., Sprenger, N., et al. (2008). Top-down systems biology integration of conditional prebiotic modulated transgenomic interactions in a humanized microbiome mouse model. *Molecular Systems Biology, 4,* 205.

64. Bukowska, H., Pieczul-Mróz, J., Jastrzebska, M., et al. (1998). Decrease in fibrinogen and LDL-cholesterol levels upon supplementation of diet with *Lactobacillus plantarum* in subjects with moderately elevated cholesterol. *Atherosclerosis, 137,* 437–438.

65. Naruszewicz, M., Johansson, M. L., Zapolska-Downar, D., & Bukowska, H. (2002). Effect of *Lactobacillus plantarum* 299v on cardiovascular disease risk factors in smokers. *The American Journal of Clinical Nutrition, 76,* 1249–1255.

66. Kiessling, G., Schneider, J., & Jahreis, G. (2002). Long-term consumption of fermented dairy products over 6 months increases HDL cholesterol. *European Journal of Clinical Nutrition, 56,* 843–849.

67. Simons, L. A., Amansec, S. G., & Conway, P. (2006). Effect of *Lactobacillus fermentum* on serum lipids in subjects with elevated serum cholesterol. *Nutrition, Metabolism, and Cardiovascular Diseases, 16,* 531–535.

68. Greany, K. A., Bonorden, M. J., Hamilton-Reeves, J. M., et al. (2008). Probiotic capsules do not lower plasma lipids in young women and men. *European Journal of Clinical Nutrition, 62,* 232–237.

69. Aaltonen, J., Ojala, T., Laitinen, K., et al. (2008). Evidence of infant blood pressure programming by maternal nutrition during pregnancy: a prospective randomized controlled intervention study. *Journal of Pediatrics, 152,* 79–84.

70. Laitinen, K., Poussa, T., & Isolauri, E. (2008). The Nutrition, Allergy, Mucosal Immunology and Intestinal Microbiota Group. Probiotics and dietary counselling contribute to glucose regulation during and after pregnancy: a randomised controlled trial. *The British Journal of Nutrition, 19,* 1–9.

71. Delzenne, N. M., Cani, P. D., & Neyrinck, A. M. (2007). Modulation of glucagon-like peptide 1 and energy metabolism by inulin and oligofructose: experimental data. *Journal of Nutrition, 137,* 2547S–2551S.

72. Trautwein, E. A., Rieckhoff, D., & Erbersdobler, H. F. (1998). Dietary inulin lowers plasma cholesterol and triacylglycerol and alters biliary bile acid profile in hamsters. *Journal of Nutrition, 128,* 1937–1943.

73. Rault-Nania, M. H., Gueux, E., Demougeot, C., et al. (2006). Inulin attenuates atherosclerosis in apolipoprotein E-deficient mice. *The British Journal of Nutrition, 96,* 840–844.

74. Reimer, R. A., & Russell, J. C. (2008). Glucose tolerance, lipids, and GLP–1 secretion in JCR: LA-cp rats fed a high protein fiber diet. *Obesity, 16,* 40–46.

75. Kok, N., Roberfroid, M., Robert, A., & Delzenne, N. (1996). Involvement of lipogenesis in the lower VLDL secretion induced by oligofructose in rats. *The British Journal of Nutrition, 76,* 881–890.

76. Beylot, M. (2005). Effects of inulin-type fructans on lipid metabolism in man and in animal models. *The British Journal of Nutrition, 93,* 163–168.

77. Daubioul, C. A., Taper, H. S., De Wispelaere, L. D., & Delzenne, N. M. (2000). Dietary oligofructose lessens hepatic steatosis, but does not prevent hypertriglyceridemia in obese zucker rats. *Journal of Nutrition, 130,* 1314–1319.

78. Daubioul, C., Rousseau, N., Demeure, R., et al. (2002). Dietary fructans, but not cellulose, decrease triglyceride accumulation in the liver of obese Zucker fa/fa rats. *Journal of Nutrition, 132,* 967–973.

79. Busserolles, J., Gueux, E., Rock, E., et al. (2003). Oligofructose protects against the hypertriglyceridemic and pro-oxidative effects of a high fructose diet in rats. *Journal of Nutrition, 133,* 1903–1908.

80. Sugatani, J., Wada, T., Osabe, M., et al. (2006). Dietary inulin alleviates hepatic steatosis and xenobiotics-induced liver injury in rats fed a high-fat and high-sucrose diet: association with the suppression of hepatic cytochrome P450 and hepatocyte nuclear factor 4 alpha expression. *Drug Metabolism and Disposition, 34,* 1677–1687.

81. Rault-Nania, M. H., Demougeot, C., Gueux, E., et al. (2008). Inulin supplementation prevents high fructose diet-induced hypertension in rats. *Clinical Nutrition, 27,* 276–282.

82. Cani, P. D., Daubioul, C. A., Reusens, B., et al. (2005). Involvement of endogenous glucagon-like peptide–1(7–36) amide on glycaemia-lowering effect of oligofructose in streptozotocin-treated rats. *The Journal of Endocrinology, 185,* 457–465.

83. Delmée, E., Cani, P. D., Gual, G., et al. (2006). Relation between colonic proglucagon expression and metabolic response to oligofructose in high fat diet-fed mice. *Life Science, 79,* 1007–1013.

84. Cani, P. D., Possemiers, S., Van de Wiele, T., et al. (2009). Changes in gut microbiota control inflammation in obese mice through a mechanism involving GLP–2-driven improvement of gut permeability [Epub ahead of print]. *Gut, 24.*

85. Letexier, D., Diraison, F., & Beylot, M. (2003). Addition of inulin to a moderately high-carbohydrate diet reduces hepatic lipogenesis and plasma triacylglycerol concentrations in humans. *The American Journal of Clinical Nutrition, 77,* 559–564.

86. Giacco, R., Clemente, G., Luongo, D., et al. (2004). Effects of short-chain fructo-oligosaccharides on glucose and lipid metabolism in mild hypercholesterolaemic individuals. *Clinical Nutrition, 23,* 331–340.

87. Daubioul, C. A., Horsmans, Y., Lambert, P., et al. (2005). Effects of oligofructose on glucose and lipid metabolism in patients with non-alcoholic steatohepatitis: results of a pilot study. *European Journal of Clinical Nutrition, 59,* 723–726.

88. Vogt, J. A., Ishii-Schrade, K. B., Pencharz, P. B., et al. (2006). L-rhamnose and lactulose decrease serum triacylglycerols and their rates of synthesis, but do not affect serum cholesterol concentrations in men. *Journal of Nutrition, 136,* 2160–2166.

89. Alliet, P., Scholtens, P., Raes, M., et al. (2007). Effect of prebiotic galacto-oligosaccharide, long-chain fructo-oligosaccharide infant formula on serum cholesterol and triacylglycerol levels. *Nutrition, 23,* 719–723.

90. Luo, J., Rizkalla, S. W., Alamowitch, C., et al. (1996). Chronic consumption of short-chain fructooligosaccharides by healthy subjects decreased basal hepatic glucosa production but had no effect on insulin-stimulated glucose metabolism. *The American Journal of Clinical Nutrition, 63,* 939–945.

91. Luo, J., Van Yperselle, M., Rizkalla, S. W., et al. (2000). Chronic consumption of short-chain fructooligosaccharides does not affect basal hepatic glucose production or insulin resistance in type 2 diabetics. *Journal of Nutrition, 130,* 1572–1577.

92. Cani, P. D., Joly, E., Horsmans, Y., & Delzenne, N. M. (2006). Oligofructose promotes satiety in healthy human: a pilot study. *European Journal of Clinical Nutrition, 60,* 567–572.

93. Abrams, S. A., Griffin, I. J., Hawthorne, K. M., & Ellis, K. J. (2007). Effect of prebiotic supplementation and calcium intake on body mass index. *Journal of Pediatrics, 151,* 293–298.

17

Probiotics and *H. pylori* Infection

Francesco Franceschi, Guido de Marco, Davide Roccarina,
Bianca Giupponi, Giovanni Gigante, and Antonio Gasbarrini
Internal Medicine, Catholic University of Rome, Italy

1. INTRODUCTION

Helicobacter pylori (*H. pylori*) is a Gram-negative bacteria, which may be considered as one of the most common infectious agents of the GI tract. While there is evidence that the *Helicobacter* species are ancient inhabitants of the human stomach that have co-evolved with the host—thus developing an excellent adaptation to humans—several studies have shown a direct role of *H. pylori* in specific gastroduodenal diseases, such as chronic gastritis and peptic ulcer. In some patients it may also cause MALT-lymphoma and gastric cancer. Furthermore, there is also evidence that *H. pylori* may play a role in different non-gastric diseases, such idiopathic thrombocytopenic purpura and sideropenic anemia, while several other diseases are now under investigation. *Helicobacter pylori*-positive patients may undergo eradicating treatment, following the Maastricht III criteria, consisting of a combination of antibiotics, such as amoxicillin or metronidazole and clarithromycin in the first line, and amoxicillin and levofloxacine in the second line, together with proton pump inhibitors. Interestingly, those antibiotics also have a strong impact on intestinal ecoflora [1].

Intestinal ecoflora, together with the mucosal barrier and local immune system, are responsible for the integrity and regular function of the entire gastrointestinal tract. In particular, they are involved in the modulation of several metabolic activities such as the proliferation and differentiation of mucosal epithelial cells, the regulation of bowel motility, the synthesis of substances including vitamins and secondary biliary acids, and eventually the regulation of the local and systemic immune systems [2]. In normal adults, microbial ecoflora are composed of a mixture of aerobic bacteria (*Streptococcus* spp., *Enterococcus* spp., *Staphylococcus* spp., *Enterobacteriaceae*), anaerobic bacteria (*Peptostreptococcus* spp., *Bifidobacterium* spp., *Lactobacillus* spp., *Clostridium* spp., *Eubacterium* spp., *Bacteroides fragilis*) and yeasts (*Saccharomyces* spp.) [2].

Probiotics are defined as live, non-pathogenic microbial feeds, or food supplements that exert a positive influence on the host by altering his/her microbial balance [3, 4]. Many microorganisms have been used or considered for use as probiotics. A microorganism can be considered for clinical application when, while innocuous, alive, and metabolically active, it is able to withstand the host's natural barriers [5]. Different biologic effects have been described for probiotics,

259

including the synthesis of antimicrobial substances such as organic fatty acids, ammonia, hydrogen peroxide, and bacteriocins, the competitive interaction with pathogens for 'space and food,' through the use of available nutrients and occupation of microbial adherence sites, the modification of toxins or toxin receptors, partial sugar digestion, and finally, immunomodulation [2–5]. Immunomodulation, in particular, is achieved through adjuvant-like effects on intestinal and systemic immunity, the enhancement of specific serologic antibody response, and a balance in the generation of pro- and anti-inflammatory cytokines [5]. The most commonly used probiotics in clinical practice, besides those best-studied, include lactic acid-producing bacteria, such as *Lactobacillus* spp. and *Bifidobacterium* spp., *Bacillus* spp. and other species such as *Escherichia coli, Saccharomyces boulardii*, and *Streptococcus thermophilus* [3–6].

Probiotics may thus play an important role in contrasting some GI infectious agents, including *H. pylori*. In particular, probiotics have been described to interact with *H. pylori* in different ways by:

- contrasting directly and indirectly with an *H. pylori* infection;
- influencing the GI changes induced by the administration of the *H. pylori* eradicating treatment;
- improving patients' compliance to eradicating therapy through the reduction of the incidence of antibiotic-related side effects;
- modulating *H. pylori*-induced inflammation;
- restabilizing a normal GI environment.

2. EFFECT OF PROBIOTICS ON *H. PYLORI*

The majority of the studies performed in this field involve lactobacilli or their metabolic products, because of their ability to adhere to the gastric mucosa and even transiently reside in the stomach. In fact, lactobacilli are predominant bacteria in the normal stomach of fasting subjects, where they may reach a concentration ranging from 0 to 103 cfu/mL of fluid [2]. The role of exogenous lactobacilli in patients with *H. pylori* infection has been widely studied.

In particular, Michetti et al. [7] tested the ability of the *Lactobacillus acidophilus (johnsonii)* La1 culture supernatant to down-regulate *H. pylori* infection. Interestingly, La1 culture supernatant has been shown to inhibit *H. pylori* growth *in vitro*. Moreover, treatment of *H. pylori*-infected subjects with a drinkable, whey-based La1 culture supernatant interferes with *H. pylori* infection as demonstrated by a significant reduction in urea breath test delta oven baseline values. In a similar study, Coconnier et al. [8] showed the *in vitro* and *in vivo* effects of a culture supernatant of *L. acidophilus* strain LB, against *H. pylori*, which were independent of pH and lactic acid levels. These findings may lead to the following conclusions:

- Although the most relevant antibacterial mechanism of action seems to be acid production, some strains of lactobacilli may also exert different antimicrobial effects;
- The anti-*H. pylori* activity is extremely strain specific, as *L. acidophilus* LB was more active than *Lactobacillus* GG, and *L. johnsonii* La1 more than La10 [7, 8].

This concept was also explored by Lorca et al. who tested the effect of 17 different *Lactobacillus* strains on *H. pylori* activity. The results from this study confirmed that the general bactericidal effect shown by lactobacilli is the result of acid production but there are some strains, such as *L. acidophilus* CRL 639, which shows other specific anti-*H. pylori* activities, including the release of a proteinaceous compound [9]. Another study by Kabir et al. [10] demonstrated that *Lactobacillus salivarius* WB 1004 may inhibit the attachment of *H. pylori* to both murine and human gastric epithelial cells and reduces IL-8 release *in vitro*. They also showed in a gnotobiotic murine model, that *L. salivarius* is able to offer after-protection from an *H. pylori* infection and contrasts the colonization of the gastric mucosa sustained by *H. pylori*. In a similar study, the same authors examined the ability of different *Lactobacillus* species to suppress *H. pylori* infection either *in vitro* or *in vivo*. Interestingly, *L. salivarius*, but not *Lactobacillus casei* or *L. acidophilus*, has been shown to produce large amounts of lactic acid inhibiting *H. pylori* [11].

Concerning *Lactobacillus reuteri*, Mukai et al. [12] showed that selected strains of this probiotic (JCM1081 and TM105) may be able to hinder *H. pylori* binding to its putative glycolipid receptors (asialo-GM1 and sulfatide), suggesting a possible use of these strains as probiotics. Some specific probiotics may also exert their antibacterial activity via the production of antibiotic compounds. This is the case with *Bacillus subtilis*, which has been shown to produce, *in vitro*, at least two antibiotics (one was named amicoumacin), which are able to inhibit *H. pylori* growth, independently of pH or organic acid concentration [13]. Based on all of the previously mentioned observations, some researchers attempted to find a clinical application for probiotics in the management of patients undergoing anti-*H. pylori* eradication treatment.

It is known that fermented milk product-based probiotic preparations potentially improve *H. pylori* eradication rates by approximately 10%. The impact on the treatment-associated adverse effects is, however, heterogeneous.

In a study conducted by Felley et al. [14], the treatment of *H. pylori*-positive patients with *L. johnsonii* La1-acidified milk (LC-1) and clarithromycin induced a decrease in *H. pylori* density, inflammation, and gastritis activity, but did not improve the eradication rate.

Based on previous results, showing that *Lactobacillus gasseri* OLL 2716 (LG21) is able to bind to gastric epithelium and to resist gastric acidity, Sakamoto et al. [15] selected this strain to be used in humans infected by *H. pylori*. In this study, *L. gasseri* OLL 2716 showed a suppression of *H. pylori* and a reduction of gastric inflammation as assessed by the serum pepsinogen levels and the results of 13C-urea breath test. Another study conducted by our group demonstrated the efficacy of adding a lyophilized and inactivated culture of *L. acidophilus* LB to a standard triple anti-*H. pylori* therapy. In particular, we observed a significant improvement in the eradication rates obtained both in intention to treat (ITT) and per-protocol analysis [16]. Similar results were obtained by Sheu et al. [17] by adding *Lactobacillus* and *Bifidobacterium*-containing yogurt to the regimen but this effect was only limited to the ITT analysis. Mi Na Kim et al. [18] demonstrated that the addition of a yogurt containing *Lactobacillus acidofilus*, *L. casei*, *Bifidobacterium longum* and *Streptococcus thermophilus* did not reduce the side-effects of standard triple therapy but increased *H. pylori* eradication rate by PP analysis.

3. EFFECTS OF PROBIOTICS ON GASTRIC FUNCTION AND IMMUNOMODULATION

Verdu et al. [19] investigated the role of probiotics in the recovery of gastric function and behavioral changes after chronic *H. pylori* infection. Mice were infected with *H. pylori* for 4 months and then treated with antibiotics or placebo for 2 weeks. Animals then received probiotics (*Lactobacillus rhamnosus* R0011 and *L. helveticus* R0052) or placebo for 2 weeks. Gastric emptying, feeding behavior and intestinal permeability were assessed in all animals. Interestingly, probiotics accelerated the recovery of paracellular permeability and delayed gastric emptying, improved the CD3 cell counts, and normalized altered post-eradication feeding patterns.

Another example of probiotic-induced immunomudulation derived from the study of Li Zhang et al. [20] in which the authors studied

H. pylori-infected C57BL/6 mice treated with *L. casei* L26, *B. lactis* B94, or no probiotics for 5 weeks, in order to test the inflammatory response, the local cytokine profile, and the humoral immune response to *H. pylori* infection. In particular, the level of IL-1β was significantly reduced in gastric tissues of mice treated with either *L. casei* L26 or *B. lactis* B94, when compared to controls, thus suggesting that both *L. casei* L26 and *B. lactis* B94 are able to reduce *H. pylori*-associated gastric inflammation. These findings suggest that the reduction in gastric inflammation resulted from an immune modulatory effect by *L. casei* L26 and *B. lactis* B94, rather than a direct inhibition of *H. pylori*. The finding that there was a significant increase in IL-10 levels in the gastric tissues of mice treated with both *L. casei* L26 and *B. lactis* as compared with the control mice, would support the above view, given that IL-10 has been shown to inhibit the production of IL-1β, IL-6, IL-8, and tumor necrosis factor (TNF)-α in human monocytes and PMN [21, 22]. The suggestion that probiotics may reduce inflammation through immune modulation is further supported by a study from Sgouras et al. [23] in which they showed that *Lactobacillus johnsonii* La1 reduced levels of macrophage inflammatory protein 2 (MIP-2, a homologue to human IL-8) in mice infected with *H. pylori* without a significant reduction in *H. pylori* colonization.

Myllyluoma et al. [24] characterized four probiotics and their combination in terms of pathogen adhesion, barrier function, cell death, and inflammatory response in *H. pylori*-infected epithelial cells. *H. pylori*-infected Caco-2 cells were pretreated with *Lactobacillus rhamnosus* GG, *Lactobacillus rhamnosus* Lc705, *Propionibacterium freudenreichii* subsp. *shermanii* Js, *Bifidobacterium* Bb99, or all four organisms in combination. Interestingly, all probiotics inhibited *H. pylori* adhesion and the combination inhibited *H. pylori*-induced cell membrane leakage. *L. rhamnosus* GG, *L. rhamnosus* Lc705, and the combination initially improved epithelial barrier function but increased the *H. pylori*-induced barrier deterioration after incubation for 24 to 42 hours. *L. rhamnosus* GG, *L. rhamnosus* Lc705, and *P. freudenreichii* subsp. *shermanii* Js inhibited *H. pylori*-induced IL-8 release, whereas *L. rhamnosus* GG, *L. rhamnosus* Lc705, and *B. breve* Bb99 suppressed PGE2 release. None of these anti-inflammatory effects persisted when the probiotics were used in combination. The combination thus increased the levels of IL-8, PGE2, and LTB4 released from *H. pylori*-infected epithelial cells.

Furthermore, other studies showed how lactobacilli may inhibit IL-8; In particular, *Lactobacillus bulgaricus* (LBG) or *Lactobacillus bulgaricus* supernatant (LBG-S) significantly attenuated the expression of TLR4, inhibited the phosphorylation of TAK1 and p38MAPK, prevented the activation of NFκB, and consequently blocked IL-8 production.

4. EFFECT OF PROBIOTICS ON ANTI-*H. PYLORI* ANTIBIOTIC-RELATED SIDE EFFECTS

It is known that the occurrence of some GI adverse events during anti-*H. pylori* therapy, mostly attributed to the use of antibiotics in moderate to high doses, may affect patients' compliance, reducing the proper performance of the therapy. Even though there is substantial evidence that some of these symptoms such as bloating, diarrhea, or constipation are directly related to a qualitative or quantitative alteration of the intestinal microecology, little is known about the link between bowel microbial balance and other common adverse events, such as taste disturbance. Anyway, the imbalance of the intestinal microenvironment during antibiotic therapies seems to be related to the permanence of unabsorbed or secreted drugs in the intestinal content, causing a reduction of normal saprophytic flora and overgrowth of potentially pathogenic antibiotic-resistant indigenous strains [25, 26]. The occurrence of these adverse events may then induce patients to discontinue the treatment, thus leading to eradication failure, and possibly increasing the risk of creating antibiotic-resistant strains. As a result, new strategies have been applied to increase the tolerability of *H. pylori* eradication therapies, which also include the use of probiotics [27]. Different studies have been reported in this field, even comparing the effect of single strains versus multistrain preparations. In particular, an open trial performed by our group in which *H. pylori*-infected patients received *Lactobacillus* GG, in addition to anti-*H. pylori* standard triple therapy, resulted in a reduction of both incidence and intensity of the main gastrointestinal antibiotic-related adverse events [28]. Afterwards, the efficacy of improving treatment tolerability by adding a *Lactobacillus* GG preparation during and after standard triple therapy, in a double blind placebo-controlled study was confirmed. In this study, in fact, diarrhea, nausea, and taste disturbance were significantly reduced in the group supplemented with *Lactobacillus* GG [29]. (relative risk = 0.1, 95% CI: 0.1–0.9; relative risk = 0.3, 95% CI: 0.1–0.9; relative risk = 0.5, 95% CI: 0.2–0.9, respectively). Moreover, an overall assessment of treatment tolerability showed a significant difference in favor of the group supplemented with *Lactobacillus* GG. In another study, *H. pylori*-positive asymptomatic patients were randomized to receive probiotics (*Lactobacillus* GG or *S. boulardii* or a combination of *Lactobacillus* spp. and bifidobacteria) or a placebo, both during a standard triple therapy and 7 days afterward. Despite an *H. pylori* eradication rate that was almost identical in the probiotic and placebo groups, a significantly lower incidence of diarrhea and taste disturbance was observed in all probiotic supplemented groups during the eradication week. Overall assessment of tolerability was significantly better in the actively treated patients than in the placebo group. Interestingly, the efficacy of probiotic

supplementation on adverse events during anti-*H. pylori* regimens seemed to be independent of the probiotic species used [30]. A reduced occurrence of epigastric pain, diarrhea, and nausea in previously asymptomatic *H. pylori*-infected patients undergoing standard triple-eradication therapy was also described in patients who received a supplementation of *Bacillus clausii* for 2 weeks, although similar results were also reported for *S. boulardii* and *L. casei* [31–33]. Finally, there are also some preliminary and unpublished data from our group on the effect of the supplementation with a combination of two different prebiotics such as inulin and butyric acid in patients undergoing *H. pylori* eradicating treatment, which caused a decrease in some antibiotic-related gastrointestinal side effects.

5. CONCLUSIONS

Both *in vitro* and *in vivo* data support the use of probiotics in *H. pylori* infection [34, 35]. In particular, probiotics may act in different ways: by direct competition with *H. pylori*, by decreasing of gastric inflammation, or by improving patients' compliance to therapy, thanks to the reduction of the incidence of antibiotic-related side effects. Although a direct effect against *H. pylori* has been described, it is only supported by animal studies or *in vitro* data and therefore probiotics cannot be considered as an alternative to standard anti-*H. pylori* treatment. On the other hand, several studies have shown that probiotics may reduce gastric inflammation and indirectly improve eradication rates by lowering the incidence of some antibiotic-related gastrointestinal side effects, thus improving patient compliance and increasing the number of subjects completing the treatment. Based on those findings, the administration of probiotics in patients undergoing anti-*H. pylori* eradication treatment should be recommended.

References

1. Malfertheiner, P., Megraud, F., O'Morain, C., et al. (2007). Current concepts in the management of *Helicobacter pylori* infection: the Maastricht III Consensus Report. *Gut, 56,* 772–781.

2. Cazzato, I. A., Candelli, M., Nista, E. C., et al. (2004). Role of probiotics in *Helicobacter pylori* infections. *Scandinavian Journal of Nutrition, 26,* 31.

3. Fuller, R. (1991). Probiotics in human medicine. *Gut, 32,* 439–442.

4. Metchnikoff, E. (1907). *The prolongation of life.* London: Heinemann.

5. Asp, N. G., & Wadstrom, T. (2004). Probiotics and health-introductory comments and aim of the conference. *Scandinavian Journal of Nutrition, 48,* 14.

6. Asp, N. G., Mollby, R., Norin, L., & Wadstrom, T. (2004). Probiotics in gastric and intestinal disorders as functional food and medicine. *Scandinavian Journal of Nutrition, 48,* 14.

7. Michetti, P., Dorta, G., Wiesel, P. H., et al. (1999). Effect of whey-based culture supernatant of *Lactobacillus acidophilus (johnsonii)* La1 on *Helicobacter pylori* infection in humans. *Digestion, 60,* 203–209.

8. Coconnier, M. H., Lievin, V., Hemery, E., & Servin, A. L. (1998). Antagonistic activity against Helicobacter infection *in vitro* and *in vivo* by the human *Lactobacillus acidophilus* strain LB. *Applied and Environmental Microbiology, 64,* 4573–4580.

9. Lorca, G. L., Wadstrom, T., Valdez, G. F., & Ljungh, A. (2001). *Lactobacillus acidophilus* autolysins inhibit. *Helicobacter pylori* in vitro. *Current Microbiology, 42,* 39–44.

10. Kabir, A. M., Aiba, Y., Takagi, A., et al. (1997). Prevention of *Helicobacter pylori* infection by lactobacilli in a gnotobiotic murine model. *Gut, 41,* 49–55.

11. Aiba, Y., Suzuki, N., Kabir, A. M., et al. (1998). Lactic acid mediated suppression of *Helicobacter pylori* by the oral administration of *Lactobacillus salivarius* as a probiotic in a gnotobiotic murine model. *The American Journal of Gastroenterology, 93,* 2097–2101.

12. Mukai, T., Asasaka, T., Sato, E., et al. (2002). Inhibition of binding of *Helicobacter pylori* to the glycolipid receptors by probiotic *Lactobacillus reuteri. FEMS Immunology and Medical Microbiology, 32,* 105–110.

13. Pinchuk, I. V., Bressollier, P., Verneuil, B., et al. (2001). *In vitro* anti-*Helicobacter pylori* activity of the probiotic strain *Bacillus subtilis* 3 is due to secretion of antibiotics. *Antimicrobial Agents and Chemotherapy, 45,* 3156–3161.

14. Felley, C. P., Corthesy-Theulaz, I., Rivero, J. L., et al. (2001). Favourable effect of an acidified milk (LC-1) on *Helicobacter pylori* gastritis in man. *European Journal of Gastroenterology & Hepatology, 13,* 25–29.

15. Sakamoto, I., Igarashi, M., Kimura, K., et al. (2001). Suppressive effect of *Lactobacillus gasseri* OLL 2716 (LG21) on *Helicobacter pylori* infection in humans. *The Journal of Antimicrobial Chemotherapy, 47,* 709–710.

16. Canducci, F., Armuzzi, A., Cremonini, F., et al. (2000). A lyophilized and inactivated culture of *Lactobacillus acidophilus* increases *Helicobacter pylori* eradication rates. *Alimentary Pharmacology & Therapeutics, 14,* 1625–1629.

17. Sheu, B. S., Wu, J. J., Lo, C. Y., et al. (2002). Impact of supplement with Lactobacillus- and Bifidobacterium-containing yogurt on triple therapy for *Helicobacter pylori* eradication. *Alimentary Pharmacology & Therapeutics, 16,* 1669–1675.

18. Mi Na Kim., Kim, N., Lee, S. H., et al. (2008). The effects of probiotics on PPI-triple therapy for *Helicobacter pylori* eradication. *Helicobacter, 13,* 261–268.

19. Verdu, E. F., Bercik, P., Xi Huang, X., et al. (2008). The role of luminal factors in the recovery of gastric function and behavioural changes after chronic *Helicobacter pylori* infection. *American Journal of Physiology. Gastrointestinal and Liver Physiology, 295,* G664–G670.

20. Zhang, L., Su, P., Henriksson, A., et al. (2008). Investigation of the immunomodulatory effects of *Lactobacillus casei* and *Bifidobacterium lactis* on *Helicobacter pylori* infection. *Helicobacter, 13,* 183–190.

21. Wang, P., Wu, P., Siegel, M. I., et al. (1995). Interleukin (IL)-10 inhibits nuclear factor kappa-B (Nf-kappa-B) activation in human monocytes–IL-10 and IL-4 suppress cytokine synthesis by different mechanisms. *The Journal of Biological Chemistry, 270,* 9558–9563.

22. Zhou, C., Ma, F.-Z., Deng, X.-J., et al. (2008). Lactobacilli inhibit interleukin-8 production induced by *Helicobacter pylori* lipopolysaccharide-activated Toll-like receptor 4. *World Journal of Gastroenterology, 14,* 5090–5095.

23. Sgouras, D. N., Panayotopoulou, E. G., Martinez-Gonzalez, B., et al. (2005). *Lactobacillus johnsonii* La1 attenuates *Helicobacter pylori*-associated gastritis and reduces levels of proinflammatory chemokines in C57BL/6 mice. *Clinical and Diagnostic Laboratory Immunology, 12,* 1378–1382.

24. Myllyluoma, E., Ahonen, A. M., Korpela, R., et al. (2008). Effects of multispecies probiotic combination on *Helicobacter pylori* infection in vitro. *Clinical and Vaccine Immunology,* 1472–1482.

25. Nord, C. E., Heimdal, A., & Kager, L. (1986). Antimicrobial induced alterations of the human oropharyngeal and intestinal microflora. *Scandinavian Journal of Infectious Diseases, 49,* 64–72.

26. Adamsson, I., Nord, C. E., Lundquist, P., et al. (1999). Comparative effects of omeprazole, amoxycillin, plus metronidazole versus omeprazole, clarithromycin plus metronidazole on the oral, gastric and intestinal microflora in *Helicobacter pylori*-infected patients. *The Journal of Antimicrobial Chemotherapy, 44,* 40.

27. Lewis, S. J., & Freedman, A. R. (1998). Review article: the use of biotherapeutic agents in the prevention and treatment of gastrointestinal disease. *Alimentary Pharmacology & Therapeutics, 12,* 807–822.

28. Armuzzi, A., Cremonini, F., Ojetti, V., et al. (2001). Effect of *Lactobacillus* GG supplementation on antibiotic-associated gastrointestinal side effects during *Helicobacter pylori* eradication therapy: A pilot study. *Digestion, 63*, 1–7.

29. Armuzzi, A., Cremonini, F., Bartolozzi, F., et al. (2001). The effect of oral administration of *Lactobacillus* GG on antibiotic-associated gastrointestinal side effects during *Helicobacter pylori* eradication therapy. *Alimentary Pharmacology & Therapeutics, 15*, 163–169.

30. Cremonini, F., Di Caro, S., Covino, M., et al. (2002). Effect of different probiotic preparations on anti-*Helicobacter pylori* therapy-related side effects: A parallel group, triple blind, placebo-controlled study. *The American Journal of Gastroenterology, 97*, 2744–2749.

31. Nista, E. C., Candelli, M., Cremonini, F., et al. (2004). *Bacillus clausii* therapy to reduce side effects of anti-*Helicobacter pylori* treatment: Randomized, double-blind, placebo controlled trial. *Alimentary Pharmacology & Therapeutics, 20*, 1181–1188.

32. Duman, D. G., Bor, S., Ozutemiz, O., et al. (2005). Efficacy and safety of *Saccharomyces boulardii* in prevention of antibiotic-associated diarrhea due to *Helicobacter pylori* eradication. *European Journal of Gastroenterology & Hepatology, 17*, 1357–1361.

33. Tursi, A., Brandimarte, G., Giorgetti, G. M., & Modeo, M. E. (2004). Effect of *Lactobacillus casei* supplementation on the effectiveness and tolerability of a new second-line 10-day quadruple therapy after failure of a first attempt to cure *Helicobacter pylori* infection. *Medical Science Monitor, 10*, CR626–CR662.

34. Di Caro, S., Tao, H., Grillo, A., et al. (2005). *Bacillus clausii* effect on gene expression pattern in small bowel mucosa using DNA microarray analysis. *European Journal of Gastroenterology & Hepatology, 17*, 951–960.

35. Franceschi, F., Cazzato, A., Nista, E. C., et al. (2007). Role of probiotics in patients with *Helicobacter pylori* infection. *Helicobacter, 12*(Suppl. 2), 59–63.

Probiotics in Neonatal Sepsis Associated with Necrotizing Enterocolitis and Meningitis

Sheng-He Huang[1] *Hong Cao*[2] *and Ambrose Jong*[1]

[1]Saban Research Institute of Childrens Hospital Los Angeles, Department of Pediatrics, University of Southern California, Los Angeles, CA, USA

[2]Department of Microbiology, School of Public Health and Tropical Medicine, Southern Medical University, Guangzhou, China

1. INTRODUCTION

Bacterial sepsis and meningitis continue to be the most common serious infection in neonates [1–3]. Neonatal sepsis is classified into two major categories: early onset (within 72 hours) sepsis, which is usually due to microorganisms that are acquired from the mother antepartum or intrapartum, and late onset (after 72 hours) sepsis caused by the pathogens that are generally acquired from the postnatal environment [3]. Severe sepsis associated with multisystem organ dysfunction has been a leading cause of death in patients hospitalized in neonatal intensive care units (NICU) [3–6]. Neonates hospitalized in the NICU, particularly preterm infants, have very high rates of late onset sepsis (also referred to as nosocomial sepsis or healthcare-associated sepsis). Late onset sepsis is generally defined as bloodstream bacterial infection that presents after 72 hours of life [3]. Several risk factors for nosocomial sepsis have been identified and classified as either intrinsic or extrinsic factors. Intrinsic risk factors include the relative immunodeficiency of the neonate, and compromised portals of entry for potential pathogens including the immature barrier function of the skin and the gastrointestinal tract [6]. Risk factors associated with medical treatments, devices, and invasive procedures are extrinsic. Strategies to prevent infections in NICU patients have evolved as the progress in science and technology has advanced our understanding of the risk factors for nosocomial sepsis. It is often caused by infection of commensal bacteria derived from mucosal or skin surfaces.

Group B *Streptococcus* (GBS) and *E. coli* are the two most common bacterial pathogens causing neonatal sepsis and meningitis (NSM) [1, 2]. GBS is a commensal organism found in the gastrointestinal and genitourinary tracts of healthy individuals. However, in certain circumstances, mostly in neonates, GBS can become a life-threatening pathogen, causing invasive infections such as sepsis and meningitis. Invasive GBS disease emerged in the 1970s as a leading cause of newborn morbidity and mortality in the USA [7]. Extensive studies have demonstrated that intrapartum prophylaxis (IP) of GBS carriers and selective administration of antibiotics to neonates decrease newborn GBS infection by as much as 80 to 95% [7–10]. However, a major concern is whether IP use of antibiotics affects the incidence and the resistance of early-onset neonatal infection with non-GBS pathogens [7–10]. Currently, the focus has shifted to *E. coli*, which is a leading cause of infection among neonates, particularly among those of very low birth weight (VLBW) [11]. *E. coli* is the most common cause of neonatal Gram-negative sepsis and meningitis [1, 2]. Premature infants, immunocompromised hosts, and children with underlying severe gastrointestinal diseases are especially prone to *E. coli* sepsis and meningitis. The estimated annual incidence of *E. coli* neonatal sepsis is thought to be one case per 1000 live births [12], with *E. coli* strains possessing the K1 capsular polysaccharide being isolated from the majority of cases [13]. The intestines of breast-fed infants become colonized with *E. coli* during the first week of life [14], while the prevalence of *E. coli* K1 rectal colonization in women of child-bearing age has been documented to be as high as 50%, with up to 30% of their newborns colonized by the second day of life [15]. Although initially most multicenter reports showed stable rates of non-GBS early onset infection with IP for GBS, other studies challenge this conclusion, suggesting an increasing incidence of early onset *E. coli* infections in low birth weight and VLBW neonates and a rising frequency of ampicillin-resistant *E. coli* infections in preterm infants [16, 17]. Widespread antibiotic use, particularly with broad-spectrum antimicrobial agents, may result in a rising incidence of neonatal infections with antibiotic resistance, which is an ecological phenomenon stemming from the response of bacteria to antibiotics [18]. Antibiotic resistance has emerged as a major public health problem during the past decade [19]. Widespread antibiotic use will certainly worsen the ongoing antimicrobial resistance crisis.

2. PROBIOTICS: ECOLOGIC APPROACHES TO NEONATAL INFECTIONS

The development of microbial infections is determined by the nature of host-microbe relationships. As most microbes form a healthy symbiotic 'superorganism' with the hosts, a holistic balance of this relationship is essential to our health [20]. In view of community ecology, our health is associated with the dynamic interactions of three microbial communities [non-pathogenic microbiota (NP), conditional pathogens (CP), and unconditional pathogens (UP)] with the hosts at three different health statuses—non-susceptibility (NS), conditional susceptibility (CS), and unconditional susceptibility (US). NP is the major microbial community that forms a healthy symbiotic relationship with the hosts. The ecology and evolution of NP-NS interaction is essential and fundamental for health. From birth to death, the inherent nature of the superorganism makes us establish and maintain a symbiotic relationship with a vast, complex, and dynamic consortium of microbes. Most of our microbial commensals reside in our gastrointestinal (GI) track packed with up to 100 trillion (10^{14}) microbes [20, 21]. The GI tract harbors a rich microbiota of >600 different bacterial species. Human intestinal samples contain members of nine divisions of bacteria (Firmicutes, Bacteroidetes, Actinobacteria, Fusobacteria, Proteobacteria, Verrucomicrobia,

Cyanobacteria, Spirochaeates, and VadinBE97) [21]. Some of these microorganisms may provide positive health benefits for their hosts. These include stimulating the immune system, protecting the host from microbial invasion, aiding digestion and modulating energy balance [20]. The GI tract is a complex ecosystem formed by the symbiotic alliance of GI mucosal epithelium, immune cells and microbiota.

The GI mucosa provides a protective interface between the internal environment and the constant external challenge from food-derived antigens and microbes. The gut mucosal immune system is able to discriminate between pathogens and benign microbes by stimulating protective immunity without disrupting the integrity of the gut mucosa. Breast-feeding is associated with protection from many infections or related conditions, including gastroenteritis, respiratory tract infection, acute otitis media, urinary tract infection, neonatal septicaemia, *H. influenzae* meningitis and necrotizing enterocolitis [22–24]. Some of the protective effects may be due to an altered mucosal colonization pattern in the breast-fed infants. DNA microarray studies have demonstrated that colonization of germ-free mice with *B. thetaiotaomicron* alters expression profiles of host genes that contribute to regulation of postnatal maturation, nutrient uptake and metabolism, processing of xenobiotics, and angiogenesis [25]. A study by Gan and colleagues showed that live *L. fermentum*, a major commensal bacterium present in the GI track of mammalians, is able to hamper the ability of *S. aureus* to cause wound infection in rats [26]. These studies suggest that microbial stimulation plays an important role in neonatal development and that beneficial microorganisms such as *Lactobacillus* enhance host defense against pathogens.

The GI microbiota is established rapidly after birth [25]. The three components of the GI ecosystem, essential for human homeostasis, have interdependent relationships. They rely on each other to achieve their normal functions and

activities [27]. The GI mucosa, as a protective barrier, provides an ecological interface between the internal environment and the constant external challenge from food-derived antigens and microbes. CP and UP are minor microbial communities that mainly contribute to the pathogenesis of microbial diseases. The distinction between the commensal and the pathogen in the CP community can be blurred because they may cause diseases under certain sub-health conditions of the hosts, or in immunocompromised hosts. For example, the Pneumococcus, Meningococcus and Haemophilus bacteria regularly exist as part of the normal microbiota of the host respiratory track and are mostly carried asymptomatically despite the fact that they can cause well-defined diseases [28, 29]. Microbes in the CP community dynamically evolve in two opposite directions, either toward the NP (more cooperative or mutualistic) or UP (more pathogenic) microbial community. Microbes with high pathogenicity belong to the UP microbial community. The three microbial communities and three statuses of the hosts are subjected to dynamic reciprocal changes driven by intraspecies, cross-species or cross-kingdom transfer of genetic materials. Extending along the dynamic continuum from conflict to cooperation, microbial infections always involve symbiosis and pathogenesis, which are two opposite but interdependent aspects of the host-microbe interactions. The most fundamental issue in ecological infectomics is how to transform situations of potential conflict (pathogenesis) into cooperation (symbiosis) by dissecting the dynamic duality relationships between symbiosis and pathogenesis in microbial infections and developing symbiotic agents (symbiotics) that favor a healthy symbiosis [30]. Symbiotics are defined as products that are beneficial to symbiotic ecology of the superorganisms consisting of microbes and their human hosts. These include microbial (e.g., probiotic bacteria and phages) and nonmicrobial agents (e.g., prebiotics) [30–33].

A number of factors may cause alterations in the composition and effect of the normal microbiota. These include use of antibiotics, immunosuppressive therapy, irradiation, other means of treatment, hygiene, and the imbalance of nutrition. As a result of all the factors mentioned, there has been a decline in the incidence of microbial stimulation that may reduce host defense and predispose the host to infectious, inflammatory, degenerative, and neoplasic diseases [25, 34]. Therefore, the introduction of beneficial microorganisms such as probiotics into our body is a very attractive rationale for modulating the microbiota, improving the symbiotic homeostasis of the superorganism, and providing a microbial stimulus to the host immune system against microbial pathogens [25, 34]. Multiple mechanisms of probiotic therapy have been postulated, including the production of antimicrobial agents, competition for space or nutrients, and immunomodulation. The microbes frequently used as probiotic agents include *Lactobacillus* and *Bifidobacterium*. For example, *Lactobacillus* spp. is able to attenuate colitis in IL-10-deficient mice; probiotic agents containing *Lactobacillus*, *Bifidobacterium*, and *Streptococcus* spp. are effective in treatment of chronic 'pouchitis,' a complication subsequent to surgical therapy for ulcerative colitis [35, 36]. The protective effects of *Lactobacillus* on both Shiga toxin-producing *E. coli* O157:H7 and enteroinvasive *E. coli* infections were demonstrated in infant rabbits and intestinal epithelial cells, respectively [37, 38]. A study by Alvarez-Olmos and Oberhelman suggests that the use of lactic acid bacteria as live vectors is a promising approach for delivering drugs, antimicrobial agents, and vaccines to defined host niches, due to their safety, ability to persist within the indigenous microbiota, adjuvant properties, and low intrinsic antigenicity [39]. Dissecting the role of probiotics as modulators of the host defense system will be challenging, and may be important for the pathogenesis and prophylaxis of neonatal microbial infections, including NSM.

3. PROBIOTICS FOR THE PREVENTION OF NEONATAL SEPSIS ASSOCIATED WITH NECROTIZING ENTEROCOLITIS

Necrotizing enterocolitis (NEC), an acute inflammatory disease, is the common GI emergency that affects the intestine of neonates resulting in intestinal necrosis, systemic sepsis and multisystem organ failure [40–43]. Most NECs are associated with prematurity as full-term newborns account for only 5–25% of all cases [43]. It is the leading cause of death and long-term disability from GI diseases in preterm infants [40]. NEC affects approximately 20% of preterm infants. Mortality (20–40%) and morbidity, including long-term neuronal developmental disorders, remain high, especially in infants with VLBW [43]. NEC has not only been one of the most serious clinical problems to affect neonates, but also one of the most challenging to treat. This disease typically develops after the onset of enteral feeds and when the intestinal tract has become colonized. Several lines of evidence suggest that the interaction between indigenous bacteria and the newborn intestine have a crucial role in the pathogenesis of NEC [40].

Probiotic bacteria have been used as live microbial supplements for the prevention of NEC [41–43]. The most frequently used probiotics are *Lactobacillus* and *Bifidobacterium*. Potential mechanisms by which probiotics may protect high risk infants from developing NEC and/or sepsis include: increased barrier to migration bacteria and their products across the mucosa; competitive exclusion of potential pathogens; modification of host response to microbial products; augmentation of GI mucosal responses; enhancement of enteral nutrition that inhibit the growth of pathogens; and up-regulation of immune responses [41]. Data for definite NEC in probiotic and placebo (control) groups were reported in seven trials, which included 1,393 neonates [43]. The rate of NEC in the control group (8 of 690, 6%) was significantly higher than that of the probiotics group (15 of 703, 2%). A combination of available data from five clinical trials ($n = 1,268$) showed a reduced risk of death due to all causes in the infants treated with probiotics, as compared with the control group [43]. No significant differences in the risk of mortality due to NEC between the probiotics and the control groups were shown by pooling of data from four clinical trials ($n = 901$) [43]. A significant reduction in the time to reach full feeds in the probiotics was suggested when compared to the control group by meta-analysis of data available from three clinical trials ($n = 316$) [43]. Overall, the data from a number of clinical trials suggest a significant reduction in the risk of NEC and in mortality after probiotic supplementation in preterm neonates with VLBW, compared with the controls [41–43].

As indicated in a number of studies, there is still considerable variation in treatment recommendations for neonates with sepsis and NEC [41–43]. These variations include type, dose, and duration of probiotic supplementation, the age of commencement, and the use of antibiotics. The optimum type of probiotic supplements, with the use of single or multiple microbes, remains to be determined. Individual organisms are known to have variable rates of colonization in different populations. The colonization rates of *Lactobacillus* are shown to range from 60 to 87% in preterm neonates [43]. Maturity of the host also plays an important role in colonization by probiotic organisms. It has been reported that the rates (25%) of colonization in neonates with VLBW are much lower (50%) than that of those infants weighing 1500–1999 g at birth [43]. Whether colonization with a particular probiotic agent may have benefits over only a specific period of postnatal life is not clear. The use of antibiotics for suspected or proven sepsis will also affect the gut colonization in preterm neonates. Specific data for the use of antibiotics during the trial has been reported by Manzoni et al., and by Mohan and colleagues, who also

investigated the gut colonization by resistant bacterial strains in neonates treated with or without antibiotics [44, 45]. No significant difference between the probiotic and control groups was observed with regard to the number of neonates colonized with antibiotic-resistant strains irrespective of antibiotic treatment. As the results of these data are limited, it is premature to make any conclusive comment on the effect of antibiotic use on the gut colonization during probiotic supplementation. There is a difference in the gut microbiota of preterm infants and normal-term neonates [43]. Neonates with VLBW usually acquire microbiota mainly from the nosocomial environment rather than from their mothers. The mode of delivery also affects the pattern of gut colonization, which may differ between neonates delivered vaginally and those delivered by cesarean section. The establishment of a stable and healthy neonatal gut microbiota may be delayed after delivery by cesarean section [43].

There is a potential risk of bacteremia secondary to enterally administered probiotic strains, although sepsis caused by the specific organisms in the probiotic supplement has not been reported in any of the clinical trials mentioned in this article. Caution is essential for the use of the prevention of sepsis and NEC in immunocompromised hosts such as preterm neonates, since neonatal *Lactobacillus* bacteremia has already been reported [46, 47].

4. PROBIOTICS FOR THE PROPHYLAXIS OF NEONATAL BACTERIAL MENINGITIS

As probiotics help to maintain ecological balance, the use of probiotics for the prophylaxis of early onset neonatal meningitic infections may overcome the major disadvantage of widespread antibiotic use, which disturbs the normal microbiota. As mentioned above, probiotics are effective in the prevention of sepsis associated with NEC in neonates. Studies using probiotics have demonstrated that atopic dermatitis of newborns can be prevented in 50% of cases if mothers take probiotics during pregnancy and newborns ingest them during the first 6 months of life [48]. Newborns fed with probiotic-enriched formula grew better than those fed with the regular one [49]. Probiotics have also been shown to decrease the frequency and duration of diarrhea caused by *E. coli* and other pathogens [50, 51]. However, it is unknown whether probiotics are effective in preventing neonatal bacterial meningitis in humans. In order to dissect this issue and develop probiotics as a better approach for the prophylaxis of NSM caused by meningitic pathogens including GBS and *E. coli* K1, we have tested the prophylactic efficacy of LGG in NSM *in vitro* (cell culture model) and *in vivo* (neonatal rat model of bacteremia and meningitis) [52].

LGG is one of the most studied probiotic strains (ATCC 53103). It was originally isolated from human intestinal flora [53]. LGG has been shown to reduce the duration and symptoms of infantile rotavirus diarrhea, to have some effect on preventing atopic diseases among infants, and to modulate immune responses [53]. LGG has been used for many years with an excellent overall safety record [39]. It is well tolerated and extremely safe, and serious adverse effects rarely occur, compared to many pharmaceutical agents [53]. Side effects were not observed in a large population receiving LGG in Finland [39]. However, *Lactobacillus bacteremia* has been reported in two high-risk groups: premature neonates and immune compromised individuals [39]. Large population studies showed that the increased use of LGG has not led to an increase in *Lactobacillus bacteremia* [54]. As LGG has an excellent track record for success and safety, this probiotic agent has been chosen for testing the efficacy of anti-meningitic infection *in vitro* and *in vivo* [52].

Caco-2, a human intestinal epithelial cell line, was used as an *in vitro* model for testing effects

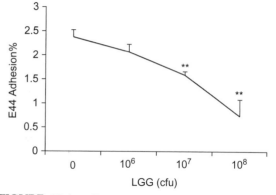

FIGURE 18.1 Effects of LGG on meningitic *E. coli* K1 (E44) adhesion to human intestinal epithelial cells (Caco-2). Epithelial cells were incubated with various doses of *Lactobacillus* for 3 hours before adding bacteria. Adhesion assays were carried out as described previously [52]. All values represent the means of triplicate determinations. The results were expressed as adhesion activities compared to that of the control without LGG. Error bars indicate standard deviations. **$p < 0.01$.

of LGG on meningitic *E. coli* adhesion to and invasion of the gut barrier since it has been one of the most relevant *in vitro* models for the studies of small intestinal epithelial cell differentiation and transport properties [55]. Competitive exclusion/adhesion inhibition assays were used to examine the ability of LGG to interfere with the adhesion of *E. coli* K1 to Caco-2 cells. In this study, Caco-2 cells were pre-incubated with different doses of LGG (10^6 to 10^8 cfu) before addition of meningitic *E. coli* K1 strain E44, a rifampin-resistant strain of a clinical isolate *E. coli* RS218 (O18:K1:H7) from the CSF of a newborn infant with meningitis [56]. As shown in Figure 18.1, E44 invasion of Caco-2 cells was competitively inhibited by LGG in a dose-dependent manner ($p < 0.01$). Blocking effects of LGG on the invasive phenotype of strain E44 into Caco-2 cells were tested utilizing competitive exclusion/invasion inhibition assays. Caco-2 cells were pre-incubated with different doses of LGG (10^7 to 10^8 cfu) before addition of E44. The intracellular pathogens were determined by the gentamicin protection assay, which is based

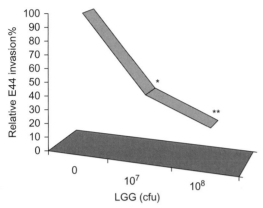

FIGURE 18.2 Inhibition of meningitic E44 invasion of Caco-2 by LGG. Caco-2 cells were incubated with various doses of *Lactobacillus* for 3 hours before adding bacteria. Invasion assays were carried out as described previously [52]. All values represent the means of triplicate determinations. The results were expressed as relative invasion activities compared to that of the control without LGG. Error bars indicate standard deviations. *$p < 0.05$; **$p < 0.01$.

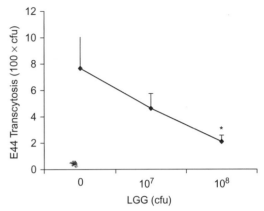

FIGURE 18.3 Effects of LGG on *E. coli* K1 translocation across Caco-2 monolayers. Epithelial cells were incubated with various doses of LGG for 3 hours before adding 10^7 cfu of E44. Transcytosis assays were carried out as described previously [52]. All values represent the means of triplicate determinations at 4 hours. Experiments were repeated three times. Error bars indicate standard deviations. *$p < 0.05$.

upon the principle that intracellular organisms are 'protected' from the bactericidal effects of gentamicin, while extracellular organisms are killed. The invasion rate of E44 at the zero-concentration of LGG was assigned as 100% and the effects of probiotic preincubation were compared to this control level (Figure 18.2). As shown in Figure 18.2, E44 invasion of Caco-2 cells was blocked by LGG in a dose-dependent manner. The invasion ability of E44 was reduced by 78% at 1×10^8 cfu of LGG ($p < 0.01$). A similar result was obtained using the rat intestinal epithelial cell line IEC6 (Data not shown).

In order to examine whether LGG influences the internalized bacteria across the monolayers of Caco-2 cells using the transcellular pathway with or without enhancement of the epithelial barrier functions, competitive exclusion/transcytosis inhibition assays were performed. In this experiment, Caco-2 cells were pre-incubated with different doses of LGG (10^7 to 10^8 cfu) before addition of meningitic *E. coli* K1 strain E44. After incubation with LGG, 1×10^7 cfu of E44 was added to the upper chamber of the

Transwell. The appearance of E44 in the bottom chamber was determined. As shown in Figure 18.3, LGG was able to significantly reduce transcytosis of E44 across the Caco-2 monolayers at 1×10^8 cfu of LGG at 4 hours ($p < 0.05$). To further determine whether LGG influenced the barrier function that led to decreased E44 crossing the Caco-2 monolayers from the apical to the basolateral side, horseradish peroxidase (HRP) assay was carried out as previously described [57]. The HRP concentration was determined spectrophotometrically at 470 nm to determine the peroxidase activity. E44 cfu in the lower chamber were significantly reduced in the experimental group (E44 + LGG) at 1×10^8 cfu of LGG compared to the control (E44 without adding LGG) ($p < 0.05$) [52]. However, stable TEER [52] and HRP activity ($25.6 \pm 1.7 \mu g/mL$ at 6 h) were observed in both groups, suggesting that the barrier function or permeability was not remarkably altered.

Our *in vitro* experiments demonstrated that the probiotic agent LGG was able to significantly block meningitic *E. coli* K1 adhesion, invasion and transcytosis. Next, the probiotics-induced blocking effects on meningitic pathogens were further examined in the neonatal rat model of *E. coli* K1 meningitis. LGG was administered orally to 2-day-old rats for 3 days before *E. coli* K1 infection. The 5-day-old rats were infected with *E. coli* E44, and the stool, blood and CSF samples were cultured for indication of intestinal colonization, bacteremia and meningitis, respectively [52]. Our results showed that the rates of E44 intestinal colonization, bacteremia and meningitis were significantly different between the experiment group with LGG and the control receiving PBS [52]. Quantitative cultures of LGG were also done with the blood samples from the pups receiving LGG. No LGG was detected. The average number of intestinal *E. coli* K1 colonies in the animals given LGG was significantly lower than that of the control group, suggesting that LGG is able to suppress *E. coli* K1 colonization in the rat intestine. No bacteremia and meningitis occurred in the animal group inoculated with LGG. In contrast, among the animals in the control group, 100% of them colonized with meningitic *E. coli* K1 and the majority (64%) of the rats had bacteremia ($>10^5$ to 10^8 cfu/mL), which is critical for the development of meningitis. Twenty-one percent of the rats in the control group developed meningitis.

Adhesion and invasion are two subsequent steps essential for microbial pathogen entry into the host cells. Enteric pathogens such as *E. coli* K1 must penetrate across two tissue barriers, the gut and the blood–brain barrier (BBB), in order to cause meningitis [1, 2]. *E. coli* K1 binding to and invasion of intestinal epithelial cells are a prerequisite for bacterial crossing of the gut barrier *in vivo* [58, 59]. Therefore, it is important to understand how probiotics suppress meningitic *E. coli* translocation through the gastrointestinal epithelium. We have examined the blocking effects of LGG on *E. coli* K1 strain E44 adhesion, invasion and transcytosis in the human colon carcinoma cell line Caco-2, which is one of the most relevant *in vitro* models

of gut epithelium for the studies of small intestinal epithelial cell differentiation, transport properties and barrier functions [58, 59]. This *in vitro* cell culture model has been successfully used for identification of *E. coli* K1, *S. fimbria* and *ibeA* as virulence factors required for efficient intestinal epithelial adhesion and invasion [58, 60]. Our results show that in the *in vitro* Caco-2 cell line experiments LGG reduces *E. coli* K1 adhesion, invasion and transcytosis. To further assess the role of LGG in the suppression of meningitic *E. coli* K1 infection, the animal study was carried out to test its biological functions using the newborn rat model of experimental hematogenous meningitis. This animal model of *E. coli* bacteremia and meningitis has been successfully established and used by us to assess the ability of pathogens to cross the gut barrier and the BBB *in vivo* [1, 2, 58, 60]. Experimental *E. coli* bacteremia and meningitis in newborn murines have important similarities to human newborn *E. coli* infection, e.g., age-dependency, hematogenous infection of meninges, without need for adjuvant or direct inoculation of bacteria into CSF [1, 2]. The availability of this animal model enables us to examine the clinical relevance of probiotics-induced protective effects on newborns against the development of NSM. We showed that LGG was able to significantly reduce the pathogen intestinal colonization and the genesis of *E. coli* K1 bacteremia. LGG was not detected in the blood samples of the animals treated with the probiotics, suggesting that LGG, which has the most extensive safety assessment record [39], exhibited a high degree of safety in the neonatal murine pups. Significant difference in the rates of meningitis was observed between the probiotic and control groups [52]. It has been previously shown that a high degree of bacteremia ($>10^5$ bacteria/mL) is a primary determinant for meningeal invasion by *E. coli* K1 (2). Our studies suggest that the significantly decreased or even abolished translocation of the pathogen across the gut barrier leads to a reduced number of bacteria or no bacteria entry into the bloodstream. This eventually results in no pathogens crossing the BBB to cause meningitis.

5. CONCLUSION

In summary, clinical or preclinical studies show that probiotics might reduce the risk of sepsis, NEC and meningitis in neonates. Despite the considerable differences in type, dose, and duration of organisms used, the age of commencement, and the use of antibiotics, the remarkable progress suggests that probiotics might be a promising way to prevent sepsis, NEC and meningitis in newborns with the choice of an effective probiotic regimen. Large well-designed trials are needed to support the routine use of probiotics in preterm and mature neonates. Prematurity, which is the most important risk factor, may impede the use of probiotic supplementation alone in preterm neonates.

SUMMARY

Probiotics have been proposed as a promising way to prevent microbial infection in neonates. Results from several clinical trials suggest that probiotics reduce the risk of sepsis associated with necrotizing enterocolitis in preterm neonates. The prophylactic efficacy of *Lactobacillus rhamnosus* GG (LGG) in meningitic infection has been examined by using *in vitro* inhibition assays with E44 (a CSF isolate from a newborn baby with *E. coli* meningitis), and the neonatal rat model of *E. coli* sepsis and meningitis. LGG was able to block E44 adhesion, invasion and transcytosis in a dose-dependent manner. A significant reduction in the levels of pathogen colonization, bacteremia and meningitis was observed in the LGG-treated neonatal rats, as assessed by viable cultures, compared to the levels in the control group. These studies suggest that probiotics could be useful to correct ecological disorders in human intestinal microbiota associated with neonatal sepsis and meningitis, and might play a protective role in excluding pathogens from the intestine and preventing infections.

References

1. Huang, S. H., Stins, M., & Kim, K. S. (2000). Bacterial penetration across the blood-brain barrier during the development of neonatal meningitis. *Microbes and Infection, 2,* 1237–1244.
2. Huang, S. H., & Jong, A. (2001). Cellular mechanisms of microbial proteins contributing to invasion of the blood-brain barrier. *Cell Microbiology, 3,* 277–287.
3. Sankar, M. J., Agarwal, R., Deorari, A. K., & Paul, V. K. (2008). Sepsis in the newborn. *Indian Journal of Pediatrics, 75,* 261–266.
4. Bu, H. F., Wang, X., Zhu, Y. Q., et al. (2006). Lysozyme-modified probiotic components protect rats against polymicrobial sepsis: role of macrophages and cathelicidin-related innate immunity. *Journal of Immunology, 177,* 8767–8776.
5. Madsen, K. (2008). Probiotics in critical ill patients. *Journal of Clinical Gastroenterology, 42,* S116–S118.
6. Saiman, L. (2006). Strategies for prevention of nosocomial sepsis in the neonatal intensive care unit. *Current Opinion in Pediatrics, 18,* 101–106.
7. Schrag, S. J., Zywicki, S., Farley, M. M., et al. (2000). Group B streptococcal disease in the era of intrapartum antibiotic prophylaxis. *New England Journal of Medicine, 342,* 15–20.
8. Daley, A. J., & Isaacs, D. (2004). Australian Study Group for Neonatal Infections. Ten-year study on the effect of intrapartum antibiotic prophylaxis on early onset group B streptococcal and *Escherichia coli* neonatal sepsis in Australasia. *Pediatric Infectious Disease Journal, 23,* 630–634.
9. Lopez Sastre, J. B., Fernandez Colomer, B., Coto Cotallo, G. D., et al. (2005). Trends in the epidemiology of neonatal sepsis of vertical transmission in the era of group B streptococcal prevention. *Acta Paediatrica, 94,* 451–457.
10. Apgar, B. S., Greenberg, G., & Yen, G. (2005). Prevention of group B streptococcal disease in the newborn. *American Family Physician, 71,* 903–910.
11. Schrag, S. J., Hadler, J. L., Arnold, K. E., et al. (2006). Risk factors for invasive, early-onset *Escherichia coli* infections in the era of widespread intrapartum antibiotic use. *Pediatrics, 118,* 570–576.
12. Mustafa, M. M., & McCracken, G. H., Jr. (1992). Perinatal bacterial diseases. In R. D. Feigin & J. D. Cherry (Eds.), *Textbook of pediatric infectious diseases* (3rd edn.) (pp. 891–924). Philadelphia, PA: W.B. Saunders.

13. Korhonen, T. K., Valtonen, M. V., Parkinen, J., et al. (1985). Serotypes, hemolysin production, and receptor recognition of *Escherichia coli* strains associated with neonatal sepsis and meningitis. *Infection and Immunity, 48,* 486–491.

14. Smith, H. W., & Crabb, W. E. (1961). The faecal bacterial flora of animals and man: its development in the young. *Journal of Pathology and Bacteriology, 82,* 53–66.

15. Sarff, L. D., McCracken, G. H., Jr., Schiffer, M. S., et al. (1975). Epidemiology of *Escherichia coli* K1 in healthy and diseased newborns. *Lancet, 1,* 1099–1104.

16. Alarcón, A., Pena, P., Salas, S., et al. (2004). Neonatal early onset *Escherichia coli* sepsis: trends in incidence and antimicrobial resistance in the era of intrapartum antimicrobial prophylaxis. *Pediatric Infectious Disease Journal, 23,* 295–299.

17. Levine, E. M., Ghai, V., Barton, J. J., & Strom, C. M. (1999). Intrapartum antibiotic prophylaxis increases the incidence of gram-negative neonatal sepsis. *Infect Disease Obstetrical Gynecology, 7,* 210–213.

18. Daley, A. J., & Garland, S. M. (2004). Prevention of neonatal group B streptococcal disease: progress, challenges and dilemmas. *Journal of Paediatrics Child Health, 40,* 664–668.

19. Furuya, E. Y., & Lowy, F. D. (2006). Antimicrobial-resistant bacteria in the community setting. *Nature Reviews Microbiology, 4,* 36–45.

20. Huang, S. H., Wang, X. N., & Jong, A. (2007). The evolving role of infectomics in drug discovery. *Expert Opinion Drug Discovery, 2,* 961–975.

21. Ley, R. E., Peterson, D. A., & Gordon, J. I. (2006). Ecological and evolutionary forces shaping microbial diversity in the human intestine. *Cell, 124,* 837–848.

22. Silfverdal, S. A., Bodin, L., & Olcen, P. (1999). Protective effect of breastfeeding: an ecologic study of *Haemophilus influenzae* meningitis and breastfeeding in a Swedish population. *International Journal of Epidemiology, 28,* 152–156.

23. Wold, A. E., & Adlerberth, I. (2000). Breast feeding and the intestinal microflora of the infant—implications for protection against infectious diseases. *Advances in Experimental Medicine and Biology, 478,* 77–93.

24. Mastretta, E., Longo, P., Laccisaglia, A., et al. (2002). Effect of *Lactobacillus* GG and breast-feeding in the prevention of rotavirus nosocomial infection. *Journal of Pediatrics Gastroenterol Nutrition, 35,* 527–531.

25. Huang, S. H., Triche, T., & Jong, A. Y. (2002). Infectomics: genomics and proteomics of microbial infections. *Functional & Integrative Genomics, 1,* 331–344.

26. Gan, B. S., Kim, J., Reid, G., et al. (2002). *Lactobacillus fermentum* RC–14 inhibits *Staphylococcus aureus* infection of surgical implants in rats. *Journal of Infectious Diseases, 185,* 1369–1372.

27. McCracken, V. J., & Lorenz, R. G. (2001). The gastrointestinal ecosystem: a precarious alliance among epithelium, immunity and microbiota. *Cell Microbiology, 3,* 1–11.

28. Falkow, S. (2006). Is persistent bacterial infection good for your health? *Cell, 124,* 699–702.

29. Kuklinska, D., & Kilian, M. (1984). Relative proportions of Haemophilus species in the throat of healthy children and adults. *European Journal of Clinical Microbiology, 3,* 249–252.

30. Van Den Driessche, M., & Veereman-Wauters, G. (2002). Functional foods in pediatrics. *Acta Gastro-Enterologica Belgica, 65,* 45–51.

31. Huang, S. H., Jong, A., & Warburton, D. (2004). Infectomics in the discovery and development of new antimicrobial agents. *Current Medicinal Chemistry–Anti-Infective Agents, 3,* 57–67.

32. Brussow, H. (2005). Phage therapy: the *Escherichia coli* experience. *Microbiology, 151,* 2133–2140.

33. Levin, B. R., & Bull, J. J. (2004). Population and evolutionary dynamics of phage therapy. *Nature Reviews Microbiology, 2,* 166–173.

34. Guarner, F., & Malagelada, J. R. (2003). Gut flora in health and disease. *Lancet, 361,* 512–519.

35. Gionchetti, P., Rizzello, F., Venturi, A., et al. (2000). Oral bacteriotherapy as maintenance treatment in patients with chronic pouchitis: a double-blind, placebo-controlled trial. *Gastroenterology, 119,* 305–309.

36. Schultz, M., Veltkamp, C., Dieleman, L. A., et al. (2002). *Lactobacillus plantarum* 299V in the treatment and prevention of spontaneous colitis in interleukin–10-deficient mice. *Inflammatory Bowel Diseases, 8,* 71–80.

37. Ogawa, M., Shimizu, K., Nomoto, K., et al. (2001). Protective effect of *Lactobacillus casei* strain Shirota on Shiga toxin-producing *Escherichia coli* O157: H7 infection in infant rabbits. *Infection and Immunity, 69,* 1101–1108.

38. Resta-Lenert, S., & Barrett, K. E. (2003). Live probiotics protect intestinal epithelial cells from the effects of infection with enteroinvasive *Escherichia coli* (EIEC). *Gut, 52,* 988–997.

39. Alvarez-Olmos, M. I., & Oberhelman, R. A. (2001). Probiotic agents and infectious diseases: a modern perspective on a traditional therapy. *Clinical Infectious Diseases, 32,* 1567–1576.

40. Sodhi, C., Richardson, W., Gribar, S., & Hackam, D. J. (2008). The development of animal models for the study of necrotizing enterocolitis. *Disease Models & Mechanisms, 1,* 94–98.

41. Alfaleh, K., & Bassler, D. (2008). Probiotics for prevention of necrotizing enterocolitis in preterm infants CD005496. *Cochrane Database of Systematic Reviews*(1).

42. Gaul, J. (2008). Probiotics for prevention of necrotizing enterocolitis. *Neonatal Network, 27,* 75–80.

43. Deshpande, G., Rao, S., & Patole, S. (2007). Probiotics for prevention of necrotising enterocolitis in preterm

neonates with very low birthweight: a systematic review of randomised controlled trials. *Lancet, 369,* 1614–1620.

44. Manzoni, P., Mostert, M., Leonessa, M. L, et al. (2006). Oral supplementation with *Lacibacillus casei* subspecies rhamnosus prevents enteric colonisation by candida species in preterm neonates: a randomised study. *Clinical Infectious Diseases, 42,* 1735–1742.

45. Mohan, R., Koebnick, C., Schildt, J., et al. (2006). Effects of *Bifidobacterium lactis* Bb12 supplementation on intestinal microbiota of preterm neonates: a double placebo controlled, randomised study. *Journal of Clinical Microbiology, 44,* 4025–4031.

46. Thompson, C., McCarter, Y. S., Krause, P. J., & Herson, V. C. (2001). *Lactobacillus acidophilus sepsis* in a neonate. *Journal of Perinatology, 21,* 258–260.

47. Broughton, R. A., Gruber, W. C., Haffar, A. A., & Baker, C. J. (1983). Neonatal meningitis due to lactobacillus. *Pediatric Infectious Diseases, 2,* 382–384.

48. Reid, G., & Kirjaivanen, P. (2005). Taking probiotics during pregnancy. Are they useful therapy for mothers and newborns? *Canadian Family Physician, 51,* 1477–1479.

49. Vendt, N., Grunberg, H., Tuure, T., et al. (2006). Growth during the first 6 months of life in infants using formula enriched with *Lactobacillus rhamnosus* GG: double-blind, randomized trial. *Journal of Human Nutrition and Dietetics, 19,* 51–58.

50. Basu, S., Chatterjee, M., Ganguly, S., & Chandra, P. K. (2007). Effect of *Lactobacillus rhamnosus* GG in persistent diarrhea in Indian children: a randomized controlled trial. *Journal of Clinical Gastroenterology, 41,* 756–760.

51. Mattar, A. F., Drongowski, R. A., Coran, A. G., & Harmon, C. M. (2001). Effect of probiotics on enterocyte bacterial translocation *in vitro*. *Pediatric Surgery International, 17,* 265–268.

52. Huang, S. H., He, L., Zhou, Y. H., et al. (2009). *Lactobacillus rhamnosus* GG suppresses meningitic *E.coli* K1 penetration across human intestinal epithelial cells *in vitro* and protects neonatal rats against experimental hematogenous meningitis [Epub online doi:10.1155/2009/647862]. *International Journal of Microbiology, 9.*

53. Reid, G. (2006). Safe and efficacious probiotics: what are they? *Trends Microbiology, 14,* 348–352.

54. Salminen, M. K., Tynkkynen, S., Rautelin, H., et al. (2002). *Lactobacillus bacteremia* during a rapid increase in probiotic use of *Lactobacillus rhamnosus* GG in Finland. *Clinical Infectious Diseases, 35,* 1155–1160.

55. Rousset, M. (1986). The human colon carcinoma cell lines HT–29 and Caco–2: two *in vitro* models for the study of intestinal differentiation. *Biochimie, 68,* 1035–1040.

56. Weiser, J. N., & Gotschlich, E. C. (1991). Outer membrane protein A (OmpA) contributes to serum resistance and pathogenicity of *Escherichia coli* K–1. *Infection and Immunity, 59,* 2252–2258.

57. Bruckener, K. E., el Baya, A., Galla, H. J., & Schmidt, M. A. (2003). Permeabilization in a cerebral endothelial barrier model by pertussis toxin involves the PKC effector pathway and is abolished by elevated levels of cAMP. *Journal of Cell Sciences, 116,* 1837–1846.

58. Pietzak, M. M.., Badger, J., Huang, S. H., et al. (2001). *Escherichia coli* K1 IbeA is required for efficient intestinal epithelial invasion *in vitro* and *in vivo* in neonatal rats. *Journal of Pediatric Gastroenterology Nutrition, 33,* 400.

59. Burns, J. L., Griffith, A., Barry, J. J., et al. (2001). Transcytosis of gastrointestinal epithelial cells by *Escherichia coli* K1. *Pediatric Research, 49,* 30–37.

60. Kim, J. W., Chakraborty, E., Huang, S., et al. (2003). Does S-fimbrial adhesin play a role in E. coli K1 bacterial pathogenesis? *Gastroenterology, 124,* A–A483.

Probiotics and Prebiotics—Prevention and Therapy in Atopic Eczema

Britta Bunselmeyer, and Kirsten Buddendick

Department of Dermatology, University Hospital Münster, Germany

1. INTRODUCTION

Atopic eczema (AE) is a chronic, inflammatory skin disorder affecting 10–25% of children in western countries [1–4]. Although the incidence of AE has increased over the past several decades, this trend is not evenly distributed throughout the population. For example, there is a genetic predisposition to develop AE if first-degree family members are already suffering from an atopic disease (AE, allergic rhinoconjunctivitis or asthma). The highest risk for newborns developing AE exists if the mother is suffering from AE, or if both parents are suffering from the same atopic disease.

In AE, a dysregulation of cellular immunity leads to an imbalance of the T-helper lymphocyte ratio (Th1/Th2) in favor of Th2, which is the predominant response in allergic patients. For both pathways there are numerous specific cytokines, with modulating allergic or non-allergic immune responses. The steady increase of AE in developed countries might be linked to hygiene improvement within the environment; children might be less exposed to infectious agents during the first months of life and might therefore develop a predominant Th2 response.

Other environmental factors are preventive: exposure to other children, infections, exclusively breast-feeding, animals and farming environments during infancy. These observations support the hygiene hypothesis, which proposes that exposure to infections, e.g. due to more siblings, an anthroposophical lifestyle, or microbial products in infancy which can favorably modify immune development towards Th1 and inhibit atopic diseases [5–7].

Standard symptomatic treatment strategies for AE include consequent emollient therapy in combination with anti-inflammatory treatments using topical steroids or calcineurin inhibitors, and, if necessary, oral immune-suppressive drugs, antimicrobial agents, phototherapy or antihistamines. Changing environmental and genetic factors is difficult. For this reason, a number of trials have been conducted to evaluate nutritional strategies for prevention and therapy of AE. Exclusively breast-feeding for the first 4 months is recommended in all newborns. If nursing is not possible, for high-risk infants there are several extensive or partial hydrolysates available, which are sufficient to reduce the incidence of AE during the first 6 years of life [8]. Additional preventive effects due to probiotic intake have been shown as primary in 2001 by Kalliomäki in a Finnish randomized, double blind placebo-controlled study [9].

2. PROBIOTICS

2.1. Immune Modulating Characteristics of Probiotics—Result of *In Vitro* and *In Vivo* Trials

In vitro trials show that probiotic lactic acid bacteria have a modulating influence on the production of certain cytokines and so can possibly influence naïve T cells in their differentiation to Th1 or Th2, respectively.

Pochard [10] and coworkers isolated mononuclear white blood cells of subjects allergic to house dust mites and stimulated these with the house dust mite antigen Dermatophagoides pteronissimus. Here they showed that a preincubation of these white blood cells with different Gram-positive lactobacilli, dependent on the dose, inhibited the production of Th2 interleukin (IL)-4 and IL-5 as well as increased the production of Th1 γ–interferon (IFN-γ). This effect does not arise from pre-incubation with Gram-negative *Escherichia coli*.

Similar findings are provided by Shida [11], who immunized mice with a hen's egg antigen (ovalbumin) and incubated the sensitized spleen cells with and without *Lactobacillus casei* with ovalbumin. There was evidence of an inhibiting effect through *Lactobacillus casei* on IL-4 and IL-5 production as well as an increase of IL-12 and IFN-γ. The authors suspect that this shift of cytokines is the reason for the reduction in total IgE as well as the allergen specific IgE against ovalbumin in their trial [11].

Pelto and coworkers [12] could show in a double blind, placebo-controlled cross-over trial that a supplementation of cows' milk with LGG (*Lactobacillus* Goldin and Gorbach) influences the unspecific immune answer in humans with and without intolerance to cows' milk in different ways. In this trial volunteers with gastrointestinal symptoms after cows' milk ingestion ($n = 8$, intolerant to milk) and a control group ($n = 9$, tolerant to milk) were challenged with milk over 1 week each. Intolerance to lactose was excluded in all volunteers in the run-up. The groups received 200 mL of pure cows' milk with or without LGG in a dose of 2.6×10^8 cfu (colony-forming units) twice a day over 1 week. After a subsequent 1-week wash-out phase the groups were switched. The expression of phagozytose receptors on neutrophil granulocytes and monocytes were measured via flow cytometry before and after the intervention phases. In milk-tolerant patients cows' milk ingestion led to a significant increase of receptor expression on neutrophil granulocytes (CRI, FcγRI, FcaR) and monocytes (CRI, CR3, FcaR). When the milk was augmented with LGG, this increased expression failed to appear. In milk-tolerant volunteers, cows' milk consumption did not lead to an increased receptor expression on neutrophil granulocytes, whereas supplementation with LGG did.

This thesis is supported by trials with non-allergic or, respectively, non-atopic adult probands. The phagocytosis activity of granulocytes was increased after a 3-week period of ingesting probiotic lactic acid bacteria *in vitro*. This effect was achieved by *Lactobacillus acidophilus* La1 (7×10^{10} cfu/day) as well as by *Bifidobacterium bifidum* Bb12 (1×10^{10} cfu/day) [13].

Schiffrin [14] described a humoral increase of specific Immunoglobulin A (IgA) against Salmonella typhi Ty2a after oral vaccination in patients after supplementation of probiotics. Probands taking each $>5 \times 10^9$ cfu *Lactobacillus acidophilus* La1 and *Bifidobacterium bifidum* Bb12, showed an IgA-Salmonella-typhi-titer increased by four times in comparison to the control group ($p = 0.04$). Secretory IgA in feces of healthy infants could be significantly increased by giving a formula augmented with *Bifidobacterium bifidum* Bb12 [15]. In healthy subjects, probiotics may act as adjuvants to the humoral immune response following oral vaccination or food antigen introduction [16], whereas bacterial strains have different effects [17].

2.2. Prevention of Atopic Diseases with Probiotics—Clinical Trials

Clinically relevant effects on infants highly at risk of developing an atopic disease were shown in the context of a randomized, double blind, placebo-controlled trial [9]. Infants are determined as at high risk if at least one first-degree relative (mother, father, sibling) already suffers from an atopic disease such as asthma, allergic rhinitis and/or atopic eczema. One hundred and fifty-nine pregnant women were randomized into two groups. The verum group was given two capsules with a total of 10^{10} cfu LGG per day 2–4 weeks before expected date of delivery until 6 months postnatally. The placebo group was also given two capsules daily, but with microcristalline cellulose. If the baby was breast-fed the mother consumed the capsules, if not, the baby was given the contents of the capsules dissolved in water. By daily ingestion of LGG the prevalence of atopic eczema at the age of 2 years was decreased by 50%. This effect continued until the age of 4 years (Table 19.1) [18]. The same study method has been used by a German team to verify these findings for Germany, but failed to show any preventive effect in the probiotic group [19]. Possible explanations might be: a different genetic background; lack of information regarding the duration of 'exclusively' breast-feeding; and/or different amounts of older siblings between the intervention groups.

The preventive effect of LGG in the Finnish trial was irrespective of the mother breast-feeding the baby or not. Presumptive, there is a correlation of the increased production of TGF-β

in breast milk of nursing women supplementing LGG, in comparison to breast-feeding mothers who ingested placebo [20]. In this context, it is important to point out that maternal colostrum naturally contains a significantly higher concentration of TGF-β than mature breast milk [21], but there is an increase of TGF-β and IgA after probiotic supplementation [22, 23].

In the course of the physiological development of tolerance within the first 6 months of life, a shift takes place from the initially intrauterine T_{H2}- to a T_{H1}-response. This is explained by the findings of Prescott and coworkers [23, 24], who detected increased INF-γ in cord blood of neonates of mothers who received probiotics, compared with the placebo group. Previous trials give reason to believe that probiotics are able to encourage a T_{H1}- response and hence a physiological development of tolerance.

Infants with allergies in western societies are reported to be less frequently colonized with infant-type *Bifidobacterium* species such as *Bifidobacterium longum* and *Bifidobacterium breve*, and more frequently colonized by *Bifidumbacterium adolescentis* and other species typical of the adult intestinal microbiota than infants without allergies [25, 26]. Exclusively prenatal probiotic administration with LGG (from 36 weeks of gestation until delivery) can influence *Bifidobacterium microbiota* development in infants with high risk of allergy [27]. These findings are in line with the outcome of less IgE-associated allergic diseases in cesarean-delivered children [28]. A summary of randomized, double blind, placebo-controlled clinical trials for prevention of AE is listed in Table 19.1.

2.3. Therapy of Atopic Eczema with Probiotics—Findings From Clinical Trials

Majamaa and Isolauri [29] showed in 1997 for the first time that probiotic bacteria are able to improve the symptoms of atopic eczema within 1 month. Twenty-seven children, aged 2.5–15.7 months with atopic eczema and verified cows' milk

TABLE 19.1 Clinical outcomes of randomized, double blind, placebo-controlled trials with pro- and prebiotic intake for prevention of atopic eczema

Reference	N (randomized, pregnant women or infants)	N (infants/children available for assessment)	Efficacy endpoint—Age of atopic eczema determination	Intervention Probiotics/prebiotics	Ingestion	Study design	Results
Kalliomäki 2001, Finland[1]	159 women, family atopy	132	2 years	LGG[2] directly ingested by breast-feeding mothers or cEHF[3] supplemented with LGG[2] versus microcrystalline cellulose (placebo)	Pregnant women and infants	2–4 weeks prenatally until 6 months postnatally; LGG[2] versus placebo	↓Prevalence of AE[4] at age of 2 years; 23% LGG[2]; 46% placebo
Kalliomäki 2003, Finland[5]		107	4 years				↓Prevalence of AE[4] at age of 4 years; 28% LGG[2]; 46% placebo
Moro 2006, Italy[6]	259 infants, parental atopy	206	6 months	wEHF[7] supplemented with GOS[8] and FOS[9] versus maltodextrin (placebo)	Infants	Start bottle feeding within the first 2 weeks of life, no breast-feeding after 6 weeks of life; 5.2–6 month study formula ad libitum	↓Prevalence of AE at age of 6 months; 10% prebiotic (GOS[8]/FOS[9]); 23% placebo
Arslanoglu 2008, Italy[10]		134	2 years				↓Prevalence of AE[4] at age of 2 years; 14% prebiotic (GOS[8]/FOS[9]); 28% placebo
Kukkonen 2007, Finland[11]	1223 women, parental atopy	925	2 years	Mixture of four different probiotic strains (including LGG[2]) and additionally GOS[8] for the infant versus microcrystalline cellulose and sugar syrup (placebo)	Pregnant women and infants	2–4 weeks prenatally until 6 months postnatally	↓Prevalence of AE[4] at age of 2 years (eczema without IgE sensitization); 26% probiotic/prebiotic (GOS[8]); AE[4] 32% placebo; AE[4] (eczema with IgE sensitization); 12.4% probiotic/prebiotic (GOS[8]); 17.7% placebo

Study	Participants	N	Intervention	Population	Duration	Results
Taylor 2007, Australia[12]	226 infants, maternal atopy	178	Lactobacillus acidophilus (LAVRI-A1) with maltodextrin versus maltodextrin (placebo)	Infants	6 months postnatally	No difference in prevalence of AE[4] at 6 months; 26% probiotic; 23% placebo. No difference in prevalence of AE[4] at 12 months; 38% probiotic; 34% placebo
Kopp 2008, Germany[13]	105 women, family atopy	94	LGG[2] versus microcrystalline cellulose (placebo)	Pregnant women and infants	4–6 weeks prenatally until 6 months postnatally (3 months breast-feeding mothers and then 3 months to the infant directly); LGG[2] versus placebo	No difference in prevalence of AE[4] at age of 2 years; 28% LGG[2]; 27% placebo
Wickens 2008, New Zealand[14]	512 women, parental atopy	446	Lactobacillus rhamnosus HN001 versus Bifidobacterium animalis subsp. lactis HN019 versus placebo (dextran, salt, yeast extract)	Pregnant women and infants	35 weeks' gestation and 6 months postnatally L. rhamnosus HN001 versus B. animalis subsp. lactis HN019 versus placebo	↓Prevalence of AE[4] at the age of 2 years in the Lactobacillus rhamnosus group. Atopic eczema (eczema with IgE sensitization); 10% L. rhamnosus HN001; 19% placebo; 13% B. animalis subsp. lactis HN019; (eczema without IgE sensitization); 5% L. rhamnosus HN001; 11% B. animalis subsp. lactis HN019; 9% placebo

(Continued)

TABLE 19.1 (Continued)

Reference	N (randomized, pregnant women or infants)	N (infants/children available for assessment)	Efficacy endpoint—Age of atopic eczema determination	Intervention Probiotics/Prebiotics	Ingestion	Study design	Results
Kuitunen 2009, Finland[15]	1223 women, parental atopy	891	5 years	Mixture of four different probiotic strains (including LGG[2]) and additionally GOS[8] for the infant versus microcrystalline cellulose and sugar syrup (placebo)	Pregnant women and infants	36 weeks' gestation probiotic mixture for mothers and 6 months postnatally probiotic mixture + GOS[8] for the infant for 6 months	No change in AE[4] prevalence at the age of 5 years. ↓Prevalence of AE[4] at 5 years of life in cesarean-delivered children 15.7 vs 30.4%

[1] Kalliomaki, M., Salminen, S., Arvilommi, H. et al. (2001). *Lancet* 357, 1076–1079.

[2] LGG: *Lactobacillus* Goldin and Gorbach.

[3] cEHF: extensive hydrolysate formula on casein basis.

[4] AE: atopic eczema.

[5] Kalliomaki, M., Salminen, S., Poussa, T. et al. (2003). *Lancet* 361, 1869–1871.

[6] Moro, G., Arslanoglu, S., Stahl, B. et al. (2006). *Archives of Disease in Childhood* 91, 814–819.

[7] wEHF: extensive hydrolysate formula on whey basis.

[8] GOS: galacto-oligosaccharides.

[9] FOS: fructo-oligosaccharides.

[10] Arslanoglu, S., Moro, G. E., Schmitt, J. et al. (2008). *J Nutr* 138, 1091–1095.

[11] Kukkonen, K., Savilahti, E., Haahtela, T. et al. (2007). *Journal of Allergy and Clinical Immunology* 119, 192–198.

[12] Taylor, A. L., Dunstan, J. A. & Prescott, S. L. (2007). *Journal of Allergy and Clinical Immunology* 119, 184–191.

[13] Kopp, M. V., Hennemuth, I., Heinzmann, A. & Urbanek, R. (2008). *Pediatrics* 121, E850–E856.

[14] Wickens, K., Black, P. N., Stanley, T. V. et al. (2008). *J Allergy Clin Immunol* 122, 788–794.

[15] Kuitunen, M., Kukkonen, K., Juntunen-Backman, K. et al. (2009). *J Allergy Clin Immunol* 123, 335–341.

allergy (CMA), received an extensive hydrolysate on the base of whey with LGG (5×10^8 cfu/g formula) or without LGG (placebo) on a randomized basis over 4 weeks. Determination of AE severity has been done by the severity scoring index for atopic dermatitis (SCORAD), which included objective and subjective symptoms of AE within a scale of 0 to 103 [30]. Clinically, the verum group showed a significant improvement of skin condition, in comparison to the placebo group (–11 points vs –2 points). There was no difference in serum concentration of inflammatory cytokines (ECP, TNF-α, IL-4 and INF-γ) in the groups, but there was a decline of tumor necrosis factor alpha (TNF-α) in the feces of the probiotic group which was not seen in the placebo group.

Similar findings were demonstrated in a randomized, double blind, placebo-controlled trial [31], which compared the effects of two different probiotic strains. Twenty-seven infants with atopic eczema took part in this trial, with an average age of 4.6 months (SCORAD at baseline between 7–25 points) which previously were exclusively breast-fed. The first group received an extensive hydrolysate on the base of casein (cEHF), augmented with LGG in a concentration of 3×10^8 cfu/g. Group 2 received the same formula with *Bifidobacterium lactis* Bb12 (1×10^9 cfu/g). The third group received the cEHF without supplementation as placebo. After an 8-week intervention phase the skin condition in both probiotic groups improved significantly ($p = 0.002$) in comparison to the placebo group.

A Danish study group [32] demonstrated in a randomized, double blind, placebo-controlled cross-over trial a therapeutic effect by giving *Lactobacillus rhamnosus* (2×10^{10} cfu/day) combined with *Lactobacillus reuteri* (2×10^{10} cfu/day) to children (1–13 years) with atopic eczema over 6 weeks. Between the intervention phases, a 6-week wash-out phase was maintained in which no supplementation took place. Fifty-six percent of patients reported an improvement of their atopic eczema after the verum phase versus 15% of patients after the placebo phase. In the total sample there was no significant difference in SCORAD, but definitely in the subgroup of sensitized patients (at least one positive reaction in the prick test and an increased total IgE). The SCORAD index declined significantly in comparison to the not sensitized patients ($p = 0.02$). Whilst here as well there was no difference in the cytokine pattern (IL-2, IL-4, IL-10 and INF-γ) to be determined, there was a significant decline of ECP in the serum of the patients after the verum phase.

No therapeutic effects could be demonstrated in patients with cows' milk allergy [9, 18, 29, 33] or pre-existing pollen-associated allergies to apple (oral allergy syndrome) [34]. There also appears to be no evidence as yet that total or allergen specific IgE *in vivo* is reduced by ingesting such microorganisms.

In summary, these trials show that a slight improvement in skin condition in children with atopic eczema with or without cows' milk allergy can be achieved by probiotic lactic acid bacteria (Table 19.2). However, this effect was only demonstrated for a few probiotic strains and only in a mild form of atopic eczema (SCORAD <40). At this point in time, the existing findings argue for a therapeutic effect expected in IgE-sensitized children, not older than 18 months of age, rather than in older patients without sensitization. A summary of the results of double blind, placebo-controlled clinical trials for therapeutic use in AE is listed in Table 19.2.

3. PREBIOTICS

Prebiotics are specific indigestible substances that facilitate growth of selective bifidobacteria and possibly other microorganisms in the colon and therefore achieve health-benefiting effects. Prebiotics employed in foods can be divided into two main groups:

1. Fructo-oligosaccharides (FOS) are medium- and long-chain fructose molecules that

TABLE 19.2 Clinical outcomes of double blind, placebo-controlled trials with pro- and prebiotic intake for therapy of atopic eczema

References	N (available for assessment)	Age	Study population	Intervention Probiotics/prebiotics	Dietary restrictions during intervention	Study duration/design	Results
Majamaa 1997, Finland[1]	27	2.5–15.7 months	AE[2] and CMA[3]	wEHF[4] with LGG[5] versus wEHF[4] (placebo)		4 weeks	Significant SCORAD[6] reduction; probiotic/LGG[5]: −11; placebo: −2
Isolauri 2000, Finland[7]	27	4.6 months (median)	AE[2]	cEHF[8] with LGG[5] or Bb12 versus cEHF[8] (placebo)		8 weeks	Significant SCORAD[6] reduction; probiotic/LGG[5]: −15; probiotic/Bb12: −16; placebo: −2.6
Rosenfeld 2003, Denmark[9]	43	1–13 years	AE[2]	L. rhamnosus 19070–2 and L. reuteri (DSM 122460) versus placebo		6 weeks (cross-over) Group A: 6 weeks probiotic 6 weeks wash-out 6 weeks placebo Group B: 6 weeks placebo 6 weeks wash-out 6 weeks probiotic	No significant difference in SCORAD[6] reduction. Note: Statistical significant reduction in SCORAD[6] was shown in the IgE sensitized probiotic subgroup
Weston 2005, Australia[10]	56	6–18 months	AE[2]	L. fermentum VRI-033 PCC versus placebo		8 weeks	Significant SCORAD[6] reduction in the probiotic group (especially in the extent)
Viljanen 2005, Finland[11]	230	1.4–11.9 months (mean 6.4 months)	AE[2] and suspected CMA	LGG[5] versus a mixture of 4 probiotic strains (LGG, L. rhamnosus LC705, Bifidobacterium breve Bbi99, Propionibacterium freudenreichii ssp. Shermanii JS) versus placebo	Elimination of cows' milk (wEHF[4])	4 weeks supplementation, 4 weeks wash-out, DBPCFC[12] with cows' milk	No difference in SCORAD[6] reduction between probiotics and placebo group after 4 weeks' intervention and 8 weeks' follow-up. No difference in prevalence of CMA[3]. Note: Statistical significant reduction in SCORAD[6] (−35.4 points) was shown in the IgE sensitized LGG[5] subgroup (n = 28)

Study	N	Condition	Age	Intervention	Diet	Duration	Results
Fölster-Holst 2006, Germany[13]	43	AE[2]	1–55 months (median 19 months)	LGG *versus* placebo		8 weeks	No difference in SCORAD between probiotic and placebo group
Passeron 2006, France[14]	39	AE[2]	2–12 years (mean 5.82 years)	*L. rhamnosus* Lcr35 *versus L. rhamnosus* Lcr35 and prebiotic preparation	No change from normal diet	3 months	Significant reduction in total and objective SCORAD[6] score in the probiotic and symbiotic group after 3 months. Probiotic: from 39 to 24; symbiotic: from 39 to 21; placebo: no data available
Brouwer 2006, Netherlands[15]	50	AE[2] and suspected CMA[3]	<5 months	wEHF[4] with *L. rhamnosus versus* wEHF[4] with LGG[5] *versus* wEHF (placebo)	wEHF[4] 3–5 weeks before intervention	3 months	No differences between probiotics and placebo group
Sistek 2006, New Zealand[16]	59	AE[2] (IgE sensitized)	1–10 years	*L. rhamnosus* and *B. lactis versus* placebo		12 weeks	No difference in SCORAD[6] between probiotic and placebo group. Significant SCORAD[6] reduction only in the food IgE sensitized children

(Continued)

TABLE 19.2 (Continued)

References	N (available for assessment)	Age	Study population	Intervention Probiotics/prebiotics	Dietary restrictions during intervention	Study duration/ design	Results
Grüber 2007, Germany[17]	102	3–12 months	AE	LGG[5] *versus* placebo		12 weeks	No difference in SCORAD[6] between probiotic and placebo group. No difference in SCORAD[6] in the IgE sensitized subgroup

[1]Majamaa, H. & Isolauri, E. (1997). *J Allergy Clin Immunol 99*, 179–185.

[2]AE: atopic eczema.

[3]Cows' milk allergy.

[4]wEHF: extensive hydrolysate formula on whey basis.

[5]*Lactobacillus* Goldin and Gorbach.

[6]SCORAD: severity scoring index for atopic dermatitis.

[7]Isolauri, E., Arvola, T., Sutas, Y. et al. (2000). *Clin Exp Allergy 30*, 1604–1610.

[8]cEHF: extensive hydrolysate formula on casein basis.

[9]Rosenfeldt, V., Benfeldt, E., Nielsen, S. D., Michaelsen, K. F. et al. (2003). *J Allergy Clin Immunol 111*, 389–395.

[10]Weston, S., Halbert, A., Richmond, P. & Prescott, S. L. (2005). *Arch Dis Child 90*, 892–897.

[11]Viljanen, M., Savilahti, E., Haahtela, T. et al. (2005). *Allergy 60*, 494–500.

[12]DBPCFC: double blind placebo-controlled food challenge.

[13]Folster-Holst, R., Muller, F., Schnopp, N. et al. (2006). *Br J Dermatol 155*, 1256–1261.

[14]Passeron, T., Lacour, J. P., Fontas, E. & Ortonne, J. P. (2006). *Allergy 61*, 431–437.

[15]Brouwer, M. L., Wolt-Plompen, S. A. A., Dubois, A. E. J. et al. (2006). *Clinical and Experimental Allergy 36*, 899–906.

[16]Sistek, D., Kelly, R., Wickens, K. et al. (2006). *Clinical and Experimental Allergy 36*, 629–633.

[17]Gruber, C., Wendt, M., Sulser, C. et al. (2007). *Allergy 62*, 1270–1276.

cannot be macerated enzymatically by the human organism. Among these are inulin and oligofructose mainly used for non-alcoholic drinks and yogurt.

2. Galacto-oligosaccharides (GOS) consist of glucose, galactose and diverse amino sugars. Galacto-oligosaccharides occur naturally, mainly in breast milk, and are augmented to baby food, primarily in combination with fructo-oligosaccharides, by the food industry.

Breast milk facilitates the development of the microflora of the colon, with bifidobacteria and lactobacilli dominating with 90% of the total flora. A possible reason for the bifidogene effect of breast milk is its high content of galacto-oligosaccharides, of which more than 130 different ones have been characterized. Prebiotics in the form of soluble fibers such as fructo- and galacto-oligosaccharides are augmented to infant food, to facilitate a bifidogene flora in the colon—as is the case in breast-fed babies [35].

3.1. Health-related Impacts

The food industry suggests a health promoting impact of prebiotics by slogans such as 'promotes the body's own intestinal flora and immune defense' or 'increases the number of useful intestinal bacteria and therefore blocks unwanted bacteria and promotes the immune defense.' Inulin and oligofructose are declared on the ingredients list as prebiotic ingredients (FOS). Declarations on dose–response refer to a significant increase of bifidobacteria in feces. Double blind, placebo-controlled trials show that this is possible by a 3–4-week diet with prebiotic baby food for mature- and premature-born babies. Mixtures of fructo- and galacto-oligosaccharides in a concentration of 0.4–1% in ready-to-drink baby food were used [35, 36]. With an assumed consumption of 500–1000 mL per day, a baby would therefore take in 2–10 g oligosaccharides, which is comparable to the intake quantity through breast milk [37].

To reach a prebiotic effect in adults, the ingestion of 4–20 g fructo-oligosaccharides per day is necessary. Prebiotic drinks for children and adults contain 0.4–0.6% inulin or 0.4–1% oligofructose and, therefore, in most cases are dosed too low in order to reach a bifidogene effect under normal eating habits.

Different to probiotics, the data situation in reference to clinically relevant questions for prebiotics is humble. It is proven that the consumption of fructo- and galacto-oligosaccharides leads, dependent on dose, to an increase of bifidobacteria in feces after 2–4 weeks. Prebiotics have (like other fibers) a direct influence on stool frequency and consistency.

Bifidobacteria are reduced in patients with atopic eczema, as well as in allergic and bottle fed children [38–40]. There is a randomized, double blind, placebo-controlled trial available, which shows a reduction in AE prevalence at the age of 6 months [41] and 2 years [42] in infants who receive a wEHF supplemented with FOS and GOS, compared to the placebo group (wEHF). The authors summarize that GOS/FOS supplementation led to a significant reduction in the plasma level of total IgE, IgG1, IgG2 and IgG3, whereas no effect on IgG4 was observed. Cows' milk protein specific IgG1 was significantly decreased. Diphtheria, tetanus, and polio specific immunglobulin levels were not affected. This study shows that GOS/FOS supplementation is able to modify the antibody profile [43]. Immunological effects after vaccinations, or a potential prevention of travel diarrhea, could not be proved so far [44, 45].

There is a correlation between the quantity of bifidobacteria in feces and the severity of atopic eczema. Patients with pronounced skin findings had significantly less bifidobacteria and more often *Staphylococcus aureus* in the feces than patients with milder forms [40].

A direct influence of prebiotics on immunological parameters is questionable, as these indigestible carbohydrates function merely as a substrate for colon bacteria. It remains unclear to what extent an indirect influence on the immune system is possible by increasing 'probiotic' colon bacteria by means of prebiotics consumption.

4. OUTLOOK

The task group 'Probiotic microorganism cultures in foods' of the Federal Ministry of Food, Agriculture and Consumer Protection points out that physiological effective metabolic achievements in bacteria are, even *in vitro*, only relevant and measurable above the value of 10^6 cfu (colony-forming units) per gram of food. This quantity is guaranteed by most foodmakers until the end of the best before date. Probiotic milk products contain between 10^3 and 10^8 cfu/g until the end of the printed best-before-date when kept refrigerated at 4°C [46].

Physiological and measurable changes *in vivo* show at an ingested quantity of at least 10^8 cfu per day, so that immune modulating effects are inducible with a daily ingestion of 100 g probiotic yogurt with 10^6 cfu per gram. To what extent this is clinically relevant, remains unanswered as yet. So far a noteworthy preventive and therapeutic effect with reference to atopic eczema was only determined for some strains, especially LGG in high concentrations (lyophilic capsule form), which cannot be achieved by intake of available supplemented foods.

The results from prevention trials are controversial. Whereas the prevention trial from Finland showed a 50% reduction in AE, the German study did not show any preventive effect with nearly the same study design. In contrast, the German authors showed that children with recurrent episodes of wheezing bronchitis were more frequent in the LGG group (versus placebo), but no difference was observed between both groups in total IgE concentrations or number of specific sensitization to inhalant allergens.

Supplementation with probiotic lactic acid bacteria can be suggested in high-risk families for pregnant and nursing women, because of the following arguments:

- LGG as specific probiotic strain reduces the prevalence of AE in infants of high-risk families at the age of 2 and 4 years in Finnish population.
- A mixture of probiotics (including LGG) and prebiotics seemed to be effective to reduce the risk of AE in cesarean-delivered children in high-risk families from Finland.
- The risk of developing AE was the same for both the probiotic and the placebo group in trials which failed to show any preventive effect.
- Exclusively breast-feeding is still highly recommended and one protective mechanism of LGG seemed to be the immunologic change of colostrum and breast milk.
- No adverse events have been reported after ingestion of probiotic strains in AE trials, neither for the pregnant or nursing women, nor for the infant, if the probiotic preparation is not heated over 37°C.
- Probiotics, which are used in the clinical trials mentioned above, are generally recognized as safe for mature infants and children without indwelling venous catheters. Even though a preventive effect is not yet proven, at least it is worth a try for families at risk.

Besides general prevention measures, at-risk families should be informed about a pre- and postnatal supplementation as an additional prevention measure. If at least one first-degree family member suffers from an atopic disease, the mother can supplement 5×10^9 cfu LGG in capsules twice a day for 2–4 weeks before expected date of delivery as well as a further 6 months postnatally, where breast-feeding is highly recommended. If breast-feeding is not possible, the probiotic lactic acid bacteria can be dissolved in sterile water, or respectively, in infant formula (<37°C) and given to the baby directly.

Therapeutically, a supplementation in the same concentration is possible for children under the age of 18 months with mild to moderate skin findings. However, it has to be noted that by giving probiotics, only a slight improvement of eczema is anticipated, so that this measure can only be supportive in atopic eczema.

The actual data situation is not sufficient for evident recommendations for prebiotics at this point in time, as confirming studies are still outstanding.

5. CONCLUSION

Food supplementation with pre- and probiotics may reduce the prevalence for the infant in high-risk families developing an atopic eczema during the first 2 years of life. Those pregnant women should be advised to take probiotics (LGG) in late pregnancy and the first 6 months postnatally during nursing. If breast-feeding is not possible, pro- or prebiotics can be supplemented to the infant. There are no known adverse reactions and it might prevent atopic eczema, especially in neonates after cesarean delivery. Therapeutic use of probiotics to improve atopic eczema is only supportive in infants <18 months and with IgE sensitization.

References

1. Williams, H., Robertson, C., Stewart, A., et al. (1999). Worldwide variations in the prevalence of symptoms of atopic eczema in the International Study of Asthma and Allergies in Childhood. *The Journal of Allergy and Clinical Immunology, 103,* 125–138.
2. Nickel, R., Lau, S., Niggemann, B., et al. (2002). Messages from the German Multicentre Allergy Study. *Pediatric Allergy and Immunology, 13* (Suppl. 15), 7–10.
3. Ninan, T. K., & Russell, G. (1992). Respiratory symptoms and atopy in Aberdeen schoolchildren: Evidence from two surveys 25 years apart. *BMJ, 304,* 873–875.
4. Schultz, L. F., Diepgen, T., & Svensson, A. (1996). The occurrence of atopic dermatitis in north Europe: an international questionnaire study. *Journal of the American Academy of Dermatology, 34,* 760–764.
5. Strachan, D. P. (1989). Hay fever, hygiene, and household size. *BMJ, 299,* 1259–1260.
6. Zirngibl, A., Franke, K., Gehring, U., et al. (2002). Exposure to pets and atopic dermatitis during the first two years of life. A cohort study. *Pediatric Allergy and Immunology, 13,* 394–401.
7. Schoetzau, A., Filipiak-Pittroff, B., Franke, K., et al. (2002). Effect of exclusive breast-feeding and early solid food avoidance on the incidence of atopic dermatitis in high-risk infants at 1 year of age. *Pediatric Allergy and Immunology, 13,* 234–242.
8. von Berg, A., Filipiak-Pittroff, B., Kramer, U., et al. (2008). Preventive effect of hydrolyzed infant formulas persists until age 6 years: Long-term results from the German Infant Nutritional Intervention Study (GINI). *The Journal of Allergy and Clinical Immunology, 121,* 1442–1447.
9. Kalliomaki, M., Salminen, S., Arvilommi, H., et al. (2001). Probiotics in primary prevention of atopic disease: A randomised placebo-controlled trial. *Lancet, 357,* 1076–1079.
10. Pochard, P., Gosset, P., Grangette, C., et al. (2002). Lactic acid bacteria inhibit TH2 cytokine production by mononuclear cells from allergic patients. *The Journal of Allergy and Clinical Immunology, 110,* 617–623.
11. Shida, K., Makino, K., Morishita, A., et al. (1998). *Lactobacillus casei* inhibits antigen-induced IgE secretion through regulation of cytokine production in murine splenocyte cultures. *International Archives of Allergy and Immunology, 115,* 278–287.
12. Pelto, L., Isolauri, E., Lilius, E. M., et al. (1998). Probiotic bacteria down-regulate the milk-induced inflammatory response in milk-hypersensitive subjects but have an immunostimulatory effect in healthy subjects. *Clinical and Experimental Allergy, 28,* 1474–1479.
13. Donnet-Hughes, A., Rochat, F., Serrant, P., et al. (1999). Modulation of nonspecific mechanisms of defense by lactic acid bacteria: Effective dose. *Journal of Dairy Science, 82,* 863–869.
14. Schiffrin, E. J., Rochat, F., Link-Amster, H., et al. (1995). Immunomodulation of human blood cells following the ingestion of lactic acid bacteria. *Journal of Dairy Science, 78,* 491–497.
15. Fukushima, Y., Kawata, Y., Hara, H., Terada, A., & Mitsuoka, T. (1998). Effect of a probiotic formula on intestinal immunoglobulin A production in healthy children. *International Journal of Food Microbiology, 42,* 39–44.
16. Rautava, S., Arvilommi, H., & Isolauri, E. (2006). Specific probiotics in enhancing maturation of IgA responses in formula-fed infants. *Pediatric Research, 60,* 221–224.
17. Paineau, D., Carcano, D., Leyer, G., et al. (2008). Effects of seven potential probiotic strains on specific immune responses in healthy adults: A double-blind, randomized, controlled trial. *FEMS Immunol Med Microbiol, 53,* 107–113.
18. Kalliomaki, M., Salminen, S., Poussa, T., et al. (2003). Probiotics and prevention of atopic disease: 4-year follow-up of a randomised placebo-controlled trial. *Lancet, 361,* 1869–1871.
19. Kopp, M. V., Hennemuth, I., Heinzmann, A., & Urbanek, R. (2008). Randomized, double-blind, placebo-controlled trial of probiotics for primary prevention: No clinical effects of *Lactobacillus* GG supplementation. *Pediatrics, 121,* E850–E856.

20. Rautava, S., Kalliomaki, M., & Isolauri, E. (2002). Probiotics during pregnancy and breast-feeding might confer immunomodulatory protection against atopic disease in the infant. *The Journal of Allergy and Clinical Immunology, 109*, 119–121.

21. Kalliomaki, M., Ouwehand, A., Arvilommi, H., et al. (1999). Transforming growth factor-beta in breast milk: A potential regulator of atopic disease at an early age. *The Journal of Allergy and Clinical Immunology, 104*, 1251–1257.

22. Huurre, A., Laitinen, K., Rautava, S., et al. (2008). Impact of maternal atopy and probiotic supplementation during pregnancy on infant sensitization: A double-blind placebo-controlled study. *Clinical and Experimental Allergy, 38*, 1342–1348.

23. Prescott, S. L., Wickens, K., Westcott, L., et al. (2008). Supplementation with *Lactobacillus rhamnosus* or *Bifidobacterium lactis* probiotics in pregnancy increases cord blood interferon-gamma and breast milk transforming growth factor-beta and immunoglobin A detection. *Clinical and Experimental Allergy, 38*, 1606–1614.

24. Prescott, S. L., Macaubas, C., Smallacombe, T., et al. (1999). Development of allergen-specific T-cell memory in atopic and normal children. *Lancet, 353*, 196–200.

25. Suzuki, S., Shimojo, N., Tajiri, Y., et al. (2007). Differences in the composition of intestinal Bifidobacterium species and the development of allergic diseases in infants in rural Japan. *Clinical and Experimental Allergy, 37*, 506–511.

26. He, F., Ouwehand, A. C., Isolauri, E., et al. (2001). Comparison of mucosal adhesion and species identification of bifidobacteria isolated from healthy and allergic infants. *FEMS Immunol Med Microbiol, 30*, 43–47.

27. Lahtinen, S. J., Boyle, R. J., Kivivuori, S., et al. (2009). Prenatal probiotic administration can influence Bifidobacterium microbiota development in infants at high risk of allergy. *The Journal of Allergy and Clinical Immunology, 123*, 499–501.

28. Kuitunen, M., Kukkonen, K., Juntunen-Backman, K., et al. (2009). Probiotics prevent IgE-associated allergy until age 5 years in cesarean-delivered children but not in the total cohort. *The Journal of Allergy and Clinical Immunology, 123*, 335–341.

29. Majamaa, H., & Isolauri, E. (1997). Probiotics: A novel approach in the management of food allergy. *The Journal of Allergy and Clinical Immunology, 99*, 179–185.

30. Anonymous. (1993). Severity scoring of atopic dermatitis: The SCORAD index. Consensus Report of the European Task Force on Atopic Dermatitis. *Dermatology, 186*, 23–31.

31. Isolauri, E., Arvola, T., Sutas, Y., et al. (2000). Probiotics in the management of atopic eczema. *Clinical and Experimental Allergy, 30*, 1604–1610.

32. Rosenfeldt, V., Benfeldt, E., Nielsen, S. D., et al. (2003). Effect of probiotic Lactobacillus strains in children with atopic dermatitis. *The Journal of Allergy and Clinical Immunology, 111*, 389–395.

33. Hol, J., van Leer, E. H., Elink Schuurman, B. E., et al. (2008). The acquisition of tolerance toward cow's milk through probiotic supplementation: A randomized, controlled trial. *The Journal of Allergy and Clinical Immunology, 121*, 1448–1454.

34. Helin, T., Haahtela, S., & Haahtela, T. (2002). No effect of oral treatment with an intestinal bacterial strain, *Lactobacillus rhamnosus* (ATCC 53103), on birch-pollen allergy: A placebo-controlled double-blind study. *Allergy, 57*, 243–246.

35. Boehm, G., Lidestri, M., Casetta, P., et al. (2002). Supplementation of a bovine milk formula with an oligosaccharide mixture increases counts of faecal bifidobacteria in preterm infants. *Archives of Disease in Childhood, 86*, 178–181.

36. Moro, G., Minoli, I., Mosca, M., et al. (2002). Dosage-related bifidogenic effects of galacto- and fructo-oligosaccharides in formula-fed term infants. *Journal of Pediatric Gastroenterology and Nutrition, 34*, 291–295.

37. Kunz, C., Rudloff, S., Baier, W., et al. (2000). Oligosaccharides in human milk: Structural, functional, and metabolic aspects. *Annual Review of Nutrition, 20*, 699–722.

38. Bjorksten, B., Sepp, E., Julge, K., et al. (2001). Allergy development and the intestinal microflora during the first year of life. *The Journal of Allergy and Clinical Immunology, 108*, 516–520.

39. Kleessen, B., Bunke, H., Tovar, K., et al. (1995). Influence of two infant formulas and human milk on the development of the faecal flora in newborn infants. *Acta Paediatrica, 84*, 1347–1356.

40. Watanabe, S., Narisawa, Y., Arase, S., et al. (2003). Differences in fecal microflora between patients with atopic dermatitis and healthy control subjects. *The Journal of Allergy and Clinical Immunology, 111*, 587–591.

41. Moro, G., Arslanoglu, S., Stahl, B., et al. (2006). A mixture of prebiotic oligosaccharides reduces the incidence of atopic dermatitis during the first six months of age. *Archives of Disease in Childhood, 91*, 814–819.

42. Arslanoglu, S., Moro, G. E., Schmitt, J., et al. (2008). Early dietary intervention with a mixture of prebiotic oligosaccharides reduces the incidence of allergic manifestations and infections during the first two years of life. *The Journal of Nutrition, 138*, 1091–1095.

43. van Hoffen, E., Ruiter, B., Faber, J., et al. (2009). A specific mixture of short-chain galacto-oligosaccharides and long-chain fructo-oligosaccharides induces a beneficial immunoglobulin profile in infants at high risk for allergy. *Allergy, 64*, 484–487.

44. Bunout, D., Hirsch, S., Pia, D.l. M., et al. (2002). Effects of prebiotics on the immune response to vaccination in the elderly. *Journal of Parenteral and Enteral Nutrition, 26*, 372–376.

45. Cummings, J. H., Christie, S., & Cole, T. J. (2001). A study of fructo oligosaccharides in the prevention of travellers' diarrhoea. *Alimentary Pharmacology & Therapeutics, 15*, 1139–1145.

46. Schillinger, U. (1999). Isolation and identification of lactobacilli from novel-type probiotic and mild yoghurts and their stability during refrigerated storage. *International Journal of Food Microbiology, 47*, 79–87.

20

Bioengineering of Bacteria: Improved Probiotics

Roy D. Sleator

Department of Biological Sciences, Corls Institute of Technology, Rossa avenue,
Bishopstown Corls, Ireland

1. INTRODUCTION

Probiotics are beneficial organisms that can be harnessed for therapeutic or prophylactic effect [1]. In acute infections, probiotics may boost the protection afforded by commensal flora through competitive interactions, direct antagonism of pathogens, and/or production of antimicrobial factors [2]. In other clinical conditions, such as chronic infections and immunosuppression, microbe-host signaling is probably more relevant to effective probiotic action. Gut homeostasis, the maintenance of a 'balanced' and beneficial flora, requires continual signaling from bacteria within the gut lumen, maintaining the mucosal barrier while at the same time priming the gut for responses to injury [3]. Given these health-promoting benefits, improving probiotic stress tolerance and the ability to grow and survive in foods prior to ingestion and subsequently within the animal host is an important clinical goal. This is particularly relevant given that many potentially beneficial probiotics often

prove to be physiologically fragile; a significant limitation in clinical applications [4].

The patho-biotechnology concept [5–7] seeks to attain this goal, ultimately leading to the development of improved probiotic strains. A primary focus of this approach involves equipping probiotic bacteria with the genetic elements necessary to overcome the many stresses encountered during the probiotic life cycle (both external and internal to the host) as well as enabling probiotics to better deal with invading pathogens [8, 9]. This strategy can be divided into three distinct approaches (Figure 20.1). The first tackles the issue of probiotic storage and delivery by cloning and expression of pathogen specific stress survival mechanisms (facilitating improved survival at extremes of temperature and water availability), thus countering reductions in probiotic numbers which can occur during manufacture and storage of delivery matrices (such as foods and tablet formulations). The second approach aims to improve host colonization by expression of host specific survival strategies (or virulence associated factors—such

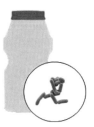
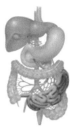
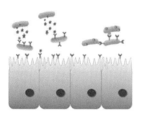

1. Delivery: Engineering
technological
robustness

2. Survival: Improved
competitiveness
in the GI tract

3. Efficacy: Improved
therapeutic/prophylactic
properties

FIGURE 20.1   The patho-biotechnology concept involves three approaches to generating improved probiotic cultures. Adapted from Sleator and Hill [29].

as the ability to cope with bile; an important component of the body's physicochemical defense system) thereby positively affecting the therapeutic efficacy of the probiotic. The final approach involves the development of so-called 'designer probiotics'; strains which specifically target invading pathogens by blocking crucial ligand-receptor interactions between the pathogen and host cell [10].

2. IMPROVING PROBIOTIC STORAGE AND DELIVERY

The most common stresses encountered during production of probiotic delivery matrices (food and/or tablet formulations) are temperature and water availability (a_w) [11]. The ability to cope with such stresses is a particularly desirable trait in the selection of commercially viable probiotic strains. A common strategy employed by a variety of microbes to deal with both low a_w and temperature stress is the accumulation of protective compounds such as betaine, carnitine and proline. These compatible solutes help to stabilize protein structure and function at low temperatures while preventing water loss from the cell and plasmolysis under low a_w conditions [12].

Improving a strain's ability to accumulate compatible solutes is thus an obvious first step in the development of more robust probiotic strains. Bacteria have evolved sophisticated mechanisms for compatible solute accumulation, including both uptake and synthesis systems [12]. Indeed, the foodborne pathogen *Listeria monocytogenes* (an extensively well-studied pathogen in terms of compatible solute accumulation [13]) possesses three distinct uptake systems (BetL, Gbu and OpuC) and at least one compatible solute synthesis system (ProBA). By placing the *betL* gene (encoding the betaine uptake system BetL [14]) under the transcriptional control of the nizin inducible promoter P*nisA* it was possible to assess the role of BetL (and thus betaine accumulation) in contributing to probiotic growth and survival under a variety of stresses likely encountered during food and/or tablet manufacture [8]. Our probiotic of choice, *Lactobacillus salivarius* UCC118, exhibits significantly lower betaine accumulation levels than *L. monocytogenes* and is correspondingly less physiologically robust than the pathogen. As expected, the *L. salivarius betL*$^+$ strain showed a significant increase in betaine accumulation compared to the wild type. Indeed, sufficient BetL was produced to confer increased salt tolerance [8], with growth of the transformed strain occurring at significantly higher salt concentrations than the parent (Figure 20.2).

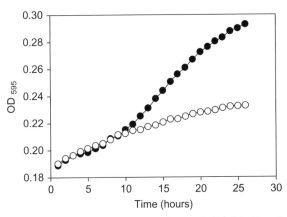

FIGURE 20.2   Growth of *Lb. salivarius* BetL$^+$ (black) and *Lb. salivarius* BetL$^-$ (white) in MRS with 7% added NaCl. Adapted from Sheehan et al. [8].

Furthermore, the presence of BetL resulted in a significant improvement in barotolerance. This is particularly significant given that high pressure processing is gaining increasing popularity as a novel non-thermal mechanism of food processing and preservation [15, 16].

3. HOST SPECIFIC COLONIZATION AND PERSISTENCE

As well as the stresses encountered during processing and storage, probiotic bacteria must also overcome the physicochemical defenses of the host in order to reach the gastrointestinal tract in sufficient numbers to exert a beneficial effect. In 2007, we demonstrated that BetL significantly improved the tolerance of the probiotic strain *Bifidobacterium breve* UCC2003 to gastric juice [9]. Interestingly, in support of this observation Termont et al. [17] also reported similar results for a *L. lactis* strain expressing the *E. coli* trehalose synthesis genes, thus suggesting a novel protective role for compatible solutes in the gastric environment. Furthermore, in line with our previous observations with

L. salivarius UCC118 [8], a significant osmoprotective effect was observed following the introduction of *betL* into *B. breve*, allowing significantly improved growth of the probiotic in conditions similar to those encountered *in vivo* (1.5% NaCl; equivalent to the osmolarity of the gut). In addition, *B. breve* strains expressing BetL were recovered at significantly higher levels than the wild type in the feces, intestines and cecum of inoculated animals. Finally, in addition to improved gastric transit and intestinal persistence (Figure 20.3A), the addition of BetL improved the clinical efficacy of the probiotic culture; mice fed *B. breve* UCC2003 (BetL$^+$) exhibited significantly lower levels of systemic infection compared to the control strain following oral inoculation with *L. monocytogenes* (Figure 20.3B). Furthermore, *in vitro* bile tolerance of *B. breve* was significantly enhanced by heterologous expression of the *L. monocytogenes* bile resistance mechanism BilE (Figure 20.4A), a phenotype which most likely explains why the *bilE$^+$* strain was recovered at significantly higher levels than the control strain from the feces and intestines of mice, following oral inoculation (Figure 20.4B). In addition, the *bilE$^+$* strain demonstrated increased clinical efficacy, reducing oral *L. monocytogenes* infection in mice (Figure 20.5). Collectively the data indicate that rational genetic manipulation of selected probiotic strains can significantly improve delivery to and colonization of the GI tract [18].

4. EXPANDING THE PATHO-BIOTECHNOLOGY CONCEPT BY DIRECTED EVOLUTION

In addition to an already existing array of useful pathogen derived stress survival systems [4] it may be possible to artificially engineer improved systems using a directed evolution approach. One such approach involves the use of the *E. coli* mutator strain XL1-Red; deficient in three of the

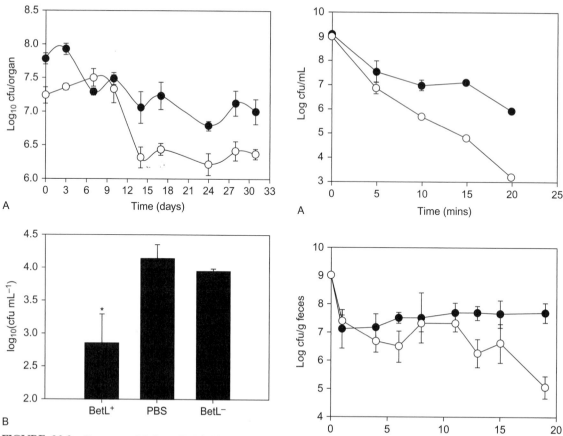

FIGURE 20.3 Recovery of *B. breve* BetL$^+$ (closed circles) and *B. breve* BetL$^-$ (open circles) from female BALB/c mice over 32 days of analysis. (A) Feces for bacteriological analysis were obtained from five mice in each treatment group and viable counts of *B. breve* BetL$^-$ derivatives were determined. (B) Listerial infection in the spleens of BALB/c mice. Animals were fed ~10^9 cfu mL^{-1} of either *B. breve* BetL$^+$ or *B. breve* BetL$^-$ for three consecutive days. The control group was fed PBS. On the fourth day, all animals were infected with ~10^{11} cfu mL^{-1} *L. monocytogenes* EGD-e. Three days post-listerial infection the animals were sacrificed and the numbers of *Listeria* were determined. Asterisks represent significant differences.

FIGURE 20.4 (A) Survival of stationary phase *B. breve* in 1% porcine bile. *B. breve* bilE$^+$ (closed circles) and *B. breve* bilE$^-$ (open circles). Overnight cultures were inoculated (3%) into GM17 and MRS broth containing 1% porcine bile. Viable cell counts were performed by serial dilution in one-quarter strength Ringer's solution followed by plating onto GM17Cm5 or RCMCm4, respectively. Standard deviations of triplicate results are represented by error bars. (B) Effect of *bilE* on the gastrointestinal persistence of *B. breve* bilE$^+$ (closed circles) and *B. breve* bilE$^-$ (open circles) were used for peroral inoculation of female BALB/c mice ($n = 5$). *B. breve* counts were determined in stools at 48-hour intervals. Adapted from Watson et al. [18].

primary DNA repair pathways (*mutS*, *mutD* and *mutT*), plasmid replication in this strain results in a mutation rate ~5000-fold higher than that of the wild type. Thus, with each successive generation, random point mutations (some of which are beneficial) are introduced into the gene of interest, creating a bank of mutant genes from which the most effective can be selected based on an improved phenotype (e.g. increased osmotolerance, etc.).

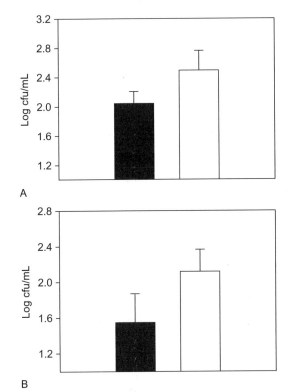

A

B

FIGURE 20.5 Improved clinical efficacy. Probiotic dosing of BALB/c mice with *B. breve bilE*⁺ (black) reduces the level of subsequent *L. monocytogenes* infection when compared to the wild type *B. breve bilE*⁻ strain. Bacterial growth was followed in (A) the liver and (B) the spleen 3 days post infection. Adapted from Watson et al. [18].

We employed this technique to engineer proline hyper-producing strains of *E. coli* with a significantly increased ability to tolerate elevated osmolarities (Figure 20.6). Bacterial proline synthesis from glutamate occurs *via* three enzymatic reactions, catalyzed by γ-glutamyl kinase (GK) (*proB* product), γ-glutamyl phosphate reductase (GPR) (*proA* product), and Δ^1-pyrroline-5-carboxylate reductase (P5C) (*proC* product). For both prokaryotic and eukaryotic systems proline synthesis from glutamate is regulated by feedback inhibition of the first enzyme in the pathway (GK). Thus, it is possible to isolate proline hyper-producing

strains by screening for isolates exhibiting reduced proline-mediated feedback inhibition of GK activity (as a consequence of single-base-pair substitutions in the *proB* gene). This was achieved by passaging the listerial *proBA* operon through *E. coli* XL1-Red thus creating a bank of randomly mutated *proBA* operons. The resulting gene bank was then transformed into *E. coli* CSH26 (a proline auxotroph) and successful transformants were screened for proline hyper-production. Three independent proline overproducing mutants were obtained (each carrying point mutations at a different location within the *proB* gene). These strains, heterologously expressing the mutated listerial *proBA* operon, were shown to be considerably more osmotolerant than strains expressing the wild type listerial *proBA* [19]. Thus, while complementation with wild type listerial *proBA* offers a significant degree of osmoprotection, the bioengineered *proBA* operon is far more effective, proving that the directed evolution approach provides a new dimension to the patho-biotechnology concept. It is of course entirely likely that this directed evolution approach may well dispense with the need for pathogens altogether as a source of stress survival systems in favor of selectively enhancing the probiotic's own gene complement.

5. DESIGNER PROBIOTICS

Faced with an emerging pandemic of antibiotic resistance clinicians and scientists alike are now struggling to find viable therapeutic alternatives to our failing antibiotic wonder drugs. Many disease-causing bacteria exploit oligosaccharides displayed on the surface of host cells as receptors for toxins and/or adhesins, enabling colonization of the host and entry of the pathogen or secreted toxins into the host cell. Blocking this adherence prevents infection, while toxin neutralization ameliorates symptoms until the

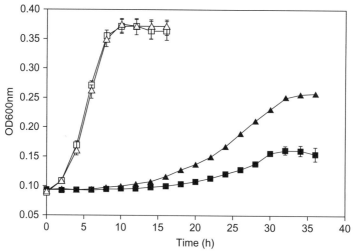

FIGURE 20.6 Growth of a proline hyper-producing strain of *E. coli* expressing a mutated version of the listerial *proB* gene relative to a wild type *E. coli* in M9 minimal medium of elevated osmolarity. Growth (as determined by turbidity using a Spectra max 340 spectrophotometer, Molecular Devices), was measured both in the presence (closed symbols) and absence (open symbols) of 4% added NaCl. (□,■) CSH26C control strain, (△,▲) CSH26proB^{mut}. Each point represents the mean value of three independent experiments.

pathogen is eventually overcome by the host's immune system. 'Designer probiotics' have been engineered to express receptor-mimic structures on their surface which fool the pathogen into thinking that the administered probiotic is in fact their target host cell [10, 20–22]. When administered orally, these engineered probiotics bind to, and neutralize toxins in, the gut lumen and interfere with pathogen adherence to the intestinal epithelium—thus essentially 'mopping up' the infection. One such construct consists of an *E. coli* strain expressing a chimeric lipopolysaccharide (LPS) terminating in a shiga toxin (Stx) receptor. One milligram (1 mg) dry weight of this recombinant strain has been shown to neutralize >100 μg of Stx1 and Stx2 (20). Paton et al. [21, 22] have also constructed probiotics with receptor-blocking potential against Enterotoxigenic *E. coli* (ETEC) toxin LT and cholera toxin (Ctx). As well as treating enteric infections, 'designer probiotics' have also been developed to combat HIV. In 2005, Rao

et al. [23] described the construction of a probiotic strain of *E. coli*, engineered to secrete HIV-gp41-haemolysin A hybrid peptides which block HIV fusion and entry into host cells. When administered orally or as a rectal suppository, this 'live microbicide' colonizes the gut mucosa and secretes the peptide *in situ*, thereby providing protection in advance of HIV exposure for up to a month. Other anti-HIV probiotics currently in development include a genetically engineered *Streptococcus gordonii* which produces cyanovirin-N, a potent HIV-inactivating protein originally isolated from cyanobacterium, and a natural human vaginal isolate of *Lactobacillus jensenii* modified to secrete two-domain CD4 which inhibits HIV entry into target cells [24].

Notwithstanding *in vitro* and *in vivo* efficacy in animal models, further refinements to the receptor-mimic probiotics might be necessary before commencement of Phase I clinical trials. Patho-biotechnology, the introduction of genes to improve resistance to stomach acid, or otherwise promote colonization or survival in the gut, for example would enable dose regimens to be substantially lowered, thus providing greater efficacy and further cost benefits.

In addition to infection control, probiotics (and other non-pathogenic bacteria) are also being engineered to function as novel vaccine delivery vehicles which can stimulate both innate and acquired immunity but lack the possibility of reversion to virulence which exists with more conventional pathogenic platforms. Guimarães et al. [25] described the construction of a *L. lactis* strain expressing *inlA*, encoding internalin A, a surface protein related to invasion in *L. monocytogenes*. In this instance, the otherwise non-invasive *L. lactis* strain is now capable of invading the small intestine and delivering molecules (DNA or protein) into mammalian epithelial cells, making it a safer and more attractive alternative to attenuated *L. monocytogenes* as an antigen delivery vehicle.

Probiotic vaccine carriers administered by the mucosal route mimic the immune response elicited by natural infection and can lead to long-lasting protective mucosal and systemic responses [26]. Mucosal vaccine delivery (those administered orally, anally or by nasal spray) also offers significant technological and commercial advantages over traditional formulations including: reduced pain and the possibility of cross contamination associated with intramuscular injection as well as the lack of a requirement for medically trained personnel to administer the vaccine [27].

However, despite their obvious clinical potential, the use of genetically modified organisms in food and medicine raises legitimate concerns about their propagation in the environment and about the dissemination of antibiotic markers or other genetic modifications to other microorganisms. At least some of these concerns might be allayed by the implementation of stringent bio-containment measures. Steidler et al. [28] identified the thymidylate synthase (*thyA*) gene as a target gene that combines the advantages of passive and active containment systems.

Thymine auxotrophy involves activation of the SOS repair system and DNA fragmentation, thereby constituting an indigenous suicide system. Thymine and thymidine growth dependence differs from most other auxotrophys in that absence of the essential component is bactericidal in the former and bacteriostatic in the latter. Thus, *thyA*-deficient bacteria cannot accumulate in the environment. This approach addresses biosafety concerns on a number of levels. Firstly, no resistance marker is required to guarantee stable inheritance of the transgene(s), thus overcoming any potential problems associated with dissemination of antibiotic resistance. Secondly, accumulation of the genetically modified organism in the environment is highly unlikely given that rapid death occurs upon thymidine starvation. Finally, should an intact *thyA* be acquired from closely related bacteria by means of homologous recombination then the transgene(s) would be lost.

6. CONCLUSION AND FUTURE PROSPECTS

Engineered probiotics thus have the potential to alleviate the symptoms of chronic gastrointestinal disorders and associated sequelae, to fight infection, modulate the immune system and act as delivery vehicles for bioactive molecules [27]. Notwithstanding these impressive health benefits, probiotic research has really only begun to achieve scientific credibility over the last decade [29], this despite the fact that Yakult launched the first probiotic fermented food drink in Japan in 1935; long before the appearance of the first commercially available antibiotics.

However, the increasing emergence of antibiotic resistance, coupled with a significant decline in production of new antibacterials, means that probiotics are finally coming of age, representing a real alternative to traditional drug-based therapies [30, 31].

ACKNOWLEDGMENTS

Roy Sleator is a Health Research Board (HRB) Principal Investigator. The author wishes to acknowledge the continued financial assistance of the HRB, and the Alimentary Pharmabiotic Centre (APC) through funding by Science Foundation Ireland (SFI).

References

1. Fuller, R. (1989). Probiotics in man and animals. *The Journal of Applied Bacteriology, 66*, 365–378.
2. Shanahan, F. (2006). Probiotics: promise, problems, and progress. *Gastroenterol Hepatol Ann Rev, 1*, 41–45.
3. Madara, J. (2004). Building an intestine: Architectural contributions of commensal bacteria. *The New England Journal of Medicine, 351*, 1685–1686.
4. Sleator, R. D., & Hill, C. (2007). Patho-biotechnology; using bad bugs to make good bugs better. *Science Progress, 90*, 1–14.
5. Sleator, R. D., & Hill, C. (2006). Patho-biotechnology; using bad bugs to do good things. *Current Opinion in Biotechnology, 17*, 211–216.
6. Sleator, R. D., & Hill, C. (2007). 'Bioengineered Bugs' a patho-biotechnology approach to probiotic research and application. *Medical Hypotheses, 70*, 167–169.
7. Sleator, R. D., & Hill, C. (2007). Improving probiotic function using a patho-biotechnology approach. *Gene Therapy & Molecular Biology, 11*, 269–274.
8. Sheehan, V., Sleator, R. D., Fitzgerald, G., & Hill, C. (2006). Heterologous expression of BetL, a betaine uptake system, enhances the stress tolerance of *Lactobacillus salivarius* UCC118. *Applied and Environmental Microbiology, 72*, 2170–2177.
9. Sheehan, V. M., Sleator, R. D., Hill, C., & Fitzgerald, G. F. (2007). Improving gastric transit, gastrointestinal persistence and therapeutic efficacy of *Bifidobacterium breve* UCC2003 using a patho-biotechnology approach. *Microbiol, 153*, 3563–3571.
10. Paton, A. W., Morona, R., & Paton, J. C. (2006). Designer probiotics for prevention of enteric infections. *Nature Reviews Microbiology, 4*, 193–200.
11. Hill, C., Cotter, P., Sleator, R. D., & Gahan, C. G. M. (2002). Bacterial stress response in *Listeria monocytogenes*: Jumping the hurdles imposed by minimal processing. *International Dairy Journal, 12*, 273–283.
12. Sleator, R. D., & Hill, C. (2002). Bacterial osmoadaptation: The role of osmolytes in bacterial stress and virulence. *FEMS Microbiology Reviews, 26*, 49–71.
13. Sleator, R. D., Gahan, C. G. M., & Hill, C. (2003). A post-genomic appraisal of osmotolerance in *Listeria monocytogenes*. *Applied and Environmental Microbiology, 69*, 1–9.
14. Sleator, R. D., Gahan, C. G. M., Abee, T., & Hill, C. (1999). Identification and disruption of BetL, a secondary glycine betaine transport system linked to the salt tolerance of *Listeria monocytogenes* LO28. *Applied and Environmental Microbiology, 65*, 2078–2083.
15. Smiddy, M., Sleator, R. D., Kelly, A., & Hill, C. (2004). A role for the compatible solutes glycine betaine and L-carnitine in listerial barotolerance. *Applied and Environmental Microbiology, 70*, 7555–7557.
16. Smiddy, M., O'Gorman, L., Sleator, R. D., et al. (2005). Greater high-pressure resistance of bacteria in oysters than in broth. *Innovation Food Science and Emerging Technologies, 6*, 83–90.
17. Tremont, S., Vandenbrouke, K., Iserentant, D., et al. (2006). Intracellular accumulation of trehalose protects *Lactococcus lactis* from freeze-drying damage and bile toxicity and increases gastric acid resistance. *Applied and Environmental Microbiology, 72*, 7694–7700.
18. Watson, D., Sleator, R. D., Hill, C., & Gahan, C. G. (2008). Enhancing bile tolerance improves survival and persistence of Bifidobacterium and Lactococcus in the murine gastrointestinal tract. *BMC microbiology, 8*, 176.
19. Sleator, R. D., Gahan, C. G. M., & Hill, C. (2001). Mutations in the listerial *proB* gene leading to proline overproduction: Effects on salt tolerance and murine infection. *Applied and Environmental Microbiology, 67*, 4560–4565.
20. Paton, A. W., Morona, R., & Paton, J. C. (2000). A new biological agent for treatment of Shiga toxigenic *Escherichia coli* infections and dysentery in humans. *Nature Medicine, 6*, 265–270.
21. Paton, A. W., Morona, R., & Paton, J. C. (2001). Neutralization of shiga toxins Stx1, Stx2c and Stx2e by recombinant bacteria expressing mimics of globotriose and globotetraose. *Infection and Immunity, 69*, 1967–1970.
22. Paton, A. W., Jennings, M. P., Morona, R., et al. (2005). Recombinant probiotics for treatment and prevention of enterotoxigenic *Escherichia coli* diarrhea. *Gastroenterology, 128*, 1219–1228.
23. Rao, S., Hu, S., McHugh, L., et al. (2005). Toward a live microbial microbicide for HIV: Commensal bacteria secreting an HIV fusion inhibitor peptide. *Proceedings of the National Academy of Sciences of the United States of America, 102*, 11993–11998.
24. Chang, T. L.Y. , Chang, C. H. , Simpson, D. A., et al. (2003). Inhibition of HIV infectivity by a natural human isolate of *Lactobacillus jensenii* engineered to express functional two-domain CD4. *Proceedings of the National Academy of Sciences of the United States of America, 100*, 11672–11677.

25. Guimarães, V. D., Gabriel, J. E., Lefèvre, F., et al. (2005). Internalin-expressing *Lactococcus lactis* is able to invade small intestine of guinea pigs and deliver DNA into mammalian epithelial cells. *Microbes and infection, 7,* 836–844.

26. Holmgren, J., & Czerkinsky, C. (2005). Mucosal immunity and vaccines. *Nature Medicine, 11,* S45–S53.

27. Sleator, R. D., & Hill, C. (2007). Probiotics as therapeutics for the developing world. *Journal of Infection Developing Countries, 1,* 7–12.

28. Steidler, L., Neirynck, S., Huyghebaert, N., et al. (2003). Biological containment of genetically modified *Lactococcus lactis* for intestinal delivery of human interleukin 10. *Nature Biotechnology, 21,* 785–789.

29. Sleator, R. D., & Hill, C. (2008). New frontiers in probiotic research. *Letters in Applied Microbiology, 46,* 143–147.

30. Sleator, R. D., & Hill, C. (2008). Battle of the bugs. *Science, 321,* 1294–1295.

31. Sleator, R. D., & Hill, C. (2008). Designer probiotics: A potential therapeutic for *Clostridium difficile? Journal of Medical Microbiology, 57,* 793–794.

Effects of Probiotics on Intestinal Transport and Epithelial Barrier Function

Ulrike Lodemann

Institute of Veterinary Physiology, Department of Veterinary Medicine, Freie Universität Berlin, Germany

1. INTRODUCTION

The intestinal mucosa or epithelium[1] represents an interface between the internal milieu and the outside world. It serves two vital functions: a transport function, such as the absorption of nutrients or secretion of electrolytes and water, and a barrier function, protecting the host against the uptake of unwanted substances, toxins and microorganisms, and against the loss of autochthonous substances or back diffusion of ions.

Transport and barrier functions in the gastrointestinal tract (GIT) can be compromised by stress, injury or by pathogenic microorganisms, which act by releasing toxins or by adhering to the epithelial cells and activating a myriad of signaling pathways. These pathways sometimes lead to severe changes in physiological functions such as: a) the disruption of tight junction

(TJ) barrier structure and function; b) the induction of fluid and electrolyte secretion; and c) the activation of the inflammatory cascade [1].

The destruction of the integrity of intercellular TJs by pathogens is generally achieved by either influencing specific TJ proteins or by affecting the cytoskeleton [1]. The increased permeability allows bacteria and foreign antigens to enter the subepithelial layers, activating the immune cells of the *lamina propria* with the consequent induction of inflammatory reactions. These include the secretion of pro-inflammatory cytokines, e.g. tumor necrosis factor (TNF), that can affect the TJ proteins and thus promote further leakiness [2, 3]. Furthermore, intestinal pathogens can dramatically change the transport properties of the epithelium by inhibiting absorptive mechanisms and by stimulating Cl^-, Na^+, and water secretion without influencing epithelial integrity [4].

The mechanisms of action of pathogenic bacteria and pathogen–epithelial crosstalk have been studied extensively over the last few years,

---

[1]In transport physiology, the term 'epithelium' is commonly used instead of mucosa.

and new perspectives for therapeutic regimens have been proposed. These perspectives include a growing interest in the role of potentially beneficial microbes in the GIT, viz., probiotics, which comprise various species such as lactobacilli, bifidobacteria, or aerobic spore-forming bacteria, or yeasts such as *Saccharomyces* [5, 6]. Probiotics have been proven to have beneficial effects in diseases involving the deterioration of transport or barrier functions as in acute infectious diarrhea in children [7], traveler's diarrhea [8], antibiotic-associated diarrhea, *Clostridium difficile* disease [9], and necrotizing enterocolitis in preterm children [10]; and they have shown promising results in the treatment of inflammatory bowel disease [11]. In most cases, however, the underlying mechanisms and signaling pathways of the effects of the probiotics are not clear or only partly understood. Results from scientific studies will be compiled here and summarized to show the current state of knowledge and to encourage proposals and suggestions for future research.

A short introduction to the physiological barrier and transport functions of epithelia and to the parameters and experimental methods used to characterize these functions is given first.

1.1. Anatomical structure of the intestinal barrier

The intestinal barrier is a function of the total mucosa rather than a defined physical structure [12], comprising not only physical or anatomical components, but also immunological components. This chapter mainly focuses on histological and electrophysiological aspects of the intestinal barrier. Immunological aspects are presented in other chapters of this book.

The structure of the intestinal barrier includes, from the lumen to the blood side: a) the indigenous microbiota; b) the mucus layer; c) epithelial cells; and d) the subepithelial compartment with a variety of cells including immune cells.

The *indigenous microbiota* contributes essentially to the intestinal barrier by preventing mucosal colonization by pathogens and by regulating immune responses, antimicrobial protein expression, and repair functions [13–15].

The protective *mucus layer* consists of secreted products such as mucin glycoproteins, trefoil peptides, and surfactant phospholipids secreted by the goblet cells. It acts both as a lubricant for the ingesta and as a barrier for microorganisms by preventing direct contact with the epithelial cells. Changes in the mucus content or structure affect barrier function [16–18].

The *intestinal epithelium* consists of a single layer of columnar epithelial cells that are interconnected by a series of intercellular junctions: TJ or *zonulae occludentes*, adherens junctions, desmosomes, and gap junctions. The most apically located TJs determine paracellular permeability. They are composed of: 1) transmembrane proteins (occludin, claudin(s) and junctional adhesion molecule-1); 2) adaptor proteins, e.g. the cytoplasmic *zonula occludens* proteins ZO-1, -2 and -3; 3) regulatory proteins, e.g. protein kinase C (PKC): and 4) transcriptional and post-transcriptional regulators, e.g. symplekin (see Figure 21.1). The transmembrane proteins seal the intercellular space and form selective paracellular pores. The adaptor proteins bind to the cytoplasmic tails of the transmembrane proteins and link the TJ to the actin cytoskeleton [3, 19, 20]. The structure of the intercellular junctions is not static, and the function of these junctions is dynamically regulated in health and disease [21].

1.2. Electrical Resistance and Transport Pathways Across Intestinal Epithelia

Two transport pathways lie across the single-layered epithelium of the intestine (see Figure 21.2): 1) a transcellular pathway across

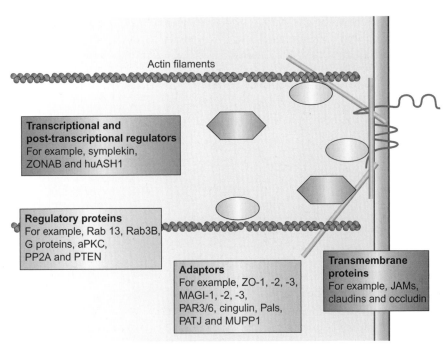

FIGURE 21.1 **The composition of tight junctions**. The biochemical composition of epithelial tight junctions (TJs) is outlined. For simplicity, the junctional components have been grouped into transmembrane proteins, adaptors, regulatory proteins, and transcriptional and post-transcriptional regulators. Although examples are given for each group, the list provided is not complete [...]. A comprehensive list of TJ components can be found in reviews by D'Atri and Citi [D'Atri, F. & Citi, S. (2002). Molecular complexity of vertebrate tight junctions (Review). *Mol Membr Biol, 19*, 103–112] and Tsukita et al. [Tsukita, S., Furuse, M. & Itoh, M. (2001). Multifunctional strands in tight junctions. *Nat Rev Mol Cell Biol, 2*, 285–293]. It should be noted that some of the components that are thought to become recruited to TJs do not localize exclusively to TJs, but can also localize to the nucleus (for example, huASH1 and ZONAB) or to other areas of the plasma membrane (for example, PTEN, PP2A and heterotrimeric G proteins). In addition, many TJ components interact directly or indirectly with actin filaments. aPKC, atypical protein kinase C; huASH1, human absent, small or homeotic discs 1; JAMs, junctional adhesion molecules; MAGI, Membrane-associated guanylate kinase inverted; MUPP1, multi-PDZ domain protein 1; Pals1, Protein associated with Lin-7 1; PAR, Partitioning defective; PATJ, Pals1-associated tight junction protein; PP2A, protein phosphatase 2A; PTEN, phosphatase and tensin homologue; ZO, zonula occludens; ZONAB, ZO-1-associated nucleic-acid binding [19].

the apical and basolateral membrane; and 2) a paracellular pathway across the TJ and the intercellular space [22].

The traditional electrophysiological parameter of epithelial barrier function is its tissue or transepithelial electrical resistance (R_t). The electrical resistance (R) is a ratio reflecting the degree to which an object opposes an electric current through it, measured in Ohms. Its inverse value is its conductance (G). R_t is composed of a paracellular resistance (R_s), which consists of the resistance of the TJ (R_{TJ}) and the resistance of the intercellular space (R_{ICS}), and a cellular resistance (R_c), which consists of the resistance of the apical membrane (R_a) and the resistance of the basolateral membrane (R_b) [22, 23].

Transcellular and paracellular fluxes across intestinal epithelia are closely controlled by membrane pumps, ion channels, and TJs, which adjust permeability to physiological needs [12].

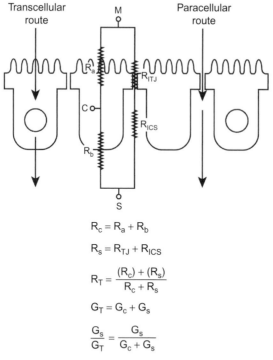

$$R_c = R_a + R_b$$

$$R_s = R_{TJ} + R_{ICS}$$

$$R_T = \frac{(R_c) + (R_s)}{R_c + R_s}$$

$$G_T = G_c + G_s$$

$$\frac{G_s}{G_T} = \frac{G_s}{G_c + G_s}$$

FIGURE 21.2 Two permeation routes across epithelia, the transcellular resistance (R_c) and resistance of paracellular shunt path (R_s), operate in parallel. R_c and R_s each contain two resistances in series: R_a and R_b are resistances of apical and basolateral cell membranes, respectively, while R_{TJ} and R_{ICS} are resistances of tight junction proper and intercellular space, respectively. Relations between resistances and conductances (G) are given by simple electrical circuit analysis [22].

1.3. Methods for the Measurement of Transport and Barrier Functions

The assessment and characterization of transport and barrier functions of epithelia make use of a variety of methods:

1. measurement of the electrophysiological parameters:
   - transepithelial electrical resistance (R_t or TEER)
   - transepithelial potential difference (PD_t)
   - short circuit current (I_{sc});
2. flux rate measurement of radioactive markers;
3. sugar tests;
4. passage of macromolecules;
5. determination of bacterial translocation.

Method 1. The classical method for *in vitro* studies on electrophysiological parameters of epithelia is the Ussing chamber technique [24]. The rationale of this method is the measurement of transport rates of ions or nutrients in the absence of passive driving forces. The usual parameters involved in this method are R_t (or TEER), PD_t, I_{sc}, and transport rates of radioactively labeled ions or nutrients. Active and passive transport mechanisms can be distinguished, and under special experimental conditions, trans- and paracellular transport rates can be differentiated. I_{sc} is a measure of the active electrogenic ion transport across the epithelium.

A common method to assess the barrier function of cell monolayers is the measurement of TEER with a voltohmmeter. The principle of this measurement is similar to that of the Ussing chamber technique but it is less elaborate, so that only information about TEER (or PD$_t$) can be obtained. For this kind of measurement, cells have to be grown on special cell culture inserts where they can develop differentially with an apical and basolateral side.

Method 2. Flux rate measurements can be conducted with radioactively labeled ions or markers for transcellular or paracellular transport, e.g. ^{36}Cl for Cl$^-$ secretion or ^{51}chromium-labeled ethylenediaminetetraacetic acid (^{51}CrEDTA) for permeability.

In uptake experiments, the uptake of a substance into cells within a defined period of time is determined, e.g. ^{3}H-glucose to assess absorptive capacities.

Method 3. Tests to measure intestinal permeability non-invasively *in vivo* have been developed [25, 26]. The basic idea behind these tests is that the urinary excretion of an orally applied probe reflects the non-mediated diffusion of that probe across the intestinal epithelium. Many substances such as monosaccharides, oligosaccharides, ^{51}CrEDTA, and polyethylene glycol (PEG) have been used for this purpose.

After administration of the test substances orally to subjects, urinary excretion over a 5-hour period is measured. Because many factors other than mucosal permeability can affect the results, the so-called dual sugar test is employed. Intestinal permeability is calculated from the urinary excretion ratio of two substances (mostly disaccharide/monosaccharide) as a percentage of the initially applied value [25].

However, only gastric and small bowel permeability can be measured by this method because lactulose and monosaccharides are fermented in the colon. In order to obtain a measure for whole gut permeability, the dual sugar test has been expanded to a triple sugar test, which is still controversial. This test includes sucralose, which is not fermented in the colon [26].

Method 4. The passage of macromolecules of various sizes can be measured by low and high molecular weight markers such as the macromolecular conjugate probe 10-kDa dextran, measured by its fluorescence, or horseradish peroxidase, measured by its enzymatic activity.

Method 5. Bacterial translocation has been measured to assess intestinal barrier integrity and is defined as the passage of bacteria from the intestine to extraintestinal sites such as the mesenteric lymph nodes or blood. Under physiological conditions, such translocation occurs at a low rate. Bacterial translocation is mainly promoted by bacterial overgrowth, defects in the integrity of the mucosal barrier, and the dysfunction of the immune response [27].

2. PROBIOTICS AND TRANSPORT

The application of probiotics in human and animal nutrition is very common, the main interest up to now being the prevention or attenuation of changes associated with pathologic processes in which amongst others absorptive function is abrogated or secretion is pathologically enhanced. However, only a small number of studies have been carried out to characterize the effects of probiotics on transport properties of the intestine. This is surprising because obvious benefits in human and animal health and improved weight gain and feed conversion in farm animals have been reported, which suggest that the underlying mechanisms of these positive effects are related to the transport properties of the intestine.

2.1. Probiotic Effects on Absorption

The positive influences of probiotics on absorptive GIT functions imply almost inherently pro-absorptive effects on nutrients and ions, e.g. on Na$^+$/glucose cotransport or Ca^{2+} absorption.

2.1.1 Na^+-coupled Glucose Transport

In pigs supplemented with the probiotics *Saccharomyces boulardii*, *Bacillus cereus* var. *toyoi*, or *Enterococcus faecium* NCIMB 10415, an enhancing effect on Na^+/glucose cotransport in the jejunum has been observed *in vitro* with the Ussing chamber technique and in uptake studies with brush border membrane vesicles [28–30].

The Na^+/glucose cotransport in weaners (young pigs between weaning and 6 months of age) fed with the probiotic *S. boulardii* for 8 days or with *B. cereus* var. *toyoi* for 21 days is significantly higher than that of controls [28, 30]. Likewise, in the jejunal epithelia from piglets aged 14, 28, 35, and 56 days supplemented with *E. faecium* NCIMB 10415, the Na^+/glucose cotransport tends to be higher [29]. However, the enhancing effect of *B. cereus* var. *toyoi* observed in weaners has not been confirmed in a study with intestine from piglets aged 14, 28, 35, and 56 days [31].

Protection of absorptive function when toxic substances are included in feed has been shown in a study with broiler chickens [32]. The addition of *Eubacterium* sp. DSM 11798 prevents the deoxynivalenol-induced decrease in Na^+-coupled glucose absorption [32].

Similarly, the decrease of Na^+-coupled glucose uptake after proximal enterectomy can be prevented by *S. boulardii*. This is paralleled by a two-fold increase in the expression of SGLT-1 protein, the main Na^+-coupled glucose transporter in the small intestine [33].

2.1.2 Na^+-coupled Amino Acid Transport

Na^+-coupled L-glutamine transport tends to be higher in the jejunum of piglets supplemented with *E. faecium* NCIMB 10415 and *B. cereus* var. *toyoi* [29, 31]. Likewise, the uptake of the amino acid alanine is increased after administration of *S. boulardii* and *B. cereus* var. *toyoi* to weaned pigs [30].

2.1.3 Na^+ Transport

Some of the effects of probiotics on absorptive function seem to be time-dependent. In a study on the time course of the effects of *S. boulardii* on pig jejunum a reduced electrogenic net ion transport, which has been attributed to the reduced Na^+ flux from the mucosal to serosal side (J_{ms} Na^+), has been observed at day 8 of probiotic supplementation [34]. However, at the other time points (3 days, 16 days) measured in this study, no such effect has been observed. This effect on the Na^+ flux has not been seen in a similar study [35].

No changes in Na^+ flux rates have been measured in pigs supplemented with *Bacillus cereus* var. *caron* or *B. cereus* var. *toyoi* for 21 days [35].

Protection against the pronounced reduction in Na^+ absorption induced by dextran sulfate sodium (DSS) is provided by *Escherichia coli* Nissle 1917 in a mouse model of colitis [36].

2.1.4 Ca^{2+} Transport

Probiotics have also been applied to optimize calcium availability from foods. *Lactobacillus salivarius* has an enhancing effect on Ca^{2+} uptake in Caco-2 cells (human epithelial intestinal cells from colorectal adenocarcinoma). Transepithelial Ca^{2+} transport and transepithelial resistance are unaffected by incubation for 6 or 24 hours with *L. salivarius*, but Ca^{2+} uptake is significantly higher after a 24-hour incubation [37], whereas *Bifidobacterium infantis* has no effect; no explanation for the discrepancy between the increase of Ca^{2+} uptake and unchanged transepithelial transport is given by the authors. A stimulation of transepithelial Ca^{2+} transport by several lactobacilli has been observed in a study with Caco-2 cells by Brassat and Vey [38]. A possible explanation for the enhancing effect on Ca^{2+} transport has been provided by Vinderola et al. [39] who have observed the enhanced expression of Ca^{2+} channels (TRPV6) in the duodenum of mice treated with supernatant from milk fermented by *Lactobacillus helveticus* R389.

2.1.5 Peptide Transport

S. boulardii and *B. cereus* var. *toyoi* have a stimulating effect on the proton-dependent dipeptide transport with glycyl-L-sarcosine and glycyl-L-glutamine in the jejunum of pigs [28].

Similar results have been obtained in a study with Caco-2 cells. A 48-hour *Lactobacillus casei* treatment resulted in a significant increase in human intestinal oligopeptide-transporter hPEPT1-mediated glycyl-sarcosine uptake, compared with the controls [40].

2.1.6 Cl^-/OH^- Exchange

Lactobacillus acidophilus and *Lactobacillus rhamnosus* dose-dependently stimulate apical Cl^-/OH^- exchange (~50%) in Caco-2 cells. The surface expression of the predominant transport protein for Cl^-/OH^- exchange, SLC26A3, increases in parallel. The filtered supernatant of *L. acidophilus* has the same effect. Other *Lactobacillus* species (*L. casei*, *Lactobacillus plantarum*) or heat-killed bacteria are ineffective [41].

2.2 Probiotic Effects on Secretion

Many enteric pathogens induce diarrhea by enhancing the secretion or inhibiting the absorption of electrolytes by enterocytes [4]. Because probiotics have shown antidiarrheal effects, for example, in acute infectious diarrhea in children [7], traveler's diarrhea [8] and *C. difficile* disease [9], studies have been designed to investigate the effects of probiotics on the secretory properties of epithelia. In the studies quoted below, the probiotics change either the basal secretion or the responses to so-called secretagogues or both. Furthermore, the probiotics prevent pathological secretion elicited by pathogenic bacteria or noxious agents. Most of the studies have been conducted in animal models or with cell culture.

In many of the studies, secretagogues have been used that act by mainly inducing Cl^- and water secretion. Secretagogues such as prostaglandin E_2 (PGE_2), vasoactive intestinal peptide (VIP), and theophylline induce receptor and forskolin non-receptor-mediated elevation of intracellular cyclic 3',5'-adenosine monophosphate (cAMP) levels. These cyclic nucleotides influence various electrolyte-transporting steps in epithelia; in the intestine, they mainly induce a rise in Cl^- secretion. Prostacyclin (PGI_2) induces Cl^- secretion *via* a change in the intracellular Ca^{2+} concentration.

2.2.1 Effects on Basal Secretion

In most studies, basal Cl^- secretion under physiological conditions is not affected by probiotic treatment. Supplementation of pigs with *S. boulardii*, *B. cereus* var. *caron*, or *B. cereus* var. *toyoi* has no effect on Cl^- secretion [34, 35]. Likewise, in T84 cells (human intestinal epithelial cells from colorectal carcinoma) pretreated with medium conditioned by *S. boulardii*[2], no effect has been observed on Cl^- fluxes [42]. In HT29/cl.19A cells (human intestinal epithelial cells from colorectal adenocarcinoma) infected with a combination of *Streptococcus thermophilus* and *L. acidophilus*, no effect has been detected on the expression of cystic fibrosis transmembrane conductance regulator (CFTR) [43]. However, Krammer and Karbach [44] have noted an acute effect of *S. boulardii in vitro*. Chloride absorption is significantly increased under basal conditions in rat jejunum or colon.

2.2.2. Effects on Secretagogue-induced Secretion

The effects of *S. boulardii* have been extensively investigated in studies of secretagogue-induced secretion. Krammer and Karbach [44] have used the yeast *in vitro* to test its acute effects. In isolated jejunum of rat, *S. boulardii* turns

---

[2]Medium conditioned by *Saccharomyces boulardii* was prepared as follows: supernatant of stationary growth cultures was cleared by centrifugation, dialyzed against succinic acid, and cryoconcentrated.

PGE_2-induced cAMP-mediated Cl^- secretion into Cl^- absorption by stimulating mucosal-to-serosal Cl^- transport. In the colon, treated with the Ca^{2+}-mediated agonist PGI_2 to stimulate Cl^- secretion, it additionally normalizes the serosa-to-mucosa Cl^- flux. Therefore, the authors have concluded that *S. boulardii* acts on Cl^- secretion by two distinct mechanisms.

T84 cells are stimulated by various agonists that induce an increase in cAMP levels, such as PGE_2, VIP, and forskolin, or that act *via* the Ca^{2+}-mediated pathway, as does carbachol. Pretreatment with medium conditioned by *S. boulardii* reduces the Cl^- secretion evoked by the cAMP pathway by 40–50% and inhibits the Cl^- secretion induced by the Ca^{2+} signaling pathway [42].

A similar effect has been seen in two feeding trials with pigs supplemented with *S. boulardii* for 8 days. The secretory response of the isolated jejunum to theophylline is attenuated by 50–60% [34, 35]. In line with an antisecretory response, studies with pigs supplemented for 21 days with *B. cereus* var. *caron* have demonstrated a significant and, with *B. cereus* var. *toyoi*, a slight decrease in the secretory response [35]. Moreover, *E. coli* Nissle 1917 supplementation to pigs reduces the forskolin-stimulated I_{sc} response by 55% compared with that in control pigs [45].

However, no effects on forskolin-stimulated I_{sc} have been seen in colons of mice treated with *E. coli* Nissle 1917 [36], in colons of mice treated with VSL#3[3] for 4 weeks [46], and in Caco-2 cells incubated with *L. plantarum* [47]. *S. thermophilus* and *L. acidophilus* have no effect on Bt2-cAMP-stimulated and on 8Br-guanosine 3′, 5′-cyclic monophosphate (cGMP)-stimulated Cl^- secretion in HT29/cl.19A, Caco-2, or T84 cells [48].

By contrast, stimulating effects of probiotics on secretory properties have also been reported. In two feeding trials with piglets supplemented

[3]A mixture of *B. longum, B. breve, B. infantis, L. casei, L. plantarum, L. acidophilus, Lactobacillus delbrueckii* subsp. *bulgaricus*, and *Streptococcus salivarius* subsp. *thermophilus*.

with either *B. cereus* var. *toyoi* or *E. faecium* NCIMB 10415 for 56 days, the PGE_2-stimulated I_{sc} in jejunal epithelia is higher in the probiotic group than in the control group around the time of weaning [29, 31]. These results are in accordance with a study by Leonhard-Marek et al. [49] who have observed a tendency for a higher I_{sc} response to forskolin in the jejunum of pigs supplemented with *E. coli* Nissle 1917, and a higher increase in I_{sc} induced by carbachol, after supplementation with *S. boulardii*.

This increase in the secretory response should not be interpreted as a negative effect because the enhancement of secretion into the intestinal lumen, as long as it remains within certain limits, can have positive effects. It facilitates the mixing of the ingesta with fluid and enzymes, with a probable beneficial effect on digestion and absorption [50], and flushes the intestine to prevent colonization by enteric pathogens [51].

2.2.3 Prevention of Secretion in Pathological States

Enteric pathogens or noxious substances use various signaling pathways to affect the secretory or absorptive properties of intestinal mucosa. These effects elicited by pathogens can be modulated by probiotics.

Infectious Pathogens

1. ***Vibrio cholera.*** Pretreatment with medium conditioned by *S. boulardii* reduces the Cl^- secretion in T84 cells stimulated with cholera toxin from *V. cholera* [42]. This toxin activates cellular adenylate cyclase, leading to a rise in intracellular cAMP levels, which induces the secretion of Cl^- [52]. An inhibitory effect on cholera-toxin-induced water and Na^+ secretion has even been observed when *S. boulardii* is added after the application of the cholera toxin in intestinal loops of rat jejunum [53]. Irradiation and heating of *S. boulardii* does not abolish its

antisecretory effect, whereas the supernatant obtained after the centrifugation of living or irradiated cell suspensions has no inhibitory effect.

2. **C. difficile toxin A.** *S. boulardii* and, equally, its filtered conditioned medium attenuates the fluid secretion induced by *C. difficile* toxin A in rat ileum [54].

3. **E. coli heat-labile toxin.** *S. boulardii* also brings about a protective effect against *E. coli* heat-labile toxin, which increases Cl^- secretion *via* cAMP activation in enterocytes. Its conditioned medium inhibits the toxin-induced increase in the cAMP level in human intestinal HT29-D4 cells [55].

4. **E. coli Abbotstown.** In a piglet model of intestinal infection, *E. coli* Abbotstown has been used to induce mild secretory diarrhea without changes in epithelial structure [45]. Supplementation of the piglets with *E. coli* Nissle 1917 for 10 days prevents all the clinical signs of diarrhea seen in animals infected solely with *E. coli* Abbotstown. In addition, jejunal epithelia from pigs infected solely with *E. coli* Abbotstown show a significantly higher secretory response upon stimulation with forskolin than the controls. Pretreatment with *E. coli* Nissle 1917 reduced the response to forskolin to that of control animals.

5. **Enteropathogenic E. coli (EPEC).** In a Caco-2 cell model, preincubation with the probiotic strain *L. plantarum* reduces the increase in I_{sc} elicited by EPEC infection [47]. This effect is diminished when the cells are coinfected with the probiotic, and no effect is seen when the probiotic is added after incubation with EPEC. The I_{sc} response induced by EPEC is caused by Cl^- secretion *and* possibly by an influx of Na^+ and amino acids into host cells.

6. **Enteroinvasive E. coli (EIEC).** Pretreatment with a combination of live *S. thermophilus* and *L. acidophilus* completely prevents the increase in Cl^- secretion induced by EIEC in HT29/cl.19A and Caco-2 cells. The EIEC-induced increase in I_{sc} is not reduced when EIEC and the probiotics are added simultaneously, or when the cells are exposed to the probiotic after infection with EIEC [56].

Model Colitis Interleukin-10 (IL-10)-deficient mice develop spontaneous colitis. The colon of these mice exhibits significant reductions of basal I_{sc} and PD_t compared with age-matched controls and a 90% reduction in I_{sc} in response to forskolin, which has been attributed by the authors to an impairment of cAMP-dependent Cl^- secretion. After 4 weeks of treatment with VSL#3, baseline I_{sc} and PD_t and I_{sc} responses to forskolin are normalized [46]. Similar results have been obtained with a mouse model in which sepsis is induced by the injection of lipopolysaccharide (LPS) and D-galactosamine. The reduced I_{sc} response to forskolin has not been observed when mice are pretreated with VSL#3 [57].

Stress In a rat model of chronic psychological stress, water-avoidance stress induces excess ion secretion and an increase of tissue conductance in the ileum and colon. The application of the combination of the strains *L. rhamnosus* and *L. helveticus* inhibits the increase in I_{sc} in the ileum but has no effect on I_{sc} in the colon [58].

Cytokines Interferon-γ (IFN-γ) inhibits forskolin-stimulated Cl^- secretion and down-regulates the protein expression of the Cl^- channel CFTR and the $Na^+-K^+-2Cl^-$ cotransporter (NKCC1) in HT29/cl.19A cells. This is prevented by live *S. thermophilus* and *L. acidophilus* or the commensal *Bacteroides thetaiotaomicron*. The latter can, however, only partially counteract transporter down-regulation [43].

3. PROBIOTICS AND BARRIER FUNCTION

The possible protective effects of probiotics on intestinal permeability have raised considerable interest, because a loss of barrier function (increase of permeability) is involved in the pathogenesis of many gastrointestinal diseases such as intestinal infections with pathogenic *E. coli*, inflammatory bowel diseases, and even sepsis.

Most of the studies of the impairment of barrier function have been conducted in animal models or cell culture. Although many clinical trials in humans have established the preventive or curative effects of probiotics on diseases involving changes in intestinal barrier integrity, only a few studies have actually measured parameters associated with intestinal permeability. Some researchers have examined the effect of probiotics *per se*, i.e. without a pathophysiological background; the majority of research has been performed on deteriorated barrier function in states of disease.

3.1. Animal Studies and Clinical Trials

3.1.1 *Per se*

Application of probiotics in the absence of a pathophysiological challenge has, in most of the studies, either an enhancing or no effect on the barrier function of intestinal epithelia (see Table 21.1).

The positive effect of probiotics, a reduced permeability, appears to be mediated by several mechanisms. On the one hand, probiotics can influence the production of mucin by goblet cells, thereby inhibiting the adhesion of pathogenic bacteria. This has been seen in the study of Caballero-Franco et al. [59] in which VSL#3 significantly stimulates colonic mucin (MUC) secretion and the expression of the MUC2 (the major secreted gel-forming mucin) gene.

Furthermore, probiotics also have a stabilizing effect on TJs, for example, by up-regulating TJ proteins. Application of *E. coli* Nissle 1917 specifically up-regulates ZO-1 expression in intestinal epithelial cells at the mRNA and protein levels in gnotobiotic mice [36].

3.1.2 *Colitis*

Colitis Models. Animal colitis models are often used to study human diseases, such as inflammatory bowel disease. They complement and expand clinical studies on patients but cannot reproduce the complexity of the diseases, merely some aspects of it.

Trinitrobenzene Sulfonic Acid (TNBS)-induced Colitis. In various studies, probiotics have had positive effects on TNBS-induced colitis as a model of Crohn's disease. Pretreatment with *Lactobacillus farciminis* reduces colonic permeability in rats as measured by ^{51}CrEDTA fluxes [60]. The translocation of endogenous microflora to mesenteric lymph nodes, liver, and spleen is decreased when mice are pretreated with *L. plantarum* NCIMB8826 (decrease by 10^5-fold) or with *Lactococcus lactis* MG1363 (decrease by 10^3-fold) [61] and when rats are pretreated with *L. casei* [62]. *L. plantarum* species 299, however, does not improve intestinal permeability, as measured by radiolabeled PEG [63]; this might be because the probiotic was administered 24 hours after the induction of colitis and not in advance, as in the other studies.

IL-10 Knockout (IL-10−/−) Model of Colitis. *L. plantarum* species 299 has been found to improve gut permeability in an IL-10 knockout mouse model of colitis, which serves as another model for human Crohn's disease (Kennedy et al., 2000 according to [64]). This effect has also been seen after 4 weeks of treatment with VSL#3, which completely normalizes formerly enhanced mannitol fluxes in IL-10-deficient mice [46].

TABLE 21.1 The effects of various probiotic strains, alone or in combination, on intestinal permeability measured in animal models

Probiotic	Experimental model	Method to assess permeability	Permeability	Reference
B. cereus var. toyoi	Rat colon	^{51}CrEDTA flux	↓	[60]
Bacteroides fragile	Rat colon loop	Mannitol flux	↓[1]	[2]
		Dextran flux	→	
E. faecium NCIMB 10415	Pig mid-jejunum	Mannitol flux	→	[29]
E. coli Nissle 1917	Pig mid-jejunum	Mannitol flux	↓	[45]
Lactobacillus brevis	Rat colon loop	Mannitol flux	↓	[2]
		Dextran	→	
L. farciminis	Pig mid-jejunum	Mannitol flux	↓	[35]
L. plantarum 299v	Rat small intestine	Mannitol flux	→	[81]
L. rhamnosus + L. helveticus	Rat distal colon	Horseradish peroxidase flux	→	[72]
S. boulardii	Pig mid-jejunum	Mannitol flux	↓	[35]
VSL#3	Mouse colon	Mannitol flux	↓	[46]
VSL#3	Mouse colon	Mannitol flux	↓	[57]

Various methods to assess permeability were used. The symbols indicate: ↓ a decrease, → no effect, and ↑ an increase of intestinal permeability.
[1]Not statistically significant.
[2]Garcia-Lafuente, A., Antolin, M., Guarner, F. et al. (2001). Modulation of colonic barrier function by the composition of the commensal flora in the rat. *Gut, 48*, 503–507.

A reduction or normalization of colonic permeability can be seen both with acute treatment (4 hours) with *B. infantis* and following long-term (4 weeks) oral application [64].

However, neither prophylactic nor therapeutic treatment with *L. salivarius* subsp. *salivarius* 433118 (UCC118) alters TEER or mannitol fluxes in the colon of IL-10 2/2 mice compared to control mice [66].

Dextran Sulfate Sodium (DSS)-induced Colitis. Administration of DSS causes acute colitis with disintegration of the epithelium and inflammatory infiltrates, which resembles the clinical and morphological features of human ulcerative colitis. *L. salivarius* subsp. *salivarius* 433118 has no effect on TEER and mannitol fluxes in DSS-treated mice [66].

E. coli Nissle 1917, however, has proved to be effective in this model. The DSS-induced increase in permeability, measured by the uptake of Evans Blue into the colonic mucosa, is much lower in DSS+*E. coli* Nissle 1917-treated mice than in DSS-treated mice. This positive effect can be explained by the observed elevation of mRNA expression of TJ protein ZO-1 in the epithelial cells of the mice treated with DSS+*E. coli* Nissle 1917; these cells also exhibit a slight increase in ZO-2 mRNA [36].

Methotrexate-induced Enterocolitis. Another barrier-enhancing effect of probiotics has been observed in methotrexate-induced enterocolitis. Methotrexate is a chemotherapeutic agent with severe side effects, such as enterocolitis. *L. plantarum* or *Lactobacillus reuteri* decrease intestinal permeability, as measured by ^{51}CrEDTA clearance, and significantly lower the magnitude of bacterial translocation to extraintestinal sites in methotrexate-induced enterocolitis in rats [67].

In the same model, a sheep-milk yogurt, containing *Lactobacillus bulgaricus* and *S. thermophilus*, and a cow yogurt, containing *Lactobacillus johnsonii*, have been shown to be capable of improving small intestinal permeability, as measured by urinary lactulose/mannitol excretion [68].

Clinical Studies

Crohn's Disease. Patients with Crohn's disease in remission have been treated with *S. boulardii*, in addition to their baseline medication.[4] After 3 months, an improvement could be observed in intestinal permeability, evaluated by the lactulose/mannitol ratio in the treatment group compared with the placebo group [69].

In a study with children suffering from Crohn's disease, the addition of *Lactobacillus* GG decreases the intestinal permeability, as measured by a double sugar permeability test (cellobiose/mannitol), at 12-week follow-up. The decrease of cellobiose levels in their urine suggests a decrease of paracellular permeability. However, after 24 weeks of treatment, intestinal permeability again shows a trend toward an increase, i.e. improved intestinal permeability is not maintained [70].

Irritable Bowel Syndrome (IBS). In patients with IBS, small bowel permeability decreased significantly after the application of probiotic fermented milk (containing *S. thermophilus, L. bulgaricus, L. acidophilus*, and *Bifidobacterium longum*), whereas colonic permeability did not improve after probiotic treatment. Intestinal permeability was measured by a triple sugar test before and after treatment [71].

[4]Baseline medication: mesalamine, azathioprine, prednisone, metronidazole, and/or thalidomide.

3.1.3 Stress-induced States

Probiotic effects on the stress-induced increase of intestinal permeability have been studied in rats. Neonatal maternal separation of rat pups causes immediate and long-term changes in intestinal physiology. The stress-induced increase in colon permeability is reduced by *L. rhamnosus* strain R0011 and *L. helveticus* R0052 [72], by *Lactobacillus paracasei* NCC362 [73], and *L. paracasei* NCC2461 combined with long-chain fatty acids and prebiotics [74], whereas *Bifidobacterium lactis* NCC362 and *L. johnsonii* NCC533 are ineffective [73].

Probiotic treatment of maternal-separated pups in neonatal life also has long-term effects: it significantly reduces the stress-induced increases in intestinal permeability in their adult life [72].

3.1.4 Critical Illness

Sepsis. In a mouse model in which LPS challenge induces a systemic reaction resulting in a sepsis-like condition, the application of VSL#3 maintains colonic barrier function, measured by mannitol fluxes, and prevents bacterial translocation [57].

Intra-abdominal Infection. In a model of abdominal infection (cecum perforation and ligation), rats were divided into two groups, one group receiving parenteral nutrition and the other group additionally *L. acidophilus*. The bacterial translocation rate and endotoxin in blood were reduced in the *L. acidophilus* group; this could be explained by enhanced occludin expression and improved intestinal TJ and microvilli integrity [75]. The findings were supported by results obtained with *L. plantarum* in a similar experimental setup [76].

Short Bowel Syndrome. The administration of *B. lactis* reduced bacterial translocation to extraintestinal sites in rat after 80% gut resection. The incidence of total bacterial translocation was 6% in the untreated control group, 87% in resesected animals, and 50% in resected animals with additional probiotic treatment [77].

Acute Pancreatitis.   Mice were injected with cerulein to induce acute pancreatitis. Pretreatment with a multispecies probiotic (*L. acidophilus, L. casei, L. salivarius, L. lactis, Bifidobacterium bifidum,* and *B. lactis*) abolished the decrease in TEER and the increase in Na$^+$-fluorescein fluxes in the ileum that were induced by the acute pancreatitis. However, the effects were only seen in the late phase of pancreatitis (3 days after the insult) [78].

Hemorrhagic Shock.   *L. rhamnosus* and *Lactobacillus fermentum* have been examined for their effects on intestinal barrier integrity in a rat model of hemorrhagic shock. Animals treated with *L. rhamnosus* show reduced levels of plasma endotoxin, bacterial translocation, and disruption of F-actin distribution in the ileum following hemorrhagic shock, compared with untreated control animals. In contrast, treatment with *L. fermentum* has no substantial effect on intestinal barrier integrity [79].

3.1.5 Infection

Probiotic supplementation also has positive effects on changes of intestinal permeability caused by bacterial or viral infection.

In a neonatal animal model, rabbit pups have been treated with either pathogenic *E. coli* K1A, *L. casei* GG, or a combination of both. *L. casei* GG decreases the frequency of *E. coli* K1A translocation by 46, 61 and 23% to mesenteric lymph nodes, spleen, and liver, respectively [80].

The impact of duration of treatment and various application modes was examined in rats that were treated with *L. plantarum* 299v by tube feeding, that had free access to probiotic-supplemented drinking water, or that received regular feed. The small intestine was exposed *in vitro* to pathogenic *E. coli* F131 and *L. plantarum* (alone or together) in an Ussing chamber. One week of pretreatment with *L. plantarum* in the drinking water abolished the *E. coli*-induced increase of mannitol passage. In contrast, tube feeding had no effect. The short-term addition of *L. plantarum* for 2 hours in Ussing chamber

studies had no effect on *E. coli*-increased mannitol fluxes. The lack of effect under tube-feeding conditions may be ascribed to the fact that rats with free access to the probiotic-supplemented drinking water consumed four times more than the amount administered to rats by tube-feeding [81].

L. casei strain GG also decreased jejunal permeability in rotavirus-induced enteritis in suckling rats [82].

3.1.6 Indomethacin-induced States

A region-specific effect of *Lactobacillus* GG on alterations in gastrointestinal permeability induced by indomethacin was observed in a study with healthy volunteers. The ingestion of live *Lactobacillus* GG had a protective effect on the indomethacin-induced increase of gastric permeability but did not change intestinal permeability [83].

3.1.7 Allergy

In a study with rat pups, a prolonged challenge with cows' milk increased intestinal permeability, but this was almost completely abolished by the application of *L. casei* strain GG, as measured by the absorption of horseradish peroxidase [84]. This observation is in agreement with results of a study where rat pups were fed with cows' milk or hydrolyzed whey formula (i.e. unhydrolyzed or hydrolyzed dietary antigens) and additionally treated with the probiotic *L. casei* strain GG. The probiotic reduced aberrant macromolecular transport and enhanced macromolecular degradation by the gut mucosa, thereby reducing the antigen load [85].

L. rhamnosus 19070-2 and *L. reuteri* DSM 12246 were administered to children with moderate and severe atopic dermatitis to determine whether probiotics could attenuate the small intestinal inflammation and reinforce barrier function. The lactulose/mannitol ratio was lower after probiotic treatment compared with placebo treatment, indicating a decrease in permeability. The lactulose/mannitol ratio and the severity of eczema were positively correlated [86].

3.1.8 Necrotizing Enterocolitis in Preterm Infants

In preterm infants, the administration of probiotics significantly reduces the risk of severe necrotizing enterocolitis and mortality, as a meta-analysis of clinical trial data could show [10]. However, in a study of Caplan et al. [87] presumably this effect is not attributable to a change in intestinal permeability [87]. In a study on rats *B. infantis* significantly reduced the incidence of neonatal necrotizing enterocolitis, but there was no effect on mucosal permeability in the period of observation (8, 24 and 48 hours) [87].

However, the administration of an infant formula supplemented with *Bifidobacterium lactis* decreases intestinal permeability in preterm infants at days 7 and 30 after birth. The incidence of sepsis and NEC was also lower in the *B. lactis* group as compared to the control group but due to small numbers this did not reach significance [88]. The protective effect on intestinal permeability is supported by a recent study conducted in a rat model of necrotizing enterocolitis, where *B. bifidum* normalized the expression and localization of ileal and TJ and adherens junctions proteins compared to rats with NEC [1].

3.2. Cell Culture Studies

3.2.1 Per se

In most studies with intestinal epithelial cell lines, probiotics improve barrier function by decreasing permeability (see Table 21.2). Klingberg et al. [89] have shown that the decrease in permeability is dependent on the dose. In many studies, a time-dependent effect on permeability has also been demonstrated. Barrier function increases after a few hours of incubation, reaches a plateau phase, later decreases to starting values or even declines further [46, 90, 91].

Possible mechanisms improving the barrier function include epithelia changes of TJ proteins and of mucin production. *S. thermophilus* in combination with *L. acidophilus* enhances the phosphorylation of the TJ proteins occludin and ZO-1 [56]. *L. plantarum* MF1298 and *L. salivarius* DC5 increase the protein expression of ZO-1 [89]. *B. infantis* increases ZO-1 and occludin expression and decreases claudin-2 expression [65]. *E. coli* Nissle 1917 increases ZO-2 mRNA and protein levels and fosters redistribution toward cellular contact sites [92].

Mucin mRNA and protein expression is induced by VSL#3 in HT29 cells [90]. In LS174T cells (human colonic adenocarcinoma cell line), mucin secretion is surprisingly only induced when the cells are incubated with conditioned media of VSL#3, not with live bacteria. Among three bacterial groups, *Bifidobacteria*, *Lactobacilli* and *Streptococci*, *Lactobacillus* species are the strongest inducer of mucin secretion [59].

3.2.2 Infection

E. coli. Because of their relevance in human medicine, many *in vitro* cell culture studies have been conducted with the enteropathogenic *E. coli* strain E2348/69 (serotype O127:H6) or the enterohemorrhagic *E. coli* (EHEC) O157:H7.

EHEC O157:H7. The drop in TEER induced by *E. coli* serotype O157:H7 in T84 cells is reduced by preincubation with the probiotic strains *L. acidophilus* R0052, *L. rhamnosus* R0011 [93], *L. rhamnosus* GG [94], and by surface-layer protein extracts of *L. acidophilus* strain LB [95]. A decreasing effect on macromolecular permeability as measured by dextran has also been observed in two studies [94, 95].

Pretreatment and viable bacteria seem to be necessary for this effect, as in some studies, coincubation [93] or incubation with non-viable bacteria [93, 94], with bacterial culture supernatant, or conditioned medium[5] [93] are inefficient.

---

[5]To prepare 'conditioned medium', T84 cells were incubated with lactobacilli for 18–24 hours, then the medium was removed and subsequently filtered, whereas 'supernatants' were obtained from the bacterial cultures in de Man, Rogosa, and Sharpe broth.

TABLE 21.2 The effects of various probiotic strains, alone or in combination, on intestinal permeability measured in cell models

Probiotic	Experimental model	Method to assess permeability	Permeability	Duration of incubation resp. time point of measurement	Reference
B. infantis	T84	TEER	↓	6–24 h	[65]
		Mannitol flux			
E. coli Nissle 1917	T84	TEER	↑	0–120 min	[92]
	Caco-2		↑		
E. coli Nissle 1917	T84	TEER	↑	<8 h	[90]
			(↑)	8–12 h	
L. acidophilus	T84	TEER	↑	18 h	[93]
L. acidophilus	Caco-2	TEER	→	6–24 h	[56]
		Low MW marker[1]	→	12 h	[56]
		High MW marker[2]	↑	12 h	[56]
L. acidophilus	HT29/cl.19a	TEER	→	6–24 h	[48, 56]
		Low MW marker	→	12 h	[56]
		High MW marker	↑	12 h	[56]
L. casei GG	Caco-2	TEER	↑	180 min	[102]
Lactobacillus lactis	Caco-2	TEER	→	4–10 h	3
		Mannitol flux	→	4 h	
L. plantarum	Caco-2	TEER	→	1–2 h	[89]
L. rhamnosus	T84	TEER	↑	18 h	[93]
L. rhamnosus GG	Caco-2	TEER	→	18 h	[91]
			←	24–48 h	
L. rhamnosus Lc705	Caco-2	TEER	→	18 h	[91]
			←	24–48 h	
L. rhamnosus GG + L. rhamnosus Lc705	Caco-2	TEER	→	18 h	[91]
			←	24–48 h	

(Continued)

TABLE 21.2   (Continued)

Probiotic	Experimental model	Method to assess permeability	Permeability	Duration of incubation resp. time point of measurement	Reference
L. salivarius	Caco-2	TEER	→	1–2 h	[89]
S. boulardii	T84	TEER	↑	0–12 h	[99]
S. thermophilus	Caco-2	TEER	→	6–24 h	[56]
		Low MW marker	→	12 h	[56]
		High MW marker	↑	12 h	[56]
S. thermophilus	HT29/cl.19a	TEER	→	6–24 h	[56]
		Low MW marker	↑	12 h	[56]
		High MW marker	↑	12 h	[56]
S. thermophilus + L. acidophilus	Caco-2	TEER	→	6–24 h	[48, 56]
				3–24 h	[56]
		Low MW marker	→	12 h	[56]
		High MW marker	↑	12 h	[56]
S. thermophilus + L. acidophilus	HT29/cl.19a	TEER	→	6–24 h	[48, 56]
		Low MW marker	→	12 h	[56]
		High MW marker	↑	12 h	[56]
S. thermophilus + L. acidophilus	T84	TEER	↑	6–24 h	[48]
VSL#3	T84	TEER	→	4–6 h	[90]
VSL#3	T84	TEER	→	5–6 h	[46]
		Mannitol flux	→	4–6 h	
Synbiotic Bifidobacterium Bb12, *Bifidobacterium* sp 420, *Lactobacillus rhamnosus* GG + *Raftiline* and *Raftilose*[4]	Caco-2	TEER	→	24 h	[111]

Various methods to assess permeability were used.

The symbols indicate: ↓ a decrease, → no effect, and ↑ an increase of permeability.

[1] Low molecular weight (MW) marker: 478 Da, fluorescein sulfonic acid.

[2] High molecular weight (MW) marker: 10 000 Da, dextran labeled with fluorescein isothiocyanate.

[3] Shao, J. & Kaushal, G. (2004). Normal flora: living vehicles for non-invasive protein drug delivery. *Int J Pharm*, 286, 117–124.

[4] Raftiline and raftilose are non-digestible oligosaccharides.

However, surface layer protein extracts from *L. helveticus* have proved to be effective [94]. MUC-2 expression, which is an important component of the physical barrier, increases if *L. acidophilus* cell extract is used to counteract *E. coli* O157:H7 effects [96]. MUC2 and MUC3 mRNA expression levels were increased when *L. plantarum* 299v was incubated with HT29 cells and is probably responsible for the inhibition of adherence of EHEC strain CL8 (serotype O157:H7) to these cells [97].

EPEC strain E2348/69 (serotype O127:H6). The decrease in TEER induced by EPEC strain E2348/69 is attenuated when T84 cells are preincubated with the probiotic strains *L. acidophilus* R0052 or *L. rhamnosus* R0011. Coincubation or incubation with non-viable bacteria, filtered bacterial culture supernatants, or conditioned medium[6] has no such effects [93].

Other probiotics even show the ability to *restore* barrier integrity. In a study with *E. coli* Nissle 1917, coincubation, or subsequent addition after removal of the pathogen has a reducing effect on the TEER drop induced by EPEC strain E2348/69 in both T84 and Caco-2 cells [92]. A similar observation has been made in studies with T84 cells co- or post-infected with *L. casei* DN-144001 [98]. The yeast *S. boulardii* also abrogates the effect of EPEC on TEER and paracellular inulin flux [99].

In some of the studies mentioned above, concomitant probiotic effects on ZO-2 mRNA and protein levels and on ZO-1 and ZO-2 distribution have been observed [92, 98, 99]. Incubation of HT29 cells with *L. plantarum* 299v increased MUC2 and MUC3 mRNA expression levels, and this was proposed as a reason for its inhibitory effect on the adherence of *E. coli* strain E2348/69 to the cells [97].

Other Pathogenic *E. coli* Strains. *Lactobacillus sobrius* DSM 16698 protects IPEC-1 cells from the disruption of TJ structure by inhibiting the delocalization of ZO-1, the reduction in the amount of occludin, the rearrangement of F-actin, and the dephosphorylation of occludin caused by enterotoxigenic *E. coli* (ETEC) strain K88 [100].

Pretreatment with a combination of live *S. thermophilus* and *L. acidophilus* prevents the decrease in TEER evoked by enteroinvasive *E. coli* (EIEC), but spent filtered medium from bacterial cultures,[7] heat-inactivated, or antibiotic-killed probiotics are inefficient. The probiotic effects depend on the time-point of addition. A partial effect is seen with coincubation. When the probiotic is added 1 hour after infection with EIEC, the decrease in TEER is only attenuated at extremely high probiotic inoculation (multiplicity of infection >5000:1). The changes of permeability for small or large molecules as measured by fluorescent probes are only prevented when cells are treated with live probiotics before infection with EIEC. Pretreatment or coincubation at higher probiotic inoculations with live *S. thermophilus* and *L. acidophilus* prevents the disruption of cytoskeletal and TJ protein localization and the phosphorylation of actinin, occludin, and ZO-1 [56].

The filtered culture supernatant of *L. acidophilus* strain LB protects Caco-2/TC7 cells against the alterations induced by *E. coli* (Afa/Dr DAEC) C1845 with regard to the expression of brush-border-associated structural and functional proteins such as F-actin, sucrose-isomaltase, dipeptidylpeptidase IV, alkaline phosphatase, and fructose transporter GLUT-5 [101].

L. casei GG inhibits *E. coli* C25 translocation across Caco-2 monolayers dose-dependently. TEER is not significantly altered by the addition of *L. casei* GG or *E. coli*; in this experimental setting, the incubation with both bacterial strains was short (120–180 min), and non-adherent probiotic bacteria were washed out before incubation with *E. coli* [102]. These findings were reproduced in another experiment, and the reduction was attributed by the authors to the up-regulated MUC2 RNA and protein expression [103].

---

[6]See footnote 5.

[7]Spent, centrifuged, and filtered medium from *S. thermophilus* and *L. acidophilus* cultures.

Pre- and coincubation with *S. boulardii* prevents the decrease of TEER in T84 cells infected with EHEC strain EDL931 [104].

Salmonella Dublin. Coincubation of T84 cells with various concentrations of VSL#3 (10^2–10^6 cfu/mL) or *E. coli* Nissle 1917 significantly reduces the *S. Dublin*-induced decrease in TEER [90]. Whereas preconditioned medium from VSL#3 has similar effects, preconditioned medium from *E. coli* Nissle 1917 has no effects on *S. Dublin*-induced alterations in TEER. When the probiotics are washed off before the challenge with *S. Dublin*, only preincubation with VSL#3, but not with *E. coli* Nissle 1917, has a protective effect on TEER. The *S. Dublin*-induced alterations in the distribution of ZO-1 are decreased when T84 cells are coincubated with VSL#3 [90].

Helicobacter pylori. The effects of multispecies probiotic bacteria (*L. rhamnosus* GG, *L. rhamnosus* Lc705, *Propionibacterium freudenreichii* supsp. *shermanii Js, Bifidobacterium breve* Bb99) alone or in combination have been tested on Caco-2 cells infected with *H. pylori*. Pretreatment with *L. rhamnosus* GG and *L. rhamnosus* Lc705 initially improves epithelial barrier function, indicated by enhanced TEER (8 hours), but, after 18 hours, potentiates the *H. pylori*-induced decrease in TEER. This is also the case for the decreasing effect of *L. rhamnosus* GG, *L. rhamnosus* Lc705, and *P. freundenreichii* supsp. *shermanii Js* on membrane leakage, measured by the release of lactate dehydrogenase [91].

Listeria monocytogenes. Preincubation with *L. plantarum* MF1298 but not with *L. salivarius* DC5 attenuates the decrease in TEER elicited by the pathogen *L. monocytogenes*. However, this effect is diminished after 8 hours of incubation, and after 24 hours the TEER is no different from that of cells treated with *L. monocytogenes* alone [89].

3.2.3 Non-infectious Pathogens

Acetylsalicylic Acid. Heat-killed *L. acidophilus* with its spent culture supernatant protects HT29 cells from damage by acetylsalicylic acid. It prevents the acetylsalicylic acid-induced downregulation in protein expression and redistribution of ZO-1 [105].

H₂O₂. Pretreatment with soluble proteins produced by *L. rhamnosus* GG reduce the H_2O_2-induced decrease in TEER and increase in inulin fluxes in a time- and dose-dependent manner. It also inhibits the H_2O_2-induced redistribution of occludin, ZO-1, E-cadherin, and β-catenin from the TJs and adherens junctions and their dissociation from the actin cytoskeleton [106].

Cytokines.* The cytokines TNF-α and IFN-γ induce a drop in TEER when added to various cell monolayers. Several probiotic strains have proved to be effective in preventing this change of TEER. Treatment with *B. infantis* prevents TNF-α- and IFN-γ-induced drops in TEER and the re-arrangement of TJ proteins in T84 cells [65]. The TNF-α-induced decrease in TEER across Caco-2 monolayers has been inhibited by *L. plantarum* [107].

Pretreatment with *S. thermophilus* and *L. acidophilus* or the commensal *B. thetaiotaomicron* prevent the decrease in TEER in Caco-2 and HT29/cl.19A cells, incubated with IFN-γ or TNF-α for 48 hours. Simultaneous treatment or treatment with heat-inactivated bacteria, spent medium[8] from bacterial cultures, or DNA has no effect. This observation has been corroborated by the measurement of epithelial permeability to a low and a high molecular weight marker in the Ussing chamber. Pretreatment and simultaneous treatment with *S. thermophilus* and *L. acidophilus* or *B. thetaiotaomicron* prevent the increase in permeability [43].

Aflatoxin.* In an *in vitro* study with Caco-2 cells, the transport of aflatoxin B1, a potent hepatocarcinogen, across cell monolayers is diminished,

[8]See footnote 7.

and the decrease in TEER induced by the myco-toxin is reduced, by coincubation with non-viable *L. rhamnosus* GG [108].

Gliadin.* In celiac disease patients, wheat gliadin induces grave intestinal symptoms and small intestine mucosal injury. *B. lactis*, but not *L. fermentum*, inhibits, dose-dependently, the gliadin-induced increase in TEER in Caco-2 monolayers. Both bacterial strains also inhibit the formation of membrane ruffles and partly preserve the pattern of ZO-1 expression after treatment with gliadin [109].

4. MECHANISMS AND SIGNALING PATHWAYS MEDIATING PROBIOTIC EFFECTS ON INTESTINAL TRANSPORT AND BARRIER FUNCTION

Although many of the mechanisms of action and signaling pathways of *pathogenic* bacteria have been characterized in recent times, our knowledge of the molecular mechanisms of probiotics is still fragmental. However, this knowledge would facilitate the differential and targeted application of probiotics in prevention and therapy.

The description of mechanisms in this section is restricted to probiotic effects on intestinal transport and barrier functions. Each probiotic microorganism has its own properties. Hence, the effects obtained with one strain cannot be extrapolated to another [110]. Sometimes, the obtained effects are even different for phylogenetically almost identical strains [100].

4.1. Mode of Application

A few points have to be considered to achieve an optimal probiotic effect on transport and barrier functions. The possible results depend on:

1. time point of application;
2. duration of treatment;
3. dose;
4. use of single strains or mixtures.

1. The time point of application, i.e. preincubation, coincubation or postincubation in cell cultures or the pretreatment or curative treatment in humans and animals, determines the outcome. In most of the studies, in which pathogens or other damaging agents have been employed, only pretreatment with the probiotic has produced the designated effect. Coincubation and, rarely, the subsequent addition of the probiotic have been shown to be effective in only a few experimental setups. In some cases, augmentation of the infection dose seems to compensate for a later time point of addition [56].

2. Probiotics can have time-dependent effects. This should be taken into account when evaluating divergent results of studies with different durations of probiotic treatment.

Some probiotics have proven to have both an effect on intestinal permeability when added *in vitro* for short-term, e.g. to the Ussing chamber, and when administered orally long-term [65]. Other preparations need long-term oral application before showing an effect [81]. The probiotic effect can change over days and weeks and, sometimes, a therapeutic effect disappears after a longer application time over weeks or months [34, 70]. A time-dependent change of permeability has also been reported in cell culture studies. After a few hours of incubation with the probiotic, a positive effect is achieved (i.e. permeability is decreased) that persists for some hours, disappears later or even turns into a negative effect [90, 91]. Some of these deteriorating effects with longer incubation time in cell culture models might be attributed to the lack of exchange of the milieu (unlike the *in vivo* situation), e.g. the pH decreases, as in the study of Madsen et al. [46]. Therefore, many researchers define a timeframe for their studies, which is, for example, orientated to the decrease of pH in the cell culture medium.

3. Dose–response studies have rarely been performed, and research is still needed in this

respect. A dose-dependent effect of probiotics has been reported in studies with animals [81] and cell lines [41, 46, 89, 101, 102, 106, 109]. However, Commane et al. [111] have observed a poor correlation between the optical density of the bacterial cultures and changes of TEER. They conclude that the concentration of specific metabolites of the bacteria is the determining factor, and not the number of bacteria.

4. The application of a single strain versus multistrain and multispecies probiotic combinations is controversial. A combination might have the advantage of developing synergistic actions or allowing the 'occupation of different niches'. On the other hand, in a probiotic combination, the strains can inhibit each other's positive actions. For example, in the study of Myllyluoma et al. [91] inflammatory effects prevailed when a multispecies probiotic combination was used. However, Madsen et al. [46] have reported that the use of the multispecies mixture VSL#3 is more effective than the use of a single *Lactobacillus* species in improving colitis and stabilizing epithelial barrier function in IL-10 gene-deficient mice.

4.2. Mechanisms of Action

The mechanisms of action can be classified into: 1) the interaction of the probiotic with (pathogenic) bacteria in the GIT; and 2) the interaction with host (effector) cells such as epithelial cells or cells of the immune system (the effects on immune cells will not be discussed here).

A better understanding of these interactions requires knowledge concerning: a) the responsible component of the probiotic; b) the receptor in the case of interaction with host cells; c) the signaling pathway; and d) the elicited response in the host cell.

A variety of techniques and experimental conditions has been used to test the effects of live or dead bacteria (killed by heat, γ-irradiation, enzymes, or antibiotics), and to study soluble components from bacterial culture supernatants, conditioned media, or bacterial DNA. Depending on the mechanism of interaction, live bacteria, soluble factors secreted by probiotic strains, DNA, or parts of bacteria such as surface layer proteins can be responsible for the probiotic effect. Resta-Lenert and Barrett [56] have concluded from their studies with *S. thermophilus* and *L. acidophilus* that both live probiotics and their secreted products can affect epithelial responses to pathogens, but that only the former can exert the full spectrum of preventive effects.

Some probiotics exert a general effect on epithelial permeability or transport [46], and others are characterized by a specific effect against pathogen-induced changes [47, 81]. Furthermore, probiotic bacteria often use not only one but several mechanisms and induce manifold intracellular signal transduction pathways [106, 112]. When affecting both cellular secretory and barrier function, the regulation can be divergent [56].

In the following section, some mechanisms of action and signaling pathways will be described, and examples are given.

4.2.1 Interaction with Bacteria

Antimicrobial Activity.   The spent supernatant of *L. acidophilus* strain LB showed dose-dependent antimicrobial activity against *E. coli* (Afa/Dr DAEC) [101]. The antibacterial substances were heat stable, of low molecular weight, and distinct from lactic acid [113].

Degradation of Toxins.   A protease, secreted by *S. boulardii,* has been identified that cleaves the *C. difficile* toxin A molecule and that inhibits its binding to the intestinal receptor, thereby inhibiting secretion induced by the toxin [114].

Eubacterium sp. DSM 11798 degrades deoxynivalenol (DON) into its non-toxic metabolite de-epoxy DON (DOM-1) (Binder et al., 1997 and 1998 according to Ref. [32]); this detoxification of DON could be the reason for the attenuated decrease of Na^+/glucose cotransport.

Binding of Toxins. A recombinant probiotic *E. coli* strain, designed to express a chimeric LPS capable of binding heat-labile enterotoxin with high affinity, provides significant *in vivo* protection against heat-labile enterotoxin-induced fluid secretion in ligated ileal loops of rabbits (Paton et al., 2005). The reduction in the aflatoxin-B1 (AFB1)-induced decrease in TEER is attributable to alterations in the availability of AFB1 because of its binding to heat-inactivated *Lactobacillus* GG, or to the subsequent sequestering of metabolites within the culture medium, or to a combination of both processes [108].

Prevention of Adhesion of Pathogenic Bacteria. The adhesion of pathogenic bacteria to mucosal surfaces is the first step in an intestinal infection and can be inhibited by physically blocking the receptor or by steric hindrance. The ability to inhibit adhesion of the pathogen depends both on the specific probiotic and the pathogen. This represents a common mechanism used by many probiotics. Some probiotics express receptors that resemble the receptors of pathogenic bacteria, for competitive binding to epithelial cells. Some *Lactobacillus* species, such as *L. helveticus*, possess so-called surface-layer proteins, located in a paracrystalline layer outside the bacterial cell wall; these proteins are thought to play a role in adherence to epithelial cells [115].

In studies with animal and cell models the adhesion of various pathogenic *E. coli* strains to intestinal epithelial cells is inhibited by *L. plantarum* [47], *S. thermophilus* and *L. acidophilus* [56], *L. helveticus* R0052 and surface-layer proteins extracted from it [93, 95], *L. sobrius* [100], and *L. rhamnosus* R0011 [93].

L. rhamnosus GG, *L. rhamnosus* Lc705, *P. freudenreichii* supsp. *shermanii Js*, and *B. breve* Bb99 alone or in combination inhibit *H. pylori* adhesion in a Caco-2 model [91].

S. thermophilus NCC2496, *L. rhamnosus* NCC 4007, *L. paracasei* NCC 2461, *B. longum* NCC 3001, and *B. lactis* NCC 2818 have the ability *in vitro* to inhibit, displace, or compete with the adhesion of *Enterobacter sakazakii*, an occasional contaminant in powdered infant formula, to mucus [116].

Prevention of Invasion. The invasion of *S. Dublin* into T84 monolayers has been inhibited by a secreted factor of VSL#3, which may either enter the cell and induce a signaling pathway to enhance barrier integrity or bind to apical surface receptors and block *S. Dublin* invasion. This inhibition of invasion has also been seen when VSL#3 itself is removed before the addition of *S. Dublin* [46].

Preincubation and coincubation with live or antibiotic-killed *S. thermophilus* and *L. acidophilus* inhibit the invasion of EIEC in Caco-2 monolayers [56].

4.2.2 Interaction with Epithelial Cells

Polyamines. Polyamines are involved in the regulation of cell growth and differentiation and are generated by most cells and bacteria in the GIT. Sources of polyamines may be endogenous or exogenous.

The (trophic) effects of *S. boulardii* are at least in part mediated by polyamines. Yeast cells contain substantial amounts of putrescine, spermidine, and spermine that can be either secreted or released as a result of catabolism. The uptake of endoluminal polyamines by brush border membrane vesicles is a selective and saturable process. Polyamine concentrations in the mucosa and the endoluminal fluid have been shown to increase after yeast treatment, and disaccharidase activities and Na^+-dependent glucose uptake in ileal brush border vesicles and in parallel SGLT-1 (Na^+/glucose cotransporter) expression is enhanced [33, 117].

Heat Shock Proteins. Heat shock proteins play a central role in the protection of cells, tissues, and organs exposed to various forms of stress and they are found in all mammalian tissues [118]. They exert manifold effects on epithelial functions, including effects on transport function and epithelial integrity [119, 120].

Hsp25 and Hsp72, which are known for their ability to maintain cytoskeletal integrity, are produced in YAMC (young adult mouse colon) cells exposed to VSL#3 or to VSL#3-conditioned medium in a dose-dependent fashion, likely mediated by proteasome inhibition [121]. Soluble low molecular weight factors of *L. rhamnosus* GG induce the expression of the same Hsps in colonic epithelial cells through the activation of several MAPKs [122].

Short-chain Fatty Acids (SCFA). Pro- and prebiotics can affect the profile of SCFAs in the lumen of the colon. SCFAs that serve as a primary energy source might enhance TJ strength via increasing energy levels. In a study of Commane et al. [111] fermentation products of various probiotics (*Bifidobacterium* Bb12, *Bifidobacterium* sp. 420, and *Lactobacillus* GG) or non-digestible oligosaccharides (Raftilose), or the SCFAs such as lactate and acetate showed similar effects on TJ integrity.

Part of the permeability changes induced by combined application of *L. plantarum* 299 and oatmeal fiber have been attributed to enhanced levels of SCFA [123].

Cytokines. Cytokine expression and secretion from epithelial cells can be influenced by probiotic strains [124]. Many cytokines have been shown to regulate TJ and the structure and function of the cytoskeleton [125]. TNF-α and IFN-γ decrease TEER by inducing the redistribution of various TJ proteins *via* internalization [126], or by regulating the transcription level of TJ proteins such as occludin [127]. IFN-γ selectively activates populations of paracellular pores, thereby increasing the flux of large molecules [128], and reduces ZO-1 levels [129].

Strategies that probiotics use to modulate barrier dysfunction might be to enhance the secretion of anti-inflammatory cytokines or to abolish the production of pro-inflammtory cytokines.

The oral pretreatment with VSL#3 inhibits the up-regulation of gene expression and the enhanced secretion of TNF-α and IFN-γ in the mouse colon in response to LPS. This is associated with the preservation of transport and barrier functions [57]. Madsen et al. [46] have attributed part of the reduction in colonic permeability in IL-10-deficient mice by VSL#3 to a diminished release of the pro-inflammatory cytokines TNF-α and IFN-γ.

L. sobrius counteracts the ETEC-induced increase in IL-8 and increases IL-10 expression in IPEC-1 cells [100], thereby protecting the epithelial barrier.

Signaling Pathways. Epithelial cells express both surface and internal receptors that can sense bacterial components able to activate various intracellular signaling cascades such as MAPK pathways, the nuclear factor κB inhibitor/nuclear factor κB (IκB/NFκB) pathway, and the phosphatidylinositol 3-kinase (PI3K)/Akt[9] pathway. Important receptors are the Toll-like receptors (TLRs), which convert the recognition of bacteria-associated molecules into signals for, amongst others, barrier enhancement or cell proliferation.

In the following, examples are given how probiotics interfere with intracellular signaling pathways.

S. boulardii. The mechanisms used by *S. boulardii* to prevent the pathogen-dependent alteration of transport and barrier functions have been examined in various studies.

A 120-kDa protein secreted by *S. boulardii* counteracts the cAMP elevation and subsequent Cl⁻ secretion induced by cholera toxin [55]. This might involve interaction with both: 1) a

[9]Akts are enzymes that are members of the serine/threonine-specific protein kinase family.

receptor coupled to a pertussis-toxin-sensitive G protein which is associated with the inhibitory subunit of adenylate cyclase; and 2) with a secretory pathway that bypasses the adenylate cyclase system [42, 55]. Possibly, *S. boulardii* interferes only with the adenylate cyclase–cAMP transduction pathway to trigger the decrease in cAMP concentration enhanced by the secretagogues VIP and PGE_2 or forskolin [42].

Secretion by the Ca^{2+}-mediated pathway is inhibited by *S. boulardii*, despite the absence of inhibition of inositol-1,4,5-triphosphate production [42]. Media conditioned by *S. boulardii* might inhibit Ca^{2+}-dependent Cl^- secretion by activating an inhibitory mechanism that dissociates increases in intracellular Ca^{2+} from Cl^- secretion. PKC might be involved in this mechanism. An elevation of the intracellular Ca^{2+} level has enhancing effects on $Na^+/K^+/2Cl^-$ and basolateral K efflux. The latter hyperpolarizes the cell to create a favorable electrical gradient for Cl^- exit across the apical surface [130].

Kinetics studies have revealed that EHEC-induced myosin light chain (MLC) phosphorylation precedes the decrease of TEER. *S. boulardii* abolishes this EHEC-induced MLC phosphorylation, which is one of the transduction pathways implicated in the control of TJ structure [104].

The activation of the pro-apoptotic protease Caspase-3 triggered by EPEC is delayed when intestinal epithelial cells are infected in the presence of *S. boulardii* [99].

Additional to these mechanisms directly influencing transport and barrier function in infected T84 cells, *S. boulardii* inhibits the invasion of EPEC by a MAPK pathway and IL-8 pro-inflammatory secretion via inhibition of the NFκB and MAPK signaling pathways [104].

S. thermophilus and L. acidophilus (in combination).

Probiotics can also activate signal transduction originating from the epidermal growth factor receptor (EGFr), which has manifold effects on ion transport and tight junction integrity [131–133]. Pretreatment with *S. thermophilus* and *L. acidophilus* prevents EGF inactivation by EIEC and reverses the inhibition of the MAPKs ERK 1 and 2, which are downstream effectors of EGFr [56].

In a further study, *S. thermophilus* and *L. acidophilus* pretreatment reverses the inhibitory effects of IFN-γ on epithelial chloride secretion and prevents the IFN-γ down-regulation of CFTR and NKCC1 levels. The MAPK p38, ERK1, 2, and the PI3K pathway mediate this effect. The protective effects of *S. thermophilus* and *L. acidophilus* on TEER and permeability involve the same pathways [43].

S. thermophilus and *L. acidophilus* also inhibit the degradation of IκB-α protein, an NFκB negative-feedback regulator, whereas a commensal bacterium (*B. thetaiotaomicron*) causes the increased phosphorylation of this protein implying NFκB activation. NFκB is a crucial target in the propagation of inflammatory responses evoked by cytokines and intestinal pathogens [43].

Some of the antagonistic effects of probiotics against IFN-γ result from the modulation of gene expression evoked by IFN-γ. The IFN-γ first activates the transcription factors STAT1 and STAT3 and later a suppressor of cytokine signaling, SOCS3. The probiotics reduce the ability of IFN-γ to increase the expression and activation of SOCS3 and to activate STAT3 [43].

VSL#3.

The increases in TEER and mucin expression, observed after incubation with VSL#3 or media conditioned with VSL#3, involve MAPKs p38 and p42/44 (= ERK1, 2) [90]. A soluble heat-labile pH-dependent protease-sensitive substance of >50 kDA has been isolated from the conditioned medium.

E. coli Nissle 1917.

The assembly and paracellular permeability of TJs are regulated by a network of signaling pathways involving PKC isoforms. PKCs are located in the cytosol near the *zonula occludens* complex; PKCζ is the only PKC that has also been located at the cellular border [134, 135]. The inhibition of PKCζ protects against the disruption of TJs caused by

EPEC infection, by preventing the removal of ZO-2 from TJs to the cytoskeleton, as only phosphorylated ZO-2 can be withdrawn from the TJ leading subsequently to their destabilization. The beneficial effect of *E. coli* Nissle 1917 on epithelial barrier function seems to be associated with a block, or at least a reduction, of PKCζ phosphorylation rendering the enzyme partially inactive. The disruption of the epithelial barrier caused by EPEC is inhibited (at coincubation) or the epithelial barrier is even restored (at postincubation) by *E. coli* Nissle 1917 [92].

These findings are supported by a study with a TLR2-agonist, the synthetic lipopeptide Pam$_3$CysSK4 in HT29 and Caco-2 cells. The binding of the specific synthetic ligand to TLR2 leads to a concentration- and time-dependent activation of specific PKC isoforms (PKCα and PKCδ), and this increases TEER. The increase in TEER correlates with the apical tightening and sealing of ZO-1 [136].

A DNA microarrray of T84 cells incubated with *E. coli* Nissle 1917 has additionally revealed the up-regulation of NFκB inhibitor [92].

L. rhamnosus GG. Two proteins, p75 and p40, isolated from *L. rhamnosus* GG supernatant promote the survival of intestinal epithelial cells by activating Akt in a PI3K-dependent manner and by inhibiting pro-apoptotic p38 MAPK. Akt promotes cell survival by the stimulation of cell proliferation (by activating cell-cycle regulators and inhibiting pro-apoptotic pathways, such as caspase-3), and thereby TNF-induced damage is significantly reduced [137, 138]. In addition to their anti-apoptotic effect, the same proteins inhibit the H$_2$O$_2$-induced decrease of TEER, an increase in inulin flux, and the redistribution of the proteins of TJs and adherens junctions in a time- and dose-dependent manner, *via* a PKC and MAPK pathway independently of one another [106].

L. rhamnosus GG and *L. rhamnosus* Lc705 prevent the activation of pro-apoptotic caspase-3 when Caco-2 cells are infected with *H. pylori* [91].

L. plantarum inhibits the TNF-α-induced decrease in TEER in Caco-2 monolayers by two pathways: the NFκB and the ERK pathway [107].

B. infantis. In T84 cells, the increase in TEER, ZO-1, and occludin and the down-regulation of claudin-2[10] after incubation with medium conditioned by *B. infantis* are associated with changes in MAPKs [65].

L. acidophilus. The stimulation of Cl$^-$/OH$^-$ exchange activity in Caco-2 cells is mediated by heat-stable soluble factors, secreted by *L. acidophilus*, via the PI3-kinase-mediated pathway [41]. PI3-kinase and its downstream effector molecules have a well-established role in intracellular trafficking. Indeed, *L. acidophilus* significantly increases the surface expression of a transport protein for Cl$^-$/HO$^-$ exchange, viz., SLC26A3, whereas total cellular SLC26A3 does not change.

Host Response to Probiotics. The underlying mechanisms of effects on transport and barrier function, such as an increase in TEER or the reduction of secretion, include changes in transporter expression (mRNA and protein) and localization (which can be modulated by intracellular trafficking), changes in the expression of TJ proteins and their distribution, and changes in mucus secretion.

Changes in the expression of transporters have been observed with *S. thermophilus* and *L. acidophilus*, which reverse the cytokine-mediated down-regulation of CFTR and NKCC1 in HT29/cl.19A cells [43], with *S. boulardii*, which enhances the expression of SGLT-1 in the rat ileum [33], and with *L. helveticus* R389, which increases the expression of Ca^{2+} channel TRPV6 in the duodenum of mice [39]. The surface expression of the transport protein for Cl$^-$/OH$^-$ exchange is increased by *L. acidophilus* in Caco-2 cells [41].

---

[10]A claudin expressing cation-selective pores and increasing permeability.

Probiotics have various effects on TJ proteins as detailed in section 4, 'Probiotics and barrier function.' *E. coli* Nissle 1917 counteracts the DSS-induced down-regulation of ZO-1 and ZO-2 expression in an animal model of colitis [36] and abrogates the decrease in ZO-2 expression and the redistribution of ZO-2 caused by EPEC [92]. *L. casei* [98] and *S. boulardii* [99] prevent the effect of EPEC on ZO-1 distribution. VSL#3 decreases the redistribution of ZO-1 induced by *S. Dublin* [90]. *S. thermophilus* and *L. acidophilus* prevent the reduction in the phosphorylation of actinin, occludin, and ZO-1 induced by EIEC [56]. *L. sobrius* inhibits the delocalization of ZO-1, the reduction in the amount of occludin, the rearrangement of F-actin, and the dephosphorylation of occludin caused by ETEC [100].

The mucin layer enforces the intestinal barrier by preventing the attachment of pathogenic bacteria. Various *Lactobacillus* strains which adhere to HT29 cells (such as *L. rhamnosus* GG and *L. plantarum* 299v) induce the up-regulation of MUC3 mRNA expression and extracellular secretion. *Lactobacillus* strains with minimal ability to ahere to epithelial cells (such as *L. acidophilus* strain DDS-1) have no such effect [139].

The ability to induce MUC3 secretion is paralleled by an inhibitory effect on the adherence of EPEC strain E2348/69 [139]. Most likely, MUC3 is not anchored but is secreted into the lumen where it interacts with or binds EPEC and is subsequently flushed out by peristaltic motions.

Incubation of HT29 cells with *L. plantarum* 299v increased MUC2 and MUC3 mRNA expression levels, and this was proposed as a reason for its inhibitory effect on the adherence of *E. coli* strain E2348/69 and EHEC strain CL8 (serotype O157:H7) to the cells [97].

MUC2 expression is also increased when *L. acidophilus* A4 cell extract is added and is considered as part of the mechanism that reduces the degree to which *E. coli* O157:H7 attaches to epithelial HT29 cells [96].

L. casei GG significantly reduces *E. coli* C25 translocation through Caco-2 monolayers. This is attributed to the up-regulation of MUC2 RNA and protein expression [103].

6. CONCLUSION

Many diseases of the GIT involve changes in the transport and barrier functions of intestinal epithelia. In clinical studies, probiotics have proven beneficial in infectious diarrhea in children, traveler's diarrhea, and *C. difficile* colitis and have shown promising effects on diseases of the inflammatory bowel complex. However, only a small number of studies have actually included experimental parameters precisely assessing the effects of probiotiocs on epithelial integrity or transport functions in order to overcome the descriptive character of the early observations. Most of the recent studies have been conducted in animal or cell models and have included the characterization of receptors and signal cascades, the regulation of genes, and the modulation of transport or TJ proteins, so that, in some cases, the mechanisms of action are exactly characterized, e.g. with regard to the effects of *S. boulardii*. Despite these efforts and some progress in the last few years, our knowledge of the mechanisms and signaling pathways used by probiotics remains limited.

The effects of probiotics, although producing similar results on transport and barrier functions, are mediated by different probiotic-specific pathways. Hence, it is hardly possible to make general conclusions. The interpretation of results from studies on probiotics is further complicated by the fact that some probiotics obviously protect or improve epithelial functions *per se*, independently of pathophysiological challenge, whereas other probiotics exert their positive effects specifically against individual pathogens. Furthermore, the dose, time, and duration of the application of probiotics have a determining impact on the effects exerted.

Future research is needed with regard to dose–response relationships and to the characterization of the signaling pathways and the mechanisms of action that mediate probiotic effects. This should help us to apply probiotics in a more targeted and efficient way against diseases involving changes in epithelial transport and barrier functions.

ACKNOWLEDGMENT

The author thanks Prof. Dr. Holger Martens for critically reading the manuscript and useful suggestions, and the Margarete Markus Charity and the DFG (FOR 438) for financial support.

References

1. Berkes, J., Viswanathan, V. K., Savkovic, S. D., & Hecht, G. (2003). Intestinal epithelial responses to enteric pathogens: effects on the tight junction barrier, ion transport, and inflammation. *Gut, 52*, 439–451.
2. Turner, J. R. (2006). Molecular basis of epithelial barrier regulation: From basic mechanisms to clinical application. *The American Journal of Pathology, 169*, 1901–1909.
3. Forster, C. (2008). Tight junctions and the modulation of barrier function in disease. *Histochemistry and Cell Biology, 130*, 55–70.
4. Field, M. (1976). Regulation of active ion transport in the small intestine. *Ciba Foundation Symposium*, 109–127.
5. Alvarez-Olmos, M. I., & Oberhelman, R. A. (2001). Probiotic agents and infectious diseases: A modern perspective on a traditional therapy. *Clinical Infectious Diseases, 32*, 1567–1576.
6. Fuller, R. (1989). Probiotics in man and animals. *The Journal of Applied Bacteriology, 66*, 365–378.
7. Van Niel, C. W., Feudtner, C., Garrison, M. M., & Christakis, D. A. (2002). Lactobacillus therapy for acute infectious diarrhea in children: A meta-analysis. *Pediatrics, 109*, 678–684.
8. McFarland, L. V. (2007). Meta-analysis of probiotics for the prevention of travelers' diarrhea. *Travel Medicine and Infectious Disease, 5*, 97–105.
9. McFarland, L. V. (2006). Meta-analysis of probiotics for the prevention of antibiotic associated diarrhea and the treatment of *Clostridium difficile* disease. *The American Journal of Gastroenterology, 101*, 812–822.
10. Alfaleh, K., & Bassler, D. (2008). Probiotics for prevention of necrotizing enterocolitis in preterm infants. *Cochrane Database of Systematic Reviews*, CD005496.
11. Fedorak, R. N., & Madsen, K. L. (2004). Probiotics and the management of inflammatory bowel disease. *Inflammatory Bowel Diseases, 10*, 286–299.
12. Baumgart, D. C., & Dignass, A. U. (2002). Intestinal barrier function. *Current Opinion in Clinical Nutrition and Metabolic Care, 5*, 685–694.
13. Ismail, A. S., & Hooper, L. V. (2005). Epithelial cells and their neighbors. IV. Bacterial contributions to intestinal epithelial barrier integrity. *American Journal of Physiology. Gastrointestinal and Liver Physiology, 289*, G779–G784.
14. Sanderson, I. R., & Walker, W. A. (1993). Uptake and transport of macromolecules by the intestine: Possible role in clinical disorders (an update). *Gastroenterology, 104*, 622–639.
15. Stecher, B., & Hardt, W. D. (2008). The role of microbiota in infectious disease. *Trends in Microbiology, 16*, 107–114.
16. Deplancke, B., & Gaskins, H. R. (2001). Microbial modulation of innate defense: Goblet cells and the intestinal mucus layer. *The American Journal of Clinical Nutrition, 73*, 1131S–1141S.
17. Kindon, H., Pothoulakis, C., Thim, L., et al. (1995). Trefoil peptide protection of intestinal epithelial barrier function: Cooperative interaction with mucin glycoprotein. *Gastroenterology, 109*, 516–523.
18. Allen, A., Leonard, A. J., & Sellers, L. A. (1988). The mucus barrier. Its role in gastroduodenal mucosal protection. *Journal of Clinical Gastroenterology, 10* (Suppl 1), S93–S98.
19. Matter, K., & Balda, M. S. (2003). Signalling to and from tight junctions. *Nature Reviews. Molecular Cell Biology, 4*, 225–236.
20. Ballard, S. T., Hunter, J. H., & Taylor, A. E. (1995). Regulation of tight-junction permeability during nutrient absorption across the intestinal epithelium. *Annual Review of Nutrition, 15*, 35–55.
21. Barrett, K. E. (2008). New ways of thinking about (and teaching about) intestinal epithelial function. *Advances in Physiology Education, 32*, 25–34.
22. Powell, D. W. (1981). Barrier function of epithelia. *The American Journal of Physiology, 241*, G275–G288.
23. Frömter, E. (1986). The paracellular shunt in leaky epithelia. *Pflug Arch Eur J Physiol* (Suppl 406), R3.
24. Ussing, H. H., & Zehran, K. (1951). Active transport of sodium as the source of electric current in the short-circuited isolated frog skin. *Acta Physiologica Scandinavica, 23*, 110–127.
25. Bjarnason, I. (1994). Intestinal permeability. *Gut, 35*, S18–S22.
26. Anderson, A. D., Jain, P. K., Fleming, S., et al. (2004). Evaluation of a triple sugar test of colonic permeability in humans. *Acta Physiologica Scandinavica, 182*, 171–177.

27. Berg, R. D. (1995). Bacterial translocation from the gastrointestinal tract. *Trends in Microbiology*, *3*, 149–154.

28. Breves, G., Walter, C., Burmester, M., & Schröder, B. (2000). *In vitro* studies on the effects of *Saccharomyces boulardii* and *Bacillus cereus* var. *toyoi* on nutrient transport in pig jejunum. *Journal of Animal Physiology and Animal Nutrition*, *84*, 9–20.

29. Lodemann, U., Hubener, K., Jansen, N., & Martens, H. (2006). Effects of *Enterococcus faecium* NCIMB 10415 as probiotic supplement on intestinal transport and barrier function of piglets. *Archives of Animal Nutrition*, *60*, 35–48.

30. Breves, G., Hattenhauer, O., Schöneberger, M., & Winckler, C. (1997). Untersuchungen zum Einfluß von Probiotika auf die intestinale Glucose- und Alaninaufnahme beim Schwein. *Proceedings of the Society of Nutrition Physiology*, *6*, 45.

31. Lodemann, U., Lorenz, B. M., Weyrauch, K. D., & Martens, H. (2008). Effects of *Bacillus cereus* var. *toyoi* as probiotic feed supplement on intestinal transport and barrier function in piglets. *Archives of Animal Nutrition*, *62*, 87–106.

32. Awad, W. A., Bohm, J., Razzazi-Fazeli, E., et al. (2004). Effects of deoxynivalenol on general performance and electrophysiological properties of intestinal mucosa of broiler chickens. *Poultry Science*, *83*, 1964–1972.

33. Buts, J. P., De Keyser, N., Marandi, S., et al. (1999). *Saccharomyces boulardii* upgrades cellular adaptation after proximal enterectomy in rats. *Gut*, *45*, 89–96.

34. Schroeder, B., Winckler, C., Failing, K., & Breves, G. (2004). Studies on the time course of the effects of the probiotic yeast *Saccharomyces boulardii* on electrolyte transport in pig jejunum. *Digestive Diseases and Sciences*, *49*, 1311–1317.

35. Winckler, C., Schroeder, B., & Breves, G. (1998). Effects of *Saccharomyces boulardii*, *Bacillus cereus* var. *caron* and *Bacillus cereus* var. *toyoi* on epithelial transport functions in pig jejunum. *Zeitschrift für Gastroenterologie*, *36*, 30–37.

36. Ukena, S. N., Singh, A., Dringenberg, U., et al. (2007). Probiotic *Escherichia coli* Nissle 1917 inhibits leaky gut by enhancing mucosal integrity. *PLoS ONE*, *2*, e1308.

37. Gilman, J., & Cashman, K. D. (2006). The effect of probiotic bacteria on transepithelial calcium transport and calcium uptake in human intestinal-like Caco–2 cells. *Current Issues in Intestinal Microbiology*, *7*, 1–5.

38. Brassat, D. & Vey, E., 1998. Patient Cooperation Treaty. *WO99/02170*.

39. Vinderola, G., Matar, C., & Perdigon, G. (2007). Milk fermentation products of *L. helveticus* R389 activate calcineurin as a signal to promote gut mucosal immunity. *BMC Immunology*, *8*, 19.

40. Neudeck, B. L., Loeb, J. M., & Faith, N. G. (2004). *Lactobacillus casei* alters hPEPT1-mediated glycylsarcosine uptake in Caco–2 cells. *Journal of Nutrition*, *134*, 1120–1123.

41. Borthakur, A., Gill, R. K., Tyagi, S., et al. (2008). The probiotic *Lactobacillus acidophilus* stimulates chloride/hydroxyl exchange activity in human intestinal epithelial cells. *Journal of Nutrition*, *138*, 1355–1359.

42. Czerucka, D., & Rampal, P. (1999). Effect of *Saccharomyces boulardii* on cAMP- and Ca^{2+}-dependent Cl$^-$ secretion in T84 cells. *Digestive Diseases and Sciences*, *44*, 2359–2368.

43. Resta-Lenert, S., & Barrett, K. E. (2006). Probiotics and commensals reverse TNF-alpha- and IFN-gamma-induced dysfunction in human intestinal epithelial cells. *Gastroenterology*, *130*, 731–746.

44. Krammer, M., & Karbach, U. (1993). Antidiarrheal action of the yeast *Saccharomyces boulardii* in the rat small and large intestine by stimulating chloride absorption. *Zeitschrift für Gastroenterologie*, *31* (Suppl 4), 73–77.

45. Schroeder, B., Duncker, S., Barth, S., et al. (2006). Preventive effects of the probiotic *Escherichia coli* strain Nissle 1917 on acute secretory diarrhea in a pig model of intestinal infection. *Digestive Diseases and Sciences*, *51*, 724–731.

46. Madsen, K., Cornish, A., & Soper, P., et al. (2001). Probiotic bacteria enhance murine and human intestinal epithelial barrier function. *Gastroenterology*, *121*, 580–591.

47. Michail, S., & Abernathy, F. (2002). *Lactobacillus plantarum* reduces the *in vitro* secretory response of intestinal epithelial cells to enteropathogenic *Escherichia coli* infection. *Journal of Pediatric Gastroenterology and Nutrition*, *35*, 350–355.

48. Resta-Lenert, S., & Barrett, K. E. (2002). Enteroinvasive bacteria alter barrier and transport properties of human intestinal epithelium: role of iNOS and COX–2. *Gastroenterology*, *122*, 1070–1087.

49. Leonhard-Marek, S., Schröder, B., & Breves, G. (2003). Effects of different probiotics on the secretory responses of pig small intestine. *Proceedings of the Society of Nutrition Physiology*, *12*, 67.

50. Barrett, K. E. (1997). Bowditch lecture. Integrated regulation of intestinal epithelial transport: intercellular and intracellular pathways. *The American Journal of Physiology*, *272*, C1069–C1076.

51. El Asmar, R., Panigrahi, P., & Bamford, P., et al. (2002). Host-dependent zonulin secretion causes the impairment of the small intestine barrier function after bacterial exposure. *Gastroenterology*, *123*, 1607–1615.

52. Vanden Broeck, D., Horvath, C., & De Wolf, M. J. S. (2007). *Vibrio cholerae*: Cholera toxin. *The International Journal of Biochemistry & Cell Biology*, *39*, 1771–1775.

53. Vidon, N., Huchet, B., & Rambaud, J. C. (1986). [Influence of *Saccharomyces boulardii* on jejunal secretion in rats induced by cholera toxin]. *Gastroentérologie Clinique et Biologique*, *10*, 13–16.

54. Pothoulakis, C., Kelly, C. P., Joshi, M. A., et al. (1993). *Saccharomyces boulardii* inhibits *Clostridium difficile* toxin

A binding and enterotoxicity in rat ileum. *Gastroenterology*, *104*, 1108–1115.

55. Czerucka, D., Roux, I., & Rampal, P. (1994). *Saccharomyces boulardii* inhibits secretagogue-mediated adenosine 3',5'-cyclic monophosphate induction in intestinal cells. *Gastroenterology*, *106*, 65–72.

56. Resta-Lenert, S., & Barrett, K. E. (2003). Live probiotics protect intestinal epithelial cells from the effects of infection with enteroinvasive *Escherichia coli* (EIEC). *Gut*, *52*, 988–997.

57. Ewaschuk, J., Endersby, R., & Thiel, D., et al. (2007). Probiotic bacteria prevent hepatic damage and maintain colonic barrier function in a mouse model of sepsis. *Hepatology*, *46*, 841–850.

58. Zareie, M., Johnson-Henry, K., Jury, J., et al. (2006). Probiotics prevent bacterial translocation and improve intestinal barrier function in rats following chronic psychological stress. *Gut*, *55*, 1553–1560.

59. Caballero-Franco, C., Keller, K., De Simone, C., & Chadee, K. (2007). The VSL#3 probiotic formula induces mucin gene expression and secretion in colonic epithelial cells. *American Journal of Physiology. Gastrointestinal and Liver Physiology*, *292*, G315–G322.

60. Lamine, F., Eutamene, H., & Fioramonti, J., et al. (2004). Colonic responses to *Lactobacillus farciminis* treatment in trinitrobenzene sulphonic acid-induced colitis in rats. *Scandinavian Journal of Gastroenterology*, *39*, 1250–1258.

61. Pavan, S., Desreumaux, P., & Mercenier, A. (2003). Use of mouse models to evaluate the persistence, safety, and immune modulation capacities of lactic acid bacteria. *Clinical and Diagnostic Laboratory Immunology*, *10*, 696–701.

62. Llopis, M., Antolin, M., & Guarner, F., et al. (2005). Mucosal colonisation with *Lactobacillus casei* mitigates barrier injury induced by exposure to trinitronbenzene sulphonic acid. *Gut*, *54*, 955–959.

63. Kennedy, R. J., Hoper, M., & Deodhar, K., et al. (2000). Probiotic therapy fails to improve gut permeability in a hapten model of colitis. *Scandinavian Journal of Gastroenterology*, *35*, 1266–1271.

64. Kennedy, R. J., Kirk, S. J., & Gardiner, K. R. (2002). Mucosal barrier function and the commensal flora. *Gut*, *50*, 441–442.

65. Ewaschuk, J. B., Diaz, H., Meddings, L., et al. (2008). Secreted bioactive factors from *Bifidobacterium infantis* enhance epithelial cell barrier function. *American Journal of Physiology. Gastrointestinal and Liver Physiology*, *295*, G1025–G1034.

66. Feighery, L. M., Smith, P., O'Mahony, L., et al. (2008). Effects of *Lactobacillus salivarius* 433118 on intestinal inflammation, immunity status and *in vitro* colon function in two mouse models of inflammatory bowel disease. *Digestive Diseases and Sciences*, *53*, 2495–2506.

67. Mao, Y., Nobaek, S., Kasravi, B., et al. (1996). The effects of *Lactobacillus* strains and oat fiber on methotrexate-induced enterocolitis in rats. *Gastroenterology*, *111*, 334–344.

68. Southcott, E., Tooley, K. L., Howarth, G. S., et al. (2008). Yoghurts containing probiotics reduce disruption of the small intestinal barrier in methotrexate-treated rats. *Digestive Diseases and Sciences*, *53*, 1837–1841.

69. Garcia Vilela, E., De Lourdes De Abreu Ferrari, M., Oswaldo Da Gama Torres, H., et al. (2008). Influence of *Saccharomyces boulardii* on the intestinal permeability of patients with Crohn's disease in remission. *Scandinavian Journal of Gastroenterology*, *43*, 842–848.

70. Gupta, P., Andrew, H., Kirschner, B. S., & Guandalini, S. (2000). Is *Lactobacillus* GG helpful in children with Crohn's disease? Results of a preliminary, open-label study. *Journal of Pediatric Gastroenterology and Nutrition*, *31*, 453–457.

71. Zeng, J., Li, Y. Q., Zuo, X. L., et al. (2008). Clinical trial: Effect of active lactic acid bacteria on mucosal barrier function in patients with diarrhea-predominant irritable bowel syndrome. *Alimentary Pharmacology & Therapeutics*, *28*, 994–1002.

72. Gareau, M. G., Jury, J., MacQueen, G., et al. (2007). Probiotic treatment of rat pups normalises corticosterone release and ameliorates colonic dysfunction induced by maternal separation. *Gut*, *56*, 1522–1528.

73. Eutamene, H., Lamine, F., Chabo, C., et al. (2007). Synergy between *Lactobacillus paracasei* and its bacterial products to counteract stress-induced gut permeability and sensitivity increase in rats. *Journal of Nutrition*, *137*, 1901–1907.

74. Garcia-Rodenas, C. L., Bergonzelli, G. E., Nutten, S., et al. (2006). Nutritional approach to restore impaired intestinal barrier function and growth after neonatal stress in rats. *Journal of Pediatric Gastroenterology and Nutrition*, *43*, 16–24.

75. Qin, H. L., Shen, T. Y., Gao, Z. G., et al. (2005). Effect of lactobacillus on the gut microflora and barrier function of the rats with abdominal infection. *World Journal of Gastroenterology*, *11*, 2591–2596.

76. Shen, T. Y., Qin, H. L., Gao, Z. G., et al. (2006). Influences of enteral nutrition combined with probiotics on gut microflora and barrier function of rats with abdominal infection. *World Journal of Gastroenterology*, *12*, 4352–4358.

77. Eizaguirre, I., Urkia, N. G., Asensio, A. B., et al. (2002). Probiotic supplementation reduces the risk of bacterial translocation in experimental short bowel syndrome. *Journal of Pediatric Surgery*, *37*, 699–702.

78. Rychter, J. W., van Minnen, L. P., Verheem, A., et al. (2009). Pretreatment but not treatment with probiotics abolishes mouse intestinal barrier dysfunction in acute pancreatitis. *Surgery*, *145*, 157–167.

79. Luyer, M. D., Buurman, W. A., Hadfoune, M., et al. (2005). Strain-specific effects of probiotics on gut barrier integrity following hemorrhagic shock. *Infection and Immunity, 73,* 3686–3692.

80. Lee, D. J., Drongowski, R. A., Coran, A. G., & Harmon, C. M. (2000). Evaluation of probiotic treatment in a neonatal animal model. *Pediatric Surgery International, 16,* 237–242.

81. Mangell, P., Nejdfors, P., Wang, M., et al. (2002). *Lactobacillus plantarum* 299v inhibits *Escherichia coli*-induced intestinal permeability. *Digestive Diseases and Sciences, 47,* 511–516.

82. Isolauri, E., Kaila, M., Arvola, T., et al. (1993). Diet during rotavirus enteritis affects jejunal permeability to macromolecules in suckling rats. *Pediatr Res, 33,* 548–553.

83. Gotteland, M., Cruchet, S., & Verbeke, S. (2001). Effect of *Lactobacillus* ingestion on the gastrointestinal mucosal barrier alterations induced by indometacin in humans. *Alimentary Pharmacology & Therapeutics, 15,* 11–17.

84. Isolauri, E., Majamaa, H., Arvola, T., et al. (1993). *Lactobacillus casei* strain GG reverses increased intestinal permeability induced by cow milk in suckling rats. *Gastroenterology, 105,* 1643–1650.

85. Pessi, T., Sutas, Y., Marttinen, A., & Isolauri, E. (1998). Probiotics reinforce mucosal degradation of antigens in rats: Implications for therapeutic use of probiotics. *Journal of Nutrition, 128,* 2313–2318.

86. Rosenfeldt, V., Benfeldt, E., Valerius, N. H., et al. (2004). Effect of probiotics on gastrointestinal symptoms and small intestinal permeability in children with atopic dermatitis. *The Journal of Pediatrics, 145,* 612–616.

87. Caplan, M. S., Miller-Catchpole, R., Kaup, S., et al. (1999). Bifidobacterial supplementation reduces the incidence of necrotizing enterocolitis in a neonatal rat model. *Gastroenterology, 117,* 577–583.

88. Stratiki, Z., Costalos, C., Sevastiadou, S., et al. (2007). The effect of a bifidobacter supplemented bovine milk on intestinal permeability of preterm infants. *Early Hum Dev, 83,* 575–579.

89. Klingberg, T. D., Pedersen, M. H., Cencic, A., & Budde, B. B. (2005). Application of measurements of transepithelial electrical resistance of intestinal epithelial cell monolayers to evaluate probiotic activity. *Applied and Environmental Microbiology, 71,* 7528–7530.

90. Otte, J. M., & Podolsky, D. K. (2004). Functional modulation of enterocytes by gram-positive and gram-negative microorganisms. *American Journal of Physiology. Gastrointestinal and Liver Physiology, 286,* G613–G626.

91. Myllyluoma, E., Ahonen, A. M., Korpela, R., et al. (2008). Effects of multispecies probiotic combination on *Helicobacter pylori* infection *in vitro. Clin Vaccine Immunol, 15,* 1472–1482.

92. Zyrek, A. A., Cichon, C., Helms, S., et al. (2007). Molecular mechanisms underlying the probiotic effects of *Escherichia coli* Nissle 1917 involve ZO–2 and PKCzeta redistribution resulting in tight junction and epithelial barrier repair. *Cell Microbiol, 9,* 804–816.

93. Sherman, P. M., Johnson-Henry, K. C., & Yeung, H. P., et al. (2005). Probiotics reduce enterohemorrhagic *Escherichia coli* O157:H7- and enteropathogenic *E. coli* O127:H6-induced changes in polarized T84 epithelial cell monolayers by reducing bacterial adhesion and cytoskeletal rearrangements. *Infection and Immunity, 73,* 5183–5188.

94. Johnson-Henry, K. C., Donato, K. A., & Shen-Tu, G., et al. (2008). *Lactobacillus rhamnosus* strain GG prevents enterohemorrhagic *Escherichia coli* O157:H7-induced changes in epithelial barrier function. *Infection and Immunity, 76,* 1340–1348.

95. Johnson-Henry, K. C., Hagen, K. E., & Gordonpour, M., et al. (2007). Surface-layer protein extracts from *Lactobacillus helveticus* inhibit enterohaemorrhagic *Escherichia coli* O157:H7 adhesion to epithelial cells. *Cell Microbiol, 9,* 356–367.

96. Kim, Y., Kim, S. H., Whang, K. Y., Kim, Y. J., & Oh, S. (2008). Inhibition of *Escherichia coli* O157:H7 attachment by interactions between lactic acid bacteria and intestinal epithelial cells. *J Microbiol Biotechnol, 18,* 1278–1285.

97. Mack, D. R., Michail, S., Wei, S., et al. (1999). Probiotics inhibit enteropathogenic *E. coli* adherence *in vitro* by inducing intestinal mucin gene expression. *The American Journal of Physiology, 276,* G941–G950.

98. Parassol, N., Freitas, M., Thoreux, K., et al. (2005). *Lactobacillus casei* DN–114 001 inhibits the increase in paracellular permeability of enteropathogenic *Escherichia coli*-infected T84 cells. *Res Microbiol, 156,* 256–262.

99. Czerucka, D., Dahan, S., Mograbi, B., et al. (2000). *Saccharomyces boulardii* preserves the barrier function and modulates the signal transduction pathway induced in enteropathogenic *Escherichia coli*-infected T84 cells. *Infection and Immunity, 68,* 5998–6004.

100. Roselli, M., Finamore, A., Britti, M. S., et al. (2007). The novel porcine *Lactobacillus sobrius* strain protects intestinal cells from enterotoxigenic *Escherichia coli* K88 infection and prevents membrane barrier damage. *Journal of Nutrition, 137,* 2709–2716.

101. Lievin-Le Moal, V., Amsellem, R., Servin, A. L., & Coconnier, M. H. (2002). *Lactobacillus acidophilus* (strain LB) from the resident adult human gastrointestinal microflora exerts activity against brush border damage promoted by a diarrhoeagenic *Escherichia coli* in human enterocyte-like cells. *Gut, 50,* 803–811.

102. Mattar, A. F., Drongowski, R. A., Coran, A. G., & Harmon, C. M. (2001). Effect of probiotics on

enterocyte bacterial translocation *in vitro*. *Pediatr Surg Int, 17,* 265–268.

103. Mattar, A. F., Teitelbaum, D. H., Drongowski, R. A., et al. (2002). Probiotics up-regulate MUC–2 mucin gene expression in a Caco–2 cell-culture model. *Pediatr Surg Int, 18,* 586–590.

104. Dahan, S., Dalmasso, G., Imbert, V., et al. (2003). *Saccharomyces boulardii* interferes with enterohemorrhagic *Escherichia coli*-induced signaling pathways in T84 cells. *Infection and Immunity, 71,* 766–773.

105. Montalto, M., Maggiano, N., Ricci, R., et al. (2004). *Lactobacillus acidophilus* protects tight junctions from aspirin damage in HT–29 cells. *Digestion, 69,* 225–228.

106. Seth, A., Yan, F., Polk, D. B., & Rao, R. K. (2008). Probiotics ameliorate the hydrogen peroxide-induced epithelial barrier disruption by a PKC- and MAP kinase-dependent mechanism. *American Journal of Physiology. Gastrointestinal and Liver Physiology, 294,* G1060–G1069.

107. Ko, J. S., Yang, H. R., Chang, J. Y., & Seo, J. K. (2007). *Lactobacillus plantarum* inhibits epithelial barrier dysfunction and interleukin–8 secretion induced by tumor necrosis factor-alpha. *World Journal of Gastroenterology, 13,* 1962–1965.

108. Gratz, S., Wu, Q. K., El-Nezami, H., et al. (2007). *Lactobacillus rhamnosus* strain GG reduces aflatoxin B1 transport, metabolism, and toxicity in Caco–2 cells. *Applied and Environmental Microbiology, 73,* 3958–3964.

109. Lindfors, K., Blomqvist, T., Juuti-Uusitalo, K., et al. (2008). Live probiotic *Bifidobacterium lactis* bacteria inhibit the toxic effects induced by wheat gliadin in epithelial cell culture. *Clinical and Experimental Immunology, 152,* 552–558.

110. Fioramonti, J., Theodorou, V., & Bueno, L. (2003). Probiotics: what are they? What are their effects on gut physiology? *Best Practice & Research. Clinical Gastroenterology, 17,* 711–724.

111. Commane, D. M., Shortt, C. T., Silvi, S., et al. (2005). Effects of fermentation products of pro- and prebiotics on trans-epithelial electrical resistance in an *in vitro* model of the colon. *Nutr Cancer, 51,* 102–109.

112. Czerucka, D., & Rampal, P. (2002). Experimental effects of *Saccharomyces boulardii* on diarrheal pathogens. *Microbes Infect, 4,* 733–739.

113. Coconnier, M. H., Lievin, V., Bernet-Camard, M. F., et al. (1997). Antibacterial effect of the adhering human *Lactobacillus acidophilus* strain LB. *Antimicrobial Agents and Chemotherapy, 41,* 1046–1052.

114. Castagliuolo, I., LaMont, J. T., Nikulasson, S. T., & Pothoulakis, C. (1996). *Saccharomyces boulardii* protease inhibits *Clostridium difficile* toxin A effects in the rat ileum. *Infection and Immunity, 64,* 5225–5232.

115. Frece, J., Kos, B., Svetec, I. K., et al. (2005). Importance of S-layer proteins in probiotic activity of *Lactobacillus*

acidophilus M92. *Journal of Applied Microbiology, 98,* 285–292.

116. Collado, M. C., Isolauri, E., & Salminen, S. (2008). Specific probiotic strains and their combinations counteract adhesion of *Enterobacter sakazakii* to intestinal mucus. *FEMS Microbiology Letters, 285,* 58–64.

117. Buts, J. P., De Keyser, N., & De Raedemaeker, L. (1994). *Saccharomyces boulardii* enhances rat intestinal enzyme expression by endoluminal release of polyamines. *Pediatric Research, 36,* 522–527.

118. Feder, M. E., & Hofmann, G. E. (1999). Heat-shock proteins, molecular chaperones, and the stress response: Evolutionary and ecological physiology. *Annual Review of Physiology, 61,* 243–282.

119. Ikari, A., Nakano, M., Kawano, K., & Suketa, Y. (2002). Up-regulation of sodium-dependent glucose transporter by interaction with heat shock protein 70. *The Journal of Biological Chemistry, 277,* 33338–33343.

120. Musch, M. W., Sugi, K., Straus, D., & Chang, E. B. (1999). Heat-shock protein 72 protects against oxidant-induced injury of barrier function of human colonic epithelial Caco2/bbe cells. *Gastroenterology, 117,* 115–122.

121. Petrof, E. O., Kojima, K., Ropeleski, M. J., et al. (2004). Probiotics inhibit nuclear factor-kappaB and induce heat shock proteins in colonic epithelial cells through proteasome inhibition. *Gastroenterology, 127,* 1474–1487.

122. Tao, Y., Drabik, K. A., Waypa, T. S., et al. (2006). Soluble factors from *Lactobacillus* GG activate MAPKs and induce cytoprotective heat shock proteins in intestinal epithelial cells. *American Journal of Physiology. Cell Physiology, 290,* C1018–C1030.

123. White, J. S., Hoper, M., Parks, R. W., et al. (2006). The probiotic bacterium *Lactobacillus plantarum* species 299 reduces intestinal permeability in experimental biliary obstruction. *Letters in Applied Microbiology, 42,* 19–23.

124. Maassen, C., Laman, J. D., Boersma, W. J. A., & Claassen, E. (2000). Modulation of cytokine expression by lactobacilli and its possible therapeutic use. In R. Fuller & G. Perdigon (Eds.), *Probiotics 3 Immunmodulation by the Gut Microflora and Probiotics* (pp. 176–193). Dordrecht: Kluwer Academic Publishers.

125. Nusrat, A., Turner, J. R., & Madara, J. L. (2000). Molecular physiology and pathophysiology of tight junctions. IV. Regulation of tight junctions by extracellular stimuli: Nutrients, cytokines, and immune cells. *American Journal of Physiology. Gastrointestinal and Liver Physiology, 279,* G851–G857.

126. Bruewer, M., Luegering, A., Kucharzik, T., et al. (2003). Proinflammatory cytokines disrupt epithelial barrier function by apoptosis-independent mechanisms. *Journal of Immunology, 171,* 6164–6172.

127. Mankertz, J., Tavalali, S., Schmitz, H., et al. (2000). Expression from the human occludin promoter is

affected by tumor necrosis factor alpha and interferon gamma. *Journal of Cell Science, 113* (Pt 11), 2085–2090.

128. Watson, C. J., Hoare, C. J., Garrod, D. R., et al. (2005). Interferon-gamma selectively increases epithelial permeability to large molecules by activating different populations of paracellular pores. *Journal of Cell Science, 118*, 5221–5230.

129. Youakim, A., & Ahdieh, M. (1999). Interferon-gamma decreases barrier function in T84 cells by reducing ZO–1 levels and disrupting apical actin. *The American Journal of Physiology, 276*, G1279–G1288.

130. Dharmsathaphorn, K., & Pandol, S. J. (1986). Mechanism of chloride secretion induced by carbachol in a colonic epithelial cell line. *The Journal of Clinical Investigation, 77*, 348–354.

131. O'Mahony, F., Toumi, F., Mroz, M. S., et al. (2008). Induction of Na+/K+/2Cl⁻ cotransporter expression mediates chronic potentiation of intestinal epithelial Cl⁻ secretion by EGF. *American Journal of Physiology. Cell Physiology, 294*, C1362–C1370.

132. McCole, D. F., Rogler, G., Varki, N., & Barrett, K. E. (2005). Epidermal growth factor partially restores colonic ion transport responses in mouse models of chronic colitis. *Gastroenterology, 129*, 591–608.

133. Raimondi, F., Santoro, P., Barone, M. V., et al. (2008). Bile acids modulate tight junction structure and barrier function of Caco–2 monolayers via EGFR activation. *American Journal of Physiology. Gastrointestinal and Liver, 294*, G906–G913.

134. Dodane, V., & Kachar, B. (1996). Identification of isoforms of G proteins and PKC that colocalize with tight junctions. *The Journal of Membrane Biology, 149*, 199–209.

135. Song, J. C., Hanson, C. M., & Tsai, V., et al. (2001). Regulation of epithelial transport and barrier function by distinct protein kinase C isoforms. *American Journal of Physiology. Cell Physiology, 281*, C649–C661.

136. Cario, E., Gerken, G., & Podolsky, D. K. (2004). Toll-like receptor 2 enhances ZO–1-associated intestinal epithelial barrier integrity via protein kinase C. *Gastroenterology, 127*, 224–238.

137. Yan, F., Cao, H., & Cover, T. L., et al. (2007). Soluble proteins produced by probiotic bacteria regulate intestinal epithelial cell survival and growth. *Gastroenterology, 132*, 562–575.

138. Yan, F., & Polk, D. B. (2002). Probiotic bacterium prevents cytokine-induced apoptosis in intestinal epithelial cells. *The Journal of Biological Chemistry, 277*, 50959–50965.

139. Mack, D. R., Ahrne, S., Hyde, L., et al. (2003). Extracellular MUC3 mucin secretion follows adherence of *Lactobacillus* strains to intestinal epithelial cells in vitro. *Gut, 52*, 827–833.

140. Khailova, L., Dvorak, K., Arganbright, K. M., Halpern, M. D., Kinouchi, T., & Yajima, M., Dvorak, B. (2009). *Bifidobacterium bifidum* improves intestinal integrity in a rat model of necrotizing enterocolitis. *American Journal of Physiology. Gastrointestinal and liver Physiology, 297*, 6940–6949.

Food Formulation to Increase Probiotic Bacteria Action or Population

Esther Sendra Nadal, Estrella Sayas-Barberá,
Juana Fernández-López and José Angel Pérez-Alvarez

Departamento de Tecnología Agroalimentaria. Universidad Miguel Hernández de Elche,
Orihuela (Alicante)-Spain

1. INTRODUCTION

Probiotic, prebiotic and symbiotic foods are a growing sector of the food industry. The most common presentation of probiotic foods is the daily-dose drink [1] (single serving 65–125 mL) which is supposed to contain an effective dose of bacteria. These daily-dose drinks are commonly fermented milks or yogurt drinks flavored with juice or juice concentrates. Other active ingredients are often added: prebiotics, plant sterols or stanol esters for lowering levels of serum cholesterol and antioxidative substances. Other foods susceptible and can be used in delivering probiotics are ice-cream, cheese, candy, chocolate and chewing gum, oat- or soy-enriched milks or directly oat- or soy-based products and a huge category of infant formula; fermented meat products are also being studied [2, 3].

Probiotic foods and supplements are covered by the Food Products Directive and Regulation (178/2000/EC), whereas nutrition and health claims of such products fall under the regulation 1924/2006/EC. Under this regulation, the use of unauthorized claims and promises is not allowed and so there is an urgent need to provide consumers with the information on the validation of the probiotic effects of commercially available probiotic foods or either revise label information of products. In order to properly inform the consumers, manufacturers should provide information on: 1) identification of the genus, species and strain of the probiotic present in the product; 2) citations of published human studies on the effectiveness of the probiotic strain in the product; 3) assurance that the product contains the effective level of the probiotic through the end of shelf life as determined in the published studies [4].

TABLE 22.1 Potentially probiotic cultures used in probiotic foods or probiotic food supplements

Genera	Species
Lactobacillus	acidophilus/johnsonii/gasseri
	delbrueckii subsp. bulgaricus[a]
	casei
	crispatus
	lactis
	paracasei
	fermentum
	plantarum
	rhamnosus
	reuteri
	salivarius
Bifidobacterium	adolescentis
	animalis/lactis
	bifidum
	breve
	essensis
	infantis
	longum
Bacillus	subtilis[b]
	clausii[b]
Enterococcus	faecalis
	faecium
Escherichia	coli strain Nissle
Pediococcus	acidilacti
Propionibacterium	freudenreichii
Saccharomyces	boulardii
Streptococcus	thermophilus[a]

[a]Yogurt starter cultures.
[b]Spores.

Regarding the probiotics bacteria used (Table 22.1), they are mainly bifidobacteria and lactobacilli, and they are often labeled and marketed with imaginative names (*Bifidobacterium digestivum*, *Lactobacillus anti-caries* …). Bifidobacteria from infant origin seem to grow better than from adult origin. They have low acid tolerance, low oxygen tolerance, and milk-based medium are suitable for their growth. Lactobacilli grow quite well in milk media. Some species of lactobacilli are acid tolerant or aciduric. Selection of probiotic strains for technological performance is needed [5]. The main technological properties of probiotics (given that they should fulfill the desired biological effect and have no toxicity) are:

- oxygen tolerance;
- acid tolerance;
- bile tolerance;
- heat tolerance;
- ability to grow in milk;
- ability to metabolize prebiotics;
- not adversely affect product quality or sensory characteristics;
- stable to commercial conditions.

There is a need to implement reliable selective enumeration media to assure the final counts of probiotic bacteria in foods, as it is widely accepted that many 'selective' or 'differential' media fail to assure selective counts of probiotic bacteria. In this case, molecular genetics provides more accurate tools for their identification.

Many reviews provide comprehensive views on probiotics and prebiotics [1, 4, 6, 7]. The most commonly used prebiotics are fructans and resistant starches. Fructans are a group of naturally occurring oligosaccharides and fructo-oligosaccharides found in milligram quantities in onions, bananas, wheat, artichokes, garlic and other whole foods. They are usually extracted from chicory or manufactured from fructose. Fructans are not a homogeneous group as they are distinct in origin, structure and fermentation characteristics. Resistant starch has been, and is being, investigated as a prebiotic ingredient. Resistant starch is found in unripe fruits (like banana), raw potatoes, cooked and cooled starchy products (retrograded starch). It is specially manufactured for the food industry and there are many types of modified starches; not all of them are resistant to digestion. The group of prebiotic ingredients will continue to expand as ingredient technology develops. Dosage of prebiotics ranges from 2.5 to 20 g resistant starch/day [4],

TABLE 22.2   Substances with proven prebiotic properties

Carbohydrate	Non-digestible	Fermentable	Selectively used
Inulin	Yes	Yes	Yes
Oligofructose	Yes	Yes	Yes
Trans-galacto-oligosaccharides	Yes	Yes	Yes
Lactulose	Yes	Yes	Yes
Isomalto-oligosaccharides	Partially	Yes	Probably
Lactosacarose	NP	Yes	Probably
Xylo-oligosaccharides	NP	Yes	Probably
Soy oligosaccharides	Yes	Yes	NP
Resistant starch[a]	Yes	Yes	NP

NP, not yet proven. Adapted from: Gibson, G. R., Probert, H. M., Van Loo, J. et al. (2004). Dietary modulation of the human colonic microbiota: Updating the concept of prebiotics. *Nutrition Research Reviews, 17*(2), 259–275.

[a]Depending on crystallinity of the polymorph (Lesmes, U., Beards, E. J., Gibson, G. R. et al. (2008). Effects of resistant starch type III polymorphs on human colon microbiota and short chain fatty acids in human gut models. *Journal of Agricultural and Food Chemistry, 56*(13), 5415–5421).

3 to 8g fructans/day [4, 8]; however, substrate specificity may be important in considering prebiotic products and dose level.

The International Scientific Association for Probiotics and Prebiotics [9] has set down that: 'Prebiotics target the microbiota already present within the ecosystem acting as a "food" for the target microbes seen as beneficial'. A good prebiotic should:

- be safe;
- have good sensory properties;
- be stable under heat and when dried;
- withstand storage at room temperature;
- resist degradation by stomach acid, mammalian enzymes or hydrolysis;
- be fermented by intestinal microbes;
- selectively stimulate the growth and/or activity of positive microorganism of the gut;
- have proved health effects by clinical studies in humans;
- be administered in adequate dose (5–8g/day for fructans).

Only bifidogenic, non-digestible oligosaccharides (particularly inulin) and its hydrolysis product (oligofructose) and trans-galacto-oligosaccharides, appear to fulfill all of the criteria for prebiotic classification (Table 22.2). They are dietary fibers with a well-established positive impact on the intestinal microflora. Some prebiotics occur naturally in foods, but to exert prebiotic effect it would be necessary to intake a large amount of these foods, so it is more popular to fortify foodstuffs with defined amounts of prebiotics. As most common prebiotics are water soluble and clear in water, they are easily incorporated in most foods and almost undetectable.

Prebiotic carbohydrates are metabolized only by selected members of the gastrointestinal (GI) tract. But given the known metabolic diversity of probiotics, there is considerable variation in prebiotic activity scores for a particular prebiotic utilized by a single probiotic strain or even strains within a single species. Utilization of prebiotics by lactic acid bacteria (LAB) and related bacteria requires the presence of specific hydrolysis and transport systems for the particular prebiotic. The selective use of prebiotics by the target probiotics may be effective *in vitro* with pure culture, but in a mixed culture may not be that efficient. It is known that in the GI tract there are commensal organisms such as *Escherichia coli*, some *Bacteroides* and others that have the ability to metabolize these sugars [6]. In addition, the metabolic process may release hydrolysis products to the extracellular space and they may cross-feed other non-fermentor species. A prebiotic assay has been developed and it has been proven that in order to formulate symbiotics there is a need to evaluate the optimized combination of pre- and probiotics [6].

Inulin-type prebiotics include fructo-oligosaccharides (FOS), oligofructose, and inulin—terms that have been used inconsistently in both the scientific literature and food applications [7]. Commercially available inulin-type prebiotics can be extracted from food (typically chicory root) or synthesized from a more fundamental molecule (typically sucrose). Depending on the starting source and degree of processing, inulin-type prebiotics can be produced with very different chemical compositions. All inulin-type prebiotics are bifidogenic—stimulating the growth of bifidobacteria species. A minimal dose of inulin-type prebiotic appears to be needed to produce a bifidogenic effect. However, there is strain dependent intra-individual response to an identical dose of the same inulin-type prebiotic.

Symbiotics are foods with prebiotics and probiotics, where the presence of prebiotics improves the survival of probiotic bacteria during the storage of the product and during the passage through the intestinal tract and may enhance the implantation of probiotics in colonic microbiota.

Other chapters of this book deal with the evaluation of probiotics and prebiotics, the preparation of probiotic cultures, probiotic dairy foods, probiotic infant formula and probiotic vegetable products. This chapter aims to review the impact of food formulation and food processing on the survival, growth and activity of probiotics and prebiotics as well as food quality and stability.

2. EFFECT OF FOOD PROCESSING ON PREBIOTIC INGREDIENTS AND PROBIOTIC BACTERIA

2.1. Effect of Food Processing on Probiotic Bacteria

Probiotic cultures are commonly included in fermented milks and it is widely accepted the need to develop foods containing probiotic bacteria in sufficient numbers (over 7 log cfu/g). Such counts may be present until the end of shelf life; however, foods pose hurdles for the survival of probiotics such as acidity, oxygen stress, competition with other microorganisms of the product, storage temperature and moisture content [10]. There is considerable strain variability for acid, bile and oxygen tolerance. For some strains and manufacturing conditions, it is possible to use only the probiotic strain as an acid producing strain, but it is more usual to use it in combination with supporter cultures. In non-dairy products, probiotics do not usually multiply, and so its stability is critical. Interactions of probiotics with starter bacteria should be evaluated prior to product development, especially metabolites released by starters: lactic acid, hydrogen peroxide and bacteriocins [11].

A first step for the manufacture of probiotic foods is the availability of commercial starter cultures. The preparation of bulk cultures is difficult, and may be reviewed in another chapter of this book; the most common presentations are freeze-dried powders, frozen concentrates and spray-dried powder. The main challenges associated with the development of dried probiotic cultures are [10]:

- *Freeze drying*: the loss of viability in this process is linked to temperature changes, phase changes and drying as all tend to damage cell membranes and proteins. The use of cryoprotectants may reduce its impact on cell viability.

- *Spray drying*: its cost is lower than that of freeze drying; some species of lactobacilli and bifidobacteria undergo successful spray drying. But many strains do not easily survive the spray-drying process: present low survival rates, low stability under storage or difficulties during rehydration. Controlled stress to stimulate cross-protection mechanisms and encapsulation may be applied to enhance bacterial survival to spray-drying stress.

Encapsulation of probiotics is a common practice [5] in order to improve their performance under heat, spray drying and gastric acid exposure. Several techniques of encapsulation have been reported: spray drying, extrusion, emulsion and phases separation. Some possibilities are the encapsulation in calcium alginate beds, starch, or mixtures as gum acacia combined with gelatin and soluble starch. In any case, the coating may be suited to the food application of the probiotics, and their protective effect against acidity, bile salts and heat has to be tested. They appear to provide significant protection, and hexopolysaccharide-producing strains of bifidobacteria may be naturally protected. Several microencapsulated probiotics have been successful in acid, bile and heat tolerance tests [12, 13].

Excellent reviews on the challenges of probiotic inclusion in foods are available [5, 8, 10–12, 14]. Even international organizations have directed efforts in this direction. The EU Commission financed a project on the processing effects on the nutritional advancement of probiotics and prebiotics [8]. The researchers demonstrated that cell viability—storage stability and probiotic properties (acid/bile tolerance)—could be influenced by fermentation technology and downstream processing. 'Viability' is the percentage of viable cultures at the end of the shelf life of a food product and 'vitality' is its ability to resist external stress conditions occurring in a food product during its shelf life, resulting in a higher survival rate during passage in the GI tract [8]. Both characteristics are relevant for the successful inclusion of probiotics in foods. We will center the efforts in food product development and so we review the related conclusions on this topic.

Critical environmental factors for probiotic survival in fermented foods are oxygen stress, acidity, osmotic pressure, storage temperature and co-culture competition. A high strain dependency has been reported on the response to such factors.

Oxygen Stress

As probiotics are anaerobic, the use of impermeable containers and the presence of *S. thermophilus*, which acts as an oxygen scavenger, enhance probiotics survival [14]. Oxygen has a direct toxicity to probiotic cells, probably due to the intracellular production of hydrogen peroxides of certain cultures, particularly *Lactobacillus delbrueckii* ssp. *bulgaricus* (*L. bulgaricus*), which is a reason that justifies the removal of this specie from the starter cultures in order to enhance the survival of probiotic bacteria [12]. The elimination of peroxide-producing strains and the addition of antioxidants (such as ascorbic acid) may be used in order to prevent oxygen derived toxicity. It has been reported that *Propionibacterium freudenreichii* produces extracellular growth stimulator(s) for bifidobacteria that effectively suppress the production of peroxide under anaerobic conditions [15]. The effects of packaging materials on the survival of probiotics have been evaluated [16]: the lower the level of oxygen the more favored the survival of probiotics is. The use of glass containers favors the survival of probiotics due to their low oxygen permeability; however, the high costs and hazards of handling make it an inappropriate packaging for dairy products. The development of multilayer packaging with selective permeability and the inclusion of oxygen scavengers in the packaging material have potential application for probiotics foods. Further research is needed to optimize its use and make this possibility technologically and economically viable.

Acidity

Over-acidification in fermented milks is mainly due to strains of *L. bulgaricus*, which is the reason why this strain is sometimes reduced or suppressed from starter cultures [12, 14]. Probiotic lactobacilli are more acid tolerant than bifidobacteria although acid tolerance is strain-dependent [12, 14, 17]. For practical application, final pH must be maintained above 4.6 to prevent the decline in bifidobacteria populations [14]. It has been suggested that over-acidification may be prevented by: i) heat shock (58°C for 5 min) to yogurt before the addition of probiotic cultures; ii) lowering storage temperature to less than 3–4°C; and iii) adding whey proteins [8] to improve buffering capacity of yogurt, as well as the proper selection of acid tolerant strains together with the reduction of even elimination of *L. bulgaricus* (to reduce over-acidification and hydrogen peroxide release). Cheeses with higher pH than fermented milks may be better vehicles for probiotic [18], low-fat Cheddar cheese confers better protection during storage and passage through the GI tract to *Lactobacillus casei* than yogurt. When matured cheeses are to be used as carriers, it must be taken into consideration that high numbers of probiotic bacteria will be alive at the time of consumption, so either the strains must be capable of growing during cheese ripening or they should be inoculated at high levels during cheese manufacture and survive the ripening period. It seems that some adaptation mechanisms to acidity occurs. It has been observed that *Lactobacillus acidophilus* suffered greater viability losses during storage of refrigerated yogurt when the probiotic was added to the yogurt prior to storage rather than when it was added at the beginning of fermentation [19].

Starter Cultures

When mixing probiotics with starter cultures, every single strain needs to be tested together with the starter to evaluate competitive growth as well as stability during storage. Microbial metabolism releases to the medium bacteriocins which may reduce the growth of unwanted microorganisms [20], as well as hydrogen peroxide and organic acids. All of them may decrease probiotic populations; but metabolism also releases vitamins, free amino-acids, and may cause oxygen depletion (*S. thermophilus*) in which case probiotics survival is enhanced [14]. The addition of lactic acid bacteria (LAB), together with probiotics, slows the growth of the probiotics [12] due to the fast growth of the LAB and the liberation of bacteriocins and other inhibitors. However, it seems that bifidobacteria perform better when it is inoculated separately from the starter cultures, whereas *L. acidophilus* performs better when it is added together with the traditional starter cultures [14]. To enhance probiotic survival, several strategies may be used [12]:

- Reduction of the inoculate starter with the risk of liberation of inhibitors from the probiotic bacteria that may inhibit the starters, or inhibit the probiotics between themselves.
- The use of starters with proteolytic or oxygen scavenging properties which may enhance bifidobacteria growth.
- The addition of soy-based substrates which enhances the growth of probiotic lactobacilli.
- Promotion of sequenced growth, as for propionibacteria following the lactic fermentation, so they may use the lactate; sometimes associations between probiotic cultures may be beneficial.
- Interactions between probiotic yeasts and starters may be of interest and need to be explored.

It is usual to avoid the inoculation of probiotics together with lactic cultures; addition of probiotics after fermentation, just before packaging, is the most common industrial practice in fermented milks [10]. Bacteriophages are not yet a big concern for probiotics, but the problem may rise if a given strain is extensively used. Preventive strategies may be: i) strain rotation, ensuring the same biological effect on health of the new strain, which is rather difficult; and ii) adding the probiotic at the very end of the manufacturing process, which is costly. Inoculation practice also affects probiotic survival: higher inoculation of conventional starter cultures will lead them to dominate the fermentation and result in lower populations of probiotics in the final product, and high numbers of inoculation (up to 10–20%) favor the growth of probiotic bacteria [14]. However, although counts of probiotic bacteria are desired to be high, low sensory scores have been reported for yogurts with excessive inoculations of *L. acidophilus* (2.33 g/100 g) as well as increased syneresis and higher a* and b* values [21].

Incubation Temperatures

Temperatures of 43°C favor starter cultures, whereas lower temperatures (37–40°C) favor the growth rate and survival of probiotic bacteria [14].

Osmotic Pressure

Osmotic pressure effects are strain specific, most studies are in the usual range of probiotic foods formulation (from 0 to 10% sucrose addition) [8]. Salt tolerance needs to be tested when matured cheeses or fermented sausages are intended to use as probiotic carriers.

Heating Effects

Heating under 45°C is not detrimental to probiotics, but over 45°C will destroy at least a fraction of the population [12]. *L. acidophilus* is quite sensitive to heating, and in general, heat treatments over 65°C are quite detrimental to probiotics. Microencapsulation or probiotic addition

previous to aseptic packaging may be good options to protect against heat damage. The possibility of pre-adapting the probiotic cells with NaCl, bile salts, heating, and hydrogen peroxide has been suggested [10]. The previous heat treatment of the milk may affect the growth of probiotics: milks heated at 85 to 95°C seem appropriate for the subsequent growth of probiotics.

High Pressure Homogenization

An interesting finding is that milk treated by high pressure homogenization when used for the manufacture of probiotic Crescenza cheese enhanced the viability of *L. acidophilus* and *Lactobacillus paracasei* [22].

Storage Temperature

It seems that the ability to survive during processing and storage are not linked [12]: Freezing does not seem to affect the ability to assimilate cholesterol, but this character can be reduced in *L. acidophilus* following storage in unfermented milk at 5°C for 21 days [12]. The effect of refrigerated storage temperature (at 2, 5 and 8°C) on the viability of probiotics (*L. acidophilus*, *Bifidobacterium animalis* subsp. *lactis* Bb12) in yogurt has been studied [23]. After 20 days, storage at 2°C resulted in the highest viability of *L. acidophilus*, whereas for *B. lactis* the highest viability was obtained when yogurt was stored at 8°C. However, although bifidobacteria are less tolerant to low temperatures than lactobacilli, low storage temperatures favor the survival of probiotics as *L. bulgaricus* growth and post-acidification are restricted [14]. Although tolerance to frozen stress is strain dependent, most lactobacilli survive well-frozen storage. Ice-cream, which is subject to freezing and has high pH, seems to be a good product for the delivery of probiotics. The survival of two probiotic (*L. acidophilus* La5 and *B. animalis* subsp. *lactis* Bb12) inoculated at 4% dose in ice-creams (4% fat) and stored at −25°C for 60 days was studied [24]. Both probiotics had final counts over 6 log cfu/g. Frozen yogurts are the ones with more difficulties as low pH, freezing injuries, high temperatures of treatment, oxygen toxicity or moisture content may reduce probiotic survival. Several solutions can be given [10]: the addition of substances with cryoprotective properties, usually present in ice-cream formulations (including casein, sucrose, fat and glycerol), or even the use of microencapsulation technologies to aid in pH protection (encapsulation in gelatin and vegetable gums). Regular ice-creams, non-fermented, have the advantage of having moderate pH.

Type of Substrate

Milk types may influence probiotics survival [12]. However, there is no conclusive data at this point. These studies have been reported primarily on cows' milk but also on sheep, goat, camel and buffalo milk. Probiotic cultures generally grow faster on synthetic media than in pure milk; that may be due to the low proteolytic activity of milk. Mixing non-proteolytic strains with a high proteolytic LAB may seem helpful but the growth of LAB may overwhelm the probiotics and so sometimes milk is supplemented with yeast extract, a combination of substances (amino acids, minerals, ribonucleotides), or casein hydrolysates. This strategy works better for lactobacilli than for bifidobacteria where other factors such as redox conditions have greater impact. Regarding yeasts, although many types of yeast are unable to grow in milk, some yeasts have the ability to become established in dairy products and act as starters (i.e. Kefir starters). The potential use of yeasts as probiotics is of great interest due to their ability to grow at low pH, low water activities, low temperature and high salt concentration. Essential variables for the propagation of microorganisms in milk and milk products are the type and quantities of available carbohydrates and the degree of hydrolysis of milk proteins and lipids [10]. Dry-cured meat products have the advantage of not suffering heat treatment and having a moderate high pH which is beneficial for the growth and survival of probiotics.

Growth Promoting Factor

Several bifidogenic factors have been reported: fructo-oligosaccharides, galacto-oligosaccharides, protein hydrolysates, and the co-culture of proteolytic species. Regarding protein hydrolysates, casein hydrolysates, yeast extracts, amino sugars, and peptides have been studied to improve the growth of bifidobacteria [10]. Some strains do not grow well in milk. In such cases the presence of plant-based ingredients may improve the growth of probiotic cultures in milk [10, 12]: tomato juice, peanut milk, soy milk, buffalo whey/soy milk, rice, carrot and cabbage juice, as well as casein peptone, whey protein, sucrose, papaya pulp, manganese and magnesium ions, simple fermentation sugars or combinations of various. Growth promoting factors in probiotic fermented milks to stimulate *L. acidophilus* are [14]: 1) the combination of casitone, casein hydrolysate and fructose; 2) whey protein concentrate, tomato juice and papaya (due to simple sugars and minerals); and 3) acetate. And to stimulate bifidobacteria: i) cysteine, acid hydrolysates, tryptone; ii) peptides and amino acids; iii) vitamins, dextrins and maltose; and iv) 0.01% baker's yeast. Finally, for both lactobacilli and bifidobacteria: microencapsulation combined with the addition of oligosaccharides.

Evidences of the beneficial prebiotic–probiotic interaction in finished foods have been reported [8]. Inulin, oligofructose and galacto-oligosaccharides were supplemented in the milk-based media for bifidobacteria. Five percent of oligofructose was the best growth promoter of bifidobacteria and also enhanced viability of bifidobacteria during the refrigerated storage of yogurts. In *in vitro* studies, it has been reported that the presence of up to 3% oligofructose improves the survival of probiotics during gastrointestinal transit but this effect was only found when yogurts were stored for 4 or more weeks. Lactitol and various types of fructose containing oligosaccharides and other potential prebiotic carbohydrates were tested for feeding rats with probiotics and evaluate the production of short-chain fatty acids by them as estimators of the capability to improve colonic health and reduce the prevalence of colonic diseases. Fructose containing oligosaccharides (FOS) performed better than lactitol as FOS metabolisms increased the release of propionic and butyric acid, whereas lactitol caused high proportions of acetic acid. The degree of polymerization and the crystallinity of the carbohydrates are of great importance for the total fermentability, as well as the short fatty acid pattern. However, the combination of the carbohydrates with certain probiotic strains may modify the fatty acid pattern.

2.2. Effect of Food Processing on Prebiotics

Regarding modification of prebiotics due to food processing, the effect of processing conditions (low pH, heating at low pH, and Maillard reaction conditions) on some commercial prebiotics (two types of fructo-oligosaccharides (FOS) and two types of inulins) have been studied [25]. Prebiotic activity was stable at low pH and Maillard reaction conditions, but heating at low pH caused some hydrolysis of the prebiotics resulting in formation of sucrose, glucose and fructose, and so no longer offering selective stimulation. This is a relevant finding for acidic foods such as yogurt, cultured dairy products, salad dressings, crackers and others.

Enzymatic modification of prebiotics in order to give probiotics a selective advantage is an interesting topic [8]. Little is known on the

enzymatic machinery for galactose utilization but glycosidases from bifidobacteria appear quite interesting. Some of them are capable of elongating oligosaccharides, others can catalyze transglycosylation reactions, and so may prepare the substrates to be utilized by probiotic strains. Using enzymes from bifidobacteria may ensure that such carbohydrates are degraded. These studies have focused on β-galactosidase and α-galactosidase from bifidobacteria. β-galactosidase has low transglycosylation activity, and α-galactosidase has a high transferase activity. These authors concluded that carbohydrate substrates containing a pyranose ring and a CH_2OH group at the C-5 of the pyranose ring are good galactose-acceptors for the α-galactosidase. The enzymes of interest may be cloned and over-expressed in other microorganisms such as *E. coli* in order to further investigate the obtention of better prebiotics [8].

Changes in processing steps may be done in food processing to enhance probiotic survival [12]: changes in incubation temperature, addition of enzymes (β-galactosidase) to enhance prebiotic use by probiotics, modifying the redox conditions (mainly by addition of L-cysteine or ascorbic acid), microencapsulation of probiotics and others.

3. SENSORY ASPECTS OF PROBIOTIC, PREBIOTIC AND SYMBIOTIC FOODS

As sensory characteristics are on the basis of consumers' choice and acceptance, it is needed to evaluate the sensory impact of probiotics and prebiotics in food. Most of the studies regarding this issue reflect that little or no effect on sensory properties is reported when probiotic bacteria are less than 10% of the total microbial population [12]. As stated previously, an excess inoculation of *L. acidophilus* impairs yogurt sensory properties [21]. In the case of soy-based probiotic foods, fermentation with probiotics improves flavor due to the ability of probiotics to reduce pentanal and n-hexanal, which are responsible for the beany taste of soya [12]. There is a need to adapt the formulation and starter inoculation of fruit fortified probiotic fermented milks to ensure optimal textural and sensory scores [26].

Most studies related to sensory impact of the inclusion of probiotics in dairy foods have been successful: the inclusion of *L. acidophilus* in Minas cheese in co-culture with conventional starters [27]; inulin and oligofructose addition to ice-cream together with *L. acidophilus* La5 and *B. animalis* Bb12 increased apparent viscosity and overrun and developed the melting properties in ice-cream during storage [28]. Inulin yielded best results regarding rheological properties whereas oligofructose was needed to ensure counts of bifidobacteria over 6 log cfu/g. A symbiotic ice-cream containing 1% of resistant starch, encapsulated *L. casei* (Lc01) and *B. animalis* subsp. *lactis* (Bb12) ensured increased survival rate of probiotic bacteria in ice-cream over an extended shelf life [29]. The addition of encapsulated probiotics had no significant effect on the sensory properties of non-fermented ice-cream containing resistant starch as prebiotic.

Chocolate products have also been tested as probiotic carriers. Chocolate mousse is an excellent vehicle for the delivery of *L. paracasei*, and the prebiotic ingredient inulin did not interfere in its viability, or in the sensory acceptability of the mousse [30]. Lyophilized probiotics (*L. casei* and *L. paracasei*) added to dark chocolate masses with different sweeteners showed that sensory attributes of these chocolates were not different from that of traditional chocolates. Counts of probiotics were within 6–7 log cfu/g after 12 months of keeping at 4 and 18°C [31].

As an example of vegetable probiotics, calcium alginate immobilized *L. acidophilus* was used in a probiotic tomato juice to overcome the loss of viability of probiotic free cells, due to the acidic pH of the tomato [32]. Cell viability was enhanced and the sensory quality of the juice was improved.

4. FOOD FORMULATION EFFECTS ON PROBIOTIC SURVIVAL AND ACTIVITY

As fermented milks are the most common vehicle for probiotics, most of the literature regarding the effect of food formulation on probiotic survival is centered in dairy products. Regular yogurts are fortified in milk non-fat solids; if they contain fruits, they have additional carbohydrates in the form of sucrose, glucose and fructose. It is commercial practice that probiotic yogurts contain higher fat, non-fat solids and have a higher pH than regular yogurt [33]. There is no evidence that the sugar used to sweeten yogurt negates the health benefits associated with the probiotics contained in the yogurt [4]. Also, regarding dairy ingredients, total solids of milk and milk-whey mixture affected the viability of *L. delbrueckii* subsp. *bulgaricus* and *L. acidophilus* [34]. Fat content does not affect probiotic stability during storage [12]. Some ingredients may influence growth of the probiotic bacteria as salts, sweeteners, aroma compounds and preservatives.

4.1. Effects of Food Ingredients on Probiotic Survival

Carbohydrates: Prebiotics and Others

Many studies report results on the effect of the inclusion of prebiotics in food formula in the survival and growth of probiotics. The metabolic capacity to form acid from dietary sugars differed significantly between probiotic strains [35]. Regarding the addition of carbohydrates to fermented yogurts and milks, the effect of chain length of inulins (short (P95), medium (GR) and long (HP) chain lengths) on the characteristics of fat-free plain yogurt manufactured with *L. casei* has been studied [36]. Flavor scores and yogurt syneresis decreased with increased chain length, although body and texture improved.

Co-culture, together with prebiotics addition, has been demonstrated to be highly beneficial by several authors. Inulin (4%) has been used as a prebiotic to improve the quality and consistency of skim milk fermented by co-cultures and pure cultures of *L. acidophilus*, *Lactobacillus rhamnosus*, *L. bulgaricus* and *B. lactis* with *S. thermophilus* [37]. It was reported that inulin addition to the milk increased in co-cultures acidification rate, favored post-acidification, exerted a bifidogenic effect, and preserved almost intact cell viability during storage. In addition, *S. thermophilus* was shown to stimulate the metabolism of the other lactic bacteria. Contrary to co-cultures, most of the effects in pure cultures were not statistically significant. The simultaneous effects of different binary co-cultures of *L. acidophilus*, *L. bulgaricus*, *L. rhamnosus* and *B. lactis* with *S. thermophilus* and of different prebiotics (4% (w/w) malto-dextrin, oligofructose and polydextrose) on the production of fermented milk was studied [38]. Fermented milk quality was strongly influenced both by the co-culture composition and the selected prebiotic. Depending on the co-culture, prebiotic addition to milk influenced to different extent kinetic acidification parameters. Polydextrose addition led to the highest post-acidification. Probiotic counts were stimulated by oligofructose and polydextrose, and among these *B. lactis* always exhibited the highest counts in all supplemented milk samples. However, other studies [39] reported that oligofructose did not show any significant influence on fermentation time, acidity, syneresis and probiotics survival of fermented milks. The highest amounts of conjugated linoleic acid (CLA) (38% higher than in the control) were found in milk fermented by *S. thermophilus–L. acidophilus* co-culture and supplemented with maltodextrin [36]. The CLA formation in yogurt containing *L. acidophilus* or *B. animalis* and/or

2% fructo-oligosaccharide (FOS) and formulated with three commercial starter cultures has been studied [40]. The addition of FOS alone did not significantly affect CLA isomer formation in yogurts. Significant increases in CLA formation were obtained by using *L. acidophilus* or *B. animalis* in yogurt manufacture. The highest increases in c9t11-CLA isomer and total CLA content were found in yogurts manufactured with *L. acidophilus* and FOS and *B. animalis* and FOS.

The addition of prebiotics to cream cheeses has been successful. The addition of inulin, oligofructose and oligosaccharides from honey to probiotic petit-suisse containing (*B. animalis* subsp. *lactis* and *L. acidophilus*) yielded high probiotic counts for all formulations but best sensory scores for the combination of inulin and oligofructose [41]. Petit-suisse cheese formulations combining candidate prebiotics (inulin, oligofructose, honey) and probiotics (*L. acidophilus*, *B. animalis* subsp. *lactis*) have been evaluated [42]. Prebiotic effect was measured by comparing bacterial changes through determination of maximum growth rates of groups, rate of substrate assimilation and production of lactate and short-chain fatty acids. Highest prebiotic effects were obtained with addition of prebiotics to a probiotic cheese. Inulin has been successfully inoculated in a probiotic fresh cream cheese (*L. paracasei*) obtaining good sensory scores [43]. Sugar and aloe vera, sugar and chocolate, and sugar and jam have been tested on probiotic sweet whey cheeses [44]. All combinations yielded high survival rates. Additives enhanced the organoleptic features of whey cheeses, and produced different textural patterns.

Proteins

The effect of the addition of 1–2% of a protein-based fat replacer on the growth and metabolic activities of yogurt starters (*S. thermophilus* and *L. delbrueckii* ssp. *bulgaricus*) and probiotics (*L. casei*, *L. acidophilus*, and *Bifidobacterium longum*) has been tested [45]. The addition of the fat replacer resulted in a significantly improved growth of *S. thermophilus* and *B. longum* but inhibited that of *L. casei*, *L. acidophilus*, and *L. delbrueckii* ssp. *bulgaricus*.

Whey protein concentrate has also shown to increase probiotic survival in foods: The viability of yogurt starter cultures and *B. animalis* in reduced-fat yogurts supplemented with 1.5% fructo-oligosaccharide or whey protein concentrate has been studied [46]. Supplementation with 1.5% whey protein concentrate in reduced-fat yogurt increased the viable counts of *S. thermophilus*, *L. delbrueckii* subsp. *bulgaricus*, and *B. animalis* by 1 log cycle in the first week of storage when compared to control sample. Similar improvement in the growth of both yogurt bacteria and *B. animalis* was also obtained in the full-fat yogurt containing 3% milk fat and no supplement.

Yeast Extracts

Yeast extracts have been successful in increasing probiotic survival: *Lactobacillus reuteri* RC-14 and *L. rhamnosus* GR-1 survival was tested on low-fat yogurt (1% fat) enriched with: 0.33% yeast extract (T1); 0.4% inulin (T2); 0.33% yeast extract and 0.4% inulin (T3); and one with no additives (T4) [47]. *L. rhamnosus* GR-1 survived better than *L. reuteri* RC-14 and that survival was highest in media including 0.33% yeast extract (T1 and T3).

Addition of Fruit Products

Several fruit ingredients seem to enhance probiotic survival: the addition of either 5 or 10 g/100 g fruit preparations had no significant effect on the viability of the probiotic strains evaluated except on *L. acidophilus* LAFTI® L10 yogurt with 10 g/100 g passion fruit or mixed berry. All yogurts presented high counts of probiotics at the end of a 35-day shelf life [48]. The addition of citrus fiber to probiotic fermented milks stimulated the growth and survival of

L. casei and *L. acidophilus*, whereas bifidobacteria was unevenly affected. The co-culture with conventional starters favored the survival of probiotics [49]. A probiotic coconut flan, with high counts of probiotics (*B. animalis* subsp. *lactis*, *L. paracasei* and *B. lactis* + *L. paracasei*) and high sensory scores was successfully developed [50].

Soy Ingredients

Soy-based foods and soy ingredients are increasingly demanded by consumers due to their healthy image: they target pre- and postmenopausal women, milk allergies or intolerants. Such ingredients are often added to dairy foods or directly processed to obtain dairy imitation products. Many studies report interactions among soy components and probiotic bacteria. The addition of skim milk powder for the manufacture of fermented soy milk supplemented with probiotic bacteria (*L. acidophilus* 4461, *L. acidophilus* 4962, *L. casei* 290 and *L. casei* 2607) increased microbial counts of probiotics and enhanced the biotransformation level of isoflavone glycosides to isoflavone aglycones [51]. *L. acidophilus* 4461, *L. acidophilus* 4962, *L. casei* 290, and *L. casei* 2607 presented higher activities to hydrolyze isoflavone glycosides to biologically active forms—isoflavone aglycones—in soy milk when 0.5% (w/v) of lactulose was added [52]. Probiotic counts were also increased. The reverse option, the supplementation of skim milk with soy protein isolate together with six probiotic organisms (*L. acidophilus* 4461, *L. acidophilus* 4962, *L. casei* 290, *L. casei* 2607, *B. animalis* subsp. *lactis* Bb12, and *B. longum* 20099), enhanced lactose utilization acetic acid production but slightly reduced the lactic acid production and the growth of probiotic microorganisms [53]. The same effect was observed for *B. animalis* A and B (54). Three probiotics: *L. acidophilus* LAFTI® L10, *Bifidobacterium lactis* LAFTI® B94, and *L. casei* LAFTI® L26, were evaluated for the manufacture of fermented soy milk and production of β-glucosidase for hydrolysis of isoflavone to aglycones. It was observed that all of them produced β-glucosidase [55]. Fermenting calcium-fortified soy milk with *L. acidophilus* ATCC 4962, ATCC 33200, ATCC 4356, ATCC 4461, *L. casei* ASCC 290, *Lactobacillus plantarum* ASCC 276, and *Lactobacillus* fermentum VRI-003 can potentially enhance the calcium bioavailability of calcium-fortified soy milk due to increased calcium solubility and bioactive isoflavone aglycone enrichment [56]. Soy and cows' milk yogurts prepared including a yogurt starter in conjunction with either the probiotic bacteria *Lactobacillus johnsonii* NCC533 (La1), *L. rhamnosus* ATCC 53103 (GG) or human derived bifidobacteria have been studied [57]. The presence of the probiotic bacteria did not affect the growth of the yogurt strains. The probiotic bacteria and the bifidobacteria were using different sugars to support their growth, depending on whether the bacteria were growing in cows' milk or soy beverage.

Non-dairy Products

Several non-dairy products may be good carriers of probiotic bacteria such as fermented vegetable drinks, fermented sausages, cereal-based fermented drinks, as well as pharmaceutical preparation containing probiotic bacteria. Non-dairy probiotics are a growing field; there is a great demand especially from those who are allergic to milk. Some examples are given: carrot juice seems to be a good substrate for the growth and survival of *B. lactis* and *B. bifidum* [58]. *L. rhamnosus* was inoculated into an apple-pear-raspberry juice and the effect of storage conditions on probiotic viability evaluated [59]. Champagne and colleagues obtained high counts of probiotics in this juice and concluded that viability losses were higher at 7°C than at 4°C and that over a few weeks of refrigerated storage good viability of *L. rhamnosus* is expected even if the bottles have been opened and the cells exposed to oxygen. In a cereal-based fermented beverage, the presence of yeast enhanced the growth of probiotic lactic acid bacteria [60]. Other food grade

formulae may also include probiotics: fruit coatings have been successfully formulated to be carriers of probiotic bacteria [61] like edible coatings for apple and papaya cuts containing *B. animalis* ssp. *lactis* Bb12 based on alginate (2% w/v) or gellan (0.5%).

Cereal-based foods are a group of fermented foods of special interest regarding formulation. The effects of the addition of β-glucan from cereals (oat and barley) on growth and metabolic activity of *B. animalis* ssp. *lactis* (Bb12) compared to unsupplemented and inulin supplemented controls have been investigated [62]. Oat β-glucan addition resulted in improved probiotic viability and stability comparable to that of inulin. It also enhanced lactic and propionic acid production. The barley β-glucan addition suppressed proteolytic activity more than that from oat. These improvements were hindered by greater syneresis likely caused by thermodynamic incompatibility. The addition of β-glucan may be possible at or below 0.24 w/w% to avoid phase separation. Oat bran, whole and white oat flour have been tested as substrates for *L. plantarum* for the production of a probiotic beverage. The highest probiotic cell concentration was observed in white flour (9.16 log cfu/mL) and the lowest in the bran sample (8.17 log cfu/mL) [63].

Some fibers (oat flour, apple fiber, wheat dextrin, polydextrose and inulin), as carriers for probiotic bacteria *L. rhamnosus*, and the stability of probiotics during freeze drying and further use in apple juice and chocolate-coated breakfast cereals have been evaluated [64]. The best storage stability was obtained with wheat dextrin and polydextrose. In the probiotic apple juice, which is an acidic food, oat flour with 20% β-glucan had a protective effect on fresh *L. rhamnosus*—this effect was not observed for freeze-dried bacteria. In chocolate-coated cereals, a low water activity food, polydextrose and wheat dextrin provided the best probiotic protection, for 7 and 3 months, respectively. It is possible to use fibers to maintain the viability and stability of probiotics, although this function seems to be application dependent (pH, food composition, water activity, etc.).

4.2. Effects of Food Formulation on Probiotic Activity

Probiotic foods should meet international standards. They should contain appropriate microorganisms in shelf stable formulations that have been shown in well-designed clinical studies to confer defined health benefits on the consumer [65], so it is crucial to prove the effect of the ingredients in the activity of probiotics and prebiotics. Prebiotic compounds may also contribute to the immunomodulatory properties of probiotic bacteria: in a study using *L. rhamnosus* GG and *B. lactis* Bb12 plus 10 g of inulin enriched with oligofructose in colon cancer patients several colorectal cancer biomarkers were altered favorably by symbiotic intervention [66, 67]. Beneficial effects of probiotics, which fermentation of mannitol, fructo-oligosaccharide and inulin favored the production of formic, lactic and butyric acids, respectively, and correlated with cholesterol removal, have been reported [68–70]. The administration of certain prebiotics, together with the probiotics, seems to be important in modulating gut microbiota and abdominal organ health. Animal studies have shown that the administration of resistant starch (which escapes small intestinal digestion by microbes) in the form of high amylase corn starch decreased intestinal pH, increased short-chain fatty acid formation, and induced an apoptotic response to a genotoxic carcinogen [71].

However, several studies have reported no enhancement of the beneficial effect by administration of symbiotics [72, 73]. A symbiotic with *L. fermentum* and fructo-oligosaccharide was investigated to alleviate mucositis in rats. *L. fermentum* BR11 consumption reduced inflammation of the upper small intestine. However, its combination with FOS did not confer any further therapeutic benefit for the alleviation of mucositis [72]. The consumption of probiotic yogurt or resistant starch (as prebiotic) in combination with high soy intake had no effect on isoflavone bioavailability; probably the gut microflora were not modified in a manner that significantly affected isoflavone bioavailability or metabolism [73].

5. CONCLUSIONS AND FUTURE PROSPECTS

The consumption of designed healthy foods is included in the trend towards long-term prevention of illness. It is in this scenario where probiotic, prebiotic and symbiotic foods fit. Probiotics need to have clinically proven health benefits and be able to withstand large-scale cultivation, concentration, incorporation and food manufacturing and storage. Prebiotics, as well as probiotics doses and types, need to be established to ensure that health benefits are accomplished, so reliable clinical data is needed to determine if the probiotic counts and prebiotic dose used are sufficient for health benefits. The influence of the carrier must be examined bearing in mind the main constraints for the survival of probiotics: low oxygen tolerance and low acidity tolerance, and the convenience of the inclusion of prebiotics or growth-promoting factors in the formulation of probiotic foods.

Future development in genomics should provide details on the physiological performance of health-promoting strains in a variety of environments that may lead to novel solutions for current and future challenges on probiotic foods development. A potential major problem of probiotics is the misuse of the term, as the term 'probiotic' should be only applied to strains fulfilling the outlines as given in the guidelines of the World Health Organization [74].

References

1. Saxelin, M. (2008). Probiotic formulations and applications, the current probiotics market, and changes in the marketplace: A European perspective. *Clinical Infectious Diseases, 46*, 76–79.

2. Pennachia, C., Vaughan, E. E., & Villani, F. (2006). Potential probiotic *Lactobacillus* strains from fermented sausages: Futher investigations on their probiotic properties. *Meat Science, 73*, 90–101.

3. Sendra, E. (2008). Application of prebiotics and probiotics in meat products. In J. Fernández-López (Ed.), *Technological strategies for functional meat products development* (pp. 117–137). Kerala, India: Transworld Research Network.

4. Douglas, L. C., & Sanders, M. E. (2008). Probiotics and prebiotics in dietetics practice. *Journal of the American Dietetic Association, 108*(3), 510–521.

5. Ross, R. P., Desmond, C., Fitzerald, G. F., & Stanton, C. (2005). A review: Overcoming the technological hurdles in the development of probiotic foods. *Journal of Applied Microbiology, 98*, 1410–1417.

6. Huebner, J., Wehling, R. L., & Hutkins, R. W. (2007). Functional activity of commercial prebiotics. *International Dairy Journal, 17*, 770–775.

7. Kelly, G. (2008). Inulin-type prebiotics—A review: Part 1. *Alternative Medicine Review, 13*(4), 315–329.

8. Ananta, E., Birkeland, S. E., Corcoran, B., et al. (2004). Processing effects on the nutritional advancement of probiotics and prebiotics. *Microbial Ecology in Health and Disease, 16*(2), 113–124.

9. International Scientific Association for Probiotics and Prebiotics (www.isapp.net). Prebiotics: A consumer guide for making smart choices (downloaded January 2009).

10. Stanton, C., Desmond, C., Coakley, M., et al. (2003). Challenges facing development of probiotic containing functional foods. In E. R. Franworth (Ed.), *Handbook of fermented functional foods* (pp. 27–58). Boca Raton, USA: CRC Press.

11. Mattila-Sandholm, T., Myllärinen, P., Critteden, R., et al. (2002). Technological challenges for future probiotic foods. *International Dairy Journal, 12*, 173–182.

12. Champagne, C. P., & Gardner, N. (2005). Challenges in the addition of probiotic cultures to foods. *Critical Reviews in Food Science and Nutrition, 45*, 61–84.

13. Ding, W. K., & Shah, N. P. (2007). Acid, bile and heat tolerance of free and microencapsulated probiotic bacteria. *Journal of Food Science, 72*(9), 446–450.

14. Lourens-Hatting, A., & Viljoen, B. C. (2001). Yogurt as probiotic carrier food. *International Dairy Journal, 11*, 1–17.

15. Mori, H., Sato, Y., Takemoto, N., et al. (1997). Isolation and structural identification of bifidogenic growth stimulator produced by *Propionibacterium freudenreichii*. *Journal of Dairy Science, 80*, 1959–1964.

16. da Cruz, A. G., Faria, J. D. A. F., & Van Dender, A. G. F. (2007). Packaging system and probiotic dairy foods. *Food Research International, 40*(8), 951–956.

17. Donkor, O. N., Henriksson, A., Vasiljevic, T., & Shah, N. P. (2006). Effect of acidification on the activity of probiotics on yogurt during cold storage. *International Dairy Journal, 16*, 1181–1189.

18. Sharp, M. D., McMahon, D. J., & Broadbent, J. R. (2008). Comparative evaluation of yogurt and low-fat cheddar cheese as delivery media for probiotic *Lactobacillus casei*. *Journal of Food Science, 73*(7), 375–377.

19. Hull, R. R., Roberts, A. V., & Mayes, J. J. (1984). Survival of *Lactobacillus acidophilus* in yoghurt. *The Australian Journal of Dairy Technology, 39*(4), 164–166.

20. Galtz, B. A. (1992). The classical propionibacteria: their past, present and future as industrial organisms. *ASM News, 58*(4), 197–201.

21. Olson, D. W., & Aryana, K. J. (2008). An excessively high *Lactobacillus acidophilus* inoculation level in yogurt lowers product quality during storage. *LWT— Food Science and Technology, 41*(5), 911–918.

22. Burns, P., Patrignani, F., Serrazanetti, D., et al. (2008). Probiotic crescenza cheese containing *Lactobacillus casei* and *Lactobacillus acidophilus* manufactured with high-pressure homogenized milk. *Journal of Dairy Science, 91*(2), 500–512.

23. Mortazavian, A. M., Ehsani, M. R., Mousavi, S. M., et al. (2007). Effect of refrigerated storage temperature on the viability of probiotic micro-organisms in yogurt. *International Journal of Dairy Technology, 60*(2), 123–127.

24. Magariños, H., Selaive, S., Costa, M., et al. (2007). Viability of probiotic micro-organisms (*Lactobacillus acidophilus* La-5 and *Bifidobacterium animalis* subsp. *lactis* Bb-12) in ice cream. *International Journal of Dairy Technology, 60*(2), 128–134.

25. Huebner, J., Wehling, R. L., Parkhurst, A., & Hutkins, R. W. (2008). Effect of processing conditions on the prebiotic activity of commercial prebiotics. *International Dairy Journal, 18*, 287–293.

26. Kaur, H., Mishra, H. N., & Kumar, P. (2009). Textural properties of mango soy fortified probiotic yoghurt: Optimisation of inoculum level of yoghurt and probiotic culture. *International Journal of Food Science and Technology, 44*(2), 415–424.

27. Souza, C. H. B., & Saad, S. M. I. (2009). Viability of *Lactobacillus acidophilus* La-5 added solely or in co-culture with a yoghurt starter culture and implications on physico-chemical and related properties of Minas fresh cheese during storage. *LWT—Food Science and Technology, 42*(2), 633–640.

28. Akalin, A. S., & Erişir, D. (2008). Effects of inulin and oligofructose on the rheological characteristics and probiotic culture survival in low-fat probiotic ice cream. *Journal of Food Science, 73*(4), 184–188.

29. Homayouni, A., Azizi, A., Ehsani, M. R., et al. (2008). Effect of microencapsulation and resistant starch on the probiotic survival and sensory properties of synbiotic ice cream. *Food Chemistry*, 111(1), 50–55.

30. Aragon-Alegro, L. C., Alarcon Alegro, J. H., Roberta Cardarelli, H., et al. (2007). Potentially probiotic and synbiotic chocolate mousse. *LWT—Food Science and Technology*, 40(4), 669–675.

31. Nebesny, E., Zyzelewicz, D., Motyl, I., & Libudzisz, Z. (2007). Dark chocolates supplemented with *Lactobacillus* strains. *European Food Research and Technology*, 225(1), 33–42.

32. King, V. A.-E., Huang, H.-Y., & Tsen, J.-H. (2007). Fermentation of tomato juice by cell immobilized *Lactobacillus acidophilus*. *Mid-Taiwan Journal of Medicine*, 12(1), 1–7.

33. Hussain, I., Attiq-ur-Rahman., & Atkinson, N. (2009). Quality comparison of probiotic and natural yogurt. *Pakistan Journal of Nutrition*, 8(1), 9–12.

34. Almeida, K. E., Tamime, A. Y., & Oliveira, M. N. (2009). Influence of total solids contents of milk whey on the acidifying profile and viability of various lactic acid bacteria. *LWT—Food Science and Technology*, 42(2), 672–678.

35. Hedberg, M., Hasslöf, P., Sjöström, I., et al. (2008). Sugar fermentation in probiotic bacteria – An *in vitro* study. *Oral Microbiology and Immunology*, 23(6), 482–485.

36. Aryana, K. J., & McGrew, P. (2007). Quality attributes of yogurt with *Lactobacillus casei* and various prebiotics. *LWT—Food Science and Technology*, 40(10), 1808–1814.

37. de Souza Oliveira, R. P., Perego, P., Converti, A., & De Oliveira, M. N. (2009). Growth and acidification performance of probiotics in pure culture and co-culture with *Streptococcus thermophilus*: The effect of inulin. *LWT—Food Science and Technology*, Article in Press, February 2009.

38. Oliveira, R. P. S., Florence, A. C. R., Silva, R. C., et al. (2009). Effect of different prebiotics on the fermentation kinetics, probiotic survival and fatty acids profiles in nonfat symbiotic fermented milk. 2009. *International Journal of Food Microbiology*, 128(3), 467–472.

39. de Castro, F. P., Cunha, T. M., Ogliari, P. J., et al. (2009). Influence of different content of cheese whey and oligofructose on the properties of fermented lactic beverages: Study using response surface methodology. *LWT—Food Science and Technology*, 42, 993–997.

40. Akalin, A. S., Toku oglu, O., Gönç, S., & Aycan, S. (2007). Occurrence of conjugated linoleic acid in probiotic yoghurts supplemented with fructo-oligosaccharide. *International Dairy Journal*, 17(9), 1089–1095.

41. Cardarelli, H. R., Buriti, F. C. A., Castro, I. A., & Saad, S. M. I. (2008). Inulin and oligofructose improve sensory quality and increase the probiotic viable count in potentially synbiotic petit-suisse cheese. *LWT—Food Science and Technology*, 41(6), 1037–1046.

42. Cardarelli, H. R., Saad, S. M. I., Gibson, G. R., & Vulevic, J. (2007). Functional petit-suisse cheese: Measure of the prebiotic effect. *Anaerobe*, 13(5–6), 200–207.

43. Buriti, F. C. A., Cardarelli, H. R., & Saad, S. M. I. (2008). Influence of *Lactobacillus paracasei* and inulin on instrumental texture and sensory evaluation of fresh cream cheese. *Revista Brasileira de Ciencias Farmaceuticas/ Brazilian Journal of Pharmaceutical Sciences*, 44(1), 75–84.

44. Madureira, A. R., Soares, J. C., Pintado, M. E., et al. (2008). Sweet whey cheese matrices inoculated with the probiotic strain *Lactobacillus paracasei* LAFTI® L26. *Dairy Science and Technology*, 88(6), 649–665.

45. Ramchandran, L., & Shah, N. P. (2008). Effect of Versagel® on the growth and metabolic activities of selected lactic acid bacteria. *Journal of Food Science*, 73(1), 21–26.

46. Akalin, A. S., Gönç, S., Ünal, G., & Fenderya, S. (2007). Effects of fructo-oligosaccharide and whey protein concentrate on the viability of starter culture in reduced-fat probiotic yogurt during storage. *Journal of Food Science*, 72(7), 222–227.

47. Hekmat, S., Soltani, H., & Reid, G. (2009). Growth and survival of *Lactobacillus reuteri* RC-14 and *Lactobacillus rhamnosus* GR-1 in yogurt for use as a functional food. *Innovative Food Science and Emerging Technologies*. Article in Press, February 2009.

48. Kailasapathy, K., Harmstorf, I., & Phillips, M. (2008). Survival of *Lactobacillus acidophilus* and *Bifidobacterium animalis* ssp. *lactis* in stirred fruit yogurts. *LWT—Food Science and Technology*, 41(7), 1317–1322.

49. Sendra, E., Fayos, P., Lario, Y., et al. (2008). Incorporation of citrus fibers in fermented milk containing probiotic bacteria. *Food Microbiology*, 25(1), 13–21.

50. Corrêa, S. B. M., Castro, I. A., & Saad, S. M. I. (2008). Probiotic potential and sensory properties of coconut flan supplemented with *Lactobacillus paracasei* and *Bifidobacterium lactis*. *International Journal of Food Science and Technology*, 43(9), 1560–1568.

51. Pham, T. T., & Shah, N. P. (2008). Skim milk powder supplementation affects lactose utilization, microbial survival and biotransformation of isoflavone glycosides to isoflavone aglycones in soymilk by Lactobacillus. *Food Microbiology*, 25(5), 653–661.

52. Pham, T. T., & Shah, N. P. (2008). Effect of lactulose on biotransformation of isoflavone glycosides to aglycones in soymilk by lactobacilli. *Journal of Food Science*, 73(3), 158–165.

53. Pham, T. T., & Shah, N. P. (2008). Fermentation of reconstituted skim milk supplemented with soy protein isolate by probiotic organisms. *Journal of Food Science*, 73(2), 62–66.

54. Pham, T. T., & Shah, N. P. (2007). Biotransformation of isoflavone glycosides by *Bifidobacterium animalis* in

soymilk supplemented with skim milk powder. *Journal of Food Science, 72*(8), 316–324.

55. Donkor, O. N., & Shah, N. P. (2008). Production of β-glucosidase and hydrolysis of isoflavone phytoestrogens by *Lactobacillus acidophilus, Bifidobacterium lactis,* and *Lactobacillus casei* in soymilk. *Journal of Food Science, 73*(1), 15–20.

56. Tang, A. L., Shah, N. P., Wilcox, G., et al. (2007). Fermentation of calcium-fortified soymilk with Lactobacillus: Effects on calcium solubility, isoflavone conversion, and production of organic acids. *Journal of Food Science, 72*(9), 431–436.

57. Farnworth, E. R., Mainville, I., Desjardins, M.-P., et al. (2007). Growth of probiotic bacteria and bifidobacteria in a soy yogurt formulation. *International Journal of Food Microbiology, 116*(1), 174–181.

58. Kun, S., Rezessy-Szabó, J. M., Nguyen, Q. D., & Hoschke, A. (2008). Changes of microbial population and some components in carrot juice during fermentation with selected Bifidobacterium strains. *Process Biochemistry, 43*(8), 816–821.

59. Champagne, C. P., Raymond, Y., & Gagnon, R. (2008). Viability of *Lactobacillus rhamnosus* R0011 in an apple-based fruit juice under simulated storage conditions at the consumer level. *Journal of Food Science, 73*(5), 221–226.

60. Kedia, G., Wang, R., Patel, H., & Pandiella, S. S. (2007). Use of mixed cultures for the fermentation of cereal-based substrates with potential probiotic properties. *Process Biochemistry, 42*(1), 65–70.

61. Tapia, M. S., Rojas-Graü, M. A., Rodríguez, F. J., et al. (2007). Alginate- and gellan-based edible films for probiotic coatings on fresh-cut fruits. *Journal of Food Science, 72*(4), 190–196.

62. Vasiljevic, T., Kealy, T., & Mishra, V. K. (2007). Effects of β-glucan addition to a probiotic containing yogurt. *Journal of Food Science, 72*(7), 405–411.

63. Kedia, G., Vázquez, J. A., & Pandiella, S. S. (2008). Fermentability of whole oat flour, PeriTec flour and bran by *Lactobacillus plantarum. Journal of Food Engineering, 89*(2), 246–249.

64. Saarela, M., Virkajärvi, I., Nohynek, L., et al. (2006). Fibers as carriers for *Lactobacillus rhamnosus* during freeze-drying and storage in apple juice and chocolate-coated breakfast cereals. *International Journal of Food Microbiology, 112*, 171–178.

65. Reid, G. (2008). Probiotics and prebiotics: Progress and challenges. *International Dairy Journal, 11*, 969–975.

66. Roller, M., Clune, Y., Collins, K., et al. (2007). Consumption of prebiotic inulin enriched with oligofructose in combination with the probiotics *Lactobacillus rhamnosus* and *Bifidobacterium lactis* has minor effects on selected immune parameters in polypectomised and colon cancer patients. *British Journal of Nutrition, 97*(4), 676–684.

67. Rafter, J., Bennett, M., Caderni, G., et al. (2007). Dietary synbiotics reduce cancer risk factors in polypectomized and colon cancer patients. *American Journal of Clinical Nutrition, 85*(2), 488–496.

68. Liong, M. T., & Shah, N. P. (2005a). Production of organic acids from fermentation of mannitol, fructo-oligosaccharide and inulin by a cholesterol removing *Lactobacillus acidophilus* strain. *Journal of Applied Microbiology, 99*(4), 783–793.

69. Liong, M. T., & Shah, N. P. (2005b). Optimization of cholesterol removal, growth and fermentation patterns of *Lactobacillus acidophilus* ATCC 4962 in the presence of mannitol, fructo-oligosaccharide and inulin: A response surface methodology approach. *Journal of Applied Microbiology, 98*(5), 1115–1126.

70. Liong, M. T., & Shah, N. P. (2005c). Optimization of cholesterol removal by probiotics in the presence of prebiotics by using a response surface method. *Applied and Environmental Microbiology, 71*(4), 1745–1753.

71. Le Leu, R. K., Brown, I. L., Hu, Y., & Young, G. P. (2003). Effect of resistant starch on genotoxin-induced apoptosis, colonic epithelium, and lumenal contents in rats. *Carcinogenesis, 24*(8), 1347–1352.

72. Smith, C. L., Geier, M. S., Yazbeck, R., et al. (2008). *Lactobacillus fermentum* BR11 and fructo-oligosaccharide partially reduce jejunal inflammation in a model of intestinal mucositis in rats. *Nutrition and Cancer, 60*(6), 757–767.

73. Larkin, T. A., Price, W. E., & Astheimer, L. B. (2007). Increased probiotic yogurt or resistant starch intake does not affect isoflavone bioavailability in subjects consuming a high soy diet. *Nutrition, 23*(10), 709–718.

74. FAO/WHO. (2002). Guidelines for the evaluation of probiotics in food. ftp://ftp.fao.org/es/esn/food/wgreport2.pdf.

23

Probiotics in Adhesion of Pathogens: Mechanisms of Action

Maria Carmen Collado[1,2], Miguel Gueimonde[2,3], and Seppo Salminen[2]

[1]Instituto de Agroquímica y Tecnología de los Alimentos (IATA-CSIC), Valencia, Spain
[2]Functional Food Forum, University of Turku, Turku, Finland
[3]Instituto de Productos Lácteos de Asturias (IPLA-CSIC), Asturias, Spain

1. PROBIOTICS: CONCEPT AND SELECTION CRITERIA

The human intestinal microbiota constitutes a complex microbial ecosystem that plays an important role in health and disease. This microbiota may be divided in commensals, symbiotic and pathogenic microorganisms. A correct individual balance of the microbiota plays a critical role in the maintenance of the health status of the host. The presence of bacterial pathogens may alter the intestinal bacterial homeostasis (microbiota composition and activity) leading to either an increased risk of disease or specific diseases. Ingested microorganisms may also be present. These exhibit specific beneficial properties through, for instance, microbiota modulation, the so-called probiotics. The protective role of probiotic bacteria against gastrointestinal pathogens and the underlying mechanisms

have received special attention. Pathogen inhibition by lactic acid bacteria might provide significant protection either as a natural barrier against exposure in the gastrointestinal tract, or as a method for the preservation or decontamination of drinking water or food. This would enhance human health and have a positive economic impact, especially in developing countries where people suffer from frequent gastrointestinal infections.

A probiotic has been defined as a 'live microorganism which, when administered in adequate amounts, confers a health benefit on the host' [1]. Specific strains of *Lactobacillus*, *Enterococcus*, *Bifidobacterium* and some *Propionibacterium* strains, among others, have been introduced as probiotics in food products due to their health-promoting effects. Often the criteria for the selection of probiotics include the tolerance to gastrointestinal conditions (gastric acid and bile), ability to adhere to the gastrointestinal mucosa, and competitive exclusion of pathogens [2, 3]. Traditionally, it has been proposed that a probiotic must fulfill the following criteria:

- Have a demonstrated beneficial effect on the host.
- Be non-pathogenic, non-toxic, and free of significant adverse side effects.
- Be able to survive through the gastrointestinal tract (*in vitro* and *in vivo*).
- Be present in the product in an adequate number of viable cells to confer the health benefit.
- Be compatible with product matrix, processing and storage conditions to maintain desired properties; and labeled accurately.

The demonstrated beneficial health effects of probiotic consumption consist of the regulation of microbiota, and stimulation and development of the intestinal barrier effect including the immune system; beneficial impact on the bioavailability of nutrients; a reduction or alleviation of symptoms of lactose intolerance; and reduction in the risk of specific microbiota-associated diseases, such as acute gastroenteritis caused by viruses or bacteria, especially in infants and children. At present, the specific live microbial food ingredients and their effects on human health are studied both within food matrices and as single or mixed culture preparations [4, 5].

Several studies and clinical applications of probiotics have been related to the regulation of parameters associated with gastrointestinal infections caused by pathogenic microorganisms. Alternative therapies to replace antibiotics based on enhancing the barrier or replacement of pathogens are considered as important due to the rapid emergence of antibiotic-resistant pathogenic strains and the adverse consequences of antibiotic therapy on the protective healthy intestinal microbiota [6]. Specific probiotics have been demonstrated to exert protective effects against different diseases caused by pathogenic bacteria [7–10]. The mechanisms by which probiotics exert their effects are largely unknown, but they are very likely to be multifactorial. Specific important mechanisms underlying these antagonistic effects include the reduction of luminal pH, competition for adhesion sites and nutritional sources, secretion of antimicrobial substances, toxin inactivation, and immune stimulation [11, 12].

2. INTESTINAL MUCOSA AND MUCUS PRODUCTION

The intestinal mucosa forms a barrier between the external and internal environment of the human body. The intestinal tract is covered by a mucus membrane. The mucosa has a large area (around 300 m^2) due to its unique structure [13], which consists of polarized epithelial cells that form a single layer of columnar cells named enterocytes. Scattered between these cells are specialized enterocytes, goblet cells, which synthesize and excrete mucus. Mucus is a gel layer covering the epithelial lining. The main function of mucus is to protect the epithelium from chemical, enzymatic, physical processes as gastric juices, digestive enzymes among others.

Mucin glycoproteins (mucins) are major macromolecular constituents of epithelial mucus and have long been implicated in health and disease. The interactions between mucus and bacteria present in the intestinal tract are important for the gut health. Commensal bacteria specifically adhere to the complex carbohydrates present in the mucus and these bacteria may prevent the adhesion of relevant pathogen strains. The production of mucus is a constant process as it is lost in feces and by bacterial degradation [14]. The mucus gel consists mainly of water (up to 95%) while the main organic components are mucus glycoproteins (mucins; up to 5%), which dictate the viscoelastic characteristics of mucus [15]. Additionally, lipids, free proteins, immunoglobulins and salts are present in the mucus gel [14]. Mucins are macromolecules with a peptide core linked to oligosaccharide chains through O-glycosidic bonds [16]. There are two types of mucins, membrane-associated and secreted. Different oligosaccharides are found in mucins including N-acetyl or N-glycolyl neuramine acids, fucose, galactose, N-acetyl glucosamine and N-acetyl galactosamine. Depending on the composition of oligosaccharides, two subtypes of mucins are described: neutral and acidic. Mucins can be classified into acidic subtypes if the chains are terminated with sulfate or sialic acid groups [17]. If these groups, sulfate or sialic acid groups are not present, mucins are classified as neutral subtypes [18]. Neutral mucins appear to be the predominant subtype expressed in the gastric mucosa, whereas acidic mucins are expressed in the intestinal tract— mainly in the large intestinal epithelium.

Mucin is also one of the most important substrates for bacterial fermentation leading to the production of fermentation products such as short-chain fatty acids (SCFAs), mainly butyrate, acetate and propionate [18]. The main role of butyrate is to fuel enterocytes, covering up to 70% of their energy needs and contributing to epithelial cell growth regulation and differentiation [19]. In addition, intestinal bacteria degrade mucin differently which, together with the differential expression of mucin genes in different gut areas, makes the mucus composition variable along the intestinal tract [20]. It is also important to assess the role of specific potentially mucus utilizing bacteria such as *Akkermansia muciniphila*, on the role of barrier effect and pathogen adhesion [21, 22].

Twenty-one different mucin genes have been identified, cloned and partially sequenced in humans [23, 24], and the majority of their homologues have been identified in mice and rats. The mucins are sub-divided into secretory and membrane-associated forms, depending on their structure and location. Secreted mucins contribute to the formation of the mucus gel but the function of membrane-associated mucins is not well characterized, despite the fact that they are located on the surface of epithelial cells

throughout the body [24]. A summary of the mucins, their tissue distribution and expression is listed in Table 23.1. Mucin is secreted by specialized cells, goblet cells, and the process is multifaceted, being regulated by a number of different factors that have been divided into two mechanisms: baseline secretion and compound exocytosis. Baseline secretion involves the constitutive release of newly produced mucin granules that move along the periphery of the apical granule mass [25].

3. MECHANISMS OF ACTION OF PROBIOTICS

The current knowledge on probiotic mechanisms of action is scarce. Mechanisms are likely to be multifactorial processes. Probiotics have specific targets and different bacterial strains are not similar with respect to their health effects. Varying levels of host–microbe interaction can be distinguished:

- Microbe–epithelium interface, including adhesion to mucosal and epithelial cells, stimulation of mucus secretion, production of defensive molecules resulting in reinforcing gut barrier function.
- Microbe–immune system interaction comprising of immune-modulation and regulation of immune responses beyond the gut.
- Microbe–microbe interaction including the exclusion and inhibition of pathogens by prevention of adhesion, inhibition of replication of pathogens mediated through secretion of antimicrobial substances, competition for nutrients necessary for pathogen survival and anti-toxin effects.

Advances on the knowledge of these mechanisms of action, the microbe–microbe interaction, are detailed in Figure 23.1.

TABLE 23.1   Characteristics of different mucin genes

MUC gene	Species	Nature	TR/cysteine	Tissue expression
MUC1	Human; rat; mouse	Membrane-associated	TR	Lung, salivary glands, esophagus, stomach, pancreas, large intestine, breast, prostate, ovary, kidney, uterus, cervix
MUC2	Human; rat; mouse	Secreted	Cysteine rich	Lung, conjunctiva, ear, stomach, small intestine, colon, nasopharyngeal tract, prostate
MUC3A	Human; rat; mouse	Membrane-associated	TR	Thymus, small intestine, colon, kidney
MUC3B	Human; rat; mouse	Membrane-associated	TR	Small intestine, colon
MUC4	Human; rat; mouse	Membrane-associated	TR	Lung, cornea, salivary glands, esophagus, small intestine, kidney
MUC5AC	Human; rat; mouse	Secreted	Cysteine rich	Lung, conjunctiva, middle ear, stomach, gall bladder, nasopharyngeal tract mucosa
MUC5B	Human; rat; mouse	Secreted	Cysteine rich	Lung, middle ear, sublingual gland, larynx, submucosal glands, esophageal glands, stomach, duodenum
MUC6	Human; rat; mouse	Secreted	Cysteine rich	Stomach, duodenum, pancreas, kidney
MUC7	Human; rat; mouse	Secreted	Cysteine poor	Lung, lachrymal glands, salivary glands, nose
MUC8	Human; rat; mouse	Secreted	Cysteine poor	Oviduct
MUC9	Human; rat; mouse	Secreted	Cysteine poor	Submandibular glands
MUC10	Rat; mouse	Membrane-associated	TR	Submandibular glands, testis
MUC11	Human; rat; mouse	Membrane-associated	TR	Lung, middle ear, thymus, small intestine, pancreas, colon, liver, kidney, uterus, prostate
MUC12	Human; rat; mouse	Membrane-associated	TR	Middle ear, pancreas, colon, uterus, prostate
MUC13	Human; rat; mouse	Membrane-associated	TR	Lung, conjunctiva, stomach, small intestine, colon, kidney
MUC14	Human; rat; mouse	Membrane-associated	TR	Ovary
MUC15	Human; rat; mouse	Membrane-associated	TR	Conjunctiva, thymus, lymph node, breast, small intestine, colon, liver, spleen, prostate, ovary, leukocytes, bone marrow
MUC16	Human; rat; mouse	Membrane-associated	TR	Conjunctiva, ovary
MUC17	Human; rat; mouse	Membrane-associated	TR	Intestinal cells, conjunctival epithelium
MUC18	Human; rat; mouse	Membrane-associated	None	Prostate

(Continued)

TABLE 23.1 (Continued)

MUC gene	Species	Nature	TR/cysteine	Tissue expression
MUC19	Human; rat; mouse	Secreted	Cysteine rich	Lung, salivary gland, kidney, liver, colon, placenta, prostate
MUC20	Human; rat; mouse	Membrane-associated	TR	Lung, liver, kidney, colon, placenta, prostate
MUC21	Human; mouse	Membrane-associated	TR	Lung, large intestine, thymus, testis

TR = tandem repeat.
Adapted from Dharmani, P., Srivastava, V., Kissoon-Singh, V. 5 & Chadee, K. (2009). Role of intestinal mucins in innate host defense mechanisms against pathogens. *J Innate Immun 1*, 123–135.

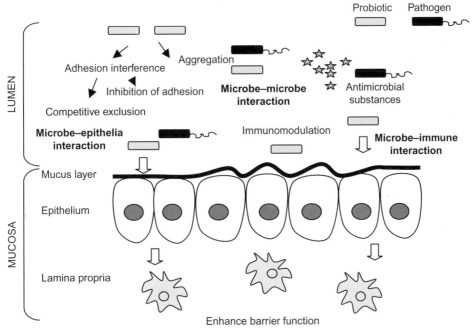

FIGURE 23.1 Mechanisms of probiotics against pathogen infection. 1. antimicrobial substances against pathogens. 2. Immunomodulation. 3. Improvement of barrier function. 4. adhesion: competitive inhibition with pathogenic bacteria, inhibition and displacement of pathogen's adhesion. 5. aggregation and coaggregation with pathogens.

3.1. Antimicrobial Substances

The antimicrobial metabolites produced by lactic acid bacteria can be divided into two groups: 1) low molecular mass compounds (<1.000 Da) such as organic acids, which have a broad spectrum of action; and 2) antimicrobial proteins, termed bacteriocins (>1.000 Da), which have a relatively narrow specificity of action against closely related organisms and other Gram-positive bacteria [26, 27].

The organic acids secreted in the fermentative metabolism of carbohydrates by probiotics have been considered to be the main antimicrobial compounds responsible for their inhibitory activity against pathogens [28, 29]. The antimicrobial activity of organic acids is due to the reduction of pH and to the presence of undissociated forms of acids. In addition, some probiotics are able to generate hydrogen peroxide in the presence of oxygen. The bactericidal effect of hydrogen peroxide is due to its oxidizing effect on bacterial cell surface. Carbon dioxide is produced by heterofermentative bacteria, and its antimicrobial activity is due to the inhibition of enzymatic decarboxylation and its accumulation in the membrane causing dysfunction in the permeability of the membrane. Carbon dioxide can inhibit the growth of many food spoilage microorganisms, especially Gram-negative psychrotrophic bacteria [30].

Bacteriocins are proteins or protein complexes that show bactericidal activity against bacterial species, which are closely related to the producer species. Bacteriocins produced by Gram-positive bacteria, usually lactic acid bacteria, inhibit strains of the same or closely related species. Bacteriocins have been subdivided into four classes: class I, the lantibiotics, comprises small (<5 kDa) heat-stable peptides that contain post-translationally modified amino acids; class II, the non-antibiotic peptides, comprises small (<10 kDa) heat-stable proteins; class III comprises large (>30 kDa) heat-labile proteins; and class IV comprises an undefined mixture of proteins, lipids, and carbohydrates [31]. In addition, the term bacteriocin-like compound has been coined to refer to antagonistic substances that are incompletely defined or do not fit the typical criteria defining bacteriocins and tend to have a broader spectrum of activity [32]. Most of the studies related to the characterization of bacteriocins or bacteriocin-like compounds from lactic acid bacteria and probiotics have been focused on species of the genera *Lactobacillus*, *Lactococcus*, *Pediococcus* and *Enterococcus*, because of the diversity of their species and their potential applications as natural preservatives in foods [27, 33]. Some

bacteriocin-like compounds have also been described for the *Bifidobacterium* species [34–36] and a unique bacteriocin, bifidocin B, from *Bifidobacterium bifidum* NCFB 1454 has been purified [37, 38]. Probiotics have exhibited antagonistic effects against different pathogenic species including *Salmonella*, *Listeria*, *Helicobacter* among others [34–36, 39, 40]. Due to the potential interest of these antimicrobial proteins in novel therapeutic developments, further studies should be carried out on their genetics, biochemistry and mechanisms of action.

3.2. Adhesion to Intestinal Mucosa

Adhesion to the intestinal mucosa is regarded as a prerequisite for colonization and is an important characteristic relating to the ability of strains to interact with the host [15, 41, 42]. Thus, adhesion has been one of the main selection criteria for new probiotic strains [43, 44]. This property is important for colonization [15, 45] and it has been related to certain beneficial effects of probiotics [46]. Adhesion is also important for the modulation of the immune system [42, 47, 48] and antagonism against pathogens [49, 50]. Using two isogenic strains of *L. crispatus*—one with aggregation phenotype and showing a high adhesion and the other non-aggregative—it was shown that this aggregation phenotype favors intestinal colonization and modulates the expression of immune receptors in the mucosa [51].

Intestinal mucus has a dual role: it protects the mucosa from certain microorganisms, while providing an initial binding site, nutrient source, and matrix on which bacteria can proliferate. Further, adherence of bacteria to intestinal epithelium is required for both temporary colonization of the gut and adherence or penetration is a prerequisite for infection by many pathogens [52]. Mucosal colonization with non-pathogenic resident microbiota is of particular importance for the protection of the host against pathogenic strains by competitive exclusion.

Non-specific Versus Specific Adhesion Mechanisms

The mechanisms of adhesion are complex and may involve non-specific and specific interactions between microorganisms and mucosal surfaces. Non-specific adhesion of bacteria is based on van der Waals and electrostatic forces between the cell and the mucosal surface, explained by the DLVO theory (Derjaguin, Landau, Verwey and Overbeek). The DLVO theory originally described the attachment of inert particles to a solid substratum but has also been applied to bacteria [53]. This theory postulates that the interaction between surfaces is given by the attracting van der Waals forces and the electrostatic repulsion. Although bacteria are negatively charged, they are still attracted to negatively charged host tissue because the attracting van der Waals forces are stronger than the electrostatic repulsion. However, it appears that the interactions between bacteria and host epithelium are too complicated to be explained only by the DLVO theory [54]. An additional explanation is based on the hydrophobic molecules on the bacterial surface, which counteract the repulsive electrostatic forces, allowing bacteria to draw near the negatively charged mucosal. This type of adhesion is considered to be weak and reversible [55, 56]. Non-specific interaction between bacteria and substratum may also be due to hydrophobic interactions or hydrogen bonding [57].

Specific adhesion has been described as a 'lock and key' interaction between bacteria and the host mucosa and is mediated by adhesins and their receptors in the epithelium [57, 58]. The matching connection between receptor and adhesin allows numerous bonds between the bacterium and host cells. In this way, the interaction is much stronger when compared to non-specific adhesion, as it is unlikely that all the adhesive bonds rupture simultaneously. Adhesion can be inhibited by altering the structure of adhesins or receptors with enzymes or other chemical compounds; or with antibodies mimicking the adhesins or their receptors [41].

Adherence of specific *Lactobacillus* strains to the human intestinal HT29 cell line induces up-regulation of mucin gene expression, and correlates with increased extracellular secretion of mucin MUC3 [59]. These *Lactobacillus* strains inhibited the adherence of enteropathogenic *E. coli* to HT29 intestinal epithelial cells via induction or over-expression of mucin [60]. In an *in vitro* cell model using Caco-2 cells, *L. rhamnosus* GG up-regulates MUC2 expression and has an inhibitory effect on bacterial translocation of the intestinal epithelium [61]. Thus, an increased expression of intestinal mucin in response to lactobacilli mediates inhibition of adherence of pathogens to intestinal cells.

Potential probiotic strains can also induce the release of defensins from epithelial cells. These small peptides/proteins are active against bacteria, fungi, and viruses, and stabilize the gut barrier function [62]. It has been shown that *E. coli* Nissle 1917 induces the human b-defensin-2 (hBD-2) gene expression in Caco-2 intestinal epithelial cells [63]. This induction was mediated by NFκB and AP-1 signaling pathways. Several strains of *E. coli*, *L. acidophilus*, *Lactobacillus fermentum*, *Lactobacillus paracasei* subsp. *paracasei*, *Pediococcus pentosaceus*, and the VSL#3 probiotic mixture were found to induce hBD-2 gene expression in Caco-2 cells [64]. This was also dependent on mitogen-activated protein kinase (MAPK), NFκB, and AP-1 signaling pathways [64]. This induction of hBD-2 may also enhance mucosal barrier function.

Probiotic strains may use both types of mechanisms when competing with pathogens for binding to the intestinal mucosa. *L. crispatus* was reported to inhibit the *in vitro* adhesion of *E. faecalis* due to the combined effect of both bactericidal activity and competition for the attachment site [65].

Host Specificity of Adhesion

Adhesion of bacterial to different surfaces has been reported to be species specific [66]. The intestinal mucosa has been widely used as an environment to test adhesion abilities of both probiotics and pathogens. Nowadays, other mucosa are being analyzed due to, their interest for health as, for example, nasal, oral and vaginal mucosa.

Adhesion, and at least temporary colonization to host tissue, is regarded as an important factor for the probiotic to induce its beneficial health effects. Therefore, host specificity has been considered as a desirable property for probiotic bacteria and it has been recommended as one of the selection criteria [43]. Host specificity was challenged earlier by Conway and coworkers [67] where they reported similar adhesion of lactobacilli to porcine and human epithelial cells and concluded that the adhesion was non-specific, suggesting that pig intestinal cells could be used *in vitro* to screen the adhesion properties of lactic acid bacteria (LAB) aimed for human consumption. Other results [68] supported the use of animal models for probiotic studies, but further studies are needed to investigate whether determinants other than mucus adhesion are required to stimulate health effects. The results may also imply that probiotic strains isolated from humans may be beneficial for animal use [69, 70]. This may have important safety implications: strains shown to be safe for humans can be fed to livestock and pets without a potential safety concern for the consumer or owner. It is a subject of additional studies to investigate whether the highly binding LAB do also initiate similar immune effects in animals as in humans.

Adhesins

It has been described that FimH alleles of fimbriae I binding to mannose with scarce affinity are expressed by commensal intestinal bacteria, whereas those binding with higher affinity are associated to uropathogenic bacteria [71]. Thus, small differences in structural genes may act as a switch from a commensal to a pathogenic lifestyle [72].

The adhesion mechanisms involve passive forces, electrostatic and hydrophobic interactions, lipoteichoic acids, and specific structures such as polysaccharides and lectins. Lipoteichoic acids are complex surface-exposed polymers in the cell structure of Gram + bacteria and are suggested to be involved in adhesion processes. These acids have been described as essential factors for *Staphylococcus aureus* adhesion on nasal mucosa [73, 74]. In addition, the lipoteichoic acid serves as adhesinc in the adherence of lactobacilli to intestinal surfaces [75, 76]. The role of exopolysaccharides produced by some probiotic strains in adhesion has also been demonstrated [77, 78].

In the intestine, the mucus layer covering the gut epithelium is rich in glycoproteins and glycolipids, providing abundantly carbohydrate moieties for bacterial adhesion [41]. The exact mechanisms of the lactic acid producing bacteria adhesion to the intestinal mucosa are not very well characterized. A *L. fermentum* strain was documented to bind to mucus glycoproteins isolated from porcine gastric mucus [79], and several lactic acid producing bacteria adhered to human ileostomy glycoproteins [54]. These findings suggest that glycoproteins in intestinal mucus can act as suitable receptors. Several reports indicate that proteinaceous components are involved in the adhesion of bacterial to intestinal cells in animal models and *in vitro* human studies [80–86]. Mub is a cell surface protein involved in the adhesion of certain lactobacilli to mucin [82, 87]. Msa is a mannose-specific adhesin of *L. plantarum*, which was found to be present in different *L. plantarum* strains [88]. The ability of probiotics to bind to mannose is of interest as probiotics with similar binding abilities may inhibit the pathogen adhesion. Bacterial lectin adhesins can be located on cell surface appendages, as in tips of the fimbriae in *E. coli* [89]. Some LAB and bifidobacteria do not commonly possess such prominent structures; although fimbriae and flagella have been identified in some vaginal LAB strains [90] and

Bifidobacterium longum [91]. Bacteria belonging to the *L. acidophilus* group are documented as having lectin-like proteins in the surface layer protein [92]. Such elements in the surface layer protein may contribute to the bacterial adhesion, as they bind to carbohydrate portions of the intestinal mucosal layer [93] and it has been reported that adhesion to human cells of some lactobacilli is mediated by surface layer proteins [81, 84, 94].

4. FACTORS AFFECTING THE ADHESION

Factors such as cell wall properties and composition, and possibly host specificity, are the most important determinants of adhesion properties. The effects of gastrointestinal conditions (pH, bile, digestive enzymes) and the effects of acid and bile resistance acquisition on the adhesion of probiotic bacteria have also been documented [44, 95]. In addition, other reports describe how the presence of different substances such as calcium ions or exopolysaccharides produced by probiotic bacteria can modify the bacterial adhesion to intestinal mucus [77, 96]. However, further studies have shown that the presence of magnesium and zinc ions did not modify the adhesion abilities of probiotics to porcine intestinal epithelial IPEC-J2 cells [96].

The presence of endogenous microbiota has no influence on the adhesion abilities of probiotics to mucus in an *in vitro* human mucus model [97, 98]. Combinations of probiotics may have synergistic effects on adhesion. In *in vitro* trials, the probiotic properties have mainly been tested alone or in combination with yogurt bacteria such as *L. delbrueckii* and *S. thermophilus* [99] but rarely combined with other probiotics. However, some studies are available on the interactions of different probiotics regarding adhesion properties in an intestinal mucus system [5, 99, 100]. These reports showed the influence of other probiotic strains in the adhesion of probiotics

and this influence may be positive (enhance the adhesion) or negative (decrease) and the adhesion with the corresponding effects on probiotic properties related to these bacteria.

5. COMPETITIVE INHIBITION OF PATHOGENS

In the case of probiotic strains, the probiotic therapy has now gained massive interest worldwide due to the potentially beneficial effects on both general and gastrointestinal health as well as being seen as an important complement to antibiotic treatments. Although the mechanisms of action are not fully understood, it is generally accepted that the ability of probiotics to aggregate with pathogens is a desired property. To be effective against oral infections, probiotic bacteria need to adhere to the oral mucosa and dental tissues as a part of the oral biofilm and compete with the growth of cariogenic bacteria and/or periodontal pathogens [101].

The adhesion levels of the probiotic and pathogen strains on intestinal mucus showed a great variability depending on the strain, species and genus [5, 39, 44, 95, 102]. Probiotic bacteria can competitively inhibit the adhesion of pathogenic microorganisms and displace the previously adhered pathogens, such as *Salmonella, Escherichia coli, Listeria monocytogenes, Staphylococcus aureus, Bacteroides vulgatus, Clostridium difficile* and *C. perfringens* [5, 44, 95, 102–104]. The adhesive properties of probiotics widely vary, depending on the strain, and high *in vitro* adherence ability in one strain does not always guarantee *in vivo* persistence and protective effect. This should always be corroborated by studies in animal models and humans [44, 104]. A direct correlation has not been found between the overall adhesion level of probiotic strains and their abilities to inhibit or displace pathogens, suggesting that different mechanisms could be implied in both processes [102, 104–106]. Probiotic strains and combinations that inhibit and displace pathogens may be excellent candidates for their use as new combinations in fermented milk products or as new therapies to prevent and treat specific diseases. In some reports [5, 39, 44, 95], all of the probiotic strains tested showed abilities to inhibit, displace and compete with pathogens. However, it is important to take into account the high specificity of these processes and the importance to properly characterize the properties of the strains in order to select the best strain or combinations to prevent or treat infection by a specific pathogen. In addition, it has been shown in animal studies that LAB populations are not exclusively dependent on genetics but rather are influenced by environmental factors. Such findings underline the effect of intestinal microbiota for studies in probiotic trials and a similar competitive role for fecal bacteria has been reported in adherence studies using Caco-2 cells [107, 108]. The specificity of adhesion properties should thus be further clarified prior to using this trait for the development of products based on the host specificity of adhesion.

5.1. Mechanisms of Exclusion of Intestinal Pathogens by Probiotics

Competitive exclusion of pathogens is thought to be one of the most important beneficial mechanisms of probiotic bacteria [80, 109, 110]. Other mechanisms as inhibitions of pathogen adhesion by probiotic strains and displacement of pre-adhered pathogens have also been described [5, 44]. Competitive exclusion by intestinal bacteria is based on a bacteria-to-bacteria interaction mediated by the competition for available nutrients and for mucosal adhesion sites. In order to gain a competitive advantage, bacteria can also modify their environment to make it less suitable for their competitors. The production of antimicrobial substances, such as lactic and acetic acid, is one example of this kind of environmental modification [111].

Several reports demonstrate that specific probiotics can competitively inhibit the adhesion of pathogens and displace them [5, 39, 44, 95, 102–104]. It has been shown that some lactobacilli and bifidobacteria share carbohydrate-binding specificities with some enteropathogens [112, 113]. This makes it possible for the strains to compete for the receptor sites on the host cell with specific pathogens [65, 114]. In general, it is considered that probiotic strains are able to inhibit the attachment of pathogenic bacteria by means of steric hindrance at enterocyte pathogen receptors. In addition, probiotic strains may reduce the pathogen colonization and possible subsequent invasion by the reduction of the viability of a pathogen by producing growth inhibitors [115].

The effect of probiotic LAB on the competitive exclusion of pathogens has been demonstrated using human mucosal material *in vitro* [50, 54], and *in vivo* in chickens [116] and pigs [117]. Hirano and colleagues [50] showed that the well-adhering strain *L. rhamnosus* was capable of inhibiting the internalization of Enterohemorrhagic *E. coli* (EHEC) to a human intestinal cell line. These results suggest that a close interaction with the host cells may have been responsible for this suppression of EHEC internalization. In Finland, the competitive exclusion method has effectively reduced the incidence of salmonellae in broiler chicken [116].

6. MODELS TO TEST ADHESION

As previously stated, the ability to adhere to intestinal mucosa has been suggested as a potential mechanism for temporary colonization. However, the difficulties involved in studying bacterial adhesion *in vivo*, specifically in humans, have led to the development of different *in vitro* model systems for the preliminary selection of potentially adherent strains.

In vitro models involving human epithelial cell lines, mostly Caco-2 and HT29, or mucus-secreting HT29-MTX cells as well as intestinal mucus isolated from feces, ileostomy or resected human intestinal tissue have been used to assess the adhesion properties of potential probiotic strains.

The advantage of the epithelial cells lines as Caco-2, HT29 and HT29-MTX is that they show the characteristics of the mature enterocytes [118]. The HT29-MTX cell line produces mucus and may mimic the conditions of the intestine. In general, adhesion of bacteria to this cellular line is higher than that obtained for other cell lines such as HT29 or Caco-2 [118]. However, the composition of mucus produced by HT29-MTX and the number and type of binding sites differ from that of the intestinal human mucus [119]. Therefore, models using human intestinal mucus have also been developed. Among them, the isolation of mucus from feces [5, 44, 68, 95, 120–122] or the use of mucus directly obtained from the mucosa [123, 124] have been the most frequently used. These intestinal mucus models allows for the testing of host-specific factors such as health status or age in adhesion studies, providing further information. Resected intestinal tissue is probably the most realistic option to test the adhesion because the normal microbiota present in the intestine mucosa is taken into account in the assay (98, 97, 105).

7. IN VITRO VERSUS IN VIVO RESULTS

The reproducibility and validity of *in vitro* adhesion tests and their correlation to *in vivo* colonization have been evaluated in several studies. Indirect evidence suggests that adhesion to intestinal cells and mucus is associated with temporary colonization. However, *in vitro* and *in vivo* results do not always correlate. *In vitro* adherence of different strains of *Bifidobacterium* to Caco-2 cells was analyzed [45] and data were compared to *in vivo* human study results. Good *in vitro* adhesion was observed for strains capable of colonization. However, in another report [125], *L. johnsonii* and *L. paracasei*, analyzed *in vitro* and *in vivo* in a mice model showed similar *in vitro* properties but different *in vivo* colonization. It is important to take into account the *in vitro* results but it is also necessary to test the properties in *in vivo* studies.

The genetic information becoming increasingly available will enable us to focus on probiotic properties that can be characterized to counteract specific microbiota disturbances. This has required thorough knowledge on both aberrancies, and the genetic information of the probiotics will be used to counteract aberrant microbiota and to support healthy microbiota development. In this way, more targeted probiotics can be identified for the future. This development underlines the focus on adhesion and adhesion interaction with pathogens and normal microbiota as a means of modulating the composition and activity of microbiota in the intestinal epithelium. It will allow future careful identification of new probiotics and probiotic combinations for targeting challenges in pathogen adhesion prevention and enhancement of the intestinal barrier functions.

8. COMBINING SPECIFIC PROBIOTICS STRAINS

Beneficial effects of probiotics are strain-dependent and strains may interact with each other in different ways. It has been suggested that specific combinations of probiotics should be selected for cases where the microbiota deviations or aberrancies are more complex. In such circumstances, combinations of probiotics may have an impact either together on specific microbiota deviations or as single strains in different parts of the gastrointestinal tract [126]. Among the possible mechanisms underlying the enhanced effects of probiotics, the combinations of different strains are currently an area of major interest. Strains used in multistrain and multispecies probiotics should be compatible or, preferably, synergistic, as the actions could be also counteracting each other's efficacy in competitive exclusion. The design and use of combinations of probiotic strains should be encouraged, reflecting the complex intestinal conditions, and the potential need to have an impact in several niche areas.

The number of scientific reports on the effects of probiotic combinations on the health of the host is increasing rapidly [127–132]. Research using single probiotics strains has been reported earlier but, at present, probiotic combinations with possibly additional health benefits are being assessed prior to use in clinical studies. It has been demonstrated that a combination of probiotic strains may complement or improve health benefits given by individual strains [128, 129, 133–136]. It is expected that combinations of different probiotics strains may be more effective than single strains of probiotics depending on the target [4]. It is clear that combinations may also be needed for counteracting complex microbiota aberrancies in adults and infants. However, the impact can be counteractive, if strains are not selected in a scientifically sound manner.

The best known probiotic combination consisting of a mixture of eight lactic acid bacterial species (VSL#3) reported as being effective in several human diseases [128, 133–136]. Some *in vitro* and *in vivo* studies have assessed other combinations such as, for example, *Lactobacillus rhamnosus*, *Propionibacterium freudenreichii* and *Bifidobacterium lactis*. This combination has then been demonstrated effectively in clinical studies on irritable bowel syndrome patients [137]. The same probiotic combination did not have an impact on the alleviation of allergy symptoms in infants, while *Lactobacillus rhamnosus* GG was previously demonstrated to be effective [138, 139]. However, when the combination was given with a galacto-oligosaccharide the resulting effect was a reduction in atopic eczema

prevention [140]. It must also be considered that, in the end, *in vivo* studies are always necessary to confirm the potential health effects of such combinations and results obtained with the independent strains should not be extrapolated to the combination.

It has been demonstrated that strain combinations can be tested *in vitro* and reasonably reliable results can be achieved. In some cases probiotic combinations show clear benefits as has been described in combinations counteracting the adhesion of pathogens [7, 100] or in adhering toxins [141, 142] and heavy metals [143, 144]. Studies on the combination of well-known probiotic strains, such as *L. rhamnosus* GG and *B. lactis* Bb12 and their effects in the pathogen adhesion to intestinal mucus system, have been reported [99, 126]. Probiotic strains and their combinations were able to significantly inhibit the adhesion of *B. vulgatus*, *C. histolyticum*, *C. difficile*, *S. aureus* [5, 7, 100]. Interestingly, in these studies, *S. enterica* serovar *Typhimurium* was inhibited significantly only by one probiotic strain, whereas all probiotic combinations were able to inhibit the pathogen [5, 7, 100]. In addition, none of the single probiotic strains was able to inhibit the adhesion of *E. coli* and *L. monocytogenes*, whereas all probiotic combinations were able to significantly inhibit the adhesion of these pathogens [5, 100] and in several cases they were more able to enhance the inhibition percentages than when the probiotic strains were tested alone. These results emphasized the potential application of probiotic combinations in the inhibition of pathogen adhesion to intestinal mucus but further studies are needed to clarify the mechanisms involved in pathogen inhibition by probiotic combinations.

Probiotic combinations that inhibit and displace pathogens may be good candidates in the case of specific microbiota aberrancies related to disease risk reduction. However, as stated previously, it is important to take into account the high specificity of these processes being necessary to characterize the properties of the strains in order to select the best combination for a specific application. The change of one strain in a combination may modify all the properties against pathogen adhesion regarding inhibition, displacement and competition mechanisms [126]. All together, these studies would allow the development of new probiotic combinations for the treatment or prevention of specific diseases by targeting the adhesion of specific pathogens. These results support the idea that the use of probiotic combinations selected for specific targets may have a major impact on the disease.

9. CONCLUSION

Probiotics are viable beneficial microorganisms with a demonstrated health impact on the host. The assessment of adhesion properties and competitive exclusion of pathogens constitutes an important point in probiotic characterization. Selection of new probiotic strains and combinations counteract both pathogen challenges against normal healthy microbiota as well as counteracting identified microbiota deviations that may predispose the subjects to later disease. Probiotic strains or combinations that inhibit and displace pathogens may be good candidates for the treatment or prevention of specific diseases caused by known pathogens or microbiota deviations related to disease risk reduction.

References

1. FAO/WHO (2002). Guidelines for the evaluation of probiotics in food. Food and Agricultural Organization of the United Nations and World Health Organization. Working Group Report 2002.
2. Collins, J. K., Thornton, G., & Sullivan, G. O. (1998). Selection of probiotic strains for human application. *International Dairy Journal, 8*, 487–490.
3. Ouwehand, A. C., Salminen, S., & Isolauri, E. (2002). Probiotics: an overview of beneficial effects. *Antonie van Leeuwenhoek, 82*, 279–289.
4. Timmerman, H. M., Koning, C. J., Mulder, L., et al. (2004). Monostrain, multistrain and multispecies probiotics—A comparison of functionality and efficacy. *International Journal of Food Microbiology, 96*, 219–233.
5. Collado, M. C., Meriluoto, J., & Salminen, S. (2007). *In vitro* analysis of probiotic strains combinations to inhibit pathogen adhesion to human intestinal mucus. *Food Res Int, 40*(5), 629–636.
6. Forestier, C., De Champs, C., Vatoux, C., & Joly, B. (2001). Probiotic activities of *Lactobacillus casei rhamnosus: in vitro* adherence to intestinal cells and antimicrobial properties. *Research in Microbiology, 152*, 167–173.
7. Collado, M. C., Isolauri, E., & Salminen, S. (2008). Role of probiotic strains and their combinations in *Enterobacter sakazakii* in vitro infection associated with powdered infant formula. *FEMS Microbiology Letters, 285*(1), 58–64.
8. Ng, S. C., Hart, A. L., Kamm, M. A., et al. (2009). Mechanisms of action of probiotics: Recent advances. *Inflammatory Bowel Diseases, 15*(2), 300–310.
9. Corr, S. C., Hill, C., & Gahan, C. G. (2009). Chapter 1 understanding the mechanisms by which probiotics inhibit gastrointestinal pathogens. *Advances in Food and Nutrition Research, 56*, 1–15.
10. Collado, M. C., Isolauri, E., Salminen, S., & Sanz, Y. (2009). The impact of probiotic on gut health. *Advances in Food and Nutrition Research, 10*(1), 68–78.
11. Fooks, L. J., Fuller, R., & Gibson, G. R. (1999). Prebiotics, probiotics and human gut microecology. *International Dairy Journal, 9*, 53–61.
12. Servin, A. L. (2004). Antagonistic activities of lactobacilli and bifidobacteria against microbial pathogens. *FEMS Microbiology Reviews, 28*, 405–440.
13. Bourlioux, P., Koletzko, B., Guarner, F., & Braesco, V. (2003). The intestine and its microflora are partners for the protection of the host: Report on the Danone Symposium 'The Intelligent Intestine,' held in Paris, June 14, 2002. *The American Journal of Clinical Nutrition, 78*(4), 183–675.
14. Neutra, M. R., & Forstner, J. F. (1987). Gastrointestinal mucus: Synthesis, secretion and function. In L. R. Johnson (Ed.), *Physiology of the Gastrointestinal Tract* (2nd edn). New York: Raven Press.
15. Juntunen, M., Kirjavainen, P. V., Ouwehand, A. C., et al. (2001). Adherence of probiotic bacteria to human intestinal mucus in healthy infants and during rotavirus infection. *Clin Diag Lab Immunol, 8*(2), 293–296.
16. López-Ferrer, A., de Bolós, C., Barranco, C., et al. (2000). Role of fucosyltransferases in the association between apomucin and Lewis antigen expression in normal and malignant gastric epithelium. *Gut, 47*(3), 349–356.
17. Deplancke, B., & Gaskins, H. R. (2001). Microbial modulation of innate defense: Goblet cells and the intestinal mucus layer. *The American Journal of Clinical Nutrition, 73*, 1131S–1141S.
18. Montagne, L., Piel, C., & Lallés, J. P. (2004). Effect of diet on mucin kinetics and composition: Nutrition and health implications. *Nutrition Reviews, 62*, 105–114.

19. Hamer, H. M., Jonkers, D., Venema, K., et al. (2008). Review article: The role of butyrate on colonic function. *Alimentary Pharmacology & Therapeutics, 27*(2), 104–119.

20. Forstner, J. F. (1978). Intestinal mucins in health and disease. *Digestion, 17*(3), 234–263.

21. Collado, M. C., Ben-Amor, K., Salminen, S., & de Vos, W. (2008). The mucin-degrader *Akkermansia muciniphila* is an important member of the human intestinal tract. *Applied and Environmental Microbiology, 74*, 1646–1648.

22. Collado, M. C., Derrien, M., Isolauri, E., et al. (2007). Intestinal integrity and *Akkermansia muciniphila*: A mucin-degrading member of the intestinal microbiota present in infants, adults and the elderly. *Applied and Environmental Microbiology, 73*(22), 7767–7770.

23. Dekker, J., Rossen, J. W., Büller, H. A., & Einerhand, A. W. (2002). The MUC family: An obituary. *Trends in Biochemical Sciences, 27*(3), 126–131.

24. Dharmani, P., Srivastava, V., Kissoon-Singh, V., & Chadee, K. (2009). Role of intestinal mucins in innate host defense mechanisms against pathogens. *Journal of Innate Immunity, 1*, 123–135.

25. Forstner, J. F., Oliver, M. G. & Sylvester, F. A., 1995. Production, structure and biologic relevance of gastrointestinal mucins. In *Infections of the Gastrointestinal Tract* (Chapter 5). New York: Raven Press.

26. Niku-Paavola, M. L., Laitila, A., Mattila-Sandholm, T., & Haikara, A. (1999). New types of antimicrobial compounds produced by *Lactobacillus plantarum*. *Journal of Applied Microbiology, 86*, 29–35.

27. Chen, H., & Hoover, D. G. (2003). Bacteriocins and their food applications. *Comprehensive Rev Food Sci Food Safety, 2*, 82–100.

28. Ibrahim, S. A., & Bezkorovainy, A. (1993). Survival of bifidobacteria in the presence of bile salt. *Journal of the Science of Food and Agriculture, 62*, 351–354.

29. Bruno, F. A., & Shah, N. P. (2002). Inhibition of pathogenic and putrefactive microorganisms by *Bifidobacterium* sp. *Milchwissenschaft, 57*, 617–621.

30. Daniels, J. A., Krishnamurthi, R., & Rizvi, S. S. H. (1985). A review of the effects of carbon dioxide on microbial growth and food quality. *Journal of Food Protection, 6*, 532–537.

31. Riley, M. A., & Wertz, E. (2002). Bacteriocins: evolution, ecology and application. *Annual Review of Microbiology, 56*, 117–137.

32. Boris, S., & Barbes, C. (2000). Role played by lactobacilli in controlling the population of vaginal pathogens. *Microbes and Infection, 2*, 543–546.

33. Klaenhammer, T. R. (1998). Functional activities of Lactobacillus probiotics: Genetic mandate. *International Dairy Journal, 8*, 497–505.

34. Touré, R., Kheardr, E., Lacroix, C., et al. (2003). Production of antibacterial substances by bifidobacterial isolates from infant stool active against *Listeria monocytogenes*. *Journal of Applied Microbiology, 95*, 1058–1069.

35. Collado, M. C., Hernández, M., & Sanz, Y. (2005). Production of bacteriocin-like inhibitory compounds by potentially probiotic bifidobacteria. *Journal of Food Protection, 68*(5), 1034–1040.

36. Collado, M. C., González, A., González, R., et al. (2005). Antimicrobial peptides are within the antagonistic metabolites produced by Bifidobacterium against *Helicobacter pylori*. *International Journal of Antimicrobial Agents, 25*, 385–391.

37. Yildirim, Z., & Johnson, M. G. (1998). Characterization and antimicrobial spectrum of bifidocin B, a bacteriocin produced by *Bifidobacterium bifidum* NCFB 1454. *Journal of Food Protection, 61*, 47–51.

38. Yildirim, Z., Winters, D. K., & Johnson, M. G. (1999). Purification, amino acid sequence and mode of action of bifidocin B produced by *Bifidobacterium bifidum* NCFB 1454. *Journal of Applied Microbiology, 86*, 45–54.

39. Lee, Y.-J., Yu, W.-K., & Heo, T.-R. (2003). Identification and screening for antimicrobial activity against *Clostridium difficile* of Bifidobacterium and Lactobacillus species isolated from healthy infant faeces. *International Journal of Antimicrobial Agents, 21*, 340–346.

40. Gagnon, M., Kheadr, E. E., Le Blay, G., & Fliss, I. (2004). *In vitro* inhibition of *Escherichia coli* O157:H7 by bifidobacterial strains of human origin. *International Journal of Food Microbiology, 92*, 69–78.

41. Beachey, E. H. (1981). Bacterial adherence: Adhesin-receptor interactions mediating the attachment of bacteria to mucosal surfaces. *Journal of Infectious Diseases, 143*, 325–345.

42. Schiffrin, E. J., Brassart, D., Servin, A. L., et al. (1997). Immune modulation of blood leukocytes in humans by lactic acid bacteria: Criteria for strain selection. *The American Journal of Clinical Nutrition, 66*, 515S–520S.

43. Salminen, S., Bouley, C., Boutron-Ruault, M.-C., et al. (1998). Functional Food science and gastrointestinal physiology and function. *The British Journal of Nutrition, 80*, S147–S171.

44. Collado, M. C., Gueimonde, M., Hernández, M., et al. (2005). Adhesion of selected *Bifidobacterium* strains to human intestinal mucus and its role in enteropathogen exclusion. *Journal of Food Protection, 68*(12), 2672–2678.

45. Crociani, J., Grill, J. P., Huppert, M., & Ballongue, J. (1995). Adhesion of different bifidobacterias strains to human enterocyte-like Caco-2 cells and comparison with *in vivo* study. *Letters in Applied Microbiology, 21*, 146–148.

46. Castagliuolo, I., Galeazzi, F., Ferrari, S., et al. (2005). Beneficial effect of auto-aggregating *Lactobacillus crispatus* on experimentally induced colitis in mice. *FEMS Immunol Med Microbiol, 43*(2), 197–204.

47. O'Halloran, F. M., Morrissey, S. D., Murphy, L., et al. (1998). Adhesion of potential probiotic bacteria to human epithelial cell lines. *International Dairy Journal, 8*, 596.

48. Perdigon, G., Maldonado Galdeano, C., Valdez, J. C., & Medici, M. (2002). Interaction of lactic acid bacteria with the gut immune system. *European Journal of Clinical Nutrition, 56*(4), S21–26.

49. Jin, L. Z., Marquardt, R. R., & Zhao, X. (2000). A strain of *Enterococcus faecium* (18C23) inhibits adhesion of enterotoxigenic *Escherichia coli* K88 to porcine small intestine mucus. *Applied and Environmental Microbiology, 66*, 4200–4204.

50. Hirano, J., Yoshida, T., Sugiyama, T., et al. (2003). The effect of *Lactobacillus rhamnosus* on enterohemorrhagic *Escherichia coli* infection of human intestinal cells in vitro. *Microbiology and Immunology, 47*, 405–409.

51. Voltan, S., Castagliuolo, I., Elli, M., et al. (2007). Aggregating phenotype in *Lactobacillus crispatus* determines intestinal colonization and TLR2 and TLR4 modulation in murine colonic mucosa. *Clinical and Vaccine Immunology, 14*(9), 1138–1148.

52. Freter, M. (1992). Factors affecting the microecology of the gut. In R. Fuller (Ed.), *Probiotics. The Scientific basis* (pp. 111–145). Glasgow: Chapman and Hall.

53. Busscher, H. J., & Weerkamp, A. H. (1987). Specific and non-specific interactions in bacterial adhesion to solid substrata. *FEMS Microbiology Reviews, 46*, 165–173.

54. Tuomola, E. M., Ouwehand, A. C., & Salminen, S. (1999). The effect of probiotic bacteria on the adhesion of pathogens to human intestinal mucus. *FEMS Immunology and Medical Microbiology, 26*, 137–142.

55. Ofek, I., & Beachey, E. H. (1980). Bacterial adherence. *Advances in Internal Medicine, 25*, 503–532.

56. Vigeant, M. A., Ford, R. M., Wagner, M., & Tamm, L. K. (2002). Reversible and irreversible adhesion of motile *Escherichia coli* cells analyzed by total internal reflection aqueous fluorescence microscopy. *Applied and Environmental Microbiology, 68*, 2794–2801.

57. An, Y. H., Dickinson, R. B., & Doyle, R. J. (2000). Mechanisms of bacterial adhesion and pathogenesis of implant and tissue infections. In Y. H. An & R. J. Friedman (Eds.), *Handbook of bacterial adhesion: Principles, Methods and Applications* (pp. 1–28). Totowa: Humana Press.

58. Dunne, C., O'Mahony, L., Murphy, L., et al. (2001). *In vitro* selection criteria for probiotic bacteria of human origin: Correlation with *in vivo* findings. *The American Journal of Clinical Nutrition, 73*, 386S–392S.

59. Mack, D. R., Ahrne, S., Hyde, L., et al. (2003). Extracellular MUC3 mucin secretion follows adherence of *Lactobacillus* strains to intestinal epithelial cells in vitro. *Gut, 52*(6), 827–833.

60. Mack, D. R., Michail, S., Wei, S., et al. (1999). Probiotics inhibit enteropathogenic *E. coli* adherence *in vitro* by inducing intestinal mucin gene expression. *The American Journal of Physiology, 276*, G941–G950.

61. Mattar, A. F., Teitelbaum, D. H., Drongowski, R. A., et al. (2002). Probiotics up-regulate MUC-2 mucin gene expression in a Caco-2 cell-culture model. *Pediatric Surgery International, 18*, 586–590.

62. Furrie, E., Macfarlane, S., Kennedy, A., et al. (2005). Synbiotic therapy (*Bifidobacterium longum*/Synergy 1) initiates resolution of inflammation in patients with active ulcerative colitis: A randomised controlled pilot trial. *Gut, 54*(2), 242–249.

63. Wehkamp, J., Harder, J., Wehkamp, K., et al. (2004). NF-κB- and AP-1-mediated induction of human b-defensin-2 in intestinal epithelial cells by *Escherichia coli* Nissle 1917: A novel effect of a probiotic bacterium. *Infection and Immunity, 72*(10), 5750–5758.

64. Schlee, M., Harder, J., Koten, B., et al. (2008). Probiotic lactobacilli and VSL#3 induce enterocyte b-defensin 2. *Clinical and Experimental Immunology, 151*(3), 528–535.

65. Todoriki, K., Mukai, T., Sato, S., & Toba, T. (2001). Inhibition of adhesion of food-borne pathogens to Caco-2 cells by *Lactobacillus* strains. *Journal of Applied Microbiology, 91*, 154–159.

66. Fuller, R. (1973). Ecological studies on the *Lactobacillus* flora associated with the crop epithelium of the fowl. *The Journal of Applied Bacteriology, 36*, 131–139.

67. Conway, P. L., Gorbach, S. L., & Goldin, B. R. (1987). Survival of lactic acid bacteria in the human stomach and adhesion to intestinal cells. *Journal of Dairy Science, 70*, 1–12.

68. Rinkinen, M., Westermarck, E., Salminen, S., & Ouwehand, A. C. (2003). Absence of host specificity for *in vitro* adhesion of probiotic lactic acid bacteria to intestinal mucus. *Veterinary Microbiology, 97*, 55–61.

69. Nikoskelainen, S., Salminen, S., Bylund, G., & Ouwehand, A. C. (2001). Characterization of the properties of human- and dairy-derived probiotics for prevention of infectious diseases in fish. *Applied and Environmental Microbiology, 67*, 2430–2435.

70. Nikoskelainen, S., Ouwehand, A. C., Salminen, S., & Bylund, G. (2001). Protection of rainbow trout (*Oncorhynchus mykiss*) from furunculosis by *Lactobacillus rhamnosus*. *Aquaculture, 198*, 229–236.

71. Le Bouguénec, C. (2005). Adhesins and invasins of pathogenic *Escherichia coli*. *International Journal of Medical Microbiology, 295*(6–I7), 471–478.

72. Weissman, S. J., Moseley, S. L., Dykhuizen, D. E., & Sokurenko, E. V. (2003). Enterobacterial adhesins and the case for studying SNPs in bacteria. *Trends Microbiol, 11*(3), 115–117.

73. Weidenmaier, C., Kokai-Kun, J. F., Kristian, S. A., et al. (2004). Role of teichoic acids in *Staphylococcus aureus* nasal colonization, a major risk factor in nosocomial infections. *Nature Medicine, 10*, 243–245.

74. Weidenmaier, C., Peschel, A., Xiong, Y. Q., et al. (2005). Lack of wall teichoic acids in *Staphylococcus aureus* leads to reduced interactions with endothelial cells and to attenuated virulence in a rabbit model of endocarditis. *The Journal of Infectious Diseases, 191*, 1771–1777.

75. Sherman, L. A., & Savage, D. C. (1986). Lipoteichoic acids in *Lactobacillus* strains that colonize the mouse gastric epithelium. *Applied and Environmental Microbiology, 52*, 302–304.

76. Granato, D., Perotti, F., Masserey, I., et al. (1999). Cell surface-associated lipoteichoic acid acts as an adhesion factor for attachment of *Lactobacillus johnsonii* La1 to human enterocyte-like Caco-2 cells. *Applied and Environmental Microbiology, 65*, 1071–1077.

77. Ruas-Madiedo, P., Gueimonde, M., Margolles, A., et al. (2006). Exopolysaccharides produced by probiotic strains modify the adhesion of probiotics and enteropathogens to human intestinal mucus. *Journal of Food Protection, 69*(8), 2011–2015.

78. Sun, J., Le, G. W., Shi, Y. H., & Su, G. W. (2007). Factors involved in binding of *Lactobacillus plantarum* Lp6 to rat small intestinal mucus. *Letters in Applied Microbiology, 44*(1), 79–85.

79. Henriksson, A., & Conway, P. L. (1996). Adhesion of *Lactobacillus fermentum* 104-S to porcine stomach mucus. *Current Microbiology, 33*, 31–34.

80. Adlerberth, I., Cerquetti, M., Poilane, I., et al. (2000). Mechanisms of colonisation and colonisation resistance of the digestive tract. *Microbial Ecology in Health and Disease, 11*, 223–239.

81. Bergonzelli, G. E., Granato, D., Pridmore, R. D., et al. (2006). GroEL of *Lactobacillus johnsonii* La1 (NCC 533) is cell surface associated: potential role in interactions with the host and the gastric pathogen *Helicobacter pylori*. *Infection and Immunity, 74*, 425–434.

82. Buck, B. L., Altermann, E., Svingerud, T., & Klaenhammer, T. R. (2005). Functional analysis of putative adhesion factors in *Lactobacillus acidophilus* NCFM. *Applied and Environmental Microbiology, 71*, 8344–8351.

83. Coconnier, M. H., Klaenhammer, T. R., Kerneis, S., et al. (1992). Protein mediated adhesion of *Lactobacillus acidophilus* BG2FO4 on human enterocyte and mucus-secreting cell lines in culture. *Applied and Environmental Microbiology, 58*, 2034–2039.

84. Granato, D., Bergonzelli, G. E., Pridmore, R. D., et al. (2004). Cell surface-associated elongation factor Tu mediates the attachment of *Lactobacillus johnsonii* NCC533 (La1) to human intestinal cells and mucins. *Infection and Immunity, 72*, 2160–2169.

85. Henriksson, A., Szewzyk, R., & Conway, P. L. (1991). Characteristics of the adhesive determinants of *Lactobacillus fermentum* 104. *Applied and Environmental Microbiology, 57*, 499–502.

86. Miyoshi, Y., Okada, S., Uchimura, T., & Satoh, E. (2006). A mucus adhesion promoting protein, MapA, mediates the adhesion of *Lactobacillus reuteri* to Caco-2 human intestinal epithelial cells. *Bioscience, Biotechnology, and Biochemistry, 70*, 1622–1628.

87. Roos, S., & Jonson, H. (2002). A high-molecular-mass cell-surface protein from *Lactobacillus reuteri* 1063 adheres to mucus components. *Microbiology, 148*, 433–442.

88. Pretzer, G., Snel, J., Molenaar, D., et al. (2005). Biodiversity-based identification and functional characterization of the mannose-specific adhesin of *Lactobacillus plantarum*. *Journal of Bacteriology, 187*, 6128–6136.

89. Thomas, W. E., Trintchina, E., Forero, M., et al. (2002). Bacterial adhesion to target cells enhanced by shear force. *Cell, 109*, 123–913.

90. McGroarty, J. A. (1994). Cell surface appendages of lactobacilli. *FEMS Microbiology Letters, 124*, 405–410.

91. Schell, M. A., Karmirantzou, M., Snel, B., et al. (2002). The genome sequence of *Bifidobacterium longum* reflects its adaptation to the human gastrointestinal tract. *Proceedings of the National Academy of Science, 99*, 14422–14427.

92. Yamada, M., Saito, T., Toba, T., et al. (1994). Hemagglutination activity of *Lactobacillus acidophilus* group lactic acid bacteria. *Bioscience, Biotechnology, and Biochemistry, 58*, 910–915.

93. Matsumura, A., Saito, T., Arakuni, M., et al. (1999). New binding assay and preparative trial of cell-surface lectin from *Lactobacillus acidophilus* group lactic acid bacteria. *Journal of Dairy Science, 82*, 2525–2529.

94. Hynönen, U., Westerlund-Wikström, B., Palva, A., & Korhonen, T. K. (2002). Identification by flagellum display of an epithelial cell- and fibronectin-binding function in the SlpA surface protein of *Lactobacillus brevis*. *Journal of Bacteriology, 184*, 3360–3367.

95. Gueimonde, M., Noriega, L., Margolles, A., et al. (2005). Ability of *Bifidobacterium* strains with acquired resistance to bile to adhere to human intestinal mucus. *International Journal of Food Microbiology, 101*, 341–346.

96. Larsen, N., Nissen, P., & Willats, W. G. (2007). The effect of calcium ions on adhesion and competitive exclusion of *Lactobacillus* ssp. and E. coli O138. *International Journal of Food Microbiology, 114*, 113–119.

97. Ouwehand, A. C., Parhiala, R., Salminen, S., et al. (2004). Influence of the endogenous mucosal microbiota on the adhesion of probiotic bacteria *in vitro*. *Microbial Ecology in Health and Disease, 16*, 202–204.

98. Ouwehand, A. C., Tuomola, E. M., Tölkkö, S., & Salminen, S. (2001). Assessment of adhesion properties of novel probiotic strains to human intestinal mucus. *International Journal of Food Microbiology, 64*, 119–126.

99. Ouwehand, A. C., Isolauri, E., Kirjavainen, P. V., et al. (2000). The mucus binding of *Bifidobacterium lactis* Bb12 is enhanced in the presence of *Lactobacillus*

GG and *Lact. delbrueckii* subsp. *bulgaricus. Letters in Applied Microbiology, 30,* 10–13.

100. Collado, M. C., Meriluoto, J., & Salminen, S. (2008). Interactions between pathogens and lactic acid bacteria: aggregation and coaggregation abilities. *Eur J Food Res Technol, 226*(5), 1065–1073.

101. Haukioja, A., Yli-Knuuttila, H., Loimaranta, V., et al. (2006). Oral adhesion and survival of probiotic and other lactobacilli and bifidobacteria *in vitro. Oral Microbiology and Immunology, 21,* 326–332.

102. Gueimonde, M., Jalonen, L., He, F., et al. (2006). Adhesion and competitive inhibition and displacement of human enteropathogens by selected lactobacilli. *Food Res Int, 39*(4), 467–471.

103. Bernet, M. F., Brassart, D., Nesser, J. R., & Servin, A. L. (1993). Adhesion of human bifidobacterial strains to cultured human intestinal epithelial cells and inhibition of enterophatogen-cell interactions. *Applied and Environmental Microbiology, 59,* 4121–4128.

104. Bibiloni, R., Perez, P. F., & de Antoni, G. L. (1999). Will a high adhering capacity in a probiotic strain guarantee exclusion of pathogens from intestinal epithelia? *Anaerobe, 5,* 519–524.

105. Ouwehand, A. C., Salminen, S., Tolkko, S., et al. (2002). Resected human colonic tissue: New model for characterizing adhesion of lactic acid bacteria. *Clinical and Diagnostic Laboratory Immunology, 9,* 184–186.

106. Ouwehand, A. C., Salminen, S., Tolkko, S., et al. (2002). Dependent adhesion of lactic acid bacteria to colonic tissue *in vitro. Microecol Ther, 29,* 95–102.

107. Haller, D., Colbus, H., Ganzle, M. G., et al. (2001). Metabolic and functional properties of lactic acid bacteria in the gastro-intestinal ecosystem: A comparative *in vitro* study between bacteria of intestinal and fermented food origin. *Systematic and Applied Microbiology, 24,* 218–226.

108. De Waard, R., Snel, J., Bokken, G. C., et al. (2002). Comparison of faecal *Lactobacillus* populations in experimental animals from different breeding facilities and possible consequences for probiotic studies. *Letters in Applied Microbiology, 34,* 105–109.

109. Rolfe, R. D. (2000). The role of probiotic cultures in the control of gastrointestinal health. *The Journal of Nutrition, 130,* 396S–402S.

110. Reid, G., & Burton, J. (2002). Use of *Lactobacillus* to prevent infection by pathogenic bacteria. *Microbes and Infection, 4,* 319–324.

111. Schiffrin, E. J., & Blum, S. (2002). Interactions between the microbiota and the intestinal mucosa. *European Journal of Clinical Nutrition, 56,* S60–S64.

112. Nesser, J.-R., Granato, D., Rouvet, M., et al. (2000). *Lactobacillus johnsonii* La1 shares carbohydrate-binding specificities with several enteropathogenic bacteria. *Glycobiology, 10,* 1193–1199.

113. Fujiwara, S., Hashiba, H., Hirota, T., & Forstner, J. F. (2001). Inhibition of the binding of enterotoxigenic *Escherichia coli* Pb176 to human intestinal epithelial cell line HCT-8 by an extracellular protein fraction containing BIF of *Bifidobacterium longum* SBT2928: Suggestive evidence of blocking of the binding receptor gangliotetraosylceramide on the cell surface. *International Journal of Food Microbiology, 67,* 97–106.

114. Mukai, T., Asasaka, T., Sato, E., et al. (2002). Inhibition of binding of *Helicobacter pylori* to the glycolipid receptors by probiotic *Lactobacillus reuteri. FEMS Immunology and Medical Microbiology, 32,* 105–110.

115. Coconnier, M. H., Bernet, M. F., Chauviere, G., & Servin, A. L. (1993). Adhering heat-killed human *Lactobacillus acidophilus*, strain LB, inhibits the process of pathogenicity of diarrhoeageic bacteria in cultured human intestinal cells. *Journal of Diarrhoeal Diseases Research, 11,* 235–242.

116. Hirn, J., Nurmi, E., Johansson, T., & Nuotio, L. (1992). Long-term experience with competitive exclusion and salmonellas in Finland. *International Journal of Food Microbiology, 15,* 281–285.

117. Genovese, K. J., Anderson, R. C., Harvey, R. B., & Nisbet, D. J. (2000). Competitive exclusion treatment reduces the mortality and fecal shedding associated with enterotoxigenic *Escherichia coli* infection in nursery-raised neonatal pigs. *Canadian Journal of Veterinary Research, 64,* 204–207.

118. Gopal, P. K., Prasad, J., Smart, J., & Gill, H. S. (2001). *In vitro* adherence properties of *Lactobacillus rhamnosus* DR20 and *Bifidobacterium lactis* DR10 strains and their antagonistic activity against an enterotoxigenic *Escherichia coli. International Journal of Food Microbiology, 67,* 207–216.

119. Lesuffleur, T., Porchet, N., Aubert, J. P., et al. (1993). Differential expression of the human mucin genes MUC1 to MUC5 in relation to growth and differentiation of different mucus-secreting HT29 cell sub-populations. *Journal of Cell Science, 106,* 771–783.

120. Kirjavainen, P. V., Ouwehand, A. C., Isolauri, E., & Salminen, S. J. (1998). The ability of probiotic bacteria to bind to human intestinal mucus. *FEMS Microbiology Letters, 167,* 185–189.

121. Aissi, E. A., Lecocq, M., Brassart, C., & Buoquelet, S. (2001). Adhesion of some Bifidobacteria strains to human enterocyte-like cells and binding to mucosal glycoproteins. *Microbial Ecology in Health and Disease, 13,* 32–39.

122. Tuomola, E. M., Ouwehand, A. C., & Salminen, S. (2000). Chemical, physical and enzymatic pretreatments of probiotic lactobacilli alter their adhesion to human intestinal mucus glycoproteins. *International Journal of Food Microbiology, 60,* 75–81.

123. Ouwehand, A. C., & Salminen, S. (2003). *In vitro* adhesion assays for probiotics and their in vivo relevance: A review. *Microbial Ecology in Health and Disease, 15,* 175–184.

124. Vesterlund, S., Paltta, J., Karp, M., & Ouwehand, A. C. (2005). Measurement of bacterial adhesion— *in vitro* evaluation of different methods. *Journal of Microbiological Methods, 60,* 225–233.

125. Ibnou-Zekri, N., Blum, S., Schiffrin, E. J., & von der Weid, T. (2003). Divergent patterns of colonization and immune response elicited from two intestinal Lactobacillus strains that display similar properties *in vitro. Infection and Immunity, 71,* 428–436.

126. Collado, M. C., Meriluoto, J., & Salminen, S. (2007). Development of new probiotics by strains combination: Is it possible to improve the adhesion to intestinal mucus? *Journal of Dairy Science, 90,* 2710–2716.

127. Femia, A. P., Luceri, C., Dolara, P., et al. (2002). Antitumorigenic activity of the prebiotic inulin enriched with oligofructose in combination with the probiotics *Lactobacillus rhamnosus* and *Bifidobacterium lactis* on azoxymethane-induced colon carcinogenesis in rats. *Carcinogenesis, 23*(11), 1953–1960.

128. Gionchetti, P., Lammers, K. M., Rizzello, F., & Campieri, M. (2005). Probiotics and barrier function in colitis. *Gut, 54*(7), 898–900.

129. Myllyluoma, E., Veijola, L., Ahlroos, T., et al. (2005). Probiotic supplementation improves tolerance to Helicobacter pylori eradication therapy—a placebo-controlled, double-blind randomized pilot study. *Alimentary Pharmacology & Therapeutics, 21*(10), 1263–1272.

130. Kajander, K., Hatakka, K., Poussa, T., et al. (2005). A probiotic mixture alleviates symptoms in irritable bowel syndrome patients: a controlled 6-month intervention. *Alimentary Pharmacology & Therapeutics, 22*(5), 387–394.

131. Olivares, M., Diaz-Ropero, M. P., Gómez, N., et al. (2006). The consumption of two new probiotic strains, *Lactobacillus gasseri* CECT 5714 and *Lactobacillus coryniformis* CECT 5711, boosts the immune system of healthy humans. *International Microbiology, 9*(1), 47–52.

132. Roselli, M., Finamore, A., Britti, M. S., & Mengheri, E. (2006). Probiotic bacteria *Bifidobacterium animalis* MB5 and *Lactobacillus rhamnosus* GG protect intestinal Caco-2 cells from the inflammation-associated response induced by enterotoxigenic *Escherichia coli* K88. *The British Journal of Nutrition, 95*(6), 1177–1184.

133. Bibiloni, R., Fedorak, R. N., Tannock, G. W., et al. (2005). VSLd3 probiotic-mixture induces remission in patients with active ulcerative colitis. *The American Journal of Gastroenterology, 100*(7), 1539–1546.

134. Kim, H. J., Vazquez Roque, M. I., Camilleri, M., et al. (2005). A randomized controlled trial of a probiotic combination VSLd3 and placebo in irritable bowel syndrome with bloating. *Neurogastroenterology and Motility, 17*(5), 687–696.

135. Gaudier, E., Michel, C., Segain, J. P., et al. (2005). The VSLd 3 probiotic mixture modifies microflora but does not heal chronic dextran-sodium sulfate-induced colitis or reinforce the mucus barrier in mice. *The Journal of Nutrition, 135*(12), 2753–2761.

136. Camilleri, M. (2006). Probiotics and irritable bowel syndrome: Rationale, putative mechanisms, and evidence of clinical efficacy. *Journal of Clinical Gastroenterology, 40*(3), 264–269.

137. Kajander, K., Myllyluoma, E., Rajilić-Stojanović, M., et al. (2008). Clinical trial: multispecies probiotic supplementation alleviates the symptoms of irritable bowel syndrome and stabilizes intestinal microbiota. *Alimentary Pharmacology & Therapeutics, 27*(1), 48–57.

138. Kalliomäki, M., Salminen, S., Arvilommi, H., et al. (2001). Probiotics in primary prevention of atopic disease: A randomised placebo-controlled trial. *Lancet, 357,* 1076–1079.

139. Kalliomäki, M., Salminen, S., Poussa, T., et al. (2003). Probiotics and prevention of atopic disease: 4-year follow-up of a randomised placebo-controlled trial. *Lancet, 361*(9372), 1869–1871.

140. Kukkonen, K., Savilahti, E., Haahtela, T., et al. (2007). Probiotics and prebiotic galacto-oligosaccharides in the prevention of allergic diseases: A randomized, double-blind, placebo-controlled trial. *The Journal of Allergy and Clinical Immunology, 119*(1), 192–198.

141. Nybom, S., Collado, M. C., Surono, I., et al. (2008). Effect of glucose in removal of microcystin-LR by commercial probiotic strains and strains isolated from dadih fermented milk. *Journal of Agricultural and Food Chemistry, 56*(10), 3714–3720.

142. Nybom, S. M., Salminen, S. J., & Meriluoto, J. A. (2008). Specific strains of probiotic bacteria are efficient in removal of several different cyanobacterial toxins from solution. *Toxicon, 52*(2), 214–220.

143. Halttunen, T., Finell, M., & Salminen, S. (2007). Arsenic removal by native and chemically modified lactic acid bacteria. *International Journal of Food Microbiology, 120*(1–2), 173–1178.

144. Halttunen, T., Collado, M. C., El-Nezami, H., et al. (2008). Mixing of lactic acid bacteria strains may reduce their toxin removal efficiency from aqueous solution. *Letters in Applied Microbiology, 46*(2), 160–165.

24

Probiotics and Fungal Colonization of Gastrointestinal Tract

Malgorzata Zwolinska-Wcislo[1], Tomasz Mach[1], and Alicja Budak[2]

[1]Department of Gastroenterology and Hepatology, Jagiellonian University, Medical College, Krakow, Poland

[2]Department of Pharmaceutical Microbiology, Jagiellonian University, Medical College, Krakow, Poland

1. INTRODUCTION

The human gastrointestinal (GI) tract constitutes the second body surface area (250–450 m^2). It includes rich microflora of more than 500 species, which makes around 10^{14} microorganisms living in the whole GI tract from the oral cavity area to the colon. These proximal and distal parts of the GI tract are the most densely colonized areas [1, 2]. GI microflora establishes during human life through time-dependent phases. This process starts after birth, when newborns are colonized by flora derived from their mothers. After a few weeks, it resembles the adult microbial flora and becomes relatively constant in adult age [1, 3].

Normal human microflora constitutes the complex ecosystem including aerobic and aneorobic microorganisms. The stomach is inhabited mainly by Gram-positive and aerobic bacteria represented by such species as *Streptococci, Staphylococci, Lactobacilli* and various fungi found in concentrations not exceeding 10^3 cfu/mL [3]. The microflora of the proximal small intestine resembles that in the stomach area. The bacteria species are dominated by Gram-positive, aerobic microorganisms. The bacterial concentration is 10^3–10^4 cfu/mL [3]. In the distal ileum, Gram-negative bacteria predominance is observed. Anaerobic bacterial species, such as *Bacteroides, Bifidobacterium, Fusobacterium* and *Clostridium* are found in substantial concentrations in that region [3]. Distally to the ileocecal sphincter, bacterial concentration increases significantly. Its concentration in the colon reaches 10^{11}–10^{12} cfu/mL. Anaerobes outnumber aerobic species by a factor of 10^2–10^4 [3]. Nearly one-third of the fecal dry weight consists of viable bacteria [3]. The most frequently isolated bacterial strains include the *Bacteroides, Bifidobacterium* and *Eubacterium*

TABLE 24.1   Prevalence of fungi in the gastrointestinal tract

Part of gastrointestinal (GI) tract, fungal species isolated from GI tract		Prevalence of fungi	Reference
Oral cavity	*Candida*	52–62%	[8]
		75% in elderly population	[10]
Stomach	*Candida* sp.	31.3%	[8]
	C. albicans,		[1]
	C. kruzei		
	C. tropicalis		[12]
	C. glabrata		
	C. lusitaniae		
	Saccharomyces sp.		[13]
Intestine	*Candida* sp.	23.1% healthy people	[1]
		38.8% IBD	[8]
Colon	*Candida* sp.	1.3% irritable bowel disease	[14]
		13.8–33.3% IBD	

species. Among anaerobic Gram-positive cocci, *Peptococci* and *Peptostreptococci* are isolated. *Clostridia*, *Enterococci* and *Enterobactriaceae* are also common [3].

Fungi are important but small fractions of human GI tract microflora. Still little is known about the composition of commensal fungal species in this region [4]. Among the yeasts, *Candida* (*C.*) dominates as a genus [1]. Some *Candida* species are not always found in different GI tract locations, so they are considered as transient flora [1]. There are reports that some *C. albicans* strains inhabit GI tract. They are based on equal strain specific characteristics of *Candida* isolated from babies and their mothers. This finding favors consideration that *C. albicans* is part of the resident GI tract microflora [1]. It is also the most prevalent fungal species isolated from that region. The *Candida* genus is comprised of about 150 fungal species, assigned to the family of deuteromycetes [5]. Some *Candida* species, such as *C. albicans*, *C. tropicalis*, *C. parapsilosis*, *C. kruzei*, *C. kefyr*, *C. glabrata*, *C. guilliermondi*, *C. lusitaniae* and *C. colliculosa* are isolated from the GI tract [1, 6, 7].

The prevalence of *Candida* in the GI tract is given in Table 24.1. Oral cavity is inhabited by yeasts mainly colonizing the surface of the tongue, palate and jaws, and is age-dependent. Carriage of *Candida* is considered as a function of the aging process [8]. *Candida* species were isolated from oral cavity in 58.3% of all cases. In people aged over 60 years *Candida* species were isolated in 52–62% of cases [1, 9]. It was isolated in 75% from oral cavities in the elderly Finnish population [10]. *Candida* colonization in the upper GI tract was reported in 31.3% of cases [8]. The main fungal species in the stomach included *C. albicans*, *C. kruzei* and *C. tropicalis*. The first two fungal species were isolated independently on the gastric acidity and were able to multiply in a pH of 2.0 [1]. *C. tropicalis* was seen more frequently in non-acidic milieu. In a pH >3.0, the *C. glabrata* and *Saccharomyces* species were also found in the stomach [1]. Previously, it was generally accepted that bacterial and yeasts overgrowth was not possible in gastric pH <4.0 [11] (Table 24.1).

Results from both *in vitro* and *in vivo* studies revealed that a variety of bacteria and yeasts are able to survive and multiply in environments as low as pH 3.0 [11]. Fluorescence microscopy investigation demonstrated the elongation of yeasts and bacterial cells at pH <5.0, as indicative of a stress response to the increasingly acidic conditions. Also, invasive fungal forms, pseudohyphae were found to be protruding to the region of bacterial colonies and aggregated with bacteria, especially *Streptococci* [11]. Results from our own studies revealed that significant fungal colonization >10^4 cfu/mL was found in 54.2% of gastric ulcer patients and 10.3% of patients with chronic gastritis compared to the control group: 4.3%. The most frequently isolated fungal species from gastric ulcers were *C. glabrata* (42.4%), *C. albicans* (38.7%); and from the stomach of chronic gastritis patients these were *C. albicans* (41.1%), *C. glabrata* (32.9%) [12]. Our *in vitro* studies on the growth of fungal strains isolated from patients with ulcer diseases and chronic gastritis in variable acidity from pH 2–8 revealed differences between the *C. albicans* and *C. tropicalis* strains, which started to grow in an acidic pH as low as 2.0, whereas *C. lusitaniae* strains started to grow from pH 3 [13].

Intestine. *Candida* species were isolated from the duodenal juice in 23.1% of healthy people. About one-third of patients with different GI diseases were colonized with *C. albicans*, *C. tropicalis* and *C. glabrata* [1]. In 38.8% of patients with inflammatory bowel diseases (IBD), fungi were found in the proximal GI tract [8].

Colon. Our previous studies revealed significant fungal colonization in 13.8–33.3% of patients with ulcerative colitis depending on the duration of disease, less and more than 5 years respectively, in comparison to irritable bowel syndrome (1.3%) [14].

1.1. Factors Influencing the GI Microflora

The prevalence of commensal microflora in GI tract in certain parts of the GI tract depends on different environmental factors including pH, motility, synergism or antagonism of microbiota

TABLE 24.2 Factors influencing the GI tract microflora

	Source
GI peristalsis	[8]
Gastric pH	[11]
Bacterial antagonism	[8]
Mucins secretion	
Age	[8]
Stress	[10]
Shortage of nutrients	
Enteral starvation within the use of parenteral nutrition	[2]
Hospitalization	[2]
Medications (antibiotics, immune-suppression)	[2]

species, age, nutrition, infections, stress, hospitalization and treatment [3, 8] (Table 24.2). Diet seems to play a role in the composition of microflora in GI tract [2]. Newborns fed with artificial food instead of being breast-fed, presented a decreased GI tract colonization with *Lactobacilli* and *Bifidobacteria* in contrast to elevated counts of *Enterococci*, *Coliformis* or *Clostridia* [2]. Fungal overgrowth is a common problem in the elderly. In this group, it appears to be associated with chronic diseases, medications, poor oral hygiene, reduced salivary flow and impairment of the immune system [10]. Stress is known to influence the composition and activity of GI tract microflora. During stress, but also enteral starvation, increased bacterial adherence to the GI tract mucosa and virulence of microbiota is observed [2]. Shortage of nutrients or enteral starvation within the use of parenteral nutrition influences the composition of intestinal microflora by reduction of *Lactobacilli*, replacing it with potentially pathogenic microorganisms [2]. Hospitalization of patients may favor GI tract colonization by specific *Escherichia* (E.) *coli* strains as well as *Clostridium difficile* associated with certain medical institutions [3]. Moreover, antibiotics may alter the GI tract microflora in a dose-dependent manner and antimicrobial spectrum [3]. Other factors that influence the GI tract microorganism composition include gastric acidity, intestinal peristalsis, immune host status, synergism and antagonism of the GI microflora, and hygiene standards. Also, chronic disorders like diabetes mellitus, alcoholism or neoplasms may affect the dynamic balance between host and physiological microflora [3, 8]. It is already known that the ecosystem of the commensal microflora in the GI tract plays an important role in preventing translocation of pathogenic microorganisms and endotoxins and makes a vital facet of the intestinal barrier mechanism [8].

2. ASPECTS OF FUNGAL PRESENCE IN THE GASTROINTESTINAL TRACT

There are a few aspects of *Candida* present in the GI tract:

1. *C. albicans* is one of the few eukaryotic microorganisms capable of achieving a non-pathogenic existence in the human GI tract and constitutes part of normal human microflora without causing illness [1, 6].
2. Fungal overgrowth may become an important risk factor in the development of dissemination.
3. An excessive increase of fungi may cause or influence different GI tract diseases [1].
4. *Candida* colonization may promote sensitization against food antigens, probably in the mechanism of affecting the mucosal barrier via release of proteinase 1 and TNF-α from mast cells [6, 14].
5. Bacterial (fungal) host interactions within the GI tract.

3. RISK FACTORS OF FUNGAL COLONIZATION

Major risk factors associated with the development of invasive candidiasis include [7]:

- usage of broad spectrum antibiotics for over 2 weeks;
- corticosteroid therapy;
- central intravenous devices (mainly Hickman catheters);
- parenteral nutrition;
- ongoing invasive ventilation over 10 days;
- fungal colonization of more than two body regions;
- haemodialysis;
- recurrent GI perforations;
- surgery for the acute pancreatitis;
- a high APACHE score >20;
- acute renal failure;
- neutropenia;
- a duration stay at an intensive care unit >9 days;
- an extensive requirement of blood transfusions.

The colonization of central venous catheters and of multiple areas is considered as the independent risk factor of invasive fungal infections in already colonized neonates [15]. A case-control study at the Cardio Thoracic Intensive Care Unit in Greece revealed that APACHE II score >30 at candidemia onset predicted *Candida* related deaths. Besides independent candidemia, predictors included ongoing invasive mechanical ventilation, for longer than 10 days, diabetes mellitus, cardiopulmonary bypass duration >120 min, hospital-acquired bacterial infection and/or bacteriemia [7]. *C. parapsilosis* fungemia was associated with lower mortality rates than non-parapsilosis candidemia [7].

Epidemiology: Disseminated candidiasis is no longer a solely characteristic disease of immunocompromised people, such as neutropenic patients. The incidence of disseminated candidiasis is growing [16]. *Candida* species are the third most frequent agent of late-onset in preterm neonates, with estimated incidence of 1.6–9% [16]. *Candida* colonization is the most important predictor of invasive diseases in this group of patients [16]. It is also an important enteric reservoir of fungal dissemination [17]. The colonization rate of intensive care units by *Candida* species ranges from 2.5–6% of cases, reaching 17% in EPIC study [16].

Disseminated candidiasis at one intensive care unit was 20.4% of all infections in a Cisterna study [7]. The mortality directly attributable to the infection itself ranged from 22–38% [15]. According to the Centers for Disease Control and Prevention, *Candida* species caused 8% of hospital-acquired bloodstream infections [7]. It independently influences the outcome of nosocomial bloodstream infection (odds ratio for mortality: 1:84) [7]. In a large 1-day point prevalence study (EPIC study) from Europe consisting of 1,317 patients from an intensive care unit, fungi was the fifth leading pathogen among the most frequently reported microorganisms: 17.1% [7]. Nosocomial candidiasis with primarily candidemia can vary between 3–15%, depending on the hospital [7].

4. FUNGI AND INTESTINAL MUCOSA INTERACTION

Pathogenesis of the fungal colonization of the GI tract mucosa is complex and involves yeast and host interaction (Fig. 24.1). The interaction between adherence, clearance, colonization and fungal-host immune competence determines different states of yeast existence within the GI tract:

1. Low level asymptomatic existence among bacterial microflora.
2. Mucosal candidiasis resulting from fungal overgrowth.
3. Tissue invasion observed in the immunocompetent as well as in the immunodeficient host [5, 15].

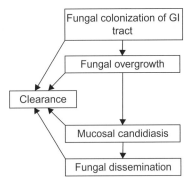

FIGURE 24.1 States of host fungus interaction within the gastrointestinal tract. Fungal colonization, fungal overgrowth, mucosal candidiasis, fungal dissemination.

Fungal colonization of the GI tract mucosa is the result of an impaired balance between external forces that limit the microbial overgrowth—such as the effects of the host immune system and intrinsic factors, including the ability of the organism to increase the number of fungi. The combined effects of the regulatory interactions maintain the balance between healthy colonization and disease [18].

4.1. Factors Contributing to Fungal Colonization of the GI Tract

Adherence of *Candida* to the human GI tract mucosa is an important pathogenic factor. It is required for the yeast colonization and contributes to persistence within the host [5]. Fungal colonization is a risk factor of the yeast dissemination [6]. Biasoli et al. found significant differences between certain *Candida* strain adherence capacities and their ability to colonize mucosal surfaces [6]. Microarray studies analyzing interactions between *C. albicans* and cultured immune cells revealed significant changes in the *C. albicans* metabolism and stress responses [19]. Studies on the antigens expressed during oral fungal infections revealed the expression of components of mitogen-activated protein (MAP) kinase transduction pathway signals, as well as

TABLE 24.3　Host defense antifungal mechanisms and factors determining mucosal candidiasis and fungal dissemination

Host defense antifungal mechanisms	Factors determining mucosal candidiasis and fungal dissemination
1. Primary defense mechanisms: mucus covering GI mucosa, mucosal barrier, defensins, secretory IgA, mucins [5].	1. Adherence to human GI tract mucosa [5].
2. Second line anti-*Candida* protection: neutrophils, eosinophils, monocytes [5].	2. Morphogenesis [5].
3. Cell-mediated immunity. Secretion of cytokines, TNF-α, IL-13 [5].	3. Hydrolytic enzymes: aspartic proteinases, lipases, phospholipases [5, 20].
4. Humoral immunity [1, 21, 23].	4. Genes encoding virulence factors: HEX1, SAP 1–4, LIP 1–10 [50]. ECE1, RBT1, RBT4 [19].

of protein Not5, required for systemic virulence [19]. Experiments on Rockland mice, orally inoculated with a suspension of yeasts, revealed that the most adherent yeasts (*C. albicans* strain) persisted longer (over 8 weeks), while less adherent *Candida* strains were eliminated from the mice GI tract within 10 days [6]. Such fungal strains as *C. albicans*, *C. tropicalis* and *C. parapsilosis* were the most frequently isolated from the human GI tract and remained in it longer at the same time [6]. *C. albicans* expresses adhesions that recognize extracellular matrix proteins, including laminin, collagen, fibrinogen, fibronectin and entactin [5]. Some surface proteins of *Candida* cell demonstrate similarity to the mammalian integrins αMβ2, αXβ2 and -5β1 [5]. The composition of *C. albicans* cell surface is dynamic (Table 24.3). *In vitro* and *in vivo* studies revealed *C. albicans* cell surface modulations dependent on the environmental factors [5]. These surface changes enable a commensal yeast strain to escape the immune surveillance [5]. Changes in surface protein glucosylation may expose hydrophobic protein structures at the cell surface and influence adherence properties [5]. *In vitro* studies demonstrated the influence of changing environmental factors on the *C. albicans* morphogenesis, which means the

switching of the *Candida* colony morphology from non-pathogenic yeast to hyphal (invasive) and pathogenic forms [5]. The hyphal form exhibits increased adherence properties, which correlate with increased expression of the α5β1-like fibronectin receptor in cells forming hyphae [5]. It also displays certain proteins that are absent or masked in the yeast form [5].

Hydrolytic enzymes, secreted by *Candida* strains, include phospholipase, hexosaminidase, aspartic proteinases and lipases, and determine their virulence. Proteinases are secreted by the most pathogenic *Candida* species, such as *C. albicans*, *C. tropicalis* and *C. parapsilosis* and demonstrates the broad spectrum specificity [5]. They seem to be involved in the degradation of mucins, which are mucosal protective glycoproteins [20]. In comparison to bacterial enzymes, the role of fungal lipases is not fully explained [21]. Bacterial lipases are involved in disrupting tissues, providing nutrients. They play an important role in modulating the immune response and inhibiting monocyte and granulocyte chemotaxis in *in vitro* studies [21]. There are some reports indicating the contribution of fungal lipases during fungal colonization [21]. The lipase genes were expressed during systemic infection and during *in vitro* infection of reconstituted human epithelial cells [21]. *C. albicans* colonization and subsequent lipase expression resulted in significant chemokine MIP-2 and KC expression performed by gene analysis, based on gene disruption, that specifically inactivated one or more genes [21]. Genes encoding virulence factors were identified, such as the hexosaminidase gene (HEX1), several genes encoding aspartic proteinases (SAP 1–4), and the lipase genes family (LIP) 1–10 [5, 21]. LIP gene expression was observed during fungal colonization at infected mucosal sites. LIP 1, 3 and 9 expressions were detected in colonized gastric tissue in a mouse model of mucosal candidiasis. The LIP 2 gene expression seemed to be important for GI tract colonization [21]. White et al. reported expression of the EFH1 gene, which regulates fungal colonization, favoring commensalisms as opposed to candidiasis [18]. It encodes the altered expression of several cell surface proteins, which may be important in fungal colonization. Expression of the Efh1p gene may influence the interaction between colonizing *C. albicans* and the altered adherence to the mucosal surface [18]. Genes ECE1, RBT1 and RBT4 expression is linked to hyphal morphogenesis [18]. Genes encoding enzymes involved in the glyoxylate cycle are highly expressed in phagocytosed fungal cells and isocitrate lyase seems to be important for systemic virulence [18]. The analysis of *C. albicans* cells invading host parenchymal tissue revealed changes in the expression of numerous genes, demonstrating that invading cells show metabolic changes and initiate responses to stresses such as iron limitation [18]. Genes that influence commensal colonization can be distinct from genes that are required for virulence [18].

4.2. Host Defense Mechanisms

The host immune defense system, together with an ecologically balanced GI microflora and physical barrier of a healthy intestinal mucosa, comprises the defense mechanisms that inhibit *C. albicans* translocation from the GI tract [22] (Table 24.3).

The primary defense mechanisms include mucus covering GI mucosa, the mucosal barrier of the GI tract, defensins with broad-spectrum antimicrobial activity, expressed in epithelium surrounding oral lesions, secretory immunoglobulin (Ig) A, which is involved in the yeast aggregation and clearance [5]. The major structural components of mucus are mucins, high molecular weight glycoproteins produced by the goblet cells of the surface epithelium. They may protect epithelial cells from microbial: bacterial and fungal microorganisms adherence, colonization, toxin delivery and invasion [20, 23]. Moreover, candidacidal properties of saliva have been described [5]. Increasing frequency of *Candida* colonization of mucosal surfaces in the elderly could be explained with hyposalivation in this group of patients [5, 11]. Nitrates contained in the saliva are converted into nitrite by oral facultative anaerobes, including *Lactobacilli* on the tongue. When swallowed, nitrite that are converted to nitric oxide (NO) are reported to exert antimicrobial effect in the stomach [11]. The second line anti-*Candida* defense is provided by phagocytes [5]. Neutrophils, eosinophils and monocytes are involved in the phagocytosis of yeasts and hyphal forms of *C. albicans*. The *Candida* surface mannoproteins are able to modulate phagocyte responses [5]. Cell-mediated immunity plays a central role in regulating immune responses to *C. albicans* by secreting cytokines that modulate the development and activity of immune effectors [22]. The account of granulocytes, NK cells, mast cells and macrophages play important roles in candidacidal activity [10]. Tumor necrosis factor (TNF)-α is highly sensitive to fungal colonization. Interleukin (IL)-1β is released into the GI tract mucosa by lamina propria activated immune cells during inflammation. IL-1β induced mucin release in the mouse duodenum [22]. Coste et al. demonstrated that IL-13 attenuated *C. albicans* colonization [24]. Humoral immunity plays a lesser role in the defense against *Candida* [5].

5. CLINICAL APPLICATIONS OF PROBIOTICS

5.1. Mechanisms of Probiotic Activity

The best protection against *Candida* colonization is the normal bacterial flora [1]. Probiotic therapy for the control and prophylaxis of intestinal candidiasis could be the alternative treatment since it avoids the adverse effects of antifungal antibiotics and diminishes the costs of antifungal therapy [25]. Probiotic definition is derived from the Greek word (pro-bios) and means 'supporting or favoring life' [26]. According to the Food and Agriculture Organization of the United Nations World Health Organization, probiotics are defined as live microorganisms which, when consumed in adequate amounts as part of food, confer a health benefit on the host [26]. These living microorganisms are able to survive in the stomach acid and bile, maintain viability throughout extended periods of storage, and are safe for human consumption [27].

It has been suggested that probiotic bacteria are promising agents for the treatment of gastrointestinal barrier disorders, including infectious colitis, antibiotic-associated diarrhea and IBD [4]. They are widely applied in the lactulose intolerance, acute gastritis and enteritis such as: acute diarrhea, traveler's diarrhea, postantibiotic diarrhea, IBD, allergies, pseudomembranous colitis, irritable bowel syndrome [28]. The clinical applications for protiotics are:

- lactose intolerance;
- gastroenteritis: acute diarrhea, antibiotic-induced diarrhea, traveler's diarrhea;
- allergies;
- inflammatory bowel disease;
- irritable bowel syndrome;
- *Clostridium difficile*-induced colitis.

5.2. Probiotics and Fungal Interaction

Antifungal activity of probiotics is given in Table 24.4. GI tract microflora plays an important role in the pathophysiology of non-specific intestinal inflammations, like ulcerative colitis or pouchitis which is a complication after ileal pouch anal anastomosis, after restorative proctocolectomy performed in patients with ulcerative colitis [4]. Predominance of potentially harmful bacteria, and the decrease of beneficial species such as *Lactobacillus* and *Bifidobacterium*, were found in patients with IBD. Establishing normal microbial-host interactions is important for host health [26]. Molecular techniques, like fluorescent *in situ* hybridization (FISH) revealed that pouchitis was associated with the loss of beneficial intestinal bacteria, especially *Lactobacilli* and *Bifidobacteria* and fall of diversity of bacterial strains. Beneficial effects of probiotic treatment with VSL#3 resulted in the maintenance of remission and the increase of diversity of bacterial strains and restoration of *Enterobacteriaceae* species, mainly *E. coli* [4]. Fungal strains diversity seemed to be inversely related to bacterial diversity. Fungal overgrowth is considered as the consequence of the imbalance between bacterial strains, following the antibiotic therapy or dietary regimen as, for example, in intensive care units. It seems to be closely related to bacterial imbalance, associated with impaired control mechanisms and reduced competition between bacterial microbiota [4]. Molecular analysis of the fungal microflora with denaturating gradient gel electrophoresis (DGGE) method revealed increased strains diversity in the active phase of pouchitis. Administration of VSL#3 probiotic preparation consisting of four strains of *Lactobacilli* (*acidophilus, bulgaricus, casei, plantarum*), three strains of *Bifidobacteria* (*breve, infantis, longum*) and *Streptococcus thermophilus*, maintained remission of pouchitis, which was accompanied with the reduction of fungal diversity and an increase of bacterial diversity in comparison with placebo treatments

TABLE 24.4 The effect of probiotic species on the fungal colonization of GI tract

Probiotic species	Effect of fungal colonization of GI tract	Reference
VSL#3	↓ of fungal diversity, ↑of bacterial diversity	[4]
	↓ of fungal overgrowth	
	↑ of mucin expression	[25]
	↑ of mucosal barrier	
	↑ IL-10	
	Maintenance of the remission of pouchitis.	[4]
Lactobacilli	Production of lactic and acetic acid	[29]
	Bacteriocins and antifungal substances synthesis	
	↑ adherence to mucosal epithelium	
	Competition of adhesion of *Candida* sp.	
	Over-expression of MUC3 mucin gene and	[22]
	↑ production of protective mucins.	
L. casei	↓ TNF induced cytokines, chemokines.	[25]
L. acidophilus	Production of H_2O_2	[32]
	↑ IL-4, ↑ IL-12, ↑ IFN-γ, ↑ NO	
	Enhanced *C. albicans* clearance	
	↓ IL-1β, ↓ TNF-α.	[12]
L. fermentum	Effect similar to *L. acidophilus* but less expressed.	
LGG	↑ mucosal IgA response	[16]
	↑ mucosal barrier	
	↓ mucosal permeability.	[25]
LGG	Modifies fungal GI ecology.	[25]
L. coryniformis	Production of antifungal substances.	[29]
L. plantarum	Production of phenyllactic and 4-hydroxyphanullactic acid	[30]
	Production of low-molecular weight substances:	
	benzoic acid, methyhydantoin, mevalonolactone	
	Production of cyclic dipeptides	[29]
	Generation of NO (improvement of motility, circulation and mucus secretion)	[2]
	Inhibition of fungal growth.	
L. acidophilus NCTH strain	Better protection of immunodeficient mice from systemic candidiasis compared with *L. acidophilus* LA-1 strain	[33]
	↑ of mice survival, suppression of weight loss,	
	↓ fungal dissemination.	
L. acidophilus LA-1 strain	Better protection of immunodeficient mice from orogastric candidiasis compared with *L. acidophilus* NCFM strain.	[33]
Bifidobacterium (B.) species	↑ antibodies to *C. albicans*	[34]
	↓ fungal dissemination	
	Suppression of weight loss	
	↓ of fungal overgrowth.	
B. infantis	More effective in antibodies production than *B. lactis*.	[34]
B. lactis	Better protection from GI candidiasis from *B. infantis*.	[34]
B. animalis	↑ inflammatory response	[28]
	↑ of polymorphonuclear cells, macrophages and lymphocytes	
	↓ of fungal overgrowth	
	↑ of T cell dependent IgA, IgG antibodies.	[34]
Saccharomyces (S.) boulardii	↓ IL-1 β, ↓ TNF-α	[21]
	↓ of inflammation intensity	
	↓ of translocation of *Candida* to mesenteric lymphnodes, liver and kidneys of immunosuppressed rats	
	↓ of GI tract fungal colonization.	

[4, 7]. Probiotic species including *Lactobacilli*, *Bifidobacteria*, *E. coli* Nissle 1917 (a non-pathogenic *E. coli* strain), *Saccharomyces boulardii*, VSL#3 are capable of modifying the microbial balance within the GI tract by reducing the overgrowth of pathogens, such as *Candida*, in different mechanisms and with different strengths [10, 26, 29]. The mechanisms that enable probiotics to maintain the GI tract microbial balance include: production of bacteriocin-like substances, competitive inhibition of pathogen and toxin adherence to the intestinal epithelium, colonization of the GI tract mucosa and reduction of the fungal overgrowth, stimulation of the mucosal and systemic immune systems, enhancing host innate immunity, increase of anti-inflammatory and suppression of pro-inflammatory cytokine production [15, 26, 29] (Table 24.4).

Lactobacilli

Certain *Lactobacilli* species are currently used as probiotics. They were evaluated for their antifungal activity in several clinical trials and experimental models. *Lactobacilli* strains vary in their capacities for host protection from infectious diseases [29]. The antimicrobial effect of *Lactobacilli* is related mainly to the production of lactic and acetic acids, but for some strains, synthesis of bacteriocins seems to be important [30]. There are many reports on the production of antibacterial substances by *Lactobacilli*, but reports on the yeast inhibition are few. Production of proteinaceous antifungal substance by *Lactobacillus coryniformis* was described [30]. Lavermicocca et al. reported isolation of the antifungal substance, phenyllactic acid and 4-hydroxyphenyllactic acid from *Lactobacillus plantarum* strains [31]. Oral supplementation with *Lactobacillus casei* subspecies *rhamnosus* (LGG) resulted in a significant reduction of gastrointestinal *Candida* colonization in the very low birth weight neonates given LGG [17]. The potential mechanism by which LGG modifies fungal ecology in the GI tract includes competitive exclusion of fungi, reduction in their ability to colonize the GI mucosa via enhanced mucosal IgA responses, as well as changes in intestinal permeability and increased gut mucosa barrier to fungi and modification of the host response to fungal products [17]. Certain *Lactobacilli* strains can adhere to the mucosal epithelium and thereby compete for adhesion sites with *Candida* [31]. Part of vaginal *Lactobacillus* strains demonstrated higher surface hydrophobicity. Moreover, *Lactobacillus* strains showed high to moderate abilities to adhere to vaginal cells. Selected strains inhibited the growth of *C. albicans* [31]. Most *Lactobacilli* were able to inhibit the growth of *C. pseudotropicalis*. Another antifungal activity of *Lactobacillus* strains is the production of H_2O_2.

It was postulated that anti-candidal activity is based on the production of hypothiocyanate from H_2O_2 [32]. Production of a broad spectrum of antifungal substances by *Lactobacillus plantarum*, isolated from grass silage, was reported by Ström et al. [30]. Fungal inhibitory substances isolated from *Lactobacillus plantarum* were identified as 3-phenyllactic acid and cyclic dipeptides [30]. *Lactobacillus plantarum* produce fungus inhibitory low molecular-weight substances, such as benzoic acid, methylhydantoin, mevalonolactone and cyclo-(Gly-L-Leu). These antifungal cyclic peptides inhibited *in vitro Candida* growth [30]. The unique feature of *Lactobacillus plantarum* is its ability to catabolize arginine and generate NO [2]. It has the ability to degrade arginine to NO on six different pathways [2]. This function is interrupted by antibiotic treatment [2]. The administration of antibiotics such as neomycin, bacitracin, polymyxin B is known to reduce activity of intraluminal enzymes such as lysine, ornithine and arginine decarboxylases [2]. NO released within the GI tract by constitutive enzymes (NO synthase) is involved in a series of important GI tract functions, such as bacteriostasis, mucus secretion, motility regulation, splanchnic circulation and stimulation of the GI immune functions [2]. Acidified nitrate in the stomach as an NO donor plays an important role in the control of *C. albicans* growth [2, 11]. *In vitro* studies performed by Mack et al. revealed that *Lactobacillus plantarum* and *rhamnosus* species enhanced the protection of the intestinal mucosal surface by inhibiting the adherence of the enteropathogenic *E. coli* strain (EPEC) to mucin producing intestinal epithelial cells. Moreover, the adherence of *Lactobacilli* species to intestinal epithelial cells with subsequent over-expression of MUC3 mucin gene and protective mucin production was observed [23]. Elahi et al. evaluated the clearance of *C. albicans* from oral cavities of mice following oral administration of *Lactobacillus acidophilus* and *Lactobacillus fermentum* isolates. *Lactobacilli* significantly shortened the duration of *Candida* colonization in the oral cavity of mice [33]. Enhanced *C. albicans* clearance from the oral cavities correlated with increased secretion of interleukin (IL)-4 from stimulated T cells and enhanced the Th1 response characterized by production of IL-12 and IFN-γ, stimulated with *Candida* antigen [33]. Rapid clearance of fungi correlated with higher levels of IFN-γ and NO in saliva [33]. The limitation of oral colonization by *C. albicans* did not involve direct interference by *Lactobacillus acidophilus*, as the live probiotic bacteria was administered into the stomach. There were differences between probiotic strains in the induction of mucosal protection. *Lactobacillus acidophilus* isolate was more effective than *Lactobacillus fermentum* in terms of protection and local production of IL-4, NO and IFN-γ [33]. In our own studies, we compared the effect of *Candida* and vehicle gastric inoculation on gastric secretion and the healing process of gastric ulcers induced by acetic acid in rats, with or without intragastric administration of *Lactobacillus acidophilus*. Fungal colonization of the stomach resulted in the fall of gastric acid output and up-regulation of mRNA for IL-1β, TNF-α in the gastric tissue as well as in the serum [12]. Probiotic bacteria vary in their capacity to protect hosts from infectious diseases. Wagner et al. demonstrated the differences in the capacity to protect immunodeficient mice bg/bg–nu/nu and bg/bg–nu/+ from candidiasis between two isolates of *Lactobacillus acidophilus*: NCFM and LA-1 [34]. *Lactobacillus acidophilus* NCFM isolate prolonged mice survival, inhibited disseminated candidiasis, and suppressed weight loss associated with *C. albicans* infection, but did not decrease the severity or the incidence of orogastric fungal colonization in gnobiotic mice [34]. *Lactobacillus acidophilus* LA-1 isolate suppressed *C. albicans* growth in the GI tract, and reduced the severity of mucosal candidiasis, but did not improve the survival rate [34]. In conclusion, *Lactobacillus acidophilus* NCFM provided better protection of immunodeficient mice from systemic endogenous candidiasis than LA-1 isolate. *Lactobacillus acidophilus* LA-1 was better able to protect the mice from mucosal orogastric candidiasis than *Lactobacillus acidophilus* NCFM [34]. Comparison of the antifungal activity of four examined probiotic strains (*Lactobacillus acidophilus*, *Lactobacillus reuteri* and *Lactobacillus casei* GG or *Bifidobacterium animalis*) demonstrated that all examined bacteria in the GI tract prolonged the survival and reduced systemic candidiasis of the athymic adult or neonatal in mice compared with mice colonized only with *C. albicans* alone [29]. *Lactobacillus casei* and *Bifidobacterium animalis* significantly reduced the numbers of *C. albicans* in the GI tract. *Lactobacillus acidophilus* and *Bifidobacterium animalis* enhanced the inflammatory response consisting of polymorphonuclear, macrophages and lymphocytes infiltrates. None of the examined probiotic bacteria provided complete protection against candidiasis [29]. *Bifidobacterium animalis* reduced the severity of candidiasis [29].

Bifidobacterium

The *Bifidobacterium* species holds much promise for providing benefits to the host. These include the protection of neonatal animals from pathogenic viruses, bacteria and fungi, production of promoting factors for the host, providing adjuvant activity for antigens of pathogenic bacteria [35]. *Bifidobacterium animalis* presents a unique capacity to stimulate T cell dependent IgA and IgG antibodies, possibly via the thymus and mucosa tissue-associated lymphoid tissues [29]. Comparison of two *Bifidobacterium* species, *Bifidobacterium infantis* and *Bifidobacterium lactis*, demonstrated that both species prolonged the survival of *C. albicans* colonized adult and neonatal mice. The *Bifidobacteria* influenced production of antibodies to *C. albicans*, inhibited disseminated candidiasis, suppressed weight loss caused by *C. albicans* infection, inhibited the growth of *C. albicans* in the alimentary tract, inhibited systemic candidiasis of endogenous origin and decreased the severity of gastric candidiasis in mice [35]. However, *Bifidobacterium infantis* was more effective in the suppression of disseminated candidiasis [35]; this could be explained by the more effective ability of *Bifidobacterium infantis* to induce antibody production in comparison with *Bifidobacterium lactis* [34], whereas *Bifidobacterium lactis* protected mice from gastric candidiasis better than *Bifidobacterium infantis* [35].

Saccharomyces boulardii is a thermophilic, non-pathogenic yeast; administered orally comprises efficacy in the treatment of acute gastrointestinal infections and antibiotic-associated diarrhea. Oral administration of *Saccharomyces boulardii* was found to inhibit *C. albicans* translocation to the mesenteric lymph nodes, liver and kidneys in immunosuppressed rats by reducing the gastrointestinal levels of *C. albicans* [22]. It also decreased serum levels of pro-inflammatory cytokines: IL-1β and TNF-α [22]. *Saccharomyces boulardii* treatment significantly decreased intensity of inflammation in the lamina propria of colon [22].

6. CONCLUSION

Gastrointestinal tract contains around 500 microbial species. Fungi are a small part of the intestinal microbiota. Many factors such as stress of modern life, reduced physical activity, processed foods, antibiotic therapies, as well as prolonged adaptation of human genes to dynamic changes in the lifestyle, seem to derange the host–microflora interplay and contribute to the development of inflammatory and/or infectious diseases. This process could be attenuated by probiotics. The mechanism that enables probiotics to maintain the balance within the intestine includes production of bacteriocin-like substances, inhibition of pathogens and toxin adherence to the intestinal epithelium, and reduction of the fungal overgrowth.

References

1. Bernhardt, H., & Knoke, M. (1997). Mycological aspects of gastrointestinal microflora. *Scandinavian Journal of Gastroenterology, 32*(222), 102–106.
2. Bengmark, S. (1998). Ecological control of the gastrointestinal tract. The role of probiotic flora. *Gut, 42*, 2–7.
3. Linskens, R. K., Huijedens, X. W., Savelkoul, P. H., et al. (2001). The bacterial flora in inflammatory bowel disease: current insights in pathogenesis and the influence of antibiotics and probiotics. *Scandinavian Journal of Gastroenterology, 234*, 29–40.
4. Kühbacher, T., Ott, S. J., Helwig, U., et al. (2006). Bacterial and fungal microbiota in relation to probiotic therapy (VSL#3) in pouchitis. *Gut, 55*, 833–841.
5. Cannon, R. D., Holmes, A. R., Mason, A. B., & Monk, B. C. (1995). Clearance, colonization or candidiasis? *Journal of Dental Research, 74*(5), 1152–1161.
6. Biasoli, S. M., Tosello, M. E., & Magaro, H. M. (2001). Adherence of *Candida* strains isolated from the human gastrointestinal tract. *Mycoses, 45*, 465–469.
7. Ruhnke, M. (2006). Epidemiology of *Candida albicans* infections and role of non-*Candida albicans* yeasts. *Current Drug Targets, 7*(4), 495–504.
8. Reddy, B. S., Gatt, M., Sowdi, R., et al. (2008). Gastric colonization predisposes to septic morbidity in surgical patients: a prospective study. *Nutrition, 24*, 632–637.
9. Lockhart, S. R., Joly, S., Vargas, K., et al. (1999). Natural defenses against *Candida* colonization breakdown in the oral cavities of the elderly. *Journal of Dental Research, 78*, 858–868.
10. Hatakka, K., Ahola, A., Yli-Knuuttila, H., et al. (2007). Probiotics reduce the prevalence of oral *Candida* in the elderly—a randomized controlled study. *Journal of Dental Research, 86*, 125–130.
11. O'May, G. A., Reynolds, N., & Macfarlane, G. T. (2005). Effect of pH on an *in vitro* model of gastric microbiota

in enteral nutrition patients. *Applied Environment of Microbiology, 71*(8), 4777–4783.

12. Brzozowski, T., Zwolinska-Wcisło, M., Konturek, P. C., et al. (2005). Influence of gastric colonization with *Candida albicans* on ulcer healing in rats: effect of ranitidine, aspirin and probiotic therapy. *Scandinavian Journal of Gastroenterology, 40*, 286–296.

13. Zwolinska-Wcisło, M., Budak, A., Bogdał, J., et al. (2001). Fungal colonization of gastric mucosa and its clinical relevance. *Medical Science Monitor, 7*, 982–988.

14. Zwolinska-Wcisło, M., Brzozowski, T., Mach, T., et al. (2006). Are probiotics effective in the treatment of fungal colonization of the gastrointestinal tract? Experimental and clinical studies. *Journal of Physiology and Pharmacology, 57*, 35–49.

15. Manzoni, P., Farina, D., Leonessa, M. L., et al. (2006). Risk factors for progression to invasive fungal infection in preterm neonates with fungal colonization. *Pediatrics, 118*, 2350–2364.

16. Munoz, P., Burillo, A., & Bouza, E. (2000). Criteria used when initiating antifungal therapy against *Candida* spp. in the intensive care unit. *International Journal of Antimicrobial Agents, 15*, 83–90.

17. Manzoni, P., Mostert, M., Leonessa, M. L., et al. (2006). Oral supplementation with *Lactobacillus casei* subspecies *rhamnosus* prevents enteric colonization by *Candida* species in preterm neonates: a randomized studies. *Clinical Infectious Diseases, 42*(15), 1735–1741.

18. White, S. J., Rosenbach, A., Lephart, P., et al. (2007). Self-regulation of *Candida albicans* population size during GI colonization. *PLoS Pathogens, 3*(12), 1866–1878.

19. Naglik, J., Fostira, F., Ruprai, J., et al. (2006). *Candida albicans HWP1* gene expression and host antibody responses in colonization and disease. *Journal of Medical Microbiology, 55*, 1323–1327.

20. De Repetigny, L., Aumont, F., Bernard, K., & Belhumeur, P. (2000). Characterization of binding of *Candida albicans* to small intestinal mucin and its role in adherence to mucosa epithelial cells. *Infection & Immunity, 68*(6), 3170–3172.

21. Schofield, D. A., Westwater, C., Warner, T., & Balish, E. (2005). Differential *Candida albicans* lipase gene expression during alimentary tract colonization and infection. *FEMS Microbiology Letters, 244*, 359–365.

22. Algin, C., Sahin, A., & Kiraz, N., et al. (2005). Effectiveness of Bombesin and *Saccharomyces boulardii* against the translocation of *Candida albicans* in the digestive tract in immunosupressed rats. *Surg Today, 35*, 869–873.

23. Mack, D. R., Ahrne, S., Hyde, L., et al. (2003). Extracellular MUC 3 mucin secretion follows adherence of *Lactobacillus* strains to intestinal epithelial cells in vitro. *Gut, 52*, 827–833.

24. Coste, A., Lagame, C., & Filipe, C.etal. (2008). IL-13 attenuates gastrointestinal candidiasis in normal and immunodeficient RAG-2 mice via peroxysome proliferator-activated receptor-γ activation. *Journal of Immunology, 180*, 4939–4947.

25. Ruiz-Sanchez, D., Calderon-Romero, L., Sanchez-Vega, J. T., & Tay, J. (2002). Intestinal candidiasis. A clinical reports and comments about this opportunistic pathology. *Mycopathologia, 156*, 9–11.

26. Vanderpool, Ch., Yan, F., & Polk, D. B. (2008). Mechanisms of probiotic action: implications for therapeutic applications in inflammatory bowel disease. *Inflammatory Bowel Diseases, 14*, 1585–1596.

27. Damaskos, D., & Kolios, G. (2008). Probiotics and prebiotics in inflammatory bowel disease: microflora 'on the scope'. *British Journal of Clinical Pharmacology, 65*, 453–467.

28. Goldin, B. R., & Gorbach, S. L. (2008). Clinical indications for probiotics: an overwiew. *Clinical Infectious Diseases, 46*, 96–100.

29. Wagner, R. D., Pierson, C., Warnere, T., et al. (1997). Biotherapeutic effects of probiotic bacteria on candidiasis in immunodeficient mice. *Infection & Immunity, 65*(10), 4165–4172.

30. Ström, K., Sjögren, J., Broberg, A., & Schnürer, J. (2002). *Lactobacillus plantarum* MiLAB 393 produces the antifungal cyclic dipeptides Cyclo (L-Phe-L-Pro) and Cyclo (L-Phe-trans-4-OH-L-Pro) and 3-Phenyllactic Acid. *Applied Environmental Microbiology, 68*(9), 4322–4327.

31. Lavermicocca, P., Valerio, F., Evidente, A., et al. (2000). Putrification and characterization of novel ant fungal compounds from the sourdough *Lactobacillus plantarum* strain 21B. *Applied Environmental Microbiology, 66*, 4084–4090.

32. Strus, M., Kucharska, A., Kukla, G., et al. (2005). The *in vitro* activity of vaginal Lactobacillus with prebiotic properties against *Candida*. *Infectious Diseases Obstetrics Gynecology, 13*, 69–75.

33. Elahi, S., Pang, G., Ashman, R., & Clansy, R. (2005). Enhanced clearence of *Candida albicans* from the oral cavities of mice following oral administration of *Lactobacillus acidophilus*. *Clinical Experimental Microbiology, 141*, 29–36.

34. Wagner, R. D., Warner, T., Roberts, L., et al. (1998). Variable biotherapeutic effects if *Lactobacillus acidophilus* isolates on orogastric and systemic candidiasis in immunodeficient mice. *Revista iberoamericana de micología, 15*, 271–276.

35. Wagner, R. D., Warner, T., Pierson, C., et al. (1998). Biotherapeutic effect of *Bifidobacterium* spp. on orogastric and systemic candidiasis in immunodeficient mice. *Revista iberoamericana de micología, 15*, 265–270.

Probiotics and Host Defense, Health Claim and Evidences

Yoichi Fukushima[1], Antonio Marcos Pupin[2], Wei Hua Cai[3], Jian Jun Chen[3], and Eva Hurt[2]

[1]Nestlé Research Center, Nestec Ltd., Lausanne, Switzerland

[2]CT-Regulatory, Nestec Ltd., Vevey, Switzerland

[3]Shanghai Rundo Biotech Japan Co. Ltd., Kobe, Hyogo, Japan

1. INTRODUCTION

Attempts to reveal the physiological function of foods and establishment of regulations on health claims has accelerated through the world. In Japan, the Ministry of Health and Welfare, the former Ministry of Health, Labor, and Welfare (MHLW), issued the Investigative Commission Report on Functional Food in 1990. The Food for Specified Health Uses (FOSHU) system was inaugurated in 1991 as the world's first approval system on health claim labeling for food products. All health claims are regulated under this system. Some probiotics have FOSHU claim approval, but the name 'probiotics' itself is not regarded as a health claim in Japan. In China, the Ministry of Health inaugurated the Foods with a Health Claim system in 1996. This system was amended in 2005, through issuing of the 'Provision for Health Foods Registration (interim)'; and the 'Regulatory for Probiotic Health Foods Application and Examination (interim)' was issued for probiotics. For the development of food products with probiotics, another regulation 'Regulation for Novel Food' is also usually involved. In Brazil, since 1999, the use of functional and/or health claims in food labels has been regulated by the National Health Surveillance Agency (ANVISA), supported by a Technical Scientific Advisory Commission on Functional Foods and Novel Foods (CTCAF). The well-defined regulation system establishes rules for the introduction of novel foods or food ingredients and another set of rules for labeling foods with functional and/or health claims. In the European Union (EU), the new Nutrition and Health Claims (NHC) Regulation, brought into force in 2007, harmonizes the requirements on claims on food products across the 27 member states. All claims have to be authorized for use after a scientific assessment of the highest possible standard and may not be false or misleading, nor refer to prevention, treatment or cure of a disease. During a transitional period until 2010 health claims based on generally accepted scientific evidence are under the central scientific evaluation, but can be made under the manufacturer's own responsibility. At the time of writing, the European Food Safety Authority (EFSA—the central body providing scientific advice to European decision-makers) was evaluating several thousand diet–health relationships, which will lead to a Community list of permitted claims.

Probiotics is defined as live microorganisms which, when administered in adequate amounts, confer a health benefit on the host [1], and the terminology was introduced in 1991 [2]. Probiotics are scientifically well-documented food components that could deliver health benefits including gut microbiota balancing, normalizing regularity, gut comfort, immune boosting, anti-infection, anti-diarrhea, anti-allergy, and skin health. Emerging science increasingly shows health benefits of food and approximately 500 scientific articles per year show the health benefits of probiotics. Probiotics and their health benefits proven by human trials [3–115] are summarized in Table 25.1.

Since the 1990s, local authorities around the world have been establishing rules for health claims on foods. The systems have been updated several times and the process is still on-going. In this review, the health claim systems currently applied in the four major areas, Japan, China, Brazil and Europe as of April 2009, are reviewed and discussed in the scope of scientific evidence and potential health claims on probiotics.

2. HEALTH CLAIM AND PROBIOTICS IN JAPAN

2.1. Health Claim Regulation in Japan

Health claim regulations on food products, known as the Food for Specified Health Uses (FOSHU) system was inaugurated in Japan in 1991. FOSHU refers to foods containing ingredients with functions for health and officially approved claims on physiological effects on the human body. FOSHU is intended to be consumed for the maintenance/promotion of health or special health uses by people who wish to control health conditions, including blood pressure and blood cholesterol. In order to sell a food as FOSHU, the assessment of the safety of the food and effectiveness of the functions for health is required, and the claim must be approved by the MHLW. FOSHU's health claim is approved by MHLW, product-by-product, based on the application by food manufacturers. FOSHU-approved products can include a seal of FOSHU approval on product packages.

In 2001, the 'Food with Health Claims' system was employed, and FOSHU was re-positioned under the category of Food with Health Claims (FHC) alongside the new category 'Food with Nutrient Function Claims (FNFC)' shown in Figure 25.1. FHC refers to foods that comply with the specifications and standards established by the MHLW and are labeled with certain nutritional or health functions. These foods are categorized into the two groups, according to differences in purpose and function: 1) FNFC, foods that are labeled with the functions of nutritional ingredients (vitamins and minerals); and 2) FOSHU, foods officially approved to claim physiological effects on the human body. FOSHU and FNFC are categorized as foods, and cannot claim any medical terms such as cure or prevention. The new regulation on 'Reduction of Disease Risk Claims' started under FOSHU in 2005, in accordance with the CODEX draft guideline, when the reduction of disease risk claims for osteoporosis and neural tube defects were allowed on products with calcium and folic acid, respectively. In addition to 'regular' FOSHU, Qualified FOSHU and Standardized FOSHU were also introduced to facilitate application for FOSHU approval.[1] Foods with a health function

---

[1]http://www.mhlw.go.jp/english/topics/foodsafety/fhc/index.html.

TABLE 25.1 Probiotics and proven health benefit in humans

Probiotic strain(s)	Strain supplier	Health claim category			Reference
		Digestive health	Protection	Others	
Single strain					
Bifidobacterium animalis Lafti B94 (CBS118.529)	DSM (Netherland)	✓			[3]
Bifidobacterium animalis spp. lactis Bb12® (BL818) (NCC2818)	Chr. Hansen (Denmark)	✓	✓a,d,f		[4–14]
Bifidobacterium animalis spp. lactis CNCM I-2494/DN-173 010	Danone (France)	✓			[15,16]
Bifidobacterium breve Yakult (BbY)	Yakult (Japan)	✓			[17–20]
Bifidobacterium infantis 35624 (Bifantis®)	Alimentary Health (Ireland)			✓h	[21]
Bifidobacterium lactis HN019 AGAL NM97/09513 (DR10)	Danisco (Denmark)	✓	✓f		[22–24]
Bifidobacterium longum BB536 (BL999) (NCC3001)	Morinaga (Japan)	✓	✓a		[25–27]
Enterococcus faecium SF68 (NCIMB 10415) (NCC2768)	Cerbios Pharma (Switzerland)		✓d		[28]
Escherichia coli Nissle 1917	Ardeypharm (Germany)			✓b	[29]
Lactobacillus acidophilus L92	Calpis (Japan)	✓	✓a		[30–33]
Lactobacillus acidophilus LA14	Danisco (Denmark)			✓j	[34]
Lactobacillus acidophilus NCFM ATCC SD5221	Danisco (Denmark)	✓			[35]
Lactobacillus casei CNCM I-1518/DN-114 001	Danone (France)		✓f,d		[36–40]
Lactobacillus casei Shirota (LcS)	Yakult (Japan)	✓	✓c,f		[41–49]
Lactobacillus fermentum CECT5716	Puleva Biotech (Spain)		✓f		[50]
Lactobacillus fermentum VRI-033 PCC (NM 02/31047)	Probiomics (Australia)		✓a		[51,52]
Lactobacillus johnsonii NCC 533 (La1) (CNCM I-2115)	Nestlé (Switzerland)	✓	✓e,f	✓i	[53–61]
Lactobacillus paracasei 33	GenMont Biotech (Taiwan)		✓a		[62]
Lactobacillus paracasei NCC 2461 (ST11) (CNCM I-2116)	Nestlé (Switzerland)		✓d,f		[63,64]
Lactobacillus paracasei spp. paracasei CRL-431	Chr. Hansen (Denmark)		✓f		[65]
Lactobacillus plantarum 299v	Probi AB (Sweden)		✓d,h		[66–68]
Lactobacillus reuteri ATCC 55730 (SD2112)	BioGaia (Sweden)		✓a,d,f	✓g,h	[69–75]
Lactobacillus rhamnosus ATCC53103 (LGG®) (LPR) (NCC4007)	Valio (Finland)	✓	✓a,d,f	✓g	[76–89]
Lactobacillus rhamnosus HN001 AGAL NM97/09514 (DR20)	Danisco (Denmark)	✓	✓a,f		[90–93]
Saccharomyces boulardii PXN68TM	Biocodex (France)		✓d		[94]
Streptococcus salivarius K12 (Blis) (ATCC BAA-1024)	BLIS Technologies (New Zealand)		✓f	✓g	[95,96]

(Continued)

TABLE 25.1   (Continued)

Probiotic strain(s)	Strain supplier	Health claim category			Reference
		Digestive health	Protection	Others	
Combination of strains					
Bifidobacterium animalis spp. lactis Bb12®	Chr. Hansen (Denmark)	✓	✓[b,d]		[97–99]
Lactobacillus acidophilus LA-5®					
Lactobacillus acidophilus LB (Lactéol)*	Axcan Pharma (France)		✓[d]		[100,101]
Lactobacillus gasseri PA16/8	Merck (USA)		✓[f]		[102–104]
Bifidobacterium bifidum MF 20/5					
Bifidobacterium longum SP07/3					
Lactobacillus gasseri CECT5714	Puleva Biotech (Spain)		✓[f]		[105–107]
Lactobacillus coryniformis CECT5711					
Lactobacillus acidophilus I-1722 (Rosell-52)	Lallemand (Canada)	✓			[108]
Bifidobacterium longum CNCM I-3470 (Rosell-175)					
Lactobacillus rhamnosus 19070-2	Chr. Hansen (Denmark)		✓[a,d]		[109–112]
Lactobacillus reuteri DSM12246					
Lactobacillus rhamnosus GR 1 (ATCC 55826)	Urex Biotech (Canada)			✓[j]	[113]
Lactobacillus reuteri RC-14 (ATCC 55845)					
Propionibacterium freudenreichii SI 41	Standa (France)	✓			[114]
Propionibacterium freudenreichii SI 26 Propio-Fidus®					
VSL#3 (eight strains mixture including lactobacilli and bifidobacteria)	Sigma-Tau (USA)			✓[b,h]	[115]

*Heat-killed bacteria, combining with Lactobacillus fermentum and Lactobacillus delbrueckii.
[a] anti-allergy.
[b] anti-inflammatory bowel diseases (IBD).
[c] anti-cancer.
[d] anti-diarrhea.
[e] anti-Helicobacter pylori.
[f] immune boosting/anti-infection.
[g] oral health.
[h] anti-irritable bowel syndrome (IBS).
[i] skin health.
[j] virginal flora/urogenital protection.

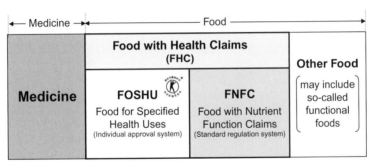

FIGURE 25.1   Food with Health Claims including FOSHU. *Seal for FOSHU approval by the Ministry of Health, Labor and Welfare.

that is not substantiated by scientific evidence, which meets the level of regular FOSHU, or a food with certain effectiveness but without an established mechanism of the effective element for the function, will be approved as Qualified FOSHU.

Foods with a Nutrient Function Claim (FNFC) refers to all foods that are labeled with the nutrient function claims specified by the MHLW. The standards and specifications for indication of nutritional function have so far been established for 17 ingredients (12 vitamins and five minerals). These foods may be freely manufactured and distributed without any permission from, or notification to, the national government, when they meet the established standards and specifications. For standards and specifications, amounts of nutritional ingredients for the recommended daily intake of the product must be within the specified range, and not only the nutrient function claims but also the warning indications must be displayed. For example, products containing vitamin C at 24 to 1000 mg/day can claim on the product package 'helps to maintain skin and mucosa healthy and has antioxidizing effect' with the mandatory alert description 'Increased intake of this product will not result in curing diseases nor promoting health. Please comply with the advisable daily intake.'

2.2. FOSHU Health Claim

FOSHU products and their health claim categories are summarized in Table 25.2. There are nine health claim categories currently approved, such as foods to modify gastrointestinal (GI) conditions, foods related to blood pressure, triacylglycerol, blood cholesterol level, blood sugar levels, osteogenesis, mineral absorption, dental hygiene, and reduction of disease risk for osteoporosis. Seven hundred and ninety-nine such products with 91 health-related components have been approved as FOSHU since November 2008, for food product categories including beverages, soups, snacks, noodles, candy, fermented milks, table sugar, cooking oil, and tablet. The target population for FOSHU is not diseased people but healthy people. The Pharmaceutical Affairs Law strictly indicates that a product aiming at influencing the function or body structure should be categorized as a drug. At the time of writing, claims for immune boosting and fatigue reduction have not been approved.

A reduction of disease risk claim was permitted under FOSHU when a reduction of disease risk is clinically and nutritionally established for an ingredient. Two ingredients, calcium for osteoporosis and folic acid for neural tube defect, were allowed with the 'Reduction of Disease

TABLE 25.2   List of FOSHU Products in Japan

Health claim (Specified Health Use) category (number of approval)	Ingredients exhibiting health functions	Health claim (example‡)
Foods for modifying gastrointestinal (GI) conditions (334)	Lactic acid bacteria (10 single and three combination of probiotic strains in Table 25.3)	This product contains [INGREDIENT]. It makes easy intake of dietary fiber for those who tend to have less dietary fiber. It adjusts GI condition and improves the bowel movement and the stool frequency./This product uses [INGREDIENT] to increase the number of bifidobacteria and thus helps maintenance of a good GI environment./[INGREDIENT] in this product reaches the intestine alive, and is useful in improving intestinal environment.
	Lactosucrose*	
	Fructo-oligosaccharides (FOS)**	
	Galacto-oligosaccharides (GOS)	
	Coffee bean manno-oligosaccharides***	
	Soybean oligosaccharides	
	Xylo-oligosaccharides	
	Isomalto-oligosaccharides	
	Raffinose	
	Lactulose	
	Indigestible dextrin	
	Indigestible dextrin + wheat bran	
	Reduced indigestible dextrin	
	Psyllium husks****	
	Degraded sodium alginate****	
	Degraded sodium alginate + corn fiber	
	Wheat bran	
	Hydrolyzed guar gum	
	Agar fiber	
	Indigestible starch	
	Polydextrose	
	Yeast fiber	
	Propionic acid	
	Whey fermented by propionic bacterium	
Foods related to blood pressure (100)	Casein dodecapeptides	This product contains [INGREDIENT]. It is suitable for those who tend to be high in blood pressure.
	Sesami peptide (LVY)	
	Royal jelly peptides (VY, IY, IVY)	
	Acetic acid	
	Eucommia leaf glycoside	
	Gamma-amino butyric acid (GABA)	
	Sardine peptides (VY)	
	Lacto-tripeptides (VPP, IPP)	
	Dried bonito oligopeptides	
	Seaweed (wakame) peptides	
	Isoleucyl-tyrosine	
	Laver seaweed (nori) oligopeptides	
	Yanron flavonoids (Hyperoside and isoquercitria)	
Foods related to blood cholesterol (125)	Phytosterol	This product contains [INGREDIENT], which helps lower the serum cholesterol level. Thus it is suitable for those who are concerned about cholesterol.
	Phytosterol ester	
	DG + phytosterol†	
	Tea catechin	
	Indigestible dextrin	
	Chitosan	
	Soy protein	
	Psyllium husks****	
	Degraded sodium alginate*****	
	Soy peptide with phospholipids	
	S-methylcystine sulfoxide from broccoli and cabbage (SMCS)	
Foods related to blood sugar level (113)	Touchi extract	This product contains [INGREDIENT] which helps to moderate the absorption of glucose. Thus it is suitable for those who are concerned about the level of blood glucose.
	L-alabinose	
	LM-alginate	
	Indigestible dextrin	
	Wheat albumin	
	Guava polyphenols	

Category	Ingredients		Claim
Foods related to triacylglycerol (56)	Globin digest (VVYP) Tea catechin Diacylglycerol (DG) DG + phytosterol† Coffee bean manno-oligosaccharides*** Medium-chain fatty acids (MCT)	Beta-conglycinin Oolong tea polymerized polyphenols EPA, DHA Touchi extract	This product contains [INGREDIENT] which is suitable for people who are concerned about body fat.\This product contains [INGREDIENT], which helps lower the neutral fat level. Thus, it is suitable for those who are concerned about their blood neutral fat.
Foods related to mineral absorption/Foods related to osteogenesis (39)	Isoflavone Vitamin K2 Milk basic protein (MBP) Fructo-oligosaccharides (FOS)** Casein phosphopeptide (CPP)	Lactosucrose* Calcium citrate malate (CCM) Poly-gamma-glutamic acid Heme iron	[INGREDIENT] helps the absorption of calcium to build strong bones.\This product contains [INGREDIENT] which helps to keep calcium in bone, and designed for its easy intake and is suitable for those who are concerned about their bone health.
Foods related to dental hygiene (37)	Casein phosphopeptide amorphous calcium phosphate nanocomplexes (CPP-ACP) Phosphorylated Ca oligosaccharides (POs-Ca) Xylitol, calcium phosphate, fnoran	Sugar alcohols + tea polyphenols etc. Maltitol Green tea flourine	This product uses sweeteners ([INGREDIENT]) which do not cause tooth decay. Also this product contains [INGREDIENT] that increase the recalcification, so it helps maintenance of strong and healthy teeth.
Reduction of Disease Risk (Osteoplosis) (6)	Ca		The product is rich in calcium. Daily physical exercise and intake of healthy diet containing an appropriate amount of calcium helps to maintain good bone health in young women, and can reduce the risk of developing osteoporosis later in life (fixed claim).
Total (799)			

As of November 2008.
*2 products claim both for 'GI condition' and 'Ca absorption.'
**A product claims both for 'GI condition' and 'Ca absorption.'
***10 products claim both for 'triacylglycerol' and 'GI condition.'
****19 products claim both for 'GI condition' and 'blood cholesterol.'
*****7 products claim both for 'blood cholesterol' and 'GI condition.'
†4 products allowed to claim 'triacylglycerol and blood cholesterol.'
‡FOSHU health claims are not fixed in general, except for Reduction of Risk Disease and Standard FOSHU, and approved not by application.

Risk Claims.' Six products are approved for calcium and osteoporosis with the fixed claim 'Intake of proper amounts of calcium contained in healthy meals with appropriate exercise may support healthy bones of young women and reduce the risk of osteoporosis when aged.' On folic acid and neural tube defects, the fixed claim 'Intake of proper amounts of folic acid contained in healthy meals may support women to bear a healthy baby by reducing the risk of neural tube defect, such as spondyloschisis, during fetal development' was allowed; however, there are no FOSHU products applying for this claim.

FOSHU approval requires a submission of the facts on effectiveness clearly proven on the human body, absence of any safety concerns (animal toxicity tests, confirmation of effects in the cases of excess intake, etc.), use of nutritionally appropriate ingredients (e.g. no excessive use of salt, etc.), a guarantee of compatibility with product specifications at the time of consumption, and established quality control methods, such as specifications of products and ingredients, processes, and methods of analysis. At least one human trial in healthy subjects on the final product published in a peer-reviewed scientific journal is required to show its efficacy, and also a human trial using three times the higher dose for several weeks should be documented as safety information. Additional human trials are required when the applicant changes the product formula or dose. 'Regular' FOSHU requires a randomized controlled human trial on the final product for efficacy confirmation. Health claims may be approved with weaker scientific evidences under Qualified FOSHU (distinguished from Regular FOSHU), and must indicate 'Qualified' in the seal of FOSHU on the product package. For Reduction of Disease Risk FOSHU and Standard FOSHU, a human trial on the product is required just as a safety confirmation but not for efficacy, where existing scientific evidence is recognized as sufficient for the claim. Standardized

FOSHU is approved when it meets the standards and specifications established for foods with sufficient FOSHU approvals and accumulation of scientific evidence. Three dietary fibers including indigestible dextrin (3–8 g/day), polydextrose (7–8 g/day), hydrolyzed guar gum (5–12 g/day) and six indigestible oligosaccharides (OS), including soy oligosaccharides (2–6 g/day), flucto-oligosaccharides (3–8 g/day), lactosucrose (2–8 g/day), galacto-oligosaccharides (2–5 g/day), xylo-oligosaccharides (1–3 g/day), and isomalto-oligosaccharides (10 g/day) are allowed to carry the fixed health claims, 'contains fiber [INGREDIENT] and maintains the GI conditions' and 'contains [INGREDIENT] OS, which increases intestinal bifidobacteria and keeps good intestinal environment, and maintains GI conditions,' respectively. The Standard FOSHU claim on products with indigestible dextrin for blood glucose levels would be approved shortly. The mechanism of action of the functional components in the product is required to be described in the FOSHU application document for Regular FOSHU; but not for Qualified FOSHU, Standard FOSHU and Reduction of Disease Risk FOSHU.

The applicants submit the FOSHU application documents with the target health claim wording and scientific evidence to the MHLW and the local health center. The MHLW then conducts a hearing session for the applicant. Two committees under MHLW composed of external scientists evaluate the application documents. The National Institute of Nutrition and Health conducts an analysis of food components, and approval for FOSHU is announced by MHLW. The whole application process takes a minimum of 6 months. Since 2003, the Food Safety Committee under the Cabinet Office have acted separately from the MHLW committee, and safety evaluation by this committee is required for FOSHU applications; in case the product contains novel functional components in FOSHU, the procedure may take an additional 6 months.

2.3. FOSHU Claims on Probiotics

A health claim category 'modify GI conditions' is a major FOSHU claim category, where FOSHU claims on products with dietary fibers, prebiotics, as well as probiotics, have been approved. As of November 2008, 73 products with 13 probiotic strains and/or combinations of strains, including eight lactobacilli and six bifidobacteria strains, have been approved under the 'modify GI conditions' claim category in FOSHU shown in Table 25.3. The FOSHU claim wording allowed on 'reaches the intestines,' 'help increase intestinal bifidobacteria and lactobacilli (or good bacillus) and decrease bad ones,' 'promotes/regulates/maintains GI conditions,' 'keeps the intestines healthy,' or 'regulates the balance of intestinal microflora,' 'useful to improve defecation,' or 'suitable for those concerned about gut health,' based on scientific evidence submitted by applicants.

The nutritional composition with the effective level of the related functional component, the approved health claim, daily standard dosage, intake manner, and caution of intake should be indicated on the package label of the FOSHU product. It is allowed to indicate 'MHLW agreed FOSHU' with a seal for FOSHU and to describe a simplified health claim 'catch copy (phrase)' where words are extracted from the approval health claim. All image and description on product label including the catch phrase is evaluated by MHLW. It is mandatory to notify for MHLW when package design for FOSHU approved product may be changed. The message, 'daily diet needs balance based on staple food, main and subsidiary dishes' has now become a mandatory description on the product label.

A FOSHU application should be done on a specific products using specific functional components. The MHLW issued guidelines for FOSHU using some functional components including indigestible oligosaccharides (OS) in 1998, in which scientific evidence that was necessary in FOSHU application documents was illustrated. There are no guidelines for probiotics; however, the criteria for government approval is based on the guideline for OS. The working criteria of human trials for products with probiotics for the FOSHU health claim is as follows:

- Improvement of intestinal flora to show an increase in beneficial bacteria such as bifidobacteria (number and/or %) and decrease in harmful bacteria such as *Clostridium perfringens* (number and/or %).
- Increase of defecation frequency per week in subjects with mild constipation, i.e. frequency less than 7 days/week before intervention.
- Detection of probiotic strain in feces.
- No side effects on general health status in excess dose study on final product.

It is well accepted by the Japanese academic community that GI conditions in healthy humans are associated with a balance of intestinal microflora, which influences the production of putrefactive (e.g. ammonia, carcinogens) or beneficial metabolites (e.g. short-chain fatty acids) in the gut. This, in turn, correlates with defecation conditions. The key measurable indicators for microflora and GI conditions are the number of fecal bifidobacteria and *Clostridium perfringens*, and defecation frequency 116–118]. For a FOSHU application, the compounds related to the functional benefit should be clearly described, and the quantity of such specific compounds should be measurable at a sufficient level in the product until the end of its shelf life. In the case of probiotics, specific methods for quantification (e.g. strain identification procedures using specific selective media and/or the PCR method using specific DNA probes) should preferably be developed.

There are some probiotic strains with health benefits proven in humans commercially available in Japan without FOSHU's approval. For instance, *B. animalis* spp. *lactis* HN019 [22–24] for immune boosting, *L. acidophilus* L-92 [32, 33] and heat-killed *L. paracasei* KW3110 [119] for anti-pollen

TABLE 25.3 FOSHU claim and probiotics in Japan

Probiotic strains in FOSHU products	Product example (Company)	Dose (min × 10⁹ cfu/day)	FOSHU health claim on products (example)
Bacillus subtilis K-2	ONAKA NATTO (ASAHIMATSU FOOD)	3.8 (spore)	This product contains *Bacillus subtilis* K-2 which helps increase the number of bifidobacteria. It helps maintenance of an excellent GI environment, and is suitable for people who are concerned about their GI condition.
Bifidobacterium breve Yakult	MIL-MIL, BIFIEL (YAKULT)	10	*B. breve* Yakult reaches the intestines in an active state. It increases useful bacteria and helps regulation of the balance of intestinal microflora that lead to maintenance of a good GI condition.
Bifidobacterium lactis Bb12	KOIWAI SEINYU 100% YOGURT (KOIWAI DAIRY)	1.0	Bifidobacteria contained in this product reaches the intestines in an active state. It improves GI condition and keeps the intestines healthy.
Bifidobacterium lactis FK120*	NOMU DENMARK YOGURT (FUKUSHIMA MILK)	1.0	Bifidobacteria contained in this product reaches the intestines in an active state. It helps growth of good bacillus and reduction of bad ones. This improves a GI condition and keeps the intestines healthy.
Bifidobacterium lactis LKM512*	ONAKA NI OISHII YOGURT (KYODO MILK)	1.0	This product helps regulation and maintenance of a comfortable GI condition.
Bifidobacterium longum BB536	BIFIDUS PLAIN YOGURT (MORINAGA MILK)	2.0	This product contains living bifidobacteria and helps growth of intestinal bifidobacteria. It helps maintenance of a good intestinal environment and regulation of the GI condition.
Lactobacillus acidophilus CK92 (L92) Lactobacillus helveticus CK60	CALPIS KIDS (DANONE JAPAN)	1.0/1.0	This product improves the GI environment and keeps the intestines healthy.
Lactobacillus casei NY1301	PILKUL (NISSHIN YORK)	15	This helps improvement of the GI environment and keeps the intestines healthy.
Lactobacillus casei Shirota YIT9029	YAKULT, JOE, SOFUHL (YAKULT)	15	*L. casei* Shirota reaches the intestines in an active state. It increases the number of useful bacteria in the intestines and helps regulation of the balance of intestinal microflora that lead to maintenance of a good GI condition.
Lactobacillus delbrueckii subsp. bulgaricus 2038 Streptococcus salivarius subsp. thermophilus 1131	MEIJI BULGARIA YOGURT LB81 (MEIJI DAIRIES)	1.0/10	This yogurt, with its *Lactobacillus* LB81, helps regulation of the balance of intestinal microflora and maintenance of a good GI condition.
Lactobacillus gasseri SBT 2055 Bifidobacterium longum SBT2928	NATURE PRO GB (NIPPON MILK COMMUNITY)	0.5/1.0	*L. gasseri* SP strain and *B. longum* SP strain contained in this product help to improve intestinal environment.
Lactobacillus johnsonii LA-1	NESTLÉ LC1 YOGURT (NESTLÉ JAPAN)	1.0	*L. johnsonii* LA-1 reaches the intestines in an active state and adheres onto intestinal wall. This decreases harmful bacteria, such as the Welch bacillus *Clostridium perfringens*, competitively in the intestines and increases beneficial bacteria such as bifidobacteria. This product helps to maintain a good GI condition.
Lactobacillus rhamnosus GG	YOGURT ONAKA-HE GG! (TAKANASHI MILK)	14	This product is a yogurt drink fermented with *Lactobacillus* GG, which reaches one's intestines in an active state so as to help growth of intestinal bifidobacteria and regulation of the GI condition.

*Same as *B. lactis* Bb12.

allergy, *L. gasseri* OLL2716 (LG21) for anti-*Helicobacter pylori* [120], and *L. salivarius* T12711 for oral health [121]. 'Probiotics' itself is not recognized as a claim in Japan, and any probiotic product is allowed to use the term 'probiotics' for product communication. However, these probiotic products cannot have any health claims nor the health benefit communication on the products. The manufacturers communicate on their probiotic products by using the image of a bland or sub-bland and/or on the probiotic strain itself using a corporate communication framework, separately from product communication. Probiotics used in FOSHU products may also have health benefits other than GI conditioning proven in human trials. For instance, natural defense (e.g. immune boosting, anti-infections/diarrhea, anti-allergy) on *B. lactis* Bb12 [5–7], *B. longum* BB536 [25–27], *L. casei* Shirota [45–49], *L. johnsonii* LA-1 [55, 56, 61], and *L. rhamnosus* GG [77–87]. However, communication on product functionality is regulated by the FOSHU system, and only FOSHU-approved claims based on GI conditioning are allowed to be used.

3. HEALTH CLAIM REGULATION AND PROBIOTICS IN CHINA

3.1. Regulatory Status in China

In 1996, the Chinese Ministry of Health (MOH) issued a 'Provision for Health Foods' to establish a registration system of foods with health claims on their labels. In 2005, the Chinese government issued a 'Provision for Health Foods Registration (interim)' with some revision of the system. Health Foods in China are divided into nutrient supplements and Foods with Health Claims; the latter is subdivided into 27 health claim categories. The claim category known as prevention of mutagenesis in the 'Provision for Health Foods' disappeared from the new health claim list issued in 2005 (Table 25.4). The application procedure is summarized in Figure 25.2. To apply for Foods with Health Claim approval, the toxicological assessment test, function assessment test, functional ingredients analysis test, stability test and hygienic test must be performed. Moreover, these tests should be performed in the State Food and Drug Administration (SFDA) designated laboratories with fixed protocols. Tests required for efficacy assessment are also shown in Table 25.5. Human trials are not required in the following seven health claim categories: enhancing immunity; sleep improvement; alleviating physical fatigue; increasing bone density; assisting in protection from irradiation hazard; protecting the liver against chemical injury; and enhancing anoxia endurance.

The SFDA in the Ministry of Health reviews the application for Health Foods approval. The Center of Disease Control (CDC) is appointed by the SFDA to evaluate the safety and efficacy of the 'Foods with Health Claim' candidates. Up to April 2009, approximately 9,000 Health Food Claim approvals had been issued: among them 5,585 approvals are still valid (5,381 domestic products and 204 overseas products); the others having expired or been revoked. On labels of the Foods with Health Claims, only certain fixed phrases can be used to describe the functions. Not only people who are able to eat the food, but also those who may not be able to eat the food must be specified on the label.

In the development of probiotics foods, another Chinese regulation is usually involved— the 'Regulation for Novel Food,' which became effective in December 2007. According to this regulation, the following materials must obtain the approval as a Novel Food from the MOH before being used even as an ordinary food. These materials include ingredients derived from animals, plants and microorganisms (e.g. probiotic strain). To apply for approval

TABLE 25.4 Health Food Categories in China

	Health Food Categories (in English)	Health Food Cate(in Chinese)	Animal test required	Human test required	Age of appropriate customers
1	Enhancing Immunity	增强免疫力	Yes	No	All
2	Antioxidative	抗氧化	Yes	Yes	Except for junior and children
3	Memory Improvement	辅助改善记忆	Yes	Yes	All
4	Alleviating Physical Fatigue	缓解体力疲劳	Yes	No	Except for junior and children
5	Weight Control	减肥	Yes	Yes	All
6	Promoting Child Growth	改善生长发育	Yes	Yes	All
7	Enhancing Anoxia Endurance	提高缺氧耐受力	Yes	No	All
8	Assisting Irradiation Hazard Protection	对辐射危害有辅助保护作用	Yes	No	All
9	Assisting Blood Lipids Reduction	辅助降血脂	Yes	Yes	Except for junior and children
10	Assisting Blood Sugar Reduction	辅助降血糖	Yes	Yes	Except for junior and children
11	Sleep Improvement	改善睡眠	Yes	No	Except for junior and children
12	Alleviating Nutritional Anemia	改善营养性贫血	Yes	Yes	All
13	Protecting Liver Against Chemical Injury	对化学性肝损伤有辅助保护作用	Yes	No	All
14	Facilitating Milk Secretion	促进泌乳	Yes	Yes	All
15	Alleviating Eye Fatigue	缓解视疲劳	No	Yes	All
16	Enhancing Lead Excretion	促进排铅	Yes	Yes	All
17	Clearing Throat	清咽	Yes	Yes	All
18	Assisting Blood Pressure Reduction	辅助降血压	Yes	Yes	Except for junior and children
19	Increasing Bone Density	增加骨密度	Yes	No	All
20	Regulating Gastrointestinal Tract Flora	调节肠道菌群	Yes	Yes	All
21	Facilitating Digestion	促进消化	Yes	Yes	All
22	Facilitating Defecation	通便	Yes	Yes	All
23	Assisting the Protection of Gastric Mucosa	对胃粘膜有辅助保护	Yes	Yes	All
24	Eliminating Acne	祛痤疮	No	Yes	Except for children
25	Eliminating Skin Chloasma	祛黄褐斑	No	Yes	Except for children
26	Improving Skin Water Content	改善皮肤水份	No	Yes	All
27	Improving Skin Oil Content	改善皮肤油份	No	Yes	All

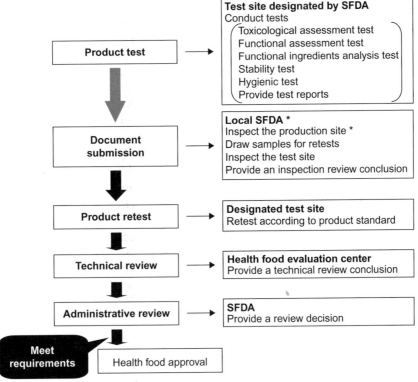

FIGURE 25.2 Health food application procedure in China. *In case of imported products, apply to central SFDA (Beijing) instead of local SFDA. Imported products have to be on market in original country for more than 1 year, and inspecting of the production site is not routine.

of a Novel Food, the following documents are necessary:

- the product development and safety test report;
- the analysis report of nutrients;
- a list of functional ingredients and toxic or harmful ingredients;
- a brief introduction of the production protocol and production flow-chart;
- the standards of product quality, information and scientific publications on the efficacy, application and safety of the product, label and leaflet; and

- other supporting materials and unopened samples of a product or 30 grams of the raw material.

If the product is made overseas, it is necessary to prove that the manufacturer has obtained production permission from the foreign government or the related material is traditionally consumed as a food in the country where the product is manufactured.

The MOH held a series of meetings in 2009, to discuss whether to issue a list of probiotics for infant foods and which probiotics should be on the list. Some parties proposed to clearly

TABLE 25.5   Probiotics for Health Food, Infant Use and Novel Food in China

	Species	Strains	Notes
Health Food	*Bifidobacterium bifidum*	–	–
	Bifidobacterium infantis	–	–
	Bifidobacterium longum	–	–
	Bifidobacterium breve	–	–
	Bifidobacterium adolescentis	–	–
	Lactobacillus delbrueckii subsp. *bulgaricus*	–	–
	Lactobacillus acidophilus	–	–
	Lactobacillus casei subsp. *casei*	–	–
	Streptococcus thermophilus	–	–
	Lactobacillus reuteri	–	–
Infant Use*	*Lactobacillus acidophilus*	NCFM/SD5221	Only for children above 1 year old
	Bifidobacterium animalis	Bb12	–
	Bifidobacterium lactis	HN019	–
	Bifidobacterium lactis	Bi-07	–
	Bifidobacterium longum	BB536	–
	Lactobacillus rhamnosus	LGG	–
	Lactobacillus rhamnosus	HN001	–
	Lactobacillus paracasei	CNCM-2116	–
	Streptococcus thermophilus	TH4	–
Novel Food	*Lactobacillus rhamnosus*	LGG/ATCC 53103	–
	Bifidobacterium animalis	Bb12 (PP011)	–
	Bifidobacterium lactis	HOWARU Bifido/HN019	–
	Bifidobacterium lactis	Bi-07/SD5220	–
	Lactobacillus acidophilus	NCFM/SD5221	Under test production, not finally approved yet
	Lactobacillus rhamnosus	HOWARU Rhamnosus/HN001	–
	Bifidobacterium animalis	BE80	Under test production, not finally approved yet
	Lactobacillus acidophilus	DSM13241	Not for children under 3 years old
	Lactobacillus paracasei	GM080	Not for children under 3 years old
	Lactobacillus paracasei	GMNL-33	Not for children under 3 years old
	Lactobacillus acidophilus	R0052	–
	Lactobacillus rhamnosus	R0011	–
	Lactobacillus plantarum	299v	Not for children under 3 years old
	Lactobacillus plantarum	CGMCC1258	–

*This list is under discussion.

define which probiotic strains (not only to the species level, as it is now) should be put on the list, while others argued that such rules would restrict the development of local enterprises which still had little R&D experience, if any. A list of probiotics for infant use proposed by the SFDA is summarized in Table 25.5. In December 2007, the 'Regulation for Novel Food' replaced the former regulation, the 'Novel Food Hygiene Regulation' issued in 1990. Some probiotic products described as 'under test production' in Table 25.5 still exist in the market, because the old Novel Food law allowed the commercialization of products prepared by test production as Novel Food 'Candidates' for 2 years. However, these would disappear soon, according to the new law prohibiting the launch of any novel food before full official approval has been received.

3.2. Probiotics and Health Claims in China

In 2005, the 'Regulatory for Probiotic Health Food Application and Examination (interim)' was issued for probiotics. Ten probiotics species, *Bifidobacterium bifidum, B. infantis, B. longum, B. breve, B. adolescentis, Lactobacillus delbrueckii* subsp. *bulgaricus, L. acidophilus, L. casei* subsp. *casei, Streptococcus thermophilus,* and *L. reuteri,* have been permitted for use in the manufacture of Foods with Health Claims as probiotic raw materials. Products made from species other than these 10 may also obtain the approval provided that the species (strain) itself passes the examination by the SFDA. Probiotic food manufacturers usually develop a new product with a new probiotic strain, and as a new strain, it must undergo Novel Food examination in China. For example, in September 2008, the SFDA issued an approval for a probiotic strain—*L. acidophilus* R0052—as a Novel Food even though *L. acidophilus* is listed in the 10 probiotic species in the 'Regulatory for Probiotic Health Foods Application and Examination (interim).' Although most of the probiotics' manufacturers emphasize

that their products are probiotic, the concept of probiotics itself is not recognized as a claim category in the Chinese Foods with Health Claim regulatory system. It is not necessary to publish in academic journals the data obtained from the required tests but the parameters and assays to be performed are fixed. To apply for a health claim on a probiotic product, the following information is required:

1. species name of the probiotics, the strain number, Latin nomenclature;
2. culture conditions (culture media, culture temperature);
3. origin of the strain, and evidences proving the safety of the strain;
4. strain identification report from the SFDA appointed institutions, Microbiology Institute, Scientific Academy Sinica;
5. safety test report;
6. storage instruction of the strain;
7. mutant genesis protocol;
8. if the probiotics product is the non-reproducing form of probiotics and/or the metabolite of probiotics, the name and related detection method of the functional factor or specific ingredient;
9. standards and technique assurance used in the manufacturing of the probiotics;
10. GMP certificate of the manufacturer.

Imported products must have been marketed in the original country for more than a year before application can be made to the SFDA. During the guarantee period of a probiotic product, the minimal viable quantity of probiotics should be above 10^6 cfu/mL (g). An example of a product package is shown in Figure 25.3. On the package, the health claim, name and number of strains, approval number, and seal of Foods with Health Claim are shown.

Until recently, 40 products using 12 probiotic species were approved under 'regulating gastrointestinal tract flora', 'enhancing immunity', 'enhancing digestion', 'facilitating defecation', and 'improving skin moisture content' claim

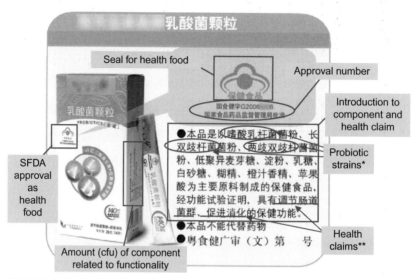

* Probiotic strains: *Lactobacillus acidophilus, Bifidobacterium longum, Bifidobacterium bifidum*
**Health claims: 'improvement of gastrointestinal (GI) conditions', and 'enhance digestion'

FIGURE 25.3   Package sample of health food in China. *Probiotic strains: *Lactobacillus acidophilus, Bifidobacterium longum, Bifidobacterium bifidum*; **Health claims: 'improvement of gastrointestinal (GI) conditions,' and 'enhance digestion'.

categories (Table 25.6). Several of the approved Food with Health Claims exist in the category of 'enhancing immunity.' In the case of applying for a Foods with Health Claim approval in this category, only animal experiments are necessary for the efficacy tests. As shown in Table 25.7, there are mainly four experiments to assess immunity in experiment animals; cellular immunity, humoral immunity, monocyte-macrophage activity, and natural killer cell activity. In an experiment assessing the immunity, three test groups at different doses and a negative control group are necessary; sometimes a positive control group is also needed. In the four categories, if assays in two or more categories show positive results, the food under examination can be regarded as effective in enhancing immunity. The result of a test on cellular immunity is graded as positive when both a Con A induced mouse splenic lymphocyte transformation test and a DTH test are positive, or two dose groups in one of these tests give positive results. The result of tests on humoral immunity

is graded as positive when both an antibody forming cell assay and serum hemolysin assay are positive or two dose groups in one of these tests give positive results. The result of tests on monocyte-macrophage activity is graded as positive when both carbon clearance assay and phagocytosis of murine macrophage show positive results, or two dose groups in one of these tests give positive results. The result of tests on NK killer activity is graded as positive when at least one dose group in either an LDH assay or ^{3}H-TdR assay shows a positive result.

4. REGULATORY STATUS OF HEALTH CLAIM AND PROBIOTICS IN BRAZIL

4.1. Regulatory Status in Brazil

ANVISA (National Health Surveillance Agency) established a systematic procedure for evaluating and approving functional and/or health claims [122–125]. Resolução No 16 (1999) approves the 'Technical regulation on procedures for registration of foods and/or new ingredients.' Resolução No 17 (1999) approves the 'Technical regulation establishing the basic guidelines for evaluation of risk and safety of foods.' Resolução No 18 (1999) approves the 'Technical regulation establishing the basic guidelines for analysis and proof of functional and/or health claims on food labels', and Resolução No 19 (1999) approves the 'Technical regulation on procedures for registration of foods with functional and/or health claims on their labels'. In Brazil, functional foods have not been defined as a category in the legislation. But functional and health claims are defined as, respectively: 'it is related to the metabolic or physiological role that the nutrient or non-nutrient plays in the growth, development, maintenance' and 'other normal functions of the human organism and states, suggests or implies the existence of a connection between the food or ingredient with a disease or condition related to health' [124]. It is forbidden to make any type of statement (e.g., labeling and advertising) indicating that a food can cure, treat or prevent any disease. The use of disease risk reduction claims may only be allowed when scientifically substantiated.

Legislation essentially requires a scientific demonstration of the safety and efficacy of novel foods (foods and ingredients with no history of use in the Brazilian diet or used at levels not normally consumed by the Brazilian population) and foods/ingredients bearing a functional or health claim on the label. All of these products should be evaluated and registered by the health authorities. Safety demonstration is a priority and should be based on risk analysis, including risk assessment, management and information. Efficacy concerning the claims should be based on scientific evidence obtained from the scientific literature or by new research and must represent scientific consensus, as has been discussed by the US Food and Drug Administration and international organizations such as International Life Science Institutes (ILSI) in several forums and in the Codex Alimentarius [126]. In order to provide scientific support to evaluate the safety and efficacy of new ingredients/foods and claims, ANVISA has appointed a Technical Scientific Advisory Commission on Functional Foods and Novel Foods (CTCAF) composed of professors and researchers coming from universities and research centers, based on their expertise in food science, nutrition and toxicology. In ANVISA's website[2] there is a list of all the ingredients, functional and health claims currently authorized to be used in the Brazilian market. It ranges from fatty acids (omega 3: EPA and DHA), carotenoids (lycopene, luteine, zeaxantin), dietary fibers (dextrin resistant, partially hydrolyzed guar gum, beta-glucan polydextrose, inulin, psiillium (psyllium), and quitosane (chitosan)), fructo-oligosaccharides (FOS), lactulose, phytosterols, polyols (mannitol, xylitol and sorbitol), probiotics and soy proteins.

Table 25.8 provides a list of claims approved by ANVISA for these functional ingredients (latest update as of July 2008). For additional detailed information such as the minimal amount required for functional ingredients to make the functional or health claim, warning phrases and latest updates, the reader should consult ANVISA's website. In 2002, in view of the need to clarify the differences between functional foods and bioactive compounds ('nutraceuticals'), the latter usually sold in pharmaceutical forms, containing mostly herbs and other botanicals, a new regulation was added to the already existing regulatory framework, covering at this time 'isolated bioactive substances and probiotics with health or functional claims' [127]. Resolução No 2 (2002) defines bioactive substance as 'nutrients and non-nutrients having a specific metabolic or physiologic activity' [128]. These substances

[2]http://anvisa.gov.br.

Table 6. Approved probiotic products with health claim(s) in China

	Approval Number	Product name (English)	Product name (Chinese)	Manufacturer name (English)
1	国食健字G20080559	President Brand Probiotic Powder	总统牌益生菌粉	MDS Parma Services (China) Inc, Beijing TRT Pharma
2	国食健字G20070320	Dier Brand Probiotic Powder	迪儿牌益生菌粉剂	Hutchison Healthcare
3	国食健字G20070367	Meidisheng Brand Probiotic Powder	美迪生牌益生菌粉剂	MDS Parma Services (China) Inc
4	国食健字G20060687	Yishengankang Brand Probiotic Capsule	怡生安康牌益生菌胶囊	Beijing YSAK Biotech Co., Ltd.
5	国食健字G20060703	Jianneng Brand Probiotic Fermented Milk	健能牌益生菌酸奶	Bright Dairy&Food Co., Ltd
6	国食健字G20060631	Guangming Brand Probiotic Fermented Milk	光明牌益生菌酸牛奶	Bright Dairy&Food Co., Ltd
7	国食健字G20060646	Time-Crystal Brand Probiotic Capsule	时间晶体牌益生菌胶囊	BJ-Timefine Biotech Inc.
8	国食健字G20060027	Only 1 R Probiotic Granule	昂立1号R益生菌颗粒	Shanghai Jiao Da Onlly Co., Ltd
9	卫食健字(2003)第0114号	Lesai Brand Probiotic Capsule	乐赛牌益生菌胶囊	BiosTime Inc.(Guangzhou)
10	国食健字G20080082	Yishengyuan Brand Probiotic Chongji	益生元牌益生菌冲剂	Dongda Technology
11	国食健字G20080146	Baoluo Brand Probiotic Capsule	保罗牌益生菌胶囊	Polo-China
12	国食健字G20080257	Baobikang Brand Probiotic Powder	葆芘康牌益生菌粉	BabyCare Ltd.
13	国食健字G20080456	Yongfutang Brand Probiotic Powder	永福堂牌益生菌粉	Guangzhou Tianhunanlu Health Foods
14	国食健字G20080503	Duoweisheng Brand Probiotic Powder	多微生牌益生菌粉	Shenzhen Duoweisheng Health Foods
15	国食健字G20080638	Jinnengyuan Brand Probiotic Capsule	金能源牌益生菌胶囊	Guangdong Yibo Health Foods
16	国食健字G20080634	Jinnengyuan Brand Probiotic Granule	金能源牌益生菌颗粒	Guangdong Yibo Health Foods
17	国食健字G20070245	Yisheng Brand Probiotic Powder	益生菌牌益生菌粉（桔子口味）	MDS Parma Services (China) Inc
18	国食健字G20070366	Meidisheng Brand Probiotic Powder	美迪生牌益生菌粉剂（桔子味）	MDS Parma Services (China) Inc
19	国食健字G20070385	Tongrentang Brand Probiotic Granule	同仁堂牌益生菌颗粒（甜橙口味）	Beijing YSAK Biotech Co., Ltd.
20	国食健字G20060738	Yishengankang Brand Probiotic Granule	怡生安康牌益生菌颗粒（水蜜桃口味）	Beijing YSAK Biotech Co., Ltd.
21	国食健字G20060307	Changneigeming R Brand B.longum, L.bulgaricus, S.thermophilus Powder	肠内革命R3三联益生菌粉剂	Inner Mongolia Shuangqi Pharmaceuticals
22	国食健字G20060397	Gaobote Brand Probiotic Granule	高博特牌普欧百奥活菌颗粒	Shanghai Cobtt Health
23	国食健字G20050834	Only 1 R Probiotic Granule	昂立1号R益菌多颗粒（女士型）	Shanghai Jiao Da Onlly Co., Ltd
24	国食健字G20040079	Yishengbao Brand Bifidobacterium Capsule	益生宝牌双歧杆菌胶囊	Shanghai Yishengbao Bioproducts
25	卫食健字(1997)第371号	Youshi R Bifidobacterium Chewing Tablet	优世R双歧口嚼片	Beijing Youshi Nutrients&Healthcare
26	国食健字G20030028	Kangdefu Brand Changweikang Drink	康德福牌长维康口服液	Nanjing Pan-asia Biotech
27	国食健字G20040261	Henglin Brand Runping Powder	恒麟牌润平粉	Harbin Hengling Biotech
28	国食健字J20060014	Probio 'Stick	民生普瑞宝牌益生菌颗粒	LALLEMAND S.A.S
29	国食健字J20060002	Biostime Probiotics Capsules	合生元牌益生菌胶囊	LALLEMAND S.A.S
30	国食健字G20060446	Yafangyimeigao Brand Lactobacilli Granule	雅芳益美高牌乳酸菌颗粒	Avon Products (China)
31	国食健字G20050323	Hailang Bifido Milk	海浪牌双叉奶	Chongqing Hailang Technology
32	国食健字G20040177	Weiquan R Active Probiotic Drink	味全R活性乳酸菌饮品	Hangzhou Dingjin Foods
33	卫食健字(2001)第0070号	Jianneng Brand Probiotic Milk	健能牌益菌奶	Bright Dairy&Food Co., Ltd
34	国食健字G20060258	Biyou Brand Daneng Fermented Milk	碧悠牌达能酸牛奶	Bright Dairy&Food Co., Ltd
35	国食健字G20070150	Longtianli Brand Longtianli Drink	龙天力牌龙天力口服液	Beijing Longtianli Biotech
36	国食健字G20041493	Yiliduo Brand Probiotic Drink	益力多牌酸菌乳饮品	Yakult China
37	国食健字G20050204	Yangleduo Brand Daitian Probiotic Drink	养乐多牌代田乳酸菌饮料	Yakult China
38	国食健字G20040361	Gongshengyuan Brand Lactobacillus acidophilus Capsule	共生源牌嗜酸乳杆菌胶囊	Guangzhou Baidi Bio-Pharma
39	国食健字G20060227	Yili R Lekang Chewing Tablet	伊利R乐康咀嚼片	Yili Dairy
40	国食健字G20080636	Benteng R Soybean Lactobacillus acidophilus Capsule	奔腾R大豆嗜酸乳杆菌胶囊	Yang Zhenhua 851 Biotech
	Number of approval		**total : 40**	

* registered as species, ** registered as strains
a) 植物乳杆菌ST-III菌株(vegetable lactobacillus): *B.breve* at 1×108 cfu/100g, *L.acidophilus* at 1×107 cfu/100g (200g×1/day)
b) 植物乳杆菌ST-III菌株(vegetable lactobacillus): *B.breve* at 1×10^6 cfu/100g, *L.acidophilus* at 1×10^8 cfu/100g (118g×1/day)
c) LP-Onlly: *B.longum* at 1×10^9 cfu/100g and *L.acidophilus* at 5.3×10^9 cfu/100g (2g ×1/day)
d) dose: 2×1.5g x2 time/day
e) LP-Onlly: *L.acidophilus* at 6.5×10^9 cfu/100g (2g ×1/day)
f) dose: 200g/day
g) 1 or 2 ×200ml/1–2 time/day
h) 植物乳杆菌ST-III菌株(vegetable lactobacillus): *B.animalis* at 3×108 cfu/100g (100g×1/day)
i) *Lactobacillus casei* Shirota at 3.4×10^{10} cfu/100ml (100 ml x2/day)

Probiotics — SFDA permitted probiotic species usable for health food*										Other strains**			Functional claims					Other information			
Bifidobacterium bifidum	*Bifidobacterium infantis*	*Bifidobacterium longum*	*Bifidobacterium breve*	*Bifidobacterium adolescentis*	*L. delbrueckii subsp. bulgaricus*	*Lactobacillus acidophilus*	*L. casei subsp. casei*	*Streptococcus thermophilus*	*Lactobacillus reuteri*	*Bifidobacteria lactis*	*Bifidobacteria animalis*	lactobacilli	Regulating Gastrointestinal Tract Flora	Enhancing Immunity	Facilitating defecation	Facilitating Digestion	Improving Skin Moisture Content	Domestic / Imported	Description for children	Approved Date	Remarks
	✓					✓							✓	✓				D		8/12/2008	
	✓					✓							✓					D	dose limitation	7/25/2007	
		✓				✓							✓	✓				D	>3Y old	9/21/2007	
			✓			✓							✓					D	>3Y old	8/1/2006	
			✓			✓									✓	✓		D		8/21/2006	a
			✓			✓							✓		✓			D		6/8/2006	b
						✓							✓					D	>3Y old	6/23/2006	
		✓				✓							✓	✓				D		1/12/2006	c
	✓			✓		✓		✓							✓	✓		D		2/13/2003	
✓		✓				✓							✓					D	>3Y old	2/3/2008	
		✓				✓	✓						✓					D		3/23/2008	
✓						✓				✓			✓					D	can take	5/7/2008	d
	✓					✓							✓					D		7/20/2008	
	✓					✓							✓					D	>3Y old	8/26/2008	
✓			✓	✓		✓		✓					✓					D	>3Y old	########	
✓	✓					✓							✓					D		########	
	✓					✓							✓	✓				D		6/19/2007	
		✓				✓							✓					D	>3Y old	9/21/2007	
			✓			✓							✓					D	>3Y old	9/21/2007	
			✓		✓			✓					✓					D		8/29/2006	
		✓						✓								✓		D	>1Y old	3/13/2006	
✓						✓							✓					D		3/23/2006	e
						✓							✓				✓	D		12/6/2005	f
	✓														✓	✓		D	dose limitation	1/9/2004	
✓						✓		✓					✓			✓		D		8/6/1997	
✓						✓							✓	✓				D		########	
							✓						✓			✓		D	dose limitation	3/17/2004	
✓	✓					✓							✓	✓				I		9/24/2006	
✓	✓					✓								✓	✓			I		1/13/2006	
					✓			✓				✓	✓			✓		D		4/4/2006	
								✓				✓	✓					D		5/10/2005	f
					✓			✓					✓			✓		D		1/21/2004	
						✓						✓			✓	✓		D		3/23/2001	g
								✓					✓		✓			D		2/27/2006	h
			✓	✓									✓	✓				D		3/9/2007	
											✓		✓	✓				D		########	i
											✓		✓	✓				D	>1Y old	3/15/2005	i
						✓							✓					D		3/17/2004	
						✓							✓					D		2/24/2006	
						✓								✓				D	>3Y old	########	
7	6	11	6	1	2	32	4	6	0	1	3	2	29	21	8	4	1	38			

TABLE 25.7 Functional assessment tests required for probiotics health food claim application in China

Functional Claims	Designated test			
	Animal test[†]		Human test	
	Test Name	Criteria	Test Name	Criteria
Regulating Gastrointestinal Tract Flora	**Body weight (BW), bacteria in mouse feces:** Bifidobacteria and/or lactobacilli *Clostridium perfringens* Enterobacteria and enterococcus	Number of bifidobacteria and/or lactobacilli significantly increased, number of *C. perfringens* decreased or didn't change significantly, number of enterobacteria and enterococcus didn't change significantly or increased significantly but less than that of bifidobacterias and lactobacillis.	**Body weight (BW), bacteria in feces:** Bifidobacteria and/ or lactobacilli *Clostridium perfringens* Enterobacteria and enterococcus	Number of bifidobacteria and/or lactobacilli significantly increased, number of *C. perfringens* decreased or didn't change significantly, number of enterobacteria and enterococcus didn't change significantly or increased significantly but less than that of bifidobacterias and lactobacillis
Enhancing Immunity	**Body weight (BW):** Weight of thymus gland/BW, weight of spleen/BW **Cellular immunity:** Con A induced mouse splenic lymphocyte transformation; (MTT assay or isotope labelling precursor incorporation assay); Delayed type hypersensitivity in mouse; (DNFB induced mouse DTH assay or SRBC induced mouse DTH assay) **Humoral immunity:** Antibody forming cell assay (also called plaque forming cell assay) using sheep erythrocyte and mouse splenocyte; Serum hemolysin assay using sheep erythrocyte and mouse splenocyte; (Hemagglutination assay or HC50 assay) **Monocyte-macrophage activity:** Mouse carbon clearance assay; phagocytosis of murine macrophage; (slide-glass assay or *in situ* assay)	In the four categories, if assays in two or more than two categories show positive results, the food under examination can be regarded as effective in enhancing immunity. Result of test at cellular immunity category is graded as positive when both Con A induced mouse splenic lymphocyte transformation test and DTH test are positive or two dosage groups in one of these tests get positive results. Result of tests at humoral immunity category is graded as positive when both antibody forming cell assay and serum hemolysin assay are positive or two dosage groups in one of these tests get positive results. Result of tests at monocyte-macrophage activity category is graded as positive when both carbon clearance assay and phagocytosis of murine macrophage show positive results or two dosage groups in one of these tests get positive results. Result of tests at NK killer activity category is graded as positive when at least one dosage group in either LDH assay or 3H-TdR assay shows positive result.	Not required	Not required

Mouse NK killer activity assay: LDH assay or 3H-TdR assay

Facilitating Defecation	**Mouse intestinal movement test; defecation time; number of feces pellets; feces weight**	The examination result is judged as positive in either of the following situations: (1) Either intestinal movement test or defecation time shows positive result; (2) either pellet number or feces weight shows positive result.	**Feces:** Frequency; bowel movement difficulty score; Bristol feces score	Defecation frequency significantly increased or bowel movement difficulty score and Bristol feces score significantly decreased
Facilitating Digestion	**Weight, food intake, food availability in rat, intestinal movement test in mouse, enzyme assay in rat**	The examination result is judged as positive when two of the three categories are positive: (1) Weight, food intake, food availability; (2) intestinal movement; (3) enzyme assay.	**Children:** Appetite, food intake, body weight, hemoglobulin **Adults:** Clinical symptom scores, stomach, intestinal movement	**Children:** If anyone of the four categories shows positive result, the food under examination can be regarded as effective **Adults:** If the clinical symptom scores are significantly improved and stomach, intestinal movement test is positive, the food under examination can be regarded as effective
Improving Skin Moisture Content	Not required	Not required	**Forehead skin moisture assay**	If forehead skin moisture assay shows significant improvement, the food under examination can be regarded as effective

†In an efficacy test, three test groups of different doses (the bodyweight-adjusted dose in one group is five (rat) or ten (mouse) times as high as the recommended dose for humans) and a negative control group are necessary, sometimes a positive control group is also needed.

TABLE 25.8   List of approved functional and health claims in Brazil

Functional ingredients	Functional or health claim
Dextrin resistant (dietary fiber) Guar gum partially hydrolyzed (dietary fiber) Dietary fibers Polydextrose (dietary fiber)	The dietary fiber helps the intestines to function normally. Its consumption should be associated with a balanced diet and healthy lifestyle.
Lactulose	The lactulose helps the intestines to function. Its consumption should be associated with a balanced diet and healthy lifestyle.
Omega-3 fatty acids (EPA; DHA)	The consumption of omega-3 fatty acids helps maintain healthy levels of triglycerides, provided it is associated with a balanced diet and healthy lifestyle.
Lycopene Lutein Zeaxantin	Lycopene (lutein, zeaxantin) has antioxidant properties that protect cells against free radicals. Its consumption should be associated with a balanced diet and healthy lifestyle.
Phytosterols	Phytosterols help to reduce the absorption of cholesterol. Its consumption should be associated with a balanced diet and healthy lifestyle.
Beta-glucan	Beta-glucan (dietary fiber) helps to reduce the absorption of cholesterol. Its consumption should be associated with a balanced diet and healthy lifestyle.
Inulin Fructo-oligosaccharides (FOS)	Inulin (FOS) helps to maintain a balanced intestinal flora. Its consumption should be associated with a balanced diet and healthy lifestyle.
Psillium (psyllium)	Psillium (dietary fiber) helps to reduce the absorption of fat. Its consumption should be associated with a balanced diet and healthy lifestyle.
Quitosane (chitosan)	Quitosane helps to reduce the absorption of fat and cholesterol. Its consumption should be associated with a balanced diet and healthy lifestyle.
Mannitol Xylitol Sorbitol	Mannitol (xylitol, sorbitol) does not form acids that damage the teeth. The consumption of the product does not replace adequate dietary and mouth hygiene habits (this claim is approved only for chewing gum without sugar).
Lactobacillus acidophilus *Lactobacillus casei* shirota *Lactobacillus casei* subsp. *rhamnosus* *Lactobacillus casei* subsp. *defensis* *Lactobacillus paracasei* *Lactococcus lactis* *Bifidobacterium bifidum* *Bifidobacterium animalis* (including subsp. *B. lactis*) *Bifidobacterium longum* *Enterococcus faecium*	The (probiotic) helps to maintain a balanced intestinal flora. Its consumption should be associated with a balanced diet and healthy lifestyle.
Soy protein	The daily consumption of at least 25 g of soy protein may help to reduce cholesterol. Its consumption should be associated with a balanced diet and healthy lifestyle.

are classified in seven different chemical groups: carotenoids, phytosterols, flavonoids, phospholipids, organosulfur compounds, polyphenols, and probiotics. These bioactive substances should be available in solid forms, semi-solid or liquids, such as tablets, pills, drugs, powders, capsules, granules, solutions and suspensions. They were included in this regulation because they are available to the consumer in non-food forms [127]. The approval process is the same as for functional foods; i.e., it is necessary to get approval from ANVISA before making the product available to the market. Bioactive substances and probiotics must carry a functional or health claim in their labeling package.

4.2. Probiotics and Health Claims in Brazil

At the time of writing, ANVISA has approved 10 microorganisms with probiotic functions (Table 25.8). There is no differentiation of claims among the different probiotics. The only health claim allowed to be used for label declaration and communication is: *'The (probiotic) helps to maintain a balanced intestinal flora. Its consumption should be associated with a balanced diet and healthy life style.'* In addition, the following information should be provided by the manufacturer:

- The minimal viable quantity of probiotics should be between 10^8 to 10^9 cfu as described in the recommended daily consumption. Lower values can be accepted once scientific data demonstrate its efficacy.
- An analytical result should be provided demonstrating the cells' viability at the end of its shelf life.
- Scientific proof should demonstrate the resistance of the probiotic to the gastric acid and the bile salts.
- The quantity of probiotics in cfu, as described in the recommended daily portion ready to eat, should be declared near the health claim.

Every new ingredient and functional or health claim needs to be approved by ANVISA in Brazil. Even functional and/or health claims already assessed by ANVISA need prior approval, once they are evaluated on a case-by-case basis, taking into account food composition, target population, efficacy on the specific food matrix, public health policies, etc. For each product, a specific and conclusive scientific dossier is necessary to support the use of the ingredient (safety) and claim (efficacy). The claims may mention general maintenance of health, the physiological role of the nutrients and the reduction of risk of diseases. Health claims that mention cures or prevention of diseases are not allowed.

The procedure for registration of foods and/or new ingredients is detailed in Resolução No 16 and should contain the following documentation presented in the 'Technical Scientific Report': name of the product, purpose of use, recommended intake indicated by the manufacturer, scientific description of the ingredients of the product according to the species of botanical, animal or mineral origin (when appropriate); the chemical composition with molecular characterization (when appropriate); and/or formulation of the product, description of the analytical methodology for evaluation of the food or ingredient that is the object of the petition; applicable scientific evidences, as appropriate, to prove safety of use; nutritional and/or physiological and/or toxicological assays in experimentation animals, biochemical assays, epidemiological studies, clinical assays, evidence of traditional use, observed in the population, without damage to health, broad evidences from scientific literature, international health organizations and internationally recognized legislation on the characteristics of the food or ingredient [122].

Resolução No 18 provides the basic guidelines for applicants who are interested in using functional and/or health claims displayed on the labels of products to be sold to consumers.

The applicant should provide the following information in the Technical Scientific report:

- recommended intake;
- chemical composition with molecular characterization (when appropriate) and/or formulation of the product;
- biochemical assays;
- nutritional and/or physiological and/or toxicological assays in experimentation animals;
- epidemiological studies;
- clinical assays;
- general evidence from scientific literature, international health organizations and internationally recognized legislation on the characteristics of the food or ingredient;
- evidence of traditional use, observed in the population, without damage to human health and documented information on approval of use of the food or ingredient in other countries, economic blocks, Codex Alimentarius and other internationally recognized organizations [124].

5. FUNCTIONAL FOOD AND HEALTH CLAIMS IN EUROPE

The term 'Functional Food' is not defined in Europe but is generally understood as 'food with a health claim.' Although the food and diet culture in Europe may be regarded as more conservative than in Asia, the relationship between nutrition and health has gained increasing public acceptance over the last decade. Consumers have become more and more health conscious and industry wishes to take advantage of the evolution in science and invest in innovation in this area.

Consequently, it is the use of health claims, not the use of functional foods, which is regulated in the EU. Since the early 1990s, the European Commission, the central institution of the EU political system, has had preliminary discussions towards securing a future claims regulatory system. It was, however, not until 2003 that an official draft was presented to the European Parliament and the Member States. Divergent views and lengthy debates, in particular on the level of scientific substantiation, data protection, and last but not least, the introduction of nutrient profiles as a condition for making nutrition and health claims, delayed the final adoption of this Regulation until late in 2006.

Before the adoption of the EU Regulation in 2006, there was a legal void with regard to health claims. The EU framework labeling legislation prohibited 'attributing to any foodstuff the property of preventing, treating or curing a human disease or referring to such properties' [129]. This was interpreted differently in each of the then 15 EU Member States. Therefore, it may have occurred that a claim, which was permitted in one country, may have been prohibited in another and vice versa [130].

The most difficult type of claim to regulate was the Disease Risk Reduction Claim. This was often regarded as a medicinal claim and therefore prohibited. It was included in the final Regulation subject to an individual application. There was a greater acceptance of so-called functional claims, although the term was not used as such, and many national lists were established with guidelines for the use of nutrition claims following Codex rules.

In the absence of a specific European legislation on health claims, the food industry became a stakeholder in self-regulatory initiatives in Sweden and in a number of EU countries in the 1990s, including the UK, France, Belgium, Netherlands, Spain, and Finland. It was observed that there was an 'underlying consistency of approach, but analysis shows that differences were sometimes minor but sometimes major' [131]. These innovative initiatives were introduced to facilitate the use of health claims. They included the adoption of guidelines and Codes of Practice in various Member States of the EU and of one industry-led European

Code of Practice by CIAA (European Food and Drink Association). In most of these countries, a partnership of industry experts, enforcement authorities and consumer representatives developed the rules for the scientific substantiation, communication and presentation of health claims to the scientific community and government authorities. The most prominent examples of these European self-regulatory systems are the Swedish Self Regulation Code and the UK Joint Health Claims Initiative.

5.1. Self-regulatory Initiatives in Europe

The Swedish Food Sector's Code of Practice

In Sweden, the use of health claims within the scope of the Food Sector's Code of Practice–Health Claims in the Labeling and Marketing of Food Products has been possible since 1990. Since its introduction, the Code, which was established in close contact with the competent authorities, has been revised three times, and the last version of the Code was launched in September 2004. Principals of the Code were the Swedish Food Federation and the Swedish Food Retailers Federation. The Swedish Nutrition Federation was the coordinating and advisory body within the Code. The Code consisted of five parts: rules, expert advice, follow-up, evaluation, and information.

Under the Swedish Health Claims Code, two probiotic claims were considered, a Fruit Drink with *Lactobacillus plantarum* 299v in 2003, and a milk-based drink containing *L. rhamnosus* GG, *L. rhamnosus* Lc-705, *P. freudenreichii* ssp. *shermani* JS, *Bifidobacterium* strain in 2007.

The Swedish Code has gradually ceased to exist in its present form. However, during the implementation of the EU Nutrition and Health Claims Regulation, parts of the Code were used as guidelines on how to apply health claims in a responsible manner on a national level.

Joint Health Claims Initiative (UK)

The Joint Health Claims Initiative (JHCI) was established in 1997 as a joint venture between consumer organizations, enforcement authorities and industry bodies to adopt a Code of Practice for the use of health claims. The initiative aimed at creating a level playing field for industry and control bodies, and to increase consumer protection by evaluating the science behind generic and innovative health claims.

The JHCI Code of Practice defined source and nature of scientific evidence requesting a systematic review of all available scientific evidence relating to the validity of the claim (Article 8.4.1). Once evaluated by the JHCI Expert Committee, the proposed claim was submitted to the JHCI Council for approval. The JHCI Directors and Council agreed in 2007 that the new EU 'Health Claims' Regulation for foods was about to supplant this area of activity (JHCI Press Release 22.3.2007). JHCI has not approved any probiotic claims.

5.2. EU Regulation on Nutrition and Health Claims (NHC) in Foodstuffs

The EU Regulation on nutrition and health made on foods (Regulation (EC) 1924/2006) lays down harmonized rules for the use of nutrition claims (such as 'low fat,' 'high fiber') and health claims (e.g. 'helps lower cholesterol') on foodstuffs based on nutrient profiles, which are to be defined at a later stage. The Health Claims Regulation will ensure that any claim made on a food label in the EU is clear, accurate and substantiated. In doing so, it will enable consumers to make informed and meaningful choices when it comes to food and drinks. This should also contribute to a higher level of health protection, as it ties in with the European Commission's campaign for healthier lifestyle choices by allowing consumers to know exactly what they are consuming.

TABLE 25.9   Classification of EU claims on foods

Nutrition claims	Health claims		
<Annex>	<Article 13.1>	<Article 13.5>	<Article 14>
• Nutrient content • Comparative • 'Other substance'	Based on generally accepted scientific evidence	Based on newly developed scientific data/intellectual property right protection	Reduction of disease risk and claims referring to children's development and health

5.3. Health Claims Under the EU Regulation

Permitted Claims

The European Regulation defines four categories of health claims and their authorization (Table 25.9): Individual authorization is needed for health claims that fall under Article 14 of the Regulation, i.e.:

- Health claims referring to the reduction of disease risk (meaning any health claim that states, suggests or implies that the consumption of a food category, a food or one of its constituents significantly reduces a risk factor in the development of human disease).
- Health claims referring to children's development and health.

Applications for authorization are subject to scientific evaluation by EFSA, prior to their inclusion in a Community list of permitted claims.

Health claims that fall under Article 13.1 of the Regulation (other than those referring to the reduction of a disease risk and to children's development and health) are generally accepted and well understood, i.e. health claims describing or referring to:

- the role of a nutrient or other substance in growth, development and the functions of the body;
- psychological and behavioral functions; or
- slimming or weight control.

These have to be included in the European Community list of permitted claims (available from 2010). The EFSA was (at the time of writing) evaluating the several thousand diet–health relationships submitted by Member States, and often prepared by EU industry associations or individual companies. This includes diet–health relationships of probiotics.

An individual application has to be filed for health claims (other than those referring to the reduction of disease risk and to children's development and health) that have not been included in the Community list of permitted claims (Article 13.5), which are based on newly developed scientific evidence, and/or which include a request for the protection of proprietary data.

Conditions for Making Claims

The Regulation contains other challenging provisions and interpretations: the introduction of Nutrient Profiles, in 2009, as a condition for making a claim has led to much debate and polemic about the role of food products in a balanced diet. The decision to classify simple 'contains' claims, such as 'contains probiotic' as a health, not a nutrition or ingredient claim, will severely limit manufacturers' ability to make claims on the benefits of probiotics because of the additional conditions which have to be fulfilled [133].

When making health claims the following labeling obligations apply:

- A statement on the label indicating the importance of a varied and balanced diet and a healthy lifestyle.
- The quantity of the food and pattern of consumption required to obtain the claimed beneficial effect.
- Where appropriate, a statement addressed to those persons who should avoid consuming the food.
- Where appropriate, a warning statement.

5.4. Scientific Substantiation in Europe

The EU NHC Regulation is silent on specific rules for the substantiation of well-established and well-understood health claims (known as 'Article 13.1 claims'). On the other hand, the technical rules for the preparation of an application for other health claims (known as 'Article 13.5' or 'Article 14 claims') are well documented [134–136].

In the EU system, scientific substantiation must include all scientific data, published and unpublished, in favor and not in favor together with a comprehensive review of the data from human studies to demonstrate that the claim is substantiated. The totality of the scientific data must be taken into account and by weighing the evidence shall demonstrate:

- how the claimed benefit is beneficial for human health;
- cause and effect relationship;
- quantity of food and pattern of consumption required;
- specific study group in which evidence was obtained.

Foods or food constituents have to be fully characterized to enable the EFSA to evaluate the relevance of the submitted studies.

The organization of pertinent data must follow the order: human data classified according to hierarchy of study design (human intervention studies, human observational studies, other human studies), non-human data (animal, *ex vivo* or *in vitro*). Data from studies in humans addressing the relationship between consumption of the food and the claimed effect is required for substantiation of a health claim. This must include a comprehensive review of the data. The framework of the health claims Regulation does not foresee a safety evaluation of the food nor a decision whether the food is classified legally as a foodstuff.

5.5. The List of Health Claims in Article 13.1

As stated previously, it was the task of the EFSA to evaluate the several thousand diet–health relationships that the 27 Member States of the EU had submitted to the European Commission based, in the main, on a list prepared by EU industry associations and screened by nutrition scientists. In January 2009, the EFSA published the list of health claims received from the European Commission for assessment. In total, the EFSA has received 4,185 main health claim entries, taking into account the conditions of use and references available for around 10,000 similar health claims. Each entry comprises of a food component, a health relationship and an example of wording.

It had been widely understood among industry that the EFSA should approach scientific substantiation on Article 13 claims in a different way to its approach to Articles 14 and 13.5. However, it would now appear that the same EFSA process of evaluation, in particular with regard to the requirement of human intervention studies, will be applied to Article 13.1 generic claims. It was very unlikely that the list of permitted health claims would be available in January 2010, foreseen in legislation due to the sheer quantity of claims submitted to the authorities and the complexity of the task.[3]

5.6. Probiotic Claims in Europe

The 27 EU member governments submitted the claims to the central scientific body EFSA based on a list prepared by EU industry associations and food and food supplement companies, including, in total, 268 proposed diet–health relationships involving probiotics after pre-screening for potential inclusion in the list of permitted claims. The most common benefit areas for probiotics are digestive health, intestinal flora, gut health, digestive system and immune system, but final evaluation of all probiotic strains and official authorization are still outstanding.

6. DISCUSSION

The health benefits of foods can now be scientifically proven, and the functional food market is expanding throughout the world. In response to this movement, authorities have implemented approval procedures to allow communication of the health advantages of some foods, if the benefit is scientifically substantiated, to allow consumers to maximize the health benefit through the consumption of such functional foods. At the same time, authorities need to regulate claims, so as not to mislead consumers, and ensure a level playing field among operators. The Health Claim Regulation systems, FOSHU in Japan and Health Food in China, were launched in 1991 and 1996, respectively. The EU launched their health claim system in 2007, and full implementation of the system was

[3]http://www.efsa.europa.eu/EFSA/efsa_locale-1178620753812_article13.htm.

targeted for completion in 2010. Brazil is one of the countries where health claims on food are most strictly regulated, and where health claims are regulated with novel food legislation since 1999. A summary of the health claim systems in Japan, China, Brazil and EU is shown in Table 25.10. In Japan, China, and Brazil, it is necessary to make an individual application for each food product for which a health claim shall be made. The application procedure and its requirements are clearly indicated by the governments in Japan and China. A unique approach is on-going in the EU, where health claims based on new science will be approved individually, but all possible health claims on food ingredients based on currently existing scientific evidences would be on a positive list, except those for children and disease risk reduction. A similar approach was taken in Japan only for vitamins and minerals, for which are allowed fixed claims on products with a certain amount of micronutrients without any specific applications, not under FOSHU but FNFC. It remains to be seen how the EU will allow health claims on food ingredients from 2010 onwards.

For all four regions, there is no doubt that scientific substantiation is necessary for claims. However, requirements for scientific substantiation are different in each region. China has the widest range of health claim categories. China has a long history of Chinese medicine and people in China as well as some Asian countries including Japan believe in the idea of food and foodstuffs having health benefits beyond those provided by nutrients. There are some unique health claim categories in the fixed 27 Chinese claim list related to Chinese medicine (e.g. immunity, sleep, fatigue, lead excretion, and milk secretion). These claims are not allowed in Japan, even if the claim systems and the popular beliefs regarding food functionality are similar. Interestingly, some health claim categories do not require human trials in China (e.g. immunity, fatigue and bone density), unlike the other three regions. In Japan,

TABLE 25.10 Summary of health claim systems in Japan, China, Brazil and EU

	Japan	China	Brazil	European Union (27 Member States)
Health claim system	Foods for Specified Health Uses (FOSHU)	Health food	ANVISA 1999	Regulation on Nutrition and Health Claims (NHC) made on foods
Year started	1991	1996	1999	2007
Definition	FOSHU is foods officially approved to claim their physiological effects on the human body.	Health food is food officially approved to claim specific health efficacy and/or replenishment of vitamins and minerals*. Among specified people, the food can regulate body function(s) but can not be supposed to cure diseases. The food should not induce any acute, sub-acute or chronic disorder.	Functional and health claims are defined as, respectively: 'it is related to the metabolic or physiological role that the nutrient or non-nutrient plays in the growth, development, maintenance' and 'other normal functions of the human organism and states, suggests or implies the existence of a connection between the food or ingredient with disease or condition related to health'.	Health claim means any claim that states, suggests or implies that a relationship exists between a food category, a food or one of its constituents and health. Categorized under 3 domains, based on generally accepted scientific evidences (Article 13.1), newly developed scientific data/IP right protection (Article 13.5) and reduction of disease risk and claims referring to children's health (Article 14).
Claim categories currently approved	GI condition, blood pressure, cholesterol, triacylglycerol, body fat, blood sugar, bone health, mineral absorption, oral health.	Immunity, physical fatigue, blood sugar, blood lipids, sleep, protecting liver against chemical injury, facilitating defecation, antioxidative, weight control, anemia, skin chloasma, bone density, clearing throat, memory, eye fatigue, anoxia endurance, hazard protection, digestion, blood pressure, lead excretion, gastrointestinal flora , child growth, skin water content, protection of gastric mucosa, eliminating acne, milk secretion, skin oil content (27 fixed claims).	Regulating gastrointestinal flora, triglyceride, teeth, bowel function, antioxidant, fat absorption, cholesterol.	Under evaluation. The scientific evaluation body EFSA has received 4,185 main health claim entries, taking into account the conditions of use and references available for around 10,000 similar health claims. Each entry comprises of a food component, a health relationship and an example of wording.

(Continued)

TABLE 25.10 (Continued)

Health claim system	Japan	China	Brazil	European Union (27 Member States)
	Foods for Specified Health Uses (FOSHU)	Health food	ANVISA 1999	Regulation on Nutrition and Health Claims (NHC) made on foods
Year started	1991	1996	1999	2007
Health claim wording	Wording freely applies.	Fixed claims.	Fixed claims.	Decision on a case-by-case basis.
Disease risk reduction claim	Allowed under FOSHU on Ca and folic acid with fixed claim.	Not allowed.	Allowed.	Allowed.
Claim on food product or ingredient/matrix	On food product.	On food product.	On food product.	Food category, food or food constituent.
Functional components	Probiotics, oligosaccharides, dietary fibers, proteins/peptides, phytochemicals, fatty acids/fat, sugar alcohols, minerals, etc.	Probiotics, dietary fibers, polysaccharides, bioactive oligosaccharides, unsaturated fatty acids, phospholipids, chlorines, antioxidants, proteins, flavones, vitamins and minerals.	Probiotics, dietary fibers, fatty acids, carotenoids, phytosterols, polyols, soy protein.	Under evaluation, EFSA has received 4,185 main health claim entries.
Claim application	Required for each product.	Required for each product.	Required for each product.	Required for health claims for Articles 13.5 and 14.
Target population	People who need specific health benefit, age is not specified.	People who need specific health benefit, age is specified.	People who need specific health benefit, age is specified.	General population, children.
Human trial for scientific substantiation	Required on each final product for efficacy and safety confirmation (Regular FOSHU). For risk reduction claim and Standard FOSHU with some specific OS and dietary fibers, just safety confirmation on product is required.	Required on final product but not for all claim categories. Animal study is also required in some categories. Trial should be conducted by the Ministry after application. Protocol is fixed.	Requires final product or similar matrix.	Required for scientific substantiation in view of inclusion in EU list of permitted claims.

No. of trials required	One.	One.	Preferable in two.	No pre-established formula.
Subjects	Local population except for oral health.	Local population.	Preferable in local population.	Preferable in one of local population.
Study protocol	Free but mostly fixed precedentally.	Fixed.	Free.	Free.
Publication on result	Required to publish in peer reviewed journal.	Not required.	Required to publish in peer reviewed journal.	Preferable.
Claim on probiotics	Approved in 'improve in GI conditions' category.	Approved in 'regulating gastrointestinal tract flora', 'enhancing immunity', 'facilitating feces excretion', 'facilitating digestion', 'improving skin water content' categories.	'Helps to maintain a balanced intestinal flora. Its consumption should be associated with a balanced diet and healthy lifestyle.'	Under evaluation, proposed benefit areas include digestive health, intestinal flora, gut health, digestive system and immune system.
Approved probiotics	10 single strain and 3 strain combinations in 73 products, as of Nov 2008.	12 species in 40 products, as of April 2009.	10 strains.	None in April 2009.
Novel food registration for probiotics	Not required.	14 probiotic strains are currently allowed to be used as Novel Food, and among them 4 strains are prohibited from infant formula.	Required for each strain. Scientific substantiation is necessary for safety and efficacy.	Not required.
Remarks	Nutrient function claim is separately ruled under Food with Nutrient Function Claims (FNFC), where 12 vitamins and 5 minerals with fixed claims are allowed without any requirement for application.	In 2005, new rules for vitamins and minerals were added, and claim categories were expanded.		Regulation will be fully applicable in 2010.

a human trial for efficacy confirmation is basically required for FOSHU claim approval. Under FOSHU, human trials for efficacy confirmation is no longer necessary for disease risk reduction claims for Ca and folic acid. This is also the case for GI conditioning claims for some oligosaccharides and dietary fibers, whose scientific evidence in humans are recognized as sufficient. However, a safety confirmation study in humans is still required for these. According to the so far very limited experience, a positive scientific evaluation by EFSA requires most likely at least one human trial in the target population. Many relationships between health benefits and food components that are allowed in Japan and China are rejected by the EFSA during discussions, because of lack of adequate scientific substantiation from the European point of view. In Japan and China, human trials are conducted on the final product. Brazil requires human trials for claim substantiation preferably conducted with the final product. Depending on the bioavailability of the functional ingredient on a specific food matrix, additional information may be required by ANVISA in case the final product is different from the one where the clinical trial was originally evaluated. In the EU, a human trial on the same food matrix is acceptable evidence, as in Brazil. There is no gold standard for scientific substantiation for food health claims as is the case for pharmaceutical products, and it finally rests on consensus of the authorities, which is influenced by academy, industry and consumers, and also by the history of any scientific approach and regulation. The discussion currently on-going in the EU would influence other regions, especially those without such health claim regulatory systems.

Novel food legislation is required for probiotics in China and Brazil. In Japan and the EU, living cultures such as lactobacilli and bifidobacteria have been consumed well before any establishment of novel foods legislation existed, and there are no regulations for probiotic use in food. 'Modify GI conditions' based on its effect on microbiota balancing is just one health claim category allowed in Japan and Brazil for probiotics. China has approved five health claim categories for products with probiotics, including immunity, skin benefit, flora regulation, facilitating digestion and fecal excretion, where the latter three categories refer to GI conditioning. Health claims and the criteria for FOSHU approval have been established through the collaboration among industries, government and academy in Japan. There was consensus to develop a common criteria to evaluate the benefit for GI conditioning in Japan. Increase in bifidobacteria in the gut connected to fecal moisturizing, fecal mass increase, and acidifying gut environment, result in an increase in defecation frequency and a decrease in harmful bacteria. Research results have been accumulated for 30 years, initiated by Prof. Mitsuoka and the Japan Bifidus Foundation collaborating with industry and academics. Interestingly, in the current discussion at EFSA, the health benefit of microflora balancing itself was questioned, resulting in some companies withdrawing claim applications. The relationship between microbiota balance, including the role of bifidobacteria and health status/disease risk, has not been clearly demonstrated compared to some other benefits filed—such as in lowering cholesterol and cardiovascular diseases. In the future, accumulation of additional scientific evidence on gut microbiota may be required in order to obtain consensus in EU authorities.

Natural defense/protection benefit, including immune reinforcement and anti-infection/diarrhea effects, is also a widely accepted health benefit of probiotics, and a similar volume of publications on the benefit of probiotics for natural defense has appeared in scientific journals in the digestive health field. In China, there is an 'enhancing immune' health claim category and 21 products with probiotics have been approved under this claim category. There were some FOSHU applications in Japan in this field, but none achieved approval because the authority considered that the field of immunity may not the territory for food but medicine. In the EU, all benefit areas are being evaluated equally under the new regulations for food health claims. Emerging science has shown that some probiotics may have anti-allergen properties [26, 32, 33, 119]. Such a claim exists nowhere in the world including in Japan, even where probiotics with anti-allergen properties has been commercialized without any claims since 2005. The EU is likely evaluating such new emerging scientific evidence for health claims.

The establishment of health claims for food is a major trend for the food industry, academics and the authorities. Probiotics is one of the most scientifically well-documented food components. Even though scientific evidence is the same, the requirement for scientific substantiation on health claims are different in Japan, China, Brazil, and the EU, which may be due to cultural and historical differences with respect to food and food policy, and hence the achievement of consensus by authorities. The final goal for health claims is for the benefit of consumers. Further scientific evidence on clearer benefits of probiotics, and more discussion on health claims with authorities in order to achieve consensus on claims should allow better communication to consumers, and thus expand the opportunity for promoting health through using probiotics.

ACKNOWLEDGMENT

We would like to express our gratitude to Dr. D. Barclay (Nestec Ltd.) Dr. Kimmo Makinen (Nestlé Research Center) and Mr. H. Watanabe (Nestlé Japan Ltd.) for reviewing this article.

References

1. Joint FAO/WHO Working Group. (2002). Guidelines for the evaluation of probiotics in food.
2. Fuller, R. (1991). Probiotics in human medicine. *Gut, 32*, 439–442.
3. Su, P., Henriksson, A., Tandianus, J. E., et al. (2005). Detection and quantification of *Bifidobacterium lactis* LAFTI B94 in human faecal samples from a consumption trial. *FEMS Microbiology Letters, 244*, 99–103.
4. Fukushima, Y., Li, S., Hara, H., et al. (1997). Effect of follow-up formula containing bifidobacteria (NAN BF) on fecal flora and fecal metabolites in healthy children. *Bioscience and Microflora, 16*, 65–72.
5. Fukushima, Y., Kawata, Y., Hara, H., et al. (1998). Probiotic formula enhances intestinal immunoglobulin A production in healthy children. *International Journal of Food Microbiology, 42*, 39–44.
6. Saavedra, J. M., Bauman, N. A., Oung, I., et al. (1994). Feeding of *Bificobacterium bificum* and *Streptococcus thermophilus* to infants in hospital for prevention of diarrhoea and shedding of rotavirus. *Lancet, 344*, 1046–1049.
7. Saavedra, J. M., Abi-Hanna, A., Moore, N., & Yolken, R. H. (2004). Long-term consumption of infant formulas containing live probiotic bacteria: tolerance and safety. *The American Journal of Clinical Nutrition, 79*, 261–267.
8. Nishida, S., Gotou, M., Akutsu, S., et al. (2004). Effect of yogurt containing *Bifidobacterium lactis* BB-12 on improvement of defecation and fecal microflora of healthy female adults. *Milk Science, 53*, 71–80.
9. Katayama, K., Hamasaki, Y., Fuchu, H., et al. (2004). Effects of yogurt containing *Bifidobacterium lactis* BB-12 on defecation and fecal microflora in healthy volunteers, and its safety. *Journal of Nutrition Food, 7*(2), 73–81.
10. Weizman, Z., Asli, G., & Alsheikh, A. (2005). Effect of a probiotic infant formula on infections in child care centers: comparison of two probiotic agents. *Pediatrics, 115*, 5–9.
11. Mao, M., Yu, T., Xiong, Y., et al. (2008). Effect of a lactose-free milk formula supplemented with bifidobacteria and streptococci on the recovery from acute diarrhoea. *Asia Pacific Journal of Clinical Nutrition, 17*, 30–34.
12. Chouraqui, J. P., Van Egroo, L. D., & Fichot, M. C. (2004). Acidified milk formula supplemented with *bifidobacterium lactis*: impact on infant diarrhea in residential care settings. *Journal of Pediatric Gastroenterology and Nutrition, 38*, 288–292.
13. Isolauri, E., Arvola, T., Sutas, Y., et al. (2000). Probiotics in the management of atopic eczema. *Clinical and Experimental Allergy, 30*, 1604–1610.
14. Wang, K. Y., Li, S. N., Liu, C. S., et al. (2004). Effects of ingesting Lactobacillus- and Bifidobacterium-containing yogurt in subjects with colonized *Helicobacter pylori*. *The American Journal of Clinical Nutrition, 80*, 737–744.
15. Bouvier, M., Meance, S., Boulev, C., et al. (2001). Effects of consumption of a milk fermented by the probiotic *Bifidobaterium animalis* DN-173 010 on colonic transit time in healthy humans. *Bioscience and Microflora, 20*, 43–48.
16. Marteau, P., Cuillerier, E., Meance, S., et al. (2002). *Bifidobacterium animalis* strain DN-173 010 shortens the

colonic transit time in healthy women: A double-blind, randomized, controlled study. *Alimentary Pharmacology & Therapeutics, 16*, 587–593.

17. Tanaka, R., Kan, T., Tejima, H., et al. (1980). Bifidobacterium Interplantation -intake for *B. bifidum* 4006 or *B. breve* 4007 (in Japanese). *Japanese Journal of Clinical Pediatrics, 33*, 2483–2492.

18. Ishikawa, H., Akedo, I., Umesaki, Y., et al. (2003). Randomized controlled trial of the effect of bifidobacteria-fermented milk on ulcerative colitis. *Journal of the American College of Nutrition, 22*, 56–63.

19. Tanaka, R. (1994). Clinical applications of Bifidobacterium in humans. In: T. Mitsuoka (Ed.), *Research of Bifidobacteria* (in Japanese, pp. 221–228). Tokyo: Japan Bifidus Foundation.

20. Nomoto, K. (2005). Prevention of infections by probiotics. *Journal of Bioscience and Bioengineering, 100*, 583–592.

21. Whorwell, P. J., Altringer, L., Morel, J., et al. (2006). Efficacy of an encapsulated probiotic *Bifidobacterium infantis* 35624 in women with irritable bowel syndrome. *The American Journal of Gastroenterology, 101*, 1581–1590.

22. Ahmed, M., Prasad, J., Gill, H., et al. (2007). Impact of consumption of different levels of *Bifidobacterium lactis* HN019 on the intestinal microflora of elderly human subjects. *The Journal of Nutrition, Health & Aging, 11*, 26–31.

23. Gill, H. S., Rutherfurd, K. J., Cross, M. L., & Gopal, P. K. (2001). Enhancement of immunity in the elderly by dietary supplementation with the probiotic *Bifidobacterium lactis* HN019. *The American Journal of Clinical Nutrition, 74*, 833–839.

24. Gill, H. S., Rutherfurd, K. J., & Cross, M. L. (2001). Dietary probiotic supplementation enhances natural killer cell activity in the elderly: An investigation of age-related immunological changes. *Journal of Clinical Immunology, 21*, 264–271.

25. Ogata, T. (1999). Effect of *Bifidobacterium longum* BB536 yogurt administration on the intestinal environment of healthy adults. *Microbial Ecology in Health and Disease, 11*, 41–44.

26. Xiao, J. Z., Kondo, S., Yanagisawa, N., et al. (2006). Probiotics in the treatment of Japanese cedar pollinosis: A double-blind placebo-controlled trial. *Clinical and Experimental Allergy, 36*, 1425–1435.

27. Odamaki, T., Xiao, J. Z., Iwabuchi, N., et al. (2007). Influence of *Bifidobacterium longum* BB536 intake on faecal microbiota in individuals with Japanese cedar pollinosis during the pollen season. *Journal of Medical Microbiology, 56*, 1301–1308.

28. Cremonini, F., Di Caro, S., Santarelli, L., et al. (2002). Probiotics in antibiotic-associated diarrhoea. *Digestive and Liver Disease, 34*(Suppl 2), S78–S80.

29. Schultz, M. (2008). Clinical use of *E. coli* Nissle 1917 in inflammatory bowel disease. Inflamm. *Bowel Disease, 14*, 1012–1018.

30. Ikeda, N., Suzuki, H., Kaneko, K., et al. (2000). Effect of lactobacillus beverage intake on fecal microflora of infants. *Journal of Nutrition Food, 3*(3), 69–74.

31. Ikeda, N., Kaneko, K., Ejiri, M., et al. (2000). Effect of lactobacillus beverage administration on defecation of healthy volunteers with constipation. *Journal of Nutrition Food, 3*(3), 59–68.

32. Ishida, Y., Nakamura, F., Kanzato, H., et al. (2005). Effect of milk fermented with *Lactobacillus acidophilus* strain L-92 on symptoms of Japanese cedar pollen allergy: A randomized placebo-controlled trial. *Bioscience, Biotechnology, and Biochemistry, 69*, 1652–1660.

33. Ishida, Y., Nakamura, F., Kanzato, H., et al. (2005). Clinical effects of *Lactobacillus acidophilus* strain L-92 on perennial allergic rhinitis: A double-blind, placebo-controlled study. *Journal of Dairy Science, 88*, 527–533.

34. Hilton, E., Isenberg, H. D., Alperstein, P., et al. (1992). Ingestion of yogurt containing *Lactobacillus acidophilus* as prophylaxis for candidal vaginitis. *Annals of Internal Medicine, 116*, 353–357.

35. Sandres, M. E., & Klaenhammer, T. R. (2001). The scientific basis of *Lactobacillus acidophilus* NCFM functionality as a probiotic. *Journal of Dairy Science, 84*, 319–331.

36. Turchet, P., Laurenzano, M., Auboiron, S., & Antoine, J. M. (2003). Effect of fermented milk containing the probiotic *Lactobacillus casei* DN-114001 on winter infections in free-living elderly subjects: A randomised, controlled pilot study. *The Journal of Nutrition, Health & Aging, 7*, 75–77.

37. Pedone, C. A., Arnaud, C. C., Postaire, E. R., et al. (2000). Multicentric study of the effect of milk fermented by *Lactobacillus casei* on the incidence of diarrhoea. *International Journal of Clinical Practice, 54*, 568–571.

38. Agarwal, K. N., Bhasin, S. K., Faridi, M. M. A., et al. (2001). *Lactobacillus casei* in the control of acute diarrhea—a pilot study. *Indian Pediatrics, 38*, 905–910.

39. Marcos, A., Wärnberg, J., Nova, E., et al. (2004). The effect of milk fermented by yogurt cultures plus *Lactobacillus casei* DN-114001 on the immune response of subjects under academic examination stress. *European Journal of Nutrition, 43*, 381–389.

40. Cobo Sanz, J. M., Mateos, J. A., & Muñoz Conejo, A. (2006). Effect of *Lactobacillus casei* on the incidence of infectious conditions in children (in Spanish). *Nutrición Hospitalaria, 21*, 547–551.

41. Tanaka, R., & Ohwaki, M. (1991). A controlled study of the effects of the ingestion of *Lactobacillus casei* fermented milk on the intestinal microflora, its microbial metabolism and the immune system of healthy humans. In: T. Mitsuoka (Ed.), *Intestinal flora and diet: Proceedings of 12th ICPR symposium on intestinal flora* (in Japanese with English summary, pp. 85–142). Tokyo: Japan Scientific Societies Press.

42. Matsumoto, K., Takada, T., Shimizu, K., et al. (2006). The effects of a probiotic milk product containing

Lactobacillus casei strain shirota on the defecation frequency and the intestinal microflora of suboptimal health state volunteers: A randomized placebo-controlled cross-over study. *Bioscience and Microflora, 25,* 39–48.

43. Ohashi, Y., Nakai, S., Tsukamoto, T., et al. (2002). Habitual intake of lactic acid bacteria and risk reduction of bladder cancer. *Urologia Internationalis, 68,* 273–280.

44. Koebnick, C., Wagner, I., Leitzmann, P., et al. (2003). Probiotic beverage containing *Lactobacillus casei* Shirota improves gastrointestinal symptoms in patients with chronic constipation. *Canadian Journal of Gastroenterology, 17,* 655–659.

45. Tamura, M., Shikina, T., Morihana, T., et al. (2007). Effects of probiotics on allergic rhinitis induced by Japanese cedar pollen: Randomized double-blind, placebo-controlled clinical trial. *International Archives of Allergy and Immunology, 143,* 75–82.

46. Nagao, F., Nakayama, M., Muto, T., & Okumura, K. (2000). Effects of a fermented milk drink containing *Lactobacillus casei* strain Shirota on the immune system in healthy human subjects. *Bioscience, Biotechnology, and Biochemistry, 64,* 2706–2708.

47. Takeda, K., & Okumura, K. (2007). Effects of a fermented milk drink containing *Lactobacillus casei* strain Shirota on the human NK-cell activity. *The Journal of Nutrition, 137*(3 Suppl 2), 791S–793S.

48. Ivory, K., Chambers, S. J., Pin, C., et al. (2008). Oral delivery of Lactobacillus casei Shirota modifies allergen-induced immune responses in allergic rhinitis. *Clinical and Experimental Allergy, 38,* 1282–1289.

49. Aso, Y., Akaza, H., Kotake, T., et al. (1995). Preventive effect of a *Lactobacillus casei* preparation on the recurrence of superficial bladder cancer in double-blind trial. *European Urology, 27,* 104–109.

50. Olivares, M., Díaz-Ropero, M. P., Sierra, S., et al. (2007). Oral intake of *Lactobacillus fermentum* CECT5716 enhances the effects of influenza vaccination. *Nutrition, 23,* 254–260.

51. Weston, S., Halbert, A., Richmond, P., & Prescott, S. L. (2005). Effects of probiotics on atopic dermatitis: A randomised controlled trial. *Archives of Disease in Childhood, 90,* 892–897.

52. Prescott, S. L., Dunstan, J. A., Hale, J., et al. (2005). Clinical effects of probiotics are associated with increased interferon-gamma responses in very young children with atopic dermatitis. *Clinical and Experimental Allergy, 35,* 1557–1564.

53. Fukushima, Y. (2007). Probiotics and natural defense function of the host. *Bioscience and Microflora, 26,* 1–10.

54. Yamano, T., Iino, H., Takada, M., et al. (2006). Improvement of the human intestinal flora by ingestion of the probiotic strain *Lactobacillus johnsonii* La1. *The British Journal of Nutrition, 95,* 303–312.

55. Link-Amster, H., Rochat, F., Saudan, K. Y., et al. (1994). Modulation of a specific humoral immune response and changes in intestinal flora mediated through fermented milk intake. *FEMS Immunology and Medical Microbiology, 10,* 55–63.

56. Schiffrin, E. J., Rochat, F., Link-Amster, H., et al. (1995). Immunomodulation of human blood cells following the ingestion of lactic acid bacteria. *Journal of Dairy Science, 78,* 491–497.

57. Michetti, P., Dorta, G., Wiesel, P. H., et al. (1999). Effect of whey-based culture supernatant of *Lactobacillus acidophilus* (johnsonii) La1 on *Helicobacter pylori* infection in humans. *Digestion, 60,* 203–209.

58. Felley, C. P., Corthesy-Theulaz, I., Rivero, J. L., et al. (2001). Favourable effect of an acidified milk (LC-1) on *Helicobacter pylori* gastritis in man. *European Journal of Gastroenterology & Hepatology, 13,* 25–29.

59. Gotteland, M., Andrews, M., Toledo, M., et al. (2008). Modulation of *Helicobacter pylori* colonization with cranberry juice and *Lactobacillus johnsonii* La1 in children. *Nutrition, 24,* 421–426.

60. Peguet-Navarro, J., Dezutter-Dambuyant, C., Buetler, T., et al. (2008). Supplementation with oral probiotic bacteria protects human cutaneous immune homeostasis after UV exposure-double blind, randomized, placebo controlled clinical trial. *European Journal of Dermatology, 18,* 504–511.

61. Fukushima, Y., Miyaguchi, S., Yamano, T., et al. (2007). Improvement of nutritional status and incidence of infection in hospitalised, enterally fed elderly by feeding of fermented milk containing probiotic *Lactobacillus johnsonii* La1 (NCC533). *The British Journal of Nutrition, 98,* 969–977.

62. Wang, M. F., Lin, H. C., Wang, Y. Y., & Hsu, C. H. (2004). Treatment of perennial allergic rhinitis with lactic acid bacteria. *Pediatric Allergy and Immunology, 15,* 152–158.

63. Sarker, S. A., Sultana, S., Fuchs, G. J., et al. (2005). *Lactobacillus paracasei* strain ST11 has no effect on rotavirus but ameliorates the outcome of non-rotavirus diarrhea in children from Bangladesh. *Pediatrics, 116,* 221–228.

64. Bunout, D., Barrera, G., Hirsch, S., et al. (2004). Effects of a nutritional supplement on the immune response and cytokine production in free-living elderly. *Journal of Parenteral and Enteral Nutrition, 28,* 348–354.

65. de Vrese, M., Rautenberg, P., Laue, C., et al. (2005). Probiotic bacteria stimulate virus-specific neutralizing antibodies following a booster polio vaccination. *European Journal of Nutrition, 44,* 406–413.

66. Niedzielin, K., Kordecki, H., & Birkenfeld, B. (2001). A controlled, double-blind, randomized study on the efficacy of *Lactobacillus plantarum* 299V in patients with irritable bowel syndrome. *European Journal of Gastroenterology & Hepatology, 13,* 1143–1147.

67. Klarin, B., Wullt, M., Palmquist, I., et al. (2008). *Lactobacillus plantarum* 299v reduces colonisation of *Clostridium difficile* in critically ill patients treated with antibiotics. *Acta Anaesthesiologica Scandinavica, 52,* 1096–1102.

68. Wullt, M., Johansson Hagslatt, M. L., Odenholt, I., & Berggren, A. (2007). *Lactobacillus plantarum* 299v enhances the concentrations of fecal short-chain fatty acids in patients with recurrent *Clostridium difficile*-associated diarrhea. *Digestive Diseases and Sciences, 52,* 2082–2086.

69. Shornikova, A. V., Casas, I. A., Mykkänen, H., et al. (1997). Bacteriotherapy with *Lactobacillus reuteri* in rotavirus gastroenteritis. *The Pediatric Infectious Disease Journal, 16,* 1103–1107.

70. Abrahamsson, T. R., Jakobsson, T., Böttcher, M. F., et al. (2007). Probiotics in prevention of IgE-associated eczema: a double-blind, randomized, placebo-controlled trial. *The Journal of Allergy and Clinical Immunology, 119,* 1174–1180.

71. Valeur, N., Engel, P., Carbajal, N., et al. (2004). Colonization and immunomodulation by *Lactobacillus reuteri* ATCC 55730 in the human gastrointestinal tract. *Applied and Environmental Microbiology, 70,* 1176–1181.

72. Tubelius, P., Stan, V., & Zachrisson, A. (2005). Increasing work-place healthiness with the probiotic *Lactobacillus reuteri*: a randomised, double-blind placebo-controlled study. *Environmental Health, 4,* 25.

73. Imase, K., Tanaka, A., Tokunaga, K., et al. (2007). *Lactobacillus reuteri* tablets suppress *Helicobacter pylori* infection—a double-blind randomised placebo-controlled cross-over clinical study. *Japanese Journal of Associate Infectious Diseases, 81,* 387–393.

74. Nikawa, H., Makihira, S., Fukushima, H., et al. (2004). *Lactobacillus reuteri* in bovine milk fermented decreases the oral carriage of mutans streptococci. *International Journal of Food Microbiology, 95,* 219–223.

75. Savino, F., Pelle, E., Palumeri, E., et al. (2007). *Lactobacillus reuteri* (American Type Culture Collection Strain 55730) versus simethicone in the treatment of infantile colic: a prospective randomized study. *Pediatrics, 119,* 124–130.

76. Hosoda, M., He, F., Hiramatsu, M., et al. (1994). Effects of *Lactobacillus* GG strains intake on fecal microflora and defication in healthy volunteers. *Bifidus, 8,* 21–28.

77. Hatakka, K., Savilahti, E., Ponka, A., et al. (2001). Effect of long-term consumption of probiotic milk on infections in children attending day care centres: double blind, randomised trial. *British Medical Journal, 322,* 1327–1329.

78. Majamaa, H., Isolauri, E., Saxelin, M., & Vesikari, T. (1995). Lactic acid bacteria in the tretment of acute rotavirus gastroenteritis. *Journal of Pediatric Gastroenterology and Nutrition, 20,* 333–339.

79. Szajewska, H., & Mrukowicz, J. Z. (2001). Probiotics in the treatment and prevention of acute infectious diarrhea in infants and children: a systematic review of published randomized, double-blind, placebo-controlled trials. *Journal of Pediatric Gastroenterology and Nutrition, 33,* S17–S25.

80. Hilton, E., Kolakowski, P., Singer, C., & Smith, M. (1997). Efficacy of *Lactobacillus* GG as a diarrheal preventive in travelers. *Journal of Travel Medicine, 4,* 41–43.

81. Kalliomäki, M., Salminen, S., Arvilommi, H., et al. (2001). Probiotics in primary prevention of atopic disease: A randomised placebo-controlled trial. *Lancet, 357,* 1076–1079.

82. Kalliomäki, M., Salminen, S., Poussa, T., et al. (2003). Probiotics and prevention of atopic disease: 4-year follow-up of a randomised placebo-controlled trial. *Lancet, 361,* 1869–1871.

83. Kalliomäki, M., Salminen, S., Poussa, T., & Isolauri, E. (2007). Probiotics during the first 7 years of life: A cumulative risk reduction of eczema in a randomized, placebo-controlled trial. *The Journal of Allergy and Clinical Immunology, 119,* 1019–1021.

84. Kawase, M., He, F., Kubota, A., et al. (2009). Effect of fermented milk prepared with two probiotic strains on Japanese cedar pollinosis in a double-blind placebo-controlled clinical study. *International Journal of Food Microbiology, 128,* 429–434.

85. Canani, R. B., Cirillo, P., Terrin, G., et al. (2007). Probiotics for treatment of acute diarrhoea in children: randomised clinical trial of five different preparations. *British Medical Journal, 335,* 340.

86. de Vrese, M., Rautenberg, P., Laue, C., et al. (2005). Probiotic bacteria stimulate virus-specific neutralizing antibodies following a booster polio vaccination. *European Journal of Nutrition, 44,* 406–413.

87. Kukkonen, K., Nieminen, T., Poussa, T., et al. (2006). Effect of probiotics on vaccine antibody responses in infancy—a randomized placebo-controlled double-blind trial. *Pediatric Allergy and Immunology, 17,* 416–421.

88. Kajander, K., Myllyluoma, E., Rajili-Stojanovi, M., et al. (2008). Clinical trial: Multispecies probiotic supplementation alleviates the symptoms of irritable bowel syndrome and stabilizes intestinal microbiota. *Alimentary Pharmacology & Therapeutics, 27,* 48–57.

89. Nase, L., Hatakka, K., Savilahti, E., et al. (2001). Effect of long-term consumption of a probiotic bacterium, *Lactobacillus rhamnosus* GG, in milk on dental caries and caries risk in children. *Caries Research, 35,* 412–420.

90. Sheih, Y. H., Chiang, B. L., Wang, L. H., et al. (2001). Systemic immunity-enhancing effects in healthy subjects following dietary consumption of the lactic acid bacterium *Lactobacillus rhamnosus* HN001. *Journal of the American College of Nutrition, 20*(2 Suppl), 149–156.

91. Sistek, D., Kelly, R., Wickens, K., et al. (2006). Is the effect of probiotics on atopic dermatitis confined to food sensitized children? *Clinical and Experimental Allergy, 36*, 629–633.

92. Tannock, G. W., Munro, K., Harmsen, H. J., et al. (2000). Analysis of the fecal microflora of human subjects consuming a probiotic product containing *Lactobacillus rhamnosus* DR20. *Applied and Environmental Microbiology, 66*, 2578–2588.

93. Wickens, K., Black, P. N., Stanley, T. V., et al. (2008). Probiotic Study Group. A differential effect of 2 probiotics in the prevention of eczema and atopy: A double-blind, randomized, placebo-controlled trial. *The Journal of Allergy and Clinical Immunology, 122*, 788–794.

94. McFarland, L. V. (2007). Meta-analysis of probiotics for the prevention of traveler's diarrhea. *Travel Medicine and Infectious Disease, 5*, 97–105.

95. Burton, J. P., Chilcott, C. N., Moore, C. J., et al. (2006). A preliminary study of the effect of probiotic *Streptococcus salivarius* K12 on oral malodour parameters. *Journal of Applied Microbiology, 100*, 754–764.

96. Power, D. A., Burton, J. P., Chilcott, C. N., et al. (2008). Preliminary investigations of the colonisation of upper respiratory tract tissues of infants using a paediatric formulation of the oral probiotic *Streptococcus salivarius* K12. *European Journal of Clinical Microbiology & Infectious Diseases, 27*, 1261–1263.

97. Wildt, S., Munck, L. K., Vinter-Jensen, L., et al. (2006). Probiotic treatment of collagenous colitis: A randomized, double-blind, placebo-controlled trial with *Lactobacillus acidophilus* and *Bifidobacterium animalis* subsp. *lactis*. *Inflammatory Bowel Diseases, 12*, 395–401.

98. Sheu, B. S., Cheng, H. C., Kao, A. W., et al. (2006). Pretreatment with Lactobacillus- and Bifidobacterium-containing yogurt can improve the efficacy of quadruple therapy in eradicating residual *Helicobacter pylori* infection after failed triple therapy. *The American Journal of Clinical Nutrition, 83*, 864–869.

99. Black, F., Einarsson, K., Lidbeck, A., et al. (1991). Effect of lactic acid producing bacteria on the human intestinal microflora during ampicillin treatment. *Scandinavian Journal of Infectious Diseases, 23*, 247–254.

100. Salazar-Lindo, E., Figueroa-Quintanilla, D., Caciano, M. I., et al. (2007). Lacteol study group. Effectiveness and safety of Lactobacillus LB in the treatment of mild acute diarrhea in children. *Journal of Pediatric Gastroenterology and Nutrition, 44*, 571–576.

101. Xiao, S. D., Zhang, D. Z., Lu, H., et al. (2003). Multicenter, randomized, controlled trial of heat-killed *Lactobacillus acidophilus* LB in patients with chronic diarrhea. *Advances in Therapy, 20*, 253–260.

102. de Vrese, M., Winkler, P., Rautenberg, P., et al. (2006). Probiotic bacteria reduced duration and severity but not the incidence of common cold episodes in a double blind, randomized, controlled trial. *Vaccine, 24*, 6670–6674.

103. de Vrese, M., Winkler, P., Rautenberg, P., et al. (2005). Effect of *Lactobacillus gasseri* PA 16/8, *Bifidobacterium longum* SP 07/3, *B. bifidum* MF 20/5 on common cold episodes: a double blind, randomized, controlled trial. *Clinical Nutrition, 24*, 481–491.

104. Winkler, P., de Vrese, M., Laue, Ch., & Schrezenmeir, J. (2005). Effect of a dietary supplement containing probiotic bacteria plus vitamins and minerals on common cold infections and cellular immune parameters. *International Journal of Clinical Pharmacology and Therapeutics, 43*, 318–326.

105. Olivares, M., Diaz-Ropero, M. P., Gomez, N., et al. (2006). The consumption of two new probiotic strains, *Lactobacillus gasseri* CECT 5714 and *Lactobacillus coryniformis* CECT 5711, boosts the immune system of healthy humans. *International Microbiology, 9*, 47–52.

106. Olivares, M., Diaz-Ropero, M. A., Gomez, N., et al. (2006). Oral administration of two probiotic strains, *Lactobacillus gasseri* CECT5714 and *Lactobacillus coryniformis* CECT5711, enhances the intestinal function of healthy adults. *International Journal of Food Microbiology, 107*, 104–111.

107. Jimenez, E., Fernandez, L., Maldonado, A., et al. (2008). Oral administration of Lactobacillus strains isolated from breast milk as an alternative for the treatment of infectious mastitis during lactation. *Applied and Environmental Microbiology, 74*, 4650–4655.

108. Diop, L., Guillou, S., & Durand, H. (2008). Probiotic food supplement reduces stress-induced gastrointestinal symptoms in volunteers: A double-blind, placebo-controlled, randomized trial. *Nutrition Research, 28*, 1–5.

109. Rosenfeldt, V., Michaelsen, K. F., Jakobsen, M., et al. (2002). Effect of probiotic Lactobacillus strains on acute diarrhea in a cohort of nonhospitalized children attending day-care centers. *The Pediatric Infectious Disease Journal, 21*, 417–419.

110. Rosenfeldt, V., Michaelsen, K. F., Jakobsen, M., et al. (2002). Effect of probiotic Lactobacillus strains in young children hospitalized with acute diarrhea. *The Pediatric Infectious Disease Journal, 21*, 411–416.

111. Rosenfeldt, V., Benfeldt, E., Valerius, N. H., et al. (2004). Effect of probiotics on gastrointestinal symptoms and small intestinal permeability in children with atopic dermatitis. *The Journal of Pediatrics, 145*, 612–616.

112. Rosenfeldt, V., Benfeldt, E., Nielsen, S. D., et al. (2003). Effect of probiotic Lactobacillus strains in children with atopic dermatitis. *The Journal of Allergy and Clinical Immunology, 111*, 389–395.

113. Reid, G. (2008). Probiotic Lactobacilli for urogenital health in women. *J Clin Gastroenterol, 42* (Suppl 3, Pt 2), S234–236.

114. Bougle, D., Roland, N., Lebeurrier, F., & Arhan, P. (1999). Effect of propionibacteria supplementation on fecal bifidobacteria and segmental colonic transit time in healthy human subjects. *Scandinavian Journal of Gastroenterology*, *34*, 144–148.

115. Chapman, T. M., Plosker, G. L., & Figgitt, D. P. (2006). VSL#3 probiotic mixture: A review of its use in chronic inflammatory bowel diseases. *Drugs*, *66*, 1371–1387.

116. Mitsuoka, T. (1969). Intestinal flora and the host. *Pharmacia*, *5*, 608–609.

117. Sakata, T. (1995). Effect of short-chain fatty acids on the proliferation of gut epithelial cells *in vivo*. In J. H. Cummings, J. L. Rombeau, & T. Sakata (Eds.), *Physiological and clinical aspects of short-chain fatty acids* (pp. 289–305). Cambridge: Cambridge University Press.

118. Visek, W. J. (1978). Diet and cell growth modulation buy ammonia. *The American Journal of Clinical Nutrition*, *31*, S216–S220.

119. Fujiwara, D., Wakabayashi, H., Watanabe, H., et al. (2005). A double-blind trial fo *Lactobacillus paracasei* strain KW3110 administration for immunomodulation in patients with pollen allergy. *Allergology International*, *54*, 143–149.

120. Sakamoto, I. M., Igarashi, K., Kimura, A., et al. (2001). Suppressive effect of *Lactobacillus gasseri* OLL2716 (LG21) on *Helicobacter pylori* infection in humans. *The Journal of Antimicrobial Chemotherapy*, *27*, 709–710.

121. Matsuoka, T., Sugano, N., Ito, K., & Koga, Y. (2005). Effect of Oral *Lactobacillus salivarius* TI 2711 (LS1) administration. *Society of Periodontology*, *47*, 194–202.

122. Resolução No 16 de 30 de Abril de 1999. Regulamento Técnico de Procedimentos para registro de Alimentos e ou Novos Ingredientes. Agência Nacional de Vigilância Sanitária, D.O.U.—Diário Oficial da União; Poder Executivo, de 03 de dezembro de 1999.

123. Resolução No 17 de 30 de Abril de 1999. Regulamento Técnico que Estabelece as Diretzrizes Básicas Avaliação de Risco e Segurança de Alimentos. Agência Nacional de Vigilância Sanitária, D.O.U.—Diário Oficial da União; Poder Executivo, de 03 de dezembro de 1999.

124. Resolução No 18 de 30 de Abril de 1999. Regulamento Técnico que Estabelece as Diretrizes Básicas para Análise e Comprovação de Propriedades Funcionais e ou de Saúde Alegadas em Rotulagem de Alimentos. Agência Nacional de Vigilância Sanitária, D.O.U.—Diário Oficial da União; Poder Executivo, de 03 de dezembro de 1999.

125. Resolução No 19 de 30 de Abril de 1999. Regulamento Técnico para Procedimento de Registro de Alimento com Alegações de Propriedades Funcionais de ou de Saúde em sua Rotulagem. Agência Nacional de Vigilância Sanitária, D.O.U.—Diário Oficial da União; Poder Executivo, de 03 de dezembro de 1999.

126. Lajolo, F. M. (2002). Functional foods: Latin American perspectives. *The British Journal of Nutrition*, *88*(Suppl 2), S145–S150.

127. Toledo, M. C. F., & Lajolo, F. M. (2008). Supplements and functional foods legislation in Brazil. In D. Bagchi (Ed.), *Nutraceutical and functional food regulations in the United States and around the world*. Academic Press.

128. Resolução No 2 de 07 de janeiro de 2002. Aprova o Regulamento Técnico de Substâncias Bioativas e Probióticos Isolados com Alegação de Propriedades Funcional e ou de Saúde. Agência Nacional de Vigilância Sanitária, D.O.U.—Diário Oficial da União, D.O.U.—Diário Oficial da União; Poder Executivo, de 09 de janeiro de 2002.

129. Regulation (EC) No 1924/2006 of the European Parliament and the Council of 20 December 2006 on nutrition and health claims made on foods.

130. Directive 2000/13/EC of the European Parliament and the Council of 20 March 2000 on the approximation of the laws of the Member States relating to the labelling, presentation and advertising of foodstuffs.

131. Hurt, E. (2002). International Guidelines and experiences on health claims in Europe. Asia-Pacific. *The Journal of Clinical Nutrition*, *11*(Suppl), S90–S93.

132. Richardson, D. P. (2003). Passclaim—Synthesis and review of existing processes. *European Journal of Nutrition*, *42*(Suppl 1), I/97.

133. Joint Health Claims Initiative (2000). JHCI Code of Practice on Health Claims on Foods.

134. Commission Regulation (EC) No 353/2008 of 18 April 2008 establishing implementing rules for applications for authorisation of health claims as provided for in Article 15 of Regulation (EC) No 1924/2006 of the European Parliament and of the Council.

135. European Food Safety Authority, Scientific and Technical Guidance for the Preparation and Presentation of the Application for Authorisation of a Health Claim, Parma, 23 July 2007.

136. EFSA Pre-Submission Guidance for Applicants intending to submit applications for authorisation of health claims made on foods, Parma, 14 March 2007, last updated 21 December 2007.

26

Probiotics and Heart Health: Reduction of Risk Factors Associated with Cardiovascular Disease and Complications Due to Foodborne Illnesses

Irene B. Hanning[1], Jody M. Lingbeck[1], and Steven C. Ricke[1,2]

[1]Center for Food Safety-IFSE and Food Science Department, University of Arkansas, Fayetteville, AR, USA

[2]Poultry Science Department, University of Arkansas, Fayetteville, AR, USA

1. INTRODUCTION

Consumers believe that certain foods can have a positive impact on long-term and current health. This has helped facilitate an acceptance of the term 'functional foods'.

'Functional foods' are foods or dietary components that may provide a health benefit beyond basic nutrition. Examples of categories of functional foods include foods that are vitamin enriched and foods that contain probiotic bacteria and/or prebiotics. Americans are becoming more aware of improved gastrointestinal health due to functional foods, especially those containing probiotics and prebiotics. In 2007, the North American market was the fastest growing for products marketed as containing probiotics. Furthermore, the market for probiotics continues to grow as awareness of their health benefits increases and more research has given probiotics scientific backing.

With nearly one in three global deaths—about 16.7 million—resulting from various forms of cardiovascular disease, many functional food products are being studied and introduced to the market to improve heart health. Global sales for heart health food and drinks are growing rapidly and are estimated to reach a total value of $7.7 billion in Europe and the USA by 2010 [1]. In 2007, the total value of the US heart health food and drinks market was $5 billion. These heart health food product sales were second only to gut health food product sales in terms of purpose categories.

Heart health can be impacted directly through an individual's diet. For example, an antioxidant called resveratrol present in red wine has been demonstrated to reduce the condition of cardiac fibrosis [2]. Cardiac fibrosis is characterized by the over-activation of fibroblasts in the heart which produce collagen. This hyper-secretion of collagen causes the heart muscle to stiffen and reduces the efficiency of the heart to pump blood, meaning the heart has to work harder. Resveratrol prevents the over-activation of fibroblasts.

Diet also indirectly impacts heart health. Poor diets containing fat and cholesterol can lead to obesity and obesity is directly linked to an increased risk of heart disease. Eating high fiber whole grains that lower blood cholesterol can result in an increase in heart health because high levels of cholesterol can result in blockages in the arteries. The link among gut health, probiotics and the health of specific systems such as the cardiac system are complex. The aim of this chapter is to explore some of these direct and indirect effects that probiotics may have on cardiac health.

2. DIRECT EFFECTS

Until the turn of the century, there appeared to be no evidence of the direct protective effects of probiotics or functional foods on the heart. However, in 2000, Oxman et al. [2, 3] reported that intravenous injection of the probiotic *Lactobacillus* conferred long-term protection to the heart against cardiac ischemia. Using male Sprague-Dawley rats, they demonstrated that *L. bulgaricus*-51 and its fermentation products (LCC), when injected intravenously 1 to 21 days before global ischemia/reperfusion, led to a decline of ventricular arrhythmia and an increase in contractility and functional recovery in LCC-treated rat hearts compared to those of control rats. The LCC-induced cardioprotection was seen 24 hours after injection and was observed for up to 21 days. In LCC hearts, prostacyclin, a tissue

protective factor during myocardial ischemia, and norepinephrine release was attenuated during reperfusion, while myocardial catalase activity and the expression of heat shock protein 70 (HSP70) were increased at ischemia and reperfusion. HSP70 is a member of heat shock proteins (HSPs) that become elevated during times of cellular stress and they help to shield cells from further insults. The level of HSP70 did not change upon injection of LCC. Only after an injection plus ischemia or reperfusion did the levels of HSP70 change, suggesting that LCC lowers the threshold of HSP expression. The over-expression of HSPs, as well as antioxidant activity [3], is thought to contribute to the cellular defense mechanism, which is attributed to LCC-induced cardioprotection.

In a follow-up study, Oxman et al. [4] investigated the effects of oral administration of LCC. Fourteen to 21-day oral administration of LCC induced similar cardioprotective effects in Sprague-Dawley rats such as reduced tachyarrhythmias and improved cardiac functional recovery without causing toxic side effects to the animal. As with the single injection of LCC, oral administration of LCC induced a delayed cardioprotection.

It has yet to be seen whether these same effects would be seen in human subjects, but these results clearly demonstrate the potential for the utilization of a functional food containing probiotic bacteria for the prevention or treatment of cardiac diseases.

3. INDIRECT EFFECTS

In humans, beneficial bacteria synthesize vitamins, break down indigestible substances, and provide protection from the colonization of pathogenic bacteria by competing for food and living space or by producing antimicrobial substances [4]. Due to its essential function, the heart is well guarded and the impacts that ingested materials can have on the heart are typically limited. However, many indirect factors exist which negatively affect the heart and we are now learning that the digestive microbiota profile can define health in nearly all the organs of the body including the heart. Probiotics may play a role in nutrient acquisition, alleviating hypertension, reducing cholesterol levels and protection against colonizing foodborne pathogens. These indirect routes can ultimately define cardiac health, which will be discussed in the following sections.

3.1. Probiotics, Cardiac Health and Obesity

The intestinal microbiota has a profound effect on nutrient acquisition. The mouse gastrointestinal tract (GIT) microbiota suppresses gene expression of factors produced by the intestinal epithelium and promotes absorption of monosaccharides, resulting in increased fat storage [5]. There is a direct link between obesity and heart disease. Because the microflora of the gut has an impact on fat deposition, probiotics are being investigated as a means to manipulate GI flora to reduce fat deposition, which could result in a reduced risk for heart disease.

Over half the American population is overweight, and nearly one quarter is obese [6]. The relationship between obesity and coronary heart disease was previously viewed as indirect through variables related to both obesity and coronary heart disease risk including hypertension and non-insulin-dependent diabetes mellitus. Although hypertension is approximately three times more common in obese than normal-weight persons [7], some obese patients without hypertension may still have heart disease [8]. Thus, the view of the relationship between heart health and obesity must be considered in light of indirect and direct impacts.

Although the classical cardiovascular risk factors such as smoking are becoming more effectively managed, the obesity rate in the United States continues to climb. The classical approaches to controlling obesity rely on four main modes of action: 1) control of food intake, mainly through modification of appetite; 2) an increase in exercise to burn calories; 3) controlling the fate of available energy produced by ingestion of food; and 4) modification of lipogenesis and lipolysis in adipose tissue. Pharamacological approaches to controlling obesity have been explored and are continuing to be developed. Much of the current research is centered on the development of drugs for neuropeptidic control of appetite, followed by controlling calorie burning mechanisms and drugs that target and reduce fat storage [9].

Consumers are becoming more attracted to natural health solutions to improve fitness and reduce obesity as opposed to pharmaceuticals. Prescription pharmaceuticals may be effective at reducing obesity, but negative side effects can occur. For example, Sibutramine keeps serotonin and norepinephrine in balance, which helps to increase metabolism and causes a feeling of fullness and increases energy levels. However, patients who discontinue the drug report significant weight gain afterwards—and common side effects include dry mouth, constipation, and insomnia with reports of increases in heart rate and blood pressure [10]. Some consumers are more attracted to 'functional foods' because of the multiple health benefits without negative side effects.

The concept that food has a role to play in the gut beyond that of a simple caloric impact on obesity has emerged as more has become known about the relationship between gut microflora and host metabolism. Several lines of evidence suggest that this relationship is relatively complex. It is not surprising that obese and lean people would have different microflora profiles since the gut microflora play such an important role in converting food into energy [5]. There is a large body of experimental evidence and empirical data showing that both antibiotics and probiotics, which modify the gut microflora profile, can act as growth promoters, increasing the size and weight of animals [11]. As growth promotants in animals, the mechanism of the growth promoting effect of antibiotics is supposedly associated with the inhibition of the gut flora of the animals by the antibiotics, but the exact mechanism is unknown [12]. Ternak [13] suggested that the widespread usage of antibiotics may be a large factor in the obesity epidemic of humans. Humans can be exposed to antibiotics not only from medicinal use, but also from drinking water and from residues in meat tissue of food animals [14]. However, considerable research is needed to clearly establish the relationship among the gut microflora, antibiotics and obesity. Historically, molecular microbiological techniques such as metagenomics, microarray analysis and density gradient gel electrophoresis combined with biochemical analysis of cellular nutrient uptake have yielded valuable insight into microbiota modifications after antibiotic and probiotic intake that can identify the modifications associated with increased size and weight [15].

Probiotics can stimulate the immune system by promoting the natural host defense systems and thus reducing the excessive need for antibiotics and perhaps weaken the link between obesity and antibiotic use. In addition, probiotics may serve as a treatment for obesity [16]. In a study by Lee et al. [17] *L. rhamnosus* PL60 was able to reduce bodyweight of obese mice without reducing energy intake. The weight loss was thought to be due to the production of conjugated linoleic acids (CLA) by *L. rhamnosus* PL60. CLA are thought to possess a number of health benefits including the reduction of body fat [18]. Similar results were seen with *L. plantarum* PL62, which also produces CLA. The culture supernatant of *L. plantarum* PL62 was able to reduce the bodyweight of white adipose tissue and overall bodyweights in mice [19]. These results, however, have not been demonstrated in humans. In a separate study, Sonnenburg et al. [20] showed that certain

combinations of probiotic bacteria increased the range of polysaccharides metabolized by germ-free mice. Finally, Martin et al. [21] administered probiotic drinks to mice with a humanized microbiome. Using spectroscopic techniques and mathematical modeling they were able to demonstrate that probiotics altered the metabolism of the mice in a variety of tissues. Thus, the consumption of probiotics may reduce the dependence on antibiotics and its association with obesity as well as act as a treatment to obesity thereby alleviating the symptoms of being overweight with heart disease.

3.2. Probiotics, Cardiac Health and Hypertension

Hypertension, or high blood pressure, contributes to heart disease by increasing the workload of the heart, which in turn causes the walls of the heart to thicken and become stiff. Hypertension arises from the conversion of angiotensin I to the potent vasoconstrictor angiotensin II by the angiotensin converting enzyme (ACE). Angiotensin II also inhibits the vasodilator bradykinin, adding an additional factor for blood pressure elevation. Dairy products fermented with probiotic bacteria, especially *Lactobacillus*, produce bioactive peptides known to inhibit the activity of ACE and thus alleviate hypertension. For example, Nakamura et al. [22], used Calpis sour milk fermented with *L. helveticus* and *S. cerevisiae* and identified two peptides, Ile-Pro-Pro and Val-Pro-Pro, both of which possessed ACE inhibitory activity *in vitro*. The authors further demonstrated that oral administration of Calpis sour milk or the peptides to spontaneously hypertensive rats (SHR) was able to lower systolic blood pressure in these animals [23]. Similar results were seen with oral administration of milk fermented with *L. helveticus* CP790 [24].

Studies in humans have also shown promise for the use of probiotic bacteria in the reduction of hypertension. In a study by Seppo et al. [25] hypertensive subjects were fed milk fermented with *L. helveticus* LBK-16H containing bioactive peptides. At the end of 21 weeks, test subjects showed a significant lowering of their blood pressure. In a separate study, Aihara et al. [26] were able to reduce blood pressure in patients with high–normal blood pressure or mild hypertension by daily feeding of tablets containing powdered milk fermented with *L. helveticus* CM4 for 4 weeks. (For a more complete evaluation of the effects of milk peptides on hypertension see the review by Jauhiainen and Korpela [27].) The results of these and other studies warrant further exploration for the use of bioactive peptides produced during probiotic bacteria fermentation for the treatment of hypertension.

3.3. Probiotics, Cardiac Health and Hypercholesterolemia

Hypercholesterolemia is another significant risk factor for cardiovascular disease. In patients with hypercholesterolemia, excess cholesterol is deposited in the arteries leading to narrowing of the arteries and restricted blood flow to the heart. Blockage of oxygen-rich blood to the heart can cause angina and lead to a heart attack. Probiotic bacteria have demonstrated the ability to reduce blood cholesterol and are thought to work by several mechanisms including assimilation of cholesterol [28], binding cholesterol and bile acids to the cell surface thus inhibiting absorption from the small intestine [29], and suppression of bile acid absorption by deconjugation of bile salts by the bacterial bile salt hydrolase activity [30, 31].

Several studies report a lowering of cholesterol levels by probiotic bacteria. For example, hypercholesterolemic hamsters consuming microencapsulated live *L. fermentum* 11976 led to a significant reduction in their serum total cholesterol and triglyceride levels as well as low density lipoprotein (LDL) cholesterol levels [32]. Similar results were seen in rats fed a high cholesterol diet supplemented with lyophilized *L. plantarum* MA2 [33]. In humans, one study by Ataie-Jafari et al. [34]

demonstrated that hypercholesterolemic patients fed probiotic yogurt containing *L. acidophilus* and *B. lactis* were able to reduce their cholesterol levels compared to cohorts who consumed ordinary yogurt. Additional reports of cholesterol lowering of probiotic bacteria are reviewed in Liong [35]. As with the antihypertensive activities of probiotic bacteria the results of these hypocholesterolemic studies warrant further exploration.

3.4. Probiotics, Cardiac Health and Foodborne Pathogens

Foodborne Disease and Cardiac Effects

Foodborne pathogens have been associated with carditis, and any heart damage as a result of infection appears to be permanent [36, 37]. Probiotics are not only a proactive preventative treatment that may reduce the risk of foodborne illness, but also a method to eliminate and fight infection due to foodborne illnesses [38]. Thus, probiotics might offer an indirect protective effect against heart damage incurred from infecting foodborne pathogens.

Typically, patients with cardiac complications as the result of foodborne bacterial infection first experience classical foodborne illness symptoms such as diarrhea, cramping, fever and nausea. Treatment in these cases is necessary and usually involves a course of antibiotics. However, there is a growing problem of antibiotic resistance in bacteria including foodborne pathogens and this may limit treatment options [39]. Thus, alternative proactive prevention and treatment with probiotics offers a promising option.

The effects of foodborne pathogens on human health are not always limited to gastrointestinal symptoms, but can have a substantial systemic impact. Secondary complications can develop from the bacterial infection and may include meningoencephalitis, endophthalmitis, osteomyelitis, brain abscesses, Guillain-Barré syndrome and peritonitis [40]. Secondary complications such as myocarditis can permanently damage the heart [41]. There has been an increase in clinical reports of carditis associated with foodborne pathogens, but whether this is due to increased awareness or an increase in virulent pathogens is not known. Regardless, the effect that these infections can have on the vital organs of the body warrants development of probiotics specifically targeted to defend and potentially prevent these illnesses.

Foodborne Pathogens and Carditis

The symptoms and severity of bacterial enteritis suffered by a patient are dependent on the health of the individual and the mechanisms of pathogenesis utilized by the bacteria. Foodborne bacterial pathogens can cause illness by one or more of three mechanisms: 1) attachment and colonization of intestinal epithelia; 2) intestinal colonization and toxin production; or 3) extraintestinal translocation of bacteria or toxins across intestinal epithelia and migration to other locations in the body [42]. Bacterial or toxin translocation can result in serious cardiac complications including endocarditis (infection of the inner layer of the heart usually involving the valves), myocarditis (infection of the heart muscle) and/or pericarditis (inflammation of the fibrous sac surrounding the heart). Cardiac complications of bacterial enteritis are well known, and mainly present as endocarditis, while myocarditis has only rarely been described [41]. Whether the carditis is caused by metastatic infections or by toxic mechanisms is not always clear [41].

Patients developing cardiac complications have reported acute chest pain subsequent to gastrointestinal symptoms. However, myocarditis can have few or no symptoms [43]. Mohanan and co-workers [44] examined the cases of 100 patients with bacteriologically or serologically documented *Salmonella* infection and found seven cases with clinical evidence of myocarditis, but as many as 46 cases with ECG abnormalities suggesting myocarditis. The next sections will discuss specific foodborne pathogens and clinical cases of cardiac complications associated with infection.

Salmonellosis

Salmonella is a Gram-negative bacterium that inhabits the gastrointestinal tract of warm-blooded animals. There are approximately 2,500 serovars of *Salmonella* and all serovars with the exception of *gallinarum* and *pullorum* can inhabit the gastrointestinal tracts of poultry without causing disease. Most human salmonellosis cases come from eating contaminated food [45], especially food of animal origin [46]. Buzby et al. [47] reported that approximately 87% of all salmonellosis cases were foodborne with only 10% attributed to person-to-person contact and 3% to pets. Frenzen et al. [48] estimated that, due to improvements in sanitation, nearly 96% of *Salmonella* cases were foodborne.

In the United States, the CDC reported 16.2 laboratory confirmed cases per 100,000 people in 2008 [49]. Contaminated poultry and eggs have been the most frequently implicated sources of human salmonellosis outbreaks [50]. After ingestion and colonization, *Salmonella* can induce an inflammatory response in the host. It has been demonstrated that colonization with *Salmonella* in mice results in alterations of the microbiota profile, mainly an overgrowth of aerotolerant bacteria [51]. It was hypothesized by Barman and co-workers [51] that the inflammatory response induced by *Salmonella* is responsible for the alterations in microbiota profile. The group also reported that these alterations were transient and the 'normal' microbiota profile returned indicating that the profile may be predetermined.

In the intestinal tract, *Salmonella* can invade the epithelial cells. After invading the epithelium, the bacterium has the ability to multiply intracellularly and can spread to mesenteric lymph nodes and throughout the body via the systemic circulation. Once the bacteria reach the circulatory system, they are taken up by the reticuloendothelial cells. The reticuloendothelial system confines and controls the spread of the organism, but depending on the serotype and the host defenses against that serovar, some serovars may infect the liver, spleen, gall bladder, bones, meninges, heart valves, myocardium, and other organs.

Salmonella endocarditis is an uncommon infection. In 1987, Cohen and co-workers [52] identified 42 cases. Of those 42 cases, the mean age of the patients was 49 years old and 42% of the patients had diarrhea prior to heart complications. The mortality rate was 69%. In 2004, Fernandez-Guerro and co-workers [53] reviewed the medical literature and reported an additional 30 cases. The mean age of patients increased to 59 years old of which 18 were over 60 years of age. Of these 30 cases, 70% were men with predisposing heart conditions. Diarrhea was reported prior to heart complications in 30% of the cases.

Although both are rare, endocarditis is more frequently reported than myocarditis in association with *Salmonella* infection. As mentioned previously, most cases of endocarditis associated with *Salmonella* infections are reported in older males, while most cases of myocarditis have been described in young males without any predisposing conditions. Another dissimilarity between the conditions is the lack of gastrointestinal symptoms prior to endocarditis, but the medical literature reviewed indicated almost all the patients with myocarditis reported gastrointestinal symptoms likely from salmonellosis. In the myocarditis cases, the time between heart complications and gastrointestinal symptoms was a few days, most likely indicative of a toxin or direct bacterial invasion effect on the heart.

Limited studies have been conducted to elucidate the mechanism of carditis by bacterial toxins. Using rats and dogs as models, it has been demonstrated that the heart becomes resistant to the stimulating action of insulin on glucose utilization following a bacterial infection [54–57]. These mechanisms of glucose resistance (i.e. sugar uptake versus glycolysis/glycogen synthesis) in the heart were further examined by Tessier and co-workers [58]. They treated rats with lipopolysaccharides prepared from *S. typhimurium*. The inflammation reaction caused by the endotoxin impaired cardiac glucose mechanisms in two ways: through the exacerbation of the counter-regulatory effect of alternative fuels on glycolysis and through a reduction in glycogen synthesis. Interestingly, Pitcher and co-workers [59] concluded that endogenous estrogen mediated a higher threshold for *Salmonella* endotoxin (LPS) tolerance in female myocardium. This finding may partially explain why males are more often afflicted than females with carditis induced by salmonellosis.

Campylobacteriosis

Campylobacter is Gram-negative, thermophilic, spiral-shaped and fastidious in nutrient and environmental requirements. The bacterium is an obligate microaerophile and is well-adapted to the preferred environment of the intestinal tract of birds. *Campylobacter* has become a leading cause of foodborne illnesses worldwide [60]. In the United States, the CDC reported 12.68 laboratory-confirmed cases per 100,000 people in 2008 [49]. However, because many campylobacteriosis cases are not reported, the actual number of cases per year is thought to be underestimated by 5 or even 10 times [61].

The infective dose is typically thought to be low (less than 500 cells), but may be dependent on various factors [62]. Like many other foodborne illnesses, the young, the elderly, and immunocompromised patients are generally more susceptible and relatively lower doses may cause illness in these patients. The disease is usually self-limiting and no treatment is required, but depending on the health of the patient and severity of the disease, antibiotics can be administered. Patients report symptoms usually lasting about 3 to 4 days. The bacteria may be shed in the feces for up to 1 month [63]. Extraintestinal complications have been reported and include reactive arthritis and Guillain-Barré syndrome (GBS). Reactive arthritis typically occurs within 3 days to 6 weeks of infection and can last for months or up to a year [64]. GBS may occur within 1 to 3 weeks of infection, but is quite rare. The disease is a progressive paralysis due to molecular mimicry between the axonal sheath and bacterial antigen. For this reason, some serotypes of *C. jejuni* are more likely to initiate GBS. Overall, patients usually recover within 2 to 3 weeks, and the mortality rate of campylobacteriosis-induced GBS is very low.

Cardiac complications can also occur, and a review of the medical literature revealed that myocarditis is the most frequently reported outcome [65]. It has been described in young adults, mostly male, and the majority of patients recovered with antibiotic therapy. The time between enteric infection and the onset of myocarditis has been reported as short as 2 to 4 days after initial enteric infection [66]. Myocardial involvement in *C. jejuni* infection has been speculated to involve either bacterial or toxin invasion of the myocardium, or an immunologically mediated inflammation. Since myocarditis seems to appear at the same time as enteric infection, infection or toxin production seem to be more likely, because a few weeks' span is needed between infection and the subsequent immune response.

Two reported cases of myocarditis associated with *C. jejuni* exhibit some unique aspects and have given insight into the mechanisms of pathogenesis. In one of these two cases, the outcome was fatal [65]. The patient had typical gastrointestinal symptoms of diarrhea, vomiting and fever and heart problems did not arise until a few days after the initial gastrointestinal symptoms. At autopsy, stool cultures were positive for *Campylobacter*; however, heart tissues were analyzed by nucleic acid detection and were negative for *Campylobacter*. It was speculated that *C. jejuni* toxin was the primary cause of myocarditis in this case due to the negative polymerase chain reaction (PCR) results and the short length of time between gastrointestinal symptoms and heart problems [65]. A second case of *C. jejuni* also presented evidence of toxin mediated myocarditis [67]. In this case, blood cultures were negative for *C. jejuni* in addition to the typical short time of gastrointestinal symptoms until severe chest pains occurred.

The fact that these two cases indicate toxin as a cause of myocarditis is very intriguing because a cytolethal distending toxin (CDT) is the only toxin identified from the entire genome sequence of *C. jejuni* [68]. However, other toxin activities of *Campylobacter* have been reported that include a shiga-like toxin, a hepatotoxin, hemolytic toxin and exotoxin. Furthermore, even CDT negative strains have been shown to have toxin effects in *in vitro* tissue culture models [69]. However, no cardiotoxin has been reported [70].

Listeriosis

Listeria monocytogenes can be found in a variety of foods. Foods most often implicated in listeriosis are processed foods that become contaminated after processing—such as deli meats, soft cheeses and hot dogs. Unpasteurized milk and raw vegetables can also be sources. The disease primarily affects persons of advanced age, pregnant women, newborns, and adults with weakened immune systems. Listeriosis is a serious foodborne illness with extraintestinal complications including septicemia, meningitis/encephalitis, and abortion that occur mostly in immune-compromised populations. According to the Bacterial Foodborne and Diarrheal Disease Surveillance report published in 2007, there were 896 cases of listeriosis recorded nationally in 2005 [71].

Endocarditis caused by *L. monocytogenes* is rare and accounts for the minority of recognized clinical syndromes caused by human listeriosis. Only 60 cases of *L. monocytogenes* infective endocarditis have been reported and of those, 15 involved a prosthetic valve [72]. Most patients with *L. monocytogenes* associated endocarditis were 50 years of age or older [73]. Men were affected more often than women and various underlying cardiac and non-cardiac conditions were present in a majority of the reported cases [72, 74]. The mortality rate for the reported cases was 50%. Most patients had typical flu-like symptoms including fever and chills. It appears that *L. monocytogenes* directly infects the heart as most patients had positive blood cultures and/or at autopsy *L. monocytogenes* was cultured from the heart valves [73].

Only a few reports of myocarditis as a complication of *L. monocytogenes* infection have been reported. In these incidents, blood cultures were positive [75, 76], indicating that infection of the heart was most likely the cause of myocarditis as opposed to toxin or immune reaction mediated. In the hearts of patients experiencing myocarditis, remodeling of the ventricle occurred as a result of chamber dilation and sphericity, resulting in a reduced left ventricular blood output. In patients with *L. monocytogenes* associated myocarditis, the reshaping of the heart was reported to be a result of extensive necrosis [76]. Like endocarditis, myocarditis was usually identified in older patients with underlying conditions. However, the condition has also been described in an immune competent patient who was 49 years old [76].

Yersiniosis

Yersinia enterolitica is an uncommon cause of foodborne illness in the United States (0.36 per 100,000) [49]. Pigs can carry *Yersinia* in the intestines and therefore pork and pork products can become contaminated with the bacteria. As with other foodborne illnesses, the population having a greater risk for yersiniosis includes the immunocompromised, very young and very old.

A summary of reports by Karachalois and coworkers in 2002 [77] reported 14 cases of *Yersinia enterolitica* endocarditis. Of those 14 cases, two had prosthetic heart valves. *Yersinia* bacteremia and septicemia are typically seen in patients with some type of predisposing factor such as diabetes, iron overload, liver disease, alcoholism, as well as in elderly patients, and nearly all the cases of endocarditis due to *Yersinia* infection had some type of predisposing condition. All cases of endocarditis had positive blood cultures for the bacterium indicating infection of the heart by bacteria as the cause of endocarditis.

Probiotics in Agricultural Animals to Reduce Foodborne Pathogens

In order to reduce foodborne illnesses, the severity of disease and the risk of secondary complications associated with cardiac health, necessitates addressing and designing intervention strategies along the farm-to-fork continuum. Probiotics offer an all-natural alternative approach and research involving the use of probiotics at all steps from production to final product have been explored. The next section will discuss probiotic uses in food production specifically aimed at reducing foodborne pathogens.

An important source of these pathogens is the mishandling or consumption of raw or undercooked meat. Agricultural food animals, including cattle, poultry and swine, can carry pathogens in their intestines without causing disease to the animal. Shedding of the pathogen in the feces causes contamination of the environment. Furthermore, if intestinal contents are ruptured during processing, contamination of the meat can occur. Pre-harvest intervention strategies, such as probiotics that reduce these foodborne pathogens, are attractive as a means of reducing human risk of illness. Therefore, considerable research has been centered on probiotic administration to these animals to prevent foodborne pathogens from colonizing the animal gut. This subject has been reviewed by Nava et al. [78], and therefore, this subject will be briefly discussed with respect to other studies.

Cattle

Cattle may carry and shed *Salmonella* and *E. coli* O157:H7 and probiotics that can reduce both of these pathogens are being explored [79]. Probiotic treatment options are appealing because they are more cost-efficient than other treatments such as sodium chlorate or bacteriophage [80]. A challenge with probiotic administration in cattle is the intermittent shedding of the pathogens, because it has been reported that *E. coli* and *Salmonella* shedding can be unpredictable and can occur in clusters of animals [81]. In feeding trials, probiotics administered on a daily basis did not completely eliminate foodborne pathogens but did reduce pathogen shedding [79, 82]. Other research indicates that, although probiotics offer some defense from colonizing pathogens, they are not completely effective and alternative probiotic cultures or other additional pre-harvest intervention strategies may be useful.

Probiotic cultures in cattle are useful because they may provide additional benefits. Chiquette and co-workers [83] demonstrated that supplementing early-lactating cows with a probiotic culture increased ruminal fermentation products and increased milk fat concentration. Magalhaes and co-workers [84] were able to improve health, minimize frequency of health treatments, and reduced the risk of morbidity and mortality in dairy calves by feeding yeast cultures. Vasconcelos and co-workers [85] were able to increase grain feed efficiency in cattle by feeding a combined culture of *Lactobacillus* and *Propionibacterium*.

Poultry

Conventional poultry association with foodborne disease and subsequent prevention has been reviewed [86]. However, the emergence of non-conventional poultry raised either as organic or pasture flocks has altered the emphasis for control measures to more natural biologicals [87]. Organic meat growers must follow the primary organic practices set forth by the USDA, which includes growing without antibiotics, coccidiostats or growth hormones and using organic feed that was grown without the use of synthetic fertilizers or pesticides. Thus, probiotics are one of the few acceptable treatments in organic production. A growing number of consumers are attracted to organic

products due to concerns of health issues related to the belief that growth hormones and antibiotics are used in conventional systems. At the time of writing, organic poultry only constitutes 2% of the total poultry market, but it is one of the fastest growing sectors in the food market. Chicken leads as an organic meat due to its short production cycle, which allows suppliers to quickly increase supply. Lower costs of production relative to other meats also means that these chicken products are only about 20% higher priced than conventional, compared to 30–40% price premiums for other meats.

The two leading causes of foodborne illnesses are *Salmonella* and *Campylobacter* and handling or consumption of poultry and poultry products are leading causes of salmonellosis and campylobacteriosis. It has been reported that nearly 98% of chicken flocks in the United States are colonized by *C. jejuni* [88]. Levels of colonization have been demonstrated to be 10^5 to 10^9 colony-forming units (cfu) per gram of intestinal contents [61]. Siemon et al. [89] reported that 44% of the farms sampled were positive for *Salmonella*. Bailey and Cosby [90] sampled a total of 135 processed free-range chickens from four different producers in 14 different lots and analyzed the carcasses for the presence of *Salmonella*. Overall, nine (64%) of 14 lots and 42 (31%) of 135 of the carcasses were positive for *Salmonella*. Esteban and co-workers [91] sampled free-range flocks in Spain and found that *Campylobacter* was the most prevalent of the four pathogens, isolated in 70.6% of the farms, followed by *L. monocytogenes* (26.5%), and *Salmonella* (2.9%).

Without the use of antibiotics, organic poultry producers face a challenge to reduce the levels of these foodborne pathogens, which are widespread in poultry. Probiotics have shown promising results in poultry production [78]. However, temporal results similar to probiotic studies for cattle are typically reported [92]. With the growing interest in organic foods, specifically poultry, it will become imperative to find probiotics and other natural treatments that are effective and acceptable for use in organic production.

Swine

The consumption and mis-handling of raw or undercooked pork can lead to infection with *Salmonella* or *Yersinia* [93]. *Salmonella* serovar *typhimurium* remains the serovar most commonly isolated from pigs [94]. The primary goal of probiotic administration in pigs is to reduce gastrointestinal colonization by pathogenic bacteria. However, because infection with *Salmonella* in pigs can result in diarrheal illness, probiotics can also serve as a treatment option.

Casey and co-workers [95] administered a combination of five lactic acid bacteria to piglets and 6 days later orally challenged the pigs with *Salmonella typhimurium*. Animals that were administered probiotics showed reduced signs of illness and the numbers of animals shedding *Salmonella* was also reduced. In the pig, probiotic effectiveness has been reported to be dependent on the strains of probiotics used. Szabo and co-workers [96] used a probiotic strain of *Enterococcus faecium* in piglets. They observed that fecal excretion and colonization of *Salmonella* in organs were significantly greater in piglets fed *E. faecium*. However, the humoral immune response against *Salmonella* (serum IgM and IgA levels) was significantly greater in the probiotic group animals than in control animals.

Probiotics in Food to Reduce Foodborne Pathogen Contamination

The level of indigenous microflora in most foods is expected to be higher than that of a pathogen on a food [97]. The growth and metabolic activity of the indigenous flora has a large influence on the intrinsic properties of the food [98]. Naturally occurring lactic acid bacteria on vegetables can inhibit pathogen growth by lowering pH, producing antimicrobial compounds, competing for nutrients, and producing H_2O_2

[99]. Therefore, it is not surprising that pathogens can grow better on foods with low background microflora [100, 101].

Lactobacilli are the most commonly used probiotic cultures as food additives because they are generally recognized as safe (GRAS), typically already present in the human GI tract and can be used without regulation [102]. They are usually present in dairy products but may be added to produce cheeses and yogurts. Lactobacilli are known to inhibit the growth of pathogenic bacteria, possibly by producing inhibitory compounds that include organic acids, hydrogen peroxide and bacteriocins [103, 104]. The added benefit of the ability of *Lactobacillus* to inhibit foodborne pathogens in these products has been reported [105]. This is especially useful for unpasteurized products as probiotic cultures could render unpasteurized cheeses safer for consumption [104].

In foods other than dairy, lactobacilli can act as spoilage organisms and possibly reduce the shelf life of the product. Nevertheless, the idea that these bacteria can inhibit or kill pathogens on food products is being explored due to consumer demands for additive- and preservative-, free foods [106, 107]. Brillet and co-workers [108] showed biopreservation of cold smoked salmon using lactic acid bacteria inhibited the growth of *L. monocytogenes* with low effect on the quality of the product. Benkerroum and co-workers [109] used lyophilized *Lactobacillus* with some success to inhibit *Listeria* in dry fermented sausages. The addition of probiotic cultures to prepared meals at the restaurant level has been explored. Rodgers [110] has reviewed this particular use of probiotics not only for the antibacterial use, but for the multiple health benefits in which consumers are interested.

Probiotics in Humans to Combat Foodborne Pathogens

Any bacteria, beneficial or pathogenic, must be able to survive passage through the acidic conditions of the stomach and colonize the intestines. Milk provides a buffering effect against the acidic conditions of the stomach and the environment of a dairy food is favorable to lactobacilli. Therefore, probiotic delivery via milk products is a proficient means to preserve cultures for shelf storage and to promote survival during administration. Evidence has been published that lactobacilli have bactericidal effect on some foodborne pathogens. Lactobacilli cultures isolated from cheese and milk products have been demonstrated to reduce *Salmonella* populations in the gut of mice and were bactericidal in *in vitro* assays [111, 112]. Jain and co-workers [113] found pre-feeding mice with *L. acidophilus* and *L. casei* ameliorated *S. enteriditis* infection by stimulating specific and non-specific immune responses. Mice fed *L. casei* prior to infection with *L. monocytogenes* had lower levels of pathogen in the gut and no translocation of the pathogen to internal organs [114].

A requirement of any pathogen invading the gut is that it must be able to compete with the indigenous microflora of the gut. In general, indigenous microflora out-compete pathogens for adhesion sites on the intestinal epithelium, essential nutrients, and may even produce bactericidal substances [115]. However, if colonization is established, the immune system plays a critical role in clearing the GI tract of the invading pathogen. Probiotic lactic acid bacteria in dairy products are known to enhance the ability of the host to fight intestinal infection through stimulation of the mucosal immune system [116]. Lactic acid bacteria can also stimulate B and T cells to produce antibodies and cytokines used to eliminate pathogens from the gut.

Search for lactic acid bacteria with immunomodulatory abilities is an important area in food science. The increase of antibiotic-resistant bacteria limits treatment options with classical drugs. In addition, foodborne pathogens can have a devastating systemic impact. Probiotics offer an approach that may not only prevent but possibly treat serious infections with foodborne pathogens.

4. CONCLUSION

The importance of the gut health of an individual is widely recognized. A more comprehensive understanding of how beneficial microorganisms shape gut health is evolving. The gut provides the essential function of nutrient uptake with microorganisms aiding in the digestion of our food. Furthermore, these bacteria play an essential role in nutrient acquisition. The presence of bacteria in the gut is critical and barriers and containments in the gut are crucial for preventing bacterial infection in other areas of the body. Molecular filters in the gut are necessary for the uptake of nutrients and prevention of toxic substances from reaching critical organs.

Due to its essential function, the heart is well guarded and the impacts that ingested materials can have on the heart are typically limited. However, many indirect factors exist which can negatively affect the heart and we are just beginning to learn and appreciate the fact that the digestive microbiota profile can define health in nearly all the organs of the body including the heart. With research, a better understanding of these complex interactions and the effects of gut microbiota on the heart will be determined and perhaps manipulation of the gut bacteria might be achieved that can result not only in improved but sustained maintenance of cardiac health.

ACKNOWLEDGMENTS

This review was funded by an American Heart Association Scientist Development Grant number 0530104N and by the Arkansas Biosciences Institute. Special thanks to Ashley Clement for her technical assistance with the preparation of this manuscript.

References

1. Anonymous. (2009). Heart Health Food and Drinks: NPD in cardiovascular health, hypertension and cholesterol reduction. *Just Foods*. <http://www.just-food.com/store/product.aspx?id = 60714>.

2. Olson, E. R., Naugle, J. E., Zhang, X., et al. (2005). Inhibition of cardiac fibroblast proliferation and myofibroblast differentiation by resveratrol. *American journal of Physiology Heart and Circulatory Physiology*, *288*, H1131–H1138.

3. Oxman, T., Shapira, M., Diver, A., et al. (2000). A new method of long-term preventive cardioprotection using Lactobacillus. *American Journal of Physiology Heart and Circulatory Physiology*, *278*, H1717–H1724.

4. Xu, J., & Gordon, J. (2003). Honor thy symbionts. *Proceedings of the National Academy of Sciences*, *100*, 10452–10459.

5. Bäckhed, F., Ding, H., Wang, T., et al. (2004). The gut microbiota as an environmental factor that regulates fat storage. *Proceedings of the National Academy of Sciences of the United States of America*, *101*, 15718–15723.

6. Eckel, R. H. (1997). Obesity and heart disease: A statement for healthcare professionals from the Nutrition Committee, American Heart Association. *Circulation*, *96*, 3248–3250.

7. Van Itallie, T. B. (1985). Health implications of overweight and obesity in the United States. *Annals of Internal Medicine*, *103*, 983–988.

8. Duflou, J., Virmani, R., Rabin, I., et al. (1995). Sudden death as a result of heart disease in morbid obesity. *American Heart Journal*, *130*, 306–313.

9. Fernández-López, J. A., Remesar, X., Foz, M., & Alemany, M. (2002). Pharmacological approaches for the treatment of obesity. *Drugs*, *62*, 915–944.

10. Tziomalos, K., Krassas, G. E., & Tzotzas, T. (2009). The use of sibutramine in the management of obesity and related disorders: An update. *Vascular Health and Risk Management*, *5*, 441–452.

11. Raoult, D. (2008). Human microbiome: Take-home lesson on growth promoters? *Nature*, *454*, 690–691.

12. Gaskins, H. R., Collier, C. T., & Anderson, D. B. (2002). Antibiotics as growth promotants: Mode of action. *Animal Biotechnology*, *13*, 29–42.

13. Ternak, G., Almasi, I., & Rakoczi, E. (2008). Hospital antibiotic management in Hungary—results of the ABS maturity survey of the ABS International group. *Wiener Klinische Wochenschrift*, *120*, 299–302.

14. Kümmerer, K. (2003). Significance of antibiotics in the environment. *The Journal of Antimicrobial Chemotherapy*, *52*, 5–7.

15. Ricke, S. C., & Pillai, S. D. (1999). Conventional and molecular methods for understanding probiotic bacteria functionality in gastrointestinal tracts. *Critical Reviews in Microbiology*, *25*, 19–38.

16. DeBaise, J. K., Zhang, H., Crowell, M. D., et al. (2008). Gut microbiota and its possible relationship with obesity. *Mayo Clinic Proceedings*, *83*, 460–469.

17. Lee, H. Y., Park, J. H., Seok, S. H., et al. (2006). Human originated bacteria, *Lactobacillus rhamnosus* PL60, produce conjugated linoleic acid and show anti-obesity effects in diet-induced obese mice. *Biochimica Biophysica Acta*, *1761*, 736–744.

18. Park, Y., Albright, K. J., Liu, W., et al. (1997). Effect of conjugated linoleic acid on body composition in mice. *Lipids*, *32*, 853–858.

19. Lee, K., Paek, K., Lee, H. Y., et al. (2007). Antiobesity effect of trans-10, cis-12-conjugated linoleic acid-producing *Lactobacillus plantarum* PL62 on diet-induced obese mice. *Journal of Applied Microbiology*, *103*, 1140–1146.

20. Sonnenburg, J. L., Chen, C. T., & Gordon, J. I. (2006). Genomic and metabolic studies of the impact of probiotics on a model gut symbiont and host. *PLoS Biolology*, *4*, e413.

21. Martin, F. P., Wang, Y., Sprenger, N., et al. (2008). Probiotic modulation of symbiotic gut microbial-host metabolic interactions in a humanized microbiome mouse model. *Molecular Systems Biology*, *4*, 157.

22. Nakamura, Y., Yamamoto, N., Sakai, K., et al. (1994). Purification and characterization of angiotensin I-converting enzyme inhibitors from sour milk. *Journal of Dairy Science*, *78*, 777–783.

23. Nakamura, Y., Yamamoto, N., Sakai, K., & Takano, T. (1995). Antihypertensive effect of sour milk and peptides isolated from it that are inhibitors of angiotensin I-converting enzyme. *Journal of Dairy Science*, *78*, 1253–1257.

24. Yamamoto, N., Akino, A., & Takano, T. (1993). Antihypertensive effects of the peptides derived from casein by an extracellular proteinase from *Lactobacillus helveticus* CP970. *Journal of Dairy Science*, *77*, 917–922.

25. Seppo, L., Jauhiainen, T., Poussa, T., & Korpela, R. (2003). A fermented milk high in bioactive peptides has a blood pressure-lowering effect in hypertensive subjects. *The American Journal of Clinical Nutrition*, *77*, 326–330.

26. Aihara, K., Kajimoto, O., Hirata, H., et al. (2005). Effect of powdered fermented milk with *Lactobacillus helveticus* on subjects with high-normal blood pressure of mild hypertension. *Journal of the American College of Nutrition*, *24*, 257–265.

27. Jauhiainen, T., & Korpela, R. (2007). Milk peptides and blood pressure. *The Journal of Nutrition*, *137*, 825S–829S.

28. Gilliland, S. E., Nelson, C. R., & Maxwell, C. (1985). Assimilation of cholesterol by *Lactobacillus acidophilus*. *Applied and Environmental Microbiology*, *49*, 377–381.

29. Danielson, A. D., Peo, E. R. J., Shahani, K. M., et al. (1989). Anticholesterolemic property of *Lactobacillus acidophilus* yoghurt fed to mature boars. *Journal of Animal Science*, *67*, 966–974.

30. De Smet, I., De Boever, P., & Versteaete, W. (1998). Cholesterol lowering in pigs through enhanced bacterial bile salt hydrolase activity. *The British Journal of Nutrition, 79*, 185–194.

31. Liong, M. T., & Shah, N. P. (2005). Bile salt deconjugation ability, bile salt hydrolase activity and cholesterol co-precipitation ability of lactobacilli strains. *International Dairy Journal, 15*, 391–398.

32. Bhathena, J., Martoni, C., Kulamarva, A., et al. (2009). Orally delivered microencapsulated live probiotic formulation lowers serum lipids in hypercholesterolemic hamsters. *Journal of Medicinal Food, 12*, 309–310.

33. Wang, Y., Xu, N., Xi, A., et al. (2009). Effects of *Lactobacillus plantarum* MA2 isolated from Tibet kefir on lipid metabolism and intestinal microflora of rats fed on high-cholesterol diet. *Applied Microbiology and Biotechnology, 84*(2), 341–7.

34. Ataie-Jafari, A., Larijani, B., Alavi Majd, H., & Tahbaz, F. (2009). Cholesterol-lowering effect of probiotic yogurt in comparison with ordinary yogurt in mildly to moderately hypercholesterolemic subjects. *Annals of Nutrition & Metabolism, 54*, 22–27.

35. Liong, M. T. (2007). Probiotics: A critical review of their potential role as antihypertensives, immune modulators, hypocholesterolemics, and perimenopausal treatments. *Nutrition Reviews, 65*, 316–328.

36. Archer, D. L., & Young, F. E. (1988). Contemporary issues: Diseases with a food vector. *Clinical Microbiology Reviews, 1*, 377–398.

37. Tarr, P. I. (1995). *Escherichia coli* O157:H7: Clinical, diagnostic, and epidemiological aspects of human infection. *Clinical Infectious Diseases, 20*, 1–8.

38. Reissbrodt, R., Hammes, W. P., dal Bello, F., et al. (2009). Inhibition of growth of Shiga toxin-producing *Escherichia coli* by nonpathogenic *Escherichia coli*. *FEMS Microbiology Letters, 290*, 62–69.

39. Centers for Disease Control and Prevention (CDC). (2008). National antimicrobial resistance monitoring system (NARMS): Enteric Bacteria. Available at: <http://www.cdc.gov/narms/>.

40. Muriana, P. & Kushwaha, K. (2006). Food pathogens of human concern: *Listeria monocytogenes*. FAPC-136. <http://www.fapc.okstate.edu/factsheets/fapc136.pdf>.

41. Wanby, P., & Olsen, B. (2001). Myocarditis in a patient with *Salmonella* and *Campylobacter enteritis*. *Scandinavian Journal of Infectious Diseases, 33*, 860–862.

42. Zheng, J., Meng, J., Zhao, S., et al. (2006). Adherence to and invasion of human intestinal epithelial cells by *Campylobacter jejuni* and *Campylobacter coli* isolates from retail meat products. *Journal of Food Protection, 69*, 768–774.

43. Franczuk, P., Rewiuk, K., & Grodzicki, T. (2007). Myocarditis related to *Salmonella enteritidis* infection. *Cardiology Journal, 14*, 589–591.

44. Mohanan, P. A., Pereira, P., & Raghuveer, C. V. (1995). Myocarditis in enteric fever. *Indian Journal of Medical Science, 49*, 28–31.

45. Helmick, C. G., Griffin, P. M., Addiss, D. G., et al. (1994). Infectious diarrheas. In J. E. Everhart (Ed.) *Digestive Diseases in the United States: Epidemiology and Impact: Vol. 3* (pp. 83–124). Washington DC: Government Printing Office.

46. Tauxe, R. V. (1991). *Salmonella*: A postmodern pathogen. *Journal of Food Protection, 54*, 563–568.

47. Buzby, J. C., Roberts, T., Lin, J.C.-T. & MacDonald, J. M. (1996). Bacterial Foodborne Disease, Medical Costs and Productivity Losses. *USDA-ERS Report, 741*.

48. Frenzen, P., Riggs, T. L., Buzby, J., et al. (1999). *Salmonella* cost estimate updated using food net data. *Food Review, 22*(2), 10–15.

49. Centers for Disease Control and Prevention (CDC). (2009). Preliminary FoodNet data on the incidence of infection with pathogens transmitted commonly through food—10 states, 2008. *Morbidity and Mortality Weekly Report, 58*, 333–337.

50. Gast, R. K., Porter, R. E., Jr., & Holt, P. S. (1997). Assessing the sensitivity of egg yolk antibody testing for detecting *Salmonella Enteritidis* infections in laying hens. *Poultry Science, 76*, 798–801.

51. Barman, M., Unold, D., Shifley, K., et al. (2008). Enteric salmonellosis disrupts the microbial ecology of the murine gastrointestinal tract. *Infection and Immunity, 76*, 907–915.

52. Cohen, J. I., Bartlett, J. A., & Corey, G. R. (1987). Extra-intestinal manifestations of *Salmonella* infections. *Medicine (Baltimore), 66*, 349–388.

53. Fernandez-Guerro, M., Aguado, M., Arribas, A., et al. (2004). The spectrum of cardiovascular infections due to *Salmonella enterica*. A review of clinical features and factors determining outcome. *Medicine, 83*, 123–138.

54. Lang, B., Wilhelm, C., Gildein, P., et al. (1990). Fetal complete heart block with myocarditis and maternal SS-A-/AA-B/antibodies. *Schweizerische Medizinische Wochenschrift, 120*, 1741–1744.

55. Shangraw, R. E., Jahoor, F., Wolfe, R. R., & Lang, C. H. (1996). Pyruvate dehydrogenase inactivity is not responsible for sepsis-induced insulin resistance. *Critical Care Medicine, 24*, 566–574.

56. Virkamäki, A., & Yki-Järvinen, H. (1994). Mechanisms of insulin resistance during acute endotoxemia. *Endocrinology, 134*, 2072–2078.

57. Raymond, R. M., McLane, M. P., Law, W. R., et al. (1988). Myocardial insulin resistance during acute endotoxin shock in dogs. *Diabetes, 37*, 1684–1688.

58. Tessier, J. P., Thurner, B., Jüngling, E., et al. (2003). Impairment of glucose metabolism in hearts from rats treated with endotoxin. *Cardiovascular Research, 60*, 119–130.

59. Pitcher, J., Wang, M., Tsai, B., et al. (2006). Endogenous estrogen mediates a higher threshold for endotoxin-induced myocardial protection in females. *American Journal of Physiology: Regional International Comparative Physiology, 290,* R27–R33.

60. Zilbauer, M., Dorrell, N., Wren, B. W., & Bajaj-Elliott, M. (2008). *Campylobacter jejuni*-mediated disease pathogenesis: An update. *Transactions of the Royal Society of Tropical Medicine and Hygiene, 102,* 123–129.

61. Lee, M. D., & Newell, D. G. (2006). *Campylobacter* in poultry: Filling an ecological niche. *Avian Diseases, 50,* 1–9.

62. Black, R. E., Levine, M. M., Clements, M. L., et al. (1988). Experimental *Campylobacter jejuni* infection in humans. *The Journal of Infectious Diseases, 157,* 472–479.

63. Skirrow, M., & Blaser, M. (2000). Clinical aspects of *Campylobacter* infection. In I. Nachamkin & M. Blaser (Eds.), *Campylobacter* (pp. 69–87). Washington, D.C: ASM Press.

64. Peterson, M. (1994). Rheumatic manifestations of *Campylobacter jejuni* and *Campylobacter fetus* infections in adults. *Canadian Journal Rheumatology, 23,* 167–170.

65. Pena, L. A., & Fishbein, M. C. (2007). Fatal myocarditis related to *Campylobacter jejuni* infection: A case report. *Cardiovascular Pathology, 16,* 119–121.

66. Hannu, T., Mattila, L., Rautelin, H., et al. (2005). Three cases of cardiac complications associated with *Campylobacter jejuni* infection and review of the literature. *European Journal of Clinical Microbiology Infectious Diseas, 24,* 619–622.

67. Reda, E., & Mansell, C. (2007). Myocarditis in a patient with *Campylobacter* infection. *New Zealand Journal of Medicine, 118,* 1–4.

68. Parkhill, J., Wren, B., Mungall, K., et al. (2000). The genome sequence of the food-borne pathogen *Campylobacter jejuni* reveals hypervariable sequences. *Nature, 403,* 665–668.

69. Gilbert, C., Hanning, I., Vaughn, B., et al. (2009). Comparison of cytolethal distending toxin and invasion abilities in *Campylobacter jejuni* isolated from clinical patients and poultry. *Journal of Food Safety, 29,* 73–82.

70. Wassenaar, T. M., Engelskirchen, M., Park, S., & Lastovica, A. (1997). Differential uptake and killing potential of *Campylobacter jejuni* by human peripheral monocytes/macrophages. *Medical Microbiology and Immunology, 186,* 139–144.

71. Centers for Disease Control and Prevention (CDC). (2007). Preliminary FoodNet data on the incidence of infection with pathogens transmitted commonly through food—10 states, 2006. *Morbidity and Mortality Weekly Report, 56,* 336–339.

72. Makaryus, A. N., Yang, R., Cohen, R., et al. (2004). A rare case of *Listeria monocytogenes* presenting as prosthetic valve bacterial endocarditis and aortic root abscess. *Echocardiography, 21,* 423–427.

73. Gallagher, P. G., & Watanakunakorn, C. (1988). *Listeria monocytogenes* endocarditis: A review of the literature 1950–1986. *Scandinavian Journal of Infectious Diseases, 20,* 359–368.

74. Speeleveld, E., Muyldermans, L., Van den Bruel, A., et al. (1994). Prosthetic valve endocarditis due to *Listeria monocytogenes*. A case report with review of the literature. *Acta Clinica Belgica, 49,* 95–98.

75. Stamm, A. M., Smith, S. H., Kirklin, J. K., & McGiffin, D. C. (1990). Listerial myocarditis in cardiac transplantation. *Reviews of Infectious Diseases, 12,* 820–823.

76. Haddad, F., Berry, G., Doyle, R. L., et al. (2007). Active bacterial myocarditis: A case report and review of the literature. *The Journal of Heart and Lung Transplantation, 26,* 745–749.

77. Karachalios, G., Bablekos, G., Karachaliou, G., et al. (2002). Infectious endocarditis due to *Yersinia enterocolitica. Chemotherapy, 48,* 158–159.

78. Nava, G. M., Bielke, L. R., Callaway, T. R., & Castañeda, M. P. (2005). Probiotic alternatives to reduce gastrointestinal infections: The poultry experience. *Animal Health Research Reviews, 6,* 105–118.

79. Tabe, E., Oloya, J., Doetkott, D., et al. (2008). Comparative effect of direct-fed microbials on fecal shedding of *Escherichia coli* O157:H7 and *Salmonella* in naturally infected feedlot cattle. *Journal of Food Protection, 71,* 539–544.

80. Dahl, K. C., Lyford, C. P., & Brashears, M. M. (2005). The cost and effectiveness of pre-harvest interventions in beef cattle. *Texas Journal of Agriculture Natural Resources, 17,* 97–110.

81. Wells, J. G., Shipman, L. D., Greene, K. D., et al. (2001). Isolation of *Escherichia coli* serotype O157:H7 and other Shiga-like toxin-producing *E. coli* from dairy cattle. *Journal of Clinical Microbiology, 29,* 985–989.

82. Stephens, T., Lonergan, G., Karunasena, E., & Brashears, M. (2007). Reduction of *Escherichia coli* O157 and *Salmonella* in feces and on hides of feedlot cattle using various doses of a direct-fed microbial. *Journal of Food Protection, 70,* 2386–2391.

83. Chiquette, J., Allison, M. J., & Rasmussen, M. A. (2008). *Prevotella bryantii* 25A used as a probiotic in early-lactation dairy cows: Effect on ruminal fermentation characteristics, milk production, and milk composition. *Journal of Dairy Science, 91,* 3536–3543.

84. Magalhães, V. J., Susca, F., Lima, F. S., et al. (2008). Effect of feeding yeast culture on performance, health, and immunocompetence of dairy calves. *Journal of Dairy Science, 91,* 1497–1509.

85. Vasconcelos, J. T., Elam, N. A., Brashears, M. M., & Galyean, M. L. (2008). Effects of increasing dose of

live cultures of *Lactobacillus acidophilus* (Strain NP 51) combined with a single dose of *Propionibacterium freudenreichii* (Strain NP 24) on performance and carcass characteristics of finishing beef steers. *Journal of Animal Science*, 86, 756–762.

86. Ricke, S. C., Kundinger, M. M., Miller, D. R., & Keeton, J. T. (2005). Alternatives to antibiotics: Chemical and physical antimicrobial interventions and foodborne pathogen response. *Poultry Science*, 84, 667–675.

87. Sirsat, S. A., Muthaiyan, A., & Ricke, S. C. (2009). Antimicrobials for foodborne pathogen reduction in organic and natural poultry production. *Journal of Applied Poultry Research*, 18, 379–388.

88. Stern, N. J., Cox, N. A., Bailey, J. S., et al. (2001). Comparison of mucosal competitive exclusion and competitive exclusion treatment to reduce *Salmonella* and *Campylobacter* spp. colonization in broiler chickens. *Poultry Science*, 80, 156–160.

89. Siemon, C. E., Bahnson, P. B., & Gebreyes, W. A. (2007). Comparative investigation of prevalence and antimicrobial resistance of *Salmonella* between pasture and conventionally reared poultry. *Avian Diseases*, 51, 112–117.

90. Bailey, J. S., & Cosby, D. E. (2005). *Salmonella* prevalence in free-range and certified organic chickens. *Journal of Food Protection*, 68, 2451–2453.

91. Esteban, J. I., Oporto, B., Aduriz, G., et al. (2008). A survey of food-borne pathogens in free-range poultry farms. *International Journal of Food Microbiology*, 123, 177–182.

92. Higgins, J. P., Higgins, S. E., Vicente, J. L., et al. (2007). Temporal effects of lactic acid bacteria probiotic culture on *Salmonella* in neonatal broilers. *Poultry Science*, 86, 1662–1666.

93. Centers for Disease Control and Prevention. (2006). Preliminary FoodNet data on the incidence of infection with pathogens transmitted commonly through food— 10 states, United States, 2005. *Morbidity and Mortality Weekly Report*, 55, 392–395.

94. Casey, P. G., Butler, D., Gardiner, G. E., et al. (2004). *Salmonella* carriage in an Irish pig herd: Correlation between serological and bacteriological detection methods. *Journal of Food Protection*, 67, 2797–2800.

95. Casey, P., Gardiner, G., Casey, G., et al. (2007). A five-strain probiotic combination reduces pathogen shedding and alleviates disease signs in pigs challenged with *Salmonella enteric* serovar *Typhimurium*. *Applied and Environmental Microbiology*, 73, 1858–1863.

96. Szabo, I., Wieler, L. H., Tedin, K., et al. (2009). Influence of a probiotic strain of *Enterococcus faecium* on *Salmonella enterica* serovar *Typhimurium* DT104 infection in a porcine animal infection model. *Applied and Environmental Microbiology*, 75, 2621–2628.

97. Sofos, J. N. (1994). Microbial growth and its control in meat, poultry and fish. Quality attributes and their measurement in meat, poultry and fish products. In A. M. Pearson & T. R. Dutson (Eds.), *Advances in Meat Research: Vol. 9* (pp. 353–403). Glasgow, United Kingdom: Chapman and Hall.

98. Francis, G., & O'Beirne, D. (1998). Effects of storage atmosphere on *Listeria monocytogenes* and competing microflora using a surface model system. *International Journal of Food Microbiology*, 33, 465–476.

99. Piard, J., & Desmazeaud, M. (1992). Inhibiting factors produced by lactic acid bacteria: Bacteriocins and other antimicrobial substances. *Lait*, 72, 113–142.

100. Aytac, S., & Gorris, L. (1994). Survival of *Aeromonas hydrophilia* and *Listeria monocytogenes* on fresh vegetables stored under moderate vacuum. *World Journal of Microbiology and Biotechnology*, 10, 670–672.

101. Carlin, F., Nguyen-the, C., & Morris, C. (1996). The influence of the background microflora on the fate of *Listeria monocytogenes* on minimally processed fresh broad leaved endive. *Journal of Food Protection*, 59, 698–703.

102. Salminen, S., von Wright, A., Morelli, L., et al. (1998). Demonstration of safety of probiotics—a review. *International Journal of Food Microbiology*, 44, 93–106.

103. Jacobsen, C. N., Rosenfeldt, N. V., Hayford, A. E., et al. (1999). Screening of probiotic activities of forty-seven strains of *Lactobacillus* spp. by *in vitro* techniques and evaluation of the colonization ability of five selected strains in humans. *Applied and Environmental Microbiology*, 65, 4949–4956.

104. Loessner, M., Guenther, S., Steffan, S., & Scherer, S. (2003). A pediocin-producing *Lactobacillus plantarum* in a multispecies cheese surface microbial ripening consortium. *Applied and Environmental Microbiology*, 69, 1854–1857.

105. Coeuret, V., Gueguen, M., & Vernoux, J. P. (2004). *In vitro* screening of potential probiotic activities of selected lactobacilli isolated from unpasteurized milk products for incorporation into soft cheese. *The Journal of Dairy Research*, 71, 451–460.

106. Liao, C., & Fett, W. (2001). Analysis of native microflora and selection of strains antagonistic to human pathogens on fresh produce. *Journal of Food Protection*, 64, 1110–1115.

107. Scheunzel, K., & Harrison, M. (2002). Microbial antagonists of foodborne pathogens on fresh, minimally processed vegetables. *Journal of Food Protection*, 65, 1909–1915.

108. Brillet, A., Pilet, M. F., Prevost, H., et al. (2005). Effect of inoculation of *Carnobacterium divergens* V41, a bioprereservative strain against *Listeria monocytogenes* risk, on the microbiological, chemical and sensory quality of cold-smoked salmon. *International Journal of Food Microbiology*, 104, 309–324.

109. Benkerroum, N., Daoudi, A., Hamraoui, T., et al. (2005). Lyophilized preparations of bacteriocinogenic *Lactobacillus curvatus* and *Lactococcus lactis* subsp. *lactis* as potential protective adjuncts to control of *Listeria monocytogenes* in dry-fermented sausages. *Journal of Applied Microbiology, 98*, 56–63.

110. Rodgers, S. (2008). Novel applications of live bacteria in food services: Probiotics and protective cultures. *Trends Food Science and Technology, 19*, 188–197.

111. Fayol-Messaoudi, D., Coconnier-Polter, M-H., Moal, V., et al. (2007). The *Lactobacillus plantarum* strain ACA-DC287 isolated from a Greek cheese demonstrates antagonistic activity *in vitro* and *in vivo* against *Salmonella enterica* serovar *Typhimurium*. *Journal of Applied Microbiology, 103*, 657–665.

112. Vinderola, G., Matar, C., & Perdigón, G. (2007). Milk fermented by *Lactobacillus helveticus* R389 and its non-bacterial fraction confer enhanced protection against *Salmonella enteritidis* serovar *Typhimurium* infection in mice. *Immunobiology, 212*, 107–118.

113. Jain, S., Yadav, H., & Sinha, P. R. (2008). Immunomodulatory potential by oral feeding of probiotic Dahi containing *Lactobacillus acidophilus* and *Lactobacillus casei* in mice. *International Journal of Probiotics and Prebiotics, 2*, 131–136.

114. De Waard, R., Garssen, J., Bokken, G. C., & Vos, J. G. (2002). Antagonistic activity of *Lactobacillus casei* strain Shirota against gastrointestinal *Listeria monocytogenes* infection in rats. *International Journal of Food Microbiology, 73*, 93–100.

115. Stavric, S., & Kornegay, E. T. (1995). Microbial probiotic for pigs and poultry. In R. J. Wallace & A. Chesson (Eds.), *Biotechnology in Animal Feeds and Animal Feeding* (pp. 205–231).

116. Erickson, K. L., & Hubbard, N. E. (2000). Probiotic immunomodulation in health and disease. *The Journal of Nutrition, 130*, 403–409.

Prebiotics and Probiotics in Infant Nutrition

Antonio Alberto Zuppa, Giovanni Alighieri, and Antonio Scorrano

Catholic University of the Sacred Heart, Division of Neonatology, Rome, Italy

1. INTRODUCTION

Prebiotics and probiotics have now gained a more central role in the nutritional scientific panorama for their important therapeutic 'alternative' role in the treatment of some pathologies that affect both adults and children, as early as the first few days of life. According to the criteria proposed in a report of the Conseil de l'Europe of 2004 entitled 'The quality of life and management of living resources program,' prebiotics and probiotics can be called 'functional foods' [1]. The term 'functional' refers to a food—not a dietary supplement—that, in addition to its intrinsic nutritional value, can also positively affect specific functions of the organism, improve a person's health and well-being, and reduce the risk of diseases [2].

1.1. Development and Physiology of the Gastrointestinal Ecosystem

The gastrointestinal bacterial flora, the intestinal epithelium and the mucosal immune system constitute a highly integrated unit called gastrointestinal ecosystem. Intrinsic disorders (genetic) and acquired alterations to any component can bring about pathological changes to the digestive system [3].

During fetal life, the intestine is sterile; at birth the gastrointestinal tract becomes progressively colonized by commensal bacteria, creating the so-called microflora that is essential to the development of intestinal structures and functions [4]. Bacteria can be classified into three groups, depending on their impact on a person's health: beneficial bacteria, potentially harmful bacteria, and bacteria that can have both pathogenic and beneficial effects [5] (Table 27.1).

Intestinal colonization is strongly influenced by genetic factors, by the type of delivery, by the maternal bacterial flora, by the type of nutrition, and by exposure to the external world [6, 7]. In babies born by spontaneous delivery, microbial colonization begins with the passage of the fetus through the birth canal. The microbial colonization pattern is the same as that of the mother's vaginal and perineal microflora (microbial heredity) [8–12]. *Enterococcus, Streptococcus,*

TABLE 27.1   Classification of indigenous intestinal bacteria

Beneficial bacteria	*Bifidobacterium* spp. *Lactobacillus* spp. *Eubacterium* spp.
Potentially harmful bacteria	*Staphylococcus* spp. *Clostridium* spp. *Proteus* spp. *Pseudomonas* (sp. *aeruginosa*)
Opportunistic bacteria	*Veillonella* spp. *Streptococcus* spp. *Bacteroides* spp. *Enterococcus* spp.

Staphylococcus and *Lactobacillus* bacteria are the first to colonize [13]. This microbial flora is transitory and its role is simply to create a favorable environment for the true intestinal flora [14]. On the contrary, the microflora of a child born through a cesarean section depends on the surrounding environment and is characterized by low levels of *Bifidobacterium* and *Bacteroides*-type bacteria, and higher levels of *Clostridium* (sp. *difficile*) [15–17].

During the first two days of a baby's life, a high oxidoreductive intestinal potential facilitates the development of facultative aerobic bacterial strains such as the more prevailing *Escherichia* (sp. *coli*) and *Streptococcus*. Only later, the progressive decrease in oxidoreductive potential, induced by the aforementioned strains, creates conditions that favor the development of obligate anaerobes belonging to the genera *Bifidobacterium*, *Bacteroides* and *Clostridium*, which after the first week of life represent about 80% of all the bacteria that make up the intestinal flora [18]. The intestinal tract of a healthy full-term infant continues to host a simple and unstable pattern of microorganisms through the first few days of life. After the first week, colonization becomes more complex but also more stable and persistent, with about 10^9–10^{10} organisms per gram of feces [8, 19].

From the second week on, and regardless of the type of delivery, the development of the gut microflora is heavily influenced by nutrition [20]. Formula-fed infants seem to develop a more complex microflora, represented mostly by anaerobes such as *Enterococcus* spp., *Klebsiella* spp., *Enterobacter* spp., *Clostridium* spp. and lesser amounts of *Bifidobacterium* spp., *Bacteroides* spp., and *Lactobacillus* spp. On the other hand, the intestinal bacterial flora of breast-fed infants is characterized by the predominant presence of *Bifidobacterium* spp. and by lesser quantities of *Staphylococcus* spp., *Streptococcus* spp., and *Lactobacillus* spp. [15, 17, 21–28]. It appears that this difference in intestinal colonization between formula-fed and breast-fed infants could be related to the influence that some breast milk components have on the microbial flora. This is especially true for oligosaccharides and some humoral mediators of the immune response, such as secretory IgAs, cytokines, and growth factors like IL-1, IL-6, IL-8, G-CSF, M-CSF, TNF-α, IFN-γ, in which breast milk is particularly rich [29].

Some data reported in the literature suggest that differential exposures to the outside world may also play an important role in the development of the endogenous flora; this is particularly important in the case of premature babies. In premature babies, delayed tube feeding, frequent wide range antibiotic treatments, and the exposure to hospital microbial flora contribute to a delayed colonization by non-pathogenic commensal bacteria and to an increased risk colonization by pathogens [8, 15, 17, 30–35]. The most prevalent genera found in the feces of preterm babies are *Enterococcus*, *Enterobacter*, *Escherichia* (sp. *coli*), *Staphylococcus*, *Streptococcus*, *Clostridium*, and *Bacteroides* [15, 36–38]. This colonization pattern, although very similar to that of formula-fed term babies, seems to persist longer in preterm infants, and *Bifidobacterium* spp. bacteria establish themselves much later and at a much slower rate in preterm infants [38, 39].

The peculiarity of a preterm baby's intestinal ecosystem is due to the fact that those bacteria, which appear early in the intestinal flora, tend to stay longer than those introduced at a later time [40–42], as well as to the fact that once this colonization pattern has established itself, it is very difficult to change it. In fact, it is believed that inappropriate colonization by pathogens plays an important role in the pathogenicity of necrotizing enterocolitis (NEC) [32].

Once the intestinal flora has become stabilized, it does not undergo any further qualitative changes [8]. As the neonatal age ends, the composition of the bacterial flora changes further at the beginning of weaning, and especially among breast-fed infants [21]. Once solid foods are introduced, the composition of the microflora gradually reaches its final pattern, which is characterized by a relatively stable prevalence of anaerobes [3]; and after the second year of life, it shows all of the characteristics typical of an adult microflora [43] (Table 27.2).

The microflora of different parts of the gastrointestinal tract differ from one another quantitatively and qualitatively (proximal-distal gradient). Anaerobes such as *Bacteroides* spp., *Eubacterium* spp., *Streptococcus* spp. and *Fusobacterium* spp. are found mostly in the large intestine and their rate reaches up to 99% in the rectum. The microflora of the colon is also horizontally stratified and shows a difference between luminal and mucosal microflora, which is further subdivided into flora of the mucosal layer, flora of the crypts, and flora that adheres to the colonocytes [44–46].

Numerous studies have shown how the 'bifidogenous flora,' which is comprised of bacteria of the genera *Bifidobacterium* and *Lactobacillus*, can benefit an individual's health by stimulating the immune system, inhibiting the development of the pathogenic flora, improving nutrients and mineral absorption, and allowing for vitamin synthesis and gas production [47–49].

The primary role of the microflora found in the colon is to obtain energy from food not digested in the upper gastrointestinal tract through fermentation. Approximately 8–10% of the total daily energy requirement derives from bacterial fermentation in the colon [50]. Short-chain fatty acids (SCFAs) such as acetic acid, butyric acid, and proprionic acid, are the main products of fermentation in the colon. Butyrate is metabolized by the epithelium of the large intestine's mucosa and plays an essential role in its trophism [51, 52].

The gut microflora also plays an important immunoregulatory role by promoting the proper development of the lymphoid tissue of the intestinal mucosa (gut associated lymphoid tissue (GALT)), as documented by studies on germ-free animals [53, 54]. The 'microbial-epithelial cross-talk' between the intestinal epithelium and commensal bacteria allows for a suitable regulation of the intestinal immune and inflammatory response [55]. The proper interaction between the microflora and the intestinal epithelium is guaranteed by the presence of an intact mucosal barrier, a suitable bacterial colonization, an adequate activation of intestinal immune defenses, and modulation of intestinal inflammation [56, 57]. On the whole, the interaction between the microflora and the intestinal immune system allows the latter to develop a 'suppressive' immune response, like oral tolerance, as well as an 'inductive' response, such as the synthesis of IgA class antibodies. The role of oral tolerance is to inhibit immune responses against food antigens and antigens of commensal bacteria, enabling one to avoid inflammatory intestinal diseases and hypersensitivity reactions to food. Meanwhile, the role of secretory IgAs is to protect the intestinal mucosa from enteropathogenic organisms and to block resident bacteria and food antigens from entering into systemic circulation. There is quite a bit of evidence that proves that, by sending signals via specific receptors, especially the toll-like receptors, intestinal bacteria can affect the function of epithelial cells, determine T cell differentiation and antibody responses to T cell dependent antigens, and regulate the intestinal immune response. The production of secretory IgAs is the primary component of the antibody response to pathogenic antigens. In addition, the

TABLE 27.2   Factors that influence the gut microflora composition

Age		
First few days of life	**After first week of life**	**After weaning**
Mode of delivery	**Type of diet**	High levels of anaerobic bacteria: *Bacteroides* spp.
		Bifidobacterium spp.
Vaginal	Breast-fed infants	*Eubacterium* spp.
Streptococcus spp.	High levels:	*Clostridium* spp.
Staphylococcus spp.	*Bifidobacterium* spp.	*Peptostreptococcus* spp.
Enterococcus spp.		*Streptococcus* spp.
Lactobacillus spp.	Low levels:	*Fusobacterium* spp.
	Straphylococcus spp.	*Veillonella* spp.
Cesarean section	*Streptococcus* spp.	
High levels:	*Lactobacillus* spp.	
Clostridium spp.		Low levels of aerobic bacteria:
	Formula-fed infants	*Escherichia* spp.
	High levels:	*Enterobacter* spp.
Low levels:	*Enterococcus* spp.	*Enterococcus* spp.
Bifidobacterium spp.	*Enterobacter* spp.	*Klebsiella* spp.
Bacteroides spp.	*Klebsiella* spp.	*Lactobacillus* spp.
	Clostridium spp.	*Proteus* spp.
		Streptococcus spp.
	Low levels:	*Straphylococcus* spp.
	Bifidobacterium spp.	
	Bacteroides spp.	
	Lactobacillus spp.	
	Preterms	
	Enterococcus spp.	
	Escherichia spp.	
	Enterobacter spp.	
	Klebsiella spp.	
	Straphylococcus spp.	
	Bacteroides spp.	
	Streptococcus spp.	
	Clostridium spp.	
	Hospitalization	
	Klebsiella spp.	
	Enterobacter spp.	
	Bacteroides spp.	
	Clostridium spp.	

colonization of the bacterial flora causes modulation of the Th2 response (pro-allergic) to a Th1 response (suppressive), which could reduce immune hyperreactivity, as occurs with allergic pathologies [58, 59].

The ability of bifidogenic flora to inhibit the growth of pathogenic microorganisms, and consequently to reduce the incidence of intestinal infections, has been documented [60, 61]. It is believed that the fundamental mechanism of this inhibitory process is directly related to a reduction of intestinal pH, caused by a substantial presence of lactic acid and acetic acid that are produced during carbohydrate fermentation. Furthermore, gut microflora cells can produce active bactericides, defined as bacteriocidins, which can attack *Clostridium* spp., *Escherichia* (sp. *coli*), and other potentially pathogenic microorganisms [62]. Given this situation, it is easy to recognize how a change in the delicate balance between intestinal resident flora, the epithelium, and GALT is essential to understanding the physiopathology of numerous gastrointestinal and systemic diseases in both pediatric and adult age [63–65].

2. PREBIOTICS

2.1. Definition

The term 'prebiotic' refers to organic substances capable of facilitating the growth of intestinal microbial flora by acting as a nutritional substrate for endogenous microorganisms. According to the definition proposed by ENDO (European Project on Non-Digestible Oligosaccharides), prebiotics are 'non-digestible oligosaccharides that can stimulate and promote the growth and/or metabolism of bifidobacteria and lactobacilli in the human intestine' [66]. Accordingly, prebiotics must possess the following characteristics:

- They cannot be hydrolyzed or absorbed in the upper gastrointestinal tract.

- They must be a selective substrate for one or a few bacteria found in the colon, such as lactobacilli and bifidobacteria.
- They must be able to change the gut microflora into a healthier and more beneficial composition to the host organism [67].
- Prebiotics should make up about 10% of the total energy requirement and about 20% of the total volume of food ingested [3] by humans.

2.2. Characteristics

Every dietary component that reaches the colon in its intact form can potentially be a prebiotic. Prebiotics include various oligosaccharides (fructo-, galacto-, isomalto-, xylo-, and soyo-oligosaccharides), lactulose and lactosucrose. When talking about prebiotic substances, the literature has focused specifically on non-digestible oligosaccharides (NDOs) [13]. Although they are part of a complex heterogeneous group of substances with different chemical compositions and prebiotic qualities, all NDOs have strong bonds that are resistant to the hydrolytic action of enzymes found at the beginning of the digestive tract, such as lactase, saccharase-isomaltase, maltase-glucoamylase, trealase, and amylase; because of this, they all arrive at the large intestine virtually untouched.

The most studied NDOs are those found in breast milk, termed human milk oligosaccharides (HMOS) and non-milk derived NDOs, such as the galacto-oligosaccharides (GOS) and the fructo-oligosaccharides (FOS), which are sold commercially. They are carbohydrates comprised of 3–10 monosaccharide units like galactose, fructose, N-acetyl-glucosamine, sialic acid; and they are linked to one another by their characteristic glucosidic bonds. Oligosaccharides are considered to be the most important prebiotic substrate because they meet all of the prebiotics' current classification criteria [68, 69].

2.3. Human Milk Oligosaccharides (HMOS)

Human milk is considered the gold standard nutrient in infant nutrition, especially during the first 6 months of life [70]. Human milk offers all of the necessary nutrients needed for a baby's healthy growth and development. The HMOS found in breast milk play their prebiotic role by facilitating an intestinal microenvironment rich with *Bifidobacterium* spp. and *Lactobacillus* spp. [71–74]. After lactose (about 6 g%) and lipids (about 4 g%), these oligosaccharides represent the third most important component of human milk. Their highest concentration is found in the colostrum (>2%). In mature milk (about 10 g/L), they stabilize at 1.2–1.4%.

HMOS are synthesized in the mammary gland by specific enzymes, the glycosyltransferases. These enzymes catalyze the sequential addition to the basic lactose molecule (Glucose–Galactose) of monosaccharide units that form linear and branched molecules thanks to the β-glycosidic bond in D-glucose molecule, D-galactose and N-acetyl-glucosamine molecules, and thanks to the α-glycosidic bond in L-fucose and sialic acid. More specifically, the L-fucose bond to the basic molecule is correlated to the secretory component of the Lewis antigen of the maternal blood group [75]. Lacto-N-tetraose is the most prominent oligosaccharide found in breast milk [76]. There is evidence indicating that the HMOS fraction is characterized by substantial structural diversity, including over 1,000 different identified molecules [77, 78]. Their concentration and composition differs among people and during the breast-feeding period. These HMOS are also present in their free form or linked to macromolecules such as glycol-proteins, glycol-lipids, or others [77–80].

Since the human gut does not release luminal enzymes that can cleave α-glycosidic or β-glycosidic bonds, HMOS become resistant to intestinal enzymatic digestion [81–83]. Because of their low digestibility, HMOS can be easily traced in the feces of breast-fed infants [84], despite the fact that some intestinal bacteria release glycosidases capable of metabolizing them [85]. Since HMOS have been identified as functional components of human milk, many efforts have been made to mimic these functions with other alternative compounds.

2.4. Non-human Milk Oligosaccharides

Oligosaccharides from Animal Milks

The concentration of oligosaccharides found in the milk of other animals is very low and by far inferior to that of human milk. In addition, oligosaccharides found in animal milks have a very simple, much less complex molecular structure than that of HMOS [77, 86]. However, the preparation of these compounds is quite difficult and mass production is not commercially available. This is why clinical trials using non-human oligosaccharides as prebiotics are not yet available.

Non-milk Oligosaccharides

Non-milk oligosaccharides can be obtained from bacteria, yeasts and plants; they can be extracted from natural sources, synthesized from monomers and/or small oligosaccharides, or produced by natural polymer hydrolysis. In fact, some NDOs, like inulin, xylo-oligosaccharides and maltose-oligosaccharides, are extracted from plant products (soy, chicory) and subsequently undergo partial enzymatic hydrolysis; others, like the FOS and GOS, are obtained from enzymatic synthesis, through glycosyltransferase, from simple sugars, such as sucrose and lactose.

The most commonly used NDOs in pediatric trials are:

- GOS, particularly the short-chain ones (scGOS);
- both short-chain and long-chain FOS (scFOS and lcFOS);
- inulin;
- lactulose;

- blends of lactulose and scGOS;
- blends of scFOS and lcFOS;
- blend of galacturonic acid oligosaccharides combined with scGOS and lcFOS;
- blends of scGOS and lcFOS [15, 87–128].

The amount of fecal bifidobacteria, their percentage compared to the total number of bacteria, and the production of SCFA, are generally used in evaluating their prebiotic effect. On the basis of these markers, there is sufficient evidence to classify only GOS, FOS and inulin as prebiotics [129, 130].

Inulin and FOS, a polymer and olygomer of fructose, respectively, are food components found as carbohydrates in nature in some plant species such as chicory, garlic, onion, leeks, radicchio, artichoke, banana and cereal. They are classified as β (2→1) fructans, a term that refers to carbohydrates that have mostly fructosyl–fructose-type glucosidic bonds. Inulin is a blend of polydisperse β-fructans, whose chains vary in length from 2 to 60 units, and has an average polymerization level equal to 10 monosaccharide units. The inulin available on the market is extracted through a hot water process from chicory root (*Cichorium intybus*), which contains 15–20% inulin and 5–10% FOS. The final product is a powder comprised of inulin with an average degree of polymerization of 10–12 monosaccharide units and a small quotient (about 6–10%) of monosaccharides and disaccharides, such as glucose, fructose and sucrose. A more refined type of inulin, a 'high performance inulin,' is now commercially available. It has an average degree of polymerization of 25 monosaccharide units and the advantage of causing less gastrointestinal side effects, such as flatulence and abdominal tension [131].

FOS can be produced in two ways: through enzymatic hydrolysis of inulin extracted from chicory, using the inulase enzyme of *Aspergillus niger*, or through enzymatic synthesis from sucrose. The resulting FOS show an average degree of polymerization of four monosaccharide units and can be made up of only fructose chains or of a combination of fructose and terminal glucose.

Meanwhile, GOS are a blend of olygominerals made up of one glucose molecule and a few galactose molecules. They are naturally found in foods such as legumes, dairy, and some fermented milk products. They are obtained from lactose biosynthesis induced by β-galactosidase of *Aspergillus oryzae* (6-galactosyl-lactose), which catalyzes trans-galactosylation reactions differently from human β-galactosidase that hydrolyzes lactose into glucose and galactose. GOS are characterized by a degree of polymerization that ranges between two and eight monosaccharide units and by β1-6 linkages. Among them are galactose β(1-6) glucose, galactose β(1-6) galactose, galactose β(1-3) glucose, and galactose β(1-2) glucose. The first two are found in yogurt and in some fermented milk products and, unlike lactose, they can resist the digestive action of human lactase because of the β(1-6) bond.

Toxicology investigations have excluded any mutagenic, carcinogenic or teratogenic action by the previously described NDOs [132]. Furthermore, inulin and FOS have been classified as food ingredients and not as additives and have obtained the GRAS acronym (Generally Recognized As Safe). GOS have also been approved as natural ingredients and are exempted from the limitations provisioned by the European Community on new foods (novel foods) [133].

Companies in both Europe and the United States tend to use more inulin, GOS and FOS, while those in Japan utilize mostly isomalto-oligosaccharides and xylo-oligosaccharides extracted from plants and synthesized from lactose or sucrose [134]. A blend of scGOS:lcFOS (9:1 ratio) has been suggested for neonatal formulas, with the intent of offering a prebiotic effect comparable to that of human milk [15, 105, 107–109, 111, 125, 134, 135].

There are many other reasons for wanting to evaluate the effectiveness of NDOs rather than single components [134]. First of all, the composition of the bacterial flora is extremely complex and therefore various substrates could be needed for its development [26]. Another reason is the great structural variability of HMOS, which seems to be necessary in order to adequately stimulate the unique intestinal flora of breast-fed babies [78].

Mechanisms of Action

The mechanisms of action of the most studied and best known prebiotics are those of the oligosaccharidic fraction of breast milk, and can be summarized as the following four main effects:

1. Biomass effect

    A number of HMOS found in the large intestine (equal to 40–60%) have a 'biomass effect' which promotes the selective development of the bifidogenous flora by reducing the percentage composition of bacteroids, clostrides and fusobacteria. The consequent fermentative metabolism determines the production of SCFAs (of which butyric acid is the most important), some amino acids (such as arginine, cysteine and glutathione), polyamines, growth factors, vitamins, and antioxidants. These substances play a crucial role in the nutritional needs of those species of bacteria that colonize the intestinal mucosa and participate in numerous metabolic processes. Even non-milk oligosaccharides, like FOS/GOS and inulin, stimulate bifidobacteria and lactobacilli's growth and activity to the detriment of bacteria of the genera *Clostridium*, *Klebsiella*, *Enterobacter*, and *Bacteroides* [136, 137]. Also, in addition to being used as a source of energy, SCFAs may have a trophic effect on the mucosa, can help reabsorb water, reduce intestinal pH, and make it less favorable for pathogenic germs to grow [5, 138, 139].

2. Fiber effect

    Many HMOS in the large intestine (equal to about 30—50% of the total) have a 'fiber effect'; they are expelled through the feces, increasing fecal mass and the number of defecations [84].

3. Immunomodulant effect

    HMOS also play an important 'immunomodulant effect.' In fact, their fermentation by anaerobes produces the previously described SCFAs, such as butyrate, that can reduce epithelial cells' glutamine requirements, in favor of immunocompetent cells [140].

4. Anti-infective effect

    The anti-infective effect is expressed through a direct and an indirect mechanism. The *direct* mechanism is linked to the chemical structure of HMOS, which is similar to that of the bonding sites recognized by the bacteria on the epithelium of the enteric mucosa. As a result, they act as 'soluble receptors,' able to competitively bind to the pathogenic agents and their toxins and blocking their actions [76]. For example, mannose-rich glycoprotein can compete for the bond with type 1 fimbriae of *Escherichia coli*, while sialo-galactoside can bind to the *S. fimbriae* of the same germ. Concerning this, protective effects of HMOS against enteropathogenic *E. coli*, *Campylobacter jejuni*, *Shigella* spp., and *Vibrio colerae* gastroenteritis have been reported [141, 142]. This protective action of the oligosaccharide fraction of breast milk is also present in the upper respiratory tract, blocking the adhesion of some strains of *S. pneumoniae* and *H. influenzae* [143]. Table 27.3 shows a number of breast milk oligosaccharides which are able to act as specific ligands (receptors) that bind to pathogenic microorganisms, both bacteria and viruses. On the other hand, the *indirect* anti-infective effect is determined by a previously described decrease in intestinal pH [140] (Figure 27.1).

TABLE 27.3 Pathogenic bacteria and oligosaccharide receptors of breast milk

Bacteria	Receptors
E. coli (type 1 fimbria)	Glycoproteins with mannose
E. coli (thermostable enterotoxin)	Fucosylated oligosaccharides
E. coli	Fucosylated tetra- and penta-saccharides
E. coli (S. fimbria)	Sialyl (α2-3) lactose and glycoproteins Mucins' sialyl (α2-3) galactosides
S. pneumoniae	Neutral oligosaccharides
Pseudomonas aeruginosa	Gal(β1-4) GlcNac o Gal (β1-3) GlcNac
C. pilory	Sialyl lactose
Streptococcus sanguis	Sialyl lactose
C. pillory	Sialyl lactose and sialyl glycoproteins
M. pneumonia	Sialyl (α2-3) glycoproteins
M. pneumoniae	Sialyl p-N-acetyl-lactosamine
Influenza virus A	Sialyl (α2-6) lactose
Influenza virus B	Sialyl (α2-6) lactose

2.5. Side Effects

A daily dose of prebiotics <20 g/day is generally well-tolerated, whereas higher doses can cause side effects such as flatulence, bloating, abdominal pain, and diarrhea [69, 126].

3. PROBIOTICS

3.1. Definition

Probiotics are defined as live microorganisms with a positive influence on their host, and with the ability to improve the intestinal microbial equilibrium [144]. According to the Food and Agriculture Organization of the United Nations (FAO) and the World Health Organization (WHO), they are defined as 'live microorganisms which when administered in adequate amounts confer a health benefit on the host' [145].

Probiotics were first introduced in the twentieth century by the Russian Nobel prize winner Ilya Mechnikov. Mechnikov suggested that the longevity of Bulgarian farmers was directly linked to their daily consumption of fermented milk products containing large amounts of live non-pathogenic bacteria like *Lactobacillus bulgaricus*, which can modify human intestinal flora in favor of microbial species useful to the host organism [146].

To be defined as probiotics, these bacteria must also meet some specific criteria listed by the European Union [47]:

- Detailed definition and typing.
- Lack of pathogenic effects (i.e., production of enterotoxins and cytotoxins, enteroinvasiveness, adhesion of pathogens, hemolysis, serological pathogenicity, presence of antibiotic-resistant genes).
- Resistance to gastric acidity and to bile.
- Ability to adhere to the intestinal epithelium.
- Ability to colonize the colon.
- Proven clinical effect on health.
- Safety [148].
- Competitive antagonism against pathogenic bacteria [13].

Some researchers suggest that probiotic bacteria need to have 'human origins' and must be administered in their live form [149, 150].

3.2. Characteristics

Bacteria used for their probiotic effects are listed in Table 27.4. Those more frequently investigated by pediatric clinical trials belong to the *Lactobacillus*, *Bifidobacterium*, and *Streptococcus* genera [51–154]. The most frequently studied probiotic agents of the *Lactobacillus* genera are LGG, *L. acidophilus*, *L. casei*, *L. johnsonii*, and *L. reuteri*. LGG is the most studied *Lactobacillus* in humans. The most frequently studied probiotic

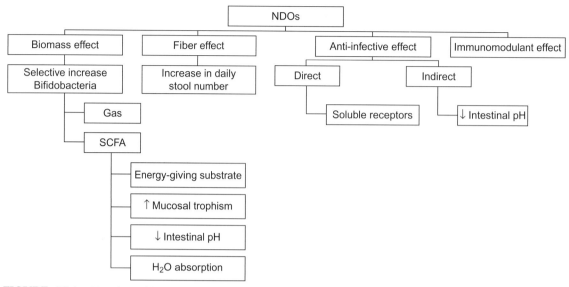

FIGURE 27.1 *Non-digestible oligosaccharides (NDOs) activity*: This figure shows the mechanisms of action of non-digestible oligosaccharides that can be summarized in the **Biomass effect** which results in a selective increase of bifidobacteria colonies; the **Fiber effect** which results in an increase of stool; the **Anti-infective effect** which results in a direct mechanism (due to the chemical structure of NDOs which results as soluble receptors for pathogenic agents) and an indirect mechanism (reduction of intestinal pH); and the **Immunomodulant effect** due to the fermentation of NDOs by anaerobes that produces SCFAs in favor of immunocompetent cells.

TABLE 27.4   Main probiotics

Lactobacilli	*Lactobacillus acidophilus*
	Lactobacillus rhamnosus GG (LGG)
	Lactobacillus shirota
	Lactobacillus bulgaricus
	Lactobacillus reuteri
	Lactobacillus brevis
	Lactobacillus plantarum
	Lactobacillus casei
Gram-positive cocci	*Streptococcus thermophilus*
	Streptococcus intermedius
	Streptococcus β-emolitico
	Streptococcus faecium
Gram-negative cocci	*Escherichia coli*
Bifidobacteria	*Bifidobacterium bifidum*
	Bifidobacterium infantum
	Bifidobacterium longum
	Bifidobacterium thermophilus
	Bifidobacterium lactis
Yeasts	*Saccharomyces boulardii*

agents of the *Bifidobacterium* genera are *B. breve*, *B. infantis*, *B. lactis*, and *B. longum*. *S. thermophilus* is the most popular organism of the *Streptococcus* genera. Besides these species of bacteria, there are also some yeasts, such as *Saccharomyces boulardii*, that act as probiotics.

Baby formulas and probiotic rich foods are widely available worldwide. In North America, a detailed description of the specific strain and the amount of probiotics contained in beverages and other foods have been well-documented for probiotics such as LGG, *L. casei* and *L. reuteri*. In baby formulas starting from birth, and which can be marketed for that specific use, *B. lactis* is the only probiotic bacteria that has undergone FDA evaluation in order to be used.

Undoubtedly, probiotic bacteria are most effective when safely and adequately integrated into one's diet. However, if used for therapeutic purposes, they should be ingested via capsules or tablets. It is important to remember that when used in pediatrics, as a preventive approach (e.g. in the case of acute diarrhea, and antibiotic-induced diarrhea and allergy) their long-term use is more practical if the chosen bacteria are incorporated in the diet through infant formula, yogurt, fermented milk, or other beverages or foods consumed during the weaning process. Relative to daily supplement use, this approach helps with compliance and it reduces costs [6]. Another problem with probiotics is their stability; some may need to be refrigerated, unlike others, such as *S. boulardii*, which are yeasts [155].

To achieve a physiological and therapeutic effect, the daily dose of probiotic needs to be in the 10^8–10^{10} cfu range [156]. It is impossible to set more specific limits since it is very difficult to estimate the number of available bacteria that will reach their targets alive. This depends largely on the technique used to prepare them. However, the quantity needed can depend on the species being used, on the target, and on the host organism.

3.3. Mechanisms of Action

The mechanisms of probiotic action on human organisms can be subdivided into direct and indirect mechanisms (Table 27.5). *Direct* mechanisms are based on the competition between good microorganisms, *Lactobacillus* spp. and *Bifidobacterium* spp., and pathogenic microorganisms, *Bacteroides* spp. and *E. coli*, by creating an unfavorable environment for colonization by pathogens [157].

The following probiotic action mechanisms support the above hypothesis: competition with pathogens for certain nutrients, competitive inhibition of pathogens' reception sites; reduced permeability of the mucosa by increasing tight junctions adhesion; inhibition of bacterial translocation; production of bacteriostatic organic acids (bacteriocidins); lower luminal pH; and change in the composition of mucins; hydrolysis

TABLE 27.5 Mechanisms of probiotic action

Direct	Competition	competition for nutrients
		competition for adhesion receptors or sites
		production of bacteriocidins
		production of zoludina
		production of SCFA
		change in mucins' composition
		↓luminal pH
		↓mucosal permeability
Indirect or immunomediated	Immune exclusion	↑production of mucus
		↑secretion of IgA and IgM
		stimulation of peristalsis
		degradation of toxin receptors
	Immune elimination	activity of complement, neutrophils and mastocytes
	Immune regulation	tolerance to foods and commensal bacteria
		↑IL-10 and TGF-β
		↓TNF

of receptors and toxins; production of IL-10 and TGF-β; and the lack of production of pro-inflammatory cytokines, such as TNF-α, IL-1, IL-6, IL-8 and IL-12 [18, 43, 158–171].

The *indirect*, or immunomediated, probiotic action mechanisms consist of increasing the intestinal barrier function and in modifying the immune response. Many tests have shown that these bacteria can positively influence the intestinal microbial composition, the barrier and permeability of the mucosa, as well as the development and selectivity of GALT [172–174].

Studies have shown that probiotics act by strengthening the three intestinal immune defenses, which are:

1. 'immune exclusion' which uses secretory IgAs and IgMs and other factors such as mucus, peristalsis, and proteolytic activity;
2. 'immune elimination' which uses the activity of complements, neutrophils, macrophages, and mastocytes;
3. 'immune regulation' which allows foods and commensal bacteria to be well tolerated, owing to a specific phenomenon of hypo-responsiveness.

Furthermore, as described in numerous *in vitro* and *in vivo* studies, probiotics have been reported to have positive effects on intestinal as well as systemic mucosal immunity. In fact, some lactobacilli strains can modulate the organism's cytokine pattern in an anti-atopic direction. Probiotics modulate intestinal inflammation by increasing the production of cytokines by T cells and macrophages, promoting the Th1 cytokine profile, increasing anti-inflammatory cytokines, and reducing the production of pro-inflammatory cytokines [175–184]. Hence, by influencing the composition of gut microflora, probiotics act on various aspects of the immune response, such as the non-specific, humoral, cell-mediated component as well as the one based on cytokine production and regulation.

3.4. Side Effects

A few cases in the literature have reported side effects produced by probiotics. There are very few cases of fungemia caused by *Saccharomyces boulardii* in severely compromised patients who were undergoing a wide spectrum antibiotic treatment [185, 186]. Probiotics that contain enterococci could be a problem for preterm infants as they can cause neonatal sepsis.

Lactobacillus spp. seem to be a safer option as they are associated with lower risks of side effects. Finally, there is a possibility that probiotics may transfer to pathogenic germs their antibiotic resistance traits, of which probiotics are often carriers. This problem does not exist with lactobacilli since their antibiotic resistance has been coded on a chromosome that cannot be transferred. Nevertheless, the risk of transferring genetic material should be investigated further [187].

4. SYMBIOTICS

Another strategy for modifying the intestinal ecosystem involves the use of symbiotics [188]. The term symbiotic refers to a 'blend of prebiotics and probiotics that benefits the host organism, improving the survival and implantation of live microbial dietary supplements in the gastrointestinal tract by selectively stimulating growth or by activating the metabolism of one or a few bacteria with beneficial effects on the health of the host organism' [67]. However, symbiotics have yet to be used in children.

There are numerous potential combinations of different bacterial species of the available probiotics and the various types of prebiotics. However, there is still not adequate clinical data describing the possible synergistic and additive activity of these combinations [189].

5. USE OF PREBIOTICS IN PEDIATRICS

In 2004, ESPGHAN's Committee on Nutrition declared that, based on current knowledge, prebiotics should not be recommended for prophylactic and therapeutic use in infants [190]. However, in the intervening few years, many studies have been conducted in order to evaluate the use of prebiotics in infants with two specific goals:

1. To verify if non-milk oligosaccharides can mimic the prebiotic effect of breast milk.
2. To verify if non-milk oligosaccharides also have a positive effect on post-natal development of the immune system, such as providing protection from infections and allergies.

5.1. Non-milk Oligosaccharides and Prebiotic Effects of Breast Milk

A few studies have demonstrated that non-milk oligosaccharides are able to mimic the prebiotic effects of breast milk by significantly increasing *Bifidobacterium* spp., by lowering fecal pH, and by increasing the production of SCFAs. Two studies conducted in 2002, one on full-term infants and the other on preterm infants, have shown a significant and dosage-dependent increase in the number of bifidobacteria whose fecal concentrations were equal to those of breast-fed infants, as well as lower fecal pH, an increased number of daily defecations, lesser fecal density, good tolerance, and no side effects [105, 125]. Both studies used a 9:1 ratio blend of GOS and FOS.

The bifidogenic effect is often associated with lower fecal pH and a change in the pattern of SCFAs [88, 103, 105, 108, 115]. Studies that used GOS or blends of scGOS/lcFOS showed lower fecal pH, while those that used only scFOS did not [87–89, 97]. In studies where infant milk formulas contained blends of scGOS/lcFOS, the SCFA pattern found in stool was similar to that of the stool of breast-fed infants [108].

A bifidogenic effect and an increased production of SCFAs were observed even when milk formulas were integrated with inulin [191, 192].

Some studies have focused on the effects of prebiotics on the development of various bifidobacteria species. These studies showed that scGOS/lcFOS blends promote the growth of *B. infantis* while reducing levels of *B. adolescentis*. A study conducted by Moro et al. on full-term infants showed how, for a period of 6 weeks during which a group of infants were breast-fed, the number of *B. adolescentis* bacteria (70%) decreased to about 20% in the first 5 days of life, while the number of *B. infantis* bacteria increased [105, 120]. Similar results were obtained in the group of infants fed formula integrated with scGOS/lcFOS prebiotics, but not in the group fed formula without prebiotics.

5.2. Non-milk Oligosaccharides and the Prevention of Infections and Allergies

Numerous studies have shown that some non-milk oligosaccharides, alone or in blends, have immunomodulant and protective effects and can significantly reduce the incidence of infections and allergies in infants. Saavedra et al. reported that supplementing weaning foods with scFOS (0.55 g/15 g of cereal; 1.2 g/day) resulted in fewer infections [90]. Firmansyah et al. reported an increase ($p < 0.05$) of plasmatic levels of IgGs after vaccination in children alimented with cereal foods integrated with scGOS/lcFOS prebiotics [102].

Moro et al. reported a lower cumulative incidence of atopic dermatitis diagnosed using international criteria (9.8 vs 23.1%; $p = 0.014$) and a lower percentage of infections (47 vs 21; $p = 0.01$) in a group of high-risk infants fed with a scGOS/lcFOS supplemented formula, compared to those fed with non-supplemented formula [105, 193].

A follow-up study carried out 2 years after the experiment further confirmed the hypothesis that prebiotics can reduce the incidence of allergic symptoms [115]. Supplementing with prebiotic blends leads to an anti-allergic immunoglobulin profile as it allows for significant reductions in blood levels of IgE, IgG1, IgG2, and IgG3, though not IgG4 [116]. In a study conducted on a population of 326 full-term newborns, the use of a formula supplemented with a blend of scGOS/lcFOS prebiotics led to a reduced incidence of infections during the first years of life (acute diarrhea, 0.13 ± 0.39 vs 0.26 ± 0.53 episodes/baby/year, $p = 0.02$; > 3 episodes of upper respiratory tract infections, 22/169 vs 36/173, $p = 0.06$; number of babies who underwent more than two cycles of antibiotics/year, 32/84 vs 59/87, $p < 0.01$) [122]. Duggan et al. did not observe any effect of scFOSs on the clinical course and incidence of diarrhea [94].

Arslanoglu et al. conducted a double blind, randomized, controlled study on 134 full-term infants with a family history of atopy. Of these 134 infants, 66 received a hypoallergenic formula supplemented with 8 g/L of a scGOS/lcFOS blend, while the remaining 68 received a placebo formula supplemented with 8 g/L of maltodextrin during the first 6 months of their lives. The goal of the study was to evaluate the incidence of allergic manifestations (atopic dermatitis, recurring episodes of wheezing, and allergic urticaria) and of infections (mostly recurring infections of the urinary tract, infections requiring antibiotics, fever) not only during the period investigated, but also later by conducting follow-up examinations during the first 2 years of life. The authors had previously demonstrated that prebiotics could significantly reduce the incidence of atopic dermatitis and infections in infants with a high risk of allergy during the treatment period. However, with this particular study, the authors not only confirmed a reduced incidence of allergies and infections, but also showed that the early use of probiotics supplemented formulas has a preventive action long after the dietary intervention. This effect was produced when the dietary intervention was commenced very early (during the second week of life) and continued for 6 months, a critical time of life when it is possible to program

long-lasting effects on the immune system (programming effect). Consequently, during the 18 months after the treatment, the following observations were made: a reduced total incidence of atopic dermatitis by over 50% (27.9% in the placebo vs 13.6% in the group treated with the scGOS/lcFOS blend) as well as a reduced incidence of other allergy related symptoms. In addition, infants who had taken scGOS/lcFOS supplements developed fewer upper respiratory infections ($p < 0.01$), fewer infections of the urinary tract ($p = 0.06$), and fewer antibiotic treatment cycles than the placebo group ($p < 0.05$). These data demonstrate that an early use of a prebiotics blend significantly reduces the incidence of infections, allergies, and use of antibiotics in the first 2 years of life [117, 120, 194].

In light of all these studies, it can be concluded that the use of prebiotics, mostly GOS/FOS blends, in young children could contribute to the priming mechanism of the intestinal immune system. This effect may be achieved by promoting mechanisms of immune tolerance, which are the basis of the lower incidence of infections and allergies in the first years of life as well as in adulthood.

5.3. Non-milk Oligosaccharides and Other Effects

A common effect of non-milk oligosaccharides is the regulation of the alvus and the production of a softer stool with a positive effect in the event of functional constipation [195]. A few studies have shown that supplementing an adolescent's diet with 16.8 g of FOS can increase calcium absorption by 12%, while the data on the positive effects of non-digestible oligosaccharides on lipid metabolism are controversial [196–200]. With regard to this issue, it has been hypothesized that fructans could inhibit the lipogenic enzymes of the liver and modulate insulinemia [201].

6. USE OF PROBIOTICS IN PEDIATRICS

The following characteristics were extrapolated from a comprehensive investigation of the literature of published works examining the use of probiotics in pediatrics:

- they are particularly numerous;
- many of the studies were randomized controlled clinical trials or meta-analyses;
- not all of the studies provide effective clinical evidence; the substantial heterogeneity of these works greatly complicates the interpretation of the results and consequently makes it difficult to draw univocal and generalizable conclusions.

Despite these obstacles, it is possible to draw some conclusions about the clinical effectiveness of probiotics by examining the most significant literature on each pathology. In particular, there is strong evidence indicating that probiotics have preventive and therapeutic effectiveness on pathologies such as acute diarrhea, antibiotic-associated diarrhea, NEC, and allergic pathology. However, current knowledge cannot confirm the safe effectiveness of probiotics in the treatment of the other pathologies.

7. ACUTE DIARRHEA

To consider diarrhea, we must examine the different clinical pictures that share similar histopathological changes in the normal equilibrium of the intestinal ecosystem, especially of the endogenous microflora. Diarrhea can result from viral or bacterial infection of the gastroenteric tract (viral or bacterial coloenteritis, traveler's diarrhea) [3, 172, 202]. The mechanisms that could explain the effectiveness of probiotics in treating acute diarrhea are:

- the promotion of the intestinal barrier function;

- inhibition of the adhesion and colonization of the mucosa by pathogenic bacteria;
- facilitation of interaction with the innate and adaptive immune systems of the host organism;
- stimulation of the production of antigen-specific IgAs [203].

Numerous clinical trials have been conducted in order to examine the role of probiotics in the treatment and prevention of acute diarrhea. LGG, *L. plantarum*, *L. casei shirota*, some strains of *Bifidobacterium* spp., and *Streptococcus thermophilus* have been the most studied probiotics in the treatment of acute diarrhea; they can significantly reduce its durations and symptoms, especially if caused by a *Rotavirus* [204–210]. Numerous meta-analyses and randomized and controlled clinical trials have shown that probiotics can significantly reduce the duration of acute diarrhea symptoms, by about one day, along with their severity and hospitalization time [209, 211–219].

LGG is the probiotic that has been subjected to the most investigations and has had the most consistent results [212, 214]. LGG significantly reduces the duration of diarrhea and the excretion of *Rotavirus* following acute diarrhea; it does so by stimulating a specific anti-*Rotavirus* immune response [220].

Interestingly, one meta-analysis showed a significant relationship between the dose given and a reduction of the duration of diarrhea. In fact, results have demonstrated how, in order to obtain a consistent therapeutic effect, the threshold dose must be higher than 10 million 'colony-forming units', making it possible to surpass 'resistance to colonization' [212, 221].

Probiotics can also be used to prevent acute diarrhea. A prospective, double blind, randomized study conducted in five centers in France investigated three different infant formulas supplemented with probiotics or symbiotics. The treatment period lasted 8 months and each infant underwent 14–16 weeks of treatment. This study demonstrated that the *B. longum* BL999 and *L. rhamnosus* LPRs blend can have a long-term effect and significantly reduce the incidence of diarrhea even 5 months after treatment [222]. The study also confirmed the safety of various blends of probiotics and prebiotics. Many other clinical trials have also shown how the use of probiotics in childhood significantly reduces the incidence of acute diarrhea [216, 217, 223–225]. Furthermore, it was demonstrated that the use of LGG and/or bifidobacteria supplements is very effective in the treatment of other types of acute diarrhea in infants, such as nosocomial associated diarrhea (and diarrhea in children from developing countries) [218, 223, 226–229].

Finally, a meta-analysis of 34 randomized and placebo-controlled trials showed that probiotics can significantly reduce the risk of contracting acute diarrhea in pediatric age by 57% (confidence interval: 35–71%), as well as the incidence of hospitalization and its duration. The protective effect of the probiotics strains *B. lacti*, LGG, *L. acidophilus* and *S. boulardii* used, can overlap [230]. The use of specific strains of *E. coli* (Nissle 1917 strain and the O83:K24: H1 strain) has been reported to prevent the occurrence of diarrhea even in preterm infants [231, 232]. In conclusion, studies reported thus far indicate that some types of probiotic bacteria, mostly LGG, can effectively treat and prevent acute diarrhea in children.

8. ANTIBIOTIC-ASSOCIATED DIARRHEA

About 20% of pediatric patients who take antibiotics can develop antibiotic-associated diarrhea (AAD) [233]. In fact, antibiotics can directly affect the resident microflora by compromising resistance to intestinal colonization by pathogens and by facilitating the growth of these microorganisms, most commonly *Clostridium* (sp. *difficile*). Surwicz et al. demonstrated that the simultaneous administration of *Saccharomyces boulardii*

with antibiotics caused a decrease in the incidence of AAD by over 50% [234, 235]. The same result was confirmed in a randomized, double blind study as well as by other subsequent meta-analyses following the use of LGG and/or other lactobacilli [226, 236, 237].

A meta-analysis of six randomized and controlled studies involving 766 infants showed that probiotics like LGG, *B. lactis*, and *S. thermophilus*, significantly reduced the risk of AAD from 28.5% (the placebo level) to 11.9% [238]. A specific subgroup of AAD is caused by *Clostridium* (sp. *difficile*); this bacterium is responsible for pseudo-membranous colitis. In 1987, Gorbach et al. conducted one of the first studies to demonstrate that LGG reduces episodes of recurring diarrhea caused by *Clostridium* (sp. *difficile*) [239].

Futhermore, LGG can help stop recidivism of the infection caused by *Clostridium* (sp. *difficile*) in both adults and children [204, 226, 236, 237, 240–248]. In conclusion, based on the cited work and on the meta-analyses conducted, it appears that probiotics can significantly reduce the risk of AAD.

9. NECROTIZING ENTEROCOLITIS

Necrotizing enterocolitis (NEC) is an intestinal inflammatory disease typical of preterm infants characterized by the loss of the integrity of the intestinal mucosa, causing tube feeding intolerance, blood in the stool and intestinal pneumatosis. It is also accompanied by systemic inflammatory response accompanied by cardio-respiratory complications and severe hemodynamic instability. The preterm infant is particularly susceptible to NEC because of the following factors: delayed intestinal colonization, colonization of environmental microbes found in the ICU, prolonged use of antibiotics, lack of exposure to the mother's normal flora and to breast-feeding, immature mucosa, and increased risk of antigenic and bacterial translocation [33]. These observations strongly support the hypothesis that composition and equilibrium of the microflora play a crucial role in the physiopathology of NEC [249, 250]. The following is a summary of the mechanisms with which probiotics could prevent NEC:

- Increase in commensal microflora and reduction of colonization and adhesion to the mucosa by pathogenic bacteria.
- Improvement in the integrity of the intestinal mucosal barrier toward the translocation of bacteria and bacterial products in to the bloodstream.
- Modulation of intestinal inflammation in response to exposure to bacterial products.
- Improvement in tolerance mechanisms.
- Anticipation in shifting toward tube feeding [29, 36, 249–252].

The potential benefits of probiotics in preventing NEC are also supported by previous studies conducted with animals [253].

In 1999, a study conducted by Hoyos was the first to show that probiotics can lower the incidence of NEC in preterm infants [151]. In this study, 1,237 patients of various NICUs in the city of Bogota (Colombia) were treated with *L. acidophilus* and *B. infantis* probiotics during their entire hospitalization. The incidence of NEC and related mortality were significantly lower ($p < 0.0002$ and $p < 0.005$, respectively) compared to the 1,282 infants hospitalized in the same units the year before, who did not receive any probiotic treatment.

Similarly, three successive randomized and controlled clinical trials investigated probiotics and their ability to reduce the risk of NEC. Two of these three trials showed a significant reduction in the incidence ($p < 0.05$) of NEC, compared to the control group, after administering *L. acidophilus* with *B. infantis* to one group and administering *B. infantis* with *S. thermophilus* and *B. bifidus* to the other group [153, 154]. In a multicentric study conducted in 2002 by Dani,

the use of LGG did not appear to significantly reduce the incidence of NEC, bacterial sepsis, or urinary tract infections [152]. However, many other studies have demonstrated that probiotics are effective in reducing NEC [171, 254–257].

A meta-analysis of randomized and controlled trials has examined probiotics' effectiveness in reducing stage 2 or higher of the NEC. The study was comprised of seven trials, involving a total of 1,393 infants. NEC occurred in 6% of infants who had received the placebo and in only 2% of those who had been treated with probiotics [258].

Therefore, a large number of studies, represented mostly by randomized and controlled clinical trials, have confirmed that some types of probiotics are extremely effective in reducing the incidence and severity of NEC in preterm and very low birth weight (VLBW) infants.

10. ALLERGY

Studies have reported that the incidence of atopic diseases in children with a family history of allergy reaches 50% by the age of 2 years old [259]. In the literature, the cumulative incidence of atopic dermatitis ranges between 13 and 44%, showing an increasing trend in recent decades. The etiology of allergic diseases is multifactorial. However, since familial history is one of the most important predictive elements, primary prevention among high-risk infants is crucial [260, 261].

Given that a low quantity of bifidobacteria and lactobacilli in the gut microbiota precedes the development of allergic diseases, it is believed that those agents that modulate gut microbiota, such as prebiotics and probiotics, could be very useful in primary prevention [117, 260–274]. Some authors believe that the high rate of allergic diseases in developed countries is due to excessive hygiene, which causes infants and babies to be less exposed to microbial stimuli, thereby facilitating type Th2 immune responses (hygiene hypothesis) [3]. In fact, the immune pathology of atopic diseases is characterized by a Th2 response against ubiquitary environmental allergens or food allergens [275]. The factors that cause an inappropriate type Th2 response, and consequently allergic diseases, are still quite unknown in early immune development. The Th2 type response is regulated by both Th1 type responses, which are usually directed against infectious agents, and by the tolerogenetic responses of regulatory T cells. Resident intestinal bacteria are important maturation signals for the development of the infant's immune system. A number of epidemiological studies have reported that changes in the composition of the infant's gut microbiota are often associated with the development of allergic diseases: before developing sensitivity to allergens, atopic babies showed lower numbers of bifidobacteria in their gut microbiota than that observed in non-atopic babies. The hypothesis is that bifidobacteria can effectively promote tolerance of non-bacterial antigens, by inhibiting primarily the development of a type Th2 response (pro-allergic) [6]. The mechanisms of action for probiotics could be summarized as follows: modulation of the initial microbial colonization, intraluminal breakdown of allergens, promotion of intestinal barrier function, promotion of immune system maturation by inducing the production of secretory IgAs, modulation of dendritic cells, and induction of regulatory T cells [276].

Numerous clinical trials that have examined the use of probiotics in the prevention and treatment of atopic dermatitis and in the treatment of allergic rhinitis have shown a significant decrease in the incidence and severity of these pathologies [263, 264, 277–288]. One of the first studies implicating probiotics in the prevention of allergic diseases in infants, which involved the infants' mothers, dates back to 2001 [263]. The goal of this double blind, placebo-controlled study was to evaluate the ability of probiotics to reduce the risks of atopic diseases in infants, by administering LGG or placebo to 159 mothers of babies with a high risk of developing an allergic disease. The treatment started 2–4 weeks prior to delivery and continued until the mothers had breast-fed their babies for the first 6 months of life. The babies of the mothers who had received the probiotic treatment showed a significant reduction in the incidence of atopic eczema in the first 2 years of life (15/64, 23% vs 31/68, 46%).

In a second clinical trial, both probiotics (administered to the mothers and the infants) and prebiotics (infants only) were used [265]. The rationale for also giving probiotics to the mothers was confirmation in a study that showed how allergic mothers have lower concentrations of TGF-β2 in their milk [289]. The TGF-β2 found in breast milk is critical because it increases the ability of the intestinal mucosa to produce IgA, and thereby induces immune tolerance in infants [290, 291]. In fact, probiotic supplementation (LGG and *B. lactis* Bb-12) increases TGF-β2 concentrations in breast milk [259, 292, 293].

Another situation in which using probiotics such as LGG, *B. lactis*, *L. fermentum*, or *L. reuteri* could be very useful in helping to acquire immunological tolerance, occurs during weaning. With respect to this, several studies have shown an improvement in atopic dermatitis and reduced serum levels of inflammatory markers [278, 280, 281, 285, 294]. Saglani et al. have reported that the typical clinical picture of adult allergy-induced asthma is already present in childhood in the form of wheezing (between the first and third years of age) [295]. Four meta-analyses have demonstrated the effectiveness of probiotics in preventing and treating atopic dermatitis and food intolerance [264, 296–298].

In conclusion, in light of the large amount of qualified work represented by both randomized and controlled studies as well as by meta-analyses, some types of probiotics have been shown to be effective in treating atopic diseases and in primary prevention among subjects at risk [299].

11. OTHER PEDIATRIC USES

11.1. Constipation

Constipation is a very common symptom in young children and at all socio-economic levels [300–302]. It is characterized by slower intestinal movement, by less amounts of/thicker stool, by sometimes painful defecation, and also by discomfort, bloating and abdominal swelling [47]. It can be distinguished into functional and organic constipation. It is estimated that functional constipation affects 12 to 30% of the general population.

The rationale for using probiotics in the treatment of constipation is based on three possible effects:

- decreased sigmoid tone;
- stimulation of colon motility;
- reduced intestinal motility time due to changes to the gut microflora [303].

A double blind, randomized, controlled study with placebo on the effectiveness of adding LGG to lactulose in the treatment of infants with constipation, did not show additional benefits [301]. However, a few other studies have demonstrated that adding probiotics to milk or yogurt can reduce the time of intestinal motility and increase the daily amount of stool in constipated patients [304–307]. Koebnik et al. described similar results [308] in a double blind, randomized, controlled study with placebo, on patients suffering from chronic constipation treated with *L. casei shirota* for a period of 4 weeks. However, the debate on the effectiveness of treating constipation with probiotics in children is ongoing.

11.2. Inflammatory Bowel Disease

Crohn's disease and ulcerative colitis are chronic and often crippling diseases, whose current treatments are not very effective and can cause many side effects. It was ascertained that changes to the function of the intestinal mucosa, which acts as a barrier, could allow endoluminal antigen bacteria to chronically activate the immune and inflammatory cascade in subjects that are genetically predisposed. In fact, some bacterial products such as peptidoglycan, lipopolysaccharide, and microbial DNA (CpG), are able to selectively bind to membrane receptors (toll-like receptors, TLR1-TLR9) or to cytoplasmic receptors (NOD1 and NOD2) capable of activating nuclear transcription factor NFκB and the transcription of pro-inflammatory, co-stimulating cytokines, and adhesion molecules. The behavior of the resistant microflora of subjects affected by inflammatory bowel disease (IBD) can vary. Hence, the inflammatory response is the result of genetic predisposition, the loss of immune tolerance, and the behavior of the mucosal microflora [309].

The role of probiotics in IBDs could be linked to:

- aggressive inhibition of the microflora;
- improvement of the functions of the mucosal and epithelial barrier;
- modulation of the mucosal immune system [310].

This is why many researchers have intensified their investigations on the possible positive effects of probiotics in the treatment of IBDs [311–320]. Numerous studies examining the effect of probiotics on Crohn's disease, on ulcerative colitis, and on pouchitis have been reported. While some positive effects have been observed in adults, pediatric studies have produced conflicting results thus far.

In two different studies Gionchetti et al. reported that the use of a blend of 8 VSL#3 probiotics (four *Lactobacillus* spp. strains, three *Bifidobacterium* spp. strains, and one *Streptococcus* spp. strain, for a total of over 10^{12} cfu) effectively prevented and treated pouchitis, if administered immediately following the closure of a temporary ileostomy [321, 322]. Pouchitis is the result of a complication of colectomy and ileostomy in ulcerative rectal colitis.

Another author reported that the risk of relapses in subjects who, after undergoing surgery for Crohn's disease, were treated for 3 months with rifaximin and then with a blend of VLS#3 probiotics for another 9 months, was cut in half compared to subjects who were treated for 12 months with only mesalazine (20 vs 40%) [323].

Another indication is the prevention of chronic pouchitis relapses after remission with metronidazole and ciprofloxacin [324, 325]. Similar effects were also obtained by administering *Lactobacillus* spp. [326, 327].

At the time of writing, only a few positive results have been obtained with pouchitis, while no significant benefits have been obtained with Crohn's disease and ulcerative rectal colitis. Thus, further studies are necessary.

11.3. Irritable Bowel Syndrome

In spite of the large number of studies in the literature, many doubts regarding the pathogenesis of irritable bowel syndrome (IBS) persist. Some researchers have hypothesized that its pathogenesis could derive from qualitative and/or quantitative changes to the flora of the colon or of the small intestine with a reduction in the number of *Bifidobacterium* spp., or to a bacterial overgrowth of the small intestine, or to changes in the interaction between intestinal flora and the host organism. Meanwhile, a possible influence of the nervous system along the SNC-intestinal axis cannot be excluded [328]. Despite the fact that few authors have confirmed these hypotheses, and report the same percentage of bacterial growth in patients affected by IBS as in the control groups, there are epidemiological, clinical, and experimental evidences that show that the occurrence and exacerbation of IBS can be linked to infections (post-infectious IBS or IBS that are concomitant to viral or bacterial gastroenteritis) or to the use of antibiotics [329–335].

The intestinal biopsies of a number of subjects affected by IBS showed changes to the fecal bacteria (reduced count of *Lactobacillus* spp. and *Bifidobacterium* spp. coliform bacteria and an increased number of the *Bacteroides*, *E. coli* strains and anaerobes) and increased production of intestinal gas [336–338]. These data could support the use of probiotics by subjects affected by IBS.

Pediatric trials published up to now have been conflicting. In fact, in one study Bausseman reported in 2005 that administration of LGG to 50 infants, for a period of 6 weeks, did not improve abdominal pain but did reduce the incidence of abdominal tension compared to the placebo [339]. But in other works it was clearly demonstrated that *L. acidophilus* did improve the symptoms in about half of the patients with IBS, that the blend of VLS#3 probiotics decreased abdominal swelling, while the combined use of *L. plantarum* and *B. breve* reduced pain intensity [340–342]. Faber administered probiotics alone (*L. acidophilus* and *B. infantis* for 4 weeks) or in combination with antibiotics (ciprofloxacin for the first week) to three different groups with IBS: one with diarrhea, one with constipation, and another with alternating diarrhea and constipation. Both therapeutic approaches have improved the quality of life and reduced symptoms in all three groups [343]. In conclusion, although the use of some types of probiotics on IBS appears promising, further studies are needed.

11.4. *Helicobacter pylori* Infection

A number of studies have reported that probiotics, especially *L. acidophilus*, *L. brevis*, LGG, and *B. lactis*, could in fact reduce possible side effects associated with traditional therapy, and signs of infection of the gastric mucosa reduced urease activity, reduced carnitine decarboxylase activity, and increased polyamine concentration [195, 344–346]. In a randomized prospective trial, one or three strains of probiotics

(*L. casei defensis, S. thermophilus,* and *L. bulgaricus*) were given to babies affected by *H. pylori* colonization. A higher percentage of *H. pylori* eradication was observed only when all three strains of probiotics were administered in conjunction with the traditional triple therapy [347]. However, currently available reports do not recommend the use of probiotics to eradicate or prevent *H. pylori* infections in pediatric patients.

11.5. Lactose Intolerance

Lactose intolerance is a clinical syndrome caused by the inability to digest lactose. Its symptoms can include abdominal pain and distention, bloating, flatulence and/or profuse watery diarrhea, and sometimes nausea and vomiting [348]. Lactose is hydrolyzed into glucose and galactose by an intestinal lactase (β-galactosidase), an essential glycoprotein of the microvillar membrane. The enzyme is located on the crypt-villus axis (mostly on the upper portion of the villus) making it very susceptible to mucosal insults.

There are two different types of lactose malabsorptions: a primary one and a secondary one. Primary lactose malabsorption is genetically linked and typical of Asian, African, African-American and Mediterranean populations [349–353]. Secondary lactose malabsorption is consequent to a variety of acquired diseases such viral gastroenteritis, celiac disease, and allergic (or eosinophilic) gastroenteritis and radiation enteritis, which damage the intestinal villi and almost always lactase.

In most people with low levels of intestinal lactase, the lactose that is not absorbed in the small intestine reaches the colon, where it undergoes bacterial fermentation by the flora, forming SCFAs and hydrogen gas. The absorption of SCFAs by the colon mucosa reduces the effects of lactose malabsorption in many lactose intolerant subjects.

Since probiotic bacteria (such as *Lactobacillus* spp. and *Bifidobacterium* spp.) increase the production of β-galactosidase (lactase), it is reasonable to suggest that they could be used in the treatment of this condition in order to improve lactose digestibility in the small intestine and alleviate symptoms associated with its malabsorption [354–356]. In addition, probiotics could potentially help people who have difficulty absorbing lactase, to digest it in two other ways: by either supplying the lactase enzyme or by restoring the normal intestinal bacterial flora in the event of secondary intolerances to viral infections or antibiotic treatments [357].

In 1985, Gilliland's study was the first to demonstrate that probiotics can improve the symptoms of lactose malabsorption [358]. In two different clinical studies, lactose-intolerant subjects showed a significant reduction of their symptoms after eating probiotics-enriched yogurt [356, 359]. In conclusion, although the work of the cited studies is quite promising, further evidence is needed to confirm the role of probiotics in the treatment of the symptoms of lactose malabsorption.

11.6. Respiratory Infections

There remains scant data on the use of probiotics in the treatment and prevention of respiratory infections. The mechanisms by which probiotics could protect respiratory pathologies are still unknown. A few studies have reported that babies treated with LGG experienced fewer incidences of otitis, sinusitis, bronchitis, and pneumonia than those not treated [360, 361]. However, a double blind placebo-controlled study reported that the administration of *B. lactis* Bb-12 or *L. reuteri* (ATCC 55730) did not have any protective effect [217]. Unfortunately, these data refer to a follow-up that lasted only 12 weeks. Therefore, further studies are needed in order to verify the effectiveness of probiotics in the prevention and treatment of respiratory infections.

11.7. Urinary Tract Infections

Probiotics could be effective in the treatment of childhood urinary tract infections (UTIs) (mostly in females), especially with preterm infants [328, 362–364]. In the early 1970s, it became clear that most pathogens affecting the female urinary tract originated from her own intestinal flora, by traveling from the perineum across the vagina and to the bladder. This is why many studies have been conducted to better understand the etiopathogenic role of *E. coli* in adult female UTIs [365–370].

The rationale behind using probiotics to prevent UTIs originates from the interesting observation that after 1-week of oral treatment with some probiotic strains (*L. rhamnosus* GR-1 and *L. fermentum* RC-14) the same probiotic strains used in the oral treatment were isolated from the vaginal mucosa. Therefore, these lactobacilli could create a very effective microbiological barrier that could interfere with vaginal colonization and consequently with the colonization of the urinary tract by pathogens.

The role of lactobacilli in reducing the incidence of UTIs was investigated for the first time in 1915. The study reported how the intravesical administration of some strains of *Lactobacillus* spp. was very successful in the treatment of women affected by cystitis [371]. The first evidence of the importance of endogenous lactobacilli in guaranteeing a urogenital microenvironment hostile to the colonization by pathogens dates back to a study conducted in 1973. This study showed that women with UTIs had a lower vaginal colonization by *Lactobacillus* spp. than women without UTIs [372].

Moreover, a few studies conducted on preterm infants showed that LGG-supplemented formula had a trend toward reducing the incidence of UTIs, but the trend did not reach significance [152]. One randomized, controlled study reported that *L. acidophilus* and low doses of trimetoprim-sulfametoxazol have the same preventive effects on UTIs of babies affected by primary vesico-ureteric reflux [373]. If *Lactobacillus* GR-1 and *L. reuteri* RC-14 are used endovaginally once a week, they can reduce recurrence of UTIs [374], and if used orally twice a day they can restore the normal vaginal flora dominated by lactobacilli [375–377]. A study conducted in 2001 reported the first clinical evidence of full remission from urogenital infections after taking probiotics orally [378]. These preliminary data could open the way to the use of probiotics in the long-term prophylaxis of UTIs, especially among children with predisposing anatomical factors such as RVU. Their use could help avoid side effects and the emergence of resistant strains associated with the long-term use of antibiotics. Further investigations are needed to confirm the effectiveness of oral prebiotics on the incidence of UTIs in children.

12. CONCLUSION

A large number of competent animal and human works examining prebiotics and probiotics have confirmed the safety and efficacy of functional foods during postnatal development of the immune system. They work by modifying the intestinal microbial population and consequently improving the protective role of the intestine, as well as by stimulating defense mechanisms and facilitating immunological tolerance.

Studies of non-milk prebiotics have reported that GOS/FOS blends in particular mimic the prebiotic effect of breast-feeding by strengthening the immune system of infants and by offering a new method of preventing infections and allergies. Studies on probiotics have reported that when used in young children, they can prevent and treat viral diarrhea, reduce the risks of NEC in preterm infants, reduce the severity of antibiotic-associated diarrhea, and modulate the host's immune response as they do with allergic diseases [379].

References

1. Conseil de l'Europe (2001–4). Lignes directrices sur la justification scientifique des allégations santé des aliments functionnels. Document technique www.coe.fr/soc-sp Arch/dav.

2. Giorgi Pier, L. (2002). Gli alimenti funzionali. *Bambini e Nutrizione*, 9(2), 57–58.

3. Premysl, Fric. (2007). Probiotics and prebiotics—renaissance of a therapeutic principle. *CEJMed*, 2(3), 237–270.

4. Underwood, M. A., Gilbert, W. M., & Sherman, M. P. (2005). Amniotic fluid: not just fetal urine anymore. *Journal of Perinatology*, 25, 341–348.

5. Gibson, G. R., et al. (1995). Dietary modulation of the human colonic microbiota: introducing the concept of prebiotics. *The Journal of Nutrition*, 125, 1401–1412.

6. Jose, M., & Saavedra, M. D. (2007). Use of probiotics in pediatrics: rationale, mechanisms of action, and practical aspects. *Nutrition in Clinical Practice*, 22, 351–365.

7. Martin, C. R., & Walker, W. A. (2008). Probiotics: role in pathophysiology and prevention in necrotizing enterocolitis. *Seminars in Perinatology*, 32, 127–137.

8. Palmer, C., Bik, E. M., Digiulio, D. B., et al. (2007). Development of the human infant intestinal microbiota. *PLoS Biol*, 5(7), e177.

9. Mandar, R., & Mikelsaar, M. (1996). Transmission of mother's microflora to the newborn at birth. *Biology of the Neonate*, 69, 30–35.

10. Bettelheim, K. A., et al. (1974). The origin of O serotypes of *Escherichia coli* in babies after normal delivery. *The Journal of Hygiene*, 72, 67–70.

11. Brook, I., et al. (1979). Aerobic and anaerobic flora of the maternal cervix and newborn gastric fluid and conjuctiva: a prospective study. *Pediatrics*, 63, 451–455.

12. Isoft, R. M., et al. (1996). Development of immune function in the intestine and its role in neonatal disease. *Pediatric Clinics of North America*, 43, 551–571.

13. Parracho, H., McCartney, A. L., & Gibson, G. R. (2007). Probiotics and prebiotics in infant nutrition. *Proceedings of the Nutrition Society*, 66, 405–411.

14. Conway, P., et al. (1997). Development of intestinal microbial. In R. I. Mackie et al. (Eds.), *Gastointestinal Microbiology: Vol. 2* (pp. 3–38). Elsevier.

15. Penders, J., This, C., Vink, C., et al. (2006). Factors influencing the composition of the intestinal microbiota in early infancy. *Pediatrics*, 118, 511–521.

16. Neut, C., Bezirtzoglou, E., Romond, C., et al. (1987). Bacterial colonization of the large intestine in newborns delivered by cesarean section. *Zentralbl Bakteriol Mikrobiol Hyg [A]*, 266, 330–337.

17. Fanaro, S., Chierici, R., Guerrini, P., & Vigi, V. (2003). Intestinal microflora in early infancy: composition and development. *Acta Paediatrica. Supplementum*, 91, 48–55.

18. Orrhage, K., & Nord, C. E. (1999). Factors controlling the bacterial colonization of the intestine in breastfed infants. *Acta Paediatrica. Supplementum*, 88, 47–57.

19. Favier, C. F., Vaughan, E. E., De Vos, W. M., & Akkermans, A. D. (2002). Molecular monitoring of succession of bacterial communities in human neonates. *Applied and Environmental Microbiology*, 68, 219–226.

20. Tissier, H., Callè, G. & Naud, C. (1900). Recherches sur la flore intestinale des nourissons (ètat normal et pathologique), Paris Thèses.

21. Stark, P. L., & Lee, A. (1982). The microbial ecology of the large bowel of breast-fed and formula-fed infants during the first year of life. *Journal of Medical Microbiology*, 15, 189–203.

22. Benno, Y., Sawada, K., & Mitsuoka, T. (1984). The intestinal microflora of infants: composition of fecal flora in breast-fed and bottle-fed infants. *Microbiology and Immunology*, 28, 975–986.

23. Harmsen, H. J. M., Wildeboer-Veloo, A. C. M., et al. (2000). Development of 16S rRNA-based probes for the Coriobacterium group and the Atopobium cluster and their application for enumeration of Coriobacteriaceae in human faeces from volunteers of different age groups. *Applied and Environmental Microbiology*, 66, 4523–4527.

24. Hopkins, M. J., Macfarlane, G. T., Furrie, E., et al. (2005). Characterisation of intestinal bacteria in infant stools using real-time PCR and northern hybridization analyses. *FEMS Microbiology Ecology*, 54, 77–85.

25. Yoshioka, H., Iseki, K., & Fujita, K. (1983). Development and differences of intestinal flora in the neonatal period in breast-fed and bottle-fed infants. *Pediatrics*, 72, 317–321.

26. Harmsen, H. J., Wildeboer-Veloo, A. C., Raangs, G. C., et al. (2000). Analysis of intestinal flora development in breast fed and formula fed infants by using molecular identification and detection methods. *Journal of Pediatric Gastroenterology and Nutrition*, 30, 61–67.

27. Balmer, S. E., & Wharton, B. A. (1989). Diet and faecal flora in the newborn: breast milk and infant formula. *Archives of Disease in Childhood*, 64, 1672–1677.

28. Penders, J., Vink, C., Driessen, C., et al. (2005). Quantification of *Bifidobacterium* spp. *Escherichia coli* and *Clostridium difficile* in faecal samples of breast-fed and formula-fed infants by real-time PCR. *FEMS Microbiology Letters*, 243, 141–147.

29. Agostoni, C., Axelsson, I., Braegger, C., et al. (2004). Probiotic bacteria in dietetic products for infants: a commentary by the ESPGHAN Committee on Nutrition. *Journal of Pediatric Gastroenterology and Nutrition*, 38, 365–374.

30. Lundequist, B., Nord, C. E., & Winberg, J. (1985). The composition of the faecal microflora in breastfed and bottle fed infants from birth to eight weeks. *Acta Paediatrica Scandinavica*, 74, 45–51.

31. Walker, W. A. (2002). Development of the intestinal mucosal barrier. *Journal of Pediatric Gastroenterology and Nutrition, 34*(Suppl. 1), 33–39.

32. Claud, E. C., & Walker, W. A. (2001). Hypothesis: inappropriate colonization of the premature intestine can cause neonatal necrotizing enterocolitis. *The FASEB Journal, 15*, 1398–1403.

33. Magne, F., Suau, A., Pochart, P., & Desjeux, J. F. (2005). Fecal microbial community in preterm infants. *Journal of Pediatric Gastroenterology and Nutrition, 41*, 386–392.

34. Agarwal, R., Sharma, N., Chaudhry, R., et al. (2003). Effects of oral *Lactobacillus* GG on enteric microflora in low-birth-weight neonates. *Journal of Pediatric Gastroenterology and Nutrition, 36*, 397–402.

35. Butel, M. J., Suau, A., Campeotto, F., et al. (2007). Conditions of bifidobacterial colonization in preterm infants: a prospective analysis. *Journal of Pediatric Gastroenterology and Nutrition, 44*, 577–582.

36. Millar, M., Wilks, M., & Costeloe, K. (2003). Probiotics for preterm infants? *Archives of Disease in Childhood. Fetal and Neonatal, 88*, 354–358.

37. Schwiertz, A., Gruhl, B., Löbnitz, M., et al. (2003). Development of the intestinal bacterial composition in hospitalized preterm infants in comparison with breast-fed, full-term infants. *Pediatric Research, 54*, 393–399.

38. Stark, P. L., & Lee, A. (1982). The bacterial colonization of the large bowel of preterm low birth weight neonates. *The Journal of Hygiene, 89*, 59–67.

39. Sakata, H., Yoshioka, H., & Fujita, K. (1985). Development of the intestinal flora in very low birth weight infants compared to normal full-term newborns. *European Journal of Pediatrics, 144*, 186–190.

40. Holman, R. C., Stehr-Green, J. K., & Zelasky, M. T. (1989). Necrotizing enterocolitis mortality in the United States, 1979–85. *American Journal of Public Health, 79*, 987–989.

41. Neu, J. (2007). Perinatal and neonatal manipulation of the intestinal microbiome: a note of caution. *Nutrition Reviews, 65*, 282–285.

42. Hooper, L. V., & Gordon, J. I. (2001). Commensal host-bacterial relationships in the gut. *Science, 292*, 1115–1118.

43. Collins, M. D., & Gibson, G. R. (1999). Probiotics, prebiotics, and synbiotics: approaches for modulating the microbial ecology of the gut. *American Journal of Clinical Nutrition, 69*, 1052–1057.

44. Rozee, K. R., Cooper, D., Lam, K., & Costerton, J. W. (1982). Microbial flora of the mouse ileum mucosa layer and epithelial surface. *App. Environmental Microbiology, 43*, 1451–1463.

45. Lee, A. (1984). Neglected niches: The microbial etiology of the gastrointestinal tract. In K. C. Marshal (Ed.), *Advances in Microbial Ecology* (pp. 115–162). New York: Plenum Press.

46. Swidsinski, A., Ladhoff, A., Pernthaler, A., et al. (2002). Mucosal flora in inflammatory bowel disease. *Gastroenterology, 122*, 44–54.

47. Salminen, S., Bouley, C., Boutron-Ruault, M. C., et al. (1998). Functional food: *Science* and gastrointestinal physiology and function. *The British Journal of Nutrition, 80*, 147–171.

48. Grizard, D., et al. (1999). Non-digestible oligosaccharides used as prebiotico agents: mode of production and beneficial effects on animal and human health. *Reproduction, Nutrition, Development, 339*, 563–588.

49. Roberfroid, M. B., et al. (2000). Prebiotics and probiotics: are they functional food? *The American Journal of Clinical Nutrition, 71*, 1682–1687.

50. Gibson, G. R., Berry-Ottaway, P., & Rastall, R. A. (2000). *Probiotics: New Developments in Functional Foods*. Oxford: Chandos Publishing Ltd.

51. Cummings, J. H. (1981). Short chain fatty acids in the human colon. *Gut, 22*, 763–779.

52. Barcenilla, A., Pryde, S. E., Martin, J. C., et al. (2000). Phylogenetic relationships of butyrate-producing bacteria from the human gut. *Applied and Environmental Microbiology, 66*, 1654–1661.

53. Sudo, N., Sawamura, S., Tanaka, K., et al. (1997). The requirement of intestinal bacterial flora for the development of an IgE production system fully susceptible to oral tolerance induction. *Journal of Immunology, 159*, 1739–1745.

54. Moreau, M. C., et al. (2001). Influence of resident intestinal microflora on the development and functions of the GALT. *Microbiol Ecology Health Dis, 13*, 65–86.

55. Vanderhoof, J. A., & Young, R. J. (2002). Probiotics in pediatrics. *Pediatrics, 109*, 956–958.

56. Caplan, M. S., & Jilling, T. (2000). Neonatal necrotizing enterocolitis: possible role of probiotic supplementation. *Journal of Pediatric Gastroenterology and Nutrition, 30*, S18–S22.

57. Millar, M., Wilks, M., & Costeloe, K. (2003). Probiotics for preterm infants? *Archives of Disease in Childhood. Fetal and Neonatal, 88*, 354–358.

58. Isolauri, E. (2004). The role of probiotics in paediatrics. *Current Paediatrics, 14*, 104–109.

59. MacDonald, T. T., & Gordon, J. N. (2005). Bacterial regulation of intestinal immune responses. *Gastroenterology Clinics of North America, 34*, 401.

60. Sandine, W. E. (1990). Roles of bifidobacteria and lactobacilli in human health. *Contemporary Nutrition, 15*, 1.

61. Koletzko, B., Aggett, P. J., Bindels, J. G., et al. (1998). Growth, development and differentiation: a functional food Science approach. *The British Journal of Nutrition, 80*(Suppl. 1), 5–45.

62. Gibson, G. R., & Wang, X. (1994). Regulatory effects of bifidobacteria on the growth of other colonic bacteria. *The Journal of Applied Bacteriology, 77*(Suppl. 4), 412–420.

63. Falk, P. G., Hooper, L. V., Mittvedt, T., & Gordon, J. I. (1998). Creating and maintaining the gastrointestinal ecosystem: what we know and need to know from

gnotobiology. *Microbiology and Molecular Biology Reviews*, *62*, 1157–1170.

64. Shanahan, F. (2002). The host-microbe interface within the gut. *Best Practice & Research. Clinical Gastroenterology*, *16*, 915–931.

65. O'Hara, A. M., & Shanahan, F. (2007). Gut microbiota: mining for therapeutic potential. *Clinical Gastroenterology and Hepatology*, *5*, 274–284.

66. Van Loo, J., Cummings, J., Delzenne, N., et al. (1999). Functional food properties of non-digestible oligosaccharides: a consensus report from the ENDO project (DGXII AIRII-CT94–1095). *The British Journal of Nutrition*, *81*(Suppl. 2), 121–132.

67. Gibson, G. R., & Roberfroid, M. B. (1995). Dietary modulation of the human colonic microflora introducing the concept of probiotics. *Journal of Nutrition*, *125*, 1401–1412.

68. Rycroft, C. E., Fooks, L. J., & Gibson, G. R. (1999). Methods for assessing the potential of prebiotics and probiotics. *Current Opinion in Clinical Nutrition and Metabolic Care*, *2*, 1–4.

69. Ouwehand, A. C., Derrien, M., de Vos, W., et al. (2005). Prebiotics and other microbial substrates for gut functionality. *Current Opinion in Biotechnology*, *16*(Suppl. 2), 212–217.

70. Cuthbertson, W. J. F. (1999). Evolution of infant nutrition. *British Journal of Nutrition*, *81*, 359–371.

71. Hamosh, M. (1996). Unravelling the mysteries of mother's milk. *Medscape Womens Health*, *16*, 4–9.

72. Goldman, A. S., Chheda, S., & Garofalo, R. (1997). Spectrum of immunomodulating agents in human milk. *IJPHO*, *4*, 491–497.

73. Garofalo, R. P., & Goldman, A. S. (1999). Expression of functional immunomodulatory and anti-inflammatory factors in human milk. *Clinics in Perinatology*, *26*, 361–377.

74. Oddy, W. H. (2002). The impact of breast milk on infant and child health. *Breastfeeding Review*, *10*, 5–18.

75. Thurl, S., Henker, J., Siegel, M., et al. (1997). Detection of four human milk groups with respect to Lewis blood group dependent oligosaccharides. *Glycoconjugate Journal*, *14*, 795–799.

76. Kunz, C., Rodriguez-Palmero, M., Koletzko, B., & Jensen, R. (1999). Nutritional and biochemical properties of human milk. *Clinics in Perinatology*, *26* (Suppl. 2), 307–333.

77. Boehm, G., & Stahl, B. (2003). Oligosaccharides. In T. Mattila-Sandholm (Ed.), *Functional Dairy Products* (pp. 203–243). Cambridge: Woodhead.

78. Bode, L. (2006). Recent advances on structure, metabolism, and function of human milk oligosaccharides. *The Journal of Nutrition*, *136*, 2127–2130.

79. Chaturvedi, P., Warren, C. D., Altaye, M., et al. (2001). Fucosylated human milk oligosaccharides vary between individuals and over the course of lactation. *Glycobiology*, *11*, 365–372.

80. Newburg, D. S., & Neubauer, S. H. (1995). Carbohydrates in milk. In R. G. Jensen (Ed.), *Handbook of milk composition* (pp. 34–123). San Diego: Academic Press.

81. Gnoth, M. J., Kunz, C., Kinne-Safrane, E., & Rudloff, S. (2000). Human milk oligosaccharides are minimally digested *in vitro*. *The Journal of Nutrition*, *130*, 3014–3020.

82. Engfer, M. B., Stahl, B., Finke, B., et al. (2000). Human milk oligosaccharides are resistant to enzymatic hydrolysis in the upper gastrointestinal tract. *The American Journal of Clinical Nutrition*, *71*, 1589–1596.

83. Rivero-Urgell, M., & Santamaria-Orleans, A. (2001). Oligosaccharides: application in infant food. *Early Human Development*, *65*, 43–52.

84. Coppa, G. V., Pierani, P., Zampini, L., et al. (2001). Characterization of oligosaccharides in milk and feces of breast-fed infants by high performance anion exchange chromatography. *Advances in Experimental Medicine and Biology*, *501*, 307–314.

85. Hill, M. J. (1995). Bacterial fermentation of complex carbohydrate in the human colon. *European Journal of Cancer Prevention*, *4*, 353–358.

86. Boehm, G., & Stahl, B. (2007). Oligosaccharides from milk. *The Journal of Nutrition*, *137*, 847–849.

87. Yahiro, M., Nishikawa, I., Murakami, Y., Yoshida, H., & Ahiko, K. (1992). Studies on application of galactosyl lactose for infant formula. II. Changes of fecal characteristics on infant fed galactosyl lactose. Reports of Research Laboratory. *Snow Brand Milk Products*, *78*, 27–32.

88. Ben, X., Zhou, X., Zhao, W., Yu, W., Pan, W., Zhang, W., Wu, S. M., Van Beusekom, C. M., & Schaafsma, A. (2004). Supplementation of milk formula with galacto-oligosaccharides improves intestinal micro-flora and fermentation in term infants. *Chinese Medical Journal*, *117*, 927–931.

89. Brunser, O., Gotteland, M., Cruchet, S., Figueroa, G., Garrido, D., & Steenhout, P. (2006). Effect of a milk formula with prebiotics on the intestinal microbiota of infants after an antibiotic treatment. *Pediatric Research*, *59*, 451–456.

90. Jose, M., Saavedra, J., Tscherina, A., Moore, N., Abi-Hanna, A., Coletta, F., Emenhiser, C., et al. (1999). Gastrointestinal function in infants consuming a weaning food supplemented with oligofructose, a prebiotic. *Journal of Pediatric Gastroenterology and Nutrition*, *29*, 513.

91. Tschernia, A., Moore, N., Abi-Hanna, A., Yolken, R., Colerts, F., Emenhiser, C., et al. (1999). Effects of long-term consumption of a weaning food supplemented with oligofructose, a prebiotic, on general infant health status. *Journal of Pediatric Gastroenterology and Nutrition*, *29*, 503.

92. Euler, A. R., Mitchell, D. K., Kline, R., & Pickering, L. K. (2005). Prebiotic effect of fructo-oligosaccharide supplemented term infant formula at two concentrations compared with unsupplemented formula and human milk. *Journal of Pediatric Gastroenterology and Nutrition, 40*, 157–164.

93. Moore, N., Chao, C., Yang, L., Storm, H., Oliva-Hemker, M., & Saavedra, J. M. (2003). Effects of fructo-oligosaccharide-supplemented infant cereal: A double-blind, randomized trial. *The British Journal of Nutrition, 90*, 581–587.

94. Duggan, C., Penny, M. E., Hibberd, P., Gil, A., Huapaya, A., Cooper, A., Coletta, F., Emenhiser, C., & Kleinman, R. E. (2003). Oligofructose supplemented infant cereal: 2 randomised, blinded, community-based trials in Peruvian infants. *The American Journal of Clinical Nutrition, 77*, 937–942.

95. Waligora-Dupriet, A. J., Campeotto, F., Nicolis, I., Bonet, A., Soulaines, P., Dupont, C., & Butel, M. J. (2007). Effect of oligofructose supplementation on gut microflora and well-being in young children attending a day care centre. *International Journal of Food Microbiology, 113*, 108–113.

96. Guesry, P. R., Bodanski, H., Tomsit, E., & Aeschlimann, J. M. (2000). Effect of 3 doses of fructo-oligosaccharides in infants. *Journal of Pediatric Gastroenterology and Nutrition, 31*, 252.

97. Bettler, J., & Euler, A. R. (2006). An evaluation of the growth of term infants fed formula supplemented with fructo-oligosaccharides. *Int J Probiotics Prebiotics, 1*, 19–26.

98. Kapiki, A., Costalos, C., Oikonomidou, C., et al. (2007). The effect of a fructo-oligosaccharide supplemented formula on gut flora of preterm infants. *Early Human Development, 83*, 335–339.

99. Nagendra, R., Viswanatha, S., Arun Kumar, K. S., et al. (1995). Effect of feeding milk formula containing lactulose to infants on faecal bifidobacterial flora. *Nutrition Research, 15*, 14–24.

100. Rinne, M., Kirjavainen, P., Salminen, S., & Isolauri, E. (2003). Lactulose—any clinical benefits beyond constipation relief? A pilot study in infants with allergic symptoms. *BioScience and Microflora, 22*, 155–157.

101. Ziegler, E., Vanderhoof, J. A., Petschow, B., et al. (2007). Term infants fed formula supplemented with selected blends of prebiotics grow normally and have soft stools similar to those reported for breast-fed infants. *Journal of Pediatric Gastroenterology and Nutrition, 44*, 359–364.

102. Firmansyah, A., Pramita, G. D., Fassler Carrie, A-L., et al. (2000). Improved humoral immune response to measles vaccine in infants receiving cereal with fructo-oligosaccharides. *Journal of Pediatric Gastroenterology and Nutrition, 31*(2), 134.

103. Fanaro, S., Jelinek, J., Stahl, B., et al. (2005). Acidic oligosaccharides from pectin hydrosylate as new component for infant formulae: effect on intestinal flora, stool characteristics, and pH. *Journal of Pediatric Gastroenterology and Nutrition, 41*, 186–190.

104. Bongers, M. E. J., de Lorijn, F., Reitsma, J. B., et al. (2007). The clinical effect of a new infant formula in term infants with constipation: a double-blind, randomized crossover trial. *Nutrition Journal, 6*, 8–15.

105. Moro, G., Minoli, I., Mosca, M., et al. (2002). Dosage-related bifidogenic effects of galacto- and fructo-oligosaccharides in formula-fed term infants. *Journal of Pediatric Gastroenterology and Nutrition, 34*, 291–295.

106. Moro, G., Stahl, B., Fanaro, S., et al. (2005). Dietary prebiotic oligosaccharides are detectable in faeces of formula fed infants. *Acta Paediatrica. Supplementum, 94*, 27–30.

107. Schmelzle, H., Wirth, S., Skopnik, H., et al. (2003). Randomized double-blind study of the nutritional efficacy and bifidogenicity of a new infant formula containing partially hydrolyzed protein, a high beta-palmitic acid level, and nondigestible oligosaccharides. *Journal of Pediatric Gastroenterology and Nutrition, 36*, 343–351.

108. Knol, J., Scholtens, P., Kafka, C., et al. (2005). Colon microflora in infants fed formula with galacto- and fructo-oligosaccharides: more like breast fed infants. *Journal of Pediatric Gastroenterology and Nutrition, 40*, 36–42.

109. Haarman, M., & Knol, J. (2005). Quantitative real-time PCR assays to identify and quantify fecal Bifidobacterium species in infants receiving a prebiotic infant formula. *Applied and Environmental Microbiology, 71*, 2318–2324.

110. Haarman, M., & Knol, J. (2006). Quantitative real-time PCR analysis of fecal Lactobacillus species in infants receiving a prebiotic infant formula. *Applied and Environmental Microbiology, 72*, 2359–2365.

111. Costalos, C., Kapiki, A., Apostolou, M., & Papathoma, E. (2008). The effect of a prebiotic supplemented formula on growth and stool microbiology of term infants. *Early Human Development, 84*, 45–49.

112. Savino, F., Cresi, F., Maccario, S., et al. (2003). 'Minor' feeding problems during the first months of life: effect of a partially hydrolyzed milk formula containing fructo- and galacto-oligosaccharides. *Acta Paediatrica, 92*(Suppl. 441), 86–90.

113. Savino, F., Maccario, S., Castangno, E., et al. (2005). Advances in the management of digestive problems during the first months of life. *Acta Paediatrica, 94*(Suppl. 449), 120–124.

114. Scholtens, P., Alles, M., Bindels, J., et al. (2006). Bifidogenic effect of solid weaning foods with added prebiotic oligosaccharides: A randomized controlled

clinical trial. *Journal of Pediatric Gastroenterology and Nutrition, 42*, 553–559.

115. Bakker-Zierikzee, A. M., Tol, E. A., Kroes, H., et al. (2006). Faecal sIgA secretion in infants fed on pre- or probiotic infant formula. *Pediatric Allergy and Immunology, 17*, 134–140.

116. Bakker-Zierikzee, A. M., Alles, M., Knol, J., et al. (2005). Effects of infant formula containing a mixture of galacto and fructo-oligosaccharides or viable *Bifidobacterium animalis* on the intestinal microflora during the first 4 months of life. *The British Journal of Nutrition, 94*, 783–790.

117. Moro, G., Arslanoglu, S., Stahl, B., et al. (2006). A mixture of prebiotic oligosaccharides reduces the incidence of atopic dermatitis during the first six months of age. *Archives of Disease in Childhood, 91*, 814–819.

118. Arslanoglu, S., Moro, G., Schmitt, J., & Boehm, G. (2007). Early dietary intervention with a mixture of prebiotic oligosaccharides reduces the allergy associated symptoms and infections during the first 2 years of life. *Journal of Pediatric Gastroenterology and Nutrition, 40*(Suppl. 1), 129.

119. van Hoffen, E., Ruiter, B., Faber, J., et al. (2009). A specific mixture of short-chain galacto-oligosaccharides and long-chain fructo-oligosaccharides induces a beneficial immunoglobulin profile in infants at risk for allergy. *Allergy, 64*, 484–487.

120. Arslanoglu, S., Moro, G., & Boehm, G. (2007). Early supplementation of prebiotic oligosaccharides protects formula-fed infants against infections during the first 6 months of life. *The Journal of Nutrition, 137*, 2420–2424.

121. Alliet, P., Scholtens, P., Raes, M., et al. (2007). An infant formula containing a specific prebiotic mixture of GOS/lc FOS leads to higher faecal secretory IgA in infants. *Journal of Pediatric Gastroenterology and Nutrition, 44*(Suppl. 1), 179.

122. Decsi, T., Arato, A., Balogh, M., et al. (2005). Randomized placebo controlled double blind study on the effect of prebiotic oligosaccharides on intestinal flora in healthy term infants (translation from Hungarian language). *Orvosi Hetilap, 146*, 2445–2450.

123. Rinne, M. M., Gueimonde, M., Kallioma'ki, M., et al. (2005). Similar bifidogenic effects of prebiotic-supplemented partially hydrolyzed infant formula and breastfeeding on infant gut microbiota. *FEMS Immunology and Medical Microbiology, 43*, 59–65.

124. Bruzzese, E., Volpicelli, M., Salvini, F., et al. (2006). Early administration of GOS/FOS prevents intestinal and respiratory infections in infants. *Journal of Pediatric Gastroenterology and Nutrition, 42*, 95.

125. Boehm, G., Lidestri, M., Casetta, P., et al. (2002). Supplementation of a bovine milk formula with an oligosaccharide mixture increases counts of faecal bifidobacteria in preterm infants. *Archives of Disease in Childhood. Fetal and Neonatal, 86*, 178–181.

126. Knol, J., Boehm, G., Lidestri, L., et al. (2005). Increase of faecal bifidobacteria due to dietary oligosaccharides induces a reduction of clinically relevant pathogen germs in the faeces of formula-fed preterm infants. *Acta Paediatrica, 94*(Suppl. 449), 31–33.

127. Mihatsch, W. A., Hoegel, J., & Pohlandt, F. (2006). Prebioitc oligosaccharides reduce stool viscosity and accelerate gastrointestinal transport in preterm infants. *Acta Paediatrica, 95*, 843–848.

128. Indrio, F., Riezzo, G., Montagna, O., et al. (2007). Effect of a prebiotic mixture of short chain galacto-oligosaccharides and long chain fructo-oligosaccharides on gastric motility in preterm infants. *Journal of Pediatric Gastroenterology and Nutrition, 44*(Suppl. 1), 217.

129. Gibson, G. R., Probert, H. M., Van Loo, J. A. E., et al. (2004). Dietary modulation of the human colonic microbiota: updating the concept of prebiotics. *Nutrition Research Reviews, 17*, 259–275.

130. Roberfroid, M. (2007). Prebiotics: the concept revisited. *The Journal of Nutrition, 137*, 830–837.

131. Frank, A. (2002). Technological functionally of inulin and oligofructose. *The British Journal of Nutrition, 87*, 287–291.

132. Carabin, I. G., & Flamm, W. G. (1999). Evaluation of safety of inulin and oligofructose as dietary fiber. *Regulatory Toxicology and Pharmacology, 30*(Suppl. 3), 268–282.

133. De Bruyn, A., Alvarez, A. P., Sandra, P., & De Leenheer, L. (1992). Isolation and identification of O-beta-D-fructofuranosyl-(2→1)-O-beta-D-fructofuranosyl-(2→1)-D-fructose, a product of the enzymic hydrolysis of the inulin from Cichorium intybus. *Carbohydrate Research, 235*, 303–308.

134. Boehm, G., Fanaro, S., Jelinek, J., et al. (2003). Prebiotic concept for infant nutrition. *Acta Paediatrica. Supplementum, 91*, 64–67.

135. Scholtens, P. A., Alles, M. S., Bindels, J. G., et al. (2006). Bifidogenic effects of solid weaning foods with added prebiotic oligosaccharides: a randomised controlled clinical trial. *Journal of Pediatric Gastroenterology and Nutrition, 42*, 553–559.

136. Langlands, S. J., Hopkins, M. J., Coleman, N., & Cummings, J. H. (2004). Prebiotic carbohydrates modify the mucosa associated microflora of the human large bowel. *Gut, 53*, 1610–1616.

137. Rastall, R. A. (2004). Bacteria in the gut: friends and foes and how to alter the balance. *The Journal of Nutrition, 134*, 2022–2026.

138. Rechkemmer, G., Rönnau, K., & von Engelhardt, W. (1988). Fermentation of polysaccharides and absorption of short chain fatty acids in the mammalian hindgut. *Comparative Biochemistry and Physiology, 90*(Suppl. 4), 563–568.

139. Cummings, J. H., Gibson, G. R., & Macfarlane, G. T. (1989). Quantitative estimates of fermentation in the

hind gut of man. *Acta Veterinaria Scandinavica, 86,* 76–82.

140. Salvini, F., et al. (2003). Le sostanze funzionali nel latte materno e nella dieta del bambino. *Doctor Pediatria, 12,* 18–23.

141. Beachey, E. H. (1981). Bacterial adherence: adhesin-receptor interactions mediating the attachment of bacteria to mucosal surface. *The Journal of Infectious Diseases, 143,* 325.

142. Mirelman, D. (1986). *Microbial lectins and agglutinins: Properties and biological activities.* New York: Wiley.

143. Andersson, B., Porras, O., Hanson, L. A., et al. (1986). Inhibition of attachment of *Streptococcus pneumoniae* and *Hemophilus influenzae* by human milk and receptor oligosaccharides. *The Journal of Infectious Diseases, 153*(Suppl. 2), 232–237.

144. Guarner, F., & Schaafsma, G. J. (1998). Probiotics. *International Journal of Food Microbiology, 39,* 237–238.

145. Food and Agriculture Organization, World Health Organization. (2001). The Food and Agriculture Organization of the United Nations and the World Health Organization Joint FAO/WHO expert consultation on evaluation of health and nutritional properties of probiotics in food including powder milk with live lactic acid bacteria. FAO/WHO Report No. 10-1-2001.

146. Zhang, L., Li, N., & Neu, J. (2005). Probiotics for Preterm Infants. *NeoReviews, 6,* 227–232.

147. Becquet, P. (2003). EU assessment of enterococci as feed additives. *International Journal of Food Microbiology, 88,* 247–254.

148. Gorbach, S. L. (2000). Probiotics and gastrointestinal health. *The American Journal of Gastroenterology, 95,* 2–4.

149. Saavedra, J. M. (2001). Clinical applications of probiotic agents. *The American Journal of Clinical Nutrition, 73,* 1147–1151.

150. Isolauri, E. (2001). Probiotics in human disease. *The American Journal of Clinical Nutrition, 73,* 1142–1146.

151. Hoyos, A. B. (1999). Reduced incidence of necrotizing enterocolitis associated with enteral administration of *Lactobacillus acidophilus* and *Bifidobacterium infantis* to neonates in an intensive care unit. *International Journal of Infectious Diseases, 3,* 197–202.

152. Dani, C., Biadaioli, R., Bertini, G., et al. (2002). Probiotics feeding in prevention of urinary tract infection, bacterial sepsis and necrotizing enterocolitis in preterm infants. A prospective double-blind study. *Biology of the Neonate, 82,* 103–108.

153. Bin-Nun, A., Bromiker, R., Wilschanski, M., et al. (2005). Oral probiotics prevent necrotizing enterocolitis in very low birth weight neonates. *Journal of Pediatrics, 147*(Suppl. 2), 192–196.

154. Lin, H. C., Su, B. H., Chen, A. C., et al. (2005). Oral probiotics reduce the incidence and severity of necrotizing

enterocolitis in very low birth weight infants. *Pediatrics, 115*(1), 1–4.

155. Charrois, T., Sandhu, G., & Vohra, S. (2006). Probiotics. *Pediatrics in Review, 27*(4).

156. Donnet-Hughes, A., Rochat, F., Serrant, P., et al. (1999). Modulation of nonspecific mechanisms of defense by lactic acid bacteria: effective dose. *Journal of Dairy Science, 82,* 863–869.

157. Ouwehand, A., Isolauri, E., & Salminen, S. (2002). The role of the intestinal microflora for the development of the immune system in early childhood. *European Journal of Nutrition, 41*(Suppl. 1), 132–137.

158. Silva, M., Jacobus, N. V., Deneke, C., & Gorbach, S. L. (1987). Antimicrobial substance from a human Lactobacillus strain. *Antimicrobial Agents and Chemotherapy, 31,* 1231–1233.

159. Wilson, K. H., & Perini, I. (1988). Role of competition for nutrients in suppression of *Clostridium difficile* by the colonic microflora. *Infection and Immunology, 56,* 2610–2614.

160. Goldin, B. R., Gorbach, S. L., Saxelin, M., et al. (1992). Survival of Lactobacillus species (strain GG) in human gastrointestinal tract. *Digestive Diseases and Sciences, 37,* 121–128.

161. Pothoulakis, C., Kelly, C. P., Joshi, M. A., et al. (1993). *Saccharomyces boulardii* inhibits *Clostridium difficile* toxin A binding and eterotoxicity in a rat ileum. *Gastroenterology, 104*(4), 1108–1115.

162. Bernet, M. F., Brassart, D., Nesser, J. R., & Servin, A. I. (1994). *Lactobacillus acidophilus* LA1 binds to human intestinal cell lines and inhibits cell attachment and cell invasion by enterovirulent bacteria. *Gut, 35,* 483–489.

163. Panigrahi, P., Gupta, S., Gewolb, I. H., & Morris, J. G., Jr. (1994). Occurrence of necrotizing enterocolitis may be dependent on patterns of bacterial adherence and intestinal colonization: Studies in Caco-2 tissue culture and weanling rabbit models. *Pediatric Research, 36,* 115–121.

164. Mack, D. R., Michail, S., Wei, S., et al. (1999). Probiotics inhibit enteropathogenic *E. coli* adherence *in vitro* by inducing intestinal mucin gene expression. *The American Journal of Physiology, 276*(4, Pt 1), 941–950.

165. Erickson, K. L., & Hubbard, N. E. (2000). Probiotic immunomodulation in health and disease. *The Journal of Nutrition, 130,* 403–409.

166. Deplancke, B., & Gaskins, H. R. (2001). Microbial modulation of innate defense: goblet cells and the intestinal mucus layer. *The American Journal of Clinical Nutrition, 73,* 1131–1141.

167. Madsen, K., Cornish, A., Soper, P., et al. (2001). Probiotic bacteria enhance murine and human intestinal epithelial barrier function. *Gastroenterology, 121*(3), 580–591.

168. Kennedy, R. J., Kirk, S. J., & Gardiner, K. R. (2002). Mucosal barrier function and the commensal flora. *Gut, 50,* 441–442.

169. Morita, H., He, F., Fuse, T., et al. (2002). Adhesion of lactic acid bacteria to caco-2 cells and their effect on cytokine secretion. *Microbiology and Immunology, 46*(4), 293–297.

170. Moretti, A., Papi, C., Koch, M., & Capurso, L. (2006). quali evidenze? Impiego dei probiotici in gastroenterologia. *Argomenti di Gastroenterologia Clinica, 19,* 31–39.

171. Stratiki, Z., Costalos, C., Sevastiadou, S., et al. (2007). The effect of a bifidobacter supplemented bovine milk on intestinal permeability of preterm infants. *Early Human Development, 83*(9), 575–579.

172. Guarino, A., & Bruzzese, E. (2001). I probiotici: indicazioni cliniche certe e potenziali meccanismi d'azione. *Prospettive Pediatria, 31,* 309–320.

173. Majamaa, H., Isolauri, E., Saxelin, M., & Vesijar, I. T. (1995). Lactic acid bacteria in the treatment of acute rotavirus gastroenteritis. *Journal of Pediatric Gastroenterology and Nutrition, 20,* 333–338.

174. Elson, C. O., & Mestecky, J. F., et al. (1995). The mucosal immune system. In M. Blaser, P. D. Smith (Eds.), *Infections of the Gastrointestinal Tract* (pp. 153–162). New York: Raven Press Ltd.

175. Sudo, N., Sawamura, S., Tanaka, K., et al. (1997). The requirement of intestinal bacterial flora for the development of an IgE production system fully susceptible to oral tolerance induction. *Journal of Immunology, 159*(4), 1739–1745.

176. Fukushima, Y., Kawata, Y., Hara, H., et al. (1998). Effect of a probiotic formula on intestinal immunoglobulin A production in healthy children. *International Journal of Food Microbiology, 42,* 39–44.

177. Schiffrin, E. J., Rochat, F., Link-Amster, H., et al. (1995). Immunomodulation of human blood cells following the ingestion of lactic acid bacteria. *Journal of Dairy Science, 78,* 491–497.

178. Weng, M., Walker, W. A., & Sanderson, I. R. (2007). Butyrate regulates the expression of pathogen-triggered IL-8 in intestinal epithelia. *Pediatric Research, 62,* 542–546.

179. Viljanen, M., Kuitunen, M., Haahtela, T., et al. (2005). Probiotic effects on faecal inflammatory markers and on faecal IgA in food allergic atopic eczema/dermatitis syndrome infants. *Pediatric Allergy and Immunology, 16*(1), 65–71.

180. Marin, M. L., Tejada-Simon, M. V., Lee, J. H., et al. (1998). Stimulation of cytokine production in clonal macrophage and T-cell models by *Streptococcus thermophilus*: comparison with *Bifidobacterium* sp. and *Lactobacillus bulgaricus*. *Journal of Food Protection, 61*(7), 859–864.

181. Murch, S. H. (2001). Toll of allergy reduced by probiotics. *Lancet, 357,* 1057–1059.

182. Klinman, D. M., Yi, A. K., Beaucage, S. L., et al. (1996). CpG motifs present in bacteria DNA rapidly induce lymphocytes to secrete interleukin 6, interleukin 12, and interferon gamma. *Proceedings of the National Academy of Sciences, 93*(7), 2879–2883.

183. Fujii, T., Ohtsuka, Y., Lee, T., et al. (2006). *Bifidobacterium breve* enhances transforming growth factor beta1 signaling by regulating Smad7 expression in preterm infants. *Journal of Pediatric Gastroenterology and Nutrition, 43*(1), 83–88.

184. Takeda, K., Suzuki, T., Shimada, S. I., et al. (2006). Interleukin-12 is involved in the enhancement of human natural killer cell activity by *Bifidobacterium breve* Shirota. *Clinical and Experimental Immunology, 146*(1), 109–115.

185. Saint-Marc, T., Rossello-Prats, L., & Touraine, J. L. (1991). Efficacité de *Saccharomyces boulardii* dans le traitment des diarrhées du SIDA. *Annales de Médecine Interne, Paris, 142,* 64–65.

186. Saint-Marc, T., Blehaut, H., Musial, Ch., & Touraine, J. L. (1995). Diarrhoenim zusammenhang mit AIDS (doppelblind studie mit *Saccharomyces Boulardii*). *Sem Hospitaux, Paris, 71,* 735–741.

187. Fontana, M., & Martelli, L. (2004). Probiotics in paediatric gastroenterology: Evidenze cliniche. *Medico e Bambino, 23,* 175–182.

188. Berg, R. D. (1998). Probiotics, prebiotics or conbiotics? *Trends in Microbiology, 6,* 89–92.

189. Roller, M., Rechkemmer, G., & Watzl, B. (2004). Prebiotic inulin enriched with oligofructose in combination with the probiotics *Lactobacillus rhamnosus* and *Bifidobacterium lactis* modulates intestinal immune functions in rats. *The Journal of Nutrition, 134,* 153–156.

190. Agostoni, C., Axelsson, I., Goulet, O., et al. (2004). Prebiotic oligosaccharides in dietetic products for infants: a commentary by the ESPGHAN Committee on Nutrition. *Journal of Pediatric Gastroenterology and Nutrition, 39*(5), 465–473.

191. Yap, K. W., Mohamed, S., Yazid, A. M., et al. (2005). Dose–response effects of inulin on fecal short-chain fatty acids content and mineral absorption of formula fed infants. *Nutr Food Sci, 35,* 208–219.

192. Kim, S. H., Lee, D. H., & Meyer, D. (2007). Supplementation of infant formula with native inulin has a prebiotic effect in formula-fed babies. *Asia Pacific Journal of Clinical Nutrition, 16,* 172–177.

193. Albers, R., Antoine, J. M., Bourdet-Sicard, R., et al. (2005). Markers to measure immunomodulation in human nutrition intervention studies. *The British Journal of Nutrition, 94*(3), 452–481.

194. Arslanoglu, S., Moro, G. E., Schmitt, J., et al. (2008). Early dietary intervention with a mixture of prebiotic oligosaccharides reduces the incidence of allergic manifestations and infections during the

first two years of life. *The Journal of Nutrition, 138,* 1091–1095.

195. Carvalho, R. S., Michail, S., Ashai-Khan, F., & Mezoff, A. G. (2008). An update on pediatric gastroenterology and nutrition: a review of some recent advances. *Current Problems in Pediatric and Adolescent Health Care, 38,* 204–228.

196. van den Heuvel, E. G., Muys, T., van Dokkum, W., & Schaafsma, G. (1999). Oligofructose stimulates calcium absorption in adolescents. *The American Journal of Clinical Nutrition, 69*(3), 544–548.

197. Pedersen, A., Sandström, B., & Van Amelsvoort, J. M. (1997). The effect of ingestion of inulin on blood lipids and gastrointestinal symptoms in healthy females. *The British Journal of Nutrition, 78*(2), 215–222.

198. van Vliet, T. (1997). A double placebo controlled, parallel trial on the effect of oligofructose intake on serum lipids in male volunteers. *Report TNO, 97,* 874.

199. Davidson, M. H., et al. (1998). Evaluation of the influence of dietary inulin on serum lipids in adults with hypercholesterolemia. *Nutrition Research, 18,* 503–517.

200. Alles, M. S. (1999). Consumption of fructo-oligosaccharides does not favourably affect blood glucose and serum lipid concentrations in patients with type 2 diabetes. *The American Journal of Clinical Nutrition, 69,* 64–69.

201. Roberfroid, M. B., & Delzenne, N. M. (1998). Dietary fructans. *Annual Review of Nutrition, 18,* 117–143.

202. Sanderson, I. R., & Walker, W. A. (1993). Uptake and transport of macromolecules by the intestine: Possible role in clinical disorders (an update). *Gastroenterology, 104,* 622–639.

203. Samuli, R. (2007). Potential uses of probiotics in the neonate. *Seminars in Fetal & Neonatal Medicine, 12,* 45–53.

204. Guandalini, S., Pensabene, L., & Zikri, M. A. (2000). *Lactobacillus* GG administered in oral rehydration solution to children with acute diarrhea: A multicenter European trial. *Journal of Pediatric Gastroenterology and Nutrition, 30,* 54–60.

205. Saavedra, J. M., Bauman, N. A., Oung, I., et al. (1994). Feeding of *Bifidobacterium bifidum* and *Streptococcus thermophilus* to infants in hospital for prevention of diarrhea and shedding of rotavirus. *Lancet, 344,* 1046–1049.

206. Costa-Ribeiro, H., Ribeiro, T. C., Mattos, A. P., et al. (2003). Limitations of probiotic therapy in acute, severe dehydrating diarrhea. *Journal of Pediatric Gastroenterology and Nutrition, 36,* 112–115.

207. Ribeiro, H., Jr. (2000). Diarrheal disease in a developing nation. *The American Journal of Gastroenterology, 95*(Suppl. 1), 14–15.

208. Kaila, M., Isolauri, E., Soppi, E., et al. (1992). Enhancement of the circulating antibody secreting cell response in human diarrhea by a human Lactobacillus strain. *Pediatric Research, 32,* 141–144.

209. Allen, S. J., Okoko, B., Martinez, E., et al. (2004). Probiotics for treating infectious diarrhoea. *Cochrane Database of Systematic Reviews, 2.*

210. Szajewska, H., Kotowska, M., Mrukowicz, J. Z., et al. (2001). Efficacy of *Lactobacillus* GG in prevention of nosocomial diarrhea in infants. *The Journal of Pediatrics, 138,* 361–365.

211. Szajewska, H., & Mrukowicz, J. Z. (2001). Probiotics in the treatment and prevention of acute infectious diarrhea in infants and children: a systematic review of published randomized, double-blind, placebo-controlled trials. *Journal of Pediatric Gastroenterology and Nutrition, 33*(Suppl. 2), 17–25.

212. Van Niel, C. W., Feudtner, C., Garrison, M. M., & Christakis, D. A. (2002). Lactobacillus therapy for acute infectious diarrhea in children: a meta-analysis. *Pediatrics, 109,* 678–684.

213. Barclay, A. R., Stenson, B., Simpson, J. H., et al. (2007). Probiotics for necrotizing enterocolitis: a systematic review. *Journal of Pediatric Gastroenterology and Nutrition, 45*(Suppl. 5), 569–576.

214. Szajewska, H., & Mrukowicz, J. Z. (2001). Probiotics in the treatment and prevention of acute infectious diarrhea in infants and children: a systematic review of published randomized, double-blind, placebo-controlled trials. *Journal of Pediatric Gastroenterology and Nutrition, 33*(Suppl. 2), 17–25.

215. Rosenfeldt, V., Michaelsen, K. F., Jakobsen, M., et al. (2002). Effect of probiotic Lactobacillus strains in young children hospitalized with acute diarrhea. *The Pediatric Infectious Disease Journal, 21*(5), 411–416.

216. Ziegler, E. E., Jeter, J. M., Drulis, J. M., et al. (2003). Formula with reduced content of improved, partially hydrolyzed protein and probiotics: infant growth and health. *Monatsschr Kinderheilkd, 1,* 565–571.

217. Weizman, Z., Asli, G., & Alsheikh, A. (2005). Effect of a probiotic infant formula on infections in child care centers: comparison of two probiotic agents. *Pediatrics, 115,* 5–9.

218. Chouraqui, J. P., Van Egroo, L. D., & Fichot, M. C. (2004). Acidified milk formula supplemented with *Bifidobacterium lactis*: impact on infant diarrhea in residential care settings. *Journal of Pediatric Gastroenterology and Nutrition, 38,* 288–292.

219. Saran, S., Gopalan, S., & Krishna, T. P. (2002). Use of fermented foods to combat stunting and failure to thrive. *Nutrition, 18,* 393–396.

220. Guarino, A., Canai, R. B., Spagnolo, M. I., et al. (1997). Oral bacterial therapy reduces the duration of symptoms and of viral excretion in children with mild diarrhea. *Journal of Pediatric Gastroenterology and Nutrition, 25,* 516–519.

221. Meucci, S. & Cannella, C. (2003). Yogurt e latti fermentati: probiotici e prebiotici. Atti 2nd Probiotics and Prebiotics, New Foods, Roma 7-9 sett. 2003, 36–44.

222. Chouraqui, J. P., Grathwohl, D., Labaune, J. M., et al. (2008). Assessment of the safety, tolerance, and protective effect against diarrhea of infant formulas containing mixtures of probiotics or probiotics and prebiotics in a randomized controlled trial. *The American Journal of Clinical Nutrition*, 87, 1365–1373.

223. Saavedra, J. M., Bauman, N. A., Oung, I., et al. (1994). Feeding of *Bifidobacterium bifidum* and *Streptococcus thermophilus* to infants in hospital for prevention of diarrhoea and shedding of rotavirus. *Lancet*, *344*, 1046–1049.

224. Sazawal, S., Dhingra, U., Sarkar, A., et al. (2004). Efficacy of milk fortified with a probiotic *Bifidobacterium lactis* (DR-10TM) and prebiotic galacto-oligosaccharides in prevention of morbidity and on nutritional status. *Asia Pacific Journal of Clinical Nutrition*, *13*(Suppl. 28).

225. Pedone, C. A., Arnaud, C. C., Postaire, E. R., et al. (2000). Multicentric study of the effect of milk fermented by *Lactobacillus casei* on the incidence of diarrhoea. *International Journal of Clinical Practice*, *54*, 568–571.

226. Szajewska, H., Kotowska, M., Mrukowicz, J. Z., et al. (2001). Efficacy of *Lactobacillus* GG in prevention of nosocomial diarrhea in infants. *The Journal of Pediatrics*, *138*(3), 361–365.

227. Oberhelman, R. A., Gilman, R. H., Sheen, P., et al. (1999). A placebo-controlled trial of *Lactobacillus* GG to prevent diarrhea in undernourished Peruvian children. *The Journal of Pediatrics*, *134*(1), 15–20.

228. Vanderhoof, J. A., Whitney, D. B., Antonson, D. L., et al. (1999). *Lactobacillus* GG in the prevention of antibiotic-associated diarrhea in children. *The Journal of Pediatrics*, *135*, 564–568.

229. Arvola, T., Laiho, K., Torkkeli, S., et al. (1999). Prophylactic *Lactobacillus* GG reduces antibiotic-associated diarrhea in children with respiratory infections. *Pediatrics*, *104*, 64.

230. Sazawal, S., Hiremath, G., Dhingra, U., et al. (2006). Efficacy of probiotics in prevention of acute diarrhoea: a meta analysis of masked, randomised, placebo-controlled trials. *The Lancet Infectious Diseases*, *6*, 374–382.

231. Lodinova-Zadnikova, R., & Sonnenborn, U. (1997). Effect of preventive administration of a nonpathogenic *Escherichia coli* strain on the colonization of the intestine with microbial pathogens in newborn infants. *Biology of the Neonate, 71*, 224–232.

232. Lodinova-Zadnikova, R., Tlaskalova-Hogenova, H., & Sonnenborn, U. (1992). Local and serum antibody response in full-term and premature infants after artificial colonization of the intestine with *E. coli*

strain Nissle 1917 (Mutaflor®). *Pediatric Allergy and Immunology*, *3*, 43–48.

233. Marteau, P., de Vrese, M., Cellier, C. J., & Schrezenmeir, J. (2001). Protection from gastrointestinal diseases with the use of probiotics. *American Journal of Clinical Nutrition*, *73*(Suppl. 2), 430–436.

234. Correa, N. B., Peret Filho, L. A., Penna, F. J., et al. (2005). A randomized formula controlled trial of *Bifidobacterium lactis* and *Streptococcus thermophilus* for prevention of antibiotic-associated diarrhea in infants. *Journal of Clinical Gastroenterology*, *39*, 385–389.

235. Walker, W. A., Goulet, O., Morelli, L., & Antoine, J. M. (2006). Progress in the *Science* of probiotics: from cellular microbiology and applied immunology to clinical nutrition. *European Journal of Nutrition*, *45*(Suppl. 1), 1–18.

236. Venderhoof, J. A., Whitney, D. B., Antonson, D. L., et al. (1999). *Lactobacillus* GG in the prevention of antibiotic associated diarrhea in children. *The Journal of Pediatrics*, *135*, 564–568.

237. Cremonini, F., Di Caro, S., Nista, E. C., et al. (2002). Meta-analysis: the effect of prebiotic administration on antibiotic-associated diarrhea. *Aliment Pharmacol Ther*, *16*(8), 1461–1467.

238. Szajewska, H., Ruszczynski, M., & Radzikowski, A. (2006). Probiotics in the prevention of antibiotic-associated diarrhea in children: a metaanalysis of randomized controlled trials. *The Journal of Pediatrics, 149*, 367–373.

239. Gorbach, S. L., Chang, T. W., & Goldin, B. (1987). Successful treatment of relapsing *Clostridium difficile* colitis with *Lactobacillus* GG. *Lancet*, *2*, 15–19.

240. Plummer, S., Weaver, M. S., Harris, J. C., et al. (2004). *Clostridium difficile* pilot study: effects of probiotic supplementation on the incidence of *C. difficile* diarrhea. *International Microbiology*, *7*, 59–62.

241. Wullt, M., Hagslätt, M. L. J., & Odenholt, I. (2003). *Lactobacillus plantarum* 299v for the treatment of recurrent *Clostridium difficile*-associated diarrhoea: a double-blind, placebo-controlled trial. *Scandinavian Journal of Infectious Disease, 35*, 365–367.

242. Szymanski, H., Pejcz, J., Jawien, M., et al. (2006). Treatment of acute infectious diarrhoea in infants and children with a mixture of three *Lactobacillus rhamnosus* strains: a randomized, double-blind, placebo-controlled trial. *Alimentary Pharmacology & Therapeutics, 23*, 247–253.

243. Sarker, S. A., Sultana, S., Fuchs, G. J., et al. (2005). *Lactobacillus paracasei* strain ST11 has no effect on rotavirus but ameliorates the outcome of non-rotavirus diarrhea in children from Bangladesh. *Pediatrics, 116*(2), 221–228.

244. Pashapour, N., & Iou, S. G. (2006). Evaluation of yogurt effect on acute diarrhea in 6–24-month-old hospitalized infants. *The Turkish Journal of Pediatrics, 48*, 115–118.

245. Kurugol, Z., & Koturoglu, G. (2005). Effects of *Saccharomyces boulardii* in children with acute diarrhoea. *Acta Paediatrica, 94,* 44–47.

246. Gaón, D., García, H., Winter, L., et al. (2003). Effect of Lactobacillus strains and *Saccharomyces boulardii* on persistent diarrhea in children. *Medicina (B Aires), 63*(4), 293–298.

247. Sudarmo, S. M., Ranuh, R. G., Rochim, A., & Soeparto, P. (2003). Management of infant diarrhea with high-lactose probiotic-containing formula. *The Southeast Asian Journal of Tropical Medicine and Public Health, 34,* 845–848.

248. Rosenfeldt, V., Michaelsen, K. F., Jakobsen, M., et al. (2002). Effect of probiotic Lactobacillus strains on acute diarrhea in a cohort of non-hospitalized children attending day-care centers. *The Pediatric Infectious Disease Journal, 21*(5), 417–419.

249. Bennet, R., Eriksson, M., Nord, C. E., & Zetterström, R. (1986). Fecal bacterial microflora of newborn infants during intensive care management and treatment with five antibiotic regimens. *Pediatric Infectious Disease, 5,* 533–539.

250. Fell, J. M. (2005). Neonatal inflammatory intestinal diseases: necrotizing enterocolitis and allergic colitis. *Early Human Development, 81,* 117–122.

251. Walker, W. A. (2000). Role of nutrients and bacterial colonization in the development of intestinal host defense. *Journal of Pediatric Gastroenterology and Nutrition, 30*(Suppl. 2), 2–7.

252. Millar, M., Wilks, M., & Costeloe, K. (2003). Probiotics for preterm infants? *Archives of Disease in Childhood. Fetal and Neonatal, 88,* 354–358.

253. Martin, C. R., & Walker, W. A. (2008). Probiotics: role in pathophysiology and prevention in necrotizing enterocolitis. *Seminars in Perinatology, 32,* 127–137.

254. Bin-Nun, A., Bromiker, R., Wilschanski, M., et al. (2005). Oral probiotics prevent necrotizing enterocolitis in very low birth weight neonates. *The Journal of Pediatrics, 147*(2), 192–196.

255. Deshpande, G., Rao, S., & Patole, S. (2007). Probiotics for prevention of necrotising enterocolitis in preterm neonates with very low birthweight: a systematic review of randomised controlled trials. *Lancet, 369,* 1614–1620.

256. Gupta, P., Andrew, H., Kirschner, B. S., & Guandalini, S. (2000). Is *Lactobacillus* GG helpful in children with Crohn's disease? Results of a preliminary, open-label study. *Journal of Pediatric Gastroenterology and Nutrition, 31*(4), 453–457.

257. Bousvaros, A., Guandalini, S., Baldassano, R. N., et al. (2005). A randomized, double-blind trial of *Lactobacillus* GG versus placebo in addition to standard maintenance therapy for children with Crohn's disease. *Inflammatory Bowel Diseases, 11*(9), 833–839.

258. Lin, P. W., Nasr, T. R., & Stoll, B. J. (2008). Necrotizing enterocolitis: recent scientific advances in pathophysiology and prevention. *Seminars in Perinatology, 32,* 70–82.

259. Rautava, S., Kalliomaki, M., & Isolauri, E. (2002). Probiotics during pregnancy and breastfeeding might confer immunomodulatory protection against atopic disease in the infant. *The Journal of Allergy and Clinical Immunology, 109,* 119–121.

260. Vandenplas, Y. (2004). Clinical overview the changing pattern of clinical aspects of allergic diseases. In E. Isolauri & W. A. Walker (Eds.), *Allergic diseases and the environment. Nestlé Nutrition Workshop Series Pediatric Program* (pp. 1–25). Basel (Switzerland): Nestec Ltd Vevey/S. Karger AG.

261. Kuehni, C. E., Davis, A., Brooke, A. M., & Silverman, M. (2001). Are all wheezing disorders in very young (preschool) children increasing in prevalence? *Lancet, 357,* 1821–1825.

262. Björksten, B., Sepp, E., Julge, K., et al. (2001). Allergy development and intestinal flora during the first year of life. *The Journal of Allergy and Clinical Immunology, 108,* 516–520.

263. Kalliomaki, M., Salminen, S., Arvilommi, H., et al. (2001). Probiotics in primary prevention of atopic disease: a randomized placebo-controlled trial. *Lancet, 357,* 1076–1079.

264. Kalliomaki, M., Salminen, S., Poussa, T., et al. (2003). Probiotics and prevention of atopic disease: 4-year follow-up of a randomised placebo-controlled trial. *Lancet, 361,* 1869–1871.

265. Kukkonen, K., Savilahti, E., Haahtela, T., et al. (2007). Probiotics and prebiotic galacto-oligosaccharides in the prevention of allergic diseases: a randomized, double-blind, placebo-controlled trial. *The Journal of Allergy and Clinical Immunology, 119,* 192–198.

266. Abrahamsson, T. R., Jakobsson, T., Bottcher, M. F., et al. (2007). Probiotics in prevention of IgE-associated eczema: a double-blind, randomized, placebo-controlled trial. *The Journal of Allergy and Clinical Immunology, 119,* 1174–1180.

267. von Berg, A., Koletzko, S., Grubl, A., et al. (2003). The effect of hydrolyzed cow's milk formula for allergy prevention in the first year of life: the German Infant Nutritional Intervention Study, a randomized double-blind trial. *The Journal of Allergy and Clinical Immunology, 111*(3), 533–540.

268. Oldaeus, G., Anjou, K., Bjorkstén, B., et al. (1997). Extensively and partially hydrolysed infant formulas for allergy prophylaxis. *Archives of Disease in Childhood, 77,* 4–10.

269. Høst, A., Koletzko, B., Dreborg, S., et al. (1999). Dietary products used in infants for treatment and prevention of food allergy. Joint Statement of the European Society for Paediatric Allergology and Clinical Immunology (ESPACI) Committee on Hypoallergenic Formulas and the European Society for Paediatric Gastroenterology, Hepatology and Nutrition (ESPGHAN) Committee on Nutrition. *Archives of Disease in Childhood, 81,* 80–84.

270. Committee on Nutrition, American Academy of Pediatrics. (2002). Hypoallergenic infant formulas. *Pediatrics, 106,* 346–349.

271. Halken, S., Hansen, K. S., Jacobsen, H. P., et al. (2000). Comparison of a partially hydrolyzed infant formula with two extensively hydrolyzed formulas for allergy prevention: a prospective, randomized study. *Pediatric Allergy and Immunology, 11*(3), 149–161.

272. Arshad, S. H., Bateman, B., Sadeghnejad, A., et al. (2007). Prevention of allergic disease during childhood by allergen avoidance: the Isle of Wight prevention study. *The Journal of Allergy and Clinical Immunology, 119,* 307–313.

273. von Berg, A., Koletzko, S., Filipiak-Pittroff, B., et al. (2007). German Infant Nutritional Intervention Study Group. Certain hydrolyzed formulas reduce the incidence of atopic dermatitis but not that of asthma: three year results of the German Infant Nutritional Intervention Study. *The Journal of Allergy and Clinical Immunology, 119,* 718–725.

274. von Berg, A. (2007). The concept of hypoallergenicity for atopy prevention. *Nestlé Nutrition Workshop Series. Paediatric Programme, 59,* 49–57, 57–62.

275. Romagnani, S. (2004). Immunologic influences on allergy and the TH1/TH2 balance. *The Journal of Allergy and Clinical Immunology, 113,* 395–400.

276. Samuli, R. (2007). Potential uses of probiotics in the neonate. *Seminars in Fetal & Neonatal Medicine, 12,* 45–53.

277. Majamaa, H., & Isolauri, E. (1997). Probiotics: a novel approach in the management of food allergy. *The Journal of Allergy and Clinical Immunology, 99,* 179–185.

278. Isolauri, E., Arvola, T., Sutas, Y., et al. (2000). Probiotics in the management of atopic eczema. *Clinical and Experimental Allergy, 30,* 1604–1610.

279. Arvola, T., Moilanen, E., Vuento, R., & Isolauri, E. (2002). Gut barrier during weaning in atopic infants. *ESPGHAN, 457.*

280. Rosenfeldt, V., Benfeldt, E., Nielsen, S. D., et al. (2003). Effect of probiotic Lactobacillus strains in children with atopic dermatitis. *The Journal of Allergy and Clinical Immunology, 111*(2), 389–395.

281. Rosenfeldt, V., Benfeldt, E., Valerius, N. H., et al. (2004). Effect of probiotics on gastrointestinal symptoms and small intestinal permeability in children with atopic dermatitis. *The Journal of Pediatrics, 145,* 612–616.

282. Kirjavainen, P. V., Salminen, S. J., & Isolauri, E. (2003). Probiotic bacteria in the management of atopic disease: underscoring the importance of viability. *Journal of Pediatric Gastroenterology and Nutrition, 36,* 223–227.

283. Pohjavuori, E., Viljanen, M., Korpela, R., et al. (2004). *Lactobacillus* GG effect in increasing IFN-gamma production in infants with cow's milk allergy. *The Journal of Allergy and Clinical Immunology, 114*(1), 131–136.

284. Wang, K. Y., Li, S. N., Liu, C. S., et al. (2004). Effects of ingesting Lactobacillus and Bifidobacterium-containing yogurt in subjects with colonized *Helicobacter pylori. The American Journal of Clinical Nutrition, 80*(3), 737–741.

285. Weston, S., Halbert, A., Richmond, P., & Prescott, S. L. (2005). Effects of probiotics on atopic dermatitis: a randomised controlled trial. *Archives of Disease in Childhood, 90,* 892–897.

286. Viljanen, M., Savilahti, E., Haahtela, T., et al. (2005). Probiotics in the treatment of atopic eczema/dermatitis syndrome in infants: a double-blind placebo-controlled trial. *Allergy, 60*(4), 494–500.

287. Peng, G. C., & Hsu, C. H. (2005). The efficacy and safety of heat-killed *Lactobacillus paracasei* for treatment of perennial allergic rhinitis induced by house-dust mite. *Pediatric Allergy and Immunology, 16,* 433–438.

288. Sistek, D., Kelly, R., Wickens, K., et al. (2006). Is the effect of probiotics on atopic dermatitis confined to food sensitized children? *Clinical and Experimental Allergy, 36,* 629–633.

289. Laiho, K., Lampi, A. M., Hamalainen, M., et al. (2003). Breast milk fatty acids, eicosanoids and cytokines in mothers with and without allergic disease. *Pediatric Research, 53,* 642–647.

290. Stavnezer, J. (1995). Regulation of antibody production and class switching by TGF-beta. *Journal of Immunology, 155,* 1647–1651.

291. Petitprez, K., Khalife, J., Cetre, C., et al. (1999). Cytokine RNA expression in lymphoid organs associated with the expression of IgA response in rat. *Scandinavian Journal of Immunology, 49,* 14–20.

292. Rinne, M., Kalliomaki, M., Arvilommi, H., et al. (2005). Effect of probiotics and breastfeeding on the bifidobacterium and lactobacillus/enterococcus microbiota and humoral immune responses. *The Journal of Pediatrics, 147,* 186–191.

293. Huurre, A., Laitinen, K., Rautava, S., et al. (2008). Impact of maternal atopy and probiotic supplementation during pregnancy on infant sensitization: a double-blind placebo-controlled study. *Clinical and Experimental Allergy, 38,* 1342–1348.

294. Rautava, S., Arvilommi, H., & Isolauri, E. (2006). Specific probiotics in enhancing maturation of IgA responses in formula-fed infants. *Pediatric Research, 60*, 221–224.

295. Saglani, S., Payne, D. N., Zhu, J., et al. (2007). Early detection of airway wall remodelling and eosinophilic inflammation in preschool wheezers. *American Journal of Respiratory and Critical Care Medicine, 176*, 858–864.

296. Osborn, D. A., & Sinn, J. K. (2007). Probiotics in infants for prevention of allergic disease and food hypersensitivity. *Cochrane Database of Systematic Reviews*(4), CD006475.

297. Rosenfeldt, V., Benfeldt, E., Nielsen, S. D., et al. (2003). Effect of probiotic Lactobacillus strains in children with atopic dermatitis. *The Journal of Allergy and Clinical Immunology, 111*, 389–395.

298. Viljanen, M., Savilahti, E., Haahtela, T., et al. (2005). Probiotics in the treatment of atopic eczema/dermatitis syndrome in infants: A double-blind placebo-controlled trial. *Allergy, 60*, 494–500.

299. Chouraqui, J. P., Dupont1, C., Bocquet, A., et al. (2008). Alimentation des premiers mois de vie et prévention de l'allergie. *Archives de Pediatrie, 15*, 431–442.

300. Ouwehand, A. C., Lagstrom, H., Suomalainen, T., & Salminen, S. (2002). Effect of probiotics on constipation, fecal azoreductase activity and fecal mucin content in the elderly. *Annals of Nutrition and Metabolism, 46*, 159–162.

301. Banaszkiewicz, A., & Szajewska, H. (2005). Ineffectiveness of *Lactobacillus* GG as an adjunct to lactulose for the treatment of constipation in children: a double-blind, placebo-controlled randomized trial. *The Journal of Pediatrics, 146*, 364–369.

302. Fernandez-Banares, F. (2006). Nutritional care of the patient with constipation. *Best Practice and Research Clinical Gastroenterology, 20*, 575–587.

303. Nader, N., & Youssef, M. D. (2007). Childhood and adolescent constipation: review and advances in management. *Current Treatment Options in Gastroenterology, 10*, 401–411.

304. Marteau, P., Cuillerier, E., Meance, S., et al. (2002). *Bifidobacterium animalis* strain DN-173 010 shortens the colonic transit time in healthy women: a double-blind, randomized, controlled study. *Alimentary Pharmacology and Therapeutics, 16*, 587–593.

305. Gutierrez, C., Marco, A., Nogales, A., & Tebar, R. (2002). Total and segmental colonic transit time and anorectal manometry in children with chronic idiopathic constipation. *Journal of Pediatric Gastroenterology and Nutrition, 35*, 31–38.

306. Mollenbrink, M., & Bruckschen, E. (1994). Treatment of chronic constipation with physiological *E. coli* bacteria. Results of a clinical trial on the efficacy and compatibility of microbiological therapy with the *E. coli*

307. strain Nissle 1917 (Mutaflor®). *Medizinische Klinik, 89*, 587–593.

307. Bruckschen, E., & Horosiewicz, H. (1994). Chronische Obstipation. Vergleich von mikrobiologischer Therapie und Laktulose. *Münchener Medizinische Wochenschrift, 16*, 241–245.

308. Koebnick, C., Wagner, I., Leitzmann, P., et al. (2003). Probiotic beverage containing *Lactobacillus casei* Shirota improves gastrointestinal symptoms in patients with chronic constipation. *Canadian Journal of Gastroenterology, 17*, 655–659.

309. Sartor, R. B. (2003). Targeting enteric bacteria in treatment of inflammatory bowel diseases: 'Why, how and when'. *Current Opinion in Gastroenterology, 19*, 358–365.

310. Sartor, R. B. (2005). Probiotic therapy of intestinal inflammation and infections. *Current Opinion in Gastroenterology, 21*, 44–50.

311. Cucchiara, S., Falconieri, P., Di Nardo, G., et al. (2002). New therapeutic approach in the management of intestinal disease: Probiotics in intestinal disease in pediatric age. *Digestive and Liver Disease, 34*(Suppl. 2), 44–47.

312. Kleesen, B., Kroesen, A. J., Buhr, H. J., & Blaut, M. (2002). Mucosal and invading bacteria in patients with inflammatory bowel disease compared with controls. *Scandinavian Journal of Gastroenterology, 37*, 1034–1041.

313. Borruel, N., Carol, M., Casellas, F., et al. (2002). Increased mucosal tumour necrosis factor alpha production in Crohn's disease can be downregulated *ex vivo* by probiotic bacteria. *Gut, 51*(5), 659–664.

314. Marteau, P., Seksik, P., & Shanahan, F. (2003). Manipulation of the bacterial flora in inflammatory bowel disease. *Best Practice & Research. Clinical Gastroenterology, 17*, 47–61.

315. Kanauchi, O., Mitsuyama, K., Arabki, Y., & Andoh, A. (2003). Modification of intestinal flora in the treatment of inflammatory bowel disease. *Current Pharmaceutical Design, 9*, 333–346.

316. Gionchetti, P., Amadini, C., Rizzello, F., et al. (2002). Probiotics role in inflammatory bowel disease. *Digestive and Liver Disease, 34*(Suppl. 2), 58–62.

317. Hart, A. L., Stagg, A. J., & Kamm, M. A. (2003). Use of probiotics in the treatment of inflammatory bowel disease. *Journal of Clinical Gastroenterology, 36*, 111–119.

318. Kuisma, J., Mentula, S., Jarvinen, H., et al. (2003). Effect of *Lactobacillus rhamnosus* GG on ileal pouch inflammation and microbial flora. *Alimentary Pharmacology & Therapeutics, 17*(4), 509–515.

319. Kwon, J., & Farrel, R. (2003). Probiotics and inflammatory bowel disease. *Bio Drug, 17*, 179–186.

320. Guandalini, S. (2002). Use of *Lactobacillus* GG in pediatric Crohn's disease. *Digestive and Liver Disease, 34*, 63–65.

321. Gionchetti, P., Rizzello, F., Helwig, U., et al. (2003). Prophylaxis of pouchitis onset with probiotic therapy: A

double-blind, placebo-controlled trial. *Gastroenterology*, *124*, 1202–1209.

322. Gionchetti, P., Rizzello, F., Lammers, K. M., et al. (2006). Antibiotics and probiotics in treatment of inflammatory bowel disease. *World Journal of Gastroenterology*, *12*(21), 3306–3313.

323. Campieri, M., Rizzello, F., & Venturi, A. (2000). Combination of antibiotic and prebiotic treatment is efficacious in prophylaxis of post-operative recurrence of Crohn's disease. *Gastroenterology*, *118*, 781.

324. Gionchetti, P., Morselli, C., Rizzello, F., et al. (2004). Management of pouch dysfunction or pouchitis with an ileoanal pouch. *Best Practice & Research. Clinical Gastroenterology*, *18*, 993–1006.

325. Gionchetti, P., Rizzello, F., Venturi, A., et al. (2000). Oral bacteriotherapy as maintenance treatment in patients with chronic pouchitis: A double-blind, placebo-controlled trial. *Gastroenterology*, *119*, 305–309.

326. Laake, K. O., Line, P. D., Aabakken, L., et al. (2003). Assessment of mucosal inflammation and circulation in response to probiotics in patients operated with ileal pouch anal anastomosis for ulcerative colitis. *Scandinavian Journal of Gastroenterology*, *38*, 409–414.

327. Kuisma, J., Mentula, S., Jarvinen, H., et al. (2003). Effect of *Lactobacillus rhamnosus* GG on ileal pouch inflammation and microbial flora. *Alimentary Pharmacology & Therapeutics*, *17*, 509–515.

328. Kassinen, A., Krogius-Kurikka, L., Mäkivuokko, H., et al. (2007). The fecal microbiota of irritable bowel syndrome patients differs significantly from that of healthy subjects. *Gastroenterology*, *133*(1), 24–33.

329. Posserud, I., Stotzer, P. O., Björnsson, E. S., et al. (2007). Small intestinal bacterial overgrowth in patients with irritable bowel syndrome. *Gut*, *56*(6), 802–808.

330. Thabane, M., Kottachchi, D. T., & Marshall, J. K. (2007). Systematic review and meta-analysis. The incidence and prognosis of postinfectious irritable bowel syndrome. *Alimentary Pharmacology & Therapeutics*, *26*, 535–544.

331. Marshall, J. K., Thabane, M., Borgaonkar, M. R., & James, C. (2007). Postinfectious irritable bowel syndrome after a food-borne outbreak of acute gastroenteritis attributed to a viral pathogen. *Clinical Gastroenterology and Hepatology*, *5*, 457–460.

332. Gwee, K. A., Leong, Y. L., Graham, C., et al. (1999). The role of psychological and biological factors in postinfective gut dysfunction. *Gut*, *44*(3), 400–406.

333. Dunlop, S. P., Jenkins, D., Neal, K. R., & Spiller, R. C. (2003). Relative importance of enterochromaffin cell hyperplasia, anxiety, and depression in postinfectious IBS. *Gastroenterology*, *125*, 1651–1659.

334. Spiller, R. C., Jenkins, D., Thornley, J. P., et al. (2000). Increased rectal mucosal enteroendocrine cells, T lymphocytes, and increased gut permeability following acute *Campylobacter enteritis* and in post-dysenteric irritable bowel syndrome. *Gut*, *47*(6), 804–811.

335. Gwee, K. A., Collins, S. M., Read, N. W., et al. (2003). Increased rectal mucosal expression of interleukin 1 beta in recently acquired post-infectious irritable bowel syndrome. *Gut*, *52*(4), 523–526.

336. Balsari, A., Ceccarelli, A., & Dubini, F. (1982). The faecal bacterial population in the irritable bowel syndrome. *Microbiologica*, *5*, 185–194.

337. Swidsinski, M. K., & Ortner, M. (1999). Alteration of bacterial concentration in colonic biopsies from patients with irritable bowel syndrome (IBS). *Gastroenterology*, *115*, A–A1.

338. King, T. S., Elia, M., & Hunter, J. O. (1998). Abnormal colonic fermentation in irritable bowel syndrome. *Lancet*, *352*, 1187–1189.

339. Bausserman, M., & Michail, S. (2005). The use of *Lactobacillus* GG in irritable bowel syndrome in children: a double-blind randomized control trial. *The Journal of Pediatrics*, *147*(2), 197–200.

340. Halpern, G. M., Prindville, T., Blankenburg, M., et al. (1996). Treatment of irritable bowel syndrome with Lacteol forte: A randomized, double-blind, crossover trial. *The American Journal of Gastroenterology*, *91*, 1579–1585.

341. Kim, H. J., Camilleri, M., McKinzie, S., et al. (2003). A randomized controlled trial of a probiotic, VSL 3, on gut transit and symptoms in diarrhoea-predominant irritable bowel syndrome. *Alimentary Pharmacology & Therapeutics*, *17*, 895–904.

342. Saggioro, A. (2004). Probiotics in the treatment of irritable bowel syndrome. *Journal of Clinical Gastroenterology*, *38*, 104–106.

343. Faber, S. M. (2000). Comparison of probiotics and antibiotics to probiotics alone in treatment of diarrhea predominant IBS (D-IBS), alternating (A-IBS) and constipation (C-IBS) patients. *Gastroenterology*, *118*, 687–688.

344. Cremonini, F., Di Caro, S., Covino, M., et al. (2002). Effect of different probiotic preparations on anti-*Helicobacter pylori* therapy-related side effects: A parallel-group, triple-blind, placebo-controlled study. *The American Journal of Gastroenterology*, *97*, 2744–2749.

345. Wang, K. Y., Li, S. N., Liu, C. S., et al. (2004). Effects of ingesting Lactobacillus- and Bifidobacterium-containing yogurt in subjects with colonized *Helicobacter pylori*. *The American Journal of Clinical Nutrition*, *80*, 737–741.

346. Linsalata, M., Russo, F., Berloco, P., et al. (2004). The influence of *Lactobacillus brevis* on ornithine decarboxylase activity and polyamine profiles in *Helicobacter pylori*-infected gastric mucosa. *Helicobacter*, *9*, 165–172.

347. Sykora, J., Valeekova, K. K. V., Amlerova, J. J. A., et al. (2004). Supplements of a one week triple drug therapy

with special probiotic *Lactobacillus casei immunitass* (strain DN 114000) and *Streptococcus thermophilus* and *Lactobacillus bulgaricus* in the eradication of *H. pylori*-colonized children: a prospective randomised trial. *Journal of Pediatric Gastroenterology and Nutrition, 39*(Suppl. 1), 400.

348. Chitkara, D. K., Montgomery, R. K., Grand, R. J. & Büller, H. A. (2007). Lactose intolerance. In B. D. Rose (Ed.). Waltham, MA: Up To Date.

349. Escher, J. C., de Koning, N. D., van Engen, C. G., et al. (1992). Molecular basis of lactase levels in adult humans. *The Journal of Clinical Investigation, 89,* 480–483.

350. Fajardo, O., Naim, H. Y., & Lacey, S. W. (1994). The polymorphic expression of lactase in adults is regulated at the messenger RNA level. *Gastroenterology, 106,* 1233–1241.

351. Troelsen, J. T. (2005). Adult-type hypolactasia and regulation of lactase expression. *Biochimica et Biophysica Acta, 1723,* 19–32.

352. Sahi, T. (1994). Genetics and epidemiology of adult-type hypolactasia. *Scandinavian Journal of Gastroenterology. Supplement, 202,* 7–20.

353. Grand, R. J., Montgomery, R. K., Chitkara, D. K., et al. (2003). Changing genes; losing lactase. *Gut, 52,* 617–619.

354. Rastall, R. A., Fuller, R., Gaskins, H. R., & Gibson, G. R. (2000). Colonic functional foods. In G. R. Gibson & C. M. Williams (Eds.), *Functional Foods* (pp. 71–89). Cambridge: Woodhead Publishing Limited.

355. Marteau, P., Pochart, P., Flourie, B., et al. (1990). Effect of chronic ingestion of a fermented dairy product containing *Lactobacillus acidophilus* and *Bifidobacterium bifidum* on metabolic activities of the colonic flora in humans. *American Journal of Clinical Nutrition, 52,* 685–688.

356. de Vrese, M., Stegelmann, A., Richter, B., et al. (2001). Probiotic: compensation for lactose insufficiency. *The American Journal of Clinical Nutrition, 73*(Suppl. 2), 421–429.

357. Grand, R. J., & Montgomery, R. K. (2008). Lactose malabsorption: current treatment options. *Gastroenterology, 11,* 19–25.

358. Gilliland, S. E. (1985). Influence of bacterial starter cultures on nutritional value of foods: improvement of lactose digestion by consuming foods containing lactobacilli. *Cultured Dairy Products Journal, 20,* 28–33.

359. Szilagyi, A. (1999). Prebiotics or probiotics for lactose intolerance: a question of adaptation. *The American Journal of Clinical Nutrition, 70,* 105–106.

360. Hatakka, K., Savilahti, E., & Ponka, A. (2001). Effect of long-term consumption of prebiotic milk on infections in children attending day care centers: double blind, randomised trial. *British Medical Journal, 322,* 1327–1331.

361. Gluck, U., & Gebbers, J. O. (2003). Ingested probiotics reduce nasal colonization with pathogenic bacteria (*Staphylococcus aureus, Streptococcus pneumoniae* and beta-hemolytic streptococci). *The American Journal of Clinical Nutrition, 77,* 517–520.

362. Reid, G. (2001). Probiotic agents to protect the urogenital tract against infection. *The American Journal of Clinical Nutrition, 73,* 437–443.

363. Probiotics. Natural Standard Monograph. Natural Standard (2005). Available at: www.naturalstandard.com.

364. Kullen, M. J., & Bettler, J. (2005). The delivery of probiotics and prebiotics to infants. *Current Pharmaceutical Design, 11,* 55–74.

365. Anderson, G. G., Palermo, J. J., Schilling, J. D., et al. (2003). Intracellular bacterial biofilm-like pods in urinary tract infections. *Science, 301,* 105–107.

366. Lane, M. C., Lockatell, V., Monterosso, G., et al. (2005). Role of motility in the colonization of uropathogenic *Escherichia coli* in the urinary tract. *Infection and Immunity, 73*(Suppl. 11), 7644–7656.

367. Marrs, C. F., Zhang, L., & Foxman, B. (2005). *Escherichia coli* mediated urinary tract infections: are there distinct uropathogenic *E. coli* (UPEC) pathotypes? *FEMS Microbiology Letters, 252*(Suppl. 2), 183–190.

368. Parham, N. J., Pollard, S. J., Desvaux, M., et al. (2005). Distribution of the serine protease autotransporters of the Enterobacteriaceae among extraintestinal clinical isolates of *Escherichia coli. Journal of Clinical Microbiology, 43*(Suppl. 8), 4076–4082.

369. Snyder, J. A., Haugen, B. J., Lockatell, C. V., et al. (2005). Coordinate expression of fimbriae in uropathogenic *Escherichia coli. Infection and Immunity, 73*(Suppl. 11), 7588–7596.

370. Usein, C. R., Damian, M., Tatu-Chitoiu, D., et al. (2003). Comparison of genomic profiles of *Escherichia coli* isolates from urinary tract infections. *Roumanian Archives of Microbiology and Immunology, l62*(Suppl. 3–4), 137–154.

371. Newman, D. (1915). The treatment of cystitis by intravesical injection of lactic bacillus cultures. *Lancet, 14,* 330–332.

372. Bruce, A. W., Chadwick, P., Hassan, A., & VanCott, G. F. (1973). Recurrent urethritis in women. *Canadian Medical Association Journal, 108,* 973–976.

373. Seung, J. L., Yoon, H. S., Su, J. C., & Jung, W. L. (2007). Probiotics prophylaxis in children with persistent primary vesicoureteral reflux. *Pediatric Nephrology, 22,* 1315–1320.

374. Reid, G., Bruce, A. W., & Taylor, M. (1995). Instillation of Lactobacillus and stimulation of indigenous organisms to prevent recurrence of urinary tract infections. *Microecol Ther, 23,* 32–45.

375. Usein, C. R., Damian, M., Tatu-Chitoiu, D., et al. (2003). Comparison of genomic profiles of *Escherichia*

coli isolates from urinary tract infections. *Roumanian Archives of Microbiology and Immunology, 62*(Suppl. 3–4), 137–154.

376. Reid, G., Hammond, J-A., & Bruce, A. W. (2003). Effect of lactobacilli oral supplement on the vaginal microflora of antibiotic treated patients: randomized, placebo-controlled study. *Nutraceut Food, 8*, 145–148.

377. Reid, G., & Bruce, A. W. (2006). Probiotics to prevent urinary tract infections: the rationale and evidence. *World Journal of Urology, 24*, 28–32.

378. Reid, G., Bruce, A. W., & Fraser, N. (2001). Oral probiotics can resolve urogenital infections FEMS. *Immunology and Medical Microbiology, 30*, 49–52.

379. Zuppa, A. A., Savarese, I., Scorrano, A., et al. (2007). Prebiotics and probiotics in infant nutrition. *Ped Med Chir, 29*, 69–83.

Microarray Analysis of Probiotics Effectiveness

Christine M. Carey and Magdalena Kostrzynska

Agriculture and Agri-Food Canada, Guelph Food Research Centre, 93 Stone Road West, Guelph, Ontario N1G 5C9, Canada

1. INTRODUCTION

Among the greater than 500 different microbial species that inhabit the human intestinal tract [1], some microorganisms, termed probiotics, can exert beneficial effects on the host by improving the intestinal microbial balance [2–4]. Probiotics are defined as live microorganisms which, when administered in adequate amounts, confer a health benefit on the host [3]. Many lactic acid bacteria (LAB) have potential probiotic properties. Probiotics include mainly species of the genera *Lactobacillus* and *Bifidobacterium* [2, 5]. Considered to be essential components of the normal intestinal microbiota, probiotics can play an important role in intestinal integrity, immunomodulation and pathogen resistance. Traditionally, many *Lactobacillus* and *Bifidobacterium* strains have been used as starter cultures in the fermentation of food and dairy products and as such, have been generally recognized as safe (GRAS) for human consumption. In addition, species of the genera *Lactobacillus* and *Bifidobacterium* have frequently been used as

health-promoting probiotic components in functional food products, such as dairy products and dietary supplements [3, 6, 7].

Probiotics have increasingly been investigated for their potential to treat or prevent human disease. Studies indicate that administration of probiotics can prevent or treat certain conditions, including atopic disease in infants, infection after surgery, acute diarrhea, symptoms associated with irritable bowel syndrome (IBS), recurring urogenital infections [8, 9], certain cancers, high serum cholesterol [10], and can have antagonistic characteristics against human pathogens [11, 12]. Probiotics may also counteract negative alterations to the normal GI microbiota, which can contribute to certain GI diseases, such as inflammatory bowel disease (IBD) [13], IBS [14] and allergies [9, 15]. Possible probiotic mechanisms promoting human health include pathogen exclusion, nutrient supply to the host and immune modulation. Characterization of the intestinal microbial community and identification of the mechanisms responsible for the beneficial effects on human and animal health is needed. Furthermore, the benefits may be specific to the probiotic bacteria strain, dose and the physiological, nutritional and immune status of the host. Consequently, in-depth research on potential probiotic strains must be comprehensive and strain specific.

The microbial intestinal community has traditionally been studied using culture-based techniques; however, these methods are labor-intensive, time-consuming, subject to erroneous interpretation [16], and can only assess approximately 40% of the gut microbiota [5]. Consequently, molecular methods have greatly increased our knowledge of the structure, diversity and factors influencing dynamics of the gut microbial community [17–21]. Within the last decade, the complete sequences of over 100 bacterial genomes have become available. Although much of this focus has been on pathogenic genomes (including foodborne pathogens), recent interest has focused on sequencing the genomes of gut commensals and symbionts, as well as food-grade bacteria. Consequently, the availability of the complete and partial sequenced genomes provides immense potential to investigate the function of bacteria within the gut, thereby contributing to new or improved functional foods. One such technology that has capitalized on this wealth of information is microarray analysis.

2. INTRODUCTION TO MICROARRAY TECHNOLOGY

Microarray analysis could be used for detection and genotyping as well as for an unbiased genome-scale examination of gene expression patterns [19, 22], and is recognized as a large-scale and high-throughput screening technique. Expression profiling of nucleic acid fragments and genes encoding proteins, antibodies, biosynthetic pathways of carbohydrates and components of tissues can be evaluated. The diverse types of microarrays have applications in clinical, environmental and food microbiology, microbial ecology, and in human, animal and plant disease diagnosis. In expression profiling experiments researchers can examine how gene expression is altered among different interconnecting systems throughout the genome, providing insight into changes occurring at the genome level. In particular, microarrays can identify which systems or genes (functions) are affected by a particular treatment and are useful when a large number of genes or small sample volumes are analyzed. Array technology is able to examine a large portion of an organism's genome (DNA microarray) or proteome (protein array) in a single assay and has become an important technique used to study the influence of probiotics on host health or intestinal microbial interactions. Microarray can be used to detect microorganisms in the gut and investigate quantitative changes in populations of specific members within the microbial community and the influence of probiotics on the structure and function of human intestinal ecosystems. As well, the influence of intestinal microorganisms on host metabolism, nutrient status, and disease through host-commensal signaling can be studied [23]. In addition, microarray can be applied to pathogen detection, characterizing microorganisms based on sequence variation among isolates and identifying the presence or absence of genes [19, 24].

DNA microarray is a nucleic acid hybridization-based technique that consists of two formats: cDNA microarray and oligonucleotide microarray. In a cDNA microarray, customized DNA probes are immobilized onto a solid surface using robotic-mediated technology. The spotted DNA can be PCR fragments, genomic fragments from a cDNA library or open reading frames from a microorganism. Each fragment represents a different gene and the array of genes more effectively represents the entire genome. In genotyping experiments DNA microarray is hybridized with labeled DNA from the test sample. Microarray-based expression profiling requires extraction of total RNA from treated and control samples, after which, both samples are reverse transcribed to form cDNA. Treated and control cDNA samples are labeled with two different fluorophores, hybridized onto the glass slide containing DNA sequences. Using specialized readers and software, the fluorescent readings can identify which fragments in the array have hybridized and thus, are either up-regulated or down-regulated.

In contrast, oligonucleotide microarray probes are designed to correspond to parts of a known or predicted sequence, thus numerous oligonucleotide design possibilities exist and reference DNA samples are not required, which are needed for amplicon-based technologies. Oligonucleotides can be either synthesized and printed onto the array or synthesized *in situ* directly onto the microarray support. Usually two separate microarrays are used to compare the two treatments, thereby increasing experimental costs. Design of short oligonucleotides improves hybridization specificity, as a single mismatched base will prevent pairing [25]; however, shorter oligonucleotides can exhibit variations in signal intensity between perfectly matched oligonucleotides of the same length but different sequences. This problem often requires a high redundancy design, where the signal of several oligonucleotides is combined and statistically normalized for analysis [26]. Short oligonucleotide microarrays also require a large number of probes, contributing to high experimental costs. Conversely, longer oligonucleotides are amenable to detection of gene families, where significant variation has occurred [25, 26].

There is growing interest in the application of microarray technology within the field of functional genomics to identify or confirm gene function related to cellular physiology, metabolic pathways, sensing and signaling, thereby identifying crucial mechanisms involved with probiotic functions. The effect of a particular treatment or microorganism on multiple pathways can be simultaneously investigated using microarrays. Analysis of microarray data can identify genes that undergo similar patterns of gene regulation and those that are affected to similar levels, as they might be co-regulated in common or converging pathways. Despite the immense possibilities associated with applications of microarray in functional genomic studies of probiotic bacteria, the use of the technique is limited to genomes that have been completely sequenced. In addition, oligonucleotide microarrays results were found to be more reliable for evaluating changes in gene expression than data from long cDNA microarrays, indicating that the microarray platform must be carefully selected for functional genomic studies.

Although capable of high-throughput detection and quantification of nucleic acids, certain DNA microarrays have low sensitivity and poor resolution at the species and subspecies levels [27]. Because species-level analyses do not necessarily provide sufficient information in clinical and environmental studies, subspecies microarray probes were found to be more reliable in these applications. Also, progress in microarray-based research is limited to organisms whose genomes have been fully sequenced and requires construction of reliable databases for gene expression. Other technical challenges include the high costs associated with duplicate oligonucleotide assays to compare two conditions, obtaining reproducible results between experiments and platforms, reducing or eliminating false positive results and obtaining high quality DNA and RNA. Handling of vast amounts of data and informatics has also confounded microarray research.

As probiotic studies commonly involve analysis in food products, the presence of inhibitors and extensive sample preparation procedures represent additional limiting factors. Moreover, food processing may degrade DNA and introduce PCR inhibitors, leading to ambiguous results. Consequently, the complexity of food samples requires stringent and possibly lengthy extraction and purification techniques to ensure efficient recovery of nucleic acids and removal of inhibitors [28], thereby increasing sample analysis time [29]. Due to difficulties associated with visual control of the oligonucleotide spotting procedure, adequate quality control system is necessary to ensure spotting uniformity. Also, the hybridization step can require extensive optimization, thus greatly increasing experimental costs associated with DNA microarray. In addition, synthesis of gene-specific primers required to amplify each gene in a genome, for spotting and labeling with fluorophores, contribute to high costs of DNA microarray.

Microarray techniques have also been used in addition to phenotypical and biochemical methods for polyphasic taxonomy of probiotic bacteria, particularly bifidobacteria. The genotyping approach has significantly enhanced our knowledge regarding phylogeny, genetics, and ecological adaptation of intestinal community. In addition, this technology has been used to provide information regarding the degree of relatedness among bifidobacterial strains, which is useful in the polyphasic identification approach [30]. Bifidobacteria are important human commensals and a number of *Bifidobacterium* spp. has been sequenced. The genomic information of *B. animalis* subsp. *lactis* Bb12 led to the generation of microarrays to study the proteome and gene expression of the organism [31].

3. APPLICATION OF MICROARRAYS TO INVESTIGATE THE COMPLEXITY OF GUT MICROBIOTA

Oligonucleotide microarrays are commonly used to study the microbial consortia of the intestinal tract. Based on lifestyle and dietary habits, composition of enteric microflora varies among individuals and specific strains provide a unique fingerprint of human microbiota. Although studies that utilize oligonucleotide microarrays to directly investigate probiotic

use, and effectiveness on intestinal microbiota are limited, the technique has been used to detect specific bacteria, including probiotic bacteria, present in fecal samples. DNA microarray technology supports a means for global gene screening of the complex bacteria-host interplay.

Membrane arrays [32] and oligonucleotide microarrays [33] were evaluated in two separate studies for the detection of 20 predominant human intestinal bacteria. Although similar in principle, membrane arrays do not require an expensive arrayer and scanner. Nylon and nitrocellulose membranes were found to give similar results; however, the color developed more quickly with nitrocellulose membranes [32]. Universal primers used in both studies were able to amplify the full size 16S rDNA from all 20 bacterial species tested. Based on hybridization results using probes specific for each bacterial species, both microarray methods were reliable for the detection of predominant intestinal bacteria and were in agreement with other studies reported on numerically important anaerobic bacteria in fecal samples [34–36]. Although PCR using specific primers for the selected bacterial species produced comparable results, membrane-array method was found to be more sensitive. These studies demonstrate the potential of oligonucleotide and membrane arrays for detecting microbial species in fecal samples, as well the cost-saving benefit of nitrocellulose arrays.

Wang et al. [37] designed an oligonucleotide microarray to identify 40 predominant intestinal bacterial species from human fecal samples. These bacteria include seven species each of *Bacteroides* and *Clostridium*, six species of *Ruminococcus*, five species of *Bifidobacterium*, four species of *Eubacterium*, two species each of *Fusobacterium*, *Lactobacillus*, and *Enterococcus* and a single species each of *Collinsella*, *Eggerthella*, *Escherichia*, *Faecalibacterium*, and *Finegoldia*. Three probes were designed to the 16S rRNA genes of each bacterial species and a positive result was defined as a positive signal from two of the three probes. The oligonucleotide microarray was a sensitive method to detect the presence of certain bacterial species. Although many common bacterial species were identified in the 11 fecal samples, no two samples were the same. Also, the oligonucleotide microarray method was found to be more sensitive than culture techniques, which did not strongly select for the bacterial species.

In another study, Harrington et al. [38] used a microarray approach to develop semi-quantitative method for detection of intestinal bacterial populations based on 16S rDNA probes. Microarray based on shorter oligonucleotides (16-21-mer) showed higher specificity than 40- and 50-mer oligonucleotides. The short oligonucleotide microarray comprising of 230 probes targeting species or groups of intestinal bacteria was found to be highly sensitive and able to detect less than 8.8×10^4 cells per gram of feces. This microarray was successfully used to obtain profiles of gut microbial communities in healthy subjects and a patient suffering from ulcerative colitis (UC). The microarray was employed to detect and quantify *Bacteroides*, lactobacilli, bifidobacteria, eubacteria, clostridia, enterobacteriaceae, ruminococci, streptococci and verrucomicrobiales and revealed differences in the types and levels of bacteria present in feces from three healthy subjects. Samples taken from a UC patient showed significant differences in the levels of *Bacteroides*, eubacteria and sulfate-reducing bacteria.

Palmer et al. [39] designed and applied a microarray based on gene sequences of the small subunit ribosomal RNA (SSU rRNA) of currently recognized bacterial species and taxonomic groups to investigate development of intestinal microbiota in infants. Authors found that the composition and temporal patterns of the microbial communities varied widely from infant to infant. Interestingly, in most babies, bifidobacteria did not appear until several months after birth, and they persisted as a minority population. By the end of the first year, the transformation of the intestinal microbiota to an adult-like pattern was observed. As such, the array can be used as a fecal screening technique, as well as monitoring changes in intestinal populations due to natural variations or response to environmental factors.

Molecular and genomics-based knowledge of the composition of the microbiota, as well as alterations in the balanced microbiota, will enhance the selection of new and specific probiotics. Furthermore, this knowledge will enable the selection of potential combinations of specific probiotics in order to reduce the risk of intestinal diseases and reconstruct specific microbial deviations.

4. MODULATION OF GUT MICROBIOTA BY PREBIOTICS AND PROBIOTICS

Prebiotics represent a promising approach to modulate intestinal microflora, whereby the addition of prebiotics within the diet has been investigated for their potential to increase the health-promoting benefits of certain aspects of the resident gut microbiota. By definition, prebiotics are non-digestible food ingredients that beneficially affect the host by selectively stimulating the growth and/or activity of one or a limited number of bacteria, such as bifidobacteria or lactobacilli, in the colon [40]. According to Gibson and Roberfroid [40], in order for a food ingredient to be classified as a prebiotic, it must be: 1) neither hydrolyzed nor absorbed in the upper part of the GI tract; 2) a selective substrate for one or a limited number of beneficial commensal bacteria in the colon, which are stimulated to grow and/or are metabolically activated; 3) consequently, able to alter the colonic microflora in favor of a healthier composition; and 4) able to induce luminal or systemic effects that are beneficial to the host health.

With the increasing evidence of the positive effects of bifidobacteria and lactobacilli on human health, these intestinal bacteria represent prime targets for use with prebiotics. Fructo-oligosaccharides (FOS) have been extensively investigated as a prebiotic. However, there is limited insight into the precise mechanism associated with how probiotics utilize fructo-oligosaccharides. Composed of a diverse family of fructose polymers with varying lengths, fructo-oligosaccharides can be a derivative of either simple fructose polymers or fructose moieties attached to a sucrose molecule. The majority of food products or nutritional supplements containing fructo-oligosaccharides are synthesized from sucrose using fructo-syltransferases derived from *Aspergillus niger* (short-chain fructo-oligosaccharides; scFOS) or extracted from chicory roots (*Cichoricum intybus*) through the partial enzymatic hydrolysis of inulin to generate FOS.

While some, but not all, lactobacilli are able to ferment scFOS, in-depth studies are needed to evaluate the oligosaccharide metabolism on an individual basis [41, 42]. Consequently, Saulnier et al. [43] used a two-color whole-genome microarray to identify differentially expressed genes when *Lactobacillus plantarum* WCFS1 was grown in the presence of scFOS or glucose as the only available carbohydrate source. Compared to *L. acidophilus* 1195, which was able to utilize both scFOS and FOS [41], *L. plantarum* WCFS1 grew only on scFOS, suggesting that different enzymes were involved with the degradation pathways of *L. acidophilus* 1195. Saulnier et al. [43] identified a group of genes that were probably involved in the transport and degradation of scFOS. These genes are predicted to encode a sucrose phosphoenolpyruvate transport system (PTS), a β-fructofuranosidase, fructokinase, α-glucosidase and a sucrose operon repressor. Pyruvate dehydrogenase was overexpressed, however, to a lesser extent. A mannose-PTS, which is a known glucose transporter in LAB, was down-regulated. In addition, genes involved in fatty acid and phospholipid metabolism and in amino acid and protein synthesis were down-regulated. Due to a slower growth rate when grown in scFOS,

down-regulation of the aforementioned genes may be explained by a lower requirement to synthesize these materials.

In a separate study, a whole-genome cDNA microarray was used to investigate transport and catabolic machinery involved in carbohydrate utilization by probiotic *Lactobacillus acidophilus* NCFM [44]. Global transcriptional profiles were obtained for *L. acidophilus* NCFM grown on glucose, fructose, sucrose, lactose, galactose, trehalose, raffinose and fructo-oilgosaccharides. Only 63 genes (3% of the genome) showed more than a 4-fold induction. These include ATP-binding cassette transporters induced in *L. acidophilus* grown on raffinose and fructo-oligosaccharides. Transporters of the phosphoeno/pyruvate sugar transferase system (PTS) were involved in the uptake of glucose, fructose, sucrose and trehalose. The genes differentially expressed in the presence of galactose and lactose were identified as LacS-permease and enzymes belonging to the Leloir pathway. Overall microarray analysis revealed that in *L. acidophilus* NCFM coordinated and regulated transcription of genes involved in carbohydrate utilization is based on the specific sugar provided.

While bifidobacteria can grow on a variety of carbon sources or prebiotics, it is important to understand the molecular systems required to metabolize the prebiotics that are necessary for the development of health-promoting food products. Based on a carbon source utilization profile, Parche et al. [45] identified 13 of 23 carbohydrates which were utilized by *Bifidobacterium longum* NCC2705. The profile indicated that *B. longum* NCC2705 had a preference towards di-, tri- and oligosaccharides. These results were supported by growth analysis, biochemical characterization of transport systems and microarray data, which illustrated the expression of transport and catabolic genes. Parche et al. [45] revealed that most genes for carbohydrate permeases from *B. longum* were also found in other closely related *Bifidobacterium* strains. This microarray study serves as a basis for further in-depth analyses of the *B. longum* nutritional requirements and lifestyle.

The use of probiotics to modulate host microbiota represents a promising therapeutic alternative in the treatment of IBS. An abundance of evidence indicates that the intestinal microbiota have an important role in the pathogenesis of IBS. However, studies indicate that the effectiveness of probiotics varies between strains. For instance, *Bifidobacterium infantis* 35624 significantly minimized IBS in two trials [46, 47], while *B. animalis* demonstrated beneficial effects only during the first portion of the study [48]. Conflicting studies have been published on the effectiveness of *Lactobacillus plantarum* 299v [48–50] in IBS treatment, whereas the combination of eight strains in VSL#3 has been more successful [51, 52]. In a previous study, Kajander et al. [53] demonstrated that a probiotic mixture containing *Lactobacillus rhamnosus* GG, *L. rhamnosus* LC705, *Bifidobacterium breve* Bb99 and *Propionibacterium freudenreichii* ssp. *shermanii* JS was effective in alleviating IBS symptoms. Subsequently, Kajander et al. [54] investigated the same multispecies probiotic supplementation on abdominal symptoms, quality of life, intestinal microbiota and inflammatory markers in IBS patients. Using a custom-made Agilent microarray HITChip, designed to cover the diversity of the human intestinal microbiota, Kajander et al. [54] demonstrated that the microbiota was stabilized with the probiotic supplementation. The similarity index increased with the probiotic supplementation (1.87 ± 3.13) and decreased with the placebo group (-2.93 ± 1.68), resulting in a significant difference between the two groups. With ongoing developments regarding diversity within the human GI tract, new bacterial phylotypes will be identified which were not included on the version of HITChip used in this study. Despite this limitation, microarray analysis is not biased for the pre-selection of bacterial species or groups to be analyzed, which is a common challenge for microbiota analysis.

Microarray has provided insight into the importance and effectiveness of prebiotics to beneficially stimulate the growth and activity of probiotic bacteria within the human host. In particular, microarray has enabled researchers to further our understanding of the metabolism of prebiotics in probiotic bacteria. Consequently, with recent advances in this field, prebiotics have become an important component of functional foods.

5. APPLICATION OF MICROARRAY TECHNOLOGY TO INVESTIGATE PROBIOTIC: HOST INTERACTIONS

Over 500 different bacterial species compose the microflora in the human gut [1]. In a healthy individual, the intestinal mucosa serves as the first line of defense against infection by providing a mechanical and immunological barrier between the host's internal milieu and gut environment. Despite an improved understanding of the components of the GI tract, from both a human and bacterial perspective, several challenges remain in characterizing the complex interactions between these components. Genomics-based approaches have recently enabled researchers to investigate probiotic interactions and expression of eukaryotic host cells, thereby providing a more complete understanding of the potential applications of probiotics and behavior in the human gut. As probiotic effects likely result from complex interactions with the intestinal microbiota and gut epithelium of the host, microarrays can provide insight into the probiotic mechanism of action and interactions with the host cell. However, studies indicate that the ability of probiotics to adhere to enterocyte-like cells is strain dependent and thus, results cannot be extrapolated to all probiotic bacteria. For this reason, the microarray represents an ideal means of characterizing the complex interactions between probiotic bacteria and intestinal epithelial cells.

Troost et al. [55] used GeneChip microarray (Affymetrix, Santa Clara, CA) to investigate the transcriptional response of human intestinal mucosa to *Lactobacillus plantarum* WCFS1 in healthy volunteers. A short (1 h) exposure to this strain induced differential expression of 669 gene reporters (225 genes were up-regulated and 444 were down-regulated). Interestingly, inhibition of fatty acid metabolism and cell cycle progression were observed. Extended (6 h) exposure to *L. plantarum* WCFS1 modulated the expression of 424 genes; 383 were up-regulated and 41 down-regulated. Particularly genes involved in lipid metabolism, cellular growth and development were up-regulated. In addition, immune responses were triggered; however, inflammatory signals were not expressed.

Di Caro et al. [56] used DNA microarray to assess the influence of *Lactobacillus rhamnosus* GG (LGG) on gene expression in the healthy duodenal mucosa of human adults. Analysis of more than 22,000 genes using the Human Genome U133A Array from Affymetrix (Santa Clara, CA) resulted in the up-regulation and down-regulation of 334 and 92 genes, respectively. Genes associated with cell adhesion (cadherins), immune response and inflammation (TGF-β and TNF family members, cytokines, nitric oxide synthase 1, defensin α-1), apoptosis, cell growth and cell differentiation, transcription, cell communication (ICAMs and integrins), defense response and cell cycle were mainly affected by LGG. Although the biological significance of these results is not well understood, DNA microarray provided a means to examine changes induced in humans taking a specific dose of LGG for a specified period of time, as well as provided insight into the mechanisms by which probiotics promote human health.

In a separate study, Di Caro et al. [57] investigated gene expression in small bowel mucosa of healthy humans exposed to *Bacillus clausii*. Microarray results were validated by real-time PCR performed on five target genes. *B. clausii* affected the expression of genes associated with immune response, apoptosis, cell signaling and adhesion, and as such, furthered the understanding of beneficial cross-talk between the host epithelial cells and probiotic bacterium. In both studies by Di Caro et al. [56, 57], probiotics affected the expression of genes involved with inflammation, immune response, cell adhesion, cell communication and apoptosis. Furthermore, these studies support the presence of bacterial-mucosal interactions. In another whole-genome microarray study of intestinal Caco-2 cells and BALB/c mice treated with the probiotic *E. coli* Nissle 1917 (EcN), pro-inflammatory genes and proteins in human and mouse intestinal epithelial cells were up-regulated [58]. Similarly, real-time RT–PCR confirmed the regulation of selected genes.

In another study, Zyrek et al. [59] used DNA microarray to investigate the underlying molecular mechanisms responsible for the beneficial effects of the probiotic *E. coli* Nissle 1917 (EcN) on the epithelial barrier function using polarized T_{84} cells in a model system. Quantitative RT–PCR was used to confirm gene expression. Differences in expression were observed following co-incubation of T_{84} cells with EcN or enteropathogenic *E. coli* (EPEC). The tight junction (TJ) protein ZO-2 was up-regulated following 2-h incubation with EcN, whereas infection with EPEC resulted in down-regulation of ZO-2. Philpott et al. [60] previously demonstrated that EPEC negatively affected ZO-2, while Zyrek et al. [59] illustrated that co-incubation with EcN resulted in a close association of ZO-2 with the cytoskeleton. The presences of ZO-2 at the cellular contact sites is known to stabilize TJ structures and help maintain cell morphology of the T_{84} cells [61]. These results support the probiotic potential of EcN and beneficial use in the treatment of inflammatory bowel diseases.

Another gastrointestinal disease, necrotizing enterocolitis (NEC), most commonly affects premature newborns and involves the infection and inflammation that causes destruction of the bowel or a portion of the bowel. Despite a poor understanding of its pathogenesis, inappropriate apoptosis of the mucosal epithelia is a suspected cause. Clinical trials have demonstrated the potential of probiotics to reduce the incidence of NEC and suppress intestinal epithelial apoptosis in cultured cells [62]. In order to elicit the mechanism of action, Lin et al. [63] used a cDNA microarray to analyze the effect of LGG on gene expression of intestinal murine cells. Results indicated that LGG up-regulated several genes which had known and likely cytoprotective effects. This study indicates that LGG may augment intestinal host defenses and cytoprotective responses. As apoptosis may be a precursor to NEC, a more thorough comprehension of the mechanism responsible for probiotic modulation of the apoptopic pathway may lead to the future development of therapies or preventive strategies that are more specific to host symptoms or disease.

Although probiotics have been shown to improve gut disorders in humans [64, 65], the exact mechanism(s) responsible for these effects remains unclear. Indigenous bacteria contribute to the development of intestinal functions, whereby segmented filamentous bacteria (SFB) play a critical role in the development of the mucosal immune system. Shima et al. [66] investigated the potential of probiotics using BALB/c mice to analyze epithelial gene expression 3 days following oral administration of the bacteria. Microarray results, which covered approximately 8,000 genes in the whole-genome, indicated that *Lactobacillus casei* Shirota and *Bifidobacterium breve* Yakult affected gene expression in ileal and colonic epithelial cells, respectively. When compared to the probiotics, SFB affected gene expression more strongly in both the small intestine and colon. Comparatively, *L. casei* Shirota enhanced gene expression involving defense/immune function, growth/development and lipid metabolism in the small intestine whereas *B. breve* Yakult stimulated genes involved with cell communication, growth/development and

metabolism in the colon. With the exception of those genes associated with structural proteins in the small intestine, SFB stimulated or suppressed genes to a greater extent than both probiotics. Shima et al. [66] suggests that the differences in gene expression between the probiotic strain- and SFB-associated mice may be attributed to the host-microorganism combination.

An additional health promoting effect of probiotic bacteria is the immunomodulatory effect of probiotics and the shift of T helper (Th)1/Th2 balance towards Th1 mediated immunity. Th1 cells are involved with activating and directing other immune cells, particularly those important to the immune system. In addition to using various immune function assays, Baken et al. [67] investigated Th1 responses and immunomodulatory capacity of orally administered *Lactobacillus casei* Shirota using microarray analysis of the mesenteric lymph nodes (MLN), spleen, liver and thymus of rats. Commonly a more sensitive and predictive method than functional tests, microarray was used as an alternative endpoint in testing immunomodulation. Using a fixed fold ratio of 1.5, three genes in the MLN were down-regulated, two genes were down-regulated in the spleen, the liver showed four down- and two up-regulated genes whereas eight up-regulated genes were observed in the liver. Based on these expression profiles, no enrichment of cellular pathways was identified and the gene expression profiles did not reflect the effects of *L. casei* Shirota on the immune response. Therefore, in this study, microarray analysis is not more predictive than immune function assays.

6. MITIGATION OF VIRULENCE AND PATHOGENICITY OF FOOD-BORNE BACTERIA BY PROBIOTICS

E. coli O157:H7 and the non-O157 Shiga toxin producing *E. coli* (STEC) are prominent food-borne pathogens that cause diarrhea, hemorrhagic colitis and hemolytic uremic syndrome. Kostrzynska et al. [68] used DNA microarray-based approach to investigate interactions between *E. coli* O157:H7 and probiotic bacteria and determined global transcriptional responses of STEC to lactobacilli and bifidobacteria. Pre-incubation of *E. coli* O157:H7 with sublethal doses of LGG resulted in down-regulation of virulence genes such as genes coding for Shiga-toxin 2 and genes encoding the expression of flagella, motility and chemotaxis. Gene encoding acid shock protein and certain genes coding for ribosomal proteins were up-regulated. As such, DNA microarray technology could be useful for investigating the mode of action of probiotics and their application to control virulence of *E. coli* O157:H7.

Salmonella enterica serovar Typhimurium, which causes gastroenteritis, can typically lead to a self-limiting disease. More severe infections can result in bacteremia, fever or death. The *Salmonella* pathogenicity island 1 (SPI1) encodes for many of the genes which are required for *Salmonella* epithelial cell invasion. One mechanism by which probiotics may antagonize intestinal pathogens is by influencing invasion gene expression. Co-expressed genes, which have similar expression profiles under different conditions, were identified by cDNA microarray-based transcript profiling of *S. enterica* serovar Typhimurium in response to the spent culture supernatant of the probiotic strain LGG [69]. In this experiment, a cluster of co-expressed *Salmonella* genes (enriched for genes known to be HilA dependent) were identified and were predicted to be down-regulated by spent culture supernatant. The study showed that the repression of *Salmonella* invasion regulatory system could be linked to a probiotic effect of *Lactobacillus rhamnosus* GG.

As normal inhabitants of the gut, probiotic bacteria may confer several benefits, including prevention against intestinal inflammation caused by pathogens. However, the exact mode of action of probiotics is not well understood.

As the primary line of defense against pathogen entry, the gut membrane barrier and probiotics may prevent pathogen-induced membrane damage by inhibiting pathogen adhesion and maintaining the correct organization of the tight junction and cytoskeleton proteins.

An entero-invasive Gram-negative bacterium, *Shigella flexneri*, causes bacillary dysentery, which is an acute recto-colitis disease responsible for lethal complications, particularly in infants and toddlers. Studies indicate that *S. flexneri* infection leads to the induction of markers associated with acute inflammation, such as the chemokines IL-8 and CCL20, which are under the control of the NFκB pathway [70]. Consequently, Tien et al. [71] used a macroarray DNA chip (1,050 genes selected) to analyze whether *L. casei* could attenuate pro-inflammatory signaling induced by *S. flexneri* invasion of intestinal epithelial cells. Results indicate that *L. casei* down-regulated the transcription of genes encoding pro-inflammatory effectors, including cytokines and chemokines, and adherence molecules which are known to be induced by invasive *S. flexneri*. Down-regulation of genes associated with the ubiquitin system appeared to be important in modulating the pro-inflammatory pathway in intestinal epithelial cells. Further investigation identified that *L. casei* specifically targets the stability of I-κBα, a specific NFκB inhibitor, which shuts down this pro-inflammatory pathway. Based on these results, *L. casei* is able to maintain intestinal homeostasis by manipulating the ubiquitin/proteasome pathway upstream of I-κBα.

As another means of investigating the preventive effect of probiotics against foodborne pathogens, Panigrahi et al. [72] investigated changes in eukaryotic gene expression of Caco-2 cells after infection with a non-pathogenic commensal strain of *Escherichia coli* and *Lactobacillus plantarum* using a high-density glass microarray, which included 19,200 genes/expressed sequence tags (EST). Real-time PCR verified microarray results of eight randomly selected genes which were expressed genes/ESTs. Compared to uninfected Caco-2 cells, a 2-hour treatment with *E. coli*, *L. plantarum* and a combined treatment resulted in two-fold changes in expression of 332, 81 and 86 genes, respectively. *E. coli* infection resulted in the up- and down-regulation of 155 and 177 genes, respectively. *L. plantarum* induced up-regulation of 45 genes and 36 genes were down-regulated. Although the combination treatment nullified stimulatory/inhibitory effects of most genes, 27 and 59 genes were up- and down-regulated, respectively. Changes in the expression of genes associated with regulation of transcription, protein biosynthesis, metabolism, cell-adhesion, ubiquitination, and apoptosis were observed. The presence of probiotic bacteria to change the expression of these genes may affect physiologic and pathologic responses triggered by pathogens in the host.

Because scientific evidence supports a correlation between the human intestinal microbiota and health status, research priorities include investigating microbe-host interactions. Consequently, research has shifted focus from pathogens to that involving commensal and probiotic bacteria and their effect on mitigating the onset of pathogen-related illnesses. Despite the limited amount of current microarray-based research to analyze host-pathogen relationships, previous studies demonstrate the immense potential within the field to increase our knowledge on the beneficial effects of probiotics in protection against pathogens. With a better understanding at the molecular level of the effect of probiotics on the expression of genes involved in pathogenesis, prophylactic treatments can be optimized individually for each probiotic formulation.

7. USE OF DNA MICROARRAYS IN CHARACTERIZING PROBIOTIC STRAINS

Microarray analysis has also been used to investigate strain characteristics, metabolic pathways and resistance of probiotics to antibiotics. Although each topic is currently in the early stage of investigation, microarray represents a method with immense possibilities to further our knowledge of characteristics and safety concerns associated with probiotic use.

Distinctive and important characteristics of probiotic bacteria can be determined through whole-genome comparisons of probiotic strains and closely related bacterial species. Whole-genome microarrays have been developed to genotype probiotic strains, to describe genetic diversity, to classify based on phylogeny and to identify polymorphism of conserved and variable regions among probiotic strains. The availability of genome sequences also provides the foundation for using microarray for functional analysis of gene and protein expression studies, which in turn, will provide information on RNA expression, protein expression and protein interactions under specific conditions. With the increasing availability of genomic sequences, classification of probiotic strains will improve; however, at the time of writing completed genomic sequence data for probiotics were still limited.

Microarray has been used in addition to multilocus sequence analysis, DNA typing and in silico whole-genome alignments to investigate similarity and differences in the *Lactobacillus acidophilus* group [73]. Microarray analysis also revealed intra-species similarities. For instance, only 17 and 5% of the genes from probiotic *L. johnsonii* strain NCC533 represented variable and strain-specific genes, respectively, when tested against four *L. johnsonii* strains. This study showed that modern whole-genome-based techniques were useful in the clarification of taxonomical relationships in *L. acidophilus* complex.

Additionally, Molenaar et al. [74] used a DNA microarray approach to genotype *L. plantarum* isolates from various sources. The authors found that genes involved in sugar transport and catabolism were highly variable between strains. Other variable regions included regions encoding biosynthesis of plantaricin and exopolysaccharide.

Genes involved in biosynthesis or degradation of proteins, lipids and DNA were conserved in all strains. The genotyping data showed that *L. plantarum* isolates clustered into two clearly distinguishable groups.

To provide an alternative in the absence of published genome sequences, Boesten et al. [75] constructed a *Bifidobacterium* Mixed Species (BSM) microarray containing over 6,000 randomly cloned genomic fragments from *B. adolescentis*, *B. animalis*, *B. bifidum*, *B. longum*, *B. pseudolongum* and *B. catenulatum*. This microarray was successfully used as a high-resolution diagnostic tool for the detection of strain- and species-specific characteristics of intestinal bifidobacteria. Interestingly, species-specific diagnostic sequences of bifidobacteria were mainly predicted to code for glycobiome and functions involving DNA metabolism. BSM microarray was also used to investigate transcriptional responses in bifidobacteria present in fecal samples [76]. This study provided insight into the metabolic activities of the bifidobacterial populations in breast- and formula-fed infants.

Microarray analysis has also been used to investigate metabolic pathways in probiotic bacteria. For instance, *Lactobacillus reuteri* can produce reuterin, a potent broad-spectrum antimicrobial agent. In *L. reuteri*, glycerol dehydratase (*gdh*) converts glycerol to reuterin, and some reuterin is converted to 1.3-propanediol by 1,3-propanediol oxidoreductase (1,3-*pdo*). Despite an understanding of the synthesis and antimicrobial effects of reuterin, little is known about the regulatory mechanisms of reuterin production. Using a two-color microarray, Spinler et al. [77] reported an increase in expression in both *L. reuteri* (ATCC 55730) and *L. reuteri* (ATCC PTA 6475) strains for a putative transcriptional regulator (TR) and a glycerol uptake facilitator, indicating that these genes might participate in reuterin production. However, these strains vary in their ability to produce and regulate reuterin production. A comparative gene expression study using TR mutants and a wild-type strain

reveal that TR controls the expression of operons involved with reuterin production and vitamin B12 synthesis for both strains. The *L. reuteri* strain 6475 insertion mutants down-regulated 1,3-*pdo*, which is produced from the conversion of reuterin. These results suggest that both reuterin production and degradation occurs in strain 6475 whereas reuterin production only occurs in strain 55730. This study demonstrates the potential of microarray for use in the characterization of mutants to enhance our understanding of the regulatory mechanisms within probiotic bacteria.

Oligonucleotide microarrays have also been used to investigate the response to acid shock and the bile stress in the probiotic strain *Lactobacillus reuteri* ATTC 55730. The response to acid shock after a severe reduction of pH resulted in up-regulation of the *clpL* gene encoding an ATPase with chaperone activity and up-regulation of several genes involved in cell envelope alterations, including gene encoding a putative esterase [78]. These genes were also involved in the bile stress response of probiotic *L. reuteri* ATTC 55730 [79].

Denou et al. [80] used a combination of genomics and transcriptome analysis and knockout mutants to identify genes associated with the long persistence of the probiotic *Lactobacillus johnsonii* NCC355 in the gut. Authors found that gene encoding a sugar phosphotransferase system (PTS) transporter annotated as mannose PTS and gene encoding putative immunoglobulin A protease were responsible for the long gut residence time of the probiotic strain NCC533.

The ability to sense and respond to environmental changes during transit through the GI tract is imperative to the survival of microorganisms. Two-component regulatory (2CR) systems are important mechanisms associated with environmental sensing and signal transduction [81]. Used extensively in yogurt, fermented foods and dietary supplements [82], the probiotic *L. acidophilus* NCFM has nine putative 2CR systems [81]. Expression profiles of a *L. acidophilus* histidine protein kinase (HPK) mutant and control, in response to ethanol and acidic conditions, were studied using a whole-genome array containing 97.4% of *L. acidophilus* annotated genes. Inactivation of 2CRs altered cell morphology, acid and ethanol sensitivity and resulted in poor acidification rates in skim milk, therefore suggesting the loss of proteolytic activity [81]. As such, microarray analysis can offer immense potential in understanding the effect of intestinal conditions on probiotic survival and effectiveness.

8. ANTIBIOTIC RESISTANCE GENES

In addition to understanding the metabolic and adaptive process of probiotic bacteria, another important criterion for the selection of probiotic bacteria for use in food products is the presence of antibiotic resistance genes and the possibility of gene transfer with pathogenic bacteria.

Multi-drug resistance has emerged among pathogenic bacteria and can affect the beneficial indigenous bacteria. Starter cultures and probiotic bacteria represent a reservoir for gene transfer to human and animal pathogens, and therefore, should be confirmed free of antibiotic resistant genes. There are various degrees of potential for the spread of antibiotic resistance genes. If the antibiotic resistance gene is carried by a mobile genetic element, transposon or self-transferable plasmid, the potential spread can be quite high. The spread can be low if the resistance gene is chromosomal, co-localized with chromosomal genetic information (increased stability) or responsible for host insensitivity and if the gene cannot be transferred *in vitro* or *in vivo* to other bacteria. PCR and hybridization analysis are commonly used to detect antibiotic resistance genes in bacteria. However, these methods are time-consuming when multiple resistance genes are investigated. In contrast, microarray represents a sensitive and specific method to screen for the presence of antibiotic resistance genes in pathogenic and commensal bacteria, as well as in proposed probiotics and starter cultures [83]. Additionally, microarrays can detect antibiotic resistance genes that are not phenotypically expressed *in vitro* [83].

A hybridization microarray was developed to detect 90 of the most prevalent and transferable antibiotic resistant genes in Gram-positive bacteria [83]. With the exception of nine antibiotic resistance genes for which only one specific oligonucleotide could be developed, each gene was detected using two different oligonucleotides, thereby providing increased specificity and sensitivity. Hybridization analysis of genomic DNA obtained from bacteria of different genera (*Bacillus*, *Clostridium*, *Enterococcus*, *Listeria*, *Staphylococcus*, *Streptococcus* and lactic acid bacteria—*Lactobacillus*, and *Lactococcus*) verified the sensitivity of 125 of 137 oligonucleotide targets and identified 71 resistance genes. Although this study did not directly evaluate the presence of resistance genes in probiotic bacteria, many lactic acid bacteria used in food preparation have probiotic properties. Using oligonucleotides provided higher hybridization specificity than PCR products, with a shorter hybridization time. With improved rapid screening of bacteria harboring antibiotic resistant genes, microarray could have future applications in food safety and surveillance programs [83].

Kastner et al. [84] examined probiotics and starter cultures used in the food industry for the presence of antibiotic resistance genes. Based on results from the disk diffusion method, 27 isolates exhibiting phenotypic resistance were screened for 90 known antibiotic resistance genes using microarray hybridization. Results were confirmed by PCR amplification or Southern hybridization. Tetracycline resistance gene was identified in five *Staphylococcus* isolates used as meat starter cultures, *Bifidobacterium lactis* DSM 10140, and *Lactobacillus reuteri* SD 2112 probiotic cultures. The study highlights the presence of antibiotic resistance genes in food bacteria and identifies the need to assess commercial starters and probiotic cultures for the presence of gene transferability. Genetic screening by microarray provides a more comprehensive analysis of antibiotic resistance genes, as compared to disk diffusion tests or methods that target single genes.

Safety is an essential component in the selection and evaluation of potential probiotics. Although probiotics can be sensitive to the majority of antibiotics, probiotics that are naturally or rendered multi-resistant can be co-administered with antibiotics in order to prevent the gastrointestinal side effects due to conventional oral antibiotic treatment. The potential to transfer antibiotic resistance genes from probiotics to bacterial pathogens represents an additional application in microarray research.

9. CONCLUSIONS

Realizing the full potential of probiotics in preventive and therapeutic applications requires a more thorough genome-based investigation of probiotic mechanisms and interactions, and their efficacy in treating gastrointestinal and relating illnesses.

DNA microarray technology has become a promising method used for comprehensive analysis of the complexity of the intestinal microbiota and its modulation by prebiotics and probiotics. Microarrays have also provided insight into the probiotic mechanism of action and interactions with the host. Additionally, microarray technology has been used to characterize probiotic strains, explore their genomic diversity, investigate metabolic pathways, and resistance to antibiotics. Consequently, microarray represents an ideal method to increase the wealth of knowledge associated with probiotic applications.

ACKNOWLEDGMENTS

Funding for this work was provided by Agriculture and Agri-Food Canada.

References

1. Malinen, E., Rinttilä, T., & Kajander, K., et al. (2005). Analysis of the fecal microbiotia of irritable bowel syndrome patients and healthy controls with real-time PCR. *American Journal of Gastroenterology, 100,* 373–382.
2. Fuller, R. (1991). Probiotics in human medicine. *Gut, 32,* 439–442.
3. Reid, G., & Hammond, J. A. (2005). Probiotics. Some evidence of their effectiveness. *Canadian Family Physician, 51,* 1487–1493.
4. Tao, Y., Drabik, K. A., Waypa, T. S., et al. (2006). Soluble factors from *Lactobacillus* GG activate MAPKs and induce cytroprotective heat shock proteins in intestinal epithelial cells. *American Journal of Physiology & Cell Physiology, 290,* C1018–C1030.
5. Tannock, G. W. (2002). In *Probiotics and Prebiotics: where are we going?* (pp. 1–39). London: Caister Academic Press.
6. Gibson, G. R., & Roberfroid, M. B. (1995). The bifidogenic nature of chicory inulin and its hydrolysis products. *Journal of Nutrition, 125,* 1401–1412.
7. Ouwehand, A., Salminen, S., & Isolauri, E. (2002). Probiotics, an overview of beneficial effects. *Antoine van Leeuwenhoek, 82,* 279–289.
8. Heselmans, M., Reid, G., Akkermans, L. M., et al. (2005). Gut flora in health and disease: potential role of probiotics. *Current Issues in Intestinal Microbiology, 6,* 1–7.
9. Schultz, M., Munro, K., Tannock, G. W., et al. (2004). Effects of feeding probiotic preparation (SIM) containing inulin on the severity of colitis and on the composition of the intestinal microflora HLA-B27 transgenic rats. *Clinical and Diagnostic Laboratory Immunology, 11,* 581–587.
10. Talwalkar, A., & Kailasapathy, K. (2004). The role of oxygen in the viability of probiotic bacteria with reference to *L. acidophilus* and *Bifidobacterium* spp. *Current Issues in Intestinal Microbiology, 5,* 1–8.
11. Gagnon, M., Kheadr, E. E., Le Blay, G., & Fliss, I. (2004). *In vitro* inhibition of *Escherichia coli* O157:H7 by bifidobacterial strains of human origin. *International Journal of Food Microbiology, 92,* 69–78.
12. Isolauri, E., Kirjavainen, P. V., & Salminen, S. (2002). Probiotics: a role in the treatment of intestinal infection and inflammation? *Gut, 50*(Suppl. 3), iii54–iii59.
13. Seksik, P., Rigottier-Gois, L., Gramet, G., et al. (2003). Alterations of the dominant fecal bacteria groups in patients with Crohn's disease of the colon. *Gut, 52,* 237–242.
14. Balsari, A., Ceccarelli, A., Dubini, F., et al. (1982). The fecal microbial population in the irritable bowel syndrome. *Microbiologica, 5,* 185–194.
15. Watanabe, S., Narisawa, Y., Arase, S., et al. (2003). Differences in fecal microflora between patients with

atopic dermatitis and healthy control subjects. *Journal of Allergy and Clinical Immunology, 111*, 587–591.

16. Matsuki, T., Watanabe, K., & Tanaka, R. (2003). Genus- and species-specific PCR primers for the detection and indentification of bifidobacteria. *Current Issues in Intestinal Microbiology, 4*, 61–69.

17. Delcenserie, V., Bechoux, N., China, B., et al. (2005). A PCR method for detection of bifidobacteria in raw milk and raw milk cheese: comparison with culture-based methods. *Journal of Microbiological Methods, 61*, 55–67.

18. Ishibashi, N., & Yamazaki, S. (2001). Probiotics and safety. *American Journal of Clinical Nutrition, 73*(Suppl.), 465s–470s.

19. Kostrzynska, M., & Bachand, A. (2006). Application of DNA microarray technology for detection, identification, and characterization of food-borne pathogens. *Canadian Journal of Microbiology, 52*, 1–8.

20. Montesi, A., Garcia-Albiach, R., Pozuelo, M. J., et al. (2005). Molecular and microbiological analysis of caecal microbiota in rats fed with diets supplemented either with prebiotics or probiotics. *International Journal of Food Microbiology, 98*, 281–290.

21. Vitali, B., Candela, M., Matteuzzi, D., & Brigidi, P. (2003). Quantitative detection of probiotic *Bifidobacterium* strains in bacterial mixtures by using real-time PCR. *Systematic and Applied Microbiology, 26*, 269–276.

22. Liu-Stratton, Y., Roy, S., & Sen, C. K. (2004). DNA microarray technology in nutraceutical and food safety. *Toxicology Letters, 150*, 29–42.

23. Hooper, L. V., Wong, M. H., Thelin, A., et al. (2001). Molecular analysis of commensal host-microbial relationships in the intestine. *Science, 29*, 881–884.

24. Haarman, M., & Knol, J. (2005). Quantitative real-time PCR assays to identify and quantify fecal *Bifidobacterium* species in infants receiving a prebiotic infant formula. *Applied and Environmental Microbiology, 71*, 2318–2324.

25. Sergeev, N., Distler, M., Courtney, S., et al. (2004). Multipathogen oligonucleotide micrarray for environmental and biodefense applications. *Biosensor and Bioelectronics, 20*, 684–698.

26. Lemarchand, K., Masson, L., & Brousseau, R. (2004). Molecular biology and DNA microarray technology for microbial quality monitoring of water. *Critical Reviews in Microbiology, 30*, 145–172.

27. Wang, Y., Barbacioru, C., Hyland, F., et al. (2006). Large scale real-time PCR validation on gene expression measurements from two commercial long-oligonucleotide microarrays. *BMC Genomics, 7*, 59–75.

28. Lipp, M., Bluth, A., Eyquem, F., et al. (2001). Validation of a method based on polymerase chain reaction for the detection of genetically modified organism in various processed foodstuff. *European Food Research and Technology, 212*, 497–504.

29. Meyer, R. (1999). Development and application of DNA analytical methods for the detection of GMOs in food. *Food Control, 10*, 391–399.

30. Ventura, M., van Sinderen, D., Fitzgerald, G. F., & Zink, R. (2004). Insights into the taxonomy, genetics and physiology of bifidobacteria. *Antonie Van Leeuwenhoek, 86*, 205–223.

31. Garrigues, C., Stuer-Lauridsen, B., & Johansen, E. (2005). Characterization of *Bifidobacterium animalis* subsp. *lactis* BB-12 and other probiotic bacteria using genomics, transcriptomics and proteomics. *Australian Journal of Dairy Technology, 60*, 84–92.

32. Wang, R. F., Kim, S. J., Robertson, L. H., & Cerniglia, C. E. (2002). Development of a membrane-array method for the detection of human intestinal bacteria in fecal samples. *Molecular and Cellular Probes, 16*, 341–350.

33. Wang, R. F., Beggs, M. L., Robertson, L. H., & Cerniglia, C. E. (2002). Design and evaluation of oligonucleotide-microarray method for the detection of human intestinal bacterial in fecal samples. *FEMS Microbiology Letters, 213*, 175–182.

34. Cerniglia, C. E., & Kotarski, S. (1999). Evaluation of veterinary drug residue in food for their potential to affect human intestinal microflora. *Regulatory Toxicology and Pharmacology, 29*, 238–261.

35. Hill, M. J., & Marsh, P. D. (Eds.) (1990). *Control of the large bowel microflora*. Florida: CRC Press (pp. 95–100).

36. Moore, W. E. C., & Moore, L. H. (1995). Intestinal floras of populations that have a high risk of colon cancer. *Applied and Environmental Microbiology, 61*, 3202–3207.

37. Wang, R. F., Beggs, M. L., Erickson, B. D., & Cerniglia, C. E. (2004). DNA microarray analysis of predominant human intestinal bacteria in fecal samples. *Molecular and Cell Probes, 18*, 223–234.

38. Harrington, C. R., Lucchini, S., Ridgway, K. P., et al. (2008). A short-oligonucleotide microarray that allows improved detection of gastrointestinal tract microbial communities. *BMC Microbiology, 8*, 195.

39. Palmer, C., Bik, M. B., DiGiulio, D. B., et al. (2007). Development of the human infant intestinal microbiota. *PloS Biology, 5*, e177.

40. Gibson, G. R., & Roberfroid, M. B. (1995). Dietary modulation of the human colonic microbiota: Introducing the concept of prebiotics. *Journal of Nutrition, 125*, 1401–1412.

41. Barrangou, R. E., Altermann, E., Hutkins, R., et al. (2003). Functional and comparative genomic analyses of an operon involved in fructo-oligosaccharide utilization by *Lactobacillus acidophilus*. *Proceedings of the National Academy of Sciences of the United States of America, 100*, 8957–8962.

42. Kaplan, H., & Hutkins, R. (2000). Fermentation of fructooligosaccharides by lactic acid bacteria and bifidobacteria. *Applied and Environmental Microbiology, 66*, 2682–2684.

43. Saulnier, D. M. A., Molenaar, D., De Vos, W. M., et al. (2007). Identification of prebiotic fructo-oligosaccharide metabolism in *Lactobacillus plantarum* WCFS1 through microarrays. *Applied and Environmental Microbiology, 73,* 1753–1765.

44. Barrangou, R., Azcarate-Peril, M. A., Duong, T., et al. (2006). Global analysis of carbohydrate utilization by *Lactobacillus acidophilus* using cDNA microarrays. *Proceedings of the National Academy of Sciences of the United States of America, 103,* 3816–3821.

45. Parche, S., Amon, J., Jankovic, I., et al. (2007). Sugar transport systems of *Bifidobacterium longum* NCC2705. *Journal of Molecular Microbiology and Biotechnology, 12,* 9–19.

46. O'Mahony, L., McCarthy, J., Kelly, P., et al. (2005). *Lactobacillus* and *Bifidobacterium* in irritable bowel syndrome: symptom responses and relationship to cytokine profiles. *Gastroenterology, 128,* 541–551.

47. Whorwell, P. J., Altringer, L., Morel, J., et al. (2006). Efficacy of an encapsulated probiotic *Bifidobacterium infantis* 35624 in women with irritable bowel syndrome. *American Journal of Gastroenterology, 101,* 1581–1590.

48. Guyonnet, D., Chassany, O., Ducrotte, P., et al. (2007). Effect of a fermented milk containing *Bifidbacterium animalis* DN-173 010 on the health-related quality of life and symptoms in irritable bowel syndrome in adults in primary care: a multicenter, randomized, double-blind, controlled trial. *Alimentary Pharmacology & Therapeutics, 26,* 475–486.

49. Niedzielin, K., Kordecki, H., & Birkenfeld, B. (2001). A controlled, double-blind, randomized study on the efficacy of *Lactobacillus plantarum* 299v in patients with irritable bowel syndrome. *European Journal of Gastroenterology & Hepatology, 13,* 1143–1147.

50. Sen, S., Mullan, M., Parker, T. J., et al. (2002). Effect of *Lactobacillus plantarum* 299v on colonic fermentation and symptoms of irritable bowel syndrome. *Digestive Diseases and Sciences, 47,* 2615–2620.

51. Kim, H. J., Camilleri, M., McKinizie, S., et al. (2003). A randomized controlled trial of a probiotic, VSL#3, on gut transit and symptoms in diarrhea-predominant irritable bowel syndrome. *Alimentary Pharmacology & Therapeutics, 17,* 895–904.

52. Kim, H. J., Vazquez Roque, M. I., Camilleri, M., et al. (2005). A randomized controlled trial of a probiotic combination VSL#3 and placebo in irritable bowel syndrome with bloating. *Neurogastroenterology and Motility, 17,* 687–696.

53. Kajander, K., Hatakka, K., Poussa, T., et al. (2005). A probiotic mixture alleviates symptoms in irritable bowel syndrome patients: a controlled 6-month intervention. *Alimentary Pharmacology & Therapeutics, 22,* 387–394.

54. Kajander, K., Myllyluoma, E., Rajilic-Stojanovics, M., et al. (2008). Clinical trial: multispecies probiotic supplementation alleviates the symptoms of irritable bowel syndrome and stabilizes intestinal microbiota. *Alimentary Pharmacology & Therapeutics, 27,* 48–57.

55. Troost, F. J., van Baarlen, P., Lindsey, P., et al. (2008). Identification of the transcriptional responses of human intestinal mucosa to *Lactobacillus plantarum* WCFS1 *in vivo. BMC Genomics, 9,* 374.

56. Di Caro, S., Tao, H., Grillo, A., et al. (2005). Effects of *Lactobacillus* GG on genes expression pattern in small bowel mucosa. *Digestive and Liver Disease, 37,* 320–329.

57. Di Caro, S., Tao, H., Grillo, A., et al. (2005). *Bacillus clausii* effect on gene expression pattern in small bowel mucosa using DNA microarray analysis. *European Journal of Gastroenterology & Hepatology, 17,* 951–960.

58. Ukena, S. N., Westendorf, A. M., Hansen, W., et al. (2005). The host response to the probiotic *Escherichia coli* strain Nissle 1917: specific up-regulation of the proinflammatory chemokine MCP-1. *BMC Medical genetics, 6,* 43–56.

59. Zyrek, A., Cichon, C., Helms, S., et al. (2007). Molecular mechanisms underlying the probiotic effects of *Escherichia coli* Nissle 1917 involve ZO-2 and PKC redistribution resulting in tight junction and epithelial barrier repair. *Cellular Microbiology, 9,* 804–816.

60. Philpott, D. J. S., Yamaoka, A., Israel, A., & Sansonetti, P. J. (2000). Invasive *Shigella flexneri* activates NF-kB through a lipopolysaccharide-dependent innate intracellular response and leads to IL-8 expression in epithelial cells. *Journal of Immunology, 165,* 903–914.

61. Chen, M. L., Pothoulakis, C., & LaMont, J. T. (2002). Protein kinase C signaling regulates ZO-1 translocation and increased paracellular flux of T84 colonocytes exposed to *Clostridium difficile* toxin. *A Journal of Biological Chemistry, 277,* 4247–4254.

62. Martin, C. R., & Walker, W. A. (2008). Probiotics: role in pathophysiology and prevention in necrotizing enterocolitis. *Seminars in Perinatology, 32,* 127–137.

63. Lin, P. W., Nasr, T. R., Berardinelli, A. J., et al. (2008). The probiotic *Lactobacillus* GG may augment intestinal host defense by regulating apoptosis and promoting cytoprotective responses in the developing murine gut. *Pediatric Research, 64,* 511–516.

64. Sartor, R. B. (2004). Therapeutic manipulation of the enteric microflora in inflammatory bowel diseases: antibiotics, probiotics and prebiotics. *Gastroenterology, 126,* 1620–1633.

65. Spiller, R. (2005). Probiotics: an ideal anti-inflammatory treatment for IBS? *Gastroenterology, 128,* 783–785.

66. Shima, T., Fukushima, S., Setoyama, H., et al. (2008). Differential effects of two probiotic strains with different bacteriological properties on intestinal gene expression,

with special reference to indigenous bacteria. *FEMS Immunology and Medical Microbiology*, *52*, 69–77.

67. Baken, K. A., Ezendam, J., Gremmer, E. R., et al. (2006). Evaluation of immunomodulation by *Lactobacillus casei* Shirota: Immune function, autoimmunity and gene expression. *International Journal of Food Microbiology*, *112*, 8–18.

68. Kostrzynska, M., Lepp, D., Ojha, S. & Carey, C. (2006). Mitigation of *E. coli* O157:H7 virulence. Federal Food Safety and Nutrition Meeting, October 11–12, 2006, Ottawa, ON, Canada.

69. De Keersmaecker, S. C. J., Marchal, K., Verhoeven, T. L. A., et al. (2005). Microarray analysis and motif detection reveal new targets of the *Salmonella enterica* serovar *Typhimurium* HilA regulatory protein, including *hilA* itself. *Journal of Bacteriology*, *187*, 4381–4391.

70. Philpott, D. J. S., Yamaoka, A., Israel, A., & Sansonetti, P. J. (2000). Invasive *Shigella flexneri* activates NF-kB through a lipopolysaccharide-dependent innate intracellular response and leads to IL-8 expression in epithelial cells. *Journal of Immunology*, *165*, 903–914.

71. Tien, M. T., Girardin, S. E., Regnault, B., et al. (2006). Anti-inflammatory effect of *Lactobacillus casei* on *Shigella*-infected human intestinal epithelial cells. *Journal of Immunology*, *176*, 1228–1237.

72. Panigrahi, P., Braileanu, G. T., Chen, H., & Stine, O. C. (2007). Probiotic bacteria changes *Escherichia coli*-induced gene expression in cultured colonocytes: implications in intestinal pathophysiology. *World Journal of Gastroenterology*, *13*, 6370–6378.

73. Berger, B., Pridmore, R. D., Barretto, C., et al. (2007). Similarity and differences in the *Lactobacillus acidophilus* group identified by polyphasic analysis and comparative genomics. *Journal of Bacteriology*, *189*, 1311–1321.

74. Molenaar, D., Bringel, F., Schuren, F. H., et al. (2005). Exploring *Lactobacillus plantarum* genome diversity using microarrays. *Journal of Bacteriology*, *187*, 6119–6127.

75. Boesten, R. J., Schuren, F. H. J., & de Vos, W. M. (2009). A *Bifidobacterium* mixed-species microarray for high resolution discrimination between intestinal bifidobacteria. *Journal of Microbiological Methods*, *76*, 269–277.

76. Klaassens, E. S., Boesten, R. J., Haarman, M., et al. (2009). Mixed-species genomic microarray analysis of fecal samples reveals differential transcriptional responses of bifidobacteria in breast- and formula-fed infants. *Applied Environmental Microbiology*, *75*, 2668–2676.

77. Spinler, J. K., Saulnier, D. M. A., Balderas, M. A., et al. (2008). Comparative genomic analyses in probiotic *Lactobacillus reuteri* strains reveal potential regulatory mechanisms for reuterin production. ASM Conference: Beneficial Microbes, October 12–16, 2008, San Diego, California, P-79A, pp. 47–48.

78. Wall, T., Bath, K., Britton, R. A., et al. (2007). The early response to acid shock in *Lactobacillus reuteri* involves the ClpL chaperone and a putative cell wall-altering esterase. *Applied and Environmental Microbiology*, *73*, 3924–3935.

79. Whitehead, K., Versalovic, J., Roos, S., & Britton, R. A. (2008). Genomic and genetic characterization of the bile stress response of probiotic *Lactobacillus reuteri* ATCC 55730. *Applied and Environmental Microbiology*, *74*, 1812–1819.

80. Denou, E., Pridmore, R. D., Berger, B., et al. (2008). Identification of genes associated with the long-gut-persistence phenotype of the probiotic *Lactobacillus johnsonii* strain NCC533 using a combination of genomics and transcriptome analysis. *Journal of Bacteriology*, *190*, 3161–3168.

81. Azcarate-Peril, M. A., McAuliffe, O., Altermann, E., et al. (2005). Microarray analysis of a two-component regulatory system involved in acid resistance and proteolytic activity in *Lactobacillus acidophilus*. *Applied Environmental Microbiology*, *71*, 5794–5804.

82. Sanders, M. E., & Klaenhammer, T. R. (2001). Invited review: the scientific basis of *Lactobacillus acidophilus* NCFM functionality as a probiotic. *Journal of Dairy Science*, *84*, 319–331.

83. Perreten, V., Vorlet-Fawer, L., Slickers, P., et al. (2005). Microarray-based detection of 90 antibiotic resistance genes of Gram-positive bacteria. *Journal of Clinical Microbiology*, *43*, 2291–2302.

84. Kastner, S., Perreten, V., Bleuler, H., et al. (2006). Antibiotic susceptibility patterns and resistance genes of starter cultures and probiotic bacteria used in food. *Systematic and Applied Microbiology*, *29*, 145–155.

Probiotics in Cancer Prevention

Alejandra de Moreno de LeBlanc,[1]
María Eugenia Bibas Bonet,[2] Jean Guy LeBlanc,[1]
Fernando Sesma[1], and Gabriela Perdigón[1,2]

[1]Centro de Referencia para Lactobacilos (CERELA-CONICET), Chacabuco 145,
San Miguel de Tucumán (T4000ILC) Tucumán, Argentina
[2]Cátedra de Inmunología. Instituto de Microbiología, Facultad de Bioquímica, Química y Farmacia,
Universidad Nacional de Tucumán, Tucumán, Argentina

1. EFFECT OF PROBIOTIC BACTERIA ON CANCER PREVENTION

1.1. Experimental and Epidemiological Studies

Probiotics have been given credit for numerous health-promoting effects; one of which is their anticarcinogenic properties [1]. Their connection with the prevention of animal and human cancers has been extensively reviewed [2, 3]. The effects of probiotics on intestinal disorders have been the most extensively studied because they can beneficially affect the intestinal microbiota, which are involved in many of these disorders. The increase of immune cell activity in the prevention of cancer by lactic acid bacteria (LAB) consumption has also been described [4, 5]. For these reasons, the effects of probiotic or fermented products containing LAB are extensively studied for colon cancer. Probiotics such as lactobacilli and bifidobacteria in fermented or culture-containing dairy foods such as yogurt may play a role in reducing the risk of colon cancer [6–8].

There are many different mechanisms by which fermented products containing viable LAB may lower the risk of colon cancer:

1. The reduction of procarcinogenic substances such as mutagenic compounds commonly found in the western meat-rich diet, that can be bound to the intestinal and lactic acid bacteria *in vitro*, has been correlated with the reduction in the mutagenicity observed after exposure to the bacterial strains [9, 10]. It is possible that the LAB supplementation can influence the uptake and excretion of mutagens by simply binding to them in the intestine.

2. Probiotics can also indirectly act by reducing the level of certain enzymes such as β-glucuronidase, azoreductase,

497

nitroreductase, among others, which convert procarcinogens to carcinogens in the intestine [6, 11, 12]. The consumption of *Lactobacillus* (*L.*) *acidophilus* in experimental animal models reduced the activity of fecal enzymes such as β-glucuronidase, azoreductase and nitroreductase [13, 14]. The products of these enzymes are known to be mutagenic and carcinogenic and their activities have been well correlated with the number of certain bacteria in the intestine. Goldin and Gorbach also studied the effect of feeding two *L. acidophilus* strains on the activity of these bacterial enzymes in 21 healthy volunteers [12]. The continuous consumption of these bacteria was necessary to maintain the effect; a reversal of the effect was observed within 10–30 days of stopping *Lactobacillus* feeding.

3. The production of short-chain fatty acids, such as butyrate and propionate, is another mechanism by which probiotics may help in the treatment for colorectal cancer [15].

4. It has also been suggested that LAB or compounds produced by these microorganisms may directly interact with tumor cells in culture and inhibit their growth, supporting the idea that they can directly produce anti-tumorigenic or anti-mutagenic compounds [16].

5. The modulation of the host immune system is one of the effects attributed to the LAB or fermented products that contain them [17]. This effect was studied against many pathologies and included different types of cancers.

Unfortunately, little epidemiologic evidence exists that relates probiotics or probiotic-containing fermented foods and cancer incidences.

A few case-controlled studies have been conducted to evaluate the effects of yogurt or fermented milks on some cancer rates. Lê Monique et al. [18] reported a study in France where an inverse relationship between frequency of yogurt consumption and risk of breast cancer was found. Peters et al. [19] found that yogurt consumption can be a protective factor in a case-controlled study of colon cancer incidences in Los Angeles. Another case-controlled study of breast cancer in the Netherlands suggested that fermented dairy products could be protective [20]. One human trial showed that the recurrence rate for superficial bladder cancer was lower for subjects receiving freeze-dried *L. casei* Shirota than a placebo [21]. Additional similar studies are important to clarify the role that probiotic products play in cancer rates.

2. YOGURT FEEDING IN THE INHIBITION OF THE DEVELOPMENT OF AN INTESTINAL TUMOR

Colon cancer inhibition by conventional yogurt (a coagulated milk product that results from the lactic acid fermentation of milk by pools of *L. delbrueckii* subsp. *bulgaricus* and *Streptococcus* (*S.*) *thermophilus* strains) was studied in an experimental model using BALB/c mice [22]. Animals were fed with yogurt for 10 consecutive days, the period of time where previously the best effects of this yogurt on the intestinal immune system were reported [23, 24]. Colon tumors were chemically induced by a dimethylhydrazine (DMH) injection and the animals were given yogurt cyclically again after tumor induction (for 10 consecutive days followed by a 1-week break and then again for 10 days) until the end of the experiment (6 months). Yogurt feeding inhibited tumor growth (yogurt-DMH-yogurt group) and decreased the large inflammatory immune response observed during tumor development in the large intestine of the mice treated only with DMH (DMH group). The administration of yogurt to DMH-injected mice resulted in an increase in the number of IgA secreting cells and CD4+ T lymphocytes in the lamina propria of the large intestine together with a decrease in the IgG+ and CD8+ cells [25] (see Table 29.1). The increase in the number of IgA secreting cells, but not of IgG+ cells, in the large intestine of the mice fed with yogurt could limit the inflammatory response, since IgA is considered as an important barrier in colonic neoplasia [26].

2.1. Relationship between Inflammation and Tumor

The association of chronic inflammation with several malignant diseases has been reported for a long time [27]. There is also evidence that this relationship would be mediated by cytokines [28] or by a reactive oxygen species generated by inflammatory phagocytes that can cause injury to target cells, thus contributing to cancer development [29].

At the intestinal level, examples of the above include intestinal cancer after intestinal chronic inflammation [30, 31]; patients with persistent ulcerative colitis have a 5 to 7 times greater incidence of colon cancer development [32]. In the relationship between inflammation and tumors, non-steroidal anti-inflammatory drugs (NSAID)—which are inhibitors of the cyclooxygenase enzyme (COX)—can delay or prevent the development and metastasis of certain cancers [33, 34]. Based on the results obtained with yogurt in DMH-injected mice, where an anti-inflammatory effect was attributed to this fermented milk, a NSAID (indometacin) was used to compare its effect with the anti-tumor activity of yogurt. Mice treated with indometacin showed that the immune cells infiltrating into the large intestine were smaller than the same observed with yogurt feeding (yogurt-DMH-yogurt group) where a great increase in the number of immune cells infiltrating the lamina propria was found [35]. This cellular infiltration also occurred in the large intestine of mice without carcinogen injection and fed yogurt continuously, suggesting that these infiltrative cells might play an important role in the antitumoral and anti-inflammatory activity of yogurt. It was also observed that the effects of the indometacin treatment were maintained when the drug was administered. When indometacin administration was stopped due to cachexia produced in the animals, the tumor developed with the same characteristics as in the DMH group in the sixth month [35]. This last observation showed different mechanisms for indometacin and yogurt, since when the yogurt feeding was stopped at the end of the experiment (6 months), the animals from the yogurt-DMH-yogurt group which was observed over a 9-month period did not develop tumors.

Most of the anti-inflammatory drugs studied by different authors and using different models exert their antitumor activities during the early stages of tumor development. It is known that the development of colon cancer presents a sequence of events that occurs in definable steps (initiation, promotion and progression).

In order to find out at which stage of the tumor process yogurt acted (initiation, promotion or progression of tumor growth), we studied whether previous feeding with yogurt was sufficient by itself in order to reach the regulatory immune response observed; or whether the cyclical administration of yogurt after DMH injections was necessary to prevent the effect of the carcinogen. The results obtained showed that previous yogurt feeding for 10 days before the DMH injections (yogurt-DMH group) only delayed tumor appearance [36]. Tumor tissue with the same characteristics as the DMH group was observed in the seventh month. Thus, yogurt administration before DMH injections was not enough to inhibit the tumor in the initiation stage. To identify if the yogurt feeding can act after tumor initiation, another group of animals did not receive yogurt previous to DMH injection but were fed cyclically with this fermented milk after tumor induction following the same protocol as the yogurt-DMH-yogurt group. This group of mice

(DMH-yogurt group) did not develop tumor and it was very similar to the yogurt-DMH-yogurt group previously described. In both groups, the number of immune cells increased in the lamina propria of the large intestine.

These results demonstrate that yogurt exerts its antitumor activity by the inhibition of tumor progression and that this effect is achieved by long-term cyclical yogurt consumption [36] (Table 29.1).

2.2. Study of Cytokines as Mediators of the Anti-inflammatory Effects of Yogurt

Different cytokines were studied using immunofluorescent methods on large intestine slices or isolated infiltrating immune cells from the large intestine taken from the different groups of mice.

Pro-inflammatory cytokines (TNFα and IFNγ) increased in cells from the large intestines of the tumor control mice (DMH group, Table 29.1) and in the groups fed with yogurt where the mice did not develop tumors (yogurt-DMH-yogurt and DMH-yogurt groups, Table 29.1) [35, 36]. Yogurt feeding itself also produced high levels of these pro-inflammatory cytokines [25]. In cells from the nodular infiltrates of the large intestine, yogurt feeding increased TNFα and IFNγ producing cells compared to the tumor control group [36]. It was shown that in this experimental model, adherent cells (macrophages/monocytes) produced increased amounts of TNFα compared

TABLE 29.1 Study of the anti-inflammatory effect of yogurt compared to an NSAID

Experimental group	Period of treatment	Number of cells positive for						
		IgA[a]	CD4[a]	CD8[a]	TNFα[b]	IFNγ[b]	IL-10[b]	iNOS[b]
DMH	2 months	60 ± 8^d	20 ± 3^d	50 ± 2^h	68 ± 4^g	$86 \pm 15^{f,g}$	$51 \pm 10^{e,g}$	23 ± 5^e
	4 months	$70 \pm 7^{d,e}$	22 ± 3^d	50 ± 3^h	155 ± 22^h	140 ± 17^h	87 ± 11^f	41 ± 5^f
	6 months	ND	36 ± 2^e	80 ± 4^i	125 ± 10^h	99 ± 22^g	$67 \pm 15^{e,f}$	25 ± 5^e
Y-DMH-Y[c]	2 months	100 ± 10^f	40 ± 2^e	30 ± 2^i	64 ± 7^g	105 ± 6^g	58 ± 13^e	$15 \pm 5^{d,e}$
	4 months	100 ± 7^f	82 ± 5^f	40 ± 2^g	$57 \pm 18^{f,g}$	$121 \pm 27^{g,h}$	88 ± 4^f	$14 \pm 4^{d,e}$
	6 months	ND	35 ± 3^d	10 ± 1^g	$75 \pm 10^{f,g}$	86 ± 7^g	40 ± 7^g	12 ± 2^d
DMH-indometacin	2 months	$76 \pm 14^{d,e,f}$	41 ± 6^e	$24 \pm 5^{e,f}$	$42 \pm 10^{e,f}$	69 ± 9^f	ND	24 ± 5^e
	4 months	106 ± 24^f	22 ± 3^d	$17 \pm 6^{d,e}$	$27 \pm 10^{d,e}$	$23 \pm 5^{d,e}$	ND	18 ± 3^e
	6 months	114 ± 22^f	32 ± 6^e	$22 \pm 5^{e,f}$	16 ± 7^d	35 ± 8^e	ND	20 ± 2^e
Yogurt basal	10 days	$84 \pm 11^{e,f}$	19 ± 3^d	10 ± 3^d	29 ± 3^e	$25 \pm 3^{d,e}$	13 ± 2^d	8 ± 2^d
Non-treatment control		65 ± 5^d	20 ± 3^d	11 ± 2^d	17 ± 2^d	21 ± 2^d	12 ± 3^d	10 ± 2^d

[a]IgA+, CD4+ and CD8+ cells were analyzed by direct immunofluorescence on large intestine tissues.
[b]The cells positive for cytokines and iNOS enzyme were analyzed by indirect immunofluorescence in the lamina propria of the large intestine tissues. Results are expressed as number of positive cells for the corresponding, immunoglobulin, marker, cytokine or protein in 10 fields of vision as seen at 1000× magnification using a fluorescence light microscope.
[c]Y-DMH-Y = yogurt-DMH-yogurt.
[d,e,f,g,h,i]Values for each column without a common letter differ significantly ($p < 0.05$).
ND = Not determined.

to non-adherent cells (fibroblast, mast cells and some T and NK cells). IFNγ was also produced for both cell populations. All of these observations showed that yogurt stimulates the activity of infiltrative cells (adherent and non-adherent), which increased cytokine production, necessary for tumor resolution.

In contrast to yogurt, mice treated with the anti-inflammatory drug (indometacin) presented fewer infiltrating cells in the large intestine with a low number of TNFα and IFNγ secreting cells (Table 29.1). When the drug treatment was stopped, both cells and pro-inflammatory cytokines increased and the tumor grew [35].

For the purpose of demonstrating that this pro-inflammatory cytokine increase in the large intestine of mice fed yogurt was not related with an inflammatory response in the gut and that these cytokines were being regulated, the inducible nitric oxide synthase (iNOS) enzyme was studied. The iNOS enzyme is induced during the course of the immune response by microbial products and/or cytokines (such as IFNγ) and plays a role in the antimicrobial mechanism of macrophages [37]. It was reported that tumor-bearing mice (DMH group) presented high amounts of iNOS+ cells, suggesting an increase in nitric oxide (NO) production by these cells. The iNOS enzyme synthesis would be induced by IFNγ which was increased in the intestinal tissue from this group. The DMH-indometacin group showed an increased number of iNOS+ cells before anti-inflammatory treatment and at the end of the study, when the tumor grew, during the anti-inflammatory treatment; this enzyme was maintained in the basal intestinal level (Table 29.1). The iNOS+ cells' increases are consistent with the increases of IFNγ+ cells in this group. In the group of mice injected with DMH and fed with yogurt, when the inflammation decreased, the iNOS+ cells also decreased; even when the IFNγ secreting cell numbers remained elevated (Table 29.1), demonstrating that yogurt would regulate the immune system by modulating the inflammatory response [35].

These results suggest that the immune mechanisms by which yogurt operates would be different from those induced with the anti-inflammatory drug indometacin, which did not show an increased activity of the infiltrative immune cells in the large intestine, where cytokine levels were lower than in the other groups and iNOS diminution was only evident during treatment.

In spite of the increased number of IFNγ+ cells, the animals fed with yogurt did not show increased NO production or presence of tumor, only cellular infiltration. The large number of positive cells for this cytokine in mice fed with yogurt could be related to the increase in the number of immune cells that produce the pro-inflammatory cytokines in the intestine which could, in turn, be regulated by other regulatory cytokines such as IL-10.

The study of IL-10 secreting cells showed significant increases of this cytokine in all the groups assayed; but it is important to note that yogurt feeding always produced more IL-10+ cells in the yogurt-DMH-yogurt group than in the DMH group [25, 35].

IL-4 was also studied as another cytokine that can regulate the response against IFNγ, but yogurt feeding did not exert any effect on the production of this cytokine in the gut immune cells.

It appears that yogurt could modulate the immune response by: 1) stimulating cytokine production when this is required; or 2) inducing down-regulation of the immune cells to avoid an exacerbated immune response. This effect would occur mainly through IL-10, which was increased in the tissue during all the assayed periods.

2.3. Other Non-immune Mechanisms Involved in the Antitumor Effect of Yogurt

The mechanisms of apoptosis, also known as programmed cell deaths, in the inhibition of tumor progression are well documented [38].

The colonic epithelium is a tissue with a high cell turnover rate. The balance between cell proliferation and cell death is important to maintain the length of the crypts and a disturbance in this balance may lead to tumor development [39], since the disruption of this type of regulation is a characteristic of the tumors.

Considering that cytokines such as TNFα could be involved in certain apoptotic pathways [40], and that an enhancement of this cytokine was observed in the experimental model described above, apoptosis induction and the relationship between mitosis and apoptosis were studied. An increase in mitosis during the first 4 weeks of tumor growth was observed in the animals treated with the carcinogen. In the mice

from the yogurt-DMH-yogurt group, a moderate cell proliferation with a significant increase in the number of apoptotic cells was reported [41] (Table 29.2).

It is also important to mention the fact that the intestinal inflammatory process preceding tumor development may be due to changes in the epithelial cells induced by the carcinogen that enters the intestine as a glucuronide, a compound synthesized and deconjugated by the gut normal microbiota. It is possible that yogurt bacteria can also affect gut flora enzymes related to colon carcinogenesis as reported for other probiotics in different animal tumors. It was demonstrated that mice injected with DMH and fed cyclically with yogurt presented lower

TABLE 29.2 Non-immune mechanisms involved in the antitumoral effect of yogurt

Experimental group	Period of treatment	Number of apoptotic cells[a]	β-glucuronidase[b]		Nitroreductase[b]	
			BGBB[c]	AGBB[d]	BGBB[c]	AGBB[d]
DMH	2 months	43 ± 5^g	3.37 ± 1.01^f	$9.38 \pm 3.24^{g,h}$	26.27 ± 5.01^i	28.51 ± 5.77^l
	4 months	$47 \pm 6^{g,h}$	26.66 ± 4.69^i	19.50 ± 4.95^i	5.30 ± 2.09^g	$6.01 \pm 1.25^{h,i}$
	5 months	ND	8.58 ± 2.05^g	17.91 ± 2.74^i	17.03 ± 2.81^h	18.26 ± 2.26^k
Y-DMH-Y[e]	2 months	110 ± 10^i	3.31 ± 1.28^f	11.25 ± 2.63^h	$18.77 \pm 5.89^{h,i}$	$22.04 \pm 5.89^{k,l}$
	4 months	60 ± 9^h	17.21 ± 1.93^h	$10.01 \pm 3.77^{g,h}$	0.72 ± 0.34^f	2.01 ± 0.88^f
	5 months	27 ± 7^f	7.35 ± 1.46^g	6.33 ± 2.18^g	1.17 ± 0.67^f	$2.89 \pm 1.01^{f,g}$
Yogurt	2 months	ND	3.89 ± 1.66^f	$5.36 \pm 2.40^{f,g}$	11.25 ± 6.14^h	$7.98 \pm 2.02^{h,i,j}$
	4 months	$50 \pm 9^{g,h}$	8.56 ± 1.55^g	7.49 ± 0.69^g	3.51 ± 0.72^g	$4.95 \pm 1.2^{g,h}$
	5 months	99 ± 12^i	4.41 ± 0.12^f	3.19 ± 0.79^f	3.22 ± 0.60^g	11.25 ± 3.15^j
Non-treatment control	2 months	24 ± 3^f	3.04 ± 1.74^f	$9.27 \pm 2.84^{g,h}$	4.17 ± 1.97^g	$8.40 \pm 1.23^{i,j}$
	4 months	22 ± 6^f	9.51 ± 2.95^g	$7.13 \pm 2.37^{g,h}$	2.32 ± 0.99^g	2.31 ± 1.15^f
	5 months	20 ± 4^f	8.03 ± 3.77^g	$13.58 \pm 4.31^{h,i}$	3.15 ± 1.01^g	$3.22 \pm 0.95^{f,g}$

[a]Apoptotic cells were analyzed on the large intestine slides with a kit based in the TUNEL method. The results are expressed as means ± SD of the number of apoptotic cells counted in 10 fields of vision at 400× of magnification (cells/10 fields).
[b]Enzyme activities were analyzed directly in the intestinal fluid before or after glass beads breaking.
[c]Before glass beads breaking.
[d]After glass beads breaking.
[e]Y-DMH-Y = yogurt-DMH-yogurt.
[f,g,h,i,j,k,l]Values in each column without a common letter differ significantly ($p < 0.01$).
ND = Not determined.

enzyme activity levels than the tumor control group, which increased the activity of these microbial enzymes contributing in this way to its mutagenic power (Table 29.2). It is important to note that the decrease of these enzyme activities was observed in the samples before and after the cells were lysed with the glass beads, showing that yogurt feeding decreases the levels of the enzymes in the intestinal fluids and prevents their induction in the interior of the cells [42].

Feeding yogurt decreased procarcinogenic enzyme levels in the large intestine contents of mice bearing colon tumor. The results of this study provide another mechanism by which yogurt starter bacteria interact with the large intestine of the mice and prevent colon cancer.

3. EFFECT OF PROBIOTIC *LACTOBACILLUS CASEI* CRL431 IN THE INHIBITION OF CHEMICAL-INDUCED FIBROSARCOMA

The effects of probiotic LAB were also reported for other non-intestinal tumors. *L. casei* CRL 431 is a probiotic strain and its modulator effects on the mucosal immune system was extensively studied. The oral administration of *L. casei* CRL 431 to mice induced an immune stimulation not only at the intestinal level, but also in bronchus and mammary glands.

The antitumor activity of *L. casei* CRL 431 was studied against a fibrosarcoma induced by methylcholantrene in mice. It was demonstrated that this probiotic strain inhibited tumor growth in a dose-dependent form. The best effect was achieved by using a low dose (2×10^9 cells) of viable bacteria [43, 44]. Hematological values and alkaline phosphatase enzyme levels, phagocytic activity, β-glucuronidase enzyme and the cytotoxic activity in peritoneal macrophages from mice bearing tumor fed and unfed with

L. casei CRL 431 were determined. TNFα levels in serum and on immune cells isolated from the spleen were also measured. It was shown that the administration of this strain caused an anti-tumor activity by stimulation of the immune system, with high levels of macrophage activation (main infiltrative cells in the tumor) measured by an increase in the phagocytic and cytotoxic activity, high levels of TNFα and with a remarkable decrease in the tumor volume. The non-preventive effect in the inhibition of the tumor observed with high doses of *L. casei* CRL 431 might be due to an auto-regulation of the immune mechanisms in the gut as a consequence of an over stimulation [45, 46].

4. USE OF GENETICALLY MODIFIED CATALASE AND SUPEROXIDE DISMUTASE PRODUCING LAB IN THE PREVENTION OF COLON CANCER

Since oxidative stress and epithelial damage are normally linked to pathologies of the gastrointestinal tract of humans such as inflammatory bowel disease (IBD), another mechanism by which LAB could prevent certain types of cancer is through the use of antioxidant enzymes that can degrade reactive oxygen species (ROS) or impair their formation.

ROS are small molecules (such as superoxide ions, free radicals and peroxides) that are formed as by-products of the normal metabolism of oxygen. The biological sources of ROS are numerous and in low quantities participate in cell signaling and regulatory pathways. When they are produced in large amounts, as is the case in inflammatory processes, they act to eliminate infectious agents by causing significant damage to cell structures and macromolecular constituents such as DNA, RNA, proteins and lipids [47]. Toxicity occurs when the concentration of ROS exceeds the capacity of cell defense systems [48]. Large amounts of H_2O_2 are produced and excreted by human tumor cells [49] and might participate in tumor invasion and proliferation. Thus, oxidative stress plays an important role in pathologies of the gastrointestinal tract of humans such as IBD and certain types of cancers [50, 51].

The normal intestinal mucosa is equipped with a network of antioxidant enzymes that neutralize ROS in a two-steps pathway. First, superoxide dismutases (SODs) convert the primary superoxide anion (O_2^-) into the more stable metabolite, hydrogen peroxide (H_2O_2). Second, H_2O_2 is converted to water by catalase (CAT) or glutathione peroxidase (GPO). The activities of these enzymes are usually balanced to maintain a low and continual steady-state level of ROS. However, the levels of these enzymes in inflammatory disease patients, such as those suffering from IBD, are frequently depleted [50, 52], highlighting the potential for increasing the local levels of these enzymes to function as a therapeutic. Probiotic LAB strains expressing high levels of SOD and CAT could increase these enzyme activities in specific locations of the gastrointestinal tract and could thus contribute to prevent oxidative epithelial damage, giving rise to potential applications for the treatment of inflammatory diseases or post-cancer drug treatments.

Since the majority of LAB are not well equipped with enzymes to detoxify oxygen-derived compounds, the insertion of genes coding for antioxidant enzymes (such as catalases or SOD) in probiotic bacteria could improve their anti-inflammatory properties beyond the modulation of the local immune-dependent inflammation response. Catalases of three lactobacilli have been successfully cloned and expressed in heterologous bacteria lacking catalase activity [53–56]. The food-grade *Lactococcus (Lc.) lactis* is a potential vector to be used as a live vehicle to deliver heterologous proteins for vaccine and pharmaceutical purposes. Since *Lc. lactis* has no catalase, Rochat et al. [57] introduced the *B. subtilis* heme catalase *KatE* gene into this industrially important microorganism,

giving rise to a strain capable of producing active catalase that can provide efficient antioxidant activity. One report has shown that this genetically engineered strain was able to prevent tumor appearance in an experimental DMH-induced colon cancer model [58]. The catalase producing the *Lc. lactis* strain used in this study was able to slightly increase catalase activity in the intestines of mice treated with dimethylhydrazine (DMH), a colon cancer-inducing drug. This increased antioxidant activity was sufficient to reduce H_2O_2 levels in the large intestines, a ROS involved in cancer promotion and progression, showing that this catalase-producing LAB could be used in novel therapeutic strategies for gastrointestinal pathologies. In 2006, the heterologous expression of a non-heme catalase in bacteria relevant to dairy industries was reported [56]. A strain of *L. casei* was constructed to offer the advantage that no heme has to be added to the culture medium for catalase activity. Although this strain was able to reduce cecal and colonic inflammatory scores, no significant differences were observed compared to the use of the native non-catalase producing strain in a dextran sulfate sodium (DSS)-induced colitis mice model [59]. This is probably due to the insufficient production of catalase by this strain in the gastrointestinal tract. These authors suggest that, in order to optimize their antioxidative strategy, evaluation of the effects of co-administration of *L. casei* strains producing high levels of catalase and SOD from *Lc. lactis* [60] will be relevant as some previous studies showed the positive impact of increased SOD activity in intestinal inflammation models [50, 61, 62].

5. EFFECT OF FERMENTED MILK ADMINISTRATION IN A BREAST CANCER MODEL

Over the past decade, considerable advances have been made towards an understanding of the molecular factors involved in breast cancer development, but for women in most western countries, breast cancer still remains a major cause of death. There are genetic and environmental factors that increase the chances of breast cancer and the most common breast cancer types are estrogen-dependent. Some of the causing factors, such as the diet, can be controlled, whereas other cannot [63, 64]. It is known that women with high fat content diets have a higher risk of developing breast cancer; an example of this is that the oriental diet has traditionally been related with a low risk of this type of cancer in these populations.

In addition to containing LAB, fermented milks can possess non-bacterial components produced during fermentation that may contribute to their immunogenicity and to properties such as their anti-tumor activities. For this reason, cultured dairy products were proposed to inhibit the growth of many types of cancers, including breast tumors. Matar et al. [65] reported different roles and functions of biologically active peptides released from fermented milks. For example, peptidic fractions released during milk fermentation with L. helveticus R389, a strain with high proteolytic activity, stimulated the immune system and inhibited the growth of an immune-dependent fibrosarcoma in a mice model [66].

The influence of the immune cells on breast cancer was reported using different models [67, 68]. A substantial proportion (up to 50%) of breast tumors is comprised of cells from the immune system that infiltrate the tumors [69]. These cells produce different biological messengers such as cytokines, which are implicated in an antitumor response.

Given the existence of a common mucosal immune system, a fermented product that enters the organisms by the oral route can exert its influence on the immune cells associated not only with the gastrointestinal tract but also with other mucosal sites and associated glands, such as mammary glands.

In this way, it was reported that the oral administration of milk fermented with the proteolytic strain L. helveticus R389 increased the number of IgA secreting cells in the small intestine as well as in the bronchus of mice. However, fermented milk obtained with the proteolytic deficient mutant strain did not show the same results [66]. Considering these previous results, the effect of milk fermented by L. helveticus R389 or its proteolytic deficient variant, L. helveticus L89 was assayed on a murine hormone-dependent breast cancer model (using the ATCC tumoral cell line 4T1 injected in the upper right mammary gland), studying the systemic and local immune responses in the mammary glands and tumors.

Mice were fed with milk fermented by L. helveticus R389 (P+) or L89 (P−), for 7 days prior to the tumor cell injection. After that, they again received the fermented milk in a cyclical basis. The results obtained showed that the administration of both fermented milks either delayed or stopped tumor development [70] (Table 29.3). When the immune mechanisms were studied, and these two groups compared with the tumor control, different cytokines were analyzed in serum, in the mammary gland tissues and in the immune cells isolated from the tumor. The study of cytokine-positive cells in mammary glands furthered the understanding of the local cell response after mice were fed with fermented milk as well as after tumor injection. In the tumor isolated cells the analysis was performed because the role of tumor-infiltrating immune cells in antitumor immunity, as well as their potential for cancer immunotherapy, has been extensively reported [71, 72].

It was observed that in serum TNFα increased significantly in the basal sample from mice receiving milk fermented by L. helveticus R389 or L89 (Table 29.3). This increase prior to tumor induction could be related to the decrease of tumor growth in both experimental groups. The P(+) group maintained the TNFα concentration at close to the basal level throughout the trial, demonstrating a regulation of this cytokine, whereas the P(−) group showed increased TNFα in the last sample (similar to the control group, Table 29.3). In the tumor control group, TNFα levels increased in the function of the time, as did the tumor volume [70]. In the cells isolated from the tumor, TNFα increased in both groups fed with fermented milk where the tumor growth was delayed, leading to an induction of the cytokine production by fermented milk, which may play a biological role in the induction of cellular apoptosis [70] (Table 29.3).

IL-6 was studied in this model because this cytokine is implicated in estrogen synthesis [73], a hormone that the tumor needs to grow. It is also a pro-angiogenic factor [74], supporting the growth of new blood vessels that are also essential for tumor growth.

The tumor control group showed elevated levels of IL-6 in the serum and that IL-6+ cells increased in mammary gland tissues and in the immune cells infiltrating the tumor for this group. However, the P(+) and P(−) groups did not show increased levels of this cytokine in serum during the study, suggesting that this IL-6 decrease could be involved as one of the mechanisms for tumor growth delay. In the mammary glands, IL-6 secreting cell numbers were constant and similar in all groups until 18 days after tumor injection (Table 29.3). This result can be explained by the relationship between this cytokine and estrogen synthesis in the mammary gland; estrogens being essential in promoting the proper growth of this tumor cell line. These cytokine-positive cells increased even more after18 days in the tumor control group, and remained unmodified in both P(+) and P(−) groups [70]. In the isolated cells, all mice fed with fermented milk showed decreases in the number of IL-6+ cells compared to the tumor control group; P(+) being the group which presented the lowest number of cells positive for this cytokine (Table 29.3).

IL-10 was the cytokine that showed differences between both groups where the tumor growth was delayed. Serum IL-10 levels were significantly increased only in the P(+) group in relation to the tumor control group. Mice fed *L. helveticus* R389 showed increased IL-10 secreting cell numbers in the mammary glands throughout the time of the entire study. These were significantly higher numbers compared to the tumor control on days 18 and 22 after tumor injection. This outcome did not seem to occur in the P(−) group, since IL-10 secreting cell numbers were not higher than those from the tumor control group (Table 29.3). Similar increases were reported for the immune cells isolated from the tumor where the mice receiving the milk fermented with the proteolytic strain showed the highest increases for IL-10 [70].

The study of the cytokines showed that the consumption of both fermented milks diminished IL-6, a cytokine that the tumor needs for growth, and this decrease could be related with the delay of the tumor growth observed in both mice fed with the proteolytic and the proteolytic deficient strain of *L. helveticus*. The increase of IL-10 in mice fed with milk fermented by *L. helveticus* R389 could explain the important difference between both fermented milks, attributed principally to the components released into the milk after the fermentation with the proteolytic strain where the regulation of the immune response was observed in the three levels studied (serum, mammary glands and tumor).

The analysis of immune B and T cells also showed differences between the mice that received both fermented milks. Only mice fed with milk fermented by *L. helveticus* R389 increased IgA+ B cells in mammary glands after tumor injection. However, this increase was not observed when a tumor was not induced, which could mean that enhancement of IgA+ cells in mammary glands needs a stronger stimulation such as that induced by tumor cells [75]. When T cells were studied in our model, it was possible to observe changes in the balance between CD4+ and CD8+ cells in mammary glands in mice from the group fed with milk fermented by *L. helveticus* R389 and injected with tumor cells. CD4+ cell numbers increased, whereas CD8+ cell numbers

TABLE 29.3 Comparative analysis of tumor volume and cytokines in serum, mammary glands and breast tumor

Experimental groups	Time (days)	Tumor volume[a]	Blood serum[b]			Mammary gland tissues[c]			Tumor infiltrating cells[d]		
			TNFα	IL-6	IL-10	TNFα	IL-6	IL-10	TNFα	IL-6	IL-10
Tumor control	Basal	ND	42.1 ± 2.1^e	$15.0 \pm 2.0^{e,f}$	121.2 ± 35.1^f	$9 \pm 3^{e,f}$	$9 \pm 3^{e,f,g}$	$6 \pm 3^{e,f}$	ND	ND	ND
	12	0.02 ± 0.01^e	$207.1 \pm 24.5^{f,g}$	12.1 ± 1.1^e	409.1 ± 113.2^g	$9 \pm 4^{e,f,g}$	15 ± 4^f	$11 \pm 3^{f,g}$	ND	ND	ND
	18	0.12 ± 0.07^f	$226.6 \pm 39.4^{f,g}$	40.4 ± 6.0^h	943.5 ± 87.3^h	21 ± 6^h	$13 \pm 6^{e,f,g}$	$14 \pm 4^{g,h}$	24 ± 2^g	29 ± 2^g	18 ± 2^g
	27	0.21 ± 0.12^f	522.7 ± 71.8^i	93.2 ± 4.1^i	50.4 ± 15.1^e	21 ± 6^h	28 ± 8^h	16 ± 3^h	13 ± 1^e	23 ± 4^g	8 ± 2^e
L. helveticus R389 (P+)	Basal	ND	$207.7 \pm 43.6^{g,h}$	17.1 ± 2.1^f	552.2 ± 69.2^g	$7 \pm 2^{e,f}$	6 ± 2^e	$7 \pm 2^{e,f}$	ND	ND	ND
	12	0.01 ± 0.01^e	176.8 ± 2.1^f	20.1 ± 2.2^g	974.5 ± 48.5^h	$13 \pm 4^{f,g,h}$	$11 \pm 3^{e,f,g}$	$15 \pm 4^{g,h}$	ND	ND	ND
	18	0.03 ± 0.03^e	248.4 ± 11.1^h	$14.0 \pm 4.1^{e,f}$	3338.9 ± 689.2^j	$12 \pm 4^{f,g,h}$	$13 \pm 4^{f,g}$	25 ± 5^i	$22 \pm 7^{f,g}$	4 ± 2^e	$14 \pm 3^{f,g}$
	27	0.04 ± 0.02^e	283.5 ± 34.74	$15.2 \pm 2.1^{e,f}$	4796.3 ± 859.5^j	$13 \pm 2^{f,g,h}$	14 ± 4^f	21 ± 5^i	13 ± 1^e	4 ± 1^e	13 ± 2^f
L. helveticus L89 (P−)	Basal	ND	256.1 ± 51.5^g	22.0 ± 2.1^g	1441.2 ± 67.2^i	5 ± 1^e	$7 \pm 2^{e,g}$	6 ± 1^e	ND	ND	ND
	12	0.01 ± 0.01^e	242.8 ± 9.9^h	$13.1 \pm 2.0^{e,f}$	1361.3 ± 155.1^i	18 ± 4^h	15 ± 5^f	$14 \pm 4^{g,h}$	ND	ND	ND
	18	0.03 ± 0.02^e	233.6 ± 18.2^h	17.1 ± 2.2^f	836.2 ± 131.2^h	$16 \pm 3^{g,h}$	14 ± 3^f	17 ± 2^h	12 ± 2^e	4 ± 1^e	$13 \pm 6^{e,f,g}$
	27	0.05 ± 0.03^e	$144.8 \pm 49.5^{f,g}$	33.2 ± 4.1^h	1556.7 ± 169.1^i	$15 \pm 2^{g,h}$	13 ± 3^f	$12 \pm 3^{f,g,h}$	$11 \pm 4^{e,f}$	13 ± 4^f	$9 \pm 3^{e,f}$

Mice fed with the milk fermented by L. helveticus R389 (strain with high proteolytic activity, P+) or by L. helveticus L89 (proteolytic deficient mutant strain, P−) were compared with the tumor control (without specific feeding).

[a] Tumor growth rate is expressed as the volume (cm³) of the tumor (cm³).

[b] For blood serum, the concentration for each cytokine was evaluated by ELISA. Results are expressed as the mean concentration of each cytokine (pg/ml) ± standard deviation.

[c] For mammary gland tissues, cytokine-positive cells were analyzed using indirect immunofluorescence. Results are expressed as means ± SD of cytokine-positive cells counted in 10 fields of vision at 1000× of magnification.

[d] For cells isolated from tumor, cytokine-positive cells were analyzed by immunoperoxidase technique and results are expressed as means ± SD of cytokine-positive cells each 100 counted cells (cells/100).

[e,f,g,h,i,j] Means in each column without a common letter differ significantly ($p < 0.05$).

ND = Not determined.

remained unmodified. This outcome was different in the tumor control group, which maintained the balance of these cells in mammary glands towards CD8+ cells more than towards CD4+ cells [75].

It is possible to conclude in this experimental model that 7 days of cyclical feeding with milk fermented by *L. helveticus* R389 or L89 delayed tumor development and consequently decreased IL-6 secreting cells. However, milk fermented by *L. helveticus* R389 induced not only a decrease of IL-6, but also an increase of the regulatory cytokine IL-10 and cell apoptosis in the tumor. These effects were observed when a local stimulus such as tumor cells was present.

6. CONCLUSIONS

There are many reports about the anticarcinogenic effect of probiotics strains and fermented product that contain them. Even when the epidemiological data and those obtained from human trails are promising, animal models are still necessary to elucidate the mechanisms by which they can act.

At the intestinal level, a fermented product can exert an antitumoral effect by several mechanisms. The studies carried out with the model of colon cancer inhibition through cyclic yogurt feeding demonstrated that yogurt modulates the immune system response and exerts its antitumor activity through its anti-inflammatory capacity with high levels of the regulatory IL-10 in the large intestine. In addition to this immunomodulator capacity, other mechanisms by which yogurt could exert the antitumor activity observed in this model would be through the activation of the apoptosis pathways and through the yogurt bacteria interaction with the intestinal microbiota inducing decreases in the certain enzyme activities involved in the development of tumors in the intestine.

The introduction of antioxidant enzyme genes (SOD and CAT) in current probiotic strains that have natural anti-inflammatory properties, such as the ability to modulate the immune-dependent anti-inflammatory processes, could generate very potent strains that could be used for the prevention of inflammatory diseases or post-cancer drug treatments. The use of other genetically modified LAB, such as the IL-10 producing strain of *Lc. lactis* [76], could be suitable for use as treatments of intestinal diseases by delivering beneficial compounds to specific sites in the gastrointestinal tract where they are required.

It can also be concluded that it is possible to obtain a beneficial effect in other mucosal sites distant to the intestine with the oral administration of a probiotic bacteria or fermented milk. Oral administration of probiotic bacteria also exerted antitumoral effects against a non-intestinal tumor such as fibrosarcoma. Fermented milk administration can regulate the response of the immune cells associated to the mammary glands and in the cells infiltrating the tumor in an estrogen-dependent breast tumor model. The regulation of the immune response can also exert an inhibitory influence on the estrogen synthesis, necessary to the tumor growth. The probiotic strain selection would play an important role in the mucosal activation observed.

The principal cause that can be attributed to the probiotic and/or fermented product against cancer is the immune surveillance, which differs according to the site where the tumor is present. In contrast to the results observed in the intestine, where the administration of the fermented products itself induces changes on the gut associated immune cells and in other immune cells as peritoneal macrophages, in the mammary glands, changes on immune cell balances were observed only when immune cells have to act against a target like tumor cells, avoiding an exacerbated immune response. This fact could be explained because at intestinal level, where there are constant stimuli on the immune system, the immune cell stimulation is maintained with the probiotic administration;

whereas at other sites, such as mammary glands, the immune system is maintained alert and when the target affects this site, the immune cells quickly react against the agent.

References

1. Kato, I. (2000). Antitumor activity of lactic acid bacteria. In R. Fuller & G. Perdigon (Eds.), *Probiotics 3: Immunomodulation by the gut microflora and probiotics* (pp. 115–138). London: Kluwer Academic Publishers.

2. Rolfe, R. D. (2000). The role of probiotic cultures in the control of gastrointestinal health. *The Journal of Nutrition, 130*, 396S–402S.

3. Hughes, R., & Rowland, I. (2003). Nutritional and microbial modulation of carcinogenesis. In R. Fuller & G. Perdigon (Eds.), *Gut flora, nutrition, immunity and health* (pp. 208–236). Oxford: Blackwell Publishing.

4. Kato, I., Yokokura, T., & Mutai, M. (1984). Augmentation of mouse natural killer cell activity by *Lactobacillus casei* and its surface antigens. *Microbiology and Immunology, 28*, 209–217.

5. Hayashi, K., & Ohwaki, M. (1989). Antitumour activity of *Lactobacillus casei* (LC 9018) in mice: T cell subset depletion. *Biotherapy, 3*, 1568–1574.

6. Fernandes, C. F., & Shahan, K. M. (1990). Anticarcinogenic and immunological properties of dietary lactobacilli. *Journal of Food Protection, 53*, 704–710.

7. Brady, L. J., Gallaher, D. D., & Busta, F. F. (2000). The role of probiotic cultures in the prevention of colon cancer. *The Journal of Nutrition, 130*, 410S–414S.

8. Wollowski, I., Rechkemmer, G., & Pool-Zobel, B. L. (2001). Protective role of probiotics and prebiotics in colon cancer. *The American Journal of Clinical Nutrition, 73*, 451S–455S.

9. Orrhage, K. M., Annas, A., Nord, C. E., et al. (2002). Effects of lactic acid bacteria on the uptake and distribution of the food mutagen Trp-P-2 in mice. *Scandinavian Journal of Gastroenterology, 37*, 215–221.

10. Morotomi, M., & Mutai, M. (1986). *In vitro* binding of potent mutagenic pyrolysates to intestinal bacteria. *Journal of the National Cancer Institute, 77*, 195–201.

11. Goldin, B. R., Swenson, L., Dwyer, J., et al. (1980). Effect of diet and *Lactobacillus acidophilus* supplements on human fecal bacterial enzymes. *Journal of the National Cancer Institute, 64*, 255–261.

12. Goldin, B. R., & Gorbach, S. L. (1984). The effect of milk and lactobacillus feeding on human intestinal bacterial enzyme activity. *The American Journal of Clinical Nutrition, 39*, 756–761.

13. Goldin, B. R., & Gorbach, S. L. (1980). Effect of *Lactobacillus acidophilus* dietary supplements on 1, 2-dimethylhydrazine dihydrochloride-induced intestinal cancer in rats. *Journal of the National Cancer Institute, 64*, 263–265.

14. Goldin, B. R., & Gorbach, S. L. (1976). The relationship between diet and rat fecal bacterial enzymes implicated in colon cancer. *Journal of the National Cancer Institute, 57*, 371–375.

15. Geier, M. S., Butler, R. N., & Howarth, G. S. (2006). Probiotics, prebiotics and synbiotics: A role in chemoprevention for colorectal cancer?. *Cancer Biology & Therapy, 5*, 1265–1269.

16. Reddy, G. V., Friend, B. A., Shahani, K. M., & Farmer, R. E. (1983). Antitumor activity of yogurt components. *Journal of Food Protection, 46*, 8–11.

17. Perdigon, G., Fuller, R., & Raya, R. (2001). Lactic acid bacteria and their effect on the immune system. *Current Issues in Intestinal Microbiology, 2*, 27–42.

18. Le, M. G., Moulton, L. H., Hill, C., & Kramar, A. (1986). Consumption of dairy produce and alcohol in a case-control study of breast cancer. *Journal of the National Cancer Institute, 77*, 633–636.

19. Peters, R. K., Pike, M. C., Garabrant, D., & Mack, T. M. (1992). Diet and colon cancer in Los Angeles County, California. *Cancer Causes Control, 3*, 457–473.

20. van't Veer, P., Dekker, J. M., Lamers, J. W., et al. (1989). Consumption of fermented milk products and breast cancer: A case-control study in The Netherlands. *Cancer Research, 49*, 4020–4023.

21. Aso, Y., & Akazan, H. (1992). Prophylactic effect of a *Lactobacillus casei* preparation on the recurrence of superficial bladder cancer. BLP study group. *Urologia Internationalis, 49*, 125–129.

22. Perdigon, G., Valdez, J. C., & Rachid, M. (1998). Antitumor activity of yogurt: Study of possible immune mechanisms. *The Journal of Dairy Research, 65*, 129–138.

23. Perdigon, G., Rachid, M., De Budeguer, M. V., & Valdez, J. C. (1994). Effect of yogurt feeding on the small and large intestine associated lymphoid cells in mice. *The Journal of Dairy Research, 61*, 553–562.

24. Valdez, J. C., Rachid, M., Bru, E., & Perdign, G. (1997). The effect of yogurt on the cytotoxic and phagocytic activity of macrophages in tumor-bearing mice. *Food and Agricultural Immunology, 9*, 299–308.

25. Perdigon, G., de Moreno de LeBlanc, A., Valdez, J., & Rachid, M. (2002). Role of yogurt in the prevention of colon cancer. *European Journal of Clinical Nutrition, 56*(Suppl. 3), S65–S68.

26. Isaacson, P. (1982). Immunoperoxidase study of the secretory immunoglobulin system and lysozyme in normal and diseased gastric mucosa. *Gut, 23*, 578–588.

27. Prescott, S. M., & Fitzpatrick, F. A. (2000). Cyclooxygenase-2 and carcinogenesis. *Biochimica et Biophysica Acta, 1470*, M69–M78.

28. Feghali, C. A., & Wright, T. M. (1997). Cytokines in acute and chronic inflammation. *Frontiers in Bioscience*, 2, d12–d26.

29. Weitzman, S. A., & Gordon, L. I. (1990). Inflammation and cancer: Role of phagocyte-generated oxidants in carcinogenesis. *Blood*, 76, 655–663.

30. Korelitz, B. I. (1983). Carcinoma of the intestinal tract in Crohn's disease: results of a survey conducted by the National Foundation for Ileitis and colitis. *The American Journal of Gastroenterology*, 78, 44–46.

31. Collins, R. H., Jr., Feldman, M., & Fordtran, J. S. (1987). Colon cancer, dysplasia, and surveillance in patients with ulcerative colitis. A critical review. *The New England Journal of Medicine*, 316, 1654–1658.

32. Ekbom, A., Helmick, C., Zack, M., & Adami, H. O. (1990). Ulcerative colitis and colorectal cancer. A population-based study. *The New England Journal of Medicine*, 323, 1228–1233.

33. Reddy, B. S., Maruyama, H., & Kelloff, G. (1987). Dose-related inhibition of colon carcinogenesis by dietary piroxicam, a nonsteroidal anti-inflammatory drug, during different stages of rat colon tumor development. *Cancer Research*, 47, 5340–5346.

34. Lala, P. K., Parhar, R. S., & Singh, P. (1986). Indomethacin therapy abrogates the prostaglandin-mediated suppression of natural killer activity in tumor-bearing mice and prevents tumor metastasis. *Cell Immunology*, 99, 108–118.

35. de Moreno de LeBlanc, A., Valdez, J., & Perdigón, G. (2004). Inflammatory immune response. *European Journal of Inflammation*, 2, 21–31.

36. de Moreno de Leblanc, A., & Perdigon, G. (2004). Yogurt feeding inhibits promotion and progression of experimental colorectal cancer. *Medical Science Monitor*, 10, BR96–BR104.

37. Bogdan, C., Rollinghoff, M., & Diefenbach, A. (2000). The role of nitric oxide in innate immunity. *Immunological Reviews*, 173, 17–26.

38. Butler, L. M., Hewett, P. J., Fitridge, R. A., & Cowled, P. A. (1999). Deregulation of apoptosis in colorectal carcinoma: theoretical and therapeutic implications. *The Australian and New Zealand Journal of Surgery*, 69, 88–94.

39. Hao, X., Du, M., Bishop, A. E., & Talbot, I. C. (1998). Imbalance between proliferation and apoptosis in the development of colorectal carcinoma. *Virchows Archiv*, 433, 523–527.

40. Sellers, W. R., & Fisher, D. E. (1999). Apoptosis and cancer drug targeting. *The Journal of Clinical Investigation*, 104, 1655–1661.

41. Rachid, M. M., Gobbato, N. M., Valdez, J. C., et al. (2002). Effect of yogurt on the inhibition of an intestinal carcinoma by increasing cellular apoptosis. *International Journal of Immunopathology and Pharmacology*, 15, 209–216.

42. de Moreno de LeBlanc, A., & Perdigon, G. (2005). Reduction of beta-glucuronidase and nitroreductase

activity by yogurt in a murine colon cancer model. *Biocell*, 29, 15–24.

43. Perdigón, G., de Jorrat, M., Valdez, J., et al. (1995). Cytolytic effect of the serum of mice fed with *Lactobacillus casei* on tumor cell. *Microbiologie-Aliments-Nutrition*, 13, 15–24.

44. Perdigón, G., de Jorrat, M., de Petrino, S., & Rachid, M. (1993). Antitumor activity of orally administered *L. casei*. Significance of its dose in the inhibition of a fibrosarcoma in mice. *Food and Agricultural Immunology*, 5, 39–49.

45. Bibas Bonet, M. E., Fontenla, S., Mesón, O., & Perdigón, G. (2005). Antitumoral effect of *L. casei* CRL 431 on different experimental tumors. *Food and Agricultural Immunology*, 16, 181–191.

46. Perdigón, G., Medici, M., de Jorrat, M., et al. (1993). Immunomodulation effect of lactic acid bacteria on mucosal and tumor immunity. *International Journal of Immunotherapy*, IX, 29–52.

47. Berlett, B. S., & Stadtman, E. R. (1997). Protein oxidation in aging, disease, and oxidative stress. *The Journal of Biological Chemistry*, 272, 20313–20316.

48. Farr, S. B., & Kogoma, T. (1991). Oxidative stress responses in *Escherichia coli* and *Salmonella typhimurium*. *Microbiological Reviews*, 55, 561–585.

49. Szatrowski, T. P., & Nathan, C. F. (1991). Production of large amounts of hydrogen peroxide by human tumor cells. *Cancer Research*, 51, 794–798.

50. Kruidenier, L., van Meeteren, M. E., Kuiper, I., et al. (2003). Attenuated mild colonic inflammation and improved survival from severe DSS-colitis of transgenic Cu/Zn-SOD mice. *Free Radical Biology & Medicine*, 34, 753–765.

51. Kruidenier, L., & Verspaget, H. W. (2002). Review article: oxidative stress as a pathogenic factor in inflammatory bowel disease—radicals or ridiculous? *Alimentary Pharmacology & Therapeutics*, 16, 1997–2015.

52. Lih-Brody, L., Powell, S. R., Collier, K. P., et al. (1996). Increased oxidative stress and decreased antioxidant defences in mucosa of inflammatory bowel disease. *Digestive Diseases and Sciences*, 41, 2078–2086.

53. Abriouel, H., Herrmann, A., Starke, J., et al. (2004). Cloning and heterologous expression of hematin-dependent catalase produced by *Lactobacillus plantarum* CNRZ 1228. *Applied and Environmental Microbiology*, 70, 603–606.

54. Knauf, H. J., Vogel, R. F., & Hammes, W. P. (1992). Cloning, sequence, and phenotypic expression of katA, which encodes the catalase *of Lactobacillus sake* LTH677. *Applied and Environmental Microbiology*, 58, 832–839.

55. Noonpakdee, W., Sitthimonchai, S., Panyim, S., & Lertsiri, S. (2004). Expression of the catalase gene katA in starter culture *Lactobacillus plantarum* TISTR850 tolerates oxidative stress and reduces lipid oxidation in fermented meat product. *International Journal of Food Microbiology*, 95, 127–135.

56. Rochat, T., Gratadoux, J. J., Gruss, A., et al. (2006). Production of a heterologous nonheme catalase by *Lactobacillus casei*: An efficient tool for removal of H2O2 and protection of *Lactobacillus bulgaricus* from oxidative stress in milk. *Applied and Environmental Microbiology*, 72, 5143–5149.

57. Rochat, T., Miyoshi, A., Gratadoux, J. J., et al. (2005). High-level resistance to oxidative stress in *Lactococcus lactis* conferred by *Bacillus subtilis* catalase KatE. *Microbiology*, 151, 3011–3018.

58. de Moreno de LeBlanc, A., LeBlanc, J. G., Perdigón, G., et al. (2008). Oral administration of a catalase-producing *Lactococcus lactis* can prevent a chemically induced colon cancer in mice. *Journal of Medical Microbiology*, 58, 100–105.

59. Rochat, T., Bermudez-Humaran, L., Gratadoux, J. J., et al. (2007). Anti-inflammatory effects of *Lactobacillus casei* BL23 producing or not a manganese-dependent catalase on DSS-induced colitis in mice. *Microbial Cell Factories*, 6, 22.

60. Sanders, J. W., Leenhouts, K. J., Haandrikman, A. J., et al. (1995). Stress response in *Lactococcus lactis*: cloning, expression analysis, and mutation of the lactococcal superoxide dismutase gene. *Journal of Bacteriology*, 177, 5254–5260.

61. Ogawa, Y., Kanatsu, K., Iino, T., et al. (2002). Protection against dextran sulfate sodium-induced colitis by microspheres of ellagic acid in rats. *Life Science*, 71, 827–839.

62. Segui, J., Gironella, M., Sans, M., et al. (2004). Superoxide dismutase ameliorates TNBS-induced colitis by reducing oxidative stress, adhesion molecule expression, and leukocyte recruitment into the inflamed intestine. *Journal of Leukocyte Biology*, 76, 537–544.

63. Divisi, D., Di Tommaso, S., Salvemini, S., et al. (2006). Diet and cancer. *Acta Bio-medica*, 77, 118–123.

64. Donaldson, M. S. (2004). Nutrition and cancer: A review of the evidence for an anti-cancer diet. *Nutrition Journal*, 3, 19.

65. Matar, C., LeBlanc, J. G., Martin, L., & Perdigon, G. (2003). Biologically active peptides released from fermented milk: Role and functions. In E. Farnworth (Ed.), *Handbook of fermented functional foods* (pp. 177–201). Boca Raton, FL: CRC Press.

66. LeBlanc, J. G., Matar, C., Valdez, J. C., et al. (2002). Immunomodulating effects of peptidic fractions issued from milk fermented with *Lactobacillus helveticus*. *Journal of Dairy Science*, 85, 2733–2742.

67. Reome, J. B., Hylind, J. C., Dutton, R. W., & Dobrzanski, M. J. (2004). Type 1 and type 2 tumor infiltrating effector cell subpopulations in progressive breast cancer. *Clinical Immunology*, 111, 69–81.

68. Zhang, G., Li, W., Holle, L., et al. (2002). A novel design of targeted endocrine and cytokine therapy for breast cancer. *Clinical Cancer Research*, 8, 1196–1205.

69. Reed, M. J., & Purohit, A. (1997). Breast cancer and the role of cytokines in regulating estrogen synthesis: An emerging hypothesis. *Endocrine Reviews*, 18, 701–715.

70. de Moreno de LeBlanc, A., Matar, C., LeBlanc, N., & Perdigon, G. (2005). Effects of milk fermented by *Lactobacillus helveticus* R389 on a murine breast cancer model. *Breast Cancer Research*, 7, R477–R486.

71. Ferrarini, M., Ferrero, E., Dagna, L. P. A., & Zocchi, M. R. (2002). Human gamma/delta T cell: A nonredundant system in the immune-surveillance against cancer. *Trends in Immunolology*, 23, 14–18.

72. Bingle, L., Brown, N. J., & Lewis, C. E. (2002). The role of tumor-associated macrophages in tumor progression: implications for new anticancer therapies. *The Journal of Pathology*, 196, 254–265.

73. Purohit, A., Newman, S. P., & Reed, M. J. (2002). The role of cytokines in regulating estrogen synthesis: Implications for the etiology of breast cancer. *Breast Cancer Research*, 4, 65–69.

74. Urban, J. L., Shepard, H. M., Rothstein, J. L., et al. (1986). Tumor necrosis factor: A potent effector molecule for tumor cell killing by activated macrophages. *Proceedings of the National Academy of Sciences of the United States of America*, 83, 5233–5237.

75. de Moreno de LeBlanc, A., Matar, C., Theriault, C., & Perdigon, G. (2005). Effects of milk fermented by *Lactobacillus helveticus* R389 on immune cells associated to mammary glands in normal and a breast cancer model. *Immunobiology*, 210, 349–358.

76. Steidler, L., Hans, W., Schotte, L., et al. (2000). Treatment of murine colitis by *Lactococcus lactis* secreting interleukin-10. *Science*, 289, 1352–1355.

The Role of Probiotics in the Treatment of Irritable Bowel Syndrome

Gareth C. Parkes

Nutritional Sciences Division, King's College London, London, UK

1. INTRODUCTION

Irritable bowel syndrome (IBS) is a gastroenterological condition characterized by a triad of abdominal pain, bloating and change in bowel habit with an absence of any overt mucosal abnormality [1]. The first modern definition of the 'irritable colon' IBS was proposed in the 1960s by Chaudhary and Truelove [2]. Since then there has been a focus to define the condition on symptom-based diagnostic criteria [1, 3, 4], the most recent of which, the Rome III classification of IBS, defines the disorder as recurrent abdominal pain at least 3 days per month in the last 3 months, with at least two of the following: improvement on defecation, onset associated with a change in stool frequency, or onset associated with a change in stool form [5]. Irritable bowel syndrome is the most frequent reason for referral to gastroenterology outpatient clinics in the developed world, affecting between 10–20% of the population [6] yet, despite its high prevalence, its pathogenesis remains poorly understood. For many years, models of IBS have focused on visceral hypersensitivity and stress and therapeutic targets within the enteric nervous system and higher centers within the central nervous system [7]). However, there is growing evidence for a role in the gastrointestinal (GI) microbiota in the etiology and treatment of IBS [8].

Probiotics are defined as 'live microorganisms, which, when administered in adequate amounts, confer a health benefit on the host' [9]. Research and clinical trials into probiotics has grown at an exponential rate. There is now evidence for their use in a wide range of GI disorders including the treatment of *Clostridium difficile* associated diarrhea [10], inflammatory bowel disease [11], acute gastroenteritis [12–14] and necrotizing enterocolitis [15]. This chapter aims to explore a mechanistic framework behind how probiotics might be of benefit in IBS. It then comprehensively reviews current clinical trials of probiotics in the treatment of IBS with a view to synthesizing guidance for the healthcare professional.

513

2. THE ROLE OF THE GASTROINTESTINAL MICROBIOTA IN IRRITABLE BOWEL SYNDROME

There are a number of factors which suggest that the GI microbiota might play a role in the pathogenesis of IBS. Alterations in the composition of the fecal and mucosa-associated microbiota, low-grade mucosal inflammation, increased incidence following acute gastroenteritis and a tentative link with small intestinal bacterial overgrowth (SIBO) have all been demonstrated.

There have been a number of studies to examine differences in the GI microbiota in patients with IBS and healthy controls. Early studies examining fecal bacteria using traditional culture methods found lower concentrations of coliforms, lactobacilli and bifidobacteria and higher numbers of pseudomonas and enterobacteria in patients with IBS [16, 17]. However, as the majority of the fecal microbiota are obligate anaerobes, these studies are limited by the use of bacterial culture which is now known to grossly underestimate fecal bacterial population [18]. A comprehensive study examined the fecal microbiota of 27 patients with IBS and 22 healthy controls using real-time PCR [19]. Comparisons were made between the phenotypic subtypes of IBS: diarrhea-predominant (IBS-D), constipation-predominant (IBS-C) and alternating IBS (IBS-A). Concentrations of lactobacilli were significantly lower in IBS-D compared to IBS-C ($p < 0.019$) although not when compared to controls. There was a trend towards lower concentrations of bifidobacteria in IBS-D compared to controls and IBS-C, albeit non-significant ($p < 0.17$). In a subsequent publication, the same group pooled the fecal samples by IBS subgroup (IBS-D, IBS-C and IBS-A) and controls, extracted the bacterial DNA and analyzed it using high throughput 16S ribosomal RNA sequencing [20]. Using population analysis, the study found significant differences between each IBS subgroup and controls. This study suggests that differing phenotypes of IBS patient appear to have a unique microbial profile. Studies such as these might be of particular importance in designing therapeutic strategies with probiotics bacteria.

One study has used endoscopic biopsies to compare the mucosa-associated microbiota in IBS [21]. Given their proximity to the GI epithelial surface changes in the bacterial population have the potential to influence the host in particular via interaction with the immune system. This study using fluorescent *in situ* hybridization (FISH) found an expansion of the mucosa-associated microbiota in IBS patients and that this was composed of the pro-inflammatory species bacteroides and clostridia. Subgroup analysis demonstrated significant reduction in bifidobacteria in IBS-D patients compared to controls and IBS-C patients.

Due to the wide range of techniques, differing patient groups and the complexity of the GI microbiota, it becomes difficult to draw firm conclusions from this series of studies. Despite these difficulties, there does appear to be a consistent theme of a relative reduction of the lactobacilli and bifidobacteria in patients with IBS and higher concentrations of species such as enterobacteriaceae, coliforms and bacteroides. However, what is less clear, without a greater understanding of the metabolic and immunological roles of the GI microbiota, is whether these changes are a primary or secondary phenomenon.

In addition to differences in the GI microbiota in IBS there is increasing evidence of an activation of the intestinal immune system in IBS. Increased concentrations of intra-epithelial lymphocytes [22, 23], mast cells [24–27] and 5-HT-secreting enterochromaffin cells [28] have been found in the mucosa of patients with IBS and in particular those with post-infectious IBS (PI-IBS) [29]. The consistent demonstration of low-grade inflammation has led to speculation regarding a link between IBS and IBD [30].

Irritable bowel syndrome may be considered as part of the spectrum of colonic inflammation, with Crohn's disease (CD) and ulcerative colitis (UC) at one end, and normality [8].

A link between acute gastroenteritis and IBS has been established for many years [2]. Between 20–30% of cases of IBS have a clear infective trigger [31], typically caused by bacterial gastroenteritis secondary to *Campylobacter jejuni*, salmonella or *Escherichia coli* (*E. coli*). A longitudinal study monitored long-term sequelae following an outbreak of gastroenteritis due to water contamination in a town in Canada resulting in over 2,300 cases of gastroenteritis [32]. Using the unaffected population as controls, this study found that over the course of 2 years the odds ratio for developing IBS in the affected population was 4.8 (confidence interval, CI, 3.4–6.8 $p < 0.001$). Gastroenteritis may lead to an increased risk of developing IBS, either through persistent activation of the host immune system or through the establishment of a dysbiosis in the host GI microbiota although there is no direct evidence of this yet.

Finally, there is controversial evidence linking SIBO and IBS. Bloating and flatulence are common symptoms of IBS [33], and bacterial fermentation of undigested carbohydrate leads to production of gases carbon dioxide, hydrogen and methane. Several authors have hypothesized a link between increased fermentation, gas production and IBS [34, 35] although other studies have suggested altered tone in the abdominal wall and diaphragm [36]. Several studies by the same group found an increased incidence of SIBO, using a lactulose hydrogen breath test (LHBT), in IBS between 78–84% [37–40]. However, when the incidence of SIBO is measured using jejunal aspiration and culture (regarded as the gold standard) the incidence has been found to be around 4% [41]. Despite these discrepancies, a number of randomized placebo-controlled trials of antibiotics to treat SIBO have been conducted based on these data

with marked success. Taken together with the evidence of an altered fecal and mucosa-associated microbiota, post-infectious IBS and an up-regulated immune system there is a consensus of data suggesting a role for the microbiota in the etiology of IBS. Furthermore, modulation of the GI microbiota, whether linked to SIBO or not, with antibiotics has been shown to be of benefit in the treatment of IBS [42, 43]. However, there is no long-term data for the efficacy of antibiotics, and given problems of drug resistance and the rising incidence of CDAD, repeated courses of antibiotics are not without risk. Therefore, using probiotic bacteria to modulate the GI microbiota in IBS is an attractive therapeutic option.

3. PROBIOTICS IN IBS

3.1. Mechanisms of Action

There is an increasing interest in the role of probiotics in IBS. Due to the widespread prevalence of the disorder there has also been a corresponding growth in advertising of probiotic products, aimed at the general public, and targeting common IBS symptoms such as slow transit and bloating. The style and the nature of this advertising, which often claims to be scientifically proven, has led many clinicians to view probiotics with some scepticism [44]. However, in a number cases, there are substantial *in vitro* and clinical trial data which set out a clear rationale for the use of species specific probiotics in IBS.

In order to be of clinical benefit, probiotic bacteria must be able to survive GI transit (e.g. gastric acid and bile acid resistance) and then be able to demonstrate functional efficacy [45]. With respect to the relieving of IBS symptoms, the functional characteristics are likely to include immune stimulation, reduction of intestinal epithelial permeability, modulation of the enteric nervous system and the suppression of enteropathogenic colonization.

There is substantial evidence demonstrating that probiotic bacteria can interact with the host GI mucosal immune system [46–51]. Given the evidence demonstrating an increase in immune cell populations in IBS, it is probable that immunomodulation by probiotics is a key constituent of their mechanism of action. Probiotics have been shown to interact with both the innate and adaptive arms of the GI immune system. Tissue culture studies have shown that specific probiotics can block the inflammatory effects of *E. coli* on colonic epithelial cells and circulating macrophages [48, 49]. Probiotic bacteria have been shown to directly interact with the immune system, increasing mucosal anti-inflammatory cytokines transforming growth factor beta (TGFβ) and interleukin-10 (IL-10) [52, 53], and reducing pro-inflammatory cytokines such as IL-12 and interferon gamma (IFNγ) [54]. Although studies have demonstrated that some of the bacteria in commercial probiotic preparations are non-viable [55], experiments have shown that even bacterial fragments have profound immunological effects [44]. Cytosine-phosphate-guanosine (CpG) motifs are common DNA sequences in bacteria not found in human DNA and act as an epitope for TLR-9 [56] found on intestinal epithelial cells, thus exerting anti-inflammatory effects. In a murine model of colitis, gamma irradiated, non-viable probiotics were shown to have an equal anti-inflammatory effect to viable probiotic bacteria [57]. Potentially target molecules could be developed with an anti-inflammatory profile, yet stable at room temperature, resistant to pH, bile salts and enzymatic degradation.

Specific probiotics also appear to directly modulate intestinal pain. *Lactobacillus acidophilus* has been shown to up-regulate μ-opioid and cannaboid receptors in colonic epithelial cell lines and in the colonic epithelium in pre-treated rats and mice [58]. Using rat, stress model of visceral hypersensitivity, pre-treatment with the probiotic ameliorated pain. Similarly, *Lactobacillus paracasei* attenuated abdominal pain and mucosal inflammation in an antibiotic induced murine model of visceral hypersensitivity [59]. In addition, the same species has been shown to attenuate colonic hypercontractility in a *Trichinella spiralis* model of P-IBS [60]. This response was specific to *L. paracasei* or its depleted culture medium (suggesting it was mediated via a secreted protein) and not seen in several other species used in the same experiment.

Probiotics have also been shown to alter the integrity of the GI mucosa. The probiotic VSL#3 (a combination of nine strains of various bifidobacteria, lactobacillus and *S. thermophilus*) has been shown to induce mucin production in the colon via up-regulation of the gene MUC2 [61]. *Escherichia coli* Nissle 1917 has been shown to repair barrier function of T84 human colonic cells following disruption by enteropathic *E. coli* by up-regulating tight junction proteins [62]. Finally, as part of a RCT of a probiotic drink containing *Streptococcus thermophilus*, *Lactobacillus bulgaricus*, *Lactobacillus acidophilus* and *Bifidobacterium longum* in patients with IBS-D, intestinal permeability was analyzed [63]. In addition to a significant improvement in global symptom score (see Table 30.1) there was a significant decrease in small intestinal permeability, measured by lactulose to mannitol urinary excretion ratios (0.038 vs 0.024, $p < 0.004$). Interestingly, there was no change in colonic permeability when measured by sucralose urinary excretion, suggesting the effects are specific to the small bowel. As several studies have shown increased GI permeability in IBS [64, 65] therapies that improve barrier function may alleviate symptoms via this mechanism. A further study using VSL#3 demonstrated that probiotic administration led to up-regulation of chloride channels in damaged rat epithelium. These channels play a vital role in water absorption in the gut [66], and their up-regulation reduces diarrhea; however, this novel mechanism of action has yet to be confirmed in human studies.

Finally, probiotics have been shown to suppress enteropathogenic colonization of the lumen and subsequent adhesion and invasion of the GI mucosa. For example, a number of *in vitro* studies have demonstrated that select probiotics inhibit enteropathogenic growth, such as pathogenic *E. coli* and *Salmonellae typhimurium* [67, 68]. This effect, termed colonization resistance, may be via direct antimicrobial action via probiotic production of antimicrobials [69] or by altering the environment such as lowering pH by production of short-chain fatty acids that lower luminal pH [70], both of which inhibit enteropathogenic growth. Given the relationship between acute gastroenteritis and IBS, this may be an important mechanism although there is little evidence to suggest a long-term colonization by pathogenic bacteria. It may be that colonization resistance may also influence the relative fecal and mucosal dysbiosis that has been demonstrated in patients with IBS. Small intestinal bacterial overgrowth, an alternative form of abnormal colonization of the GI tract, has been controversially linked to IBS [39, 71]. A small trial of *Lactobacillus shirota* in 14 patients with concomitant IBS and positive LHBT normalized the breath test in 64% of patients studied and significantly retarded the initial rise in breath hydrogen ($p = 0.03$). However, potentially due to the size of the study, there was not a significant improvement in IBS symptoms. Given the data supporting the use of antibiotics in IBS, it would be interesting to see the effects of probiotics on GI fermentation in IBS in larger studies.

3.2. Clinical Trials

Numerous trials have investigated the therapeutic benefit of probiotics in IBS albeit with contrasting results, and more recently there have been two systematic reviews [72, 73] and two meta-analyses [74, 75]. Common to many trials of probiotics, studies of probiotics in IBS have a marked heterogeneity in dosing regimens, species used and clinical endpoints. A number of the trials are of 'synbiotics,' preparations containing both a probiotic and a prebiotic in order to improve colonization of the probiotic in the gut. Prebiotics are selectively fermented short-chain carbohydrates that allow specific changes, both in the composition and/or activity in the GI microbiota, that confers a health benefit [76]. It is beyond the scope of this chapter to review the literature on prebiotics and IBS and thus the focus is on the evidence for probiotic bacteria. Finally, many of the trials have been hampered by large placebo effects, a common feature of many trials in IBS [77, 78]. Table 30.1 summarizes the important RCTs over the last 10 years, highlighting the species used, the trial design and results. Several trials have been excluded from this list for failure to compare with placebo [79], re-analysis of old data [80], unclear endpoints [81] or the use of multiple interventions [82].

Many early studies were small single-centered trials [78, 83–86] although a number of much larger multi-centered trials have also been undertaken, reflecting the growing interest in the area [87–90]. There are three studies using a liquid form of *Lactobacillus plantarum* with two studies showing some benefit [85, 91] and one with no significant benefit however significantly underpowered [86]. However, these initial results have never been followed up in larger multi-centered studies. Trials of *Lactobacillus* GG (LGG), a species which has had significant efficacy in the treatment of infectious diarrhea in children [13], have had some success in treating childhood IBS and recurrent abdominal pain [83, 92]. However, a Cochrane review of dietary intervention in functional bowel disorders in children found insufficient evidence to support its use [93]. A single trial of 54 patients with IBS *Lactobacillus reuteri* ATCC 55730 over a period of 6 months demonstrated an improvement in the global symptom scores (GSS) from baseline

TABLE 30.1   Summary of recent randomized controlled trials of probiotics in IBS

References	n	Intervention (daily dose)	Duration (weeks)	Result
Kajander et al [122]	103	*Lactobacillus GG, L. rhamnosus* LC705, *B. breve* Bb99, *Propionibacterium freudenreichii* spp. *shermanii* JS	26	Significant reduction in GSS $p < 0.015$
Kim et al [84]	48	VSL#3 (10^{11})	4	Failed to show improvement in bloating scores (PEP) $p < 0.19$ Reduction in flatulence scores $p < 0.01$
Bausserman et al [83]	50	*L.* GG (10^{10})	6	Failed to show reduction in GSS over placebo $p < 0.77$ (children)
Niv et al [78]	54	*L. reuteri* ATCC 55730 (10^8)	26	Failed to show benefit in GSS over placebo
O'Mahony et al [101]	67	*B. infantis* 35624 (10^{10}) *L. salivarius* UCC4331	8	*B. infantis* showed significant improvement in GSS over placebo $p < 0.05$, *L. salivarius* failed to show benefit
Tsuchiya et al [114]	68	*L. helviticus, L acidophilus, Bifidobacterium* (10^9)	12	Global assessment 80% vs 10% $p < 0.01$
Kim et al [98]	25 IBS-D	VSL#3 (10^{11})	8	No difference in transit or GSS, reduction in bloating $p < 0.046$)
Sens et al [86]	12	*L. plantarum* 299V (10^7)	4	Failed to show reduction in GSS over placebo
Niedzielin [85]	40	*L. plantarum* 299V (10^7)	4	PEP defined as resolution of pain: 100% vs 55% $p < 0.001$
Nobaek et al [91]	60	*L. plantarum* 299V (10^{10})	4	Improved flatulence only $p < 0.05$
Enck et al [88]	298	*E. coli* DSM17252 (10^7–10^8)	8	Complete remission 18.4% vs 4.7% $p < 0.001$
Williams et al [115]	52	*L. acidophilus* (NCIMB 30157) and (NCIMB 30156), *B. lactis* (NCIMB 30172) *and B. bifidum* (NCIMB 30153) (10^{10})	8	Significant improvement in GSS over placebo $p < 0.02$
Andriulli et al [87]	267	*Lactobacillus paracasei* B21060 (10^{10}) + prebiotic vs prebiotic alone	12	Failure to show improvement over placebo in GSS
Drouault-Holowacz et al [104]	100	*B. longum* LA 101 (29%), *L. acidophilus* LA 102 (29%), *L. lactis* LA 103 (29%) and *S. thermophilus* LA 104 (13%) (10^{10})	4	Failure to show improvement over placebo in GSS
Sinn et al [113]	40	*L. acidophilus* SDC 2012,2013 (10^9)	4	Significant reduction in abdominal pain $p = 0.011$
Kajander et al [123]	86	*L.* GG, *L. rhamnosus* LC705, *B. breve* Bb99, *Propionibacterium freudenreichii* spp. *shermanii* JS	20	Significant reduction in GSS $p < 0.008$

TABLE 30.1 (Continued)

References	n	Intervention (daily dose)	Duration (weeks)	Result
Guynonnet et al [77]	274 IBS-C	*B. animalis* DN 173 010	6	Although significant improvement over baseline, no benefit over placebo
Whorwell et al [90]	362	*B. infantis* 35624 (10^8)	4	Reduction in pain score (PEP) $p < 0.03$
				Reduction in GSS $p < 0.01$
Gawronska et al [48, 92]	37[*]	*L.* GG (10^9)	4	GSS 33% vs 5.1% $p < 0.04$ (children)

[*]Sub-group analysis of IBS in a larger cohort of functional abdominal pain disorders. (PEP – Primary endpoint; GSS – Global symptom score).

but due to a large placebo effect failed to show any benefit over controls [78]. The combination probiotic VSL#3 has been used in a number of trials for the treatment of ulcerative colitis (UC) [94] and pouchitis [95, 96] and has extensive *in vitro* data demonstrating immunomodulatory action [97] and enhanced epithelial barrier function [66]. However, trials of VSL#3 in the treatment of IBS, although well designed, have had mixed results. An initial trial of 25 patients with IBS-D used colonic transit (measured by scintography) as the primary endpoint with reduction in symptom scores as secondary targets [98]. However, there was no significant reduction in GI transit in the study group and the only significant symptom score reduction was in abdominal bloating. Therefore, a second, larger trial was designed with 48 patients with a reduction in abdominal bloating as the primary endpoint and colonic transit and other symptoms as secondary endpoints. Although there was only a non-significant reduction in abdominal bloating in the study group versus placebo (31.3 ± 3.1 vs 38.5 ± 3.1, $p = 0.22$) there was a significant reduction in flatulence (29.7 ± 2.6 vs 39.5 ± 2.6, $p = 0.01$). In addition, VSL#3 significantly retarded colonic transit ($p = 0.05$) although without a corresponding change in stool frequency or form. Thus there is only weak evidence supporting the use of VSL#3 in IBS at present.

In contrast to VSL#3, which appears to have greater efficacy in UC than in IBS, *Bifidobacteria infantis* 35624 was a probiotic species, specifically designed to work in UC with robust *in vitro* data behind it [50, 99]. Despite this, an international multi-center trial of maintenance of steroid-induced remission in UC failed to show efficacy of *B. infantis* over placebo [100]. However, in a trial of 77 patients with IBS randomized to either *B. infantis* or *Lactobacillus salivarius* or placebo, *B. infantis* significantly reduced pain, bloating and bowel satisfaction scores in comparison to placebo as well as composite scores [101]. In addition, patients with IBS were shown to have abnormal IL-12/IL-10 cytokine ratios at baseline suggesting a pro-inflammatory state; these ratios were normalized in the patients taking *B. infantis*. These data have been supported in a large multi-center dose finding trial of *B. infantis* in 362 female patients with IBS, randomized to four groups taking doses of 10^6 or 10^8 or 10^{10} cfu per day or placebo [90]. The group taking *B. infantis* 10^8 cfu per day scored significantly better than placebo in all symptom groups including a global assessment of IBS relief which was the primary endpoint (62.3 ± 6.2 vs 42.0 ± 6.4, $p < 0.02$). Interestingly, although the original trial had used a dose of 10^{10} cfu in a liquid preparation in this second study, the group taking 10^{10} performed worse than placebo; this was later found to be due to problems with a novel capsule formulation.

Two trials by the same group have used a multi-species probiotic containing *L. rhamnosus* GG, *L. rhamnosus* LC705, *Bifidobacterium breve, Propionibacterium freudenreichii spp.* and *shermanii* JS [102, 103]. The first single-center trial of 103 patients with IBS found that at the end of a 6-month treatment regimen there was a mean difference in reduction of the total symptom scores (the primary endpoint) of 7.7 points ($p = 0.015$). The second follow-up study of 86 patients confirmed benefit, with a difference in reduction in GSS of 11 points ($p < 0.01$) between treatment group and control. However, there were marked differences in baseline severity scores between treatment groups and controls, with the treatment group having greater symptom severity and therefore more likely to improve. In addition, a high proportion of both control and treatment arms were prescribed antibiotics in the treatment period (22%) although significantly different between arms. This study examined inflammatory cytokines and C-reactive protein (CRP) levels but found no significant differences between baseline and the end of the trial. A notable feature in these trials was the longer treatment period of 5 and 6 months, respectively, with a consistent GSS improvement over the treatment course; however, there is no data to suggest whether this response is sustained after cessation of probiotic intake.

In 2007 and 2008, there were several well-designed, large, multi-center trials of probiotics in IBS that have failed to demonstrate benefit, again often in part due to a high placebo response [77, 87, 104]. The trial of *B. animalis* DN 173010 in 274 primary care patients with IBS-C did demonstrate significant symptomatic relief compared to baseline in its primary endpoint (improvement in a functional bowel disorder quality of life score) but not over placebo [77]. However sub-group analysis of patients with less than three bowel motions a week ($n = 19$) at baseline showed a significant rise in stool frequency compared to controls ($p < 0.001$). Potentially recruiting from primary rather than secondary care meant that overall patients had less severe symptoms and therefore benefit was harder to achieve. One of these trials used a symbiotic preparation Flortec®, a combination of prebiotic (xylo-oligosaccharide) and probiotic (*L. paracasei* B21060) in its treatment arm and prebiotic alone in the control arm [87]. The improvement in global relief scores was almost identical in the study and control arm. However, one placebo-controlled trial of different prebiotic product, trans-galacto-oligosaccharide in the treatment of IBS, demonstrated significant reduction in GSS over placebo [105]. Thus, the lack of efficacy over placebo in the trial of *L. paracasei* may be due in part to a beneficial effect of the prebiotic in the control arm.

A small single-center study of 40 IBS patients randomized to *L. acidophilus* SDC 2012 and 2013 or placebo showed significant benefit over placebo. Using any reduction in abdominal pain scores as a primary endpoint comparing *L. acidophilus* to placebo there was a 23.8% (15.3–32.3) versus 0.2% (-14.3–14.7) reduction in pain ($p = 0.003$). However, this study did not use a global symptom relief score as an endpoint, and using any reduction in pain as 'a responder' is questionable. It is interesting that there appeared to be no appreciable placebo effect in this trial conducted in South Korea in contrast to many of the studies mentioned in this chapter. A study which used *L. acidophilus* (NCIMB 30157 and 30156) in combination with *B. lactis* (NCIMB 30172) and *B. bifidum* (NCIMB 30153) also demonstrated benefit. At the end of the 8-week trial of 52 IBS patients randomized to the probiotic combination (sold as LAB4®) or placebo there was a significant drop in the symptom severity score in the study arm over controls (133 vs 80, $p < 0.05$). However, once again the study arm had a higher baseline severity score than placebo and this effect was negated two weeks after stopping the probiotic.

Finally, a primary care-based, placebo-controlled trial in IBS of 298 patients diagnosed by primary care criteria [106] were randomized to either *E. coli* DSM 17252 only or placebo. In this study, response was defined as 'clinical remission' with complete resolution of IBS symptoms. In comparison to placebo the treatment arm achieved complete remission in 18.4 vs 4.6% ($p < 0.0004$) of patients studied (intention to treat analysis). In addition, there was a 50% drop in abdominal pain scores of 18.9 vs 6.7% in treatment and placebo groups, respectively ($p = 0.001$). This trial was based on a much earlier trial of *E. coli* DSM 17252 in combination with *Enterococcus faecalis* DSM 16440 originally published in the early nineties [107], and then re-analyzed [80] by re-defining the clinical endpoints to give a GSS in accordance with modern guidelines. This had demonstrated a response rate (defined by a drop in GSS by 50%) was significantly better in the treatment arm than placebo (68.5 vs 37.8%, $p < 0.001$) [80] (data not included in Table 30.1). Although both of these trials failed to use Rome or Manning definitions in their inclusion criteria, they were otherwise large and well designed. Data from primary, rather than secondary, care are particularly useful given that probiotics are freely available to the general public.

4. DISCUSSION

Irritable bowel syndrome remains one of the more difficult gastroenterological conditions to treat. Despite its widespread prevalence and extensive research into novel pharmaceutical therapies most clinicians rely on traditional therapies such as anti-spasmodics, anti-diarrheals, laxatives and fiber [108]. Although initially promising, new therapies such as tegaserod [109] and alosetron [110] are costly, and meta-analysis has demonstrated only modest benefit as well as the potential for complications [111].

Therefore, probiotics, given their impressive safety profile and relatively low cost, are an attractive proposition.

Perhaps the biggest obstacle to new therapies in IBS is the heterogeneous nature of the disorder. Although some of the clinical trials examined benefited in only IBS-D or IBS-C subgroups the majority did not. Differing probiotic species are likely to cause different effects on GI transit and stool composition. Defining IBS by sub-groups is only the beginning of a process of differentiation by a clinician. Some patients clearly have psycho-social issues likely to respond to therapies that directly address this whereas others may have a primary neuromotility disorder. The focus for much of the research into novel therapies in the past decade has focused on the brain–gut axis and pharmacological targets within the enteric nervous system and relatively little attention paid to the contents of the GI tract. However, the evidence for alterations into the GI microbiota in IBS such as differences in concentrations of fecal bacteria, PI-IBS, and SIBO supports its therapeutic manipulation.

Based on current evidence, the probiotics with the most robust data for efficacy in treating IBS are *B. infantis* 35624 and *E. coli* DSM 17252. Both of these probiotics have had initial successful trials supported by larger studies [80, 88, 90, 101]. In the case of *B. infantis* there are a number of *in vitro* studies supporting its mechanism of action and furthermore data in human studies demonstrating anti-inflammatory effects. One reservation with regard to the second, larger study of *B. infantis* is that it was only conducted in women and, therefore, there is less evidence to support its use in men. The probiotic combination of *L. rhamnosus* GG, *L. rhamnosus* LC705, *B. breve*, *Propionibacterium freudenreichii* spp. and Shermanii JS has also demonstrated significant benefit in two sequential trials [89, 112]. However, both trials recruited from a single center and were conducted by the same investigators. A larger, ideally multi-national, trial would be helpful before making stronger recommendations. Many other products have been hampered by a large placebo effect; in particular, a large trial of *B. animalis* DN 173010 [77]. However, given the sub-group analysis showing benefit in patients with a stool frequency of less than 3 a week, the use of *B. animalis* DN 173010 could be cautiously recommended in patients with severe IBS-C although clearly further data are needed. There are obviously a number of smaller trials that demonstrated benefit [113–115] but given the limited numbers and lack of supporting evidence it is difficult to recommend their use at this stage. Single-center, pilot data suggesting benefit for a probiotic agent in treating IBS, should be supported by data from larger multi-centered trials.

One systematic review on probiotics in IBS concluded that *B. infantis* 35624 had the strongest evidence for efficacy in the treatment of IBS [73], although it is worth mentioning that the most recent trial of *E. coli* DSM 17252 had only just been published at the time of writing [88]. Three meta-analyses all agreed that probiotics were beneficial to varying degrees: McFarland et al. relative risk (RR) of not improving GSS 0.77 (95% confidence interval (95% CI) 0.62–0.94) [74], Moayeddi et al. RR not improving GSS 0.72 (95% CI 0.57–0.88) [72] and Hoveyda et al. odds ratio (OR) of symptomatic improvement 1.63 (95% CI 1.23–2.17) [75]. These data are encouraging, particularly as all three analyses appear to concur to some degree; however, meta-analysis of trials of probiotics in any clinical condition is difficult. Efficacy of a probiotic species in one disease process cannot be extrapolated to another. Similarly, results suggesting a specific species of *Lactobacillus* is beneficial in the treatment of IBS does not mean that alternative lactobacilli will be equally efficacious. Each probiotic product needs to be rigorously trialed and preferably initially in the laboratory in either cellular or animal models of IBS. Meta-analysis or systematic reviews which group disparate species of probiotics together, risk diluting

evidence of successful trials with studies using entirely different species and vice versa.

Like any therapeutic agent, probiotics can have adverse side effects although in the main these have been relatively minor in trials treating IBS. Probiotics have been used safely and effectively in a variety of patient groups without harmful effects, including neonates with necrotizing enterocolitis [116], human immunodeficiency virus [117] and chemotherapy induced neutropenia [118]. However, there are a number of case reports of sepsis following probiotic [119], although all within an inpatient hospital setting. Guidelines have divided risk factors for adverse events following probiotic use into major (immune compromise, premature infant) and minor (central venous catheter, impaired intestinal barrier function, administration via jejunostomy, probiotics with known pathogenic factors, cardiac valvular disease, and the use of antibiotics to which the probiotic is resistant) [119]. A further important safety consideration is that antibiotic resistance genes should not be transferable to other gastrointestinal microbiota [120]. A randomized controlled trial of a multi-species probiotic in patients with acute severe pancreatitis found that patients in the study arm had a higher mortality rate than the placebo arm (RR 2.53; 95% CI 1.22–5.25) [121]. Clearly, acute pancreatitis carries a significant morbidity and mortality in its own right and there are few parallels between this condition and IBS. However, it does highlight that probiotics can be much more than just 'nutritional' supplements and should be treated as so.

Therefore, given that the vast majority of IBS treatments are conducted in either primary care, secondary care, outpatient, or probiotics are safe to use. This chapter has explored the ways in which probiotics are likely to work and given guidance on which probiotics have proven efficacy in the treatment of IBS. Selecting which patients are likely to respond remains a difficult dilemma. Novel methods of identifying those likely to benefit from manipulation of the GI microbiota as opposed to psychological or neuromotility therapy are needed. Furthermore, as our understanding of the interaction between the host and the GI microbiota improves, new probiotic strains and new mechanisms of action are likely to be discovered.

5. CONCLUSIONS

There is now sufficient evidence to suggest the use of certain, species specific, probiotics in the treatment of IBS. Based on the trials reviewed in this chapter *B. infantis* 35624 and *E. coli* DSM 17252 have shown in more than one trial to significantly reduce symptom burden in IBS. In addition, there is limited evidence for the use of the combination probiotic containing *L. rhamnosus* GG, *L. rhamnosus* LC705, *B. breve*, *Propionibacterium freudenreichii* spp. and Shermanii JS. Probiotics offer a safe, sustainable method of manipulating the GI microbiota in IBS and producing symptomatic relief.

References

1. Thompson, W. G., Longstreth, G. F., Drossman, D. A., et al. (1999). Functional bowel disorders and functional abdominal pain. *Gut, 45*(Suppl. 2), II43–II47.
2. Chaudhary, N. A., & Truelove, S. C. (1962). The irritable colon syndrome. A study of the clinical features, predisposing causes, and prognosis in 130 cases. *The Quarterly Journal of Medicine, 31*, 307–322.
3. Manning, A. P., Thompson, W. G., Heaton, K. W., & Morris, A. F. (1978). Towards positive diagnosis of the irritable bowel. *British Medical Journal, 2*, 653–654.
4. Thompson, W. G., Creed, F., & Drossman, D. A. (1992). Functional bowel disorders and functional abdominal pain. *Gastroenterology International, 5*, 75–91.
5. Longstreth, G. F., Thompson, W. G., Chey, W. D., et al. (2006). Functional bowel disorders. *Gastroenterology, 130*, 1480–1491.
6. Bommelaer, G., Poynard, T., Le, P. C., et al. (2004). Prevalence of irritable bowel syndrome (IBS) and variability of diagnostic criteria. *Gastroentérologie Clinique et Biologique, 28*, 554–561.
7. Kellow, J. E., Azpiroz, F., Delvaux, M., et al. (2006). Applied principles of neurogastroenterology: Physiology/motility sensation. *Gastroenterology, 130*, 1412–1420.
8. Parkes, G. C., Brostoff, J., Whelan, K., & Sanderson, J. D. (2008). Gastrointestinal microbiota in irritable bowel syndrome: their role in its pathogenesis and treatment 2. *American Journal of Gastroenterol, 103*, 1557–1567.
9. Food and Agriculture Organization of the United Nations and World Health Organization Expert Consultation Report (2001). Evaluation of health and nutritional properties of probiotics in food, including powder milk with the live lactic acid bacteria. http://www.who.int/foodsafety/publications/fs_management/en/probiotics.pdf.
10. Parkes, G. C., Sanderson, J. D., & Whelan, K. (2009). The mechanisms and efficacy of probiotics in the prevention of *Clostridium difficile*-associated diarrhea. *Lancet Infectious Diseases, 9*, 237–244.
11. Kruis, W., Fric, P., Pokrotnieks, J., et al. (2004). Maintaining remission of ulcerative colitis with the probiotic *Escherichia coli* Nissle 1917 is as effective as with standard mesalazine. *Gut, 53*, 1617–1623.
12. Van Niel, C. W., Feudtner, C., Garrison, M. M., & Christakis, D. A. (2002). Lactobacillus therapy for acute infectious diarrhea in children: A meta-analysis. *Pediatrics, 109*, 678–684.
13. Szajewska, H., Skorka, A., Ruszczynski, M., & Gieruszczak-Bialek, D. (2007). Meta-analysis: *Lactobacillus* GG for treating acute diarrhea in children. *Alimentary Pharmacology & Therapeutics, 25*, 871–881.
14. Szajewska, H., Skorka, A., & Dylag, M. (2007). Meta-analysis: *Saccharomyces boulardii* for treating acute diarrhea in children. *Alimentary Pharmacology & Therapeutics, 25*, 257–264.
15. Alfaleh, K., & Bassler, D. (2008). Probiotics for prevention of necrotizing enterocolitis in preterm infants. *Cochrane Database of Systematic Reviews*, CD005496.
16. Balsari, A., Ceccarelli, A., Dubini, F., et al. (1982). The fecal microbial population in the irritable bowel syndrome. *Microbiologica, 5*, 185–194.
17. Si, J. M., Yu, Y. C., Fan, Y. J., & Chen, S. J. (2004). Intestinal microecology and quality of life in irritable bowel syndrome patients. *World Journal of Gastroenterol, 10*, 1802–1805.
18. Suau, A., Bonnet, R., Sutren, M., et al. (1999). Direct analysis of genes encoding 16S rRNA from complex communities reveals many novel molecular species within the human gut. *Applied and Environmental Microbiology, 65*, 4799–4807.
19. Malinen, E., Rinttila, T., Kajander, K., et al. (2005). Analysis of the fecal microbiota of irritable bowel syndrome patients and healthy controls with real-time PCR. *The American Journal of Gastroenterology, 100*, 373–382.
20. Kassinen, A., Krogius-Kurikka, L., Makivuokko, H., et al. (2007). The fecal microbiota of irritable bowel

syndrome patients differs significantly from that of healthy subjects. *Gastroenterology*, *133*, 24–33.

21. Parkes, G. C., Rayment, N. B., Hudspith, B. N. & et al. (2009). Sub-groups of irritable bowel syndrome have a distinct colonic mucosa-associated microbiota, Gut, 58(Suppl):A157–A172.

22. Spiller, R. C., Jenkins, D., Thornley, J. P., et al. (2000). Increased rectal mucosal enteroendocrine cells, T lymphocytes, and increased gut permeability following acute *Campylobacter enteritis* and in post-dysenteric irritable bowel syndrome. *Gut*, *47*, 804–811.

23. Chadwick, V. S., Chen, W., Shu, D., et al. (2002). Activation of the mucosal immune system in irritable bowel syndrome. *Gastroenterology*, *122*, 1778–1783.

24. Chadwick, V. S., Chen, W., Shu, D., et al. (2002). Activation of the mucosal immune system in irritable bowel syndrome. *Gastroenterology*, *122*, 1778–1783.

25. Guilarte, M., Santos, J., de Torres, I., et al. (2007). Diarrhoea-predominant IBS patients show mast cell activation and hyperplasia in the jejunum. *Gut*, *56*, 203–209.

26. O'Sullivan, M., Clayton, N., Breslin, N. P., et al. (2000). Increased mast cells in the irritable bowel syndrome. *Neurogastroenterology and Motility*, *12*, 449–457.

27. Weston, A. P., Biddle, W. L., Bhatia, P. S., & Miner, P. B., Jr. (1993). Terminal ileal mucosal mast cells in irritable bowel syndrome. *Digestive Diseases and Sciences*, *38*, 1590–1595.

28. Spiller, R. C., Jenkins, D., Thornley, J. P., et al. (2000). Increased rectal mucosal enteroendocrine cells, T lymphocytes, and increased gut permeability following acute *Campylobacter enteritis* and in post-dysenteric irritable bowel syndrome. *Gut*, *47*, 804–811.

29. Spiller, R. C., Jenkins, D., Thornley, J. P., et al. (2000). Increased rectal mucosal enteroendocrine cells, T lymphocytes, and increased gut permeability following acute *Campylobacter enteritis* and in post-dysenteric irritable bowel syndrome. *Gut*, *47*, 804–811.

30. Bradesi, S., McRoberts, J. A., Anton, P. A., & Mayer, E. A. (2003). Inflammatory bowel disease and irritable bowel syndrome: Separate or unified? *Current Opinion in Gastroenterology*, *19*, 336–342.

31. Spiller, R. C., Jenkins, D., Thornley, J. P., et al. (2000). Increased rectal mucosal enteroendocrine cells, T lymphocytes, and increased gut permeability following acute *Campylobacter enteritis* and in post-dysenteric irritable bowel syndrome. *Gut*, *47*, 804–811.

32. Marshall, J. K., Thabane, M., Garg, A. X., et al. (2006). Incidence and epidemiology of irritable bowel syndrome after a large waterborne outbreak of bacterial dysentery. *Gastroenterology*, *131*, 445–450.

33. Hungin, A. P., Whorwell, P. J., Tack, J., & Mearin, F. (2003). The prevalence, patterns and impact of irritable bowel syndrome: an international survey of 40,000 subjects. *Alimentary Pharmacology & Therapeutics*, *17*, 643–650.

34. Houghton, L. A., Lea, R., Agrawal, A., et al. (2006). Relationship of abdominal bloating to distention in irritable bowel syndrome and effect of bowel habit. *Gastroenterology*, *131*, 1003–1010.

35. Koide, A., Yamaguchi, T., Odaka, T., et al. (2000). Quantitative analysis of bowel gas using plain abdominal radiograph in patients with irritable bowel syndrome. *The American Journal of Gastroenterology*, *95*, 1735–1741.

36. Perez, F., Accarino, A., Azpiroz, F., et al. (2007). Abdominal bloating: Distinctive features of organic versus functional disorder. *Gut*, *56*, A39.

37. Hasler, W. L. (2003). Lactulose breath testing, bacterial overgrowth, and IBS: Just a lot of hot air? *Gastroenterology*, *125*, 1898–1900.

38. Mishkin, D. & Mishkin, S. (2001). Re: Pimentel et al., Eradication of small intestinal bacterial overgrowth reduces symptoms of irritable bowel syndrome. *The American Journal of Gastroenterology*, *96*, 2505–2506.

39. Riordan, S. M., McIver, C. J., Duncombe, V. M., et al. (2001). Small intestinal bacterial overgrowth and the irritable bowel syndrome. *The American Journal of Gastroenterology*, *96*, 2506–2508.

40. Walters, B., & Vanner, S. J. (2005). Detection of bacterial overgrowth in IBS using the lactulose H2 breath test: Comparison with 14 C-D-xylose and healthy controls. *The American Journal of Gastroenterology*, *100*, 1566–1570.

41. Posserud, I., Stotzer, P. O., Bjornsson, E. S., et al. (2007). Small intestinal bacterial overgrowth in patients with irritable bowel syndrome. *Gut*, *56*, 802–808.

42. Sharara, A. I., Aoun, E., bdul-Baki, H., et al. (2006). A randomized double-blind placebo-controlled trial of Rifaximin in patients with abdominal bloating and flatulence. *The American Journal of Gastroenterology*, *101*, 326–333.

43. Pimentel, M., Park, S., Mirocha, J., et al. (2006). The effect of a nonabsorbed oral antibiotic (rifaximin) on the symptoms of the irritable bowel syndrome: A randomized trial. *Annals of Internal Medicine*, *145*, 557–563.

44. Atlas, R. M. (1999). Probiotics: snake oil for the new millennium? *Environmental Microbiology*, *1*, 377–382.

45. Food and Agriculture Organization of the United Nations and World Health Organization Expert Consultation Report (2001). Evaluation of health and nutritional properties of probiotics in food, including powder milk with the live lactic acid bacteria.http://www. who.int/foodsafety/publications/fs_management/ en/probiotics.pdf.

46. Drakes, M., Blanchard, T., & Czinn, S. (2004). Bacterial probiotic modulation of dendritic cells. *Infection and Immunity*, *72*, 3299–3309.

47. Fujii, T., Ohtsuka, Y., Lee, T., et al. (2006). *Bifidobacterium breve* enhances transforming growth factor beta1

signaling by regulating Smad7 expression in preterm infants. *Journal of Pediatric Gastroenterology and Nutrition, 43,* 83–88.

48. Helwig, U., Lammers, K. M., Rizzello, F., et al. (2006). Lactobacilli, bifidobacteria and *E. coli* nissle induce pro- and anti-inflammatory cytokines in peripheral blood mononuclear cells. *World Journal of Gastroenterology, 12,* 5978–5986.

49. Hudspith, B. N., Rouzard, G., Gibson, G. R., et al. (2006). Probiotic bacteria inhibit epithelial cell IL-8 production: Role of TLR receptor engagement. *Gut, 55,* A38.

50. O'Hara, A. M., O'Regan, P., Fanning, A., et al. (2006). Functional modulation of human intestinal epithelial cell responses by *Bifidobacterium infantis* and *Lactobacillus salivarius. Immunology, 118,* 202–215.

51. Schlee, M., Wehkamp, J., Altenhoefer, A., et al. (2007). Induction of human {beta}-defensin 2 by the probiotic *Escherichia coli* Nissle 1917 is mediated through flagellin. *Infection and Immunity, 75,* 2399–2407.

52. Calcinaro, F., Dionisi, S., Marinaro, M., et al. (2005). Oral probiotic administration induces interleukin-10 production and prevents spontaneous autoimmune diabetes in the non-obese diabetic mouse. *Diabetologia, 48,* 1565–1575.

53. Lammers, K. M., Brigidi, P., Vitali, B., et al. (2003). Immunomodulatory effects of probiotic bacteria DNA: IL-1 and IL-10 response in human peripheral blood mononuclear cells. *FEMS Immunology and Medical Microbiology, 38,* 165–172.

54. Chen, C. C., Louie, S., Shi, H. N., & Walker, W. A. (2005). Preinoculation with the probiotic *Lactobacillus acidophilus* early in life effectively inhibits murine *Citrobacter rodentium* colitis. *Pediatric Research, 58,* 1185–1191.

55. Hamilton-Miller, J. M., Shah, S., & Winkler, J. T. (1999). Public health issues arising from microbiological and labelling quality of foods and supplements containing probiotic microorganisms. *Public Health Nutrition, 2,* 223–229.

56. Pedersen, G., Andresen, L., Matthiessen, M. W., et al. (2005). Expression of Toll-like receptor 9 and response to bacterial CpG oligodeoxynucleotides in human intestinal epithelium. *Clinical and Experimental Immunology, 141,* 298–306.

57. Rachmilewitz, D., Katakura, K., Karmeli, F., et al. (2004). Toll-like receptor 9 signaling mediates the anti-inflammatory effects of probiotics in murine experimental colitis. *Gastroenterology, 126,* 520–528.

58. Rousseaux, C., Thuru, X., Gelot, A., et al. (2007). *Lactobacillus acidophilus* modulates intestinal pain and induces opioid and cannabinoid receptors. *Nature Medicine, 13,* 35–37.

59. Verdu, E. F., Bercik, P., Verma-Gandhu, M., et al. (2006). Specific probiotic therapy attenuates antibiotic induced visceral hypersensitivity in mice. *Gut, 55,* 182–190.

60. Verd, E. F., Bercik, P., Bergonzelli, G. E., et al. (2004). Lactobacillus paracasei normalizes muscle hypercontractility in a murine model of postinfective gut dysfunction. *Gastroenterology, 127,* 826–837.

61. Caballero-Franco, C., Keller, K., De, S. C., & Chadee, K. (2007). The VSL#3 probiotic formula induces mucin gene expression and secretion in colonic epithelial cells. *American Journal of Physiology. Gastrointestinal and Liver Physiology, 292,* G315–G322.

62. Zyrek, A. A., Cichon, C., Helms, S., et al. (2007). Molecular mechanisms underlying the probiotic effects of *Escherichia coli* Nissle 1917 involve ZO-2 and PKCzeta redistribution resulting in tight junction and epithelial barrier repair. *Cellular Microbiology, 9,* 804–816.

63. Zeng, J., Li, Y. Q., Zuo, X. L., et al. (2008). Clinical trial: effect of active lactic acid bacteria on mucosal barrier function in patients with diarrhea-predominant irritable bowel syndrome. *Alimentary Pharmacology & Therapeutics, 28,* 994–1002.

64. Dunlop, S. P., Hebden, J., Campbell, E., et al. (2006). Abnormal intestinal permeability in subgroups of diarrhea-predominant irritable bowel syndromes. *The American Journal of Gastroenterology, 101,* 1288–1294.

65. Marshall, J. K., Thabane, M., Garg, A. X., et al. (2004). Intestinal permeability in patients with irritable bowel syndrome after a waterborne outbreak of acute gastroenteritis in Walkerton, Ontario. *Alimentary Pharmacology & Therapeutics, 20,* 1317–1322.

66. Madsen, K., Cornish, A., Soper, P., et al. (2001). Probiotic bacteria enhance murine and human intestinal epithelial barrier function. *Gastroenterology, 121,* 580–591.

67. Ma, D., Forsythe, P., & Bienenstock, J. (2004). Live *Lactobacillus reuteri* is essential for the inhibitory effect on tumor necrosis factor alpha-induced interleukin–8 expression. *Infection and Immunity, 72,* 5308–5314.

68. Tuomola, E. M., & Salminen, S. J. (1998). Adhesion of some probiotic and dairy Lactobacillus strains to Caco-2 cell cultures. *International Journal of Food Microbiology, 41,* 45–51.

69. Corr, S. C., Gahan, C. G. M., & Hill, C. (2007). Impact of selected *Lactobacillus* and *Bifidobacterium* species on *Listeria monocytogenes* infection and the mucosal immune response. *FEMS Immunology and Medical Microbiology, 50,* 380–388.

70. Wullt, M., Johansson Hagslatt, M. L., Odenholt, I., & Berggren, A. (2007). Lactobacillus plantarum 299v enhances the concentrations of fecal short-chain fatty acids in patients with recurrent clostridium difficile-associated diarrhea. *Digestive Diseases and Sciences, 52,* 2082–2086.

71. Pimentel, M., Chow, E. J., & Lin, H. C. (2000). Eradication of small intestinal bacterial overgrowth reduces symptoms of irritable bowel syndrome. *The American Journal of Gastroenterology, 95,* 3503–3506.

72. Moayyedi, P., Ford, A. C., Talley, N. J., & et al. (2008). The efficacy of probiotics in the therapy of irritable bowel syndrome: a systematic review. *Gut* (e-pub ahead of print).

73. Brenner, D. M., Moeller, M. J., Chey, W. D., & Schoenfeld, P. S. (2009). The utility of probiotics in the treatment of irritable bowel syndrome: A systematic review. *The American Journal of Gastroenterology, 104*, 1033–1049.

74. McFarland, L. V., & Dublin, S. (2008). Meta-analysis of probiotics for the treatment of irritable bowel syndrome. *World Journal of Gastroenterology, 14*, 2650–2661.

75. Hoveyda, N., Heneghan, C., Mahtani, K. R., et al. (2009). A systematic review and meta-analysis: Probiotics in the treatment of irritable bowel syndrome. *BMC Gastroenterology, 9*, 15.

76. Gibson, G. R., Probert, H. M., Van de Loo, J., et al. (2004). Dietary modulation of the human colonic microbiota: Updating the concept of prebiotics. *Nutrition Research Reviews, 17*, 259–275.

77. Guyonnet, D., Chassany, O., Ducrotte, P., et al. (2007). Effect of a fermented milk containing *Bifidobacterium animalis* DN-173010 on the health-related quality of life and symptoms in irritable bowel syndrome in adults in primary care: a multicenter, randomized, double-blind, controlled trial. *Alimentary Pharmacology & Therapeutics, 26*, 475–486.

78. Niv, E., Naftali, T., Hallak, R., & Vaisman, N. (2005). The efficacy of *Lactobacillus reuteri* ATCC 55730 in the treatment of patients with irritable bowel syndrome—a double blind, placebo-controlled, randomized study. *Clinical Nutrition, 24*, 925–931.

79. Hun, L. (2009). *Bacillus coagulans* significantly improved abdominal pain and bloating in patients with IBS. *Postgraduate Medicine, 121*, 119–124.

80. Enck, P., Zimmermann, K., Menke, G., et al. (2008). A mixture of *Escherichia coli* (DSM 17252) and *Enterococcus faecalis* (DSM 16440) for treatment of the irritable bowel syndrome—a randomized controlled trial with primary care physicians. *Neurogastroenterology and Motility, 20*, 1103–1109.

81. Bittner, A. C., Croffut, R. M., & Stranahan, M. C. (2005). Prescript-assist(TM) probiotic-prebiotic treatment for irritable bowel syndrome: A methodologically oriented, 2-week, randomized, placebo-controlled, double-blind clinical study. *Clinical Therapeutics, 27*, 755–761.

82. Long, Z. R., Yu, C. H., Yang, Y., et al. (2006). Clinical observation on acupuncture combined with microorganism pharmaceutical preparations for treatment of irritable bowel syndrome of constipation type. *Zhongguo Zhen Jiu, 26*, 403–405.

83. Bausserman, M., & Michail, S. (2005). The use of *Lactobacillus* GG in irritable bowel syndrome in children: A double-blind randomized control trial. *The Journal of Pediatrics, 147*, 197–201.

84. Kim, H. J., Vazquez Roque, M. I., Camilleri, M., et al. (2005). A randomized controlled trial of a probiotic combination VSL# 3 and placebo in irritable bowel syndrome with bloating. *Neurogastroenterology and Motility, 17*, 687–696.

85. Niedzielin, K., Kordecki, H., & Birkenfeld, B. (2001). A controlled, double-blind, randomized study on the efficacy of *Lactobacillus plantarum* 299 V in patients with irritable bowel syndrome. *European Journal of Gastroenterology & Hepatology, 13*, 1143–1147.

86. Sen, S., Mullan, M. M., Parker, T. J., et al. (2002). Effect of *Lactobacillus plantarum* 299v on colonic fermentation and symptoms of irritable bowel syndrome. *Digestive Diseases and Sciences, 47*, 2615–2620.

87. Andriulli, A., Neri, M., Loguercio, C., et al. (2008). Clinical trial on the efficacy of a new symbiotic formulation, Flortec, in patients with irritable bowel syndrome: a multicenter, randomized study. *Journal of Clinical Gastroenterology, 42*(Suppl. 3, Pt. 2), S218–S223.

88. Enck, P., Zimmermann, K., Menke, G., & Klosterhalfen, S. (2009). Randomized controlled treatment trial of irritable bowel syndrome with a probiotic E. coli preparation (DSM17252) compared to placebo. *Zeitschrift für Gastroenterologie, 47*, 209–214.

89. Kajanda, K., Myllyluoma, E., Rajilic-Stojanovic, M., et al. (2008). Clinical trial: Multispecies probiotic supplementation alleviates the symptoms of irritable bowel syndrome and stabilizes intestinal microbiota. *Alimentary Pharmacology & Therapeutics, 27*, 48–57.

90. Whorwell, P. J., Altringer, L., Morel, J., et al. (2006). Efficacy of an encapsulated probiotic *Bifidobacterium infantis* 35624 in women with irritable bowel syndrome. *The American Journal of Gastroenterology, 101*, 1581–1590.

91. Nobaek, S., Johansson, M. L., Molin, G., et al. (2000). Alteration of intestinal microflora is associated with reduction in abdominal bloating and pain in patients with irritable bowel syndrome. *The American Journal of Gastroenterology, 95*, 1231–1238.

92. Gawronska, A., Dziechciarz, P., Horvath, A., & Szajewska, H. (2007). A randomized double-blind placebo-controlled trial of *Lactobacillus* GG for abdominal pain disorders in children. *Alimentary Pharmacology & Therapeutics, 25*, 177–184.

93. Huertas-Ceballos, A. A., Logan, S., Bennett, C., & Macarthur, C. (2009). Dietary interventions for recurrent abdominal pain (RAP) and irritable bowel syndrome (IBS) in childhood. *Cochrane Database of Systematic Reviews* CD003019.

94. Miele, E., Pascarella, F., Giannetti, E., et al. (2009). Effect of a probiotic preparation (VSL[num]3) on induction and maintenance of remission in children with ulcerative colitis. *American Journal of Gastroenterology, 104*, 437–443.

95. Gionchetti, P., Rizzello, F., Venturi, A., et al. (2000). Oral bacteriotherapy as maintenance treatment in patients with chronic pouchitis: A double-blind, placebo-controlled trial. *Gastroenterology, 119,* 305–309.

96. Gionchetti, P., Rizzello, F., Helwig, U., et al. (2003). Prophylaxis of pouchitis onset with probiotic therapy: a double-blind, placebo-controlled trial. *Gastroenterology, 124,* 1202–1209.

97. Hart, A. L., Lammers, K., Brigidi, P., et al. (2004). Modulation of human dendritic cell phenotype and function by probiotic bacteria. *Gut, 53,* 1602–1609.

98. Kim, H. J., Camilleri, M., McKinzie, S., et al. (2003). A randomized controlled trial of a probiotic, VSL#3, on gut transit and symptoms in diarrhea-predominant irritable bowel syndrome. *Alimentary Pharmacology & Therapeutics, 17,* 890–895.

99. McCarthy, J., O'Mahony, L., O'Callaghan, L., et al. (2003). Double blind, placebo controlled trial of two probiotic strains in interleukin 10 knockout mice and mechanistic link with cytokine balance. *Gut, 52,* 975–980.

100. Shanahan, F., Guarner, F., Von Wright, A., et al. (2006). A one year, randomised, double-blind, placebo controlled trial of a lactobacillus or a bifidobacterium probiotic for maintenance of steroid-induced remission of ulcerative colitis. *Gastroenterology, 130*(Suppl. 2), A44.

101. O'Mahony, L., McCarthy, J., Kelly, P., et al. (2005). Lactobacillus and bifidobacterium in irritable bowel syndrome: Symptom responses and relationship to cytokine profiles. *Gastroenterology, 128,* 541–551.

102. Kajander, K., Hatakka, K., Poussa, T., et al. (2005). A probiotic mixture alleviates symptoms in irritable bowel syndrome patients: A controlled 6-month intervention. *Alimentary Pharmacology & Therapeutics, 22,* 387–394.

103. Kajander, K., Myllyluoma, E., Rajilic-Stojanovic, M., et al. (2008). Clinical trial: Multispecies probiotic supplementation alleviates the symptoms of irritable bowel syndrome and stabilizes intestinal microbiota. *Alimentary Pharmacology & Therapeutics, 27,* 48–57.

104. Drouault-Holowacz, S., Bieuvelet, S., Burckel, A., et al. (2008). A double-blind randomized controlled trial of a probiotic combination in 100 patients with irritable bowel syndrome. *Gastroentérologie Clinique et Biologique, 32,* 147–152.

105. Silk, D. B., Davis, A., Vulevic, J., et al. (2009). Clinical trial: The effects of a trans-galacto-oligosaccharide prebiotic on fecal microbiota and symptoms in irritable bowel syndrome. *Alimentary Pharmacology & Therapeutics, 29,* 508–518.

106. Smith, G. D., Steinke, D. T., Kinnear, M., et al. (2004). A comparison of irritable bowel syndrome patients managed in primary and secondary care: The Episode IBS study. *The British Journal of General Practice, 54,* 503–507.

107. Panijel, M., & Burkhard, I. (1993). Pro-symbioflor for the treatment of irritable colon. *Jatros Naturheilkunde, 2*(3), 1–4.

108. Ford, A. C., Talley, N. J., Spiegel, B. M., et al. (2008). Effect of fibre, antispasmodics, and peppermint oil in the treatment of irritable bowel syndrome: Systematic review and meta-analysis. *BMJ, 337,* a2313.

109. Prather, C. M., Camilleri, M., Zinsmeister, A. R., et al. (2000). Tegaserod accelerates orocecal transit in patients with constipation-predominant irritable bowel syndrome. *Gastroenterology, 118,* 463–468.

110. Camilleri, M., Mayer, E. A., Drossman, D. A., et al. (1999). Improvement in pain and bowel function in female irritable bowel patients with alosetron, a 5-HT3 receptor antagonist. *Alimentary Pharmacology & Therapeutics, 13,* 1149–1159.

111. Ford, A. C., Brandt, L. J., Young, C., & et al. (2009). Efficacy of 5-HT(3) antagonists and 5-HT(4) agonists in irritable bowel syndrome: systematic review and meta-analysis. *The American Journal of Gastroenterology, 104*(7):1831–43.

112. Kajanda, K., Hatakka, K., Poussa, T., et al. (2005). A probiotic mixture alleviates symptoms in irritable bowel syndrome patients: A controlled 6-month intervention. *Alimentary Pharmacology & Therapeutics, 22,* 387–394.

113. Sinn, D. H., Song, J. H., Kim, H. J., et al. (2008). Therapeutic effect of *Lactobacillus acidophilus*-SDC 2012, 2013 in patients with irritable bowel syndrome. *Digestive Diseases and Sciences, 53,* 2714–2718.

114. Tsuchiya, J., Barreto, R., Okura, R., et al. (2004). Single-blind follow-up study on the effectiveness of a symbiotic preparation in irritable bowel syndrome. *Chinese Journal of Digestive Diseases, 5,* 169–174.

115. Williams, E., Stimpson, J., Wang, D., & et al. (2008). Clinical trial: a multistrain probiotic preparation significantly reduces symptoms of irritable bowel syndrome in a double-blind placebo-controlled study. *Alimentary Pharmacology & Therapeutics, 29*(1):97–103.

116. Deshpande, G., Rao, S., & Patole, S. (2007). Probiotics for prevention of necrotising enterocolitis in preterm neonates with very low birthweight: A systematic review of randomised controlled trials. *The Lancet, 369,* 1614–1620.

117. Minna, K. S., Soile, T., Rautelin, H., et al. (2004). The efficacy and safety of probiotic *Lactobacillus rhamnosus* GG on prolonged, noninfectious diarrhea in HIV patients on antiretroviral therapy: A randomized, placebo-controlled, crossover study. *HIV Clinical Trials, 5,* 183–191.

118. Mego, M., Ebringer, L., Drgona, L., et al. (2005). Prevention of febrile neutropenia in cancer patients by probiotic strain *Enterococcus faecium* M–74. Pilot study phase I. *Neoplasma, 52,* 159–164.

119. Boyle, R. J., Robins-Browne, R. M., & Tang, M. L. (2006). Probiotic use in clinical practice: What are the risks? *The American Journal of Clinical Nutrition, 83*, 1256–1264.

120. Zhou, J. S., Pillidge, C. J., Gopal, P. K., & Gill, H. S. (2005). Antibiotic susceptibility profiles of new probiotic Lactobacillus and Bifidobacterium strains. *International Journal of Food Microbiology, 98*, 211–217.

121. Besselink, M. G., van Santvoort, H. C., Buskens, E., et al. (2008). Probiotic prophylaxis in predicted severe acute pancreatitis: A randomised, double-blind, placebo-controlled trial. *The Lancet, 371*, 651–659.

122. Kajander, K., Hatakka, K., Poussa, T., et al. (2005). A probiotic mixture alleviates symptoms in irritable bowel syndrome patients: A controlled 6-month intervention. *Alimentary Pharmacology & Therapeutics, 22*, 387–394.

123. Kajander, K., Myllyluoma, E., Rajilic-Stojanovic, M., et al. (2008). Clinical trial: multispecies probiotic supplementation alleviates the symptoms of irritable bowel syndrome and stabilizes intestinal microbiota. *Alimentary Pharmacology & Therapeutics, 27*, 48–57.

ANIMAL MODELS TO STUDY PROBIOTICS

Human Flora-associated Animals as a Model for Studying Probiotics and Prebiotics

Kazuhiro Hirayama

Laboratory of Veterinary Public Health, Department of Veterinary Medical Science,
Graduate School of Agricultural and Life Sciences, The University of Tokyo,
Bunkyo, Tokyo, Japan

1. INTRODUCTION

It is now well established that the intestinal microbiota play an important role in human health and disease. There is an increasing interest in the consumption of functional foods, particularly probiotics and prebiotics, to improve gastrointestinal microbiota and confer favorable effects on the host. However, it is often difficult to study the effects of probiotics and prebiotics *in vivo*. This is largely due to the difficulties of studying the human intestinal microbiota; e.g. difficulties of controlling genetics and environmental and dietary conditions of humans. Thus, the results of studies with human volunteers are often not clear. There are also ethical problems associated with utilizing pathogens, carcinogens or toxic substances in human volunteers. In addition, it must be kept in mind that the composition and metabolic activities of the intestinal microbiota of experimental animals are significantly different from those of humans

[1], making extrapolation of results from animal studies to the human system questionable. To find a solution to this problem, germfree animals associated with human fecal microbiota, i.e. human flora-associated (HFA) animals, have been considered as a tool for studying the ecology and metabolism of intestinal bacteria of humans [2].

2. PRODUCTION OF HFA ANIMALS

By inoculating feces from various species of animals and humans, the fecal bacteria of the donor animals can be transferred to germfree animals [3–7]. Hirayama et al. [1, 8] inoculated germfree mice with the fecal suspension of different healthy human adults and the major composition of human microbiota could be transferred into HFA mice. However, bifidobacteria were eliminated from some of the HFA mouse groups [1]. Interestingly, the elimination of bifidobacteria seemed to be dependent on the composition of the microbiota in the inoculated samples.

Studies exploiting modern molecular biology-based methods also demonstrated that transplantation of intestinal microbiota from a human to germfree animals produced a donor-like microbial community with minor modification [9, 10], while some studies raised questions about the adequacy of HFA animals as a model to study the ecology of the human intestinal tract [11, 12].

3. METABOLIC ACTIVITIES OF INTESTINAL MICROBIOTA OF HFA ANIMALS

Mallett et al. [13] demonstrated that certain cancer related enzymic activities of human fecal microbiota can be simulated in rats associated with human intestinal bacteria. Hirayama et al. [1] reported that the activities of some enzyme activities of intestinal flora in HFA mice were similar to those in humans and different from those in conventional mice, while the others were not. The concentrations of putrefactive products in the feces of HFA mice were much lower than those in human feces and similar to those in conventional mice, while *p*-cresol, which is detected in human feces but not in conventional mice, was detected in most of the HFA mouse groups, and the concentration of fecal indole in some of the HFA mouse groups was significantly higher than that in conventional mice [1]. Although the concentration of fecal short-chain fatty acids (SCFAs) in HFA mice was significantly lower than that in humans and similar to that in conventional mice, the composition of SCFAs in HFA mice was closer to that in humans than that in conventional mice [1].

Thus, bacterial metabolism in the intestine of HFA mice reflected that of human feces with respect to some metabolic activities but not others, even though the bacterial composition of the feces of HFA mice was similar to that of the inocula.

4. STABILITY OF INTESTINAL MICROBIOTA OF HFA ANIMALS

The intestinal microbiota established in the intestines of HFA animals can be maintained for a long time [14], and the composition and metabolic activities of the intestinal microbiota of HFA mice can be reproduced in the intestines of the offspring of the HFA mice without any remarkable changes [1, 15]. Most of the intestinal bacteria of mother HFA mice colonized in the intestines of the offspring within 3 weeks after birth and the compositions of the microbiota of offspring were similar to those of their mothers. Molecular biology-based methods also demonstrated that, although a higher variation in fecal microbiota over time was observed for HFA than for SPF rats, the variation over time was less significant than that variation between individuals [16].

However, the development of intestinal flora in the offspring of HFA mice is similar to that of conventional mice but not to that of human infants [15]. In human infants, bifidobacteria become the most predominant bacteria within 1 week after birth [17, 18], but bifidobacteria never became the most predominant bacteria in the infant HFA mice, even though the mother HFA mice harbored a large population of bifidobacteria [15]. On the other hand, Pang et al. [10] reported that the microbial succession with aging of HFA piglets was similar to that observed in humans.

The intestinal microbiota of the HFA mice was also reproduced in ex-germfree mice by transferring germfree mice into the cages of HFA mice and allowing them to be colonized with the human intestinal microbiota [19]. These studies demonstrated that the human intestinal microbiota once established in HFA mice can be maintained for a long period.

5. APPLICATION OF HFA ANIMALS TO STUDIES ON HUMAN INTESTINAL MICROBIOTA AND ITS EFFECTS ON THE HOST

The intestinal microbiota has direct effects on the host and the effects of the human intestinal microbiota on the host have been investigated *in vivo* using HFA animals. The architecture of the colonic epithelial mucus layer was affected by the colonization of a human microbiota in rats [20]. Production and distribution of mucin were significantly different from those of germfree rats when the germfree rats were inoculated with a human microbiota [21, 22]. Human microbiota associated in the rat intestine significantly altered the number of the goblet cells and goblet cell glycoconjugates [20, 23]. An HFA animal study also demonstrated that microbial-diet interactions can affect the numbers of enteroendocrine cells [24].

The metabolism of dietary components by the human intestinal microbiota can be investigated using HFA animals [25–28]. The role of human intestinal microbiota in modification on the physiological and morphological properties of the host has also been demonstrated in studies with HFA animals. For example, an important role of human intestinal microbiota has been reported in the effects of dietary components on mucosal architecture and the biosynthesis, secretion, and degradation of mucin [20, 22, 23, 29]. Studies using HFA animals have also demonstrated that the human intestinal microbiota influences the effects of dietary components on some hepatic xenobiotic metabolizing enzymes [30, 31]. Roland et al. [32] indicated the different effects of different types of dietary fiber on hepatic and intestinal drug-metabolizing enzymes using rats inoculated with the human whole fecal microbiota. Rumney et al. [33] demonstrated that hepatic S9 fraction from HFA rats fed diet with different cancer risk-associated macrocomponents have different activities in *in vitro* activation of dietary mutagens. The authors further suggested that risk-related dietary components interact with the human intestinal microbiota to modulate the production of endogenous DNA-adducting and cross-linking substances.

Immunological studies have employed HFA animals as an experimental tool and demonstrated the immunomodulatory activities of dietary components [34–36]. HFA animals have also been used in nutritional studies [37, 38].

Comparisons between HFA animals and conventional animals often demonstrate that the effects of human intestinal microbiota are different from those of laboratory rodents [39]. Thus, HFA animals can be a useful tool for studying the human intestinal microbiota and its effects on the host *in vivo*.

6. APPLICATION OF HFA ANIMALS TO STUDIES ON THE EFFECTS OF PROBIOTICS, PREBIOTICS AND OTHER DIETARY COMPONENTS ON HUMAN INTESTINAL MICROBIOTA

HFA animals have often been used to investigate the effects of dietary supplements, such as probiotics [40] and prebiotics [19, 41–45], and changes in dietary macrocomponents [19, 33, 46] on the composition and metabolism of human intestinal microbiota. For example, Djouzi et al. [40] demonstrated that milk fermented with *Lactobacillus casei* significantly increased the amount of indigenous bifidobacteria in the feces of HFA rats. Rowland and Tanaka [41] reported an increase in the cecal concentration of total bacteria, lactobacilli and bifidobacteria by feeding transgalactosylated oligosaccharides to HFA rats. Their results were consistent with those obtained in a human volunteer study [47] although there was no change in total bacteria. Djouzi and Andrieux [42] found that feeding of β-galacto-oligosaccharides and β-fructo-oligosaccharides significantly increased the numbers of *Bifidobacterium* in feces but did not change the total numbers of anaerobic bacteria in HFA rats. These effects have also been observed previously in human subjects [47–49]. They then compared the effects of three different oligosaccharides in HFA rats and found differences among the different oligosaccharides in their effects on the intestinal microbiota.

Although some studies utilizing human volunteers report significant changes in the fecal microbiota with changes in dietary composition [50], others [51, 52] report only minor effects. Thus, influences of different dietary components on human microbiota may be detected more clearly with HFA animals rather than with human volunteers. Furthermore, study with HFA mice suggested the beneficial effects of fructo-oligosaccharides on the intestinal microbiota at doses equivalent to those usually given to humans, which are far lower than the doses used in animal experiments [19].

HFA animals have also been used to compare, under controlled conditions, responses to dietary components of human intestinal microbiota of differing compositions or from different sources [6, 53, 54]. Silvi et al. [53] investigated the effects of resistant starch, which is a portion of starch undigested by pancreatic amylase in the small intestine, on the intestinal microbiota of HFA rats inoculated with feces from Italian or United Kingdom donors and indicated that different human microbiota may respond in different ways to dietary change. Andrieux et al. [54] prepared HFA rat groups inoculated with human microbiota with different levels of methane production and showed that the effects of dietary seaweed on some of the metabolism of intestinal were different among the HFA groups.

7. APPLICATION OF HFA ANIMALS TO SIMULATION OF CONDITIONS IN THE HUMAN INTESTINAL TRACT

Using HFA animals, the survival and activity of administered bacterial strains, which are necessary to have a probiotic effect, have been investigated [55–58]. Oozeer et al. [55] demonstrated that an inoculated lactic acid bacterial strain could survive and synthesize proteins in the intestinal environment. Lan et al. [56] investigated the survival and metabolic activity of *Propionibacterium freudenreichii*, which has been identified as potential probiotics, within the gastrointestinal tract of HFA rats, and its influence on intestinal microbiota composition and metabolism. Martin et al. [57] measured and mapped the transgenomic metabolic effects of exposure to probiotic strains in ex-germfree mice colonized with human baby microbiota. Probiotic exposure exerted microbiome modification and resulted in altered hepatic lipid metabolism coupled with lowered plasma lipoprotein levels and apparent stimulated glycolysis. Probiotic treatments also altered a diverse range of pathways outcomes, including amino-acid metabolism, methylamines and SCFAs.

The effects of therapeutic doses of antibiotics on the human intestinal microbiota have been investigated with HFA animals [59–63]. Barc et al. [64] evaluated the influence of the administration of probiotic *Saccharomyces boulardii* on the composition of the fecal microbiota in antibiotic treated HFA mouse model. After the antibiotic treatment was discontinued, the intestinal microbiota returned to the initial level more rapidly in the *S. boulardii*-treated mice than in the control mice. They suggested that this quicker recovery of normal intestinal microbiota equilibrium after antibiotic therapy could be a mechanism for *S. boulardii*'s preventive effect on antibiotic-associated diarrhea in humans. Furthermore, HFA animals have been employed as a model for evaluating the impact of drug residues in food on the human intestinal microbiota [62, 65, 66].

Tuohy et al. [67] investigated the transfer of plasmids from genetically modified microorganisms *in vivo* and demonstrated that the HFA rat model provides data of real relevance to the purported risks of DNA transfer from food-borne genetically modified microorganisms. Nijsten et al. [68] investigated the *in vivo* transfer of antibiotic resistance plasmids using a rat model associated with the intestinal microbiota of various origins including humans, and showed that the *in vivo* transfer of resistance plasmids is possible among the rat and human intestinal microbiota. Interestingly, the human intestinal microbiota appeared to permit better transfer of antibiotic resistance via plasmids than an intestinal microbiota derived from either pigs or rats.

8. HFA ANIMALS AS A MODEL FOR STUDIES WHICH ARE IMPOSSIBLE WITH HUMAN VOLUNTEERS

HFA animals are useful models for studies that are impossible or difficult to perform with human volunteers. For example, there are ethical issues associated with human studies of colonization resistance against pathogenic bacteria or the effects of inoculated toxic chemicals and carcinogens.

HFA animals have been used as a new model to investigate the influence of the human intestinal microbiota on mutagenic/carcinogenic substances *in vivo*. Rumney et al. [69] reported metabolism of dietary mutagen by the intestinal microbiota to 7-keto derivative, which is a direct-acting mutagen in the *Salmonella* mutagenicity test, while the mother compound requires S9 activation. They also demonstrated that the use of HFA rats produces results particularly relevant to humans, especially when the animals are fed human diets. This conversion was enhanced in HFA rats fed a high-risk diet for colon cancer [46] and decreased by ingestion of an indigestible sugar [70]. Hirayama et al. [71] found that the capacity of human feces to increase or decrease mutagenic activities of chemicals could be transferred into HFA mice. The presence of the intestinal microbiota was essential for the activity of feces against the mutagens. HFA mice were then administered dietary and environmental mutagens orally and DNA adduct formation was investigated as an *in vivo* biomarker of cancer risk. These results with HFA mice clearly showed that the human intestinal microbiota has an active role in DNA adduct formation. Using the same model, Horie et al. [72] indicated that the probiotic mixture could decrease the DNA adduct formation in the colonic epithelium induced by 2-amino-9H-pyrido[2,3-*b*]indole. Scheepers et al. [73, 74] also demonstrated with HFA rats that the metabolic activity of the human intestinal microbiota is an essential step in hemoglobin and DNA adduct formation.

The strong impact of human intestinal microbiota on the genotoxic effects of dietary mutagens measured by Comet assay has been demonstrated using HFA rats [75, 76]. Furthermore, the protective effects of dietary factors, including probiotics and prebiotics, against the genotoxic effects of carcinogens in the Comet assay have been demonstrated in HFA animal studies [31, 70]. The formation of aberrant crypt foci and chemically induced colon cancer has also been investigated in HFA animals [76–78].

Edwards et al. [79] consequently developed a rat model associated with human breast-fed infant microbiota maintained on a modified infant formula to investigate the ability of the human microbiota to inhibit adhesion of pathogens to mucosal cells, as well as effects on the indigenous bacterial populations and bacterial metabolism. HFA animals have also been used for studying the influence of diet on colonization resistance [6, 80, 81].

9. USEFULNESS AND PROBLEMS OF HFA ANIMALS AS A MODEL

Thus, HFA animals provide stable models for studying the ecosystem and metabolism of the human intestinal microbiota in conditions similar to those found in humans. It has been reported that the composition and metabolic activities of the human intestinal microbiota differs from that of experimental animals. Also, studies have demonstrated that the role of the intestinal microbiota suggested in experiments with HFA animals is significantly different from that obtained from conventional animal experiments [23, 34, 69, 71, 75, 78, 82].

HFA animals are also a useful substitute for human volunteers. It is possible to control the experimental conditions of HFA animals including genetic, environmental, and dietary conditions, which are often quite difficult to control in human studies. Furthermore, HFA animal experiments can be performed with a sufficient number of animals for statistical analysis and, if necessary, be repeated under the same conditions. HFA animals can be challenged with pathogens or toxic substances that cannot be used ethically in human studies. Also, intestinal contents, except for feces, or tissue samples cannot be obtained easily from healthy human subjects without application of invasive techniques that cannot be justified for ethical reasons.

HFA animals, however, have some of the same limitations as other animal models. For example, bacterial metabolism in the intestine of HFA mice reflects that of human feces with respect to some metabolic activities but not to others. Some bacterial groups are occasionally eliminated from HFA animals while other dominant bacterial groups remain constant. We have reported that bifidobacteria are eliminated from some HFA mouse groups, probably due to the composition of microbiota in the inoculated sample [1]. Therefore, these HFA animals without bifidobacteria cannot be used to study the effects of bifidogenic dietary factors. On the other hand, such bifidobacteria-free HFA animals might be useful for studying the importance of bifidobacteria in the human intestinal microbiota.

Caution also should be exercised in extrapolating the results from HFA animal experiments when a group of HFA animals is given the intestinal microbiota from just one individual. Further studies should be conducted to 'standardize' the human intestinal microbiota of HFA animals as an 'average' human microbiota. For example, Silvi et al. [53] chose to inoculate germ-free rats with pooled fecal suspensions rather than utilizing individual fecal samples to provide results of more general applicability.

A laboratory rodent diet is different from the normal human diet. Rumney et al. [69] reported that the rate of conversion of potential mutagens to direct-acting mutagenic derivatives by intestinal bacteria is dependent on diets, and that the results obtained with HFA rats were particularly relevant to humans when the animals were fed a human diet. Thus, development of a special diet for HFA animals is required in order to establish HFA animals as a suitable model for studying the human intestinal microbiota.

In spite of the above limitations, studies using HFA animals provide much needed information of relevance concerning the role of the human intestinal microbiota. HFA animals will undoubtedly continue to contribute to investigations concerning the effects of probiotics, prebiotics, diet, antibiotics, and drugs on the human intestinal microbiota and its relationships with the human host.

10. CONCLUSIONS

HFA animals provide stable models for studying the ecosystem and metabolism of the human intestinal microbiota in conditions similar to those found in humans. HFA animals also are a useful substitute for human volunteers. HFA animals, however, have some limitations as a model. In spite of these limitations, studies using HFA animals will provide much needed information on the role of human intestinal microbiota and the effects of probiotics, prebiotics and other dietary components on human intestinal microbiota and on human health and disease.

References

1. Hirayama, K., Itoh, K., Takahashi, E., & Mitsuoka, T. (1995). Comparison of composition of fecal microbiota and metabolism of fecal bacteria among 'human-flora-associated' mice inoculated with feces from six different human donors. *Microbial Ecology in Health and Disease, 8,* 199–211.

2. Hirayama, K. (1999). Ex-germfree mice harboring intestinal microbiota derived from other animal species as an experimental model for ecology and metabolism of intestinal bacteria. *Experimental Animals, 48,* 219–227.

3. Raibaud, P., Ducluzeau, R., Dubos, F., et al. (1980). Implantation of bacteria from the digestive tract of man and various animals into gnotobiotic mice. *The American Journal of Clinical Nutrition, 33,* 2440–2447.

4. Hazenberg, M. P., Bakker, M., & Verschoor-Burggraaf, A. (1981). Effects of the human intestinal flora on germ-free mice. *The Journal of Applied Bacteriology, 50,* 95–106.

5. Maejima, K., Sasaki, J., Shimoda, K., & Kurosawa, T. (1981). Bacterial flora of ex-germfree mice after oral inoculation of feces from various species of conventional animals. *Experimental Animals, 30,* 157–160.

6. Ducluzeau, R., Ladiré, M., & Raibaud, P. (1984). Effect of bran ingestion on the microbial fecal floras of human donors and of recipient gnotobiotic mice, and on the barrier effects exerted by these floras against various potentially pathogenic microbial strains. *Annals of Microbiology, 135A,* 303–318.

7. Debure, A., Colombel, J. F., Flourie, B., et al. (1989). Comparison of the implantation and metabolic activity of human and rat fecal flora administered to axenic rats. *Gastroentérologie Clinique et Biologique, 13,* 25–31.

8. Hirayama, K., Kawamura, S., & Mitsuoka, T. (1991). Development and stability of human fecal flora in the intestine of ex-germ-free mice. *Microbial Ecology in Health and Disease, 4,* 95–99.

9. Licht, T. R., Madsen, B., & Wilcks, A. (2007). Selection of bacteria originating from a human intestinal microbiota in the gut of previously germ-free rats. *FEMS Microbiology Letters, 277,* 205–209.

10. Pang, X. Y., Hua, X. G., Yang, Q., et al. (2007). Inter-species transplantation of gut microbiota from human to pigs. *The ISME Journal, 1,* 156–162.

11. Wong, W. C., Hentges, D. J., & Dougherty, S. H. (1996). Adequacy of the human faecal microbiota associated mouse as a model for studying the ecology of the human intestinal tract. *Microbial Ecology in Health and Disease, 9,* 187–198.

12. Kibe, R., Sakamoto, M., Yokota, H., et al. (2005). Movement and fixation of intestinal microbiota after administration of human feces to germfree mice. *Applied and Environmental Microbiology, 71,* 3171–3178.

13. Mallett, A. K., Bearne, C. A., Rowland, I. R., et al. (1987). The use of rats associated with a human fecal flora as a model for studying the effects of diet on the human gut microflora. *The Journal of Applied Bacteriology, 63,* 39–45.

14. Alpert, C., Sczesny, S., Gruhl, B., & Blaut, M. (2008). Long-term stability of the human gut microbiota in two different rat strains. *Current Issues in Molecular Biology, 10,* 17–24.

15. Hirayama, K., Miyaji, K., Kawamura, S., et al. (1995). Development of intestinal flora of human-floral-associated (HFA) mice in the intestine of their offspring. *Experimental Animals, 44,* 219–222.

16. Bernbom, N., Norrung, B., Saadbye, P., et al. (2006). Comparison of methods and animal models commonly used for investigation of fecal microbiota: effects of time, host and gender. *Journal of Microbiological Methods, 66,* 87–95.

17. Mitsuoka, T., & Hayakawa, K. (1972). Die Darmflora bei Menschen. I. Mitteilung. Die Zusammensetzung der Faekalflora der verschiedenen Altergruppen. *Zbl Bakteriol Parasitenkd Infektionskr Hyg I Orig A 233,* 333–352.

18. Benno, Y., & Mitsuoka, T. (1986). Development of intestinal microflora in human and animals. *Bifidobacteria Microflora, 5,* 13–25.

19. Hirayama, K., Mishima, M., Kawamura, S., et al. (1994). Effects of dietary supplements on the composition of fecal flora of human-flora-associated (HFA) mice. *Bifidobacteria Microflora, 13,* 1–7.

20. Kleessen, B., Hartmann, L., & Blaut, M. (2003). Fructans in the diet cause alterations of intestinal mucosal architecture, released mucins and mucosa-associated bifidobacteria in gnotobiotic rats. *The British Journal of Nutrition, 89,* 597–606.

21. Sharma, R., & Schumacher, U. (1995). Morphometric analysis of intestinal mucins under different dietary conditions and gut flora in rats. *Digestive Diseases and Sciences, 40,* 2532–2539.

22. Fontaine, N., Meslin, J.-C., Lory, S., & Andrieux, C. (1996). Intestinal mucin distribution in the germ-free rat and in the heteroxenic rat harboring a human bacterial

flora: effect of inulin in the diet. *The British Journal of Nutrition*, 75, 881–892.

23. Sharma, R., & Schumacher, U. (1995). The influence of diets and gut microflora on lectin binding patterns of intestinal mucins in rats. *Laboratory Investigation*, 73, 558–564.

24. Sharma, R., & Schumacher, U. (1996). The diet and gut microflora influence the distribution of enteroendocrine cells in the rat intestine. *Experientia*, 52, 664–670.

25. Rouzaud, G., Rabot, S., Ratcliffe, B., & Duncan, A. J. (2003). Influence of plant and bacterial myrosinase activity on the metabolic fate of glucosinolates in gnotobiotic rats. *The British Journal of Nutrition*, 90, 395–404.

26. Roland, N., Nugon-Baudon, L., Andrieux, C., & Szylit, O. (1995). Comparative study of the fermentative characterists of inulin and different types of fiber in rats inoculated with a human whole fecal flora. *The British Journal of Nutrition*, 74, 239–249.

27. Gérard, P., Béguet, F., Lepercq, P., et al. (2004). Gnotobiotic rats harboring human intestinal microbiota as a model for studying cholesterol-to-coprostanol conversion. *FEMS Microbiology Ecology*, 47, 337–343.

28. Bowey, E., Adlercreutz, H., & Rowland, I. (2003). Metabolism of isoflavones and lignans by the gut microflora: a study in germ-free and human flora associated rats. *Food and Chemical Toxicology*, 41, 631–636.

29. Meslin, J.-C., Andrieux, C., Hibert, A., et al. (1999). Effects of ingestion of a green seaweed, *Ulva lactuca*, upon caecal and colonic mucosas in the germ-free rat and in the heteroxenic rat harboring a human bacterial flora. *Journal of the Science of Food and Agriculture*, 79, 727–732.

30. Lhoste, E. F., Ouriet, V., Bruel, S., et al. (2003). The human colonic microflora influences the alterations of xenobiotic-metabolizing enzymes by catechins in male F344 rats. *Food and Chemical Toxicology*, 41, 695–702.

31. Humblot, C., Lhoste, E. F., Knasmüller, S., et al. (2004). Protective effects of Brussels sprouts, oligosaccharides and fermented milk towards 2-amino-3-methylimidazo[4,5-f]quinoline (IQ)-induced genotoxicity in the human flora associated F344 rat: role of xenobiotic metabolizing enzymes and intestinal microflora. *Journal of Chromatography*, 802, 231–237.

32. Roland, N., Nugon-Baudon, L., Flinois, J. P., & Beaune, P. (1994). Hepatic and intestinal cytochrome P-450, glutathione-S-transferase and UDP-glucuronosyl transferase are affected by six types of dietary fiber in rats inoculated with human whole fecal flora. *The Journal of Nutrition*, 124, 1581–1587.

33. Rumney, C. J., Rowland, I. R., Coutts, T. M., et al. (1993). Effects of risk-associated human dietary macro-components on processes related to carcinogenesis in human-flora-associated (HFA) rats. *Carcinogenesis*, 14, 79–84.

34. Sudo, N., Aiba, Y., Takaki, A., et al. (2000). Dietary nucleic acids promote a shift in Th1/Th2 balance toward Th1–dominant immunity. *Clinical and Experimental Allergy*, 30, 979–987.

35. Sandré, C., Gleizes, A., Forestier, F., et al. (2001). A peptide derived from bovine β-casein modulates functional properties of bone marrow-derived macrophages from germfree and human flora-associated mice. *The Journal of Nutrition*, 131, 2936–2942.

36. Gaboriau-Routhiau, V., Raibaud, P., Dubuquoy, C., & Moreau, M. C. (2003). Colonization of gnotobiotic mice with human gut microflora at birth protects against *Escherichia coli* heat-labile enterotoxin-mediated abrogation of oral tolerance. *Ped Res*, 54, 739–746.

37. Dufour-Lescoat, C., Le Coz, Y., & Szylit, O. (1991). Nutritional effects of wheat bran and beet fiber in germ-free rats and in heteroxenic rats inoculated with human flora. *Sci Aliment*, 11, 397–408.

38. Grolier, P., Borel, P., Duszka, C., et al. (1998). The bioavailability of α- and β-carotene is affected by gut microflora in the rat. *The British Journal of Nutrition*, 80, 199–204.

39. Martin, F. P. J., Dumas, M. E., Wang, Y. L., et al. (2007). A top-down systems biology view of microbiome-mammalian metabolic interactions in a mouse model. *Molecular Systems Biology*, 3, 112.

40. Djouzi, Z., Andrieux, C., Degivry, M.-C., et al. (1997). The association of yogurt starters with *Lactobacillus casei* DN 114.001 in fermented milk alters the composition and metabolism of intestinal microflora in germ-free rats and in human flora-associated rats. *The Journal of Nutrition*, 127, 2260–2266.

41. Rowland, I. R., & Tanaka, R. (1993). The effects of transgalactosylated oligosaccharides on gut flora metabolism in rats associated with a human fecal microflora. *The Journal of Applied Bacteriology*, 74, 667–674.

42. Djouzi, Z., & Andrieux, C. (1997). Compared effects of three oligosaccharides on metabolism of intestinal microflora in rats inoculated with a human fecal flora. *The British Journal of Nutrition*, 78, 313–324.

43. Kikuchi, H., Andrieux, C., Riottot, M., et al. (1996). Effect of two levels of transgalactosylated oligosaccharide intake in rats associated with human fecal microflora on bacterial glycolytic activity, end-products of fermentation and bacterial steroid transformation. *The Journal of Applied Bacteriology*, 80, 439–446.

44. Kleessen, B., Hartmann, L., & Blaut, M. (2001). Oligofructose and long-chain inulin: Influence on the gut microbial ecology of rats associated with a human fecal flora. *The British Journal of Nutrition*, 86, 291–300.

45. Humblot, C., Bruneau, A., Sutren, M., et al. (2005). Brussels sprouts, inulin and fermented milk alter the faecal microbiota of human microbiota-associated rats as shown by PCR-temporal temperature gradient

gel electrophoresis using universal, *Lactobacillus* and *Bifidobacterium* 16S rRNA gene primers. *The British Journal of Nutrition*, 93, 677–684.

46. Hambly, R. J., Rumney, C. J., Fletcher, J. M. E., et al. (1997). Effects of high- and low-risk diets on gut microflora-associated biomarkers of colon cancer in human flora-associated rats. *Nutrition and Cancer*, 27, 250–255.

47. Ito, M., Deguchi, Y., Miyamori, A., et al. (1990). Effect of administration of galacto-oligosaccharides on the human fecal microflora, stool weight and abdominal sensation. *Microbial Ecology in Health and Disease*, 3, 285–292.

48. Ito, M., Deguchi, Y., Matsumoto, K., et al. (1993). Influence of galactooligosaccharides on the human fecal microflora. *Journal of Nutritional Science and Vitaminology*, 39, 635–640.

49. Gibson, G. R., Beatty, E. R., Wang, X., & Cummings, J. H. (1995). Selective stimulation of bifidobacteria in the human colon by oligofructose and inulin. *Gastroenterol*, 108, 975–982.

50. Reddy, B. S., Weisburger, J. H., & Wynder, E. L. (1975). Effects of high risk and low risk diets for colon carcinogenesis on fecal microflora and steroids in man. *The Journal of Nutrition*, 105, 878–884.

51. Drasar, B. S., Jenkins, D. J. A., & Cummings, J. H. (1976). The influence of a diet rich in wheat fiber on the human fecal flora. *Journal of Medical Microbiology*, 9, 423–431.

52. Hentges, D. J., Maier, B. R., Burton, G. C., et al. (1977). Effect of a high-beef diet on the fecal bacterial flora of humans. *Cancer Research*, 37, 568–571.

53. Silvi, S., Rumney, C. J., Cresci, A., & Rowland, I. R. (1999). Resident starch modifies gut microflora and microbial metabolism in human flora-associated rats inoculated with feces from Italian and UK donors. *Journal of Applied Microbiology*, 86, 521–530.

54. Andrieux, C., Hibert, A., Houari, A.-M., et al. (1998). Ulva lactuca is poorly fermented but alters bacterial metabolism in rats inoculated with human fecal flora from methane and non-methane producers. *Journal of the Science of Food and Agriculture*, 77, 25–30.

55. Oozeer, R., Goupil-Feuillerat, N., Alpert, C. A., et al. (2002). *Lactobacillus casei* is able to survive and initiate protein synthesis during its transit in the digestive tract of human flora-associated mice. *Applied and Environmental Microbiology*, 68, 3570–3574.

56. Lan, A., Bruneau, A., Philippe, C., et al. (2007). Survival and metabolic activity of selected strains of *Propionibacterium freudenreichii* in the gastrointestinal tract of human microbiota-associated rats. *The British Journal of Nutrition*, 97, 714–724.

57. Martin, F. P. J., Wang, Y., Sprenger, N., et al. (2008). Probiotic modulation of symbiotic gut microbial-host metabolic interactions in a humanized microbiome mouse model. *Molecular Systems Biology*, 4, 157.

58. Mater, D. D. G., Drouault-Holowacz, S., Oozeer, R., et al. (2006). β-Galactosidase production by *Streptococcus thermophilus* is higher in the small intestine than in the caecum of human-microbiota-associated mice after lactose supplementation. *The British Journal of Nutrition*, 96, 177–181.

59. Tancrède, C., Andremont, A., & Kherbiche, A. M. (1981). Germfree mice associated with human flora as a means of bacteriological surveillance of neutropenic patients in sterile environments. In S. Sasaki, A. Ozawa, & K. Hashimoto (Eds.), *Recent Advances in Germfree Research* (pp. 755–758). Tokyo, Japan: Tokai University Press.

60. Andremont, A., Raibaud, P., & Tancrède, C. (1983). Effect of erythromycin on microbial antagonisms: a study in gnotobiotic mice associated with a human fecal flora. *The Journal of Infectious Diseases*, 148, 579–587.

61. Gismondo, M. R., Drago, L., Lombardi, A., et al. (1995). Impact of rufloxacin and ciprofloxacin on the intestinal microflora in a germ-free mice model. *Chemother*, 41, 281–288.

62. Perrin-Guyomard, A., Cottin, S., Corpet, D. E., et al. (2001). Evaluation of residual and therapeutic doses of tetracycline in the human-flora-associated (HFA) mice model. *Regulatory Toxicology and Pharmacology*, 34, 125–136.

63. Barc, M. C., Bourlioux, F., Rigottier-Gois, L., et al. (2004). Effect of amoxicillin-clavulanic acid on human fecal flora in a gnotobiotic mouse model assessed with fluorescence hybridization using group-specific 16S rRNA probes in combination with flow cytometry. *Antimicrob Agents Chemother*, 48, 1365–1368.

64. Barc, M. C., Charrin-Sarnel, C., Rochet, V., et al. (2008). Molecular analysis of the digestive microbiota in a gnotobiotic mouse model during antibiotic treatment: influence of *Saccharomyces boulardii*. *Anaerobe*, 14, 229–233.

65. Corpet, D. E. (1993). Current status of models for testing antibiotic residues. *Veterinary and Human Toxicology*, 35, 37–46.

66. Cerniglia, C. E., & Kotarski, S. (1999). Evaluation of veterinary drug residues in food for their potential to affect human intestinal microflora. *Regulatory Toxicology and Pharmacology*, 29, 238–261.

67. Tuohy, K., Davies, M., Rumsby, P., et al. (2002). Monitoring transfer of recombinant and non-recombinant plasmids between *Lactococcus lactis* strains and members of the human gastrointestinal microbiota *in vivo*—impact on donor cell number and diet. *Journal of Applied Microbiology*, 93, 954–964.

68. Nijsten, R., London, N., van den Bogaard, A., & Stobberingh, E. (1995). *In vivo* transfer of resistance plasmids in rat, human or pig-derived intestinal flora using a rat model. *The Journal of Antimicrobial Chemotherapy*, 36, 975–985.

69. Rumney, C. J., Rowland, I. R., & O'Neill, I. K. (1993). Conversion of IQ to 7-OHIQ by gut microflora. *Nutrition and Cancer, 19*, 67–76.

70. Rowland, I. R., Bearne, C. A., Fischer, R., & Pool-Zobel, B. L. (1996). The effect of lactulose on DNA damage induced by DMH in the colon of human flora-associated rats. *Nutrition and Cancer, 26*, 37–47.

71. Hirayama, K., Baranczewski, P., Åkerlund, J.-E., et al. (2000). Effects of human intestinal flora on mutagenicity of and DNA adduct formation from food and environmental mutagens. *Carcinogenesis, 21*, 2105–2111.

72. Horie, H., Zeisig, M., Hirayama, K., et al. (2003). Probiotic mixture decreases DNA adduct formation in colonic epithelium induced by the food mutagen 2-amino-9H-pyrido[2,3-*b*]indole in a human-flora associated mouse model. *European Journal of Cancer Prevention, 12*, 101–107.

73. Scheepers, P. T. J., Strätemans, M. M. E., Koopman, J. P., & Bos, R. P. (1994). Nitroreduction and formation of hemoglobin adducts in rats with a human intestinal microflora. *Environmental Health Perspectives, 102* (Suppl. 6), 39–41.

74. Scheepers, P. T. J., Velders, D. D., Steenwinkel, M. J. S. T., et al. (1994). Role of the intestinal microflora in the formation of DNA and haemoglobin adducts in rats treated with 2-nitrofluorene and 2-aminofluorene by gavage. *Carcinogenesis, 15*, 1433–1441.

75. Kassie, F., Rabot, S., Kundi, M., et al. (2001). Intestinal microflora plays a crucial role in the genotoxicity of the cooked food mutagens 2-amino-3-methylimidazo[4,5-*f*]-quinoline (IQ). *Carcinogenesis, 22*, 1721–1725.

76. Knasmüller, S., Steinkellner, H., Hirschl, A. M., et al. (2001). Impact of bacteria in dairy products and of the intestinal microflora on the genotoxic and carcinogenic effects of heterocyclic aromatic amines. *Mutation Research, 480–481*, 129–138.

77. Hambly, R. J., Rumney, C. J., Cunninghame, M., et al. (1997). Influence of diets containing high and low risk factors for colon cancer on early stages of carcinogenesis in human flora-associated (HFA) rats. *Carcinogenesis, 18*, 1535–1539.

78. Tache, S., Peiffer, G., Millet, A. S., & Corpet, D. E. (2000). Carrageenan gel and aberrant crypt foci in the colon of conventional and human flora-associated rats. *Nutrition and Cancer, 37*, 193–198.

79. Edwards, C. A., Rumney, C., Davies, T., et al. (2003). A human flora-associated rat model of the breast-fed infant gut. *Journal of Pediatric Gastroenterology and Nutrition, 37*, 168–177.

80. Hentges, D. J., Marsh, W. W., Petschow, B. W., et al. (1995). Influence of a human milk diet on colonization resistance mechanisms against *Salmonella typhimurium* in human fecal bacteria-associated mice. *Microbial Ecology in Health and Disease, 8*, 139–149.

81. Hentges, D. J., Marsh, W. W., Petschow, B. W., et al. (1992). Influence of infant diets on the ecology of the intestinal tract of human flora-associated mice. *Journal of Pediatric Gastroenterology and Nutrition, 14*, 146–152.

82. Ward, F. W., Coates, M. E., Cole, C. B., & Fuller, R. (1990). Effect of dietary fats on endogenous formation of N-nitrosamines from nitrate in germ-free and conventional rats and rats harboring a human flora. *Food Additives & Contaminants, 7*, 597–604.

32

Probiotics and Other Microbial Manipulations in Fish Feeds: Prospective Health Benefits

F.J. Gatesoupe

INRA-Ifremer, UMR1067 Nutrition Aquaculture et Génomique, Plouzané, France

1. INTRODUCTION

Aquaculture was considered as a marginal activity until recently, but the situation changed at the turn of the century, with the always-increasing demand for seafood, while fisheries captures have stagnated. Besides the international and governmental efforts to regulate fisheries resources, the share of seafood produced by aquaculture will continue to increase inescapably [1]. The contribution of fish farming was already estimated at 47% of the total amount of fish available for human consumption in 2006 [2]. This fast increase exerts a striking impact on the environment and public health. It implies rearing intensification, which may cause fish disease outbreaks, including bacterial infections. The risk of food-borne diseases caused by seafood consumption is concurrently increasing [3, 4], and there is a risk of the emergence of new human pathogens. For example, freshwater fish have now been identified as a source of *Laribacter hongkongensis*, a bacterium associated with gastroenteritis [5]. Fish farming may also pose a risk to the spread of antimicrobial resistance [6].

The use of medicines is now strictly regulated for aquaculture practices [7], and there is a need for alternative sustainable treatments [8]. A variety of such treatments has been proposed, although the state of knowledge about microbiota in the digestive tract of farmed fish is still very limited. The available information is briefly reviewed in this chapter. Also presented here are the numerous probiotic candidates that have been tested empirically in fish, with some insight into their modes of action, which are becoming better understood. The emerging prospects for prebiotics and other dietary manipulations that can regulate gastrointestinal microflora is also discussed. Finally, besides these practical aspects relevant to public health, a less expected benefit from the research on fish microbiota is introduced, since fish appeared as an interesting model for investigating the basic features of the host–microbe interaction.

2. MICROBIOTA IN THE DIGESTIVE TRACT OF FARM FISH

Ley et al. [9] distinguished the microbial communities associated with vertebrates from those associated with invertebrates, as these were considered as being closer to environmental samples. In particular, they found similarities between the microbial communities living either in saline or non-saline habitats, and the communities associated with the invertebrates that live in the same habitat, respectively. This does not exclude the fact that some primitive metazoans seem able to exert a high selective pressure on their associated microbiota [10]. The demarcation drawn by Ley et al. [9] between vertebrates and invertebrates should also be moderated since the data concerning fish were based on one previous study of the gut microbiota in zebrafish [11].

Fish have particular features, as compared with land animals. The aquatic environment facilitates microbial influx and renewal. Fish are poikilothermic, and seasonal changes have been observed in their intestinal microbiota [12]. Their immune response is somewhat primitive, with limited antibody capability [13]. These characteristics combine to stress the differences that can be expected in the microbial ecology of fish gut, as compared with that of higher vertebrates.

A wide diversity of anatomical peculiarities can be observed among the digestive tracts of fish, and that reflects the variety of ecological niches offered to different microbial communities. Some herbivorous species may host 10^{11} cfu g^{-1}, with high fermentative activity, mainly in the posterior intestine [14]. Most aquacultured species are carnivores, whose short intestine may be extended with pyloric ceca in variable numbers [15]. The intestinal transit time is relatively brief in carnivorous fish reared in cold or temperate water (e.g. 12 hours) [16], thus limiting the potential for direct contribution of bacteria to the host's digestive activity. However, there are also some herbivorous species that are important for aquaculture; like mullets (fitted with a relatively long intestine), and carps (which are devoid of stomachs, but whose pharyngeal teeth facilitate the digestion of vegetable feeds) [17].

Moderate counts of aero-tolerant cultivable bacteria are generally retrieved from the intestine of farm fish (10^4–10^7 cfu g^{-1}) [18]. Obligate anaerobes seem present at similar levels, but they have been seldom studied [19–21]. Sakata [22] schematized the intestinal microflora as dominated by Gram-negative bacteria, with *Vibrio* and *Photobacterium* as the most ordinary genera retrieved in marine fish; *Aeromonas*, *Plesiomononas*, and *Enterobacteriaceae* in freshwater fish; and *Pseudomonas*, *Clostridium*, and *Bacteroidaceae* in both environments. Though hindgut microbiota in humans is different [23], some similarities appear at the genus level, especially among obligate anaerobes such as *Bacteroides*, *Clostridium*, *Fusobacterium* [18, 21]. Gram-positive bacteria are also present in fish, with some genera common to humans and fish, for example: *Eubacterium* [18], *Lactobacillus*, and *Streptococcus* [24]. Though rarely reported, *Bifidobacterium* is occasionally recovered from common carp and shrimp intestines [25, 26]. Besides bacteria, yeasts are frequently isolated from fish gut, more especially in freshwater [27].

The variability in fish microbiota is not necessarily related to diet or environmental conditions. For example, cod larvae fed mainly on natural zooplankton in a flow-through rearing unit were sampled individually from day 16 to day 23 after hatching [28]. In this experiment, the phenotypic profiles of culturable bacteria were found to be quite different among the individual samples.

In human and land animals, the unique features of the bacterial community in each individual has been well established. Fecal microbiota seems to be relatively stable even in weaning piglets, from 28 to 49 days of age [29]. No such temporal study has been done on fish, but one can suppose that the resilience to a hypothetical individual steady state may be compromised by the perpetual fluctuations in the aquatic environment. Ringø and Birkbeck referred to Savage's list of criteria for testing the autochthony of microorganisms found in the gastrointestinal tract of fish: 'Autochthonous (indigenous) microorganisms: 1) are found in healthy individuals; 2) colonize early stages and persist throughout life; 3) are found in both free-living and hatchery-cultured fish; 4) can grow anaerobically; and 5) are found associated with the epithelial mucosa in the stomach, small intestine or large intestine' [30, 31]. The second criterion—early colonization and long-term persistence—is essential to the definition, but it is difficult to validate, as well as the third one, which would require the comparison with wild fish. In practice, these two criteria are omitted, and in this acceptance, it is common to hear about 'autochthonous' gut microbiota in fish, though the association to mucosa may be temporary.

In view of the quantitative and qualitative limitations presented above, the nutritional impact of gut microbiota on farm fish cannot yet be clearly delineated. Bacteria isolated from fish gut produce a variety of digestive enzymes like amylase, cellulase, lipase, protease [32], and chitinase [33], but their actual contribution to the digestive process remains to be evaluated. The digestion of cellulose may be mostly attributable to microbes in the intestine of fish, which do not seem to produce endogenous cellulase, even if the issue is still in discussion [34]. Besides possibly contributing to digestion, microbiota can synthesize *de novo* some nutrients that are essential to fish; for example, vitamin B_{12} [35], amino acids [36, 37] (further references in [38]), fatty acids, especially eicosapentaenoic acid [39, 40], and docosahexaenoic acid [41, 42]. The actual transfer of these nutrients from bacteria to the host has not been evaluated, but a renewal of interest in this field may be called for because of the replacement of fishmeal and fish oil by vegetable sources in aquafeeds, due to the shortage of fisheries resources.

The importance of microbiota for the development of the digestive system was evidenced by comparing germ-free and conventionally reared zebrafish larvae. Germ-free larvae had poorly differentiated intestinal epithelium [43], and the up-regulation of some genes indicated a compromised ability to use nutrients [11]. The reintroduction of microbiota could restore normal development, and the genes marking nutrient metabolism responded both to 'conventional' and atypical consortia [44]. Heat-killed microbes or bacterial lipopolysaccharides were sufficient to stimulate intestinal brush border alkaline phosphatase activity, but no other features of gut maturation, showing that there are several concurrent pathways [43]. A possible mode of action may be initiated by the production of polyamines like spermine and spermidine by microbes, as suggested with larval European sea bass [45–47].

O'Hara and Shanahan spoke of 'gut flora as a forgotten organ' to emphasize the essential role of intestinal microbes in eliciting the mucosal immune system [48]. This role was also evidenced with germ-free zebrafish larvae [11]. Some genes used as biomarkers of the innate immune response were specifically up-regulated with 'conventional' microbiota [44], but innate immunity may also be stimulated in fish larvae by a variety of purified compounds, for instance 'high-M' alginate, which is rich in mannuronic acid polymer [49]. Adaptive immunity in the gut-associated lymphoid tissue is obviously dependent on bacterial colonization, but it appears later than innate immunity, and the onset is relatively slow especially in marine fish as compared with freshwater species like carp, rainbow trout or zebrafish [50–52].

3. PROBIOTICS IN FISH

In spite of many unanswered questions about gut microbiota in fish, the empirical application of probiotics to fish has progressed, mainly over the last decade (Figure 32.1). For extended information, there are many reviews on the subject [53–72].

To the author's knowledge, the first trial explicitly referring to probiotics for fish appeared in 1981. This was an internal report, which dealt with the limitation of mortality in Japanese eel elvers medicated with spores of *Bacillus toyoi*, a bacterium of soil origin, commercialized as a probiotic for land animals [73]. A second report on the same probiotic used as a growth promoter in the yellowtail appeared in 1984 [74]. Later, it was tested on larval European turbot, via the live food organism *Brachionus plicatilis* [75]. Lactic acid bacteria used as probiotics for terrestrial animals were also tested on marine fish larvae [76, 77]. Antagonisms among fish gut bacteria have been known for some time (e.g. Ref. [78]), but bacteriophages were first proposed to inhibit

infection with fish-pathogenic bacteria [79] (further references in [8]). Then in the late 1980s, the screening of bacteria capable of inhibiting fish viruses appeared [80], though their application for biocontrol was not evaluated. 'Autochthonous' bacteria with antagonistic behavior to fish pathogens were extensively studied in the early 1990s [8, 81]. The colonization potential is an important feature for the candidate probiotics, and it was examined simultaneously [82]. The capacity of some allochthonous microbes to persist long after inoculation was thus demonstrated in the intestine of fish. For example, a probiotic strain of *Vibrio alginolyticus* obtained from an Ecuadorian shrimp survived at least 21 days in the intestine of Atlantic salmon reared in fresh water [83], and the yeast *Debaryomyces hansenii* isolated from rainbow trout in fresh water was retrieved in significant

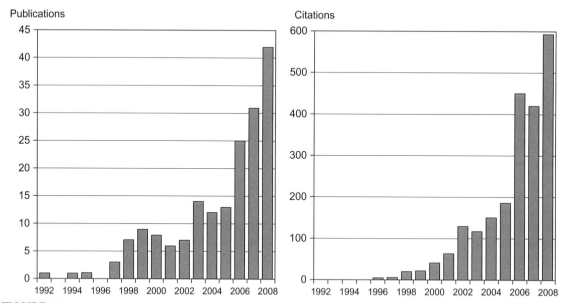

FIGURE 32.1 A bibliometric view of publications dealing explicitly with probiotics for fish. The numbers of items published (left), and their subsequent citations in each year (right), were re-drawn with the kind permission of Thomson Reuters Web of Science® after the following citation report: topics 'probiotic*' and 'fish*' were crossed on 28 November 2008, and the items were further screened to keep only those dealing with finfish, or the live food organisms, rotifers and *Artemia*. The view was obviously not exhaustive, but sufficient to illustrate the trend of fast increase in the recent years.

numbers in the intestine of turbot 11 days after inoculation [84]. The official agreement of microbial preparation as a feed additive may be facilitated when the strains are selected among the species 'generally recognized as safe' in the USA [85], or registered in the European list of 'qualified presumption of safety' [86]. For example, many lactic acid bacteria have been tested in fish because of their qualification for human use, like *Lactobacillus rhamnosus* and *Bifidobacterium lactis* [87, 88], or for animal use, like *Pediococcus acidilactici* and *Enterococcus faecium* [89, 90].

An original feature of probiotic treatment in fish is that the route of administration may not be necessarily oral. Bath methods are also convenient, because of the intimate contact with the aqueous environment. Smith and Davey [91] demonstrated the competitive exclusion of *Aeromonas salmonicida* from asymptomatically infected Atlantic salmon, after bathing in *Pseudomonas fluorescens* suspension, and stress induction. It seemed that the inhibition was due to the competition for iron, which may take place on external surfaces. This extension led several authors to consider probiotic microbes that enhance the quality of water for fish, mainly by decreasing ammonia and nitrite concentrations, and thus indirectly improving fish welfare and health. The genus *Bacillus* seemed particularly interesting in this regard [92], especially due to the possible combination with antagonistic properties [93]. It may seem rather artificial to amalgamate into the same term 'probiotics,' microbes that can act on microbiota or on the host, either directly or indirectly by improving water quality, but the main advantage of probiotics over traditional treatments lies in their potential to inhibit the infection by a variety of modes of action, which does not leave any chance to the pathogen to develop resistance (Figure 32.2).

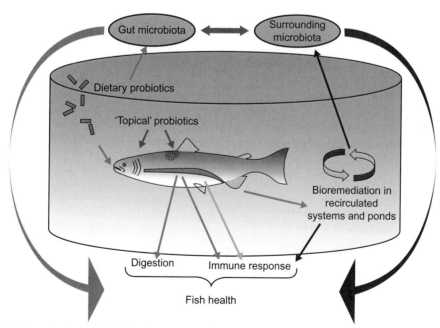

FIGURE 32.2 Complex interrelationship between probiotic treatments—either dietary, or 'topical' by bath immersion, or intended for bioremediation of water quality—and their effects on fish health and microbiota—either gut-associated or those surrounding in the culture system. The water environment may thus justify an extended concept of 'probiotics,' in comparison to that commonly accepted for man and land animals.

The complex consortia have been proposed as providing the widest available range of expected effects, like the preparation of live *Bacillus subtilis*, *Lactobacillus acidophilus*, *Clostridium butyricum*, and *Saccharomyces cerevisiae*, used to act on water quality in recirculated systems, while simultaneously improving the immune response and disease resistance in fish [94, 95]. The multiplicity of agents makes interpretation difficult, and this should require further investigation to discriminate the role of each strain, and the possible synergies.

Stimulation of the immune defenses of the host is one of the most promising modes of action. After the first evaluation in rainbow trout by Irianto and Austin [96], the number of relevant studies in this field has rapidly increased [97], thus showing the interest of the scientific community. Most of the effects concerned innate immunity [97], but the synthesis of IgM also seemed to be stimulated in the head kidney of gilthead seabream fed *D. hansenii* [98]. The viability of the cells was proved essential for some instances, in which their effect should not be confused with that of classical immunostimulants [96, 99, 100].

4. PREBIOTICS AND OTHER DIETARY MANIPULATIONS

The first attempt to use prebiotics in fish appeared in 1995 [101], contemporaneously to the introduction of the concept by Gibson and Roberfroid [102]. Although Kihara et al. [103] did not refer explicitly to prebiotics, their experiment was matched with the concept. Intestinal microbiota from red seabream fermented lactosucrose *in vitro*, and the introduction of 1% dietary lactosucrose increased the thickness of the muscular intestinal layer in fish. In spite of this early trial, there was some delay before further application. A high dose of inulin (15% of dry diet) caused abnormal vacuolization

in enterocytes, and it damaged microvilli in the pyloric ceca and hindgut of Arctic charr [103]. Microbiota was also affected [104]. Some hypertrophy of the external muscular layer was observed in the intestine of Atlantic salmon fed a lower dose of inulin (7.5%), but it did not cause damage to the intestinal mucosa, while reducing bacterial diversity [105]. Fructo-oligosaccharides derived from inulin increased the growth rate of weaning European turbot, and it affected gut microbiota [106]. There are other products called 'prebiotics' that have not been proved to correspond to the definition of Gibson and Roberfroid. This was the case with a 'dairy-yeast prebiotic,' a complex commercial mixture called Grobiotic™ [107, 108], until its effect on fish microbiota was considered [109]. The preparation seemed firstly to stimulate the immune system of the host, in the same way as mannan oligosaccharides [110, 111]. It would be interesting to combine immunomodulation with the selective stimulation of health-promoting gut microbes, and there is a need for further investigation on such effects of non-starch oligosaccharides in fish [112]. Starch and non-starch polysaccharides can stimulate fermentation in Nile tilapia and European sea bass, at least *in vitro* [113]. The combination of immunomodulatory and antimicrobial effects can also be obtained by using herb medicines, and there is growing interest for their application to fish [8, 114]. Many compounds may provide medicinal properties to plant preparations and, among those involved in the immune response of fish, one can cite as examples polysaccharides from *Astragalus membranaceus* [115], quillaja saponin [116], and anthraquinone from rhubarb [117]. The stimulation may not be limited to innate immunity, since *Achyranthes aspera* enhanced the specific antibody response in the Indian carp *Catla catla* [118]. Besides, the antimicrobial effects of herb medicines against fish pathogens have been largely studied, with some identification of active compounds, like gallic acid [119] or gossypol [120]. The main difficulty is to find the right combination of herbs, and the right dose to administer, depending on the sensitivity of each species to compounds that become harmful at high concentration.

5. RELEVANCE OF FISH AS MODEL SPECIES

At the time of writing, zebrafish is the current animal model as it is useful to many applications in embryology, genetics, and human pathology [121]. Large-scale screening is feasible at low experimental costs, and the possibility to work in gnotobiotic conditions is particularly precious to study intestinal microbiota. On the one hand, Rawls et al. [11] put forward several arguments in favor of this model in their first paper on gnotobiotic zebrafish. They revealed a number of responses to gut microbiota that were similar to those of mammals, and some of them were specifically caused by microbes. The transparency of the larvae was another argument, since it facilitated the observation of fluorescent *in situ* hybridization and protein expression in microbes, and the subsequent physiological responses in the digestive tract [43, 122, 123]. On the other hand, the model has obvious limitations as regards projection to human situation. In zebrafish, there is no acidic environment in the stomach, nor are there Paneth cells in the intestine [121], and the reciprocal transplantation of gut microbiota from mice and zebrafish lead to the conclusion of high specificity in the effects on the host's gene expression [44]. Another major difference between mammals and fish is the state of development when the digestive tract is colonized. In spite of these discrepancies, the model could work in many cases. For example, the likely role of polyamine release by *Saccharomyces boulardii* in the stimulating effects on gut maturation in weaning rats [124] was retrieved in sea bass larvae fed *Debaryomyces hansenii* [46].

6. CONCLUSION

Though most of these treatments are still experimental, fish health management may benefit as well from medical advances in probiotics as from traditional herbs and other soft medicines. In return, it now seems possible to obtain some basic information about the host–microbe interaction by experimenting on fish.

The development of new tools in molecular biology, especially the metagenomic approach, should help to fill the gap still remaining in our knowledge on fish gut microbiota [125]. The detection of specific bacterial genomic DNA does not necessarily mean that the bacterium is active in the gut, and complementary DNA may provide further insight into activity. This is crucial for understanding the modes of action of probiotics, about which there are some examples of effects that are not always conditioned by viability [126, 127]. Direct observations by confocal imaging and electron microscopy are essential to visualize what happens *in situ* [128]. Combined with these tools, the regain of interest for applying gnobiotic studies to the larval stages of farm fish may lead to significant advances in understanding the roles of probiotics and microbiota in species of interest for aquaculture [129].

References

1. Cressey, D. (2009). Future fish, the only way to meet the increasing demand for fish through aquaculture. *Nature, 458,* 398–400.
2. FAO Fisheries Department. (2009). *The State of World Fisheries and Aquaculture—2008 (SOFIA)*. Rome: FAO, p. 3.
3. Das, B., Manna, S. K., Sarkar, P., & Batabyal, K. (2009). Occurrence of *Vibrio parahaemolyticus* in different finfish and shellfish species. *Journal of Food Safety, 29,* 118–125.
4. Novotny, L., Dvorska, L., Lorencova, A., et al. (2004). Fish: a potential source of bacterial pathogens for human beings. *Veterinarni Medicina, 49,* 343–358.
5. Woo, P. C. Y., Lau, S. K. P., Teng, J. L. L., et al. (2004). Association of *Laribacter hongkongensis* in community-acquired gastroenteritis with travel and eating fish: a multicentre case-control study. *The Lancet, 363,* 1941–1947.

6. Reilly, A., & Käferstein, F. (1999). Food safety and products from aquaculture. *Journal of Applied Microbiology, 85,* 249S–257S.

7. Costello, M. J., Grant, A., Davies, I. M., et al. (2001). The control of chemicals used in aquaculture in Europe. *Journal of Applied Ichthyology, 17,* 173–180.

8. Gatesoupe, F. J. (2008). Different methods to reduce antibiotic use in farmed fish. In O. Lie (Ed.), *Improving Farmed Fish Quality and Safety* (pp. 199–237). Cambridge: Woodhead Publishing Ltd.

9. Ley, R. E., Lozupone, C. A., Hamady, M., et al. (2008). Worlds within worlds: evolution of the vertebrate gut microbiota. *Nature Reviews Microbiology, 6,* 776–788.

10. Fraune, S., & Bosch, T. C. G. (2007). Long-term maintenance of species-specific bacterial microbiota in the basal metazoan *Hydra. Proceedings of the National Academy of Sciences of the United States of America, 104,* 13146–13151.

11. Rawls, J. F., Samuel, B. S., & Gordon, J. I. (2004). Gnotobiotic zebrafish reveal evolutionarily conserved responses to the gut microbiota. *Proceedings of the National Academy of Sciences of the United States of America, 101,* 4596–4601.

12. Al-Harbi, A. H., & Uddin, M. N. (2004). Seasonal variation in the intestinal bacterial flora of hybrid tilapia (*Oreochromis niloticus* × *Oreochromis aureus*) cultured in earthen ponds in Saudi Arabia. *Aquaculture, 229,* 37–44.

13. Ellis, A. E. (1999). Immunity to bacteria in fish. *Fish & Shellfish Immunology, 9,* 291–308.

14. Clements, K. D. (1997). Fermentation and gastrointestinal microorganisms in fishes. In R. I. Mackie, & B. A. White, (Eds.), *Gastrointestinal Microbiology: Vol. 1* (pp. 156–198). New York: Chapman & Hall.

15. Guillaume, J., & Choubert, G. (2001). Digestive physiology and nutrient digestibility in fishes. In J. Guillaume, S. Kaushik, P. Bergot, & R. Métailler (Eds.), *Nutrition and Feeding of Fish and Crustaceans* (pp. 27–57). London: Springer.

16. Bucking, C., & Wood, C. M. (2006). Water dynamics in the digestive tract of the freshwater rainbow trout during the processing of a single meal. *Journal of Experimental Biology, 209,* 1883–1893.

17. Stevens, C. E., & Hume, I. D. (1998). Contributions of microbes in vertebrate gastrointestinal tract to production and conservation of nutrients. *Physiological Reviews, 78,* 393–427.

18. Cahill, M. M. (1990). Bacterial flora of fishes: A review. *Microbial Ecology, 19,* 21–41.

19. Trust, T. J., Bull, L. M., Currie, B. R., & Buckley, J. T. (1979). Obligate anaerobic bacteria in the gastrointestinal microflora of the grass carp (*Ctenopharyngodon idella*), goldfish (*Carassius auratus*), and rainbow trout (*Salmo gairdneri*). *Journal of the Fisheries Research Board of Canada, 36,* 1174–1179.

20. Sakata, T., Sugita, H., Mitsuoka, T., et al. (1980). Isolation and distribution of obligate anaerobic bacteria from the intestines of freshwater fish. *Bulletin of the Japanese Society of Scientific Fisheries, 46,* 1249–1255.

21. Ramirez, R. F., & Dixon, B. A. (2003). Enzyme production by obligate intestinal anaerobic bacteria isolated from oscars (*Astronotus ocellatus*), angelfish (*Pterophyllum scalare*) and southern flounder (*Paralichthys lethostigma*). *Aquaculture, 227,* 417–426.

22. Sakata, T. (1990). Microflora in the digestive tract of fish and shell-fish. In R. Lésel (Ed.), *Microbiology in Poecilotherms* (pp. 171–176). Amsterdam: Elsevier.

23. Hume, I. D. (1997). Fermentation in the hindgut of mammals. In R. I. Mackie, & B. A. White, (Eds.), *Gastrointestinal Microbiology: Vol. 1* (pp. 84–115). New York: Chapman & Hall.

24. Ringo, E., & Gatesoupe, F. J. (1998). Lactic acid bacteria in fish: a review. *Aquaculture, 160,* 283–303.

25. Wang, H. N., He, M. Q., Liu, P., et al. (1994). Study on the intestinal microflora of carp in freshwater culture ponds. *Acta Hydrobiologica Sinica, 18,* 354–359.

26. Yin, J. X., Shen, W. Y., & Li, P. (2004). Study on the influence of water temperature on the intestinal microflora of *Penaeus vannamei. Marine Sciences/Haiyang Kexue, 28,* 33–36.

27. Gatesoupe, F. J. (2007). Live yeasts in the gut: Natural occurrence, dietary introduction, and their effects on fish health and development. *Aquaculture, 267,* 20–30.

28. Fjellheim, A. J., Playfoot, K., Klinkenberg, G., et al. (2005). Characterization of the dominant and the antagonistic bacterial flora of cod (*Gadhus morhua* L.) larvae reared under different conditions. In: Lessons from the Past to Optimise the Future, B. R. Howell and R. Flos, Eds., Special Publication No. 35 (pp. 201–202). European Aquaculture Society, Oostende, Belgium.

29. Simpson, J. M., McCracken, V. J., Gaskins, H. R., & Mackie, R. I. (2000). Denaturing gradient gel electrophoresis analysis of 16S ribosomal DNA amplicons to monitor changes in fecal bacterial populations of weaning pigs after introduction of *Lactobacillus reuteri* strain MM53. *Applied Environmental Microbiology, 66,* 4705–4714.

30. Ringø, E., & Birkbeck, T. H. (1999). Intestinal microflora of fish larvae and fry. *Aquaculture Research, 30,* 73–93.

31. Savage, D. C. (1977). Microbial ecology of the gastrointestinal tract. *Annual Review of Microbiology, 31,* 107–133.

32. Bairagi, A., Ghosh, K. S., Kumar, S., et al. (2002). Enzyme producing bacterial flora isolated from fish digestive tracts. *Aquaculture International, 10,* 109–121.

33. Sugita, H., & Ito, Y. (2006). Identification of intestinal bacteria from Japanese flounder (*Paralichthys olivaceus*) and their ability to digest chitin. *Letters in Applied Microbiology, 43,* 336–342.

34. Krogdahl, Å., Hemre, G. I., & Mommsen, T. P. (2005). Carbohydrates in fish nutrition: digestion and absorption in postlarval stages. *Aquaculture Nutrition, 11*, 103–122.

35. Sugita, H., Miyajima, C., & Deguchi, Y. (1991). The vitamin B_{12}–producing ability of the intestinal microflora of freshwater fish. *Aquaculture, 92*, 267–276.

36. Syvokiene, J., Jankevicius, K., & Lubianskiene, V. (1977). Role of microorganisms of the digestive tract in the nourishment of pond fish (19. Free amino acids synthesized by digestive tract bacteria of grass carp and tench, fed on artificial food). *Trudy Instituta Fiziologii, Akademiia Nauk Gruzinsko SSR, Ser. C, 3*, 79–87.

37. Lesauskiene, L., Jankevicius, K., & Syvokiene, J. (1974). The role of the digestive tract microorganisms in the nutrition of pondfishes (6. Content of free amino acids in the body of second-year fish and their synthetization by the digestive tract microoganisms). *Trudy Abademiia Nauk Litovsksi SSR, Biologiya, 2*, 127–135.

38. Lésel, R. (1981). Microflore bactérienne du tractus digestif. In: Nutrition des Poissons, M. Fontaine, Ed., Actes Coll. CNERNA, Paris, May 1979 (pp. 89–100). CNRS, Paris, France.

39. Yazawa, K., Araki, K., Watanabe, K., et al. (1988). Eicosapentaenoic acid productivity of the bacteria isolated from fish intestines. *Nippon Suisan Gakkaishi, 54*, 1835–1838.

40. Ringø, E., Jøstensen, J. P., & Olsen, R. E. (1992). Production of eicosapentaenoic acid by freshwater *Vibrio. Lipids, 27*, 564–566.

41. DeLong, E. F., & Yayanos, A. A. (1986). Biochemical function and ecological significance of novel bacterial lipids in deep-sea procaryotes. *Applied Environmental Microbiology, 51*, 730–737.

42. Yano, Y., Nakayama, A., & Yoshida, K. (1997). Distribution of polyunsaturated fatty acids in bacteria present in intestines of deep-sea fish and shallow-sea poikilothermic animals. *Applied Environmental Microbiology, 63*, 2572–2577.

43. Bates, J., Mittge, E., Kuhlman, J., et al. (2006). Distinct signals from the microbiota promote different aspects of zebrafish gut differentiation. *Developmental Biology, 297*, 374–386.

44. Rawls, J., Mahowald, M., Ley, R., & Gordon, J. I. (2006). Reciprocal gut microbiota transplants from zebrafish and mice to germ-free recipients reveal host habitat selection. *Cell, 127*, 423–433.

45. Péres, A., Cahu, C. L., & Zambonino Infante, J. L. (1997). Dietary spermine supplementation induces intestinal maturation in sea bass (*Dicentrarchus labrax*) larvae. *Fish Physiology and Biochemistry, 16*, 479–485.

46. Tovar, D., Zambonino, J., Cahu, C., et al. (2002). Effect of live yeast incorporation in compound diet on digestive enzyme activity in sea bass (*Dicentrarchus labrax*) larvae. *Aquaculture, 204*, 113–123.

47. Tovar-Ramírez, D., Zambonino Infante, J., Cahu, C., et al. (2004). Influence of dietary live yeast on European sea bass (*Dicentrarchus labrax*) larval development. *Aquaculture, 234*, 415–427.

48. O'Hara, A., & Shanahan, F. (2006). The gut flora as a forgotten organ. *EMBO Reports, 7*, 688–693.

49. Skjermo, J., Størseth, T. R., Hansen, K., et al. (2006). Evaluation of β-(1→3, 1→6)-glucans and high-M alginate used as immunostimulatory dietary supplement during first feeding and weaning of Atlantic cod (*Gadus morhua* L.). *Aquaculture, 261*, 1088–1101.

50. Magnadottir, B., Lange, S., Gudmundsdottir, S., et al. (2005). Ontogeny of humoral immune parameters in fish. *Fish & Shellfish Immunology, 19*, 429–439.

51. Zapata, A., Diez, B., Cejalvo, T., et al. (2006). Ontogeny of the immune system of fish. *Fish & Shellfish Immunology, 20*, 126–136.

52. Corripio-Miyar, Y., Bird, S., Treasurer, J. W., & Secombes, C. J. (2007). RAG-1 and IgM genes, markers for early development of the immune system in the gadoid haddock, *Melanogrammus aeglefinus*, L. *Fish & Shellfish Immunology, 23*, 71–85.

53. Ringø, E., & Gatesoupe, F. J. (1998). Lactic acid bacteria in fish: a review. *Aquaculture, 160*, 283–303.

54. Gatesoupe, F. J. (1999). The use of probiotics in aquaculture. *Aquaculture, 180*, 147–165.

55. Gomez-Gil, B., Roque, A., & Turnbull, J. F. (2000). The use and selection of probiotic bacteria for use in the culture of larval aquatic organisms. *Aquaculture, 191*, 259–270.

56. Hansen, G. H. (2000). Use of probiotics in marine aquaculture. *Feed Mix, 8*, 32–34.

57. Irianto, A., Roberwen, P. A. W., & Austin, B. (2000). The use of probiotics in aquaculture. *Recent Resuslts in Developmental Microbiology, 4*, 557–567.

58. Verschuere, L., Rombaut, G., Sorgeloos, P., & Verstraete, W. (2000). Probiotic bacteria as biological control agents in aquaculture. *Microbiology and Molecular Biology Reviews, 64*, 655–671.

59. Irianto, A., & Austin, B. (2002). Probiotics in aquaculture. *Journal of Fish Diseases, 25*, 633–642.

60. Abidi, R. (2003). Use of probiotics in larval rearing of new candidate species. *Aquaculture Asia Magazine, 7*, 15–16.

61. Maeda, M. (2004). Interactions of microorganisms and their use as biocontrol agents in aquaculture. *La Mer, 42*, 1–19.

62. Burr, G., Gatlin, D., & Ricke, S. (2005). Microbial ecology of the gastrointestinal tract of fish and the potential application of prebiotics and probiotics in finfish aquaculture. *Journal of the World Aquaculture Society, 36*, 425–436.

E. ANIMAL MODELS TO STUDY PROBIOTICS

63. Gatesoupe, F. J. (2005). Probiotics and prebiotics for fish culture, at the parting of the ways. *Aqua Feeds: Formulation & Beyond*, 2, 3–5.

64. Gram, L., & Ringø, E. (2005). Prospects of fish probiotics. In W. H. Holzapfel & P. J. Naughton (Eds.), *Microbial Ecology in Growing Animals* (pp. 379–417). Edinburgh: Elsevier.

65. Ringø, E., Schillinger, U., & Holzapfel, W. (2005). Antimicrobial activity of lactic acid bacteria isolated from aquatic animals and the use of lactic acid bacteria in aquaculture. In W. H. Holzapfel & P. J. Naughton (Eds.), *Microbial Ecology in Growing Animals* (pp. 418–453). Edinburgh: Elsevier.

66. Balcázar, J. L., de Blas, I., Ruiz Zarzuela, I., et al. (2006). The role of probiotics in aquaculture. *Veterinary Microbiology*, 114, 173–186.

67. Vine, N. G., Leukes, W. D., & Kaiser, H. (2006). Probiotics in marine larviculture. *FEMS Microbiology Reviews*, 30, 404–427.

68. Gatesoupe, F. J. (2008). Updating the importance of lactic acid bacteria in fish farming: natural occurrence and probiotic treatments. *Journal of Molecular Microbiology and Biotechnology*, 14, 107–114.

69. Gómez, G. D., & Balcázar, J. L. (2008). A review on the interactions between gut microbiota and innate immunity of fish. *FEMS Immunology and Medical Microbiology*, 52, 145–154.

70. Kesarcodi Watson, A., Kaspar, H., Lategan, M. J., & Gibson, L. (2008). Probiotics in aquaculture: The need, principles and mechanisms of action and screening processes. *Aquaculture*, 274, 1–14.

71. Tinh, N. T. N., Dierckens, K., Sorgeloos, P., & Bossier, P. (2008). A review of the functionality of probiotics in the larviculture food chain. *Marine Biotechnology*, 10, 1–12.

72. Wang, Y. B., Li, J. R., & Lin, J. (2008). Probiotics in aquaculture: Challenges and outlook. *Aquaculture*, 281, 1–4.

73. Shimizu, T., Nogami, M., & Watanabe, N. (1981). Trial of feeding with Toyocerin for improvement of mortality in the young eels (elvers). *Internal Report V-17*. Tokyo: Toyo Jozo Co., Ltd 5 pp.

74. Sasagawa, T., Inoue, H., & Kitamura, H. (1984). Trial of Toyocerin for growth promotion in cultured yellowtails. *Internal report V-22*. Tokyo: Toyo Jozo Co., Ltd 3 pp.

75. Gatesoupe, F. J. (1989). Further advances in the nutritional and antibacterial treatments of rotifers as food for turbot larvae, *Scophthalmus maximus* L. In N. De Pauw, E. Jaspers, H. Ackefors, & N. Wilkins (Eds.), *Aquaculture—A Biotechnology in Progress* (pp. 721–730). Belgium: Eur Aquacult Soc, Bredene.

76. Gatesoupe, F. J., Arakawa, T., & Watanabe, T. (1989). The effect of bacterial additives on the production rate and dietary value of rotifers as food for Japanese flounder, *Paralichthys olivaceus*. *Aquaculture*, 83, 39–44.

77. Gatesoupe, F. J. (1991). The effect of three strains of lactic bacteria on the production rate of rotifers, *Brachionus plicatilis*, and their dietary value for larval turbot, *Scophthalmus maximus*. *Aquaculture*, 96, 335–342.

78. Schrøder, K., Clausen, E., Sandberg, A. M., & Raa, J. (1979). Psychrotrophic *Lactobacillus plantarum* from fish and its ability to produce antibiotic substances. In J. J. Connell (Ed.), *Advances in Fish Science and Techology* (pp. 480–483). Farnham, England: Fishing News Books Ltd.

79. Wu, J., Lin, H., Jan, L., et al. (1981). Biological control of fish bacterial pathogen, *Aeromonas hydrophila* by bacteriophage AH 1. *Fish Pathology*, 15, 271–276.

80. Kamei, Y., Yoshimizu, M., Ezura, Y., & Kimura, T. (1987). Screening of bacteria with antiviral activity against infectious hematopoietic necrosis virus (IHNV) from estuarine and marine environments. *Nippon Suisan Gakkaishi*, 53, 2179–2185.

81. Westerdahl, A., Olsson, J. C., Kjelleberg, S., & Conway, P. L. (1991). Isolation and characterization of turbot (*Scophthalmus maximus*)-associated bacteria with inhibitory effects against *Vibrio anguillarum*. *Applied Environmental Microbiology*, 57, 2223–2228.

82. Olsson, J. C., Westerdahl, A., Conway, P. L., & Kjelleberg, S. (1992). Intestinal colonization potential of turbot (*Scophthalmus maximus*)- and dab (*Limanda limanda*)-associated bacteria with inhibitory effects against *Vibrio anguillarum*. *Applied Environmental Microbiology*, 58, 551–556.

83. Austin, B., Stuckey, L. F., Robertson, P. A. W., et al. (1995). A probiotic strain of Vibrio alginolyticus effective in reducing diseases caused by *Aeromonas salmonicida*, *Vibrio anguillarum* and *Vibrio ordalii*. *Journal of Fish Diseases*, 18, 93–96.

84. Andlid, T., Juárez, R. V., & Gustafsson, L. (1995). Yeast colonizing the intestine of rainbow trout (*Salmo gairdneri*) and turbot (*Scophthalmus maximus*). *Microbial Ecology*, 30, 321–334.

85. Mattia, A., & Merker, R. (2008). Regulation of probiotic substances as ingredients in foods: Premarket approval or 'Generally Recognized as Safe' notification. *Clinical Infectious Diseases*, 46, S115–S118.

86. Cocconcelli, P. S., Järvinen, A., Klein, G., et al. (2008). Scientific opinion of the panel on biological hazards on a request from EFSA on the maintenance of the QPS list of microorganisms intentionally added to food or feed. *The EFSA Journal*, 923, 1–48.

87. Nikoskelainen, S., Salminen, S., Bylund, G., & Ouwehand, A. C. (2001). Characterization of the properties of human- and dairy-derived probiotics for prevention of infectious diseases in fish. *Applied Environmental Microbiology*, 67, 2430–2435.

88. Chabrillón, M., Ouwehand, A. C., Díaz Rosales, P., et al. (2006). Adhesion of lactic acid bacteria to mucus

of farmed gilthead seabream, and interactions with fish pathogenic microorganisms. *Bulletin of the European Association of Fish Pathologists*, 26, 202–210.

89. Aubin, J., Gatesoupe, F. J., Labbé, L., & Lebrun, L. (2005). Trial of probiotics to prevent the vertebral column compression syndrome in rainbow trout (*Oncorhynchus mykiss* Walbaum). *Aquaculture Research*, 36, 758–767.

90. Wang, Y. B., Tian, Z. Q., Yao, J. T., & Li, W. F. (2008). Effect of probiotics, *Enteroccus faecium*, on tilapia (*Oreochromis niloticus*) growth performance and immune response. *Aquaculture*, 277, 203–207.

91. Smith, P., & Davey, S. (1993). Evidence for the competitive exclusion of *Aeromonas salmonicida* from fish with stress-inducible furunculosis by a fluorescent pseudomonad. *Journal of Fish Diseases*, 16, 521–524.

92. Chen, C. C., & Chen, S. N. (2001). Water quality management with *Bacillus* spp. in the high-density culture of red-parrot fish *Cichlasomia citrinellum* × *C. synspilum*. *North American Journal of Aquaculture*, 63, 66–73.

93. Lalloo, R., Ramchuran, S., Ramduth, D., et al. (2007). Isolation and selection of *Bacillus* spp. as potential biological agents for enhancement of water quality in culture of ornamental fish. *Journal of Applied Microbiology*, 103, 1471–1479.

94. Taoka, Y., Maeda, H., Jo, J. Y., et al. (2006). Growth, stress tolerance and non-specific immune response of Japanese flounder *Paralichthys olivaceus* to probiotics in a closed recirculating system. *Fish Science*, 72, 310–321.

95. Taoka, Y., Maeda, H., Jo, J. Y., et al. (2006). Use of live and dead probiotic cells in tilapia *Oreochromis niloticus*. *Fisheries Science*, 72, 755–766.

96. Irianto, A., & Austin, B. (2002). Use of probiotics to control furunculosis in rainbow trout, *Oncorhynchus mykiss* (Walbaum). *Journal of Fish Diseases*, 25, 333–342.

97. Gómez, G. D., & Balcázar, J. L. (2008). A review on the interactions between gut microbiota and innate immunity of fish. *FEMS Immunology and Medical Microbiology*, 52, 145–154.

98. Reyes-Becerril, M., Salinas, I., Cuesta, A., et al. (2008). Oral delivery of live yeast *Debaryomyces hansenii* modulates the main innate immune parameters and the expression of immune-relevant genes in the gilthead seabream (*Sparus aurata* L.). *Fish & Shellfish Immunology*, 25, 731–739.

99. Villamil, L., Tafalla, C., Figueras, A., & Novoa, B. (2002). Evaluation of immunomodulatory effects of lactic acid bacteria in turbot (*Scophthalmus maximus*). *Clinical and Diagnostic Laboratory Immunology*, 9, 1318–1323.

100. Panigrahi, A., Kiron, V., Puangkaew, J., et al. (2005). The viability of probiotic bacteria as a factor influencing the immune response in rainbow trout *Oncorhynchus mykiss*. *Aquaculture*, 243, 241–254.

101. Kihara, M., Ohba, K., & Sakata, T. (1995). Trophic effect of dietary lactosucrose on intestinal tunica muscularis and utilization of this sugar by gut microbes in red seabream *Pagrus major*, a marine carnivorous teleost, under artificial rearing. *Comparative Biochemistry and Physiology*, 112A, 629–634.

102. Gibson, G., & Roberfroid, M. (1995). Dietary modulation of the human colonic microbiota: introducing the concept of prebiotics. *Journal of Nutrition*, 125, 1401–1412.

103. Olsen, R. E., Myklebust, R., Kryvi, H., et al. (2001). Damaging effect of dietary inulin on intestinal enterocytes in Arctic charr (*Salvelinus alpinus* L.). *Aquaculture Research*, 32, 931–934.

104. Ringø, E., Sperstad, S., Myklebust, R., et al. (2006). The effect of dietary inulin on aerobic bacteria associated with hindgut of Arctic charr (*Salvelinus alpinus* L.). *Aquaculture Research*, 37, 891–897.

105. Bakke-McKellep, A. M., Penn, M. H., Salas, P. M., et al. (2007). Effects of dietary soyabean meal, inulin and oxytetracycline on intestinal microbiota and epithelial cell stress, apoptosis and proliferation in the teleost Atlantic salmon (*Salmo salar* L.). *British Journal of Nutrition*, 97, 699–713.

106. Mahious, A. S., Gatesoupe, F. J., Hervi, M., et al. (2006). Effect of dietary inulin and oligosaccharides as prebiotics for weaning turbot, *Psetta maxima* (Linnaeus, C. 1758). *Aquaculture International*, 14, 219–229.

107. Sink, T. D., & Lochmann, R. T. (2008). Preliminary observations of mortality reduction in stressed, *Flavobacterium columnare*-challenged golden shiners after treatment with a dairy-yeast prebiotic. *North American Journal of Aquaculture*, 70, 192–194.

108. Li, P., & Gatlin, D. M. (2004). Dietary brewers yeast and the prebiotic Grobiotic™ AE influence growth performance, immune responses and resistance of hybrid striped bass (*Morone chrysops* × *M. saxatilis*) to *Streptococcusiniae* infection. *Aquaculture*, 231, 445–456.

109. Burr, G., Hume, M., Ricke, S., et al. (2008). A preliminary *in vitro* assessment of GroBiotic®-A, brewer's yeast and fructo-oligosaccharide as prebiotics for the red drum *Sciaenops ocellatus*. *Journal of Environmental Science Health*, 43B, 253–260.

110. Staykov, Y., Spring, P., Denev, S., & Sweetman, J. (2007). Effect of a mannan oligosaccharide on the growth performance and immune status of rainbow trout (*Oncorhynchus mykiss*). *Aquaculture International*, 15, 153–161.

111. Torrecillas, S., Makol, A., Caballero, M. J., et al. (2007). Immune stimulation and improved infection resistance in European sea bass (*Dicentrarchus labrax*) fed mannan oligosaccharides. *Fish & Shellfish Immunology*, 23, 969–981.

112. Grisdale-Helland, B., Helland, S. J., & Gatlin, D. M. (2008). The effects of dietary supplementation with mannanoligosaccharide, fructo-oligosaccharide or galacto-oligosaccharide on the growth and feed utilization of Atlantic salmon (*Salmo salar*). *Aquaculture, 283*, 163–167.

113. Leenhouwers, J. I., Pellikaan, W. F., Huizing, H. F. A., et al. (2008). Fermentability of carbohydrates in an in vitro batch culture method using inocula from Nile tilapia (*Oreochromis niloticus*) and European sea bass (*Dicentrarchus labrax*). *Aquaculture Nutrition, 14*, 523–532.

114. Direkbusarakom, S. (2004). Application of medicinal herbs to aquaculture in Asia. *Walailak Journal of Science & Technology, 1*, 7–14.

115. Ardó, L., Yin, G., Xu, P., et al. (2008). Chinese herbs (*Astragalus membranaceus* and *Lonicera japonica*) and boron enhance the non-specific immune response of Nile tilapia (*Oreochromis niloticus*) and resistance against *Aeromonas hydrophila*. *Aquaculture, 275*, 26–33.

116. Ninomiya, M., Hatta, H., Fujiki, M., et al. (1995). Enhancement of chemotactic activity of yellowtail (*Seriola quinqueradiata*) leucocytes by oral administration of quillaja saponin. *Fish & Shellfish Immunology, 5*, 325–328.

117. Xie, J., Liu, B., Zhou, Q. L., et al. (2008). Effects of anthraquinone extract from rhubarb *Rheum officinale* Bail on the crowding stress response and growth of common carp *Cyprinus carpio* var. *Jian*. *Aquaculture, 281*, 5–11.

118. Chakrabarti, R., & Vasudeva, R. Y. (2006). *Achyranthes aspera* stimulates the immunity and enhances the antigen clearance in *Catla catla*. *International Immunopharmacology, 6*, 782–790.

119. Li, A. J., Chen, J. X., Zhu, W. M., et al. (2007). Antibacterial activity of gallic acid from the flowers of *Rosa chinensis* Jacq. against fish pathogens. *Aquaculture Research, 38*, 1110–1112.

120. Yildirim-Aksoy, M., Lim, C., Dowd, M. K., et al. (2004). *In vitro* inhibitory effect of gossypol from gossypol-acetic acid, and (+)- and (–)-isomers of gossypol on the growth of *Edwardsiella ictaluri*. *Journal of Applied Microbiology, 97*, 87–92.

121. Lieschke, G., & Currie, P. (2007). Animal models of human disease: zebrafish swim into view. *Nature Reviews. Genetics, 8*, 353–367.

122. Cheesman, S. E., & Guillemin, K. (2007). We know you are in there: Conversing with the indigenous gut microbiota. *Research in Microbiology, 158*, 2–9.

123. Rawls, J. F., Mahowald, M. A., Goodman, A. L., et al. (2007). *In vivo* imaging and genetic analysis link bacterial motility and symbiosis in the zebrafish gut. *Proceedings of the National Academy of Sciences of the United States of America, 104*, 7622–7627.

124. Buts, J. P., de Keyser, N., & de Raedemaeker, L. (1994). *Saccharomyces boulardii* enhances rat intestinal enzyme expression by endoluminal release of polyamines. *Pediatric Research, 36*, 522–527.

125. Dinsdale, E. A., Edwards, R. A., Hall, D., et al. (2008). Functional metagenomic profiling of nine biomes. *Nature, 452*, 629–632.

126. Irianto, A., & Austin, B. (2003). Use of dead probiotic cells to control furunculosis in rainbow trout, *Oncorhynchus mykiss* (Walbaum). *Journal of Fish Diseases, 26*, 59–62.

127. Frouël, S., Le Bihan, E., Serpentini, A., et al. (2008). Preliminary study of the effects of commercial Lactobacilli preparations on digestive metabolism of juvenile sea bass (*Dicentrarchus labrax*). *Journal of Molecular Microbiology and Biotechnology, 14*, 100–106.

128. Salinas, I., Myklebust, R., Esteban, M. A., et al. (2008). *In vitro* studies of *Lactobacillus delbrueckii* subsp. *lactis* in Atlantic salmon (*Salmo salar* L.) foregut: Tissue responses and evidence of protection against *Aeromonas salmonicida* subsp. *salmonicida* epithelial damage. *Veterinary Microbiology, 128*, 167–177.

129. Marques, A., Ollevier, F., Verstraete, W., et al. (2006). Gnotobiotically grown aquatic animals: opportunities to investigate host-microbe interactions. *Journal of Applied Microbiology, 100*, 903–918.

GI Bacteria Changes in Animal Models Due to Prebiotics

Philippe Gérard and Sylvie Rabot

INRA, UR 910 Ecologie et Physiologie du Système Digestif, Jouy-en-Josas, France

1. DIETARY FIBERS

Dietary fibers (DF), as an indigestible portion of plant food, play an important role in human nutrition due to their beneficial effects on health. They are responsible for fecal bulking, enhancing gut motility and lowering transit time. Indigestible in the small intestine, they reach the colon where they are metabolized by the gut microbiota. Chemically, DF consist of non-starch polysaccharides such as cellulose and many other plant components such as pectins, dextrins, lignins, β-glucans, etc.

Studies using a mixed fiber diet have emphasized the strong impact of DF on gut microbiota. As an example, a high-fiber diet containing 40% soya cake, 20% crude potato starch, 19% wheat bran, and 5% each of apple pectin and carob gum, given for 4 weeks to rats, led to a daily fecal output of anaerobes 71 times higher than a fiber free diet. Similarly, daily excretion of total fermentation products was 20 times higher, with an increase of propionate and butyrate proportions [1].

Nevertheless, the specific effect of each type of fiber can only be scrutinized using a diet with one source of DF. Therefore, diets supplemented with barley flour, oatmeal flour, cellulose, coffee fiber or barley β-glucans have been used to assess their prebiotic effects. It was observed that the diet containing barley β-glucans of high viscosity produced large changes in microbiota profiles relative to the other diets in rats. This was mainly due to a specific stimulation of species belonging to the *Lactobacillus acidophilus* group [2]. An increase in *Lactobacillus* populations was also obtained with different barley-rich diets [3] which also resulted in coliforms and *Bacteroides* decreases. This was accompanied by a greater concentration of total short-chain fatty acids (SCFA) in cecal[1] contents and feces, with higher butyrate and lower propionate proportions [4]. The same increase in butyrate proportion was observed in the cecum of rats fed wholewheat flour diets, but propionate proportion was not affected, while acetate proportion decreased [5]. Conversely, coffee fiber led to an increase in SCFA concentrations

[1]The cecum in rats and mice is extremely developed and considered as the equivalent of proximal colon in humans.

in the cecum without changes in their proportions [6]. The amounts and proportions of secondary bile acids were markedly reduced in rats fed barley β-glucans diets, probably due to lower intestinal pH values, inhibiting the bacterial 7α-dehydroxylase. Concurrently, the microbial conversion of cholesterol to coprostanol was enhanced by the dietary fiber-rich barley based diets [7]. Similar results were obtained with different cereal flour diets that induced higher neutral sterol output, and notably that of coprostanol [5]. This likely reflects a more active metabolism of cholesterol by the microbiota in moderately acidic pH conditions.

It has been estimated that apples could provide 10–30% of the daily intake of fiber. Using a diet containing 100g of apple fiber/kg, it has been shown that soluble dietary fiber (SDF) (mainly pectin) excreted in feces of rats was 10.9% of the SDF ingested, which suggests a low resistance to fermentation of this fraction, while only 43% of the ingested insoluble fiber was fermented [8]. A pectin containing diet led to an increase in the SCFA pool in the cecum with a higher acetate molar ratio [6, 9]. An accumulation of galacturonate and succinate [9] and an increase in butyrate and isobutyrate concentrations [6] were also observed in the cecum. This was accompanied by a rise in *Bacteroides*, fusobacteria and enterobacteria in the cecal contents while an increase in *Bacteroides*, eubacteria, clostridia, lactobacilli, enterobacteria and streptococci in the feces of mice was obtained in response to pectin supplementation [10].

Pectin also caused an increase in polyamines concentrations, especially cadaverine, in the cecal contents of rats [11]. Most of the DF components remain in pomace during the usual juice preparation. Using fluorescent *in situ* hybridization (FISH), it has been observed that bacteria belonging to the *Eubacterium rectale* cluster and that *Bacteroides* genus were increased in cecal contents, whereas only *Bacteroides* were increased in the feces of rats receiving apple pomace extraction juices [12]. Cecal concentrations

of acetate and propionate were two times higher, suggesting a microbial fermentation of pectin and arabinogalactan. These results are in accordance with the known capability of the *Bacteroides* species to degrade these polysaccharides [13]. A two-step procedure using complex enzyme preparations has been proposed to extract juices with higher DF contents [14]. More total SCFA were measured in the cecal contents of rats fed extraction juices from apple, grape and red beet pomaces prepared according to this method due to an increase in acetate concentration [15]. Significantly more lactobacilli and bifidobacteria were found in feces of rats of the apple group, whereas extraction juice from red beets resulted merely in higher counts of lactobacilli. An increase in cholesterol metabolites such as coprostanol was also observed in feces of rats that received extraction juices, whereas the proportion of secondary bile acids was reduced.

Guar gum, also called guaran, is a water-soluble galactomannan frequently used in the food industry as an emulsifier or stabilizer. A major bifidogenic effect of a guar gum-containing diet (100g/kg) has been observed in the cecum of rats, while *Bacteroides*, fusobacteria and enterobacteria were also increased. Concurrently, this diet stimulated the bacterial synthesis of polyamines by decarboxylation of the amino acids ornithine, arginine and lysine [11]. It was suggested that the increase in the *Fusobacterium* population was responsible for the concomitant rise in polyamines. Similarly to guar gum, Konjac glucomannan, which derives from the tuber of *Amorphophallus* konjac, increased bifidobacteria, and was also found to decrease cecal *Clostridium perfringens* in mice [16]. Conversely, a diet containing gum arabic had no bifidogenic effect [17].

The impact of diets containing 50g/kg of either guar, karaya, tragacanth, gellan, xanthan or psyllium on microbiota metabolism has been studied in rats. Guar and karaya increased the total SCFA concentrations in the cecum while xanthan produced the opposite effect. Tragacanth and guar significantly reduced, whereas gellan increased, the molar proportion of acetate. Psyllium increased the proportion of propionate and decreased the proportion of butyrate [18], as previously shown for soybean fiber, which contains chiefly insoluble hemicelluloses [19]. A psyllium diet also dramatically decreased a cholesterol-to-coprostanol conversion, whereas diets enriched in pectin, alfalfa or mixed fibers increased coprostanol percentages in the feces. Psyllium and alfalfa diets also altered bacterial production of secondary bile acids, whereas pectin and mixed fiber diets did not [20].

The effects of five DF from different sources (carrot, wheat bran, cocoa seed, pea hull, and oat husks) have been assessed in human microbiota-associated (HMA) rats [21]. HMA rats are initially germ-free rats colonized after weaning with the fecal microbiota of a healthy human volunteer. Use of this animal model is justified by the phylogenetic and metabolic differences between rat and human microbiota and the knowledge that HMA rodents globally retain the characteristics of the human donor microbiota [22–24]. All of the diets contained 100 g fiber/kg and were given for 8 weeks. Both carrot and cocoa led to a higher proportion of acetate and a lower proportion of propionate in the cecum, and to a large production of methane. The concentration of lactate was significantly higher in rats fed on the carrot-fiber diet.

Altogether, these results revealed that different types or sources of DF led to different or even opposite effects.

2. RESISTANT STARCHES

Starch has been considered mainly as an energy and carbon source in the human diet. However, it can also have properties similar to dietary fiber and exert an important role in colonic physiology and functions. Starches are polymers of glucose, which are either straight chains (amylose) or branched (amylopectin). RS is defined as starch that escapes digestion by pancreatic amylases in the small intestine and provides a source of fermentable substrate for cecal and colonic microbiota, resulting in the production of SCFA and gases. RS can be classified into four different groups: type I, representing physically inaccessible starch found in vegetables or in whole or partly milled grains; type II, representing starch with a granular structure such as raw potato or corn; type III, representing retrograded starch obtained through feed processing; type IV, representing selected starches that have been chemically treated (etherization, esterization, cross-bonding). Table 33.1 outlines a summary of the different types of RS, their classification criteria and food sources. Unlike RS types I and IV, RS types II and III have been widely used in animal models to assess their effects on gut microbiota composition and metabolism.

Potato tubers are rich in starch packed in characteristic spherical and semi-spherical granules with an amylase:amylopectin ratio of approximately 1:3 (RS type II). These granules show strong resistance to α-amylase *in vitro* which suggests they can enter the colon and be used as substrates for fermentation by the colonic microbial community. As a consequence, stepwise additions of raw potato starch (RPS) at the expense of maize starch led to an increased ileal output of starch in rats [25]. It was then calculated that 72% of starch from a high RPS diet (240 g/kg) escaped small-bowel digestion but disappeared within the large bowel. This suggests that the fermentative capacity of the cecum is able to cope effectively with RPS over a wide range of intakes. This was confirmed by a linear increase in total SCFA concentration as RPS intake increased [25]. Acetate was always the major SCFA present and increased linearly with RPS intakes. Similar results were obtained by Le Blay et al. [26] who showed that giving a diet containing RPS (90 g/kg) for 2 weeks mainly resulted in an increase in acetate in the cecum. This was also confirmed by Andrieux et al. [27]

TABLE 33.1   Classification of types of resistant starch

Resistant starch	Description	Food sources	Resistance reduced by
Type I	Physically protected.	Whole- or partly milled grains and seeds, legumes, pasta.	Milling, chewing.
Type II	Ungelatinized resistant granules with B-type crystallinity.	Raw potatoes, green bananas, some legumes, high-amylose starches.	Food processing and cooking.
Type III	Retrograded starch formed during the cooling of gelatinized, high-amylose starch and consisting of small aggregates of hydrogen-bonded amylose.	Cooked and cooled potatoes, peas, beans, bread, corn.	Processing conditions.
Type IV	Selected chemically modified starches owing to cross-bonding with chemical reagents, ethers, esters, etc.	This type of modified resistant starch is a novel food, not yet approved by the EU.	Less susceptible to digestibility *in vitro*.

Source: Nugent, A.P. (2005). Health properties of resistant starch. *Nutrition Bulletin, 30,* 27–54.

who used a diet containing up to 480 g RPS/kg. Conversely, Berggren et al. [28] observed that the relative proportions of SCFA were not changed in cecal contents of rats given a diet with 100 g RPS/kg over 5 days. The proportion of propionate remained unchanged in all studies. Including 80 or 90 g RPS/kg in the diet resulted in a notable increase in the cecal butyrate proportion but higher RPS intakes led to lower butyrate proportions. RPS intake also yielded an increase in lactate pools in the cecum and to a much greater extent in the distal colon [26, 27]. These data suggest that RPS fermentation occurs not only in the cecum but is distributed throughout the colon. Molar proportions of the minor SCFA (isobutyrate, isovalerate and valerate) diminished in the cecum with increased RPS intakes [25, 27]. This may be due to a reduced amino acid fermentation or utilization of these SCFA for bacterial protein synthesis. All studies also found that animals fed with RPS exhibited increased cecal weight and decreased pH.

Only a few studies have analyzed the microbiota changes due to RPS in animal models. Using denaturing gradient gel electrophoresis (DGGE) of PCR amplified bacterial 16S rRNA genes, Licht et al. [29] observed that a diet containing 150 g RPS/kg affected the profile of the gut microbiota. Nevertheless, no differences were found in counts of cultivable coliforms, enterococci, or lactic acid bacteria in fecal samples of rats receiving diets with or without RPS. Le Blay et al. [26] also found no change in bacterial counts of fecal samples from rats on a diet containing 90 g RPS/kg but revealed an increase in the numbers of Gram-positive cocci, lactic acid bacteria and lactobacilli in the cecum and proximal colon. Such changes are in accordance with the known capability of lactobacilli and Gram-positive cocci to ferment or grow on starch [30, 31]. However, a diet containing 100 g RPS/kg induced no change, over a 5-month feeding period, in fecal and cecal bacterial counts in rats [32] so that the effect of RPS on gut microbiota is still inconclusive.

RPS diets have also been shown to modify bile acids bacterial metabolism with decreased conversions of β-muricholic and cholic acids into hyodeoxycholic and deoxycholic acids, respectively, and increased ω-muricholic acid formation [27]. It was suggested that these effects resulted from the decrease in cecal pH. Nevertheless, when RPS ingestion was stopped, the cecal pH returned to its initial value whereas bile acid conversions remained affected, indicating that the bacterial populations responsible for these conversions were durably affected.

Amylomaize starch constitutes the other main representative of RS type II which has been studied in animal models. Andrieux and Sacquet [33] have first demonstrated that it is not totally digested by germ-free rats, whereas it is totally degraded by the conventional rat, revealing that at least a part of amylomaize starch is fermented by the gut microbiota. The impact of amylomaize starch on bacterial metabolism has been assessed and indicated, contrary to potato starch, an increase in propionate concentration in the cecum and to a lesser extent in butyrate, whereas the concentration of acetate was reduced by one-third [27, 34]. Amylomaize starch ingestion also led to an increase in lactate concentration in the cecum of rats. Nevertheless, these effects may depend on the experimental design. Indeed, if total SCFA were also found significantly higher in another study involving rats fed an amylomaize starch diet (640 g/kg), the percentages of acetate, propionate and butyrate were not significantly changed compared to control diet [35]. Amylomaize starch also led to an increase in *Clostridium* and *Propionibacterium* fecal populations, whereas *Bacteroides* concentration decreased. Different results were obtained in mice showing that adding 300 g or more of amylomaize starch/kg of diet results in higher levels of *Bifidobacterium* and coliform population in feces [36].

An amylomaize starch diet was also found to reduce bacterial β-D-glucuronidase, N-acetyl-β-D-glucosaminidase, N-acetyl-β-D-galactosaminidase and β-D-galactosidase activities, while β-D-glucosidase and α-L-fucosidase activities were not affected [34]. Amylomaize starch also caused similar changes of bile acid bacterial metabolism as RPS [27].

RS type III is resistant to digestion in the small intestine but is fermented by the cecal microbiota to a lesser extent than RS type II. Nevertheless, it was shown that different types of retrograded starch were able to modify gut microbiota and its metabolism in animal models, causing significantly enhanced total SCFA levels in cecum and colon. This effect appeared to raise a maximum with retrograded maltodextrins, leading to an increase in butyrate and a decrease in propionate proportions [37]. The same changes in SCFA proportions were obtained with a diet enriched in freeze-dried, cooked haricot beans which starch is mainly retrograded amylose [38], whereas higher molar proportions of acetate and lower proportions of propionate were observed with a diet containing freeze-dried, cooked peas [39]. Retrograded potato starch ingestion also resulted in increased SCFA production but without any change in their proportions [32, 37]. Molar proportions of branched chains fatty acids (BCFA) were reduced with all diets containing RS type III, suggesting their greater utilization for *de novo* amino acid and, hence, bacterial protein synthesis, or reduced amino acid fermentations.

The effect of RS type III on microbiota composition has been analyzed using classical culture techniques only. The cecal microbiota of rats fed a diet containing retrograded potato starch displayed higher numbers of lactobacilli, streptococci, *Bacteroides* and enterobacteria than rats fed a control diet or a diet containing RPS, indicating that little modification in the chemical structure of starch has the potential for changing the composition of the gut microbiota [32]. Biochemical identification of species following plating revealed that *Lactobacillus cellobiosus* was the main species stimulated by a diet containing retrograded potato starch. Different leguminous-(pea, chickpea, common bean, lentil) containing diets with similar RS type III content decreased *Enterobacter* and *Bacteroides* populations, while lactobacilli and clostridia were not affected. A bifidogenic effect was only achieved with pea and chickpea-containing diets [40].

The impact of a retrograded amylose starch on human gut microbiota has been considered in HMA rats, colonized with microbiota from UK or Italian subjects [41]. Consumption of the diet increased the numbers of lactobacilli and bifidobacteria and decreased enterobacteria in both the UK and Italian microbiota. However, *Bacteroides* and streptococci were not altered by the diet in Italian microbiota-associated rats, but were reduced or enhanced, respectively, in UK microbiota-associated rats. Moreover, staphylococci increased in the UK but decreased in the Italian microbiota-associated rats, which indicates that different human microbiota may respond in different ways to dietary changes. In spite of this, the diet was associated with the same changes in the SCFA profiles in both groups, with a marked increase in the proportion of butyrate and a corresponding decrease in propionate. Cecal ammonia concentration was also significantly decreased, while β-glucosidase activity was increased in both groups. This increase could be a consequence of the stimulation of bifidobacteria and lactobacilli, which possess high levels of β-glucosidase activity.

RS type III also lowered the fecal excretion of total neutral steroids, especially of coprostanol, indicating that bacterial reduction of cholesterol was depressed [42]. In addition, the bacterial formation of hyodeoxycholic acid was partly suppressed by RS type III, while formation of ω-muricholic and lithocholic acids increased [37, 42].

3. INULIN-TYPE FRUCTANS

Inulin-type fructans are storage carbohydrates comprising fructose molecules linked or not to a terminal sucrose molecule. They are particularly abundant in the root of plant species from the *Asteraceae* family such as chicory (*Cichorium intybus* var. *sativum*) or Jerusalem artichoke (*Helianthus tuberosus*). Inulin (INU) is a generic term to cover all β−2,1 linear fructans and chicory INU, for example, is a complex mixture of linear β fructans with a degree of polymerization (DP) ranging from 2 to 60 (average

DP: 12). Through partial enzymatic hydrolysis, an oligofructose (OF) or fructo-oligosaccharide (FOS) fraction may be obtained with a DP of 2–8 (average DP: 4), whereas specific separation technologies yield long-chain INU fractions (DP 10–60, average DP: >20). Specific products have been designed by blending long-chain INU and OF fractions [43]. The aim of this reformulation is to optimize the rate of fermentation by providing OF—readily fermented in the proximal colon—on the one hand, and long-chain INU—supposed to be less rapidly fermented, hence more available in the distal colon—on the other hand [44].

In the past two decades, several studies have been undertaken in laboratory animal models, with the aim to explore how native INU, long-chain or OF fractions, or blends of these fractions, modified the intestinal microbiota composition and influenced the glycolytic activities and the fermentation characteristics within the large intestine. Most investigations used conventional rats fed a standard chow or a semi-purified diet, sometimes formulated to mimic Western human type diet characteristics, e.g. inclusion of cooked starch and animal fats [45], increase of fat content and reduction of calcium concentration [46, 47], increase of protein content and manipulation of anion and cation proportions to promote latent metabolic acidosis [48]. Introduction of the inulin-type fructan in the diet was generally at the expense of a part of the digestive carbohydrate fraction (e.g. glucose, sucrose, cereal starch) and/or, sometimes, at the expense of the cellulose fraction.

In short-term studies (about 2 weeks long), in which diets containing 3–6% of OF, FOS or INU were distributed to rats, qPCR analysis of feces or cecal contents revealed an increase of bifidobacteria populations by about 2 $\log_{10}$ cfu/g [46, 47, 49]. On the other hand, selective cultivation of these bacteria from cecal contents indicated no effect of a 6% FOS-containing diet given for the same duration [50]. Longer consumption, for 4 weeks or 6 months, of lower dosages of FOS or INU (1–2% of the diet) led to an increase of bifidobacteria populations by 1 to 2 $\log_{10}$ cfu/g, as analyzed by selective cultivation [51, 52]. In the 4 week study performed in rats, DGGE fingerprinting of the cecal contents using specific primers targeting the genus *Bifidobacterium* showed that these bacteria became predominant, confirming the increase observed by the culture techniques [51]. In the 6 month study performed in mice, the increase of bifidobacteria counts was quickly reverted, within 1 week, by return to a basal diet, suggesting that a continuous FOS- or INU-enriched diet must be followed to maintain a bifidogenic effect in the gut lumen [52]. Consumption of a high-fat diet has been shown to dramatically reduce cecal *Bifidobacterium* counts in mice [53]. Interestingly, inclusion of a high level of FOS (10%) in such a high-fat diet nullified this deleterious effect, restoring *Bifidobacterium* populations to the level of chow-fed control mice [54]. In all of above studies, alterations of other populations were inconsistent, depending obviously on the experimental design, though no correlation can be clearly established between the type of effect and experimental design parameters such as feeding duration, amount of fructan in the diet, animal model species, or method of bacterial enumeration (culture vs qPCR). Some 2 week long studies in rats and the 6 month study in mice indicate an increase of fecal or cecal lactobacilli counts [26, 46, 52], while other 2 week long studies and the 4 week study in rats could not detect any change in the amount of this population [47, 49–51]. Similarly, enterobacteria counts were found to be either increased [46, 47], decreased [51, 55], or unaffected [26, 52]. Enterobacteria and lactobacilli are subdominant populations and their concentrations in control groups were highly variable, from 10^6 to 10^9 cfu/g, depending on the study. The inconsistent effect of treatments with inulin-type fructans on these populations may be linked to these variations, suggesting that the effect may depend upon the initial level of the population in the animal gut. Other bacterial populations, in particular the strictly anaerobic groups, which are predominant in the gut microbiota, have received comparatively less attention. Cultivable *Bacteroides* counts were either unchanged [26, 52] or decreased [51]; as for *Clostridium* counts, the two studies that analyzed them concluded a decrease of their populations [51, 52]. Licht et al. [29] used an unusual high level of FOS or INU, namely 15%, for 5 weeks in rats. Selective cultivation from feces of these animals revealed a greater amount of lactic acid bacteria and a lower amount of enterobacteria, regardless of the inulin-type fructan included in the diet. However, DGGE fingerprinting resulted in completely different phylogenetic profiles in the animals fed FOS versus those fed INU. Furthermore, in INU-fed rats, comparison of DNA-based and RNA-based DGGE profiles showed that two species within the phylum *Bacteroidetes*, although they were not abundant in numbers, were highly metabolically active.

The main gut microbiota metabolic markers that have been analyzed are: i) glycolytic activities, mainly α- and β-glucosidase, α- and β-galactosidase and β-glucuronidase; ii) the end-products of carbohydrate fermentation, i.e. SCFA; iii) lactate as a typical fermentation product of bifidobacteria and lactobacilli; and iv) ammonia and BCFA as markers of protein fermentation. In short-term studies (up to 3 weeks) in which 4–10% of OF, FOS or native or long-chain INU were included in the diet of rats, the most constant effect was a 1.5- to 6-fold increase of the total SCFA cecal pool [26, 50, 56, 57] or concentration [56–58]. This dramatic increase was also consistently observed in longer term studies (up to 27 weeks) using the same amounts of inulin-type fructans [48, 58–63], and in those using greater levels of inclusion such as 15 or 20% [29, 56, 64, 65]. Taken together, these findings reflect a quick and substantial increase of the microbiota fermentation activity in the cecal compartment, regardless of the chain length of the inulin-type fructan and of the consumption duration. However, a threshold level of inclusion seems necessary to induce a significant increase of the fermentation activity. Indeed, in an experiment decreasing the INU concentration from 5 to 1% in 6 weeks, Juskiewicz et al. [61] could not obtain an increase of the SCFA pool or concentration, contrary to rats that were concomitantly fed increasing levels, from 1 to 5%, of the same INU. Among SCFA, an increase of the butyrate [57–65] and propionate proportions [46, 59–65] was consistently observed, at the expense of acetate whose proportion decreased significantly in some studies [46, 59–61, 63]. Lactate is the main fermentation product of bifidobacteria and lactobacilli, which are reported to be the main target populations of inulin-type fructans. Therefore, and although it is an intermediate fermentation metabolite, its concentration in the cecum or feces of rats consuming inulin-type fructans has been measured on several occasions. An increase, either of the concentration or of the pool, was usually observed [26, 46, 48, 56, 58, 64]. This observation is consistent with the increase of the populations of lactic acid bacteria, at least in the studies where these populations were analyzed concurrently [26, 46]. Protein fermentation was also altered, as shown by Van Craeyveld et al. [49], who observed a reduction of the cecal ammonia concentration in rats consuming FOS or long-chain INU (4%, 2 weeks), and a specific reduction of the cecal BCFA concentration in those consuming FOS. A reduction of ammonia concentration also occurred with long-chain INU given at 5% for 4 weeks [59] or native INU given at 15% for 3 weeks [65]. When rats were offered a lower amount of INU (1% for 6 weeks), no alteration of the ammonia concentration was observed [61], suggesting that, likewise SCFA, a threshold concentration is required to trigger an alteration of this marker. Decreasing of cecal ammonia concentration may reflect either an increase of ammonia utilization for bacterial protein synthesis, allowed by a greater level of energy, or an increased absorption

of this compound. Indeed, Younes et al. [57], using FOS at 7.5% for 3 weeks, showed an increase of the ammonia flux from the cecal lumen to the cecal venous blood, as did Levrat et al. [65], using native INU at 15% for 3 weeks. With regard to glycolytic enzyme activities, all results arise from Juskiewicz's group who studied the impact of inulin-type fructans in various experimental protocols. Results varied from no alteration following consumption of long-chain INU at 1 to 5% for 6 weeks [61] to a selective 3- to 4-fold increase of β-glucosidase following consumption of long-chain INU at 5 or 10% for 4 weeks [63]. However, a non-specific 1- to 4-fold increase of α- and β-glucosidase and α- and β-galactosidase occurred in a similar protocol using a lower dietary level of long-chain INU, namely 4–5% [59, 60].

The globally enhancing effect of inulin-type fructans on gut microbiota hydrolytic and fermentation activities systematically resulted in acidification of the cecal content [29, 48, 50, 56, 57, 60, 61, 63–65] or feces [46], ranging from −0.51-to −1.7 pH unit, a weight increase of the cecal content or of the fecal output, ranging from 1.5- to 5-fold, and an increase of the cecal wall weight, ranging from 1.5- to 3-fold [26, 29, 48, 50, 56–65]. Latter observations reflect both a bulking effect and a trophic effect of inulin-type fructans on the gut mucosa.

Because of their stimulating effect on the growth of resident lactic acid bacteria and their promotion of butyrate and lactate production, inulin-type fructans have been considered as a potential primary or adjuvant maintenance therapy for chronic inflammatory bowel diseases or colorectal carcinogenesis. In this respect, some authors have administered OF, FOS or INU to rats developing colitis, either spontaneously due to a genetic modification [66] or following a chemical treatment with, for example, trinitrobenzenesulfonic acid [67]. In these models, administration of FOS [67] or of a blend of OF and long-chain INU [66], starting prior to the development of inflammation and continuing for several weeks, induced an increase of lactic acid bacteria counts, as determined by selective cultivation of cecal contents [67], or by FISH using specific primers targeting the genera *Bifidobacterium* and *Lactobacillus* [66]. In addition, FISH indicated that the concentration of enterococci and of predominant anaerobic populations, namely the phylum *Bacteroidetes* and the *Clostridium* group XIVa, remained unchanged; nevertheless, DGGE profiles of inulin-type fructan-treated rats differed from those of chow-fed counterparts, indicating a rearrangement of the dominant population profile [66]. Biochemical analyses gave inconsistent results, showing no alteration of the cecal SCFA concentration [66] or a specific increase of butyric and lactic acids, accompanied by an acidification of the cecal content [67]. Taken together, these results suggest that increasing lactic acid bacteria counts in the gut may indeed be involved in the alleviating effect of inulin-type fructans on the tone of intestinal inflammation. However, the mechanisms supporting the effect of lactic acid bacteria are still unclear. Other authors have studied the effect of inulin-type fructans in rats chemically treated to develop aberrant crypt foci, which are used as biomarkers of colon carcinogenesis. FOS or INU included in the diet at 5 to 15% were given to these animal models for 3 to 12 weeks, starting the feeding treatment before [6, 68] or after administration of the chemical carcinogen [6, 69–71]. Just like in healthy rats, FOS induced an increase of cecal bifidobacteria counts by about 1 $\log_{10}$ cfu/g, as determined by selective cultivation [69, 70]; a slight decrease of enterobacteria [69] or enterococci [70] was concurrently observed. Cecal biochemistry was also altered. As expected, FOS, native INU and long-chain INU feeding increased cecal SCFA concentration [6] or pool [70] by 2.5- to 5-fold, butyrate production being particularly stimulated. As several studies have shown that ammonia is a tumor promoter and that colon cancer risk inversely correlates with cecal/fecal β-glucuronidase activity [72–74], most authors have focused on these

metabolic markers. Yet, results are inconclusive. Indeed, ammonia concentration remained steady upon FOS or long-chain INU feeding at 5% for 3 weeks [68], or decreased by about 30% upon long-chain INU feeding at 5% for 12 weeks [71]. Similarly, β-glucuronidase activity was unchanged in the former study while it decreased by about 40% in the latter. It is noticeable that native INU given at a higher level, 10%, for the same 12 week duration did not alter cecal β-glucuronidase activity [6].

Andrieux and Szylit's group in the 1990s and Blaut's group in the following decade, have undertaken a series of investigations using HMA rats in order to characterize the effect of inulin-type fructans on gut microbiota in experimental conditions closer to the human situation. Using culture techniques, Djouzi et al. [75] showed that a 4-week consumption of FOS at 4% in the diet increased the fecal bifidobacteria concentration by 2 $\log_{10}$ cfu/g while other bacterial groups including *Bacteroides*, *Clostridium*, enterobacteria and enterococci remained steady. Surprisingly, using FISH analysis, Kleessen et al. [24] could not show a bifidogenic effect of FOS at the same dietary level; they even observed a reduction of 1 $\log_{10}$ cfu/g in the cecal *Bifidobacterium* population when rats were fed on long-chain INU. It must be emphasized that their experiment was particularly short, 1 week only. Nevertheless, this duration was long enough to reduce by 1-$\log_{10}$ cfu/g of the *Clostridium histolyticum* and *Clostridium lituseburense* groups in the cecum and feces of rats fed on FOS or on a blend of FOS and long-chain INU. In the latter rats, a 1-$\log_{10}$ cfu/g increase of the *C. coccoides-E. rectale* cluster in the cecum and feces also occurred, together with a 1.5-$\log_{10}$ cfu/g increase of cecal lactobacilli. Concentrations of other groups, *Bacteroides-Prevotella*, *Enterococcus* and *Enterobacteriaceae* did not change. The absence of bifidogenic effect in Kleessen et al.'s experiment may be due to the initially high level of bifidobacteria in the human fecal inoculum they used (9.0 $\log_{10}$ cfu/g wet feces). As a matter of fact, in a longer study (4 weeks) using the same level of FOS and long-chain INU mix, they once again did not observe any increase of bifidobacteria in the distal colonic content of HMA rats displaying an initial high level of bifidobacteria (9.4 $\log_{10}$ cfu/g wet weight) [76]. However, prebiotic feeding significantly increased the mucosal bifidobacteria, from 4.0 to 5.4 $\log_{10}$ cells/mm² mucosal surface in the colon. Such findings support the idea that bacterial populations that occupy the mucosal niche are distinct from those in the lumen and, hence, are likely to respond differently to a dietary manipulation. In addition, as a stimulation of mucosal bifidobacteria may contribute to stabilize the gut mucosal barrier, this result opens new perspectives for health benefits conferred by inulin-type fructans. As a matter of fact, a challenge of the above rats with *Salmonella enterica* subsp. *enterica* serovar Typhimurium reduced the number of Salmonella cells present in the Peyer's patches, compared with control counterparts fed on rat chow [77]. With regard to metabolic characteristics, observations in HMA rats corroborated those of conventional animals. Consumption of FOS, native INU, long-chain INU, or blends of these products, increased the total SCFA cecal concentration [21, 45, 75, 76, 78] or pool [78] by about 20 to 100% and doubled the relative proportion of butyrate, regardless of the dietary level (4 to 12%) and the feeding duration (1 to 8 weeks). Similarly, the cecal content was acidified (−0.3 to −1.0 pH unit) and the cecal content and wall were heavier. In addition, Andrieux and Szylit's group have examined the effects of inulin-type fructans on the production of fermentation gases, depending on the phenotype of the human donor. In rats colonized with a non-methane producing microbiota, native INU at 10% for 3 weeks dramatically increased the excretion of dihydrogen, from 0.05 to 2.74 mL/24h/10g of food intake/

100g body wt [45]. In rats colonized with a methane-producing microbiota, FOS and INU also dramatically increased dihydrogen excretion, by 3- to 25-fold [21, 45, 75], while the effect on methane excretion was contrasting, ranging from a nearly nullification [21, 45] to a 1.5-fold increase [75].

The same group has studied the effects of FOS in an animal model simulating necrotizing enterocolitis (NEC). NEC is one of the most common serious gastrointestinal diseases in neonatal intensive care units. In healthy full-term babies fed breast milk, bifidobacteria colonization of the gut appears in the first days of life. In contrast, this colonization is often delayed in pre-term infants, thus favoring high levels of *Clostridium* sp., e.g. *C. butyricum*, *C. perfringens* and *C. paraputrificum*, implicated in the etiology of NEC. This has prompted studies on how to stimulate bifidobacteria colonization in those infants. To study the pathogenesis and dietary prevention of NEC, gnotobiotic alactasic animal models, i.e. quails (they naturally do not possess intestinal lactase), were designed; when fed on a lactose-containing diet and associated with bacterial strains isolated from patients with NEC, these animals develop cecal inflammation whose characteristics are close to NEC lesions [79]. Catala et al. [80] have studied the impact of FOS feeding (3% for 3 weeks) on the gut microbiota balance in quails associated with fecal microbiota collected from different preterm neonates. In all cases, the *Bifidobacterium* population, analyzed by selective cultivation, increased by 1 to 2 $\log_{10}$ cfu/g; concurrently, *E. coli* and *Clostridium* populations, including the pathogen *C. perfringens*, were markedly reduced. It is noticeable that no modification of the SCFA production and, hence, no acidification of the cecal content, occurred in these experiments. Nevertheless, this work showed that FOS can favor gut colonization with bifidobacteria, thus contributing to a resistance against NEC-associated pathogens.

4. GALACTO-OLIGOSACCHARIDES

Several edible plants, including grains, cruciferous vegetables and, above all, legumes contain high levels of α-galacto-oligosaccharides (α-GalOS). α-GalOS are tri- to pentasaccharides with α-1,6 linkages, sharing the following structure: galactose$(1,6)_n$-sucrose, with $n = 1$ being raffinose, $n = 2$ stachyose and $n = 3$ verbascose. Since mammals are deficient in the enzyme α-galactosidase, α-GalOS are not digested in the small intestine and reach the large intestine where they are extensively fermented by the resident microbiota. Other types of indigestible but fermentable galacto-oligosaccharides have been obtained artificially. Thus, transgalactosylated oligosaccharides (TOS) are mixtures of β-galacto-oligosaccharides synthesized enzymatically from lactose by the action of β-galactosidase from *Aspergillus oryzae* and *Streptococcus thermophilus* [81]. Their structural formula is galactose- $(galactose)_n$-glucose ($n = 1–4$) and they consist of trisaccharides and branched or unbranched chains of tetra-, penta- and hexasaccharides with β-1,6, β-1,4 and β-1,3 linkages.

A diet containing 3% raffinose led to an increase in total SCFA production without changes in SCFA proportions when given to rats for 1 week [82], and to a specific increase in acetate and lactate concentrations when given for 3 weeks [83]. Conversely, a diet containing 10% raffinose given for 1 week resulted in an increase in butyrate proportion in the cecum [4]. Bacterial counts revealed a stimulation of lactobacilli but decreased numbers of streptococci [82], while FISH demonstrated an increase in lactobacilli and bifidobacteria and a reduction of the *Clostridium coccoides* group [83]. Other assays in rats receiving α-GalOS-enriched pea or lupin extracts at 4–5% for 2 weeks showed a modest increase of the total SCFA cecal pool (pea extract), a greater cecal ammonia concentration, and a stimulation of α- and β-galactosidase, α-glucosidase and β-glucuronidase activities (lupin extract) [84]. Finally, a low dosage (1%) of soybean α-GalOS given for 6 months to mice altered the composition of their hindgut microbiota, as ascertained by selective cultivation. Main features were a marked reduction of sulfite-reducing clostridia and a slight increase of bifidobacteria.

Modification of the gut microbiota balance was also recorded following TOS feeding. Culture of feces or cecal contents in HMA rats indicated a 1- to 2-$\log_{10}$ cfu/g increase of bifidobacteria [75, 85], a slight increase of lactobacilli [84] and a marked 2-$\log_{10}$ cfu/g reduction of enterobacteria [85], while *Bacteroides*, *Clostridium* and *Enterococcus* counts remained unchanged [75, 85], following a 4 week exposure to a diet containing 4–5% TOS. Metabolic analysis of the microbiota after consumption of TOS generally gave results close to those obtained with raffinose or inulin-type fructans. TOS at 4–10% for 4–7 weeks increased the total SCFA cecal pool [62] or concentration [75, 81, 86] in conventional and HMA rats, usually with a particularly enhancing effect on butyrate, and decreased the cecal ammonia concentration [75, 81]. If β-galactosidase activity was logically considerably stimulated [75, 81, 85], the impact of TOS on other glycolytic activities was inconsistent [75, 81, 84]. Interestingly, Rowland and Tanaka [85] also showed that dietary TOS was associated with decreased conversion, by cecal contents of HMA rats, of the food-borne carcinogen 2-amino-3-methylimidazo[4,5-*f*]quinoline (IQ) to its mutagenic 7-hydroxy derivative.

5. OTHER OLIGOSACCHARIDES AND SUGAR-ALCOHOLS

5.1. Gluco-oligosaccharides

α-Gluco-oligosaccharides (GOS) contain tri- to hexasaccharides with α-1,6 linkages $(glucose(1,6)_n$-maltose), and tetra- to heptasaccharides with α-1,2 and α-1,6 linkages (glucose(1,2)-glucose(1,6)$_n$-maltose). GOS feeding of HMA rats at 2–4% for 3–4 weeks led to contrasting results. Valette et al. [87] found no change in the total SCFA cecal concentration but the BCFA proportion was reduced, suggesting some decrease of the microbiota proteolytic activity. On the other hand, Djouzi et al. [75] reported an increase of the total SCFA cecal concentration, the proportion of acetate being increased at the expense of propionate and butyrate. Gas analysis led to similar discrepancies, ranging from a drop in dihydrogen excretion accompanied by an increase of methane excretion [75] to an increase of both gases [87]. These differences may reflect a specific impact of GOS, depending on the phylogenetic and metabolic profile of the gut microbiota; indeed, as these studies were performed by the same group but at a 4-year interval, it is very likely that human microbiota used in the two protocols were not the same. Therefore, additional studies are mandatory to conclude on the modulating effects of GOS on gut microbiota.

5.2. Xylo-oligosaccharides

Xylo-oligosaccharides (XOS) consist of β-1, 4-linked xylose units with an average DP of 2-3 (xylobiose and xylotriose). Fed to mice at 1% for 6 months, they caused an increase of cecal bifidobacteria and lactobacilli, and a decrease of sulfite-reducing clostridia [52]. Cecal bifidobacteria were also consistently increased in rats fed 4–6% XOS for 2–5 weeks [49, 50, 69]. Chemical modification of the xylo-oligosaccharide backbone, such as mono- or disubstitution with arabinose residues giving rise to arabinoxylo-oligosaccharides (AXOS) did not alter this bifidogenic effect [49]. XOS also increased the total SCFA cecal pool by 2- to 4-fold [50, 57, 88]. Depending on the study, this increase affected all three major SCFA [50] or only acetate [57, 88]. As for AXOS, they specifically reduced the BCFA concentration. XOS and AXOS reduced the cecal ammonia concentration [49, 57]. Furthermore,

XOS increased the rate of ammonia absorption from cecal lumen to cecal venous blood [57]. As with inulin-type fructans, gross consequence of these metabolic modifications was a cecal acidification (−0.3 to −1.0 pH unit) [50, 57, 69]; a heavier weight of cecal content and wall was also generally reported [50, 57, 69, 88].

5.3. Sugar-alcohols

Sorbitol, a naturally occurring polyol, is widely used in the food industry as a sweetener, humectant and texturizing agent. In 1986, it was shown that sorbitol changed the fecal microbiota of rats with a displacement from Gram-negative to Gram-positive bacteria [89]. In 2007, molecular techniques revealed that sorbitol exerted a strong influence on gut microbiota of rats, and particularly raised the *Lactobacillus reuteri* population. Concurrently, sorbitol led to a specific increase in butyrate concentrations in colonic and cecal contents of rats [90].

5.4. Unclassified Oligosaccharides

Di-D-fructofuranose-1,2′:2,3′-dianhydride (DFA III) is found in chicory tubers and can be produced using inulinase II from *Arthrobacter* sp. H65-7. It is a non-digestible oligosaccharide being developed as a functional food. When DFA III was given to rats, studies using conventional culture techniques displayed an increase in the lecithinase-negative clostridia in the cecum [91]. Later, molecular techniques showed that DFA III administration stimulates the growth of dominant bacteria in the rat intestine such as *Bacteroides* spp. and *Ruminococcus productus* [92]. A lowering of pH and an increase in SCFA, especially acetate, were also observed in cecal contents.

The active hexose correlated compound (AHCC) is a product prepared from the mycelium of edible Basidiomycete fungi that contains α-1,4-glucan type of oligosaccharides. When administered to rats with induced colitis,

AHCC normalized aerobic, clostridial, and lactic acid bacterial counts. In addition, AHCC increased the count of bifidobacteria [93].

The effect of two heterogeneous oligosaccharides, which have been developed for dietary use, galactosylsucrose and xylosylfructoside, has also been assessed in rats. After 1 week of administration, galactosylsucrose led to a higher lactate concentration in the cecum, whereas xylosylfructoside shifted fermentation end-products from SCFA to succinate [94].

6. PHYTOCHEMICALS

Phytochemicals are plant-derived chemical compounds, some of which have health-promoting properties. They are regular constituents of human foods although they are not essential nutrients and are not required by the human body for sustaining life. After ingestion, some of them are poorly absorbed and directly reach the colon. Some others are absorbed, conjugated in the liver, before a partial re-excretion in the bile. The part of these compounds entering the colon is then extensively metabolized by the gut microbiota, leading to microbial metabolites that may modify their health effects [95]. Concurrently, these compounds may modulate the composition and activity of the intestinal microbiota. As an example, dietary condensed tannins (proanthocyanidins) altered fecal bacterial populations in the rat [96]. Molecular fingerprinting indicated a shift in the microbiota profiles towards tannin-resistant Gram-negative *Enterobacteriaceae* and *Bacteroides* species, while the *Clostridium leptum* group decreased. A metabolic fingerprinting also revealed a change in the functional activity of the microbiota while tannins were present in the diet [96]. Similarly, red wine polyphenols (a mix of anthocyanins, flavanols, flavonols, phenolic acids and tannins) administered to rats for 16 weeks had a very strong effect on the average percentage counts of the main genera of bacteria in the feces, with a considerable decrease in *Clostridium* and a significant increase in the *Lactobacillus* populations [97]. By contrast, xanthohumol, the main flavonoid found in hop and to a smaller extent in beer, did not affect the composition of rat intestinal microbiota [98] although it is poorly absorbed after oral administration.

To assess the impact of apple polyphenols on cecal fermentations, a diet containing 0.7 g/kg of polyphenols was administered to rats for 3 weeks. Total SCFA concentration was increased in the cecum, mainly due to raised butyrate concentration. Bile acid and sterol secretions were not affected by the polyphenols [9]. Dietary grape seed tannins also raised SCFA concentrations in the cecum, with increased acetate and decreased propionate proportions. They also reduced the activity of bacterial β-glucosidase, β-glucuronidase, mucinase and nitroreductase [99] while a 0.3% grapefruit polyphenol diet was shown to decrease bacterial β-glucosidase, and β- and α-galactosidase activities [63]. Grapefruit polyphenols also caused a considerable accumulation of cecal digesta and, therefore, a large increase in the SCFA pool, with increased acetate and decreased butyrate proportions [63].

Effects of either the flavonoid quercetin or its glycoside rutin on bacterial xenobiotic metabolizing enzymes have been studied in female mice [100]. Quercetin-fed mice exhibited higher β-glucuronidase levels, whereas these levels were reduced in rutin-fed animals. However, rutin led to induction of both β-glucosidase and nitrate reductase activities.

Few studies have concerned the impact of phytochemical-containing vegetables on the intestinal microbiota. As an example, the effects of *Brassica* vegetables, which are rich in glucosinolates, have been assessed in HMA rats. A diet containing 100 g/kg of freeze-dried Brussels sprouts was therefore administered to the animals for 4 weeks. The Brussels sprouts diet did not modify the total concentration of SCFA in the cecum but specifically increased the proportion of acetate [101]. Moreover, molecular methods revealed that the dominant fecal bacterial community was altered by the diet, displaying an extensive reorganization of the *Lactobacillus* population [102].

References

1. Maczulak, A. E., Wolin, M. J., & Miller, T. L. (1993). Amounts of viable anaerobes, methanogens, and bacterial fermentation products in feces of rats fed high-fiber or fiber-free diets. *Applied and Environmental Microbiology, 59*, 657–662.
2. Snart, J., Bibiloni, R., Grayson, T., et al. (2006). Supplementation of the diet with high-viscosity beta-glucan results in enrichment for lactobacilli in the rat cecum. *Applied and Environmental Microbiology, 72*, 1925–1931.
3. Dongowski, G., Huth, M., Gebhardt, E., & Flamme, W. (2002). Dietary fiber-rich barley products beneficially affect the intestinal tract of rats. *The Journal of Nutrition, 132*, 3704–3714.
4. Berggren, A. M., Bjorck, I. M. E., Nyman, E., & Eggum, B. O. (1993). Short-chain fatty-acid content and pH in cecum of rats given various sources of carbohydrates. *Journal of the Science of Food and Agriculture, 63*, 397–406.
5. Adam, A., Levrat-Verny, M. A., Lopez, H. W., et al. (2001). Whole wheat and triticale flours with differing viscosities stimulate cecal fermentations and lower plasma and hepatic lipids in rats. *The Journal of Nutrition, 131*, 1770–1776.
6. Rao, C. V., Chou, D., Simi, B., et al. (1998). Prevention of colonic aberrant crypt foci and modulation of large bowel microbial activity by dietary coffee fiber, inulin and pectin. *Carcinogenesis, 19*, 1815–1819.
7. Dongowski, G., Huth, M., & Gebhardt, E. (2003). Steroids in the intestinal tract of rats are affected by dietary-fibre-rich barley-based diets. *The British Journal of Nutrition, 90*, 895–906.
8. Bravo, L., Saura-Calixto, F., & Goni, I. (1992). Effects of dietary fibre and tannins from apple pulp on the composition of faeces in rats. *The British Journal of Nutrition, 67*, 463–473.
9. Aprikian, O., Duclos, V., Guyot, S., et al. (2003). Apple pectin and a polyphenol-rich apple concentrate are more effective together than separately on cecal fermentations and plasma lipids in rats. *The Journal of Nutrition, 133*, 1860–1865.
10. Tamura, M., Nakagawa, H., Tsushida, T., et al. (2007). Effect of pectin enhancement on plasma quercetin and fecal flora in rutin-supplemented mice. *Journal of Food Science, 72*, S648–S651.
11. Noack, J., Kleessen, B., Proll, J., et al. (1998). Dietary guar gum and pectin stimulate intestinal microbial polyamine synthesis in rats. *The Journal of Nutrition, 128*, 1385–1391.
12. Sembries, S., Dongowski, G., Jacobasch, G., et al. (2003). Effects of dietary fibre-rich juice colloids from apple pomace extraction juices on intestinal fermentation products and microbiota in rats. *The British Journal of Nutrition, 90*, 607–615.
13. Van Laere, K. M., Hartemink, R., Bosveld, M., et al. (2000). Fermentation of plant cell wall derived polysaccharides and their corresponding oligosaccharides by intestinal bacteria. *Journal of Agricultural and Food Chemistry, 48*, 1644–1652.
14. Will, F., Mehrlander, K., Dietrich, H., et al. (2003). Enzymatic liquefaction of apple mash by a two-step process. *Fruit Proceedings, 13*, 429–432.
15. Sembries, S., Dongowski, G., Mehrlander, K., et al. (2006). Physiological effects of extraction juices from apple, grape, and red beet pomaces in rats. *Journal of Agricultural and Food Chemistry, 54*, 10269–10280.
16. Chen, H. L., Fan, Y. H., Chen, M. E., & Chan, Y. (2005). Unhydrolyzed and hydrolyzed konjac glucomannans modulated cecal and fecal microflora in Balb/c mice. *Nutrition, 21*, 1059–1064.
17. Howard, M. D., Gordon, D. T., Garleb, K. A., & Kerley, M. S. (1995). Dietary fructooligosaccharide, xylooligosaccharide and gum arabic have variable effects on cecal and colonic microbiota and epithelial cell proliferation in mice and rats. *The Journal of Nutrition, 125*, 2604–2609.
18. Edwards, C. A., & Eastwood, M. A. (1995). Caecal and faecal short-chain fatty acids and stool output in rats fed on diets containing non-starch polysaccharides. *The British Journal of Nutrition, 73*, 773–781.
19. Levrat, M. A., Behr, S. R., Remesy, C., & Demigne, C. (1991). Effects of soybean fiber on cecal digestion in rats previously adapted to a fiber-free diet. *The Journal of Nutrition, 121*, 672–678.
20. Vahouny, G. V., Khalafi, R., Satchithanandam, S., et al. (1987). Dietary fiber supplementation and fecal bile acids, neutral steroids and divalent cations in rats. *The Journal of Nutrition, 117*, 2009–2015.
21. Roland, N., Nugon-Baudon, L., Andrieux, C., & Szylit, O. (1995). Comparative study of the fermentative characteristics of inulin and different types of fibre in rats inoculated with a human whole faecal flora. *The British Journal of Nutrition, 74*, 239–249.
22. Rumney, C. J., & Rowland, I. R. (1992). *In vivo* and *in vitro* models of the human colonic flora. *Critical Reviews in Food Science and Nutrition, 31*, 299–331.
23. Imaoka, A., Setoyama, H., Takagi, A., et al. (2004). Improvement of human faecal flora-associated mouse

model for evaluation of the functional foods. *Journal of Applied Microbiology, 96,* 656–663.

24. Kleessen, B., Hartmann, L., & Blaut, M. (2001). Oligofructose and long-chain inulin: Influence on the gut microbial ecology of rats associated with a human faecal flora. *The British Journal of Nutrition, 86,* 291–300.

25. Mathers, J. C., Smith, H., & Carter, S. (1997). Dose-response effects of raw potato starch on small-intestinal escape, large-bowel fermentation and gut transit time in the rat. *The British Journal of Nutrition, 78,* 1015–1029.

26. Le Blay, G. M., Michel, C. D., Blottiere, H. M., & Cherbut, C. J. (2003). Raw potato starch and short-chain fructo-oligosaccharides affect the composition and metabolic activity of rat intestinal microbiota differently depending on the caecocolonic segment involved. *Journal of Applied Microbiology, 94,* 312–320.

27. Andrieux, C., Gadelle, D., Leprince, C., & Sacquet, E. (1989). Effects of some poorly digestible carbohydrates on bile acid bacterial transformations in the rat. *The British Journal of Nutrition, 62,* 103–119.

28. Berggren, A. M., Bjorck, I. M. E., Nyman, E., & Eggum, B. O. (1995). Short-chain fatty-acid content and pH in cecum of rats fed various sources of starch. *J Sci of Food Agric, 68,* 241–248.

29. Licht, T. R., Hansen, M., Poulsen, M., & Dragsted, L. O. (2006). Dietary carbohydrate source influences molecular fingerprints of the rat faecal microbiota. *BMC Microbiol, 6,* 98.

30. Kandler, O., & Weiss, N. (1986). Genus *Lactobacillus* Beijerinck 1901, 212AL. In: P. H. A. Sneath, N. S. Mair, M. E. Sharpe, J. G. Holt (Eds.), *Bergey's manual of systematic bacteriology* (Vol. 2, pp. 1209–1234).

31. Schleifer, K. H. (1986). Gram-positive cocci. In: P. H. A. Sneath, N. S. Mair, M. E. Sharpe, J. G. Holt (Eds.), *Bergey's manual of systematic bacteriology* (Vol. 2, pp. 999–1103).

32. Kleessen, B., Stoof, G., Proll, J., et al. (1997). Feeding resistant starch affects fecal and cecal microflora and short-chain fatty acids in rats. *Journal of Animal Science, 75,* 2453–2462.

33. Andrieux, C., & Sacquet, E. (1986). Effects of amylomaize starch on mineral metabolism in the adult rat: Role of the microflora. *The Journal of Nutrition, 116,* 991–998.

34. Andrieux, C., Pacheco, E. D., Bouchet, B., et al. (1992). Contribution of the digestive tract microflora to amylomaize starch degradation in the rat. *The British Journal of Nutrition, 67,* 489–499.

35. Cresci, A., Orpianesi, C., Silvi, S., et al. (1999). The effect of sucrose or starch-based diet on short-chain fatty acids and faecal microflora in rats. *Journal of Applied Microbiology, 86,* 245–250.

36. Wang, X., Brown, I. L., Khaled, D., et al. (2002). Manipulation of colonic bacteria and volatile fatty acid production by dietary high amylose maize (amylomaize) starch granules. *Journal of Applied Microbiology, 93,* 390–397.

37. Dongowski, G., Jacobasch, G., & Schmiedl, D. (2005). Structural stability and prebiotic properties of resistant starch type 3 increase bile acid turnover and lower secondary bile acid formation. *Journal of Agricultural and Food Chemistry, 53,* 9257–9267.

38. Key, F. B., & Mathers, J. C. (1995). Digestive adaptations of rats given white bread and cooked haricot beans (*Phaseolus vulgaris*): Large-bowel fermentation and digestion of complex carbohydrates. *The British Journal of Nutrition, 74,* 393–406.

39. Goodlad, J. S., & Mathers, J. C. (1992). Digestion of complex carbohydrates and large bowel fermentation in rats fed on raw and cooked peas (*Pisum sativum*). *The British Journal of Nutrition, 67,* 475–488.

40. da S. Queiroz-Monici, K., Costa, G. E., da Silva, N., et al. (2005). Bifidogenic effect of dietary fiber and resistant starch from leguminous on the intestinal microbiota of rats. *Nutrition, 21,* 602–608.

41. Silvi, S., Rumney, C. J., Cresci, A., & Rowland, I. R. (1999). Resistant starch modifies gut microflora and microbial metabolism in human flora-associated rats inoculated with faeces from Italian and UK donors. *Journal of Applied Microbiology, 86,* 521–530.

42. Verbeek, M. J., De Deckere, E. A., Tijburg, L. B., et al. (1995). Influence of dietary retrograded starch on the metabolism of neutral steroids and bile acids in rats. *The British Journal of Nutrition, 74,* 807–820.

43. Roberfroid, M. B. (2005). Introducing inulin-type fructans. *The British Journal of Nutrition, 93,* S13–S25.

44. Van Loo, J. (2004). The specificity of the interaction with intestinal bacterial fermentation by prebiotics determines their physiological efficacy. *Nutrition Research Reviews, 17,* 89–98.

45. Andrieux, C., Lory, S., Dufour-Lescoat, C. R., et al. (1991). Physiological effects of inulin in germ-free rats and in heteroxenic rats inoculated with a human flora. *Food Hydrocolloids, 5,* 49–56.

46. Bovee-Oudenhoven, I. M. J., ten Bruggencate, S. J. M., Lettink-Wissink, M. L. G., & van der Meer, R. (2003). Dietary fructo-oligosaccharides and lactulose inhibit intestinal colonisation but stimulate translocation of salmonella in rats. *Gut, 52,* 1572–1578.

47. Ten Bruggencate, S. J. M., Bovee-Oudenhoven, I. M. J., Lettink-Wissink, M. L. G., & Van der Meer, R. (2003). Dietary fructo-oligosaccharides dose-dependently increase translocation of salmonella in rats. *The Journal of Nutrition, 133,* 2313–2318.

48. Demigne, C., Jacobs, H., Moundras, C., et al. (2008). Comparison of native or reformulated chicory fructans, or non-purified chicory, on rat cecal fermentation and mineral metabolism. *European Journal of Nutrition, 47,* 366–374.

49. Van Craeyveld, V., Swennen, K., Dornez, E., et al. (2008). Structurally different wheat-derived arabinoxylooligosaccharides have different prebiotic and fermentation properties in rats. *The Journal of Nutrition, 138,* 2348–2355.

50. Campbell, J. M., Fahey, G. C., Jr., & Wolf, B. W. (1997). Selected indigestible oligosaccharides affect large bowel mass, cecal and fecal short-chain fatty acids, pH and microflora in rats. *The Journal of Nutrition, 127,* 130–136.

51. Montesi, A., Garcia-Albiach, R., Pozuelo, M. J., et al. (2005). Molecular and microbiological analysis of caecal microbiota in rats fed with diets supplemented either with prebiotics or probiotics. *International Journal of Food Microbiology, 98,* 281–289.

52. Santos, A., San Mauro, M., & Diaz, D. M. (2006). Prebiotics and their long-term influence on the microbial populations of the mouse bowel. *Food Microbiology, 23,* 498–503.

53. Cani, P. D., Amar, J., Iglesias, M. A., et al. (2007). Metabolic endotoxemia initiates obesity and insulin resistance. *Diabetes, 56,* 1761–1772.

54. Cani, P. D., Neyrinck, A. M., Fava, F., et al. (2007). Selective increases of bifidobacteria in gut microflora improve high-fat-diet-induced diabetes in mice through a mechanism associated with endotoxaemia. *Diabetologia, 50,* 2374–2383.

55. Azorin-Ortuno, M., Urban, C., Ceron, J. J., et al. (2009). Effect of low inulin doses with different polymerisation degree on lipid metabolism, mineral absorption, and intestinal microbiota in rats with fat-supplemented diet. *Food Chemistry, 113,* 1058–1065.

56. Levrat, M. A., Remesy, C., & Demigne, C. (1991). High propionic-acid fermentations and mineral accumulation in the cecum of rats adapted to different levels of inulin. *The Journal of Nutrition, 121,* 1730–1737.

57. Younes, H., Garleb, K., Behr, S., et al. (1995). Fermentable fibers or oligosaccharides reduce urinary nitrogen-excretion by increasing urea disposal in the rat cecum. *The Journal of Nutrition, 125,* 1010–1016.

58. Le Blay, G., Michel, C., Blottiere, H. M., & Cherbut, C. (1999). Prolonged intake of fructo-oligosaccharides induces a short-term elevation of lactic acid-producing bacteria and a persistent increase in cecal butyrate in rats. *The Journal of Nutrition, 129,* 2231–2235.

59. Juskiewicz, J., Glazka, I., Krol, B., & Zdunczyk, Z. (2006). Effect of chicory products with different inulin content on rat caecum physiology. *Journal of Animal Physiology and Animal Nutrition, 90,* 200–207.

60. Juskiewicz, J., & Zdunczyk, Z. (2004). Effects of cellulose, carboxymethylcellulose and inulin fed to rats as single supplements or in combinations on their caecal parameters. *Comparative Biochemistry and Physiology Part A, 139,* 513–519.

61. Juskiewicz, J., Zdunczyk, Z., & Frejnagel, S. (2007). Caecal parameters of rats fed diets supplemented with inulin in exchange for sucrose. *Archives of Animal Nutrition, 61,* 201–210.

62. Sakaguchi, E., Sakoda, C., & Toramaru, Y. (1998). Caecal fermentation and energy accumulation in the rat fed on indigestible oligosaccharides. *The British Journal of Nutrition, 80,* 469–476.

63. Zdunczyk, Z., Juskiewicz, J., & Estrella, I. (2006). Cecal parameters of rats fed diets containing grapefruit polyphenols and inulin as single supplements or in a combination. *Nutrition, 22,* 898–904.

64. Remesy, C., Levrat, M. A., Gamet, L., & Demigne, C. (1993). Cecal fermentations in rats fed oligosaccharides (inulin) are modulated by dietary calcium level. *The American Journal of Physiology, 264,* G855–G862.

65. Levrat, M. A., Remesy, C., & Demigne, C. (1993). Influence of inulin on urea and ammonia nitrogen fluxes in the rat cecum—consequences on nitrogen-excretion. *The Journal of Nutritional Biochemistry, 4,* 351–356.

66. Hoentjen, F., Welling, G. W., Harmsen, H. J. M., et al. (2005). Reduction of colitis by prebiotics in HLA-1327 transgenic rats is associated with microflora changes and immunomodulation. *Inflammatory Bowel Diseases, 11,* 977–985.

67. Cherbut, C., Michel, C., & Lecannu, G. (2003). The prebiotic characteristics of fructooligosaccharides are necessary for reduction of TNBS-induced colitis in rats. *The Journal of Nutrition, 133,* 21–27.

68. Hughes, R., & Rowland, I. R. (2001). Stimulation of apoptosis by two prebiotic chicory fructans in the rat colon. *Carcinogenesis, 22,* 43–47.

69. Hsu, C. K., Liao, J. W., Chung, Y. C., et al. (2004). Xylooligosaccharides and fructooligosaccharides affect the intestinal microbiota and precancerous colonic lesion development in rats. *The Journal of Nutrition, 134,* 1523–1528.

70. Poulsen, M., Molck, A. M., & Jacobsen, B. L. (2002). Different effects of short- and long-chained fructans on large intestinal physiology and carcinogen-induced aberrant crypt foci in rats. *Nutrition and Cancer, 42,* 194–205.

71. Rowland, I. R., Rumney, C. J., Coutts, J. T., & Lievense, L. C. (1998). Effect of *Bifidobacterium longum* and inulin on gut bacterial metabolism and carcinogen-induced aberrant crypt foci in rats. *Carcinogenesis, 19,* 281–285.

72. Goldin, B. R., & Gorbach, S. L. (1976). Relationship between diet and rat fecal bacterial enzymes implicated in colon cancer. *Journal of the National Cancer Institute, 57,* 371–375.

73. Kulkarni, N., & Reddy, B. S. (1994). Inhibitory effect of *Bifidobacterium longum* cultures on the azoxymethane-induced aberrant crypt foci formation and fecal bacterial beta-glucuronidase. *Proceedings of the Society for Experimental Biology and Medicine, 207,* 278–283.

74. Visek, W. J. (1978). Diet and cell growth modulation by ammonia. *The American Journal of Clinical Nutrition, 31,* S216–S220.

75. Djouzi, Z., & Andrieux, C. (1997). Compared effects of three oligosaccharides on metabolism of intestinal microflora in rats inoculated with a human faecal flora. *The British Journal of Nutrition, 78,* 313–324.

76. Kleessen, B., Hartmann, L., & Blaut, M. (2003). Fructans in the diet cause alterations of intestinal mucosal architecture, released mucins and mucosa-associated bifidobacteria in gnotobiotic rats. *The British Journal of Nutrition, 89,* 597–606.

77. Kleessen, B., & Blaut, M. (2005). Modulation of gut mucosal biofilms. *The British Journal of Nutrition, 93,* S35–S40.

78. Fontaine, N., Meslin, J. C., Lory, S., & Andrieux, C. (1996). Intestinal mucin distribution in the germ-free rat and in the heteroxenic rat harbouring a human bacterial flora: Effect of inulin in the diet. *The British Journal of Nutrition, 75,* 881–892.

79. Szylit, O., Butel, M.-J., & Rimbault, A. (1997). An experimental model of necrotising enterocolitis. *Lancet, 350,* 33–34.

80. Catala, I., Butel, M. J., Bensaada, M., et al. (1999). Oligofructose contributes to the protective role of bifidobacteria in experimental necrotising enterocolitis in quails. *Journal of Medical Microbiology, 48,* 89–94.

81. Kikuchi, H., Andrieux, C., Riottot, M., et al. (1996). Effect of two levels of transgalactosylated oligosaccharide intake in rats associated with human faecal microflora on bacterial glycolytic activity, endproducts of fermentation and bacterial steroid transformation. *The Journal of Applied Bacteriology, 80,* 439–446.

82. Tortuero, F., Fernandez, E., Ruperez, P., & Moreno, M. (1997). Raffinose and lactic acid bacteria influence caecal fermentation and serum cholesterol in rats. *Nutrition Research, 17,* 41–49.

83. Dinoto, A., Suksomcheep, A., Ishizuka, S., et al. (2006). Modulation of rat cecal microbiota by administration of raffinose and encapsulated Bifidobacterium breve. *Applied and Environmental Microbiology, 72,* 784–792.

84. Juskiewicz, J., Zdunczyk, Z., Wroblewska, M., & Gulewicz, K. (2003). Influence of oligosaccharide extracts from pea and lupin seeds on caecal fermentation in rats. *Journal of Animal and Feed Sciences, 12,* 289–298.

85. Rowland, I. R., & Tanaka, R. (1993). The effects of transgalactosylated oligosaccharides on gut flora metabolism in rats associated with a human fecal microflora. *The Journal of Applied Bacteriology, 74,* 667–674.

86. Meslin, J. C., Andrieux, C., Sakata, T., et al. (1993). Effects of galacto-oligosaccharide and bacterial status on mucin distribution in mucosa and on large intestine fermentation in rats. *The British Journal of Nutrition, 69,* 903–912.

87. Valette, P., Pelenc, V., Djouzi, Z., et al. (1993). Bioavailability of new synthesized glucooligosaccharides in the intestinal-tract of gnotobiotic-rats. *Journal of the Science of Food and Agriculture, 62,* 121–127.

88. Imaizumi, K., Nakatsu, Y., Sato, M., et al. (1991). Effects of xylooligosaccharides on blood-glucose, serum and liver lipids and cecum short-chain fatty-acids in diabetic rats. *Agricultural and Biological Chemistry, 55,* 199–205.

89. Salminen, S., Salminen, E., Bridges, J., & Marks, V. (1986). The effects of sorbitol on the gastrointestinal microflora in rats. *Zeitschrift für Ernährungswissenschaft, 25,* 91–95.

90. Sarmiento-Rubiano, L. A., Zuniga, M., Perez-Martinez, G., & Yebra, M. J. (2007). Dietary supplementation with sorbitol results in selective enrichment of lactobacilli in rat intestine. *Research in Microbiology, 158,* 694–701.

91. Saito, K., & Tomita, F. (2000). Difructose anhydrides: Their mass-production and physiological functions. *Bioscience, Biotechnology, and Biochemistry, 64,* 1321–1327.

92. Minamida, K., Shiga, K., Sujaya, I. N., et al. (2005). Effects of difructose anhydride III (DFA III) administration on rat intestinal microbiota. *Journal of Bioscience and Bioengineering, 99,* 230–236.

93. Daddaoua, A., Martinez-Plata, E., Lopez-Posadas, R., et al. (2007). Active hexose correlated compound acts as a prebiotic and is anti-inflammatory in rats with hapten-induced colitis. *The Journal of Nutrition, 137,* 1222–1228.

94. Hoshi, S., Sakata, T., Mikuni, K., et al. (1994). Galactosylsucrose and xylosylfructoside alter digestive tract size and concentrations of cecal organic acids in rats fed diets containing cholesterol and cholic acid. *The Journal of Nutrition, 124,* 52–60.

95. Scalbert, A., Morand, C., Manach, C., & Remesy, C. (2002). Absorption and metabolism of polyphenols in the gut and impact on health. *Biomedicine & Pharmacotherapy, 56,* 276–282.

96. Smith, A. H., & Mackie, R. I. (2004). Effect of condensed tannins on bacterial diversity and metabolic activity in the rat gastrointestinal tract. *Applied and Environmental Microbiology, 70,* 1104–1115.

97. Dolara, P., Luceri, C., De Filippo, C., et al. (2005). Red wine polyphenols influence carcinogenesis, intestinal microflora, oxidative damage and gene expression profiles of colonic mucosa in F344 rats. *Mutation Research, 591,* 237–246.

98. Hanske, L., Hussong, R., Frank, N., et al. (2005). Xanthohumol does not affect the composition of rat intestinal microbiota. *Molecular Nutrition & Food Research, 49,* 868–873.

99. Tebib, K., & Rouanet, J. M. (1996). Effects of dietary grape seed tannins on rat cecal fermentation and colonic bacterial enzymes. *Nutrition Research, 16,* 105–110.

100. Alldrick, A J., Lake, B. G., Mallett, A. K., & Rowland, I. R. (1988). Modulation of hepatic-phase I and gut-microflora xenobiotic metabolizing enzymes by dietary flavonoids. In: A. R. Liss (Ed.), *Plant flavonoids in biology and medicine II: Biochemical, cellular, and medicinal properties* (pp. 139–142).

101. Humblot, C., Lhoste, E., Knasmuller, S., et al. (2004). Protective effects of Brussels sprouts, oligosaccharides and fermented milk towards 2-amino-3-methylimidazo[4,5-f]quinoline (IQ)-induced genotoxicity in the human flora associated F344 rat: Role of xenobiotic metabolising enzymes and intestinal microflora. *Journal of Chromatography. B, Analytical Technologies in the Biomedical and Life Sciences, 802,* 231–237.

102. Humblot, C., Bruneau, A., Sutren, M., et al. (2005). Brussels sprouts, inulin and fermented milk alter the faecal microbiota of human microbiota-associated rats as shown by PCR-temporal temperature gradient gel electrophoresis using universal, *Lactobacillus* and *Bifidobacterium* 16S rRNA gene primers. *The British Journal of Nutrition, 93,* 677–684.

Probiotic Treatment of Colitis in Animal Models and People

Leo R. Fitzpatrick and Kelly Dowhower Karpa

Pennsylvania State University College of Medicine, Department of Pharmacology, Hershey, PA, USA

1. INFLAMMATORY COLITIS

The pathogenesis of inflammatory bowel disease (IBD) most likely involves interplay between genetics, immune responses, and microorganisms within the intestinal milieu [1–5]. Specifically, in susceptible individuals, inappropriate immune responses are believed to be triggered or perpetuated by bacteria (or bacterial derived antigens), thus leading to the inflammatory manifestations exhibited in human diseases such as ulcerative colitis (UC) and Crohn's disease (CD). Animal models of colitis, which mimic human colitis conditions to a certain degree, provide a platform for testing the efficacy of novel pharmacological agents.

There is compelling evidence from animal models of inflammatory colitis and from clinical observations of UC and CD that bacterial factors play a prominent role in IBD pathogenesis [6]. Therefore, studies of host–microflora interactions and identification of factors that ameliorate inflammatory responses invoked by gut flora has become a focus for development of novel therapeutic modalities aimed at suppressing manifestations of IBD. Appropriately, the intent of several therapeutic approaches currently under investigation for management of IBD involves modification of intestinal flora. This may be best accomplished through administration of probiotics [1–3].

Probiotics are live microorganisms which, when ingested, can confer health benefits [7]. Typically, probiotics include various strains of the Lactobacillus and/or Bifidobacteria species. They exist as either single entities or as combination products (e.g., VSL#3) [1, 2, 7]. Other known probiotics include certain non-pathogenic *Escherichia coli* (*E. coli*) strains like Nissle 1917 and M-17 [8, 9].

Mechanisms explaining the potential role of probiotics as anti-colitis therapies have been reviewed in detail elsewhere [1, 2, 10]. Immunomodulatory actions, such as reduction of pro-inflammatory cytokines (e.g., TNF-α, IFN-γ), and increased secretion of regulatory cytokines (e.g., IL-10), have also been suggested to be operative [1, 2, 8, 10].

2. ANIMAL MODELS OF COLITIS AND ILEITIS

Various rodent models of inflammatory colitis have evolved over the past 20 years which have provided an opportunity to test new therapeutic agents that may have efficacy in management of IBD. These models have unique characteristics, as well as distinct advantages and disadvantages, which have been reviewed previously [11–15]. Two common models of IBD involve administration of chemical agents to rodents. Specifically, dextran sulfate sodium (DSS) or trinitrobenzene sulfonic acid (TNBS) is often used to induce colitis. Another commonly used model relies upon spontaneous colitis that develops in mice deficient in the immunoregulatory cytokine, IL-10 (i.e., IL-10 knockout mice). These models of colitis have been used extensively for IBD drug testing, including the testing of probiotic efficacy.

2.1. Animal Model: DSS-induced Colitis

The pathogenesis of DSS-induced colitis involves a defect in epithelial barrier function, which is related to direct cytotoxic actions of DSS [13, 16]. Changes in epithelial barrier function, as measured by loss of the tight junction protein ZO-1 and increased permeability to Evan's blue dye, can be found early during the time course of DSS-induced colitis [17, 18]. This alteration in colonic mucosal barrier subsequently leads to influx of various inflammatory cells, macrophage activation and pro-inflammatory cytokine production in a model that is somewhat reminiscent of the human condition of UC. The acute version of the model is generally thought to be T lymphocyte independent, while repeated administration of DSS in drinking water leads to chronic colitis that involves T cells [13, 14, 16].

Various probiotics have shown evidence of efficacy in the acute DSS colitis model. Examples of published studies are summarized in Table 34.1 [8, 19, 20]. Mechanistically, investigations from our laboratory have demonstrated that administration of *E. coli* strain M-17 (Probactrix®) reduces inflammation in part through interference with nuclear translocation of the p65 subunit of nuclear factor-kappa B (NFκB), as well as via decreased production of associated cytokines (IL-12, IL-6, and IL-1β) [8]. Based on these *in vitro* and *in vivo* data with *E. coli* M-17, we propose the following putative mechanism of action for attenuating inflammation (Figure 34.1). As shown in this figure, in the presence of live (but not heat-killed) *E. coli* strain M-17, there was a direct interaction of the probiotic bacteria with macrophages (step 1). Our current theory is that live *E. coli* M-17 secrete an immunomodulin into the macrophage (step 2). This process results in inhibition of the LPS-induced activation of the NFκB signal-transduction system (step 3). Subsequently, inhibition of NFκB results in attenuation of pro-inflammatory cytokine (IL-1β, TNF-α, IL-6) secretion (step 4) [8]. The putative immunomodulin responsible for the anti-inflammatory effects of *E. coli* strain M-17 remains to be determined (step 2). Similar anti-inflammatory effects were found for this probiotic in a murine model of DSS-induced colitis [8].

It should be noted that most of the studies listed in Table 34.1 utilized the acute DSS colitis paradigm. Moreover, most used probiotics as agents of *prophylaxis*. It is of interest, however, to also consider potential effects of probiotics in the chronic form of DSS-induced colitis where intestinal inflammation has already been established. To this regard, preliminary results from our laboratory found *E. coli* M-17 had therapeutic benefits in the chronic murine DSS colitis model as well [21].

TABLE 34.1 Effects of probiotics on DSS-induced colitis in rodents

Probiotic	Summary	Investigator (Reference)
Bifidobacterium infantis	Improved DAI in rats	[82]
Lactobacillus brevis	Efficacy for acute murine colitis	[83]
Lactobacillus casei (Shirota)	Efficacy for chronic murine colitis	[32]
Lactobacillus crispatus	Efficacy for acute murine colitis	[84]
Lactobacillus fermentum	Efficacy for acute murine colitis	[84]
	Improved acute colitis in rats	[82]
	Improved DAI in rats	[85]
Lactobacillus plantarum	Improved acute colitis in rats	[82, 86]
	Efficacy for acute murine colitis	[83]
Lactobacillus reuteri	Efficacy for acute murine colitis	[87]
Lactobacillus rhamnosus GG	Efficacy for chronic murine colitis	[88]
VSL#3	Efficacy for acute murine colitis	[19]
	Improved colitis in weanling rats	[20]
E. coli M-17	Efficacy for acute murine colitis	[8]
E. coli Nissle 1917	Efficacy for acute murine colitis	[89]
	Efficacy for acute murine colitis	[90]
	Efficacy for acute murine colitis	[91]
Eubacterium limosum	Efficacy for acute murine colitis	[92]

2.2. Animal Model: TNBS-induced Colitis and Related Chemical Models

Another animal model of colonic inflammation relies upon TNBS and closely mimics human CD [11–13]. This hapten-dependent model of IBD is T lymphocyte dependent and involves activation of both Th1 and Th17 CD4+ T cells [22]. As with the DSS colitis model, both acute and chronic forms of the model exist, which were succinctly summarized in a recent review paper [23]. Probiotics have demonstrated efficacy in TNBS-induced colitis in rodents and many relevant studies are summarized in Table 34.2 [19]. As in the related DSS colitis studies, the results in Table 34.2 primarily reflect work with an acute TNBS colitis paradigm. Most of these studies also utilized pre-treatment, prophylactic, regimens. Additional study of probiotic effects

in chronic forms of this hapten-induced colitis model, once the colitis has been firmly established, is warranted [23].

Probiotic efficacy has been explored in two other chemical models of IBD that utilize iodoacetamide or dinitrobenzene sulfonic acid (DNBS). Specifically, Shibolet and colleagues studied the effects of VSL#3 and *Lactobacillus* strain GG [24]. These probiotics were effective against iodoacetamide-induced colitis, but not in DNBS-induced colitis. The differential probiotic effects are likely explained by differences in underlying pathologies manifested by these colitis models. Iodoacetamide-induced colitis involves depletion of protective mucosal sulfhydryl groups and associated injury occurs through production of reactive oxygen species [25]. In contrast, the DNBS colitis model is mechanistically similar to the aforementioned TNBS model of colitis and

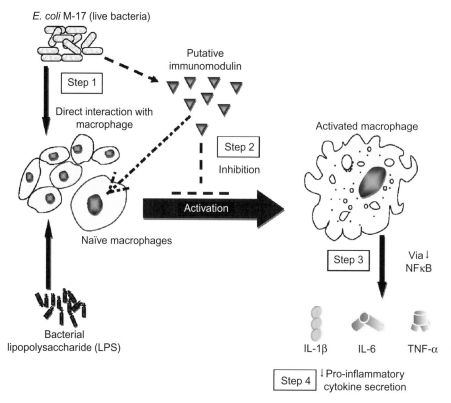

FIGURE 34.1   Attenuation of inflammation by *E. coli* strain M-17. This probiotic *E. coli* strain inhibits the production of LPS-stimulated pro-inflammatory cytokines by a four-step mechanism: 1) a direct interaction of live *E. coli* M-17 with macrophages; 2) release of an unidentified immunomodulin into the macrophage; 3) inhibition of nuclear factor-kappa B (NFκB) inside the host cell; and 4) attenuation of IL-1β, TNF-α and IL-6 secretion.

produces a transmural immunological-based injury to the colon [25]. It has been suggested that in the DNBS colitis model, VSL#3 could not prevent the more severe transmural injury. However, these results seem to contrast those of Rachmilewitz et al., who found that VSL#3 derived DNA could nearly completely limit the induction of TNBS-induced colitis in mice [19]. The reasons for the seemingly discrepant results are presently unclear.

2.3. Animal Model: IL-10 deficiency

Several studies have tested probiotics in IL-10 deficient mice. These animals develop a Th1

mediated chronic colitis if kept in conventional housing conditions [12–14]. This IBD model offers a unique opportunity to treat mice with probiotics over a prolonged period of time, relative to more acute chemical models of colitis [26]. Some published results from this spontaneous, non-chemical model of IBD are shown in Table 34.3 [26, 27].

In addition to the studies highlighted by Table 34.3, Etling and colleagues demonstrated that probiotic efficacy in mice may be age-dependent and may change across the lifespan [28]. Administration of the multi-strain probiotic VSL#3 to pre-treat IL-10 deficient young mice (10 to 12 weeks of age) prior to transfer into

TABLE 34.2 Effects of probiotics on TNBS-induced colitis in rodents

Probiotic	Summary	Investigator (Reference)
Bifidobacterium lactis	Improved acute colitis in rats	[93]
Lactobacillus farciminis	Efficacy for acute colitis in rats	[94]
Lactobacillus fermentum	Efficacy for acute colitis in rats	[95]
	Efficacy for acute murine colitis	[96]
Lactobacillus reuteri	Efficacy for acute colitis in rats	[95]
Lactobacillus GG	Efficacy for acute colitis in rats	[97]
Lactobacillus salivarius	Efficacy for acute murine colitis	[98]
	Efficacy for acute murine colitis	[99]
	Efficacy for acute colitis in rats	[100]
VSL#3	Probiotic DNA improved colitis	[19]

TABLE 34.3 Effects of probiotics on colitis in IL-10 knockout mice

Probiotic	Summary	Investigator (Reference)
Bifidobacterium infantis	Efficacy for many parameters of colitis	[101]
Lactobacillus plantarum	Improvement of colitis	[27]
Lactobacillus salivarius	S.C. injections improved colitis	[102]
	Efficacy for many parameters of colitis	[101]
E. coli Nissle 1917	Efficacy for many parameters of colitis	[91]
VSL#3	Probiotic DNA improved colitis	[103]
	Efficacy for many parameters of colitis	[26]

conventional housing, provided protection from the rapid onset of colitis usually experienced by IL-10 mice [28]. In contrast, VSL#3 pre-treatment of older mice (postnatal age of 28 to 30 weeks) was ineffective in preventing the transient colitis symptoms that occur in these aged animals. Investigators suggested that because the character and kinetics of intestinal inflammation can vary with age, loss of probiotic efficacy in older mice was not entirely unexpected [28]. These results may have relevance in clinical situations. In this regard, applied research that establishes the ideal niche for probiotics in pediatric, adult, and aging populations of patients with IBD across the lifespan warrants further investigation. To this end, see the pediatric colitis section in this chapter, for a review of two studies that utilized VSL#3 in pre-adult animal and human populations.

Lactobacillus plantarum 299v has also been investigated for efficacy in IL-10 deficient mice with established colitis [27]. Using a 4-week treatment paradigm, probiotic treated mice showed significant reductions in colonic and cecal histology scores, as well as IL-12 and IFN-γ production. These results are particularly significant, because therapeutic efficacy of the investigational probiotic agent was clearly demonstrated in a situation where inflammation was already established.

2.4. Animal Models: Other

Other rodent models of IBD also exist. Dieleman et al. found that the probiotic *Lactobacillus rhamnosus* GG prevented the recurrence of colitis in HLA-B27 transgenic rats that had been previously treated with antibiotics [29]. However, transient treatment with either antibiotics (impinem/neomycin) or *Lactobacillus rhamnosus* GG alone did not prevent the occurrence of colitis. In addition, using a CD4+ T cell transfer model of colitis, Schultz and co-workers found that the non-pathogenic *E. coli* strain Nissle 1917 attenuated histological evidence of intestinal inflammation and also reduced levels of pro-inflammatory cytokines (IFN-γ and IL-6) [30]. Various *Lactobacillus* species have, likewise, demonstrated efficacy in the T cell transfer model of colitis [25].

Finally, SAMP1/Yit mice develop a spontaneous ileitis with many features similar to human Crohn's disease. This mouse line was generated by brother-sister mating (>20 generations) of the original senescence-accelerated mouse (SAM) line. This colitis model has the advantage of developing spontaneously without gene targeting or immunological manipulations [31]. In these mice, administration of *Lactobacillus casei* strain Shirota has been shown to improve altered ileal histopathology [32]. On the basis of benefits observed with probiotic bacterial species in many animal models of intestinal inflammation, probiotic bacteria have been studied clinically for their effects in CD and UC.

3. CLINICAL USES OF PROBIOTICS IN IBD

3.1. Crohn's Disease

Over a decade ago, the use of *E. coli* (strain Nissle 1917) was first tested for ability to maintain remission in patients with *colonic* CD [33]. Patients with active disease were first treated with prednisolone to induce remission. Subsequently, those in whom remission was attained were then supplied with either *E. coli* or placebo for a period of 1 year. All patients receiving the supplement were entirely able to discontinue the steroid within 6 months, which was not the case with those randomized to placebo. In addition, those supplemented with the biotherapy were less likely to relapse compared to those assigned placebo (33 vs 64%). Nonetheless,

TABLE 34.4   Clinical trials using probiotics to maintain remission in patients with Crohn's disease

Probiotic	Number that completed study	Duration of study	Investigator (Reference)
E. coli Nissle 1917	23	1 year	[33]
Lactobacillus rhamnosus GG	4	6 months	[34, 35]
Lactobacillus rhamnosus GG	75	2 years or until relapse	[36]
Lactobacillus rhamnosus GG	11	6 months	[37]
Bifidobacterium breve Lactobacillus casei Bifidobacterium longum and 3.3 grams *psyllium*	10	13 ± 4.5 months	[38]

outcomes for this study were not statistically significant due to the small number of patients that completed the trial ($n = 23$) (Table 34.4). It was also suggested that since *E. coli* is a colonic inhabitant and rarely found in upper parts of the gastrointestinal tract, perhaps this particular probiotic bacterium might only be beneficial in those whose disease is limited to the colon [33]. Therefore, other probiotic-containing regimens containing species expected to influence small bowel disease have also been investigated in patients with CD.

One such regimen involves use of lactobacilli, but use of this genus alone has led to disappointing clinical results. Despite preliminary data from an open label study in which three of four children with mild-to-moderately active CD were able to decrease steroid dosages by 50% when *Lactobacillus rhamnosus* GG was added to their treatment regimens [34, 35], double blind placebo-controlled trials using this probiotic have not found benefits in maintaining remission among individuals with CD [36, 37].

On the other hand, use of combinations of lactobacilli and bifidobacteria which simultaneously colonize both the small intestine and large intestine might provide some benefits in alleviating Crohn's disease symptoms. However, based upon currently-available data, it is impossible to be certain. Although Fujimori et al. [38] concluded that a combination of high dose probiotics containing three different lactobacilli and bifidobacteria strains effectively induced remission in patients with active CD, there was no placebo group with which to compare these effects. In addition, enrolled patients were simultaneously receiving other medications including corticosteroids and/or aminosalicylates and dosages of these medications fluctuated throughout the study. Furthermore, the dosage of probiotic used by patients was inconsistent during the trial. Thus, at the time of writing, limitations to study design make it impossible to draw firm conclusions about potential benefits from lactobacilli and bifidobacteria in human CD.

3.2. Ulcerative Colitis: Maintaining Remission

Similar to CD, the earliest investigations into use of probiotics for management of UC relied upon *E. coli* Nissle 1917 as a therapeutic agent. The bacteriotherapy was found to be at least as efficacious as mesalamine for maintaining remission (Table 34.5) [33, 39]. However, the significance of that finding has been questioned because the efficacy of mesalamine itself has been called under scrutiny [41].

Lactic acid-producing bacteria have also been studied for efficacy in maintaining remission among patients with ulcerative colitis. Studies have included both single species lactobacilli products as well as combinations of *Lactobacillus* and *Bifidobacterium*. Among patients in remission, *Lactobacillus rhamnosus* GG significantly

TABLE 34.5 Clinical trials using probiotics to maintain remission in patients with ulcerative colitis

Probiotic	Number that completed study	Duration of study	Investigator (Reference)
E. coli Nissle 1917	103	3 months	[39]
E. coli Nissle 1917	222	12 months	[40]
E. coli Nissle 1917	21	12 months	[41]
Lactobacillus rhamnosus GG	187	12 months	[42]
Lactobacillus casei *Lactobacillus plantarum* *Lactobacillus acidophilus* *Lactobacillus delbrueckii* *Bifidobacterium longum* *Bifidobacterium breve* *Bifidobacterium infantis* *Streptococcus thermophilus*	19	12 months	[43]
Bifidobacterium breve *Bifidobacterium bifidum* *Lactobacillus acidophilus* YIT 0168	21	12 months	[44]

prolonged the relapse-free period compared to mesalamine alone [42]. An open label study using a high-dose probiotic cocktail containing 8 different bacterial species (*L. casei, L. plantarum, L. acidophilus, L. delbrueckii, B. longum, B. breve, B. infantis, S. thermophilus*) demonstrated that among patients who could not tolerate mesalamine derivatives, 15 of 20 individuals remained in remission after 1 year of treatment [43]. Similarly, another small year-long study using a mixture of lactobacilli and bifidobacteria administered via a yogurt beverage described fewer relapses among those drinking the supplement (3 of 11 versus 9 of 10; $p = 0.018$). However, even at baseline, those assigned to the control group appeared to have more severe disease [44], which, along with the small number of patients enrolled, calls the validity of these results into question until they can be duplicated in larger trials.

3.3. Ulcerative Colitis: Treatment of Active Disease

A variety of probiotic therapies have been used in an attempt to induce remission in patients experiencing active ulcerative colitis flares. However, these studies are difficult to interpret as patients were usually permitted to continue other medications (i.e. antibiotics, mesalamine derivatives, corticosteroids) simultaneously with bacteriotherapies. In addition, several studies were conducted in an open label fashion which introduces the possibility of bias. Some studies lacked a placebo group, and others were unable to demonstrate statistically significant clinical benefits despite reductions in mucosal inflammatory markers (Table 34.6) [45–49]. Furthermore, it is impossible to directly compare the different probiotic regimens studied, as trials enrolled patients with differing disease severity and relied upon disparate outcome measures.

Overall, clinical use of probiotics in management of CD or UC has recently received a 'C' recommendation. This rating acknowledges that although the possibility exists that *E. coli*, lactobacilli, and/or bifidobacteria may have some benefits in certain patients with these inflammatory conditions, the efficacy results from trials have been variable, studies have enrolled only small numbers of patients, and/or studies were conducted in an open label fashion or possessed

other serious methodological design flaws. At the time of writing, despite positive benefits observed with probiotics in most animal models of IBD, the scarcity of strong clinical data precludes a stronger recommendation for use of probiotics in humans with CD or UC [50].

TABLE 34.6 Clinical trials using probiotics to induce remission from ulcerative colitis exacerbations

Probiotic	Number that completed study	Duration of study	Investigator (Reference)
Lactobacillus casei *Lactobacillus plantarum* *Lactobacillus acidophilus* *Lactobacillus delbrueckii* *Bifidobacterium longum* *Bifidobacterium breve* *Bifidobacterium infantis* *Streptococcus thermophilus*	32	6 weeks	[45]
Bifidobacterium longum 6 g fructo-oligosaccharide inulin	13	4 weeks	[46]
Bifidobacterium breve strain *Yakult* *Bifidobacterium bifidum* strain *Yakult* *Lactobacillus acidophilus*	19	12 weeks	[47]
E. coli Nissle 1917	24	4 weeks	[48]
Streptococcus faecalis T-110 *Clostridium butyricum* TO-A *Bacillus mesentericus* TO-A	20	4 weeks	[49]

3.4. Pouchitis

Pouchitis is a complication that arises in many IBD patients who undergo surgical resection for their inflamed bowel. Specifically, pouchitis is characterized by inflammation of the ileal pouch that is surgically created as a reservoir for stool. A surgical model of pouchitis has been established in rats [51, 52]. This model seems to have certain characteristics that make it relevant to human pouchitis [51, 52], including responsiveness to metronidazole treatment [51]. However, recently DSS administration has been employed in conjunction with ileal pouch formation in order to increase inflammation in the pouch, as well as create intestinal symptoms such as diarrhea and rectal bleeding that are characteristic of clinical pouchitis in humans [52, 53]. Moreover, this model involves an increased ratio of anaerobic to aerobic bacteria in the ileal pouch, which is suggestive of bacterial dysbiosis [53]. Atila and colleagues demonstrated that administration of partially hydrolyzed guar gum improved various parameters of experimental pouchitis in rats [53]. Specifically, guar gum administration improved weight loss, diarrhea and rectal bleeding in rats with pouchitis. Moreover, colonic MPO (myeloperoxidase) activity and intestinal histology was significantly improved in animals receiving the partially hydrolyzed guar gum. Interestingly this dietary fiber/prebiotic therapeutic approach also significantly altered bacterial populations in the ileal pouch [53]. Indirectly, these results imply that a probiotic could also show utility in this model. However, at the time of writing this *in vivo* model has not been utilized to investigate the efficacy of probiotic agents. Clearly, this should be a goal of future probiotic-related research.

Nonetheless, probiotics are already being used clinically to treat pouchitis, with some success. Clinically, pouchitis has been classified into three distinct categories based upon patient response to antibiotics: a) antibiotic-responsive; b) antibiotic-dependent; or c) antibiotic-refractory [54]. While antibiotic responsiveness may influence response to probiotic therapies, few studies using the bacteriotherapies have attempted to differentiate patients into these sub-classifications.

In clinical studies, a mixture of 600 billion probiotic organisms (*L. casei, L. plantarum, L. acidophilus, L. delbrueckii, B. longum, B. breve, B infantis, S. thermophilus*) demonstrated efficacy for maintaining remission from pouchitis for up to 1 year (Table 34.7) [55, 56]. Furthermore, this same probiotic prevented development of acute pouchitis during the first year after creation of the surgical pouch in 18 of 20 (90%) patients versus 12 of 20 (60%) patients receiving placebo [57]. Similarly, Kaplan-Meier analysis demonstrated that *Lactobacillus rhamnosus* GG also may delay the time to first onset of pouchitis by more than 3 years when a daily dose of the probiotic is ingested (7 vs 29%; $p = 0.011$) [58]. However, benefits may be limited to a subset of patients that are *not* affected by antibiotic-*dependent* pouchitis. When individuals with antibiotic-*dependent* pouchitis were specifically recruited for study, even the high-cell count VLS#3 probiotic cocktail was not effective for maintaining remission [54].

In terms of inducing remission from active pouchitis, use of probiotics has met with discrepant results, which might be explained partly by the differences in probiotic strains, doses and/or dissimilarities in the underlying disease processes [59–63].

Presently, probiotic therapies have been given an 'A' recommendation for use in preventing initial episodes of pouchitis when used immediately after pouch surgery and for maintaining remission after antibiotic induction [50]. However, the bacteriotherapy approach may not be effective in those whose condition is dependent upon antibiotics. Furthermore, there is currently insufficient evidence to establish a higher rating than a 'C' level of recommendation for use of bacteriotherapies to induce remission in patients with active pouchitis [50].

TABLE 34.7   Clinical trials using probiotics to maintain remission or prevent initial episodes of pouchitis

Probiotic	Number that completed study	Duration of study	Treatment paradigm	Investigator (Reference)
Lactobacillus casei *Lactobacillus plantarum* *Lactobacillus acidophilus* *Lactobacillus delbrueckii* *Bifidobacterium longum* *Bifidobacterium breve* *Bifidobacterium infantis* *Streptococcus thermophilus*	40	9 months	Maintain Remission	[55]
Lactobacillus casei *Lactobacillus plantarum* *Lactobacillus acidophilus* *Lactobacillus delbrueckii* *Bifidobacterium longum* *Bifidobacterium breve* *Bifidobacterium infantis* *Streptococcus thermophilus*	35	12 months	Maintain Remission	[56]
Lactobacillus casei *Lactobacillus plantarum* *Lactobacillus acidophilus* *Lactobacillus delbrueckii* *Bifidobacterium longum* *Bifidobacterium breve* *Bifidobacterium infantis* *Streptococcus thermophilus*	40	12 months	Prevention	[57]
Lactobacillus rhamnosus GG *Lactobacillus casei* *Lactobacillus plantarum* *Lactobacillus acidophilus* *Lactobacillus delbrueckii* *Bifidobacterium longum* *Bifidobacterium breve* *Bifidobacterium infantis* *Streptococcus thermophilus*	117 6	>3 years 8 months	Prevention Maintain Remission	[58] [54]

4. COMBINATION THERAPIES FOR THE TREATMENT OF COLITIS

4.1. Animal Models

In clinical management of colitis, it is not uncommon for pharmacologic agents to be used in various combinations. Unfortunately, relatively few animal models of colitis have investigated combination therapies that include probiotics. Our laboratory tested the efficacy of the probiotic *E. coli* strain M-17 in combination with metronidazole (which does not kill this bacterial strain at relevant concentrations) in the DSS model of colitis [8]. The combination of EC-M17 plus metronidazole reduced pro-inflammatory cytokine production more than either treatment alone. Specifically, the combination therapy significantly reduced IL-1β compared with EC-M17 alone. Additionally, the combined treatment regimen improved colonic histology scores compared with metronidazole alone [8].

Schultz et al. tested the efficacy of a prebiotic/probiotic formulation consisting of *Lactobacillus acidophilus, Bifidobacterium lactis* Bb12, and inulin in combination with metronidazole using the HLA-B27 transgenic rat model of spontaneous colitis [64]. Interestingly, the prebiotic/probiotic formulation effectively attenuated colonic inflammation, while combination with metronidazole did not provide any added benefit compared to treatment with the antibiotic or prebiotic/probiotic formulation alone. Of note, the authors speculated that the prebiotic component likely accounted for the anti-colitis effect, since the probiotic bacteria could not be detected in the rat cecum [64]. Other investigators found that administration of a prebiotic formulation (oligofructose and inulin) plus a *Bifidobacterium infantis* probiotic strain attenuated DSS-induced colitis in rats [65]. However, the efficacy profile of the combined prebiotic and probiotic therapy was similar to that observed with either treatment alone. Using a T cell transfer model of colitis, Møller et al. found that the ingestion of two *Lactobacillus* strains *(reuteri* and *rhamnosus)* plus antibiotics improved histopathology compared to control groups of mice receiving either no treatment or receiving only antibiotics [66]. Finally, Souza and colleagues tested the efficacy of combined local treatment with a corticosteroid (budesonide) and a probiotic formulation (*Lactobacillus acidophilus* and *Bifidobacterium lactis* formulation) on acetic acid induced colitis in rats [67]. The combination treatment regimen did not significantly improve macroscopic and microscopic injury in rats. However, there was enhanced DNA content in the colon of animals with the combination therapy, suggesting a possible accelerated repair of colonic injury with the combined topical steroid and probiotic treatment [67].

Clearly, studies looking at the combination of probiotics and traditional anti-colitis drugs (sulfasalazine, 5-aminosalicylates, corticosteroids) as well as combinations of probiotics and prebiotics are lacking. Such studies represent a fertile area of research with potential clinical ramifications and should be the focus of future studies in rodent colitis models.

4.2. Human Studies

Clinically, combination therapeutic approaches incorporating probiotics have begun to be investigated in patients with ulcerative colitis and diverticular inflammation. *Bifidobacterium longum* in combination with the prebiotics fructo-oligosaccharide and inulin improved inflammatory markers of mucosal inflammation (i.e. TNF-α, IL-1), without demonstrating any improvement on clinical outcomes [46]. In the future, similar studies should enroll larger numbers of patients and treat for a longer duration time to truly ascertain whether synbiotic approaches may be beneficial.

Treatment of active intestinal inflammation often necessitates the use of steroids to suppress symptoms. Corticosteroids in conjunction with multistrain probiotics for managing diverticular colitis was explored in 2005 [68]. Similarly, use of the aminosalicylate derivative balsalazide along with a probiotic cocktail was also explored in patients with ulcerative colitis and diverticulitis [69]. On the basis of these preliminary results, a probiotic/aminosalicylate combination may help patients achieve remission from mild-to-moderate ulcerative colitis faster than aminosalicylates alone. Additional studies will be needed to truly delineate the role of probiotics when used adjunctively with conventional therapies.

5. PROBIOTICS IN PEDIATRIC POPULATIONS OF COLITIS

5.1. Animal Study

Our laboratory examined the efficacy of VSL#3 in weanling rats during the early post-natal period (day 14 to day 28). Pre-treatment of these animals with this probiotic agent for 1 week before the induction of colitis at the time of weaning (day 21) and concomitant initiation of 2% DSS administration, resulted in significant reductions in colitis [20]. Specifically, VSL#3 administration improved symptoms of colitis (diarrhea, rectal bleeding), as well as colonic histology, MPO activity, and the colonic IL-1β content. Administration of this probiotic agent also partially normalized the altered signaling of the NFκB signaling pathway in these animals, by limiting colonic IκB-α degradation [20]. We suggested that our study might provide the impetus for the more frequent use of probiotics in the treatment of pediatric IBD. Indeed, at the time of writing, a clinical report of this kind had just been published [70].

5.2. Human Study

In a pilot study, the clinical efficacy associated with adding VSL#3 to standard treatment regimens (i.e. corticosteroids, mesalamine) of patients with mild to moderate acute ulcerative colitis was evaluated in a pediatric population [70]. Eighteen patients between the ages of 3 and 17 years had either VSL#3 or placebo added to their existing therapeutic regimen for 8 weeks. Clinical and laboratory markers of ulcerative colitis were monitored to determine efficacy. Thirteen patients completed the study. Clinical remission was achieved in 10 of these patients, while two other patients showed evidence of clinical improvement [70]. Various laboratory parameters were improved in patients receiving the probiotic treatment. Interestingly, in responding patients, there was evidence of change in bacterial taxonomy. Based on these positive results, follow-up studies with probiotics in pediatric patients with IBD are warranted. The pre-clinical and clinical studies cited herein demonstrate ways in which animal studies and human trials of probiotic agents may synergize in ways that may ultimately lead to improved clinical management of intestinal inflammation [20, 70].

6. PROBIOTICS AS DRUG DELIVERY AGENTS FOR EXPERIMENTAL COLITIS

A potentially exciting niche for probiotics may be as drug delivery agents for novel therapeutic agents. This therapeutic approach has been examined in several rodent colitis studies. One novel pharmacological approach used genetically modified bacteria to deliver a regulatory cytokine to the colon. Specifically, investigators utilized a *Lactococcus lactis* secreting IL-10 strain to successfully treat chronic DSS-induced colitis in mice, as well as to prevent colitis in IL-10 deficient mice [71]. This specific approach is currently being utilized in an ongoing clinical trial for CD [72]. Moreover, the same investigators utilized a related approach to deliver cytoprotective and mucosa repair-promoting peptides (trefoil factors) to the murine colon. This localized peptide delivery resulted in prevention and healing of DSS-induced colitis [72]. Furthermore, this novel pharmacological approach also was successful in improving established chronic colitis in IL-10$^{-/-}$ mice [72].

In addition, Carroll and colleagues tested the efficacy of *Lactobacillus gasseri* expressing manganese superoxide for improving colitis in IL-10 deficient mice. This innovative colonic delivery of an antioxidant reduced the severity of murine colitis [73]. It is apparent from these studies that novel drug delivery approaches may find a niche for the treatment of intestinal inflammation in humans. Relevant probiotic carrier organisms may include the aforementioned *Lactobacillus* strains, as well as *E. coli* Nissle 1917 [74].

7. ANTIBIOTIC-RELATED COLITIS: *SACCHAROMYCES BOULARDII* IN ANIMAL MODELS AND HUMANS

Treatment with antibiotics often causes diarrhea. During severe instances of antibiotic-associated diarrhea, the toxin-producing bacterium *Clostridium difficile* is often identified as the underlying cause. Relevant studies examining probiotics in animal models of *Clostridium difficile* colitis are generally sparse. Most of these studies have involved administration of the yeast probiotic agent, *Saccharomyces boulardii*. Some of these studies were conducted over 20 years ago. Toothaker and Elmer showed that oral administration of the yeast before clindamycin exposure significantly decreased mortality rates in hamsters [75]. Similar results were also reported by other investigators [76]. Martins et al. found that another yeast strain (*Saccharomyces cerevisiae* 905) effectively colonized the distal murine gastrointestinal tract and improved cecal and colonic inflammation following an oral *Clostridium difficile* challenge in mice [77].

In clinical practice, *Saccharomyces boulardii* may have a unique place in therapy. When used as an adjunct to antibiotics, particularly in patients that have experienced recurrent episodes of *C. difficile*-associated diarrhea (CDAD), this strain decreases the likelihood of recurrent diarrhea [78–81]. Mechanistically, *Saccharomyces boulardii* produces a protease that appears to inactivate *C. difficile* toxin receptors. It is conceivable that once the toxin receptors have been acted upon by the protease, even re-growth of the *C. difficile* bacterium is incapable of producing disease because bacterial toxins cannot attach to inactivated receptor sites. Evidence for *Saccharomyces boulardii* as a means of preventing *C. difficile* recurrences appears to be strongest when the yeast probiotic is used in conjunction with high-dose vancomycin therapy. These positive clinical results demonstrate the value of simultaneous use of conventional and alternative medicinal approaches (integrative medicine) in health and wellness.

8. LESSONS LEARNED AND FUTURE DIRECTIONS

Based upon our current understanding of probiotic efficacy for treatment of intestinal colitis conditions, it should not be assumed that all microorganisms marketed as 'probiotics' are equally efficacious. In addition, the heterogeneity of the various IBD clinical disorders suggests that strain-specific properties may be required for different patient categories. The optimal probiotic composition, dose, and length of treatment in disparate IBD conditions need to be determined by large, well-designed, prospective trials.

It is likely that the discrepant results observed in clinical studies conducted thus far can be explained by: different bacterial species, disparate doses, small numbers of patients, probiotics used to maintain remission versus treatment of active disease, or different disease manifestations among enrolled patients (e.g. inflammatory versus stricturing Crohn's disease; antibiotic-responsive, -resistant, or -refractory pouchitis). In the future, clinical studies should strive to enroll sufficient numbers of patients such that significant differences of clinical relevance are capable of being identified—if differences truly exist—among homogenous patient populations. Rationally-selected dosages and probiotic regimens should be utilized. Some experts believe that a single strain of probiotic is unlikely to elicit important modifications in the gastrointestinal microecology [55]; and, thus, multistrain probiotics, using strains with synergistic activities, may offer the best chance for efficacy, as bacterial re-population may be necessary in both the small bowel and the colon.

9. CONCLUSION

At the present time, despite positive data from rodent colitis models, adequate evidence for use of probiotics in IBD exists only for *preventing* pouchitis and *maintaining remission* from pouchitis exacerbations. Nonetheless, continued development and study of probiotics in rodent models and humans appears rational given the role that bacteria seem to play in the underlying etiology of inflammatory bowel diseases. The possibility of using probiotic bacteria as a drug delivery tool has only begun to be explored. Additional preclinical and clinical studies will likely shed more light on this intriguing treatment option.

References

1. Fedorek, R. N., & Madsen, K. L. (2004). Probiotics and the management of inflammatory bowel disease. *Inflammatory Bowel Diseases, 10*, 286–299.
2. Shanahan, F. (2005). Physiological basis for novel drug therapies to treat the inflammatory bowel diseases: I. Pathophysiological basis and prospects for probiotic therapy in inflammatory bowel disease. *American Journal of Physiology: Gastrointestinal and Liver Physiology, 288*, G417–G421.
3. Mach, T. (2006). Clinical usefulness of probiotics in inflammatory bowel diseases. *Journal of Physiology and Pharmacology, 57*(Suppl. 9), 23–33.
4. Steed, H., Macfarlane, G. T., & Macfarlane, S. (2008). Probiotics, synbiotics and inflammatory bowel disease. *Molecular Nutrition and Food Research, 52*, 898–905.
5. Guarner, R. (2007). Prebiotics in inflammatory bowel diseases. *British Journal of Nutrition, 98*(Suppl. 1), S85–S89.
6. Farrell, R. J., & LaMont, J. T. (2002). Microbial factors in inflammatory bowel disease. *Gastroenterology Clinics of North America, 31*, 41–62.
7. Petrof, E. O., Kojima, K., Ropeleski, M. J., et al. (2004). Probiotics inhibit nuclear factor-kappaB and induce heat shock proteins in colonic epithelial cells through proteasome inhibition. *Gastroenterology, 127*, 1474–1487.
8. Fitzpatrick, L. R., Small, J., Hoerr, R. A., et al. (2008). *In vitro* and *in vivo* effects of the probiotic *Escherichia coli* strain M–17: Immunomodulation and attenuation of murine colitis. *British Journal of Nutrition, 100*, 530–541.
9. Schultz, M. (2008). Clinical use of *E. coli* Nissle 1917 in inflammatory bowel disease. *Inflammatory Bowel Disease, 14*, 1012–1018.
10. O'Hara, A. M., & Shanahan, F. (2007). Mechanism of action of probiotics in intestinal diseases. *The Scientific World Journal, 7*, 31–46.
11. Wirtz, S., & Neurath, M. F. (2007). Mouse models of inflammatory bowel disease. *Advanced Drug Delivery Reviews, 59*, 1073–1083.
12. Pizarro, T. T., Arseneau, K. O., Bamias, G., & Cominelli, F. (2003). Mouse models for the study of Crohn's disease. *TRENDS in Molecular Medicine, 9*, 218–222.
13. Strober, W., Fuss, I. J., & Blumberg, R. S. (2002). The immunology of mucosal models of inflammation. *Annual Review of Immunology, 20*, 495–549.
14. Boismenu, R., & Chen, Y. (2000). Insights from mouse models of colitis. *Journal of Leukocyte Biology, 67*, 267–278.
15. Elson, C. O., Cong, Y., Brandwein, S., et al. (1998). Experimental models to study molecular mechanisms underlying intestinal inflammation. *Annuals of the New York Academy of Sciences, 859*, 85–95.
16. Egger, B., Bajaj-Elliott, M., MacDonald, T. T., et al. (2000). Characterization of acute murine dextran sodium sulphate colitis: Cytokine profile and dose dependency. *Digestion, 62*, 240–248.
17. Kitajima, S., Takuma, S., & Morimoto, M. (1999). Changes in colonic mucosal permeability in mouse colitis induced with dextran sulfate sodium. *Experimental Animals, 48*, 137–143.
18. Poritz, L. S., Garver, K. I., Green, C., et al. (2007). Loss of the tight junction protein ZO–1 in dextran sulfate sodium induced colitis. *Journal of Surgical Research, 140*, 12–19.
19. Rachmilewitz, D., Katakura, K., Karmeli, F., et al. (2004). Toll-Like receptor 9 signaling mediates the anti-inflammatory effects of probiotics in murine experimental colitis. *Gastroenterology, 126*, 520–528.
20. Fitzpatrick, L. R., Hertzog, K. L., Quatse, A. L., et al. (2007). Effects of the probiotic formulation VSL#3 on colitis in weanling rats. *Journal of Pediatric Gastroenterology and Nutrition, 44*, 561–570.
21. Fitzpatrick, L. R., Small, J., & Bostwick, E. et al. (2006). Effects of the probiotic *E. coli* strain M–17 on chronic dextran sulfate sodium induced colitis in mice. *Gastroenterology, 130*, A313.
22. Alex, P., Zachos, N. C., Nguyen, T. et al., (2008). Distinct cytokine patterns identified from multiplex profiles of

murine DSS and TNBS-induced colitis. *Inflammatory Bowel Diseases* (published online).

23. te Velde, A. A., Verstege, M. I., & Hommes, D. W. (2006). Critical appraisal of the current practice in murine TNBS-induced colitis. *Inflammatory Bowel Diseases, 12,* 995–999.

24. Shibolet, O., Karmeli, F., Eliakim, R., et al. (2002). Variable response to probiotics in two models of experimental colitis in rats. *Inflammatory Bowel Diseases, 11,* 399–406.

25. Møller, P. L., Paerregaard, A., Gad, M., et al. (2005). Colitic scid mice fed *Lactobacillus* spp. show an ameliorated gut histopathology and an altered cytokine profile by local T cells. *Inflammatory Bowel Diseases, 11,* 814–819.

26. Madsen, K., Cornish, A., Soper, P., et al. (2001). Probiotic bacteria enhance murine and human intestinal epithelial barrier function. *Gastroenterology, 121,* 580–591.

27. Schultz, M., Veltkamp, C., Dieleman, L. A., et al. (2002). *Lactobacillus plantarum* 299V in the treatment and prevention of spontaneous colitis in interleukin–10-deficient mice. *Inflammatory Bowel Diseases, 8,* 71–80.

28. Etling, M. R., Davies, S., Campbell, M., et al. (2007). Maturation of the mucosal immune system underlies colitis susceptibility in interleukin-10-deficient (IL-10$^{-/-}$) mice. *Journal of Leukocyte Biology, 82,* 311–319.

29. Dieleman, L. A., Goerres, M. S., Arends, A., et al. (2003). *Lactobacillus* GG prevents recurrence of colitis in HLA-B27 transgenic rats after antibiotic treatment. *Gut, 52,* 370–376.

30. Schultz, M., Strauch, U. G., Linde, H. J., et al. (2004). Preventive effects of *Escherichia coli* strain Nissle 1917 on acute and chronic intestinal inflammation in two different murine models of colitis. *Clinical and Diagnostic Laboratory Immunology, 11,* 372–378.

31. Pizarro, T. T., Arseneau, K. O., & Cominelli, F. (2000). Lessons from genetically engineered animal models XI. Novel mouse models to study pathogenic mechanisms of Crohn's disease. *American Journal of Physiology: Gastrointestinal and Liver Physiology, 278,* G665–G669.

32. Matsumoto, S., Hara, T., Hori, T., et al. (2005). Probiotic Lactobacillus-induced improvement in murine chronic inflammatory bowel disease is associated with the down-regulation of pro-inflammatory cytokines in lamina propria mononuclear cells. *Clinical and Experimental Immunology, 140,* 417–426.

33. Malchow, H. A. (1997). Crohn's disease and *Escherichia coli*: A new approach in therapy to maintain remission of colonic Crohn's disease? *Journal of Clinical Gastroenterology, 25,* 653–658.

34. Gupta, P., Andrew, H., Kirschner, B. S., & Guadalini, S. (2000). Is *Lactobacillus* GG helpful in children with Crohn's disease? Results of a preliminary, open-label study. *Journal of Pediatric Gastroenterology and Nutrition, 31,* 453–457.

35. Guadalini, S. (2002). Use of *Lactobacillus* GG in paediatric Crohn's disease. *Digestive and Liver Disease, 34,* S63–S65.

36. Bousvaros, A., Guandalini, S., Baldassano, R. N., et al. (2005). A randomized, double-blind trial of *Lactobacillus* GG versus placebo in addition to standard maintenance therapy for children with Crohn's disease. *Inflammatory Bowel Diseases, 11,* 833–839.

37. Schultz, M., Timmer, A., Herfarth, H. H., et al. (2004). *Lactobacillus* GG in inducing and maintaining remission of Crohn's disease. *BMC Gastroenterol, 4,* 5.

38. Fujimori, S., Tatsuguchi, A., Gudis, K., et al. (2007). High dose probiotic and probiotic cotherapy for remission induction of active Crohn's disease. *Journal of Gastroenterology and Hepatology, 22,* 1199–1204.

39. Kruis, W., Schutz, E., Fric, P., et al. (1997). Double-blind comparison of an oral *Escherichia coli* preparation and mesalamine in maintaining remission of ulcerative colitis. *Alimentary Pharmacology and Therapeutics, 11,* 853–858.

40. Kruis, W., Fric, P., Pokrotnieks, J., et al. (2004). Maintaining remission of ulcerative colitis with the probiotic *Escherichia coli* Nissle 1917 is as effective as with standard mesalazine. *Gut, 53,* 1617–1623.

41. Rembracken, B. J., Snelling, A. M., Hawkey, P. M., et al. (1999). Non-pathogenic *Escherichia coli* versus mesalamine for the treatment of ulcerative colitis: a randomized trial. *Lancet, 354,* 635–639.

42. Zocco, M. A., Dal Verme, L. Z., Cremonini, F., et al. (2006). Efficacy of *Lactobacillus* GG in maintaining remission of ulcerative colitis. *Alimentary Pharmacology and Therapeutics, 23,* 1567–1574.

43. Venturi, A., Gionchetti, P., Rizzello, F., et al. (1999). Impact on the composition of the fecal flora by a new probiotic preparation: preliminary data on maintenance treatment of patients with ulcerative colitis. *Alimentary Pharmacology and Therapeutics, 13,* 1103–1108.

44. Ishikawa, H., Akedo, I., Umesaki, Y., et al. (2002). Randomized controlled trial of the effect of Bifidobacteria-fermented milk on ulcerative colitis. *Journal of the American College of Nutrition, 22,* 56–63.

45. Bibiloni, R., Fedorak, R. N., Tannock, G. W., et al. (2005). VSL#3 probiotic-mixture induces remission in patients with active ulcerative colitis. *The American Journal of Gastroenterology, 100,* 1539–1546.

46. Furrie, E., Macfarlane, S., Kennedy, A., et al. (2005). Synbiotic therapy (*Bifidobacterium longum*/Synergy 1) initiates resolution of inflammation in patients with active ulcerative colitis: a randomized controlled pilot trial. *Gut, 54,* 242–249.

47. Kato, K., Mizuno, S., Umesaki, Y., et al. (2004). Randomized placebo-controlled trial assessing the effect of bifidobacteria-fermented milk on active ulcerative

colitis. *Alimentary Pharmacology and Therapeutics, 20,* 1133–1141.

48. Guslandi, M., Giolo, P., & Testoni, P. A. (2003). A pilot trial of *Saccharomyces boulardii* in ulcerative colitis. *European Journal of Gastroenterology & Hepatology, 15,* 697–698.

49. Tsuda, Y., Yoshimatsu, Y., Aoki, H., et al. (2007). Clinical effectiveness of probiotics therapy (BIO-THREE) in patients with ulcerative colitis refractory to conventional therapy. *Scandinavian Journal of Gastroenterology, 42,* 491–501.

50. Floch, M. H., Walker, W. A., Guandalini, S., et al. (2008). Recommendations for probiotic use – 2008. *Journal of Clinical Gastroenterology, 42,* S104–S108.

51. Lichtman, S. N., Wang, J., Hummel, B., et al. (1998). A rat model of ileal pouch-rectal anastomosis. *Inflammatory Bowel Diseases, 4,* 187–195.

52. Chen, C. N., McVay, L. D., Batlivala, Z. S., et al. (2002). Anatomic and functional characteristics of the rat ileal pouch. *American Journal of Surgery, 183,* 464–470.

53. Atila, K., Terzi, C., Canda, A. E., et al. (2008). Partially hydrolyzed guar gum attenuates the severity of pouchitis in a rat model of Ileal J pouch-anal anastomosis. *Digestive Diseases and Sciences* (published online).

54. Shen, B., Brzezinski, A., Fazio, V. W., et al. (2005). Maintenance therapy with a probiotic in antibiotic-dependent pouchitis: Experience in clinical practice. *Alimentary Pharmacology and Therapeutics, 22,* 721–728.

55. Gionchetti, P., Rizzello, F., Venturi, A., et al. (2000). Oral bacteriotherapy as maintenance treatment in patients with chronic pouchitis: A double-blind, placebo-controlled trial. *Gastroenterology, 119,* 305–309.

56. Mimura, T., Rizzello, F., Helwig, U., et al. (2004). Once daily high dose initiates resolution on inflammation in patients with active ulcerative colitis: A randomized controlled pilot trial. *Gut, 54,* 242–249.

57. Gionchetti, P., Rizzello, F., Helwig, U., et al. (2003). Prophylaxis of pouchitis onset with probiotic therapy: A double-blind, placebo-controlled trial. *Gastroenterology, 124,* 1202–1209.

58. Gosselink, M. P., Schouten, W. R., van Lieshout, L. M., et al. (2004). Delay of the first onset of pouchitis by oral intake of the probiotic strain *Lactobacillus rhamnosus* GG. *Diseases of the Colon and Rectum, 47,* 876–884.

59. Gionchetti, P., Rizzello, F., Morselli, C., et al. (2007). High-dose probiotics for the treatment of active pouchitis. *Diseases of the Colon and Rectum, 50,* 2075–2084.

60. Laake, K. O., Bjorneklett, A., Aamodt, G., et al. (2005). Outcome of four week's intervention with probiotics on symptoms and endoscopic appearance after surgical reconstruction with a J-configurated ileal-pouch-anal-anastomosis in ulcerative colitis. *Scandinavian Journal of Gastroenterology, 40,* 43–51.

61. Laake, K. O., Line, P. D., Grzyb, K., et al. (2004). Assessment of mucosal inflammation and blood flow in response to four weeks' intervention with probiotics in patients operated with a J-configuration ileal-pouch-anal-anastomosis (IPAA). *Scandinavian Journal of Gastroenterology, 39,* 1228–1235.

62. Laake, K. O., Line, P. D., Aabakken, L., et al. (2003). Assessment of mucosal inflammation and circulation in response to probiotics in patients operated with ileal pouch anal anastomosis for ulcerative colitis. *Scandinavian Journal of Gastroenterology, 38,* 409–414.

63. Kuisma, J., Mentula, S., Jarvinen, H., et al. (2003). Effect of *Lactobacillus rhamnosus* GG on ileal pouch inflammation and microbial flora. *Alimentary Pharmacology and Therapeutics, 17,* 509–513.

64. Schultz, M., Munro, K., Tannock, G. W., et al. (2004). Effects of feeding a probiotic preparation (SIM) containing inulin on the severity of colitis and on the composition of the intestinal microflora in HLA-B27 transgenic rats. *Clinical and Diagnostic Laboratory Immunology, 11,* 581–587.

65. Osman, N., Adawi, D., Molin, G., et al. (2006). *Bifidobacterium infantis* strains with and without a combination of oligofructose and inulin (OFI) attenuate inflammation in DSS-induced colitis in rats. *BMC Gastroenterology, 6,* 31.

66. Møller, P. L., Paerregaard, A., Gad, M., et al. (2005). Colitic scid mice fed *Lactobacillus* spp. show an ameliorated gut histopathology and an altered cytokine profile by local T cells. *Inflammatory Bowel Diseases, 11,* 814–819.

67. Souza, M. M., Aguilar-Nascimento, J. E., & Dock-Nascimento, D. B. (2007). Effects of budesonide and probiotics enemas on the systemic inflammatory response of rats with experimental colitis. *Acta Cirúrgica Brasileira, 22*(Suppl. 1), 40–45.

68. Tursi, A., Brandimarte, G., Giorgetti, G. M., & Elisei, W. (2005). Beclomethasone Dipropionate plus VSL#3 for the treatment of mild to moderate diverticular colitis: An open, pilot study: Letter to the Eitor. *Journal of Clinical Gastroenterology, 39,* 644–654.

69. Tursi, A. (2008). Balsalazide plus high-potency probiotic preparation (VSL#3) in the treatment of mild-to-moderate ulcerative colitis and uncomplicated diverticulitis of the colon. *Journal of Clinical Gastroenterology, 42,* S119–S122.

70. Huynh, H.Q., Debruyn, J., Guan, L., et al. (2008). Probiotic preparation VSL#3 induces remission in children with mild to moderate acute ulcerative colitis: A pilot study. *Inflammatory Bowel Diseases* (published online).

71. Steidler, L., Hans, W., Schotte, L., et al. (2008). Treatment of murine colitis by *Lactococcus lactis* secreting interleukin-10. *Science, 289,* 1352–1355.

72. Vandenbroucke, K., Hans, W., Van Huysse, J., et al. (2004). Active delivery of trefoil factors by genetically modified *Lactococcus lactis* prevents and heals acute colitis in mice. *Gastroenterology, 127,* 502–513.

73. Carroll, I. M., Andrus, J. M., Bruno-Bárcena, J. M., et al. (2007). Anti-inflammatory properties of *Lactobacillus gasseri* expressing manganese superoxide dismutase using the interleukin 10-deficient mouse model of colitis. *American Journal of Physiology: Gastrointestinal and Liver Physiology, 293,* G729–G738.

74. Westendorf, A. M., Gunzer, F., Deppenmeier, S., et al. (2005). Intestinal immunity of *Escherichia coli* NISSLE 1917: A safe carrier for therapeutic molecules. *FEMS Immunology and Medical Microbiology, 43,* 373–384.

75. Toothaker, R. D., & Elmer, G. W. (1984). Prevention of clindamycin-induced mortality in hamsters by *Saccharomyces boulardii. Antimicrobial Agents and Chemotherapy, 26,* 552–556.

76. Corthier, G., Dubos, F., & Ducluzeau, R. (1986). Prevention of *Clostridium difficile* I induced mortality in gnotobiotic mice by *Saccharomyces boulardii. Canadian Journal of Microbiology, 32,* 894–896.

77. Martins, F. S., Nardi, R. M., Arantes, R. M., et al. (2005). Screening of yeasts as probiotic based on capacities to colonize the gastrointestinal tract and to protect against enteropathogen challenge in mice. *The Journal of General and Applied Microbiology, 51,* 83–92.

78. Surawicz, C. M., McFarland, L. V., Elmer, G., & Chinn, J. (1989). Treatment of recurrent *Clostridium difficile* colitis with vancomycin and *Saccharomyces boulardii. American Journal of Gastroenterology, 84,* 1285–1287.

79. Kimmey, M. B., Elmer, G. W., Surawicz, C. M., & McFarland, L. V. (1990). Prevention of further recurrences of *Clostridium difficile* colitis with *Saccharomyces boulardii. Digestive Diseases and Science, 35,* 897–901.

80. McFarland, L. V., Surawicz, C. M., Greenberg, R. N., et al. (1994). A randomized placebo-controlled trial of *Saccharomyces boulardii* in combination with standard antibiotics for *Clostridium difficile* disease. *The Journal of the American Medical Association, 271,* 1913–1918.

81. Surawicz, C. M., McFarland, L. V., Greenberg, R. N., et al. (2000). The search for a better treatment for recurrent *Clostridium difficile* disease: use of high-dose vancomycin combined with *Saccharomyces boulardii. Clinical Infectious Diseases, 31,* 1012–1017.

82. Osman, N., Adawi, D., Ahrne, S., et al. (2004). *Digestive Diseases and Sciences, 49,* 320–327.

83. Lee, H. S., Han, S. Y., Bae, E. A., et al. (2008). *International Immunopharmacology, 8,* 574–580.

84. Voltan, S., Martines, D., Elli, M., et al. (2008). *Gastroenterology, 135,* 1216–1227.

85. Geier, M. S., Butler, R. N., Giffard, P. M., & Howarth, G. S. (2007). *International Journal of Food Microbiology, 114,* 267–274.

86. Osman, N., Adawi, D., Ahrne, S., et al. (2008). *Digestive Diseases and Sciences, 53,* 2464–2473.

87. van der Kleij, H., O'Mahony, C., Shanahan, F., et al. (2008). *American Journal of Physiology: Regulatory, Integrative and Comparative Physiology, 295,* R1131–R1137.

88. Moon, G., Myung, S. J., Jeong, J. Y., et al. (2004). *Korean Journal of Gastroenterology, 43,* 234–245.

89. Grabig, A., Paclik, D., Guzy, C., et al. (2006). *Infection and Immunology, 74,* 4075–4082.

90. Ukena, S. N., Singh, A., Dringenberg, U., et al. (2008). *PLoS ONE, 2,* e1308.

91. Kamada, N., Inoue, N., Hisamatsu, T., et al. (2005). *Inflammatory Bowel Diseases, 11,* 455–463.

92. Kanauchi, O., Fukuda, M., Matsumoto, Y., et al. (2006). *World Journal of Gastroenterology, 12,* 1074–1077.

93. Peran, L., Camuesco, D., Comalada, M., et al. (2007). *Journal of Applied Microbiology, 103,* 836–844.

94. Lamine, F., Eutamène, H., Fioramonti, J., et al. (2004). *Scandinavian Journal of Gastroenterology, 39,* 1250–1258.

95. Peran, L., Sierra, S., Comalada, M., et al. (2007). *The British Journal of Nutrition, 97,* 96–103.

96. Zoumpopoulou, G., Foligne, B., Christodoulou, K., et al. (2008). *International Journal of Food Microbiology, 121,* 18–26.

97. Amit-Romach, E., Uni, Z., & Reifen, R. (2008). *Diseases of the Colon and Rectum, 51,* 1828–1836.

98. Foligne, B., Nutten, S., Grangette, C., et al. (2007). *World Journal of Gastroenterology, 13,* 236–243.

99. Daniel, C., Poiret, S., Goudercourt, D., et al. (2006). *Applied and Environmental Microbiology, 72,* 5799–5805.

100. Peran, L., Camuesco, D., Comalada, M., et al. (2005). *World Journal of Gastroenterology, 11,* 5185–5192.

101. McCarthy, J., O'Mahony, L., O'Callaghan, L., et al. (2003). *Gut, 52,* 975–980.

102. Sheil, B., MacSharry, J., O'Callaghan, L., et al. (2006). *Clinical and Experimental Immunology, 144,* 273–280.

103. Jijon, H., Backer, J., Diaz, H., et al. (2004). *Gastroenterology, 126,* 1358–1373.

E. ANIMAL MODELS TO STUDY PROBIOTICS

Prebiotics and Probiotics in Experimental Models of Rodent Colitis: Lessons in Treatment or Prevention of Inflammatory Bowel Diseases

Julio Gálvez[1], Mònica Comalada[2], and Jordi Xaus[3]

[1]CIBER-EHD, Department of Pharmacology, University of Granada, Granada, Spain

[2]Department of Physiology, University of Veterinary, Ramon y Cajal Program of the Spanish Ministry of Science and Technology, Barcelona, Spain

[3]Drug Development and Clinical Research, Palau Pharma, Palau-Solità I Plegamans, Barcelona, Spain

1. INTRODUCTION

The term inflammatory bowel disease (IBD) usually refers to two closely related intestinal conditions, namely ulcerative colitis (UC) and Crohn's disease (CD), characterized by chronic and spontaneously relapsing inflammation of the gut. UC affects only the large bowel, whereas CD may affect any part of the gastrointestinal tract, from the mouth to the anorectum, but the most frequent location is within the ileocecal region [1]. In UC, the inflammatory process is confined to the mucosa, as opposed to CD, in which the inflammation affects the entire bowel wall, even leading to the formation of abscesses and fistulas (abnormal connections between the lumen of the bowel and other organs of the surface of the skin); it may also present with bowel obstruction [2].

Although the etiology of IBD is not completely known, the most accepted hypothesis states that an abnormal exacerbated immune response to otherwise innocuous stimuli occurs, and this is not properly counteracted by the feedback system [3]. It has been reported that mucosal injury in IBD may be a consequence of an immunoinflammatory response generated by persistent and inappropriate mucosal T cell activation, which results in early histological and functional changes as well as late permanent tissue destruction [4, 5]. Inflammation is amplified and propagated as a result of the recruitment of different cell types of the immune system [3] and by an up-regulation of the synthesis and release of a variety of pro-inflammatory mediators [6]. Moreover, most of these mediators can induce the biosynthesis and release of some others, generating a 'vicious cycle' that may result in the propagation and perpetuation of the inflammatory response.

But, what is the initial stimulus that triggers the inflammatory status in the gut? There is increasing experimental and clinical evidence to support a role for luminal microorganisms in the initiation and progression of these intestinal conditions. Although different specific microorganisms, including *Mycobacterium paratuberculosis*, *Listeria monocytogenes*, *Chlamydia pneumoniae*, *Escherichia coli*, and cytomegalovirus [7–10], have been proposed to act as implicating factors in the etiopathogenesis of IBD, at the time of writing, it has been not possible to establish a definitive causative effect with any of them. Most probably, the development of intestinal lesions and/ or the impaired resolution of the lesions leading to chronic intestinal disease may occur in genetically susceptible individuals after the hyperresponsiveness to the commensal intestinal microflora rather than to single bacteria [5]. For this reason, it has been suggested that the local tolerance mechanisms towards the autologous microflora are abrogated in IBD.

It is well known that different cells located in the intestinal mucosa, including epithelial and dendritic cells, continuously monitor the gut flora and, in normal conditions, recognize potential pathogens, and differentiate from those commensal, transferring signals to other immune cells that trigger inflammation or help to avoid inadequate stimulation [5]. Two major host pattern recognition receptor systems are involved in this function: the Toll-like receptors (TLRs) and the nucleotide oligomerization domain (NOD), which are able to interact with different bacterial products, including lypopolysaccharide (LPS), peptidoglycan (PGN), flagellin, etc. Different studies have revealed that a different expression pattern of TLRs on intestinal epithelial cells occurs in IBD patients in comparison with healthy controls [11]. Similarly, several groups have proposed that three variants of the NOD2/CARD15 gene are strongly linked with CD [12, 13], whereas there is poor linkage to UC [14].

The hypothesis that suggests a role for the intestinal microflora in the pathogenesis of IBD is further supported by several observations: most inflammation occurs in areas with the highest density of intestinal bacteria; broad spectrum antibiotics improve chronic intestinal inflammation; there is an increased mucosal secretion of IgG antibodies against commensal bacteria in patients with IBD; and surgical diversion of the fecal stream can prevent recurrence of CD [15]. Moreover, the participation of enteric microflora antigens in the development of the intestinal damage have also been confirmed in many experimental models of IBD in laboratory animal, since colitis does not appear in germ-free bred IL-10 gene-deficient mice or HLA-B27 transgenic rats, or this is clearly attenuated in chemically-induced models, like those using trinitrobenzene sulfonic acid or dextran sulfate sodium in rodents, when these animals are raised in sterile conditions [16, 17].

Furthermore, the existence of differences in the fecal and mucosal microbiota between healthy subjects and IBD patients has been reported [18]. Most of the studies have revealed the higher biodiversity of species in healthy subjects [19], and dominant species, with a relevant role for Firmicutes, comprising about 90% of the total bacterial population; whereas in IBD patients biodiversity is lower and there is a high percentage (almost 30%) of 'unusual' species [20, 21]. Tamboli et al. [22] introduced the term dysbiosis to suggest that the equilibrium between protective and harmful bacteria in healthy people is broken in IBD, thus resulting in chronic intestinal inflammation [22]. Moreover, in patients suffering from IBD, modifications not only in the diversity of bacteria but also in their intestinal distribution and adhesion to the mucosal surface have also been described [23].

In consequence, and considering all the above, a possible therapeutic approach in IBD therapy is the restoration of the altered intestinal microflora balance towards a more beneficial bacterial population, thus reducing or preventing intestinal inflammation. This can be achieved through administration of probiotic microorganisms, or prebiotics or the combination of both, i.e. synbiotics, to these patients. However, there are many different probiotics and prebiotics where it is difficult to directly predict its efficacy in IBD patients without the development of corresponding preclinical studies, which initially implies the use of experimental models in laboratory animals.

2. EXPERIMENTAL MODELS OF RODENT COLITIS

The development of experimental models of IBD in rodents has certainly contributed to the understanding of the mechanisms that participate in the pathogenesis of human IBD, and they have been considered as important tools in the discovery of new potential targets and strategies to obtain more efficient and safer treatments, including probiotics and prebiotics. However, it is important to consider that there is no ideal animal model for the study of human IBD since they cannot show a complete etiologic and pathologic coincidence with human IBD. For this reason, and in order to obtain an accurate profile in the intestinal anti-inflammatory effects of a given probiotic and/or prebiotic, it is interesting to establish the major characteristics of the different experimental models. With this aim, in this section we have summarized the colitis experimental models and collected them into two main categories: chemically-inducible and spontaneous colitis.

2.1. Chemically-inducible Colitis Models

Initially introduced in the 1980s, different inductor substances have been used, including chemical agents (sulfate polysaccharides or bacterial immunocomplexes), to initiate an intestinal inflammation in susceptible animal species

(see Table 35.1). One of the first offending agents used to induce colonic inflammation was acetic acid, as originally described by Macpherson and Pfeiffer [24]. The colitis is induced by intrarectal instillation to rodents of diluted acetic acid in water (4–50%), which induces an acute inflammation accompanied by necrosis of colonic segment [25]. However, the chemically-induced IBD models most currently used are those based on trinitrobenzene sulfonic acid (TNBS) and dextran sulfate sodium (DSS).

The TNBS-induced colitis was initially described in 1989 by Morris et al. in rats [26], although its use has also been extended to mice. Basically, it consists of the application of an enema of TNBS dissolved in a solution of ethanol/water, at different doses depending on the laboratory animal used: 10 to 30 mg in rats or 0.5 to 4 mg in mice. The role of ethanol is to promote the destruction of the intestinal barrier, thus allowing the access of TNBS to the intestinal lamina propria, which exhibits a direct toxic effect and acts as a hapten which activates the host immune response of the intestine to colonic autologous or microbiota proteins. The inflammatory process induced has many of the characteristics of human CD, including severe transmural inflammation associated with diarrhea, rectal prolapse, anorexia, and weight loss. Moreover, it has been proposed to display a Th1 mediated response, since it has been associated with elevated pro-inflammatory cytokine production (TNFα, IL-12 and IFNγ), similar to that reported to occur in human CD [27]. Although there are differences between human IBD and TNBS colitis in rodents, its simplicity and reproducibility clearly contribute to its extensive use in the evaluation of novel strategies in human IBD.

The DSS model of colitis was originally described by Okayasu et al. in 1990 [28]. It consists of the administration of DSS polymers dissolved in drinking water, at different concentrations (1–5%), to mice, rats, hamsters or guinea pigs. Although the exact mechanisms involved

TABLE 35.1 Chemically-inducible colitis models

Experimental model	Laboratory animal	Involved area	Inflammation	Type of response	Type of damage	Bacterial influence	Resemblance	Reference
Acetic acid	Rat, mouse, rabbit, guinea pig	Distal colon and rectum	Acute	Production of pro-inflammatory mediators, histamine and PAF.	Transmural	NO	UC	[15]
PS-PG	Rat	Proximal colon and cecum	Acute	Macrophage and T cell activation. Production of pro-inflammatory mediators.	Transmural	YES	CD	[31]
TNBS	Rat, mouse, rabbit	Colon	Acute/Chronic	Macrophage and T cell activation. Th1 cytokines production.	Transmural	YES	CD	[26]
DSS	Rat, mouse, hamster, guinea pig	Colon	Acute/Chronic	Epithelial erosion with macrophage activation. Th1/Th2 cytokines production.	Mucosa and submucosa	YES	UC	[28]
Oxazolone	Rat, mouse	Distal colon	Acute/Chronic	Contact hypersensitivity reaction. Th2 cytokines production.	Mucosa > submucosa	?	UC	[34]
Iodacetamide	Rat	Colon	Acute/Chronic	Reduction of antioxidant defences. Th1 cytokines production.	Mucosa and submucosa	?	UC	[32]
Indometacin	Rat, mouse, dog	Small bowel and colon	Chronic	Inhibition of PGE_2 and PGI_2 production.	Transmural	YES	CD	[33]

PAF, platelet activating factor; PS-PG, peptidoglycan-polysaccharide; TNBS, trinitrobenzene sulfonic acid; DSS, dextran sulfate sodium; UC, ulcerative colitis; CD, Crohn's disease; PG, prostaglandin.

have not been completely elucidated, it is believed that DSS exerts a direct toxic effect to gut epithelial cells affecting the integrity of the mucosal barrier, thus allowing luminal bacterial translocation and the subsequent infiltration of granulocytes and mononuclear immune cells. The main manifestations of the colonic insult are animal bodyweight loss, diarrhea and rectal bleeding. Similarly to that described above with the TNBS model of colitis, the lesions observed during this phase have been associated with increased production of macrophage-derived pro-inflammatory cytokines, including IL-1β, IL-6 and TNFα. A critical role has been attributed to luminal bacteria in the pathogenesis of DSS, since the treatment with clinically effective antibiotics in human IBD, like metronidazol or ciprofloxacin, results in amelioration in the intestinal inflammatory process induced by this polymer [29], and this supports the importance of commensal bacteria in the development of colitis in this experimental model [30].

Other experimental models of chemically-induced colitis are those performed after the administration of the polysaccharide-peptidoglycan (PS-PG) [31], the sulfhydryl blocker iodoacetamide [32], indometacin [33] or even oxazolone [34] (Table 35.1). In these models, the colitic status is also characterized by diarrhea and inhibition of weight gain, associated with colonic dilation, adhesion and mucosal damage of different intensity depending on the compound and dose used. Some of these models are also valuable to elucidate the contribution of the antioxidant defenses in this pathology [32] or the involvement of the immune Th2 compartment [34].

2.2. Spontaneous Colitis Models

The experimental models of spontaneous colitis represent a good approximation for studying the different factors involved in human IBD, as well as the impact of a given therapeutic strategy.

In these models, mutations of several genes that have been mainly implicated in the regulation of the immune system led to intestinal inflammatory status resembling human IBD (see Table 35.2). In this sense, Sundberg et al. reported that the C3H/HeJBir mice, a sub-strain of C3H/HeJ mice, under certain housing conditions, can spontaneously develop right-sided colitis [35], which peaks at 3–6 weeks and resolves by 3 months of age. It has been shown that these mice develop B cell and Th1 cell responses to antigens of the commensal bacteria, and it is associated with increased production of pro-inflammatory cytokines including IL-2 and IFNγ. This model has been particularly useful in supporting the role of an abnormal immune reactivity to enteric bacterial flora in the pathogenesis of IBD [36]. However, although the list of potential antigens is numerous, only a small, highly selected number of enteric bacterial antigens (e.g. bacterial flagellins), are responsible for the development of colitis in this model [37].

Similarly, the SAMP1/Yit mice and the SAMP1/YitFc sub-strain comprise models of spontaneous intestinal inflammation quite similar to CD, since inflammation is primarily localized in the terminal ileum, the primary location of CD lesions [38]. These mice displayed established ileitis at 10 weeks of age, and the intestinal lesions were characterized by transmural involvement, with prominent muscular hypertrophy, granulomas, and alterations in epithelial morphology [39].

On the other hand, the transgenic and knock-out (KO) methodologies have also been used to develop several genetically engineered models, which have clearly contributed to the understanding of the role of key immune-related molecules in the pathogenesis of chronic intestinal inflammation (see Table 35.2). This is the case of transgenic rats for human HLA-B27 and β2-microglobulin, which develop a spontaneous intestinal inflammation that affects all of the segments of the gastrointestinal tract [40]. The different assays performed in this model have

TABLE 35.2   Animal models of spontaneous colitis

Experimental model	Laboratory animal	Involved area	Inflammation	Type of response	Bacterial influence	Resemblance	Reference
HLA-B27 Tg	Rat	Small bowel and colon	Acute/Chronic	Activation of Th1 T cells.	YES	CD	[40]
IL-10 KO	Mouse	Small bowel and colon	Chronic	Macrophage and Th1 T cell activation. High production of pro-inflammatory mediators.	YES	UC	[43]
TCRα Tg	Mouse	Colon	Chronic	Increased numbers of Th2 T cells. Production of IL-4.	YES	UC	[45]
IL-2 KO	Mouse	Colon	Acute/Chronic	High infiltration of T and B cells. Elevated immunoglobulin secretion.	?	UC	[46]
C3H/HeJBir	Mouse	Cecum/Colon	Acute/Chronic	B and Th1 cell responses to antigens of the commensal bacteria.	YES	---	[35]
T CD4+ cells CD45RB/SCID	Mouse	Colon>Ileum	Chronic/>Acute	High Th1 cytokines production. Involvement of IL-10 and TGFβ.	YES	CD	[44, 47]
SAMP1/Yit	Mouse	Terminal ileum/Cecum	Acute/Chronic	Mixed inflammatory cell infiltrate. Th1/Th2 cytokines production.	YES	CD	[38, 48]
STAT4 Tg	Mouse	Terminal ileum and colon	Chronic	High production of Th1 cyokines. Low levels of Th2 cytokines.	YES	CD	[49]
TNFΔARE	Mouse	Ileum>Colon	Chronic	High production of Th1 cytokines. Activation of CD8+ T cells.	?	CD	[50]

KO, *knock-out*; Tg, transgenic; UC, ulcerative colitis; CD, Crohn's disease; IL, interleukin; TGFβ, transforming growth factor.

supported the important role attributed to commensal intestinal bacteria in the pathogenesis of the acute and chronic stages of gastrointestinal inflammation. In fact, when HLA-B27 transgenic rats are raised in a germ-free environment, they also fail to develop intestinal inflammation, whereas colitis develops within 1 month after they have been transferred to a non-sterile environment [41]. In addition, the treatment of these rats with broad-spectrum antibiotics is effective in preventing and/or ameliorating disease [29, 42].

Moreover, several experimental models in mice with mutations in genes coding for cytokines have also been developed (resumed in Table 35.2), which have clearly contributed further knowledge on the implications of the altered immune response in IBD. One of the most used models is the IL-10 KO mice, in which animals spontaneously developed inflammation in the whole intestine, mainly in the duodenum, proximal jejunum and ascending colon with massive infiltration of lymphocytes, activated macrophages and neutrophils [43].

Finally, a 'non-classical' spontaneous colitis model is that developed in mice with severe combined immunodeficiency (SCID) mice, characterized by a spontaneous mutation that results in a deficiency of both B and T cells (Table 35.2). These mice have an intact innate immune system and they survive under specific pathogen-free conditions. The immune system of these mice can be completely reconstituted by adoptive transfer of B cells and T cells. Adoptive transfer of CD4$^+$CD45RB^{hi} into SCID mice results in colonic transmural inflammation, which does not appear following CD4$^+$CD45RB^{lo} transfer to these mice, primarily in the proximal colon 5–10 after cell transfer [44]. In consequence, this model provides two important clues in the pathogenesis of IBD. First, normal T cells contain pathogenic cells that can originate intestinal inflammation, and second, this inflammation is prevented in normal subjects by the effects of regulatory T cells.

Nowadays it is accepted that studies with experimental models of rodent colitis have allowed a better understanding of the patho-physiological mechanisms involved in human IBD, and they are currently considered as valuable tools in the development of new therapeutic strategies in the treatment of these intestinal conditions. However, it is evident that no single animal experimental model of colitis comprises all the pathogenic and clinical features of human IBD and, for this reason, new potential therapeutic strategies should be evaluated using different models. This would allow better characterization of their intestinal anti-inflammatory activity, as they are very important for their future validation when the corresponding assays in the human being are developed.

3. INTESTINAL ANTI-INFLAMMATORY ACTIVITY OF PROBIOTICS IN EXPERIMENTAL MODELS OF INTESTINAL INFLAMMATION

Probiotics are defined as living microorganisms that, upon ingestion in adequate amounts, confer a health benefit to the host beyond inherent general nutrition [51]. In 1907, Metchnikoff was the first researcher to establish that ingested bacteria, in the form of yogurt and other fermented foods, could exert beneficial effects to the human being [52]. Since then, a great variety of microorganisms have been proposed to be considered as probiotics—most of them members of the genera *Lactobacillus* and *Bifidobacterium*, although other genera of bacteria are also used as well as some yeasts (Table 35.3).

Several mechanisms have been proposed to participate in the gastrointestinal beneficial effects exerted by some species of probiotics (Figure 35.1). In this sense, probiotics could suppress the growth or mucosal adhesion and

TABLE 35.3 Probiotic microorganisms

Lactobacilli	Bifidobacteria	Other
L. acidophilus	B. bifidum	Lactococcus lactis ssp. lactis
L. casei var. Shirota	B. longum	Lactococcus lactis ssp. cremoris
L. johnsonii	B. infantis	Enterococcus faecium
L. fermentum	B. brevis	Saccharomyces boulardii
L. gasseri	B. adolescentis	Escherichia coli Nissle 1917
L. casei		Pediococcus acidilactici
L. crispatus		Propionibacterium freudenreichii
L. reuteri		Clostridium butiricum
L. rhamnosus (Lactobacillus GG)		
L. plantarum		
L. bulgaricus		
L. cellobiosus		
L. curvatus		
L. lactis cremoris		
L. salivarius		

infectiveness of enteric pathogenic bacteria; competing with them for the nutrients present in the gut and for their space/localization. Other factors that can contribute to this effect are related, firstly, with the ability of the probiotics to decrease luminal pH via production of short-chain fatty acids (SCFA) [53], or to promote the secretion of bacteriocins or hydrogen peroxide [54, 55]. Secondly, probiotics positively affect the intestinal barrier function by decreasing mucosal permeability [56] and/or stimulating mucin production by epithelial cells [57]. Finally, probiotics have also been reported to exert immunoregulatory activities, either by inducing protective cytokines, like IL-10 and TGFβ, or by suppressing pro-inflammatory cytokines, like TNFα, in the intestinal mucosa [58, 59]. However, the detailed mechanisms by which these bacteria

mediate their effects are not fully understood (Figure 35.1).

3.1. Studies of Probiotics in Experimental Models of Rodent Colitis

Over the last two decades, encouraging results have been obtained with probiotic therapy in different experimental models of colitis (see Table 35.4).

One of the first studies describing the role of microbiota in these intestinal conditions and the potential beneficial effects of lactobacilli was reported by Fabia et al. [60], who established the existence of similar changes in the colonic mucosa-associated microflora both in UC patients and in rats with acetic acid-induced experimental colitis. In comparison with healthy rats, they showed a significant decrease in the number of Lactobacillus sp. in the intestinal contents in colitic rats 4 days after acetic acid colonic instillation, and suggested that the administration of Lactobacillus sp. with the aim to restore the altered equilibrium in the microbiota would be beneficial [61].

From these initial studies, several claimed probiotic strains have been tested in animal models of colitis. Holma et al. [62] reported that the rat strain Lactobacillus reuteri R2LC, but not the human strain Lactobacillus rhamnosus GG, showed beneficial effects in reducing the severity of the inflammatory process induced with acetic acid in rats. Based on these studies and other similar observations, it has been accepted that the most important factor to attenuate experimental colitis is not the total amount of lactobacilli but the particular species or strain. In this sense, the most studied probiotic strains in the treatment of IBD mainly include representatives of the L. reuteri, L. salivarius, L. rhamnosus, L. fermentum, E. coli and L. casei species, among others (see Table 35.4).

Lactobacillus reuteri has been shown to significantly reduce inflammation in different experimental models of rodent colitis including those

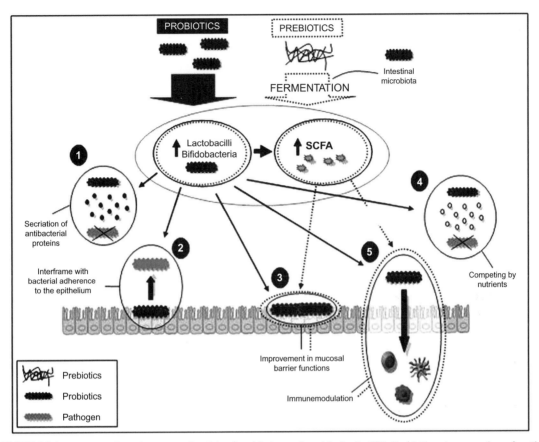

FIGURE 35.1 Suggested mechanisms of action of prebiotics and probiotics in IBD. Probiotic microorganisms (continuous line) may exert their action through a modulation of the intestinal bowel microbiota, which may result from the production of anti-microbial proteins (1), inhibition of epithelial adherence and translocation by pathogens (2), positively affect the intestinal barrier function by decreasing mucosal permeability (3), and also compete with metabolic interactions with potential pathogens. Finally, probiotics have been also reported to exert immunoregulatory activities (5). The effect of prebiotics (broken line) could be due indirectly by stimulating the selective growth of the intestinal lactobacilli and bifidobacteria, and thus acting similarly to the probiotics; or directly by the production of short chain fatty acids (SCFA) which could improve mucosal barrier funtions (3) or modulate the immune system (5).

that have been chemically induced and spontaneously developed. This probiotic effectively prevented the colonic damage induced after TNBS administration to rats, an effect which was associated with a significant reduction in the colonic production of the pro-inflammatory cytokine TNFα, down-regulation in the expression of inducible nitric oxide synthase (iNOS) and a restoration in the colonic lactobacilli

count [63]. Furthermore, *Lactobacillus reuteri* was also effective in inhibiting colitis in IL-10 KO mice [64]. The beneficial effect of *Lactobacillus reuteri* DSM-12246 was also assessed in SCID mice transplanted with CD4 T blast cells, since the association of the probiotic to antibiotic treatment (vancomycin/meropenem) was able to ameliorate the severity of the colitis, an effect which was not obtained when only antibiotics

TABLE 35.4   Probiotics used in IBD animal studies

Prebiotic	Animal model	Results	References
Lactobacillus reuteri	Acetic-induced colitis in rats	Reduced inflammation.	[60]
	IL-10 KO mice	Prevention of development of the spontaneous colitis.	[61]
	Acetic-induced colitis in rats	Reduced inflammation.	[62]
	Spontaneous colitis SCID mice	Prevention of development of the spontaneous colitis.	[65]
	TNBS-induced colitis in rats	Comparation between *L. fermentum* vs *L.reuteri*. Better anti-inflammatory effects exerted by *L. fermentum*.	[69]
Lactobacillus salivarius	IL-10 KO mice	Reduced inflammation (reduction of Th1 cytokine expression).	[68]
	TNBS-induced colitis in rats	Reduced inflammation (reduction of inflammatory cytokines, MPO, iNOS). Restoration of gluthatione levels.	[66]
	TNBS-induced colitis in mice	Reduced inflammation.	[67]
Lactobacillus casei	Spontaneous colitis SAMP1/Yit mice	Reduced inflammation (down-regulation of pro-inflammatory cytokines such as IL-6 and IFNγ).	[71]
	TNBS-induced colitis in rats	Reduced inflammation (inhibition of ICAM-1 expression).	[72]
	TNBS-induced colitis in rats	Moderate reduction of inflammation.	[69]
	DSS-induced colitis in mice	Reduced inflammation (reduction of MPO and IL-12).	[70]
Lactobacillus rhamnosus	DNBS-induced colitis in rats	Reduced inflammation (reduction of PGE$_2$, MPO, and NO).	[74]
	Spontaneous colitis SCID mice	Prevention of development of the spontaneous colitis.	[65]
Lactobacillus fermentum	TNBS-induced colitis in rats	Reduced inflammation (reduction of pro-inflammatory cytokines, MPO and iNOS). Restoration of antioxidant levels.	[78]
	TNBS-induced colitis in mice	Reduced inflammation.	[79]
Escherichia coli Nissle 1917	DSS-induced colitis in mice	Reduced inflammation (reduction of IFNγ and IL-6).	[84]
	TNBS-induced colitis in rats	Reduced inflammation (reduction of MPO and pro-inflammatory cytokines).	[83]
Bifidobacterium infantis	IL-10 KO mice	Reduced inflammation (reduction of Th1 cytokines while levels of TGFβ are maintained).	[68]
Bifidobacterium bifidum	T CD4+ cells CD45RB/SCID	Reduced inflammation (reduction of pro-inflammatory cytokines such as IFNγ and MCP-1).	[88]

TNBS, trinitrobenzene sulfonic acid; DNBS, dinitrobenzene sulfonic acid; DSS, dextran sulfate sodium; KO, *knock-out*; Tg, transgenic; PG, prostaglandin; MPO, myeloperoxidase; NO, nitric oxide; iNOS, inducible nitric oxide synthase; IFN, interferon; IL, interleukin; MCP-1, monocyte chemoattractant protein-1; TGFβ, transforming growth factor; ICAM-1, intercellular adhesion molecule-1.

were administered to these mice [65], thus demonstrating the immunomodulatory properties of this lactobacilli strain.

Different strains of *L. salivarius* have also been reported to exert an intestinal anti-inflammatory effect in different experimental models. Thus, *L. salivarius* ssp. *salivarius* CECT5713 has shown beneficial effects in the TNBS model of rat colitis [66], *L. salivarius* Ls-33 displayed preventive effect in the TNBS model in mice [67], and *L. salivarius* ssp. *salivarius* UCC118 attenuated colitis in IL-10 KO mice [68]. These studies also revealed that the immunomodulatory properties of this probiotic can account for its beneficial effects.

The probiotic is able to down-regulate TNFα and IL-12 production in colitic rodents, and this was correlated with a decreased neutrophil infiltration in the inflamed tissue [66].

Similarly, the immunomodulatory properties of *L. casei* can definitively account for the intestinal anti-inflammatory effect shown in different experimental models of colitis, namely TNBS model in rats [69], DSS in mice [70], or in the spontaneous model of colitis in SAMP1/Yit mice [71]. One of the proposed actions for this probiotic is related to the modulation of leukocyte recruitment into the inflamed intestine. This was evidenced histologically, biochemically by a reduction of the marker of neutrophil infiltration, colonic myeloperoxidase (MPO) activity, or by intravital microscopy showing a reduction in the increased number of adherent leukocytes to the venular wall in the colonic microcirculation associated with the induction of colitis [72]. This effect could be related to the abrogation of the colonic ICAM-1 up-regulation which occurs in the TNBS model [72]. Finally, when the intestinal anti-inflammatory effect of *Lactobacillus casei* was evaluated in the DSS model of colitis in TLR-4 KO mice, an attenuation of the beneficial effect was observed, thus suggesting that the TLR-4 signaling pathway may play a key role in the effect showed by this probiotic [70].

The probiotic *Lactobacillus rhamnosus* GG has been used for the treatment of acute diarrheic processes in humans for some time [73], also showing a clear beneficial effect in experimental models of colitis. In this way, this probiotic attenuates TNBS colonic-induced damage in rats [74] and ameliorates the severity of colitis in SCID mice transplanted with CD4 T cells, with a similar efficacy to that shown by *Lactobacillus reuteri* DSM-12246 [65]. The administration of *Lactobacillus rhamnosus* GG to transgenic HLA-B27 rats did not prevent the development of colitis or ameliorated the disease once it has been established. However, when the probiotic treatment was initiated after oral administration of

vancomycin and imipenem for 2 weeks, it effectively prevented colitis relapse, as evidenced by a significant reduction in gross and histological score damage. This effect was associated with a decreased activity of cecal MPO, down-regulation of IL-1β and TNFα production and increased production of the anti-inflammatory cytokine IL-10, effects that were not achieved with *Lactobacillus plantarum* 299v [42]. Moreover, it has been proposed that *Lactobacillus rhamnosus* GG may be capable of producing soluble molecules that inhibit TNFα production in activated macrophages, altering the TNFα/IL-10 balance, thus contributing to the beneficial effects in intestinal inflammation [75]. In addition, *Lactobacillus rhamnosus* has been reported to improve intestinal barrier function by inhibition of apoptosis of intestinal epithelial cells and/or by inducing cyclooxygenase-2 expression [76, 77].

Two different strains of *Lactobacillus fermentum*, ACA-DC 179 and CECT5716, have been shown to exert intestinal anti-inflammatory effects in the TNBS model of colitis in mice and rats, respectively [78, 79]. These beneficial effects were associated with an inhibition in the production and release of pro-inflammatory mediators, like TNFα and nitric oxide. Moreover, other studies have revealed that viable *L. fermentum* and the supernatant of *L. fermentum* cultures, but not the heat-killed bacteria, inhibited IL-8 secretion of HeLa cells triggered by *Yersinia enterocolitica*; an effect most probably mediated by a secreted phospholipid [80]. Nevertheless, other properties attributed to this probiotic can clearly also contribute to its beneficial effects in IBD. In this sense, it has been described that *L. fermentum* CECT5716 is able to secrete different compounds with antioxidant properties, like glutathione, which can ameliorate the deleterious effects on the intestinal mucosa exerted by the increased production of reactive oxygen metabolites during intestinal inflammation [78]. In addition, both *L. fermentum* ACA-DC 179 and CECT5716 have been shown to possess antimicrobial activity towards a broad range of microorganisms, including pathogenic bacteria [63, 78, 79]. Finally, it is important to note that the intestinal anti-inflammatory effect shown by this probiotic is not restricted to the large intestine, since it has been demonstrated that *L. fermentum* BR11 ameliorates jejunal inflammation in a model of intestinal mucositis induced with 5-fluorouracil in rats [81].

Non-pathogenic *Escherichia coli* strain Nissle 1917 (O6:K5:H1) has also been successfully used for the treatment of various human diseases of the digestive tract, including diarrhea, diverticulitis and IBD [82]. Its intestinal anti-inflammatory effect has also been described in several experimental models of colitis induced by TNBS in rats [83] or by DSS in mice [84], being associated with the inhibition of the production of pro-inflammatory cytokines. Different mechanisms of action have been proposed to participate in the intestinal anti-inflammatory effects exerted by this probiotic including the inhibition of bacterial invasion [85], or the induction of the secretion of β-defensin 2 [86]. Furthermore, it has been reported that this probiotic may reinforce the mucosal barrier through the specifically up-regulation of the zonula occludens (ZO)-1 and ZO-2 mRNA expression in intestinal epithelial cells [57].

Although these lactobacilli strains represent the most studied type, similar conclusions have been obtained with other probiotics, including other lactobacilli strains or even yeasts like *Saccharomyces boulardii*, using the same models of experimental colitis [78].

The potential effect of bifidobacteria has been less evaluated, although some of them have shown beneficial effects, in which their immunomodulatory activity also plays a role (Table 35.4). The supplementation of *Bifidobacterium infantis* 35624 significantly attenuated colitis in IL-10 KO mice, which was associated with a reduced ability to produce Th1-type pro-inflammatory cytokines, like TNFα and IFNγ

in the colonic tissue, while maintaining the levels of the anti-inflammatory cytokine TGFβ [68]. *Bifidobacterium bifidum* BGN4, a probiotic with a prominent adhesive capacity for intestinal epithelial cells [87], was able to significantly ameliorate the intestinal inflammatory response in the CD4+ CD45RBhigh T cell transfer model, an effect associated with a significant reduction in the inflammatory cell infiltration and in the inflammatory cytokine productions in the inflamed large intestine [88].

Finally, and mainly based on clinical trials performed in human IBD, several probiotic mixtures have been tested in animal models in an attempt to improve their activity. However, in contrast to that observed in humans, no clear differences were observed in the efficacy of probiotic treatments with single bacterial strains or in combinations or mixtures, VSL#3 being the most effective probiotic combination tested up to date [56, 74, 89].

The lack of a higher efficacy of probiotic mixtures in comparison to single probiotic treatments in animal models, and the high activity observed with single probiotic treatments, may respond to the simplification of the pathology in the animal models. In animal models, such as chemically-induced and genetically-driven models, the pathology is induced by a reduced number of factors or alterations, and thus, it could be more easily counteracted than that observed in humans. In this sense, most of the probiotics tested in animal models act through the regulation of the inflammatory immune response, reduction of the inflammatory cell recruitment, and restoration of the barrier function. Moreover, it is important to take into consideration that probiotics are not equally beneficial, since each may have individual mechanisms of action, and host characteristics may determine which probiotic species and even strain may be optimal. For this reason, it would be interesting to establish the most important characteristics reported for the probiotics in the different experimental models, in order to establish the best profile in a given setting and to further understand this new concept for the therapy of IBD.

4. INTESTINAL ANTI-INFLAMMATORY ACTIVITY EXERTED BY PREBIOTICS IN EXPERIMENTAL MODELS OF INTESTINAL INFLAMMATION

The term 'prebiotic' was initially proposed by Gibson and Roberfroid [90] and refers to 'a non-digestible food ingredient that beneficially affects the host by selectively stimulating the growth and/or activity of one or a limited number of bacteria in the colon, and thus improves host health.' The prebiotic definition does not emphasize or target any specific bacterial group. However, it is generally assumed that a prebiotic should increase the number and/or activity of bifidobacteria and lactobacilli.

Prebiotics are isolated from plants (e.g. chicory root) or industrially synthesized (e.g. enzymatically from sucrose), and can be incorporated into many foodstuffs, thus receiving high commercial interest. Moreover, due to their excellent safety profile and lack of serious side effects, the prebiotic therapeutic applications invite clinical trials on how to prevent various gastrointestinal disorders. Of note, although the prebiotic market is mostly restricted to a handful of nutritional companies, new products are expected to be incorporated due to the increasing interests shown by pharmaceutical companies.

Nowadays, the prebiotics used in Europe and the United States are limited so far to inulin, oligofructose (also named fructo-oligosaccharides or FOS) and galacto-oligosaccharides (GOS), mainly as food ingredients. Lactulose, a semi-synthetic disaccharide made from lactose, is also considered to be a prebiotic but is considered more as a medicinal product than a prebiotic food supplement [91]. It is important to note that some dietary fibers, like *Plantago ovata* seeds, germinated barley foodstuff and rice bran, have also been demonstrated to exert prebiotic functions [92]. Moreover, there is a growing list of potential synthetic candidates to prebiotics such as polydextrose, soybean oligosaccharides, isomalto-oligosaccharides, gluco-oligosaccharides, xylo-oligosaccharides, palatinose, gentio-oligosaccharides and sugar alcohols (such as lactitol, sorbitol and maltitol) (Table 35.5).

Since 1995, when the prebiotic concept was first used, there have been several studies evaluating the beneficial role of prebiotics in gastrointestinal health. The administration of these compounds has been shown to increase fecal biomass and water content of the stools, thus improving bowel habits [93]. Other studies have demonstrated other positive effects for prebiotics, like serum lipid-lowering activity and enhancing immune system effectiveness [94].

The described mechanisms by which the prebiotics promote their effects on intestine function are mainly based on two indirect effects by: 1) the modulation of bacteria counts, and thus acting in a similar way to probiotics; and 2) producing high amounts of short-chain fatty acids (SCFA) (Figure 35.1). In this sense, inulin and oligofructose fed supplementation for 2 weeks increases the number of bifidobacteria and lactobacilli in the mucosa-associated communities of the human colon [95]. Moreover, the increased counts of indigenous lactobacilli in the cecal lumen by oral administration of inulin are associated to a reduction in the intracolonic pH, most probably caused by increased SCFA production and to a selective stimulation of bifidobacteria growth. This would induce important changes in the composition of gut microbiota, increasing the potentially health-promoting bacteria and reducing the potentially harmful species [96].

Because bifidobacteria and lactobacilli are presumed to be antagonistic to pathogenic bacteria

TABLE 35.5　Different types of prebiotics

	Prebiotic name	Origin/Manufacturing procedure	Fermentable
Polysaccharides	Inulin	Extracts obtained from cereals, vegetables and legumes	YES
	Resistant starch	Extracts obtained from cereals, vegetables and legumes	YES
	Plantago ovata peel	Plant source	Partially
	Plantago ovata seeds	Plant source	Partially
	Germinated barley foodstuff (GBF)	Plant source	Partially
	Rice bran	Plant source	Partially
Oligosaccharides	Fructo-oligosaccharides (FOS)	Plants (legumes, vegetables, extracts)/ hydrolysis of cereals/synthesized	YES
	Galacto-oligosaccharides (GOS)	Synthesized/milk	YES
	Soybean oligosaccharides	Hydrolysis of soybean	NA
	Xylo-oligosaccharides	Plant source	NA
	Short-chain fructo-oligosaccharides (SC-FOS)	Hydrolysis of inulin	YES
	Trans-galacto-oligosaccharides	Lactose synthetic	?
Disaccharides	Lactulose	Lactose synthetic	?
	Lactitol	Lactose synthetic	NA

?, preliminary data but further research still needed; NA, data not available.

and to promote non-specific stimulation of the immune system, it is possible that the mechanisms by which inulin and derived compounds confer beneficial effects on the host will include immunomodulatory effect. Nevertheless, there have been few reports on the effect of dietary FOS or other prebiotics on the mucosal immune system. It has been demonstrated that dietary FOS enhanced the development of the gut-associated lymphoid tissue, and up-regulated the fecal IgA content in the adult mouse. Finally, this prebiotic also increases the intestinal IgA response and pIgR expression in the small intestine as well as the colon in infant mice [97, 98].

In the large bowel, the anaerobic bacteria ferment prebiotics in order to produce SCFA, mainly acetate, propionate and butyrate. There are good candidates to explain not only the gastrointestinal improvements, but also some of their systemic effects [99]. Among them, butyrate is considered as the major energy substrate for colonocytes, which also promotes key functions of the intestinal epithelium, including cell proliferation and differentiation, tight junction permeability and epithelial restitution [100]. It seems that butyrate protects against carcinogenesis [101], at least in rats, and this is probably related to its ability to induce inhibition of histones phosphorylation [102]. In addition, it has been suggested that butyrate plays an important role in mucosal repair in inflammatory conditions, through the inhibition of the production and release of inflammatory mediators, including cytokines. In this sense, different studies have shown that topical SCFA treatment can effectively be used to treat human IBD and experimental bowel inflammation in rats [103–105]. In consequence, butyrate could actively participate in promoting the epithelium regeneration that may occur after colonic damage.

4.1. Studies of Prebiotics in Experimental Models of Rodent Colitis

Similar to that previously commented with the probiotics, the experimental models of colitis have also provided valuable information about the mechanisms of action implicated in the anti-inflammatory effects of prebiotics, supporting their potential role in the treatment of human IBD. The prebiotics have been mainly tested in the TNBS and DSS chemically-induced models of colitis, but data from HLA-B27 transgenic rats or IL-10 gene-deficient mice have also been reported (see Table 35.6).

The dietary supplementation with *Plantago ovata* seeds leads to an improvement in the inflammatory status in two colitis experimental models: TNBS model and HLA-B27 transgenic rats [106, 107]. This intestinal anti-inflammatory effect was associated with a significant reduction in TNFα levels in the inflamed colon, when compared with non-treated colitic rats [106]. Moreover, in both models, the intestinal contents from fiber-treated colitic rats showed a significantly higher production of SCFA, butyrate and propionate, than non-treated colitic animals. The increased production of these SCFA may contribute to the recovery of the damaged colonic mucosa because they constitute substrates for the colonocyte and, additionally, they can inhibit the production of pro-inflammatory mediators, like TNFα.

Moreover, it has been suggested that the butyrate generated from the bacterial fermentation of germinated barley foodstuff (GBF), an insoluble mixture of glutamine-rich protein and hemicellulose-rich dietary fiber, clearly contributes to the intestinal anti-inflammatory effect observed in the spontaneous colitis induced in HLA-B27 transgenic rats and in the DSS models

of colitis in mice [108, 109] and rats [109, 110]. Furthermore, it has been demonstrated that resistant starch also showed anti-inflammatory activity in the DSS and TNBS models of murine colitis [111–113].

Other studies have reported the beneficial effects obtained with soluble dietary fiber in different experimental models of rodent colitis. Treatment with oral inulin to rats exposed to DSS resulted in the amelioration of damaged mucosa and a decreased severity of crypt destruction, an effect associated with a significant reduction in tissue MPO activity and in the mucosal release of inflammatory mediators [114, 115]. Moreover, FOS supplementation has been shown to attenuate TNBS-induced colitis in rats, promoting the growth of beneficial lactic acid bacteria and increasing colonic butyrate levels [116]. However, another study has reported that no beneficial effect was observed in the DSS-induced colitis model in rats [111]. Holma et al. have reported a similar inefficacy of galacto-oligosaccharides in TNBS-colitis rats [117], although the lack of efficacy has not been consistent with other studies. For instance, DSS-colitis rats fed goat's milk oligosaccharides showed a beneficial preventive effect evidenced by maintenance in bodyweight, a decreased colonic MPO activity, and milder clinical symptoms, as well as an increased MUC-3 compared with the control group [118]. In consequence, further studies are necessary to elucidate the mechanism involved in the beneficial effect of these compounds in intestinal function and their implication in human intestinal inflammation.

Interesting results have been obtained when short-chain fructo-oligosaccharides (SC-FOS), obtained by hydrolysis and purification procedures from inulin, are used as prebiotics. These prebiotics, in spite of being preferentially fermented in the upper part of the large intestine, seem to be as effective as other longer chain FOS in the amelioration of distal colonic inflammation. Thus, administration of SC-FOS to rats significantly ameliorated the extent of severity

TABLE 35.6　Prebiotics used in IBD animal studies

Prebiotic	Animal model	Results	References
Plantago ovata seeds	TNBS-induced colitis in rats	Reduced inflammation (reduction of MPO, TNFα and NO). Increased SCFA production.	[106]
	HLA-B27 Tg rats	Reduced inflammation (reduction of MPO, TNFα, NO and LTB$_4$). Increased SCFA production.	[107]
Germinated barley foodstuff (GBF)	DSS-induced colitis in rats	Reduced inflammation (improve intestinal barrier function). Increased butyrate production.	[108]
	DSS-induced colitis in rats	Reduced inflammation. Increased butyrate production.	[109]
	DSS-induced colitis in mice	Reduced inflammation. Increased butyrate production and adsorption of bile acids.	[110]
Resistant starch	DSS-induced colitis in rats	Reduced inflammation. Increased butyrate production.	[111]
	DSS-induced colitis in rats	Reduced inflammation. Increased butyrate uptake and its oxidation.	[112]
	TNBS-induced colitis in rats	Reduced inflammation (reduction of colonic permeability). Increased butyrate production.	[113]
Inulin	DSS-induced colitis in rats	Reduced inflammation (reduction of MPO and eicosanoids). Increased lactobacilli counts.	[114]
	DSS-induced colitis in rats	Reduced inflammation (reduction of MPO and IL-1β). Increased butyrate production.	[115]
Fructo-oligosaccharides (FOS)	DSS-induced colitis in rats	Moderate reduction of inflammation. Increased butyrate production.	[115]
	DSS-induced colitis in rats	Inefficacy in experimental colitis. Increased butyrate production.	[111]
	TNBS-induced colitis in rat	Reduced inflammation (reduction of MPO). Increased lactate and butyrate production and lactobacilli counts.	[116]
Short-chain fructo-oligosaccharides (SC-FOS)	TNBS-induced colitis in rat	Reduced inflammation (reduction of MPO, LTB$_4$ and NO). Increased SCFA production and lactobacilli/bifidobacteria counts.	[119]
Galacto-oligosaccharides (GOS)	TNBS-induced colitis in rat	Inefficacy in experimental colitis. Increased bifidobacteria counts.	[117]
	DSS-induced colitis in rat	Reduced inflammation (reduction of MPO and restoration of mucine-3 gene expression).	[118]
Lactulose	IL-10 KO mice	Prevention of development of the spontaneous colitis. Normalization of lactobacilli counts.	[64]
	DSS-induced colitis in rat	Reduced inflammation (reduction of MPO).	[121]
	TNBS-induced colitis in rat	Reduced inflammation (reduction of MPO, TNFα and NO). Increased lactobacilli and bifidobacteria counts.	[120]

TNBS, trinitrobenzene sulfonic acid; DSS, dextran sulfate sodium; Tg, transgenic; KO, *knock-out*; MPO, myeloperoxidase; NO, nitric oxide; TNF, tumor necrosis factor; SCFA, short-chain fatty acids; LTB$_4$, leukotriene B$_4$; PAF, platelet activating factor; PG, prostaglandin; IL, interleukin.

in the colonic damage in the TNBS model of rat colitis has been demonstrated [119]. This beneficial effect was associated with a reduction of colonic MPO activity, LTB_4 production and iNOS expression. Moreover, the prebiotic role of SC-FOS was also evident, since the decrease in colon lactobacilli and bifidobacteria caused by TNBS treatment in colitic rats fed the SC-FOS diet was not observed.

The effects of the prebiotic lactulose have also been tested in different animal models of intestinal inflammation. Lactulose supplementation facilitates the recovery of the inflamed tissue in the TNBS model of rat colitis, an effect that is associated with the amelioration in the production of some of the mediators involved in the inflammatory response of the intestine, like TNFα and NO (Table 34.6). This beneficial effect could again be ascribed to its prebiotic effect, by increasing the lactobacilli and bifidobacteria counts in comparison with non-treated colitic rats, thus attenuating the exacerbated immune response evoked by the colonic instillation of the hapten TNBS in rats [120]. Lactulose has also demonstrated a dose-dependent beneficial effect in DSS-induced colitis in rats, including improvements of colonic ulceration areas, body-weight changes, diarrhea, bloody stools and a reduction of MPO activity and microscopic colitis [121]. Likewise, protective effects of lactulose have been demonstrated in IL-10 KO mice [64].

Finally, several prebiotic mixtures and combinations between prebiotics/probiotics have been tested in animal models in order to improve their activity. Thus, the combination of fructo-oligosaccharides and inulin showed anti-inflammatory activity in spontaneous colitis in HLA-B27 rats [122]. The effects of oligofructose or inulin alone or in combination with probiotics have also been tested in the DSS model of rodent colitis [115], showing an improved colonic MPO activity, as well as reduced expression of inflammatory mediators. A similar study performed in HLA-B27 transgenic rats reported the effects of the symbiotic 'SIM', a combination

of lactobacilli, bifidobacteria and the prebiotic inulin, although the beneficial effects were mainly attributed to the inulin rather than to the presence of the probiotics in the combination [84].

One of the common characteristics reported in most of these studies performed with prebiotics is the fact that the beneficial effects could be associated with the increased production of SCFA in the intestinal lumen. Of note, it has been suggested that intracellular butyrate oxidation is impaired in patients with ulcerative colitis [123]. Moreover, decreased β-oxidation in colonic epithelial cells, similar to that observed in ulcerative colitis [124], was shown in the murine model of DSS-induced colitis [125]. Thus, the energetic deficit in the colonocytes observed during IBD could be counteracted by prebiotic treatment. In this sense, FOS treatment in TNBS-induced colitis increased the concentration of lactate and butyrate as well as the counts of lactic acid bacteria in the cecal contents. Since the direct intracecal infusion of lactic acid bacteria together with SCFAs was able to reproduce the intestinal anti-inflammatory effects of FOS in the TNBS-induced colitis, it has been suggested that fermentation of the prebiotic by lactic acid bacteria was the principal mechanism mediating their anti-inflammatory effect [116].

In addition to their effects on the metabolic function of the epithelial cells and on the modulation of microflora content in the gut lumen, the increased production of SCFAs associated to prebiotic intake may result in other different actions, which definitively also contribute to the intestinal anti-inflammatory effect evidenced in experimental models. These beneficial effects were associated to a reduction in the production of pro-inflammatory cytokines, including IL-6, IL-8, IL-1β and TNFα [106–109, 110], and even to enhance the expression of regulatory type cytokines like TGFβ [122]. However, the direct mechanism of action produced by prebiotics in the immune system has not been totally elucidated.

5. CONCLUSIONS

In conclusion, there is increasing evidence supporting the pivotal role that probiotics and prebiotics may have in the prevention and management of various gastrointestinal disorders, although this will depend on the bacteria and/ or prebiotic used, as well as the type and severity of the intestinal condition to be treated. These 'pharmabiotics' constitute a heterogeneous group with different properties and biological effects on gut physiology and pathophysiology. In addition, similar bacteria do not share similar therapeutic activity. Further work with well-designed randomized control clinical trials is necessary in order to understand the undoubted role of these agents in the management of gut physiology in health and disease. Meanwhile the use of validated experimental models has allowed the selection and exploration of potential therapeutical candidates previously to their translation to the human beings.

References

1. Gassull, M. A., & Cabré, E. (1994). Clinical guidelines for the diagnosis of IBD. In M. Gassull (Ed.), *Management of Inflammatory Bowel Disease* (pp. 7–12). Barcelona: Prous Science.
2. Gasche, C. (2000). Complications of inflammatory bowel disease. *Hepatogastroenterol, 47*, 49–56.
3. Laroux, F. S., Pavlick, K. P., Wolf, R. E., & Grisham, M. B. (2001). Dysregulation of intestinal mucosal immunity: Implications in inflammatory bowel disease. *News in Physiological Sciences, 16*, 272–277.
4. Neurath, M. F., Finotto, S., Fuss, I., et al. (2001). Regulation of T-cell apoptosis in inflammatory bowel disease: To die or not to die, that is the mucosal question. *Trends in Immunology, 22*, 21–26.
5. Bamias, G., Nyce, M. R., De La Rue, S. A., & Cominelli, F. (2005). New concepts in the pathophysiology of inflammatory bowel disease. *Annals of Internal Medicine, 143*, 895–904.
6. Katz, J. A., Itoh, J., & Fiocchi, C. (1999). Pathogenesis of inflammatory bowel disease. *Current Opinion in Gastroenterology, 15*, 291–297.
7. El-Zaatari, F. A., Osato, M. S., & Graham, D. Y. (2001). Etiology of Crohn's disease: The role of Mycobacterium avium paratuberculosis. *Trends in Molecular Medicine, 7*, 247–252.
8. Muller, S., Arni, S., Varga, L., et al. (2006). Serological and DNA-based evaluation of *Chlamydia pneumoniae* infection in inflammatory bowel disease. *European Journal of Gastroenterology & Hepatology, 18*, 889–894.
9. Ohkusa, T., Nomura, T., & Sato, N. (2004). The role of bacterial infection in the pathogenesis of inflammatory bowel disease. *Internal Medicine, 43*, 534–539.
10. Criscuoli, V., Rizzuto, M. R., & Cottone, M. (2006). Cytomegalovirus and inflammatory bowel disease: is there a link? *World Journal of Gastroenterology, 12*, 4813–4818.
11. Cario, E., & Podolsky, D. K. (2000). Differential alteration in intestinal epithelial cell expression of toll-like receptor 3 (TLR3) and TLR4 in inflammatory bowel disease. *Infection and Immunity, 68*, 7010–7017.
12. Hampe, J., Cuthbert, A., Croucher, P. J., et al. (2001). Association between insertion mutation in NOD2 gene and Crohn's disease in German and British populations. *Lancet, 357*, 1925–1928.
13. Hugot, J. P. (2006). CARD15/NOD2 mutations in Crohn's disease. *Annals of the New York Academy of Sciences, 1072*, 9–18.
14. Brant, S. R., Wang, M. H., Rawsthorne, P., et al. (2007). A population-based case–control study of CARD15 and other risk factors in Crohn's disease and ulcerative colitis. *The American Journal of Gastroenterology, 102*, 313–323.
15. Macpherson, A., Khoo, U. Y., Forgacs, I., et al. (1996). Mucosal antibodies in inflammatory bowel disease are directed against intestinal bacteria. *Gut, 38*, 365–375.
16. Sellon, R. K., Tonkonogy, S., Schultz, M., et al. (1998). Resident enteric bacteria are necessary for development of spontaneous colitis and immune system activation in interleukin–10-deficient mice. *Infection and Immunity, 66*, 5224–5231.
17. Taurog, J. D., Richardson, J. A., Croft, J. T., et al. (1994). The germfree state prevents development of gut and joint inflammatory disease in HLA-B27 transgenic rats. *The Journal of Experimental Medicine, 180*, 2359–2364.
18. Tannock, G. W. (2007). What immunologists should know about bacterial communities of the human bowel. *Seminars in Immunology, 19*, 94–105.
19. Ott, S. J., Musfeldt, M., Wenderoth, D. F., et al. (2004). Reduction in diversity of the colonic mucosa associated bacterial microflora in patients with active inflammatory bowel disease. *Gut, 53*, 685–693.
20. Manichanh, C., Rigotier-Gois, L., Bonnaud, E., et al. (2006). Reduced diversity of faecal microbiota in Crohn's disease revealed by a metagenomic approach. *Gut, 55*, 205–211.
21. Sokol, H., Seksik, P., Rigottier-Gois, L., et al. (2006). Specificities of the fecal microbiota in inflammatory bowel disease. *Inflammatory Bowel Diseases, 12*, 106–111.

22. Tamboli, C. P., Neut, C., Desreumaux, P., & Colombel, J. F. (2004). Dysbiosis in inflammatory bowel disease. *Gut*, *53*, 1–4.

23. Swidsinski, A., Weber, J., Loening-Baucke, V., et al. (2005). Spatial organization and composition of the mucosal flora in patients with inflammatory bowel disease. *Journal of Clinical Microbiology*, *43*, 3380–3389.

24. MacPherson, B. R., & Pfeiffer, C. J. (1978). Experimental production of diffuse colitis in rats. *Digestion*, *17*, 135–150.

25. Elson, C. O., Sartor, R. B., Tennyson, G. S., & Riddell, R. H. (1995). Experimental models of inflammatory bowel disease. *Gastroenterology*, *109*, 1344–1367.

26. Morris, G. P., Beck, P. L., Herridge, M. S., et al. (1989). Hapten-induced model of chronic inflammation and ulceration in the rat colon. *Gastroenterology*, *96*, 795–803.

27. Fuss, I. J., Boirivant, M., Lacy, B., & Strober, W. (2002). The interrelated roles of TGF-beta and IL–10 in the regulation of experimental colitis. *Journal of Immunology*, *168*, 900–908.

28. Okayasu, I., Hatakeyama, S., Yamada, M., et al. (1990). A novel method in the induction of reliable experimental acute and chronic ulcerative colitis in mice. *Gastroenterology*, *98*, 694–702.

29. Podolsky, D. K. (2002). The current future understanding of inflammatory bowel disease. *Best Practice & Research Clinical Gastroenterology*, *16*, 933–943.

30. Rath, H. C., Schultz, M., Freitag, R., et al. (2001). Different subsets of enteric bacteria induce and perpetuate experimental colitis in rats and mice. *Infection and Immunity*, *69*, 2277–2285.

31. Sartor, R. B., Bond, T. M., & Schwab, J. H. (1988). Systemic uptake and intestinal inflammatory effects of luminal bacterial cell wall polymers in rats with acute colonic injury. *Infection and Immunity*, *56*, 2101–2108.

32. Satoh, H., Sato, F., Takami, K., & Szabo, S. (1997). New ulcerative colitis model induced by sulfhydryl blockers in rats and the effects of antiinflammatory drugs on the colitis. *Japanese Journal of Pharmacology*, *73*, 299–309.

33. Yamada, T., Deitch, E., Specian, R. D., et al. (1993). Mechanisms of acute and chronic intestinal inflammation induced by indomethacin. *Inflammation*, *17*, 641–662.

34. Boirivant, M., Fuss, I. J., Chu, A., & Strober, W. (1998). Oxazolone colitis: A murine model of T helper cell type 2 colitis treatable with antibodies to interleukin 4. *The Journal of Experimental Medicine*, *188*, 1929–1939.

35. Sundberg, J. P., Elson, C. O., Bedigian, H., & Birkenmeier, E. H. (1994). Spontaneous, heritable colitis in a new substrain of C3H/HeJ mice. *Gastroenterology*, *107*, 1726–1735.

36. Brandwein, S. L., McCabe, R. P., Cong, Y., et al. (1997). Spontaneously colitic C3H/HeJBir mice demonstrate selective antibody reactivity to antigens of the enteric bacterial flora. *Journal of Immunology*, *159*, 44–52.

37. Lodes, M. J., Cong, Y., Elson, C. O., et al. (2004). Bacterial flagellin is a dominant antigen in Crohn disease. *The Journal of Clinical Investigation*, *113*, 1296–1306.

38. Matsumoto, S., Okabe, Y., Setoyama, H., et al. (1998). Inflammatory bowel disease-like enteritis and caecitis in a senescence accelerated mouse P1/Yit strain. *Gut*, *43*, 71–78.

39. Kosiewicz, M. M., Nast, C. C., Krishnan, A., et al. (2001). Th1-type responses mediate spontaneous ileitis in a novel murine model of Crohn's disease. *The Journal of Clinical Investigation*, *107*, 695–702.

40. Hammer, R. E., Maika, S. D., Richardson, J. A., et al. (1990). Spontaneous inflammatory disease in transgenic rats expressing HLA-B27 and human beta 2m: an animal model of HLA-B27-associated human disorders. *Cell*, *63*, 1099–1112.

41. Rath, H. C., Herfarth, H. H., Ikeda, J. S., et al. (1996). Normal luminal bacteria, especially Bacteroides species, mediate chronic colitis, gastritis, and arthritis in HLA-B27/human beta2 microglobulin transgenic rats. *The Journal of Clinical Investigation*, *98*, 945–953.

42. Dieleman, L. A., Goerres, M. S., Arends, A., et al. (2003). *Lactobacillus* GG prevents recurrence of colitis in HLA-B27 transgenic rats after antibiotic treatment. *Gut*, *52*, 370–376.

43. Kühn, R., Löhler, J., Rennick, D., et al. (1993). Interleukin–10-deficient mice develop chronic enterocolitis. *Cell*, *75*, 263–274.

44. Morissey, P. J., Charrier, K., Braddy, S., et al. (1993). CD4+ T cells that express high levels of CD45RB induce wasting disease when transferred into congenic severe combined immunodeficient mice. Disease development is prevented by cotransfer of purified CD4+ T cells. *The Journal of Experimental Medicine*, *178*, 237–244.

45. Mombaerts, P., Mizoguchi, E., Grusby, M. J., et al. (1993). Spontaneous development of inflammatory bowel disease in T cell receptor mutant mice. *Cell*, *75*, 274–282.

46. Sadlack, B., Merz, H., Schorle, H., et al. (1993). Ulcerative colitis-like disease in mice with a disrupted interleukin–2 gene. *Cell*, *75*, 253–261.

47. Leach, M. W., Bean, A. G., Mauze, S., et al. (1996). Inflammatory bowel disease in C.B–17 scid mice reconstituted with the CD45RBhigh subset of CD4+ T cells. *The American Journal of Pathology*, *148*, 1503–1515.

48. Rivera-Nieves, J., Bamias, G., Vidrich, A., et al. (2003). Emergence of perianal fistulizing disease in the SAMP1/YitFc mouse, a spontaneous model of chronic ileitis. *Gastroenterology*, *124*, 972–982.

49. Wirtz, S., Finotto, S., Kanzler, S., et al. (1999). Cutting edge: Chronic intestinal inflammation in STAT–4 transgenic mice: Characterization of disease and adoptive transfer by TNF- plus IFN-gamma-producing CD4+ T cells that respond to bacterial antigens. *Journal of Immunology*, *162*, 1884–1888.

50. Kontoyiannis, D., Pasparakis, M., Pizarro, T. T., et al. (1999). Impaired on/off regulation of TNF biosynthesis in mice lacking TNF AU-rich elements: implications for joint and gut-associated immunopathologies. *Immunity*, *10*, 387–398.

51. Guarner, F., & Schaafsma, G. J. (1998). Probiotics. *International Journal of Food Microbiology*, *39*, 237–238.

52. Metchnikoff, E. (1907). *The prolongation of life. Optimistic studies*. London: William Heinemann.

53. Morrison, D. J., Mackay, W. G., Edwards, C. A., et al. (2006). Butyrate production from oligofructose fermentation by the human faecal flora: What is the contribution of extracellular acetate and lactate? *The British Journal of Nutrition*, *96*, 570–577.

54. Lievin, V., Peiffer, I., Hudault, S., et al. (2000). Bifidobacterium strains from resident infant human gastrointestinal microflora exert antimicrobial activity. *Gut*, *47*, 646–652.

55. Boris, S., Jimenez-Diaz, R., Caso, J. L., & Barbes, C. (2001). Partial characterization of a bacteriocin produced by *Lactobacillus delbrueckii* subsp. *lactis* UO004, an intestinal isolate with probiotic potential. *Journal of Applied Microbiology*, *91*, 328–333.

56. Madsen, K., Cornish, A., Soper, P., et al. (2001). Probiotic bacteria enhance murine and human intestinal epithelial barrier function. *Gastroenterology*, *121*, 580–591.

57. Zyrek, A. A., Cichon, C., Helms, S., et al. (2007). Molecular mechanisms underlying the probiotic effects of *Escherichia coli* Nissle 1917 involve ZO–2 and PKCzeta redistribution resulting in tight junction and epithelial barrier repair. *Cellular Microbiology*, *9*, 804–816.

58. Chen, C. C., Louie, S., Shi, H. N., & Walker, W. A. (2005). Preinoculation with the probiotic *Lactobacillus acidophilus* early in life effectively inhibits murine *Citrobacter rodentium* colitis. *Pediatric Research*, *58*, 1185–1191.

59. Schultz, M., Linde, H. J., Lehn, N., et al. (2003). Immunomodulatory consequences of oral administration of *Lactobacillus rhamnosus* strain GG in healthy volunteers. *The Journal of Dairy Research*, *70*, 165–173.

60. Fabia, R., Ar'Rajab, A., Johansson, M. L., et al. (1993). Impairment of bacterial flora in human ulcerative colitis and experimental colitis in the rat. *Digestion*, *54*, 248–255.

61. Fabia, R., Ar'Rajab, A., Johansson, M. L., et al. (1993). The effect of exogenous administration of *Lactobacillus reuteri* R2LC and oat fiber on acetic acid-induced colitis in the rat. *Scandinavian Journal of Gastroenterology*, *28*, 155–162.

62. Holma, R., Salmenperä, P., Lohi, J., et al. (2001). Effects of *Lactobacillus rhamnosus* GG and *Lactobacillus reuteri* R2LC on acetic acid-induced colitis in rats. *Scandinavian Journal of Gastroenterology*, *36*, 630–635.

63. Peran, L., Sierra, S., Comalada, M., et al. (2007). A comparative study of the preventative effects exerted by two probiotics, *Lactobacillus reuteri* and *Lactobacillus fermentum*, in the trinitrobenzenesulfonic acid model of rat colitis. *The British Journal of Nutrition*, *97*, 96–103.

64. Madsen, K. L., Doyle, J. S., Jewell, L. D., et al. (1999). Lactobacillus species prevents colitis in interleukin 10 gene-deficient mice. *Gastroenterology*, *116*, 1107–1114.

65. Møller, P. L., Paerregaard, A., Gad, M., et al. (2005). Colitic scid mice fed *Lactobacillus* spp. show an ameliorated gut histopathology and an altered cytokine profile by local T cells. *Inflammatory Bowel Diseases*, *11*, 814–819.

66. Peran, L., Camuesco, D., Comalada, M., et al. (2005). Preventative effects of a probiotic, *Lactobacillus salivarius* ssp. *salivarius*, in the TNBS model of rat colitis. *World Journal of Gastroenterology*, *11*, 5185–5192.

67. Daniel, C., Poiret, S., Goudercourt, D., et al. (2006). Selecting lactic acid bacteria for their safety and functionality by use of a mouse colitis model. *Applied and Environmental Microbiology*, *72*, 5799–5805.

68. McCarthy, J., O'Mahony, L., O'Callaghan, L., et al. (2003). Double blind, placebo controlled trial of two probiotic strains in interleukin 10 knockout mice and mechanistic link with cytokine balance. *Gut*, *52*, 975–980.

69. Peran, L., Camuesco, D., Comalada, M., et al. (2007). A comparative study of the preventative effects exerted by three probiotics, *Bifidobacterium lactis*, *Lactobacillus casei* and *Lactobacillus acidophilus*, in the TNBS model of rat colitis. *Journal of Applied Microbiology*, *103*, 836–844.

70. Chung, Y. W., Choi, J. H., Oh, T. Y., et al. (2008). *Lactobacillus casei* prevents the development of dextran sulphate sodium-induced colitis in Toll-like receptor 4 mutant mice. *Clinical and Experimental Immunology*, *151*, 182–189.

71. Matsumoto, S., Hara, T., Hori, T., et al. (2005). Probiotic Lactobacillus-induced improvement in murine chronic inflammatory bowel disease is associated with the down-regulation of pro-inflammatory cytokines in lamina propria mononuclear cells. *Clinical and Experimental Immunology*, *140*, 417–426.

72. Angulo, S., Llopis, M., Antolín, M., et al. (2006). *Lactobacillus casei* prevents the upregulation of ICAM–1 expression and leukocyte recruitment in experimental colitis. *American Journal of Physiology. Gastrointestinal and Liver Physiology*, *291*, G1155–G1162.

73. Marteau, P. R., de Vrese, M., Cellier, C. J., & Schrezenmeir, J. (2001). Protection from gastrointestinal diseases with the use of probiotics. *The American Journal of Clinical Nutrition*, *73*, 430S–436S.

74. Shibolet, O., Karmeli, F., & Eliakim, R. et al. (2002). Variable response to probiotics in two models of experimental colitis in rats. *Inflammatory Bowel Diseases*, *8*, 399–406.

75. Peña, J. A., & Versalovic, J. (2003). *Lactobacillus rhamnosus* GG decreases TNF-alpha production in

lipopolysaccharide-activated murine macrophages by a contact-independent mechanism. *Cellular Microbiology, 5,* 277–285.

76. Gotteland, M., Cruchet, S., & Verbeke, S. (2001). Effect of Lactobacillus ingestion on the gastrointestinal mucosal barrier alterations induced by indometacin in humans. *Alimentary Pharmacology & Therapeutics, 15,* 11–17.

77. Korhonen, R., Kosonen, O., Korpela, R., & Moilanen, E. (2004). The expression of COX2 protein induced by *Lactobacillus rhamnosus* GG, endotoxin and lipoteichoic acid in T84 epithelial cells. *Letters in Applied Microbiology, 39,* 19–24.

78. Peran, L., Camuesco, D., Comalada, M., et al. (2006). *Lactobacillus fermentum*, a probiotic capable to release glutathione, prevents colonic inflammation in the TNBS model of rat colitis. *International Journal of Colorectal Disease, 21,* 737–746.

79. Zoumpopoulou, G., Foligne, B., Christodoulou, K., et al. (2008). *Lactobacillus fermentum* ACA-DC 179 displays probiotic potential *in vitro* and protects against trinitrobenzene sulfonic acid (TNBS)-induced colitis and Salmonella infection in murine models. *International Journal of Food Microbiologyl, 121,* 18–26.

80. Frick, J. S., Schenk, K., Quitadamo, M., et al. (2007). *Lactobacillus fermentum* attenuates the proinflammatory effect of *Yersinia enterocolitica* on human epithelial cells. *Inflammatory Bowel Diseases, 13,* 83–90.

81. Smith, C. L., Geier, M. S., Yazbeck, R., et al. (2008). *Lactobacillus fermentum* BR11 and fructo-oligosaccharide partially reduce jejunal inflammation in a model of intestinal mucositis in rats. *Nutrition and Cancer, 60,* 757–767.

82. Schultz, M. (2008). Clinical use of *E. coli* Nissle 1917 in inflammatory bowel disease. *Inflammatory Bowel Diseases, 14,* 1012–1018.

83. Arribas, B., Rodríguez-Cabezas, M. E., Comalada, M., et al. (2009). Evaluation of the preventative effects exerted by *Lactobacillus fermentum* in an experimental model of septic shock induced in mice. *The British Journal of Nutrition, 101,* 51–58.

84. Schultz, M., Strauch, U. G., Linde, H. J., et al. (2004). Preventive effects of *Escherichia coli* strain Nissle 1917 on acute and chronic intestinal inflammation in two different murine models of colitis. *Clinical and Diagnostic Laboratory Immunology, 11,* 372–378.

85. Boudeau, J., Glasser, A. L., Julien, S., et al. (2003). Inhibitory effect of probiotic *Escherichia coli* strain Nissle 1917 on adhesion to and invasion of intestinal epithelial cells by adherent-invasive *E. coli* strains isolated from patients with Crohn's disease. *Alimentary Pharmacology & Therapeutics, 18,* 45–56.

86. Wehkamp, J., Fellermann, K., Herrlinger, K. R., et al. (2005). Mechanisms of disease: Defensins in gastrointestinal diseases. *Nature Clinical Practice. Gastroenterology & Hepatology, 2,* 406–415.

87. Kim, I., Park, M., & Ji, G. (2003). Characterization of adhesion of *Bifidobacterium* sp. BGN4 to human enterocyte-like caco–2 cells. *Journal of Microbiology and Biotechnology, 13,* 276–281.

88. Kim, N., Kunisawa, J., Kweon, M. N., et al. (2007). Oral feeding of *Bifidobacterium bifidum* (BGN4) prevents CD4(+) CD45RB(high) T cell-mediated inflammatory bowel disease by inhibition of disordered T cell activation. *Clinical Immunology, 123,* 30–39.

89. Mennigen, R., Nolte, K., Rijcken, E. M., et al. (2009). Probiotic mixture VSLd3 protects the epithelial barrier by maintaining tight junction protein expression and preventing apoptosis in a murine model of colitis. *American Journal of Physiology Gastrointestinal and Liver Physiology, 296,* G1140–G1149.

90. Gibson, G. R., & Roberfroid, M. B. (1995). Dietary modulation of the human colonic microbiota: Introducing the concept of prebiotics. *The Journal of Nutrition, 125,* 1401–1412.

91. Lara-Villoslada, F., Olivares, M., Bañuelos, O., et al. (2006). New trends in prebiotics: The need for more specific compounds. *Nutrafoods, 5,* 5–12.

92. Galvez, J., Rodríguez-Cabezas, M. E., & Zarzuelo, A. (2005). Effects of dietary fiber on inflammatory bowel disease. *Molecular Nutrition & Food Research, 49,* 601–608.

93. Nyman, M. (2002). Fermentation and bulking capacity of indigestible carbohydrates: The case of inulin and oligofructose. *The British Journal of Nutrition, 87,* S163–S168.

94. Pereira, D. I., & Gibson, G. R. (2001). Effects of consumption of probiotics and prebiotics on serum lipids levels. *Critical Reviews in Biochemistry and Molecular Biology, 37,* 259–281.

95. Langlands, S. J., Hopkins, M. J., Coleman, N., & Cummings, J. H. (2004). Prebiotic carbohydrates modify the mucosa associated microflora of the human large bowel. *Gut, 53,* 1610–1616.

96. Kolida, S., Tuohy, K., & Gibson, G. R. (2002). Prebiotic effects of inulin and oligofructose. *The British Journal of Nutrition, 87,* S193–S197.

97. Hosono, A., Ozawa, A., Kato, R., et al. (2003). Dietary fructooligosaccharides induce immunoregulation of intestinal IgA secretion by murine Peyer's patch cells. *Bioscience, Biotechnology, and Biochemistry, 67,* 758–764.

98. Nalaamura, Y., Nosalsa, S., Suzulai, M., et al. (2004). Dietary fructooligosaccharides up-regulate immunoglobulin. A response and polymerie immunoglobulin receptor expression in intestives of infant mice. *Clinical and Experimental Immunology, 137,* 52–58.

99. Davidson, M. H., & Maki, K. C. (1999). Effects of dietary inulin on serum lipids. *The Journal of Nutrition, 129,* 1474S–1477S.

100. Comalada, M., Bailón, E., de Haro, O., et al. (2006). The effects of short-chain fatty acids on colon epithelial

proliferation and survival depend on the cellular phenotype. *Journal of Cancer Research and Clinical Oncology*, *132*, 487–497.

101. Young, G. P., McIntyre, A., Albert, V., et al. (1996). Wheat bran suppresses potato starch-potentiated colorectal tumorigenesis at the aberrant crypt stage in a rat model. *Gastroenterology*, *110*, 508–514.

102. Whitlock, J. P., Jr., Augustine, R., & Schulman, H. (1980). Calcium-dependent phosphorylation of histone H3 in butyrate-treated HeLa cells. *Nature*, *287*, 74–76.

103. Scheppach, W., Sommer, H., Kirchner, T., et al. (1992). Effect of butyrate enemas on the colonic mucosa in distal ulcerative colitis. *Gastroenterology*, *103*, 51–56.

104. Butzner, J. D., Parmar, R., Bell, C. J., & Dalal, V. (1996). Butyrate enema therapy stimulates mucosal repair in experimental colitis in the rat. *Gut*, *38*, 568–573.

105. D'Argenio, G., Cosenza, V., Sorrentini, I., et al. (1994). Butyrate, mesalamine, and factor XIII in experimental colitis in the rat: Effects on transglutaminase activity. *Gastroenterology*, *106*, 399–404.

106. Rodríguez-Cabezas, M. E., Gálvez, J., Lorente, M. D., et al. (2002). Dietary fiber down-regulates colonic tumor necrosis factor alpha and nitric oxide production in trinitrobenzenesulfonic acid-induced colitic rats. *The Journal of Nutrition*, *132*, 3263–3271.

107. Rodríguez-Cabezas, M. E., Gálvez, J., Camuesco, D., et al. (2003). Intestinal anti-inflammatory activity of dietary fiber (Plantago ovata seeds) in HLA-B27 transgenic rats. *Clinical Nutrition*, *22*, 463–471.

108. Kanauchi, O., Iwanaga, T., Mitsuyama, K., et al. (1999). Butyrate from bacterial fermentation of germinated barley foodstuff preserves intestinal barrier function in experimental colitis in the rat model. *Journal of Gastroenterology and Hepatology*, *14*, 880–888.

109. Fukuda, M., Kanauchi, O., Araki, Y., et al. (2002). Prebiotic treatment of experimental colitis with germinated barley foodstuff: A comparison with probiotic or antibiotic treatment. *International Journal of Molecular Medicine*, *9*, 65–70.

110. Kanauchi, O., Serizawa, I., Araki, Y., et al. (2003). Germinated barley foodstuff, a prebiotic product, ameliorates inflammation of colitis through modulation of the enteric environment. *Journal of Gastroenterology*, *38*, 134–141.

111. Moreau, N. M., Martin, L. J., Toquet, C. S., et al. (2003). Restoration of the integrity of rat caeco-colonic mucosa by resistant starch, but not by fructo-oligosaccharides, in dextran sulfate sodium-induced experimental colitis. *The British Journal of Nutrition*, *90*, 75–85.

112. Moreau, N. M., Champ, M. M., Goupr, S. M., et al. (2004). Resistant starch modulates in vivo colonic butyrate uptake and its oxidation in rats with dextran sulfate sodium-induced colitis. *The Journal of Nutrition*, *134*, 493–500.

113. Morita, T., Tanabe, H., Sugiyama, K., et al. (2004). Dietary resistant starch alters the characteristics of colonic mucosa and exerts a protective effect on trinitrobenzene sulfonic acid-induced colitis in rats. *Bioscience, Biotechnology, and Biochemistry*, *68*, 2155–2164.

114. Videla, S., Vilaseca, J., Antolín, M., et al. (2001). Dietary inulin improves distal colitis induced by dextran sodium sulfate in the rat. *The American Journal of Gastroenterology*, *96*, 1486–1493.

115. Osman, N., Adawi, D., Molin, G., et al. (2002). *Bifidobacterium infantis* strains with and without a combination of oligofructose and inulin (OFI) attenuate inflammation in DSS-induced colitis in rats. *Gastroenterology*, *37*, 1042–1047.

116. Cherbut, C., Michel, C., & Lecannu, G. (2003). The prebiotic characteristics of fructooligosaccharides are necessary for reduction of TNBS-induced colitis in rats. *The Journal of Nutrition*, *133*, 21–27.

117. Holma, R., Juvonen, P., Asmawi, M. Z., et al. (2002). Galacto-oligosaccharides stimulate the growth of bifidobacteria but fail to attenuate inflammation in experimental colitis in rats. *Scandinavian Journal of Gastroenterology*, *37*, 1042–1047.

118. Lara-Villoslada, F., Debras, E., Nieto, A., et al. (2006). Oligosaccharides isolated from goat milk reduce intestinal inflammation in a rat model of dextran sodium sulfate-induced colitis. *Clinical Nutrition*, *25*, 477–488.

119. Lara-Villoslada, F., de Haro, O., Camuesco, D., et al. (2006). Short-chain fructo-oligosaccharides, in spite of being fermented in the upper part of the large intestine, have anti-inflammatory activity in the TNBS model of colitis. *European Journal of Nutrition*, *45*, 418–425.

120. Camuesco, D., Peran, L., Comalada, M., et al. (2005). Preventative effects of lactulose in the trinitrobenzenesulphonic acid model of rat colitis. *Inflammatory Bowel Diseases*, *11*, 265–271.

121. Rumi, G., Tsubouchi, R., Okayama, M., et al. (2004). Protective effect of lactulose on dextran sulfate sodium-induced colonic inflammation in rats. *Digestive Diseases and Sciences*, *49*, 1466–1472.

122. Hoentjen, F., Welling, G. W., Harmsen, H. J., et al. (2005). Reduction of colitis by prebiotics in HLA-B27 transgenic rats is associated with microflora changes and immunomodulation. *Inflammatory Bowel Diseases*, *11*, 977–985.

123. Vernia, P., Caprilli, R., Latella, G., et al. (1988). Fecal lactate and ulcerative colitis. *Gastroenterology*, *95*, 1564–1568.

124. Den Hond, E., Hiele, M., Evenepoel, P., et al. (1998). *In vivo* butyrate metabolism and colonic permeability in extensive ulcerative colitis. *Gastroenterology*, *115*, 584–590.

125. Ahmad, M. S., Krishnan, S., Ramakrishna, B. S., et al. (2000). Butyrate and glucose metabolism by colonocytes in experimental colitis in mice. *Gut*, *46*, 493–499.

Index